ROGERS' HANDBOOK OF PEDIATRIC INTENSIVE CARE

FIFTH EDITION

ROGERS' HANDBOOK OF PEDIATRIC INTENSIVE CARE

FIFTH EDITION

Editors

Wynne Morrison, MD, MBE

Critical Care and Palliative Care
Director
Pediatric Advanced Care Team
The Children's Hospital of Philadelphia
Associate Professor
Department of Anesthesiology and Critical Care
Perelman School of Medicine
University of Pennsylvania
Philadelphia, Pennsylvania

Kristen Nelson McMillan, MD

Assistant Professor
Pediatric Critical Care
Departments of Anesthesiology and Critical Care Medicine and Pediatrics
Division of Pediatric Anesthesia and Critical Care Medicine
Director of Pediatric Cardiac Critical Care
Medical Director of Pediatric Ventricular Assist Device Program
Johns Hopkins University School of Medicine Baltimore, Maryland

Donald H. Shaffner, MD

Associate Professor
Departments of Anesthesiology and Critical Care Medicine and Pediatrics
Division of Pediatric Anesthesiology and Critical Care Medicine
Johns Hopkins University School of Medicine
Baltimore, Maryland

Wolters Kluwer

Philadelphia • Baltimore • New York • London
Buenos Aires • Hong Kong • Sydney • Tokyo

Acquisitions Editor: Keith Donellan
Development Editor: Franny Murphy
Marketing Manager: Dan Dressler
Production Project Manager: Bridgett Dougherty
Design Coordinator: Teresa Mallon
Manufacturing Coordinator: Beth Welsh
Prepress Vendor: S4Carlisle Publishing Services

5th edition

9 8 7 6 5 4 3

Printed in China

Library of Congress Cataloging-in-Publication Data

Names: Morrison, Wynne, editor. | McMillan, Kristen Nelson, 1970– editor. | Shaffner, Donald H., editor.
Title: Rogers' handbook of pediatric intensive care / [edited by] Wynne Morrison, Kristen Nelson McMillan, and Donald H. Shaffner McMillan.
Other titles: Handbook of pediatric intensive care | Digest of (expression): Rogers' textbook of pediatric intensive care. 5th ed.
Description: Fifth edition. | Philadelphia: Wolters Kluwer Health, [2017] | Digest of: Rogers' textbook of pediatric intensive care / editors, David G. Nichols and Donald H. Shaffner; section editors, Andrew C. Argent [and 25 others]. Fifth edition. 2016. | Includes bibliographical references and index.
Identifiers: LCCN 2016029105 | ISBN 9781496347534
Subjects: | MESH: Critical Care | Infant | Child | Emergencies | Handbooks
Classification: LCC RJ370 | NLM WS 39 | DDC 618.92/0028—dc23 LC record available at https://lccn.loc.gov/2016029105

LWW.com

CONTRIBUTORS

Nicholas S. Abend, MD
Assistant Professor
Department of Neurology and Pediatrics
The Children's Hospital of Philadelphia
Perelman School of Medicine
University of Pennsylvania
Philadelphia, Pennsylvania

Mateo Aboy, PhD
Professor
Department of Electronics Engineering and Technology
Oregon Institute of Technology
Portland, Oregon

Iki Adachi, MD
Associate Surgeon
Congenital Heart Surgery
Co-Director, Mechanical Support
Texas Children's Hospital
Assistant Professor
Michael E. DeBakey Department of Surgery and Pediatrics
Baylor College of Medicine
Houston, Texas

P. David Adelson, MD, FACS, FAAP
Director
Diane and Bruce Halle Endowed Chair in Pediatric Neurosciences
Chief
Pediatric Neurosurgery
Barrow Neurological Institute
Phoenix Children's Hospital
Professor and Chief Neurological Surgery
Department of Child Health
University of Arizona College of Medicine
Adjunct Professor
Ira A. Fulton School of Biological and Health Systems Engineering
Arizona State University
Phoenix, Arizona

Rachel S. Agbeko, FRCPCH, PhD
Consultant Paediatric Intensivist
Great North Children's Hospital
Royal Victoria Infirmary
London, United Kingdom

Jeffrey B. Anderson, MD
Associate Professor
Department of Pediatrics
Chief Quality Officer
The Heart Center
Division of Pediatric Cardiology
Cincinnati Children's Hospital Medical Center
Cincinnati, Ohio

Linda Aponte-Patel, MD, FAAP
Assistant Professor
Department of Pediatrics
Columbia University Medical Center
Division of Pediatric Critical Care Medicine
Department of Pediatrics
Columbia University College of Physicians and Surgeons
New York, New York

John H. Arnold, MD
Professor
Department of Anesthesia (Pediatrics)
Harvard Medical School
Senior Associate
Anesthesia and Critical Care
Medical Director
Respiratory Care/ECMO
Children's Hospital
Boston, Massachusetts

Stephen Ashwal, MD
Distinguished Professor
Department of Pediatrics
Loma Linda University School of Medicine
Attending Physician
Division of Child Neurology
Department of Pediatrics
Loma Linda Children's Hospital
Loma Linda, California

Swapnil S. Bagade, MD
Fellow
Mallinkrodt Institute of Radiology
Washington University
Fellow
Department of Pediatric Radiology
St. Louis Children's Hospital
St. Louis, Missouri

John S. Baird, MS, MD
Associate Professor
Department of Pediatrics
Columbia University Medical Center
Columbia University
New York, New York

Adnan M. Bakar, MD
Assistant Professor
Department of Pediatrics
Section Head
Pediatric Cardiac Critical Care
Cohen Children's Medical Center of New York
New Hyde Park, New York

Kenneth J. Banasiak, MD, MS
Pediatrician
Division of Pediatric Critical Care
Connecticut Children's Medical Center
Hartford, Connecticut

Arun Bansal, MD, MRCPCH, MAMS
Additional Professor
Department of Pediatrics
Advance Pediatric Centre
Postgraduate Institute of Medical Education and Research
Chandigarh, India

Aarti Bavare, MD, MPH
Assistant Professor
Department of Pediatrics
Baylor College of Medicine
Houston, Texas

Hülya Bayir, MD
Professor
Department of Critical Care Medicine
Department of Environmental and Occupational Health
Director of Research
Pediatric Critical Care Medicine
Associate Director
Center for Free Radical and Antioxidant Health
Safar Center for Resuscitation Research
University of Pittsburgh
Pittsburgh, Pennsylvania

Michael J. Bell, MD
Professor
Critical Care Medicine
Neurological Surgery and Pediatrics
Director
Pediatric Neurotrauma Center
Pediatric Neurocritical Care
Associate Director
Safar Center for Resuscitation Research
University of Pittsburgh School of Medicine
Pittsburgh, Pennsylvania

Kimberly S. Bennett, MD, MPH
Associate Professor
Pediatric Critical Care
University of Colorado School of Medicine
Aurora, Colorado

Robert A. Berg, MD, FAAP, FCCM, FAHA
Russell Raphaely Endowed Chair
Division Chief
Critical Care Medicine
The Children's Hospital of Philadelphia
Professor of Anesthesia and Critical Care Medicine
Professor of Pediatrics
Perelman School of Medicine
University of Pennsylvania
Philadelphia, Pennsylvania

Rachel P. Berger, MD, MPH
Associate Professor
Department of Pediatrics
Associate Director
Safar Center for Resuscitation Research
University of Pittsburgh School of Medicine
Division Chief
Child Advocacy Center
Children's Hospital of Pittsburgh
Pittsburgh, Pennsylvania

Monica Bhatia, MD
Associate Professor
Department of Pediatrics
Director
Pediatric Stem Cell Transplantation Program
Columbia University Medical Center
New York, New York

Katherine V. Biagas, MD
Associate Professor
Department of Pediatrics
Columbia University Medical Center
New York, New York

Michael T. Bigham, MD, FAAP, FCCM
Medical Director of Critical Care Transport
Assistant Director of Patient Safety
Division of Pediatric Critical Care
Akron Children's Hospital
Associate Professor of Pediatrics
Northeast Ohio Medical University
Akron, Ohio

Clifford W. Bogue, MD
Professor and Interim Chair
Department of Pediatrics
Yale School of Medicine
New Haven, Connecticut

Desmond Bohn, MB, FRCPC
Professor
Department of Anesthesia and Pediatrics
University of Toronto
Chief
Department of Critical Care Medicine
The Hospital for Sick Children
Toronto, Canada

Christopher P. Bonafide, MD, MSCE
Assistant Professor
Department of Pediatrics
Perelman School of Medicine
University of Pennsylvania
Division of General Pediatrics
The Children's Hospital of Philadelphia
Philadelphia, Pennsylvania

Geoffrey J. Bond, MBBS
Assistant Professor
Department of Surgery
University of Pittsburgh
Pediatric Transplant Surgery/Pediatric General Thoracic Surgery
Children's Hospital of Pittsburgh at UPMC
Pittsburgh, Pennsylvania

Rebecca Hulett Bowling, MD
Assistant Professor
Mallinkrodt Institute of Radiology
Washington University
Staff Radiologist
Department of Pediatric Radiology
St. Louis Children's Hospital
St. Louis, Missouri

Kenneth M. Brady, MD
Associate Professor
Departments of Anesthesiology and Pediatrics
Texas Children's Hospital
Houston, Texas

Patrick W. Brady, MD, MSc
Assistant Professor
Department of Pediatrics
University of Cincinnati College of Medicine
Attending Physician
Division of Hospital Medicine
Cincinnati Children's Hospital Medical Center
Cincinnati, Ohio

Richard J. Brilli, MD, FAAP, FCCM
Professor
Department of Pediatrics
Division of Pediatric Critical Care Medicine
The Ohio State University College of Medicine
Chief Medical Officer
Nationwide Children's Hospital
Columbus, Ohio

Ronald A. Bronicki, MD
Associate Professor
Department of Pediatrics
Baylor College of Medicine
Associate Medical Director
Cardiac Intensive Care Unit
Department of Pediatrics
Texas Children's Hospital
Houston, Texas

Kate L. Brown, MRCPCH, MPH
Consultant
Cardiac Intensive Care Unit
Great Ormond Street Hospital for Children
Institute for Cardiovascular Science
University College London
London, United Kingdom

Werther Brunow de Carvalho, MD
Full Professor of Intensive Care/Neonatology
Department of Pediatrics
Federal University of São Paulo
São Paulo, Brazil

Warwick W. Butt, MD
Director
Intensive Care
Royal Children's Hospital
Associate Professor
Department of Paediatrics
University of Melbourne
Group Leader
Clinical Sciences Theme
Murdoch Children's Research Institute
Melbourne, Australia

James D. Campbell, MD, MS
Department of Pediatrics
Center for Vaccine Development
University of Maryland School of Medicine
Baltimore, Maryland

Michael F. Canarie, MD
Clinical Instructor
Department of Pediatrics
Yale University School of Medicine
New Haven, Connecticut

G. Patricia Cantwell, MD, FCCM
Professor and Chief
Pediatric Critical Care Medicine
Department of Pediatrics
University of Miami Miller School of Medicine
Holtz Children's Hospital
Miami, Florida

Joseph A. Carcillo, MD, FCCM
Associate Professor
Critical Care Medicine and Pediatrics
Children's Hospital of Pittsburgh
University of Pittsburgh Medical
Center
Pittsburgh, Pennsylvania

Todd Carpenter, MD
Associate Professor
Department of Pediatrics
Section of Pediatric Critical Care
University of Colorado School of Medicine
Aurora, Colorado

Elena Cavazzoni, MB, ChB, PhD, FCICM
Staff Specialist
Paediatric Intensive Care Unit
Children's Hospital at Westmead
Sydney, Australia

Dominic Cave, MBBS, FRCPC
Medical Director
Pediatric Cardiac Intensive Care
Stollery Children's Hospital
Associate Clinical Professor
Department of Anesthesiology and Pain Management
Associate Clinical Professor
Department of Pediatrics
University of Alberta
Edmonton, Alberta, Canada

Paul A. Checchia, MD, FCCM, FACC
Director
Cardiovascular Intensive Care Unit
Professor of Pediatrics
Sections of Critical Care Medicine and Cardiology
Texas Children's Hospital
Baylor College of Medicine
Houston, Texas

Ira M. Cheifetz, MD, FCCM, FAARC
Professor
Department of Pediatrics
Chief
Pediatric Critical Care Medicine
Director
Pediatric Critical Care Services
DUHS
Duke Children's Hospital
Durham, North Carolina

Nataliya Chorny, MD
Assistant Professor
Hofstra North Shore-LIJ School of Medicine
Attending Physician
Department of Pediatric Nephrology
Cohen Children's Medical Center
New Hyde Park, New York

Wendy K. Chung, MD, PhD
Associate Professor of Pediatrics and Medicine
Columbia University
New York, New York

Robert S. B. Clark, MD
Professor
Critical Care Medicine and Pediatrics
University of Pittsburgh School of Medicine
Chief
Pediatric Critical Care Medicine
Children's Hospital of Pittsburgh of UPMC
Pittsburgh, Pennsylvania

Erin Coletti
Undergraduate Student in Biology
Harriet L. Wilkes Honors College
Florida Atlantic University
Jupiter, Florida

Steven A. Conrad, MD, PhD, MCCM
Professor of Emergency Medicine
Internal Medicine and Pediatrics
Louisiana State University Health Sciences Center
Director
Extracorporeal Life Support Program
University Health System
Shreveport, Louisiana

Arthur Cooper, MD, MS
Professor of Surgery
Columbia University College of Physicians and Surgeons
Director of Trauma and Pediatric Surgical Services
Harlem Hospital Center
New York, New York

Fernando F. Corrales-Medina, MD
Pediatrics Hematology/Oncology Fellow
Department of Pediatrics
University of Texas MD Anderson Cancer Center
Houston, Texas

Jose A. Cortes, MD
Assistant Professor
Department of Pediatrics
University of Texas MD Anderson Cancer Center
MD Anderson Children's Cancer Hospital
Houston, Texas

John M. Costello, MD, MPH
Associate Professor
Department of Pediatrics
Northwestern University Feinberg School of Medicine
Director
Inpatient Cardiology
Medical Director
Regenstein Cardiac Care Unit
Ann and Robert H. Lurie Children's Hospital of Chicago
Chicago, Illinois

Jason W. Custer, MD
Assistant Professor
Department of Pediatrics
Division of Pediatric Critical Care
University of Maryland School of Medicine
Baltimore, Maryland

Richard J. Czosek, MD
Associate Professor
Department of Pediatrics
The Heart Center
Division of Pediatric Cardiology
Cincinnati Children's Hospital Medical Center
Cincinnati, Ohio

Heidi J. Dalton, MD
Professor
Department of Child Health
University of Arizona College of Medicine
Phoenix, Arizona

Sally L. Davidson Ward, MD
Chief
Division of Pediatric Pulmonology and Sleep Medicine
Associate Professor of Pediatrics
Children's Hospital Los Angeles
Keck School of Medicine of the University of Southern California
Los Angeles, California

Allan de Caen, MD, FRCP
Clinical Professor/Pediatric Intensivist
Pediatric Critical Care Medicine
Edmonton Clinic Health Academy
University of Alberta
Stollery Children's Hospital
Edmonton, Alberta, Canada

Artur F. Delgado, PhD
Chief
Pediatric Intensive Care Unit
Department of Pediatrics
University Federal de São Paulo
São Paulo, Brazil

Denis J. Devictor, MD, PhD
Assistance Publique–Hopitaux de Paris
Paris SUD University
Pediatric Intensive Care Unit
Hopital de Bicetre Le Kremlin Bicetre
Paris, France

Troy E. Dominguez, MD
Consultant
Cardiac Intensive Care Unit
Great Ormond Street Hospital for Children
NHS Foundation Trust
London, United Kingdom

Aaron J. Donoghue, MD, MSCE
Associate Professor
Department of Pediatrics and Critical Care Medicine
Perelman School of Medicine
University of Pennsylvania
Emergency Medicine
The Children's Hospital of Philadelphia
Philadelphia, Pennsylvania

Lesley Doughty, MD
Associate Professor
Critical Care Medicine
Cincinnati Children's Hospital Medical Center
Cincinnati, Ohio

Laurence Ducharme-Crevier, MD
Pediatric Intensivist
Department of Pediatrics
CHU Sainte-Justine
Montreal, Quebec, Canada

Jonathan P. Duff, MD, Med, FRCPC
Associate Professor
Department of Pediatrics
University of Alberta
Edmonton, Alberta, Canada

Jennifer G. Duncan, MD
Assistant Professor
Program Director
Critical Care Fellowship
Department of Pediatrics
Washington University School of Medicine
Seattle, Washington

Genevieve DuPont-Thibodeau, MD
Pediatric Intensivist
Department of Pediatrics
CHU Sainte-Justine
Montreal, Quebec, Canada

R. Blaine Easley, MD
Fellowship Director
Pediatric Anesthesiology
Division Director
Anesthesiology Critical Care
Texas Children's Hospital
Houston, Texas

Janeth C. Ejike, MBBS, FAAP
Associate Professor
Department of Pediatrics
Loma Linda University
Loma Linda, California

Conrad L. Epting, MD, FAAP
Assistant Professor
Department of Pediatrics
Northwestern University Feinberg School of Medicine
Attending Physician
Division of Pediatric Critical Care
Ann and Robert H. Lurie Children's Hospital
Chicago, Illinois

Maria C. Esperanza, MD
Associate Chief
Division of Pediatric Critical Care Medicine
North Shore LIJ Health System
Cohen Children's Medical Center
New Hyde Park, New York

Ori Eyal, MD
Assistant Professor
Sackler Faculty of Medicine
Tel Aviv University
Clinical Director
Department of Pediatric Endocrinology
Tel Aviv Medical Center
Tel Aviv, Israel

Tracy B. Fausnight, MD
Associate Professor
Department of Pediatrics
Penn State College of Medicine
Division Chief
Division of Allergy and Immunology
Penn State Hershey Children's Hospital
Hershey, Pennsylvania

Edward Vincent S. Faustino, MD, MHS
Associate Professor
Department of Pediatrics
Yale School of Medicine
New Haven, Connecticut

Kathryn A. Felmet, MD
Department of Pediatrics
Division of Pediatric Critical Care Medicine
Oregon Health and Science University
Portland, Oregon

Jeffrey R. Fineman, MD
Professor
Department of Pediatrics
Investigator
Cardiovascular Research Institute
UCSF Benioff Children's Hospital
San Francisco, California

Ericka L. Fink, MD, MS
Associate Professor
Division of Pediatric Critical Care Medicine
Children's Hospital of Pittsburgh of UPMC
Pittsburgh, Pennsylvania

Douglas S. Fishman, MD
Director
Gastrointestinal Endoscopy
Texas Children's Hospital
Associate Professor of Pediatrics
Baylor College of Medicine
Houston, Texas

Julie C. Fitzgerald, MD, PhD
Assistant Professor
Department of Anesthesia and Critical Care Medicine
Perelman School of Medicine
University of Pennsylvania
The Children's Hospital of Philadelphia
Philadelphia, Pennsylvania

George L. Foltin, MD
Department of Pediatrics
SUNY Downstate Medical Center
Brooklyn, New York

Marcelo Cunio Machado Fonseca, MD, MSc
Department of Pediatrics
University Federal de São Paulo
São Paulo, Brazil

Jim Fortenberry, MD, FCCM, FAAP
Pediatrician in Chief
Children's Healthcare of Atlanta
Professor of Pediatric Critical Care
Emory University School of Medicine
Atlanta, Georgia

Alain Fraisse, MD, PhD
Consultant and Director
Paediatric Cardiology Service
Royal Brompton Hospital
London, United Kingdom

Charles D. Fraser, Jr, MD, FACS
Surgeon-in-Chief
Texas Children's Hospital
Professor of Pediatrics and Surgery
Baylor College of Medicine
Houston, Texas

Philippe S. Friedlich, MD, MS Epi, MBA
Professor of Clinical Pediatrics and Surgery
Keck School of Medicine of USC
Interim Center Director and Division Chief
Center for Fetal and Neonatal Medicine
USC Division of Neonatal Medicine
Department of Pediatrics
Children's Hospital Los Angeles
Los Angeles, California

James J. Gallagher, MD, FACS
Assistant Professor
Department of Surgery
Weill Cornell Medical College
New York, New York

Cynthia Gauger, MD
Division of Pediatric Hematology and Oncology
Nemours Children's Specialty Care
Jacksonville, Florida

Jonathan Gillis, MB, BS, PhD, FRACP, FCICM
Clinical Associate Professor
Department of Pediatrics and Child Health
University of Sydney
New South Wales, Australia

Brahm Goldstein, MD, MCR, FAAP, FCCM
Professor of Pediatrics
University of Medicine and Dentistry of New Jersey
Robert Wood Johnson Medical School
New Brunswick, New Jersey

Salvatore R. Goodwin, MD
Department of Anesthesiology
Office of the Vice President Quality and Safety
Nemours Children's Specialty Care
Associate Professor of Anesthesiology
Mayo Clinic
Jacksonville, Florida

Alan S. Graham, MD
Pediatric Critical Care
Cardon Children's Medical Center
Mesa, Arizona

Bruce M. Greenwald, MD
Professor
Department of Pediatrics
Weill Cornell Medical College
New York, New York

Gabriel G. Haddad, MD
Distinguished Professor
Department of Pediatrics and Neuroscience
Chairman
Department of Pediatrics
University of California
Physician-in-Chief and Chief Scientific Officer
Rady Children's Hospital
San Diego, California

Mark W. Hall, MD, FCCM
Division Chief
Critical Care Medicine
Nationwide Children's Hospital
Columbus, Ohio

E. Scott Halstead, MD, PhD
Assistant Professor
Department of Pediatrics
Pennsylvania State University College of Medicine
Hershey, Pennsylvania

Donna S. Hamel, RCP
Assistant Director
Clinical Trial Operations
Duke Clinical Research Unit
Duke University Medical Center
Durham, North Carolina

William G. Harmon, MD
Associate Professor
Department of Pediatrics
Director
Pediatric Critical Care Services
University of Virginia Children's Hospital
Charlottesville, Virginia

Z. Leah Harris, MD
Division Director
Pediatric Critical Care Medicine
Posy and John Krehbiel Professor of Critical Care Medicine
Professor
Department of Pediatrics
Northwestern University Feinberg School of Medicine
Ann & Robert H. Lurie Children's Hospital
Chicago, Illinois

Silvia M. Hartmann, MD
Assistant Professor
Pediatric Critical Care Medicine
Seattle Children's Hospital
University of Washington
Seattle, Washington

Abeer Hassoun, MD
Assistant Professor of Clinical Pediatrics
Department of Pediatrics
Columbia University
Attending Physician
Department of Pediatrics
Children's Hospital of New York
New York, New York

Masanori Hayashi, MD
Johns Hopkins University
Baltimore, Maryland

Mary F. Hazinski, RN, MSN, FAAN, FAHA, FERC
Professor
Vanderbilt University School of Nursing
Clinical Nurse Specialist
Monroe Carrell Jr. Children's Hospital at Vanderbilt
Nashville, Tennessee

Gregory P. Heldt, MD
Professor
Department of Pediatrics
University of California
San Diego, California

Mark J. Heulitt, MD
Professor
Department of Pediatrics
Physiology and Biophysics College of Medicine
University of Arkansas for Medical Sciences
Little Rock, Arkansas

Siew Yen Ho, MD
Professor of Cardiac Morphology
Imperial College
National Heart and Lung Institute
London, United Kingdom

Julien I. Hoffman, MD
Professor Emeritus
Department of Pediatrics
UCSF Medical Center
San Francisco, California

Aparna Hoskote, MRCP, MD
Consultant in Cardiac Intensive Care and ECMO
Honorary Senior Lecturer
University College London
Institute of Child Health
Great Ormond Street Hospital for Children
NHS Foundation Trust
London, United Kingdom

Joy D. Howell, MD, FAAP, FCCM
Associate Professor of Clinical Pediatrics
Pediatric Critical Care Medicine
Fellowship Director
Weill Cornell Medical College
Department of Pediatrics
New York, New York

Winston W. Huh, MD
Associate Professor
Division of Pediatrics
University of Texas MD Anderson Cancer Center
Houston, Texas

Tomas Iölster, MD
Associate Professor
Department of Pediatrics
Hospital Universitario Austral Pilar
Buenos Aires, Argentina

Narayan Prabhu Iyer, MBBS, MD
Attending Neonatalogist
Children's Hospital Los Angeles
Los Angeles, California

Ronald Jaffe, MB, BCh
Professor
Department of Pathology
University of Pittsburgh School of Medicine
Pathologist
Department of Pediatric Pathology
Children's Hospital of Pittsburgh
Pittsburgh, Pennsylvania

M. Jayashree, MD, DNB Pediatrics
Additional Professor
Department of Pediatrics
Advanced Pediatrics Centre
Postgraduate Institute of Medical Education and Research
Chandigarh, India

Larry W. Jenkins, PhD
Professor
Safari Center
University of Pittsburgh
Pittsburgh, Pennsylvania

Lulu Jin, PharmD, BCPS
Pediatric Clinical Pharmacist
UCSF Benioff Children's Hospital
Assistant Clinical Professor
UCSF School of Pharmacy
San Francisco, California

Sachin S. Jogal, MD
Assistant Professor of Pediatrics
Division of Pediatric Hematology/Oncology/BMT
Medical College of Wisconsin
Milwaukee, Wisconsin

Cintia Johnston, MD
Department de Medicina e Pediatria
University Federal de São Paulo
São Paulo, Brazil

Philippe Jouvet, MD, PhD
Full Professor
Director of the Pediatric Intensive Care Unit
Department of Pediatrics
CHU Sainte-Justine
Montreal, Quebec, Canada

Sushil K. Kabra, MD, DNB
Professor
Department of Pediatrics
All India Institute of Medical Sciences
New Delhi, India

Siripen Kalayanarooj, MD
Professor
Queen Sirikit National Institute of Child Health
College of Medicine
Rangsit University
Bangkok, Thailand

Rebecca J. Kameny, MD
Adjunct Assistant Professor
Pediatric Critical Care
University of California
San Francisco, California

Oliver Karam, MD, MSc
Associate Professor
Attending Physician
Pediatric Critical Care Unit
Geneva University Hospital
Department of Pediatrics
Geneva University
Geneva
Switzerland

Ann Karimova, MD
Consultant
Cardiac Intensive Care and ECMO
Honorary Senior Lecturer
University College London
Institute of Child Health
Great Ormond Street Hospital for Children
NHS Foundation Trust
London, United Kingdom

Todd J. Karsies, MD
Clinical Assistant Professor of Pediatrics
Pediatric Critical Care
The Ohio State University College of Medicine/Nationwide Children's Hospital
Columbus, Ohio

Thomas G. Keens, MD
Professor of Pediatrics
Physiology and Biophysics
Keck School of Medicine of USC
Division of Pediatric Pulmonology and Sleep Medicine
Children's Hospital Los Angeles
Los Angeles, California

Andrea Kelly, MD
Attending Physician
Pediatric Endocrinology
The Children's Hospital of Philadelphia
Assistant Professor of Pediatrics
Perelman School of Medicine
University of Pennsylvania
Philadelphia, Pennsylvania

Praveen Khilnani, MD, FCCM
Department of Pediatrics
Indraprastha Apollo Hospital
New Delhi
India

Apichai Khongphatthanayothin, MD, MPPM
Chief
Department of Pediatric Cardiology
Bangkok Heart Hospital
Professor of Pediatrics
Faculty of Medicine
Chulalongkorn University
Bangkok, Thailand
Professor of Clinical Pediatrics
LAC-USC Medical Center
Keck School of Medicine of USC
Los Angeles, California

Fenella Kirkham, FRCPCH
Paediatric Neurologist
University Hospital Southampton
Southampton, Hampshire, United Kingdom

Niranjan "Tex" Kissoon, MD, RCP(C), FAAP, FCCM, FACPE
Vice President
Medical Affairs
BC Children's Hospital and Sunny Hill Health Centre for Children
Professor–Global Child Health
University of British Columbia and BC Children's Hospital
Vancouver, British Columbia, Canada

Nigel J. Klein, MB, BS, BSc, PhD
Professor of Infection and Immunity
UCL Institute of Child Health
London, United Kingdom

Monica E. Kleinman, MD
Associate Professor of Anesthesia (Pediatrics)
Division of Critical Care Medicine
Department of Anesthesia
Boston Children's Hospital
Harvard Medical School
Boston, Massachusetts

Timothy K. Knilans, MD
Professor
Department of Pediatrics
The Heart Center
Division of Pediatric Cardiology
Cincinnati Children's Hospital Medical Center
Cincinnati, Ohio

Patrick M. Kochanek, MD, MCCM
Ake N. Grenvik Professor of Critical Care Medicine
Professor and Vice Chairman
Department of Critical Care Medicine
Professor of Anesthesiology
Pediatrics, Bioengineering, and Clinical and Translational Science
Director
Safar Center for Resuscitation Research
University of Pittsburgh School of Medicine
Pittsburgh, Pennsylvania

Nikoleta S. Kolovos, MD
Associate Professor of Pediatrics
Division of Pediatric Critical Care Medicine
Washington University School of Medicine
Quality and Outcomes Physician
BJC Healthcare
St. Louis, Missouri

Karen L. Kotloff, MD
Professor
Department of Pediatrics
University of Maryland School of Medicine
Baltimore, Maryland

Sheila S. Kun, RN, MS
Keck School of Medicine of USC
Division of Pediatric Pulmonology
Children's Hospital Los Angeles
Los Angeles, California

Jacques Lacroix, MD, FRCPC
Professor
Department of Pediatrics
Universite de Montreal
CHU Sainte-Justine
Montreal, Quebec, Canada

Miriam K. Laufer, MD
Associate Professor
Department of Pediatrics
Center for Vaccine Development
University of Maryland School of Medicine
Baltimore, Maryland

Matthew B. Laurens, MD, MPH
Associate Professor
Department of Pediatrics
University of Maryland School of Medicine
Baltimore, Maryland

Jan H. Lee, MBBS, MRCPCH
Consultant
Children's Intensive Care Unit
Department of Paediatric Subspecialties
KK Women's and Children's Hospital
Adjunct Assistant Professor
Duke-NUS Graduate School of Medicine
Singapore, Singapore

Heitor P. Leite, MD
Affiliate Professor
Department of Pediatrics
Federal University of São Paulo
São Paulo, Brazil

Daniel J. Licht, MD
Associate Professor of Neurology and Pediatrics
Division of Neurology
The Children's Hospital of Philadelphia
Perelman School of Medicine
University of Pennsylvania
Philadelphia, Pennsylvania

Fangming Lin, MD, PhD
Division of Pediatric Nephrology
Department of Pediatrics
Columbia University College of Physicians and Surgeons
New York, New York

Rakesh Lodha, MD
Additional Professor
Department of Pediatrics
All India Institute of Medical Sciences
New Delhi, India

David M. Loeb, MD, PhD
Assistant Professor
Department Oncology and Pediatrics
Johns Hopkins University
Bunting Blaustein Cancer Research Building
Baltimore, Maryland

Laura L. Loftis, MD, MS, FAAP
Associate Professor
Department of Pediatrics and Medical Ethics
Baylor College of Medicine
Pediatric Critical Care Medicine
Texas Children's Hospital
Houston, Texas

Anne Lortie, MD, FRCPc
Professor Agrege de Clinique, Neurologie
Department of Pediatrics
Faculty of Medicine
CHU Sainte-Justine
Montreal, Quebec, Canada

Naomi L. C. Luban, MD
Director of the E.J. Miller Blood Donor Center
Division of Laboratory Medicine
Children's National Medical Center
Vice Chair of Academic Affairs
Department of Pediatrics
George Washington University School of Medicine and Health Sciences
Washington, District of Columbia

Graeme MacLaren, MBBS, FCICM, FCCM
Paediatric ICU Physician
Royal Children's Hospital
Melbourne, Australia
Director
Cardiothoracic Intensive Care
National University Heart Centre
Singapore, Singapore

Mioara D. Manole, MD
Assistant Professor
Division of Emergency Medicine
Department of Pediatrics
University of Pittsburgh School of Medicine
Children's Hospital of Pittsburgh
Pittsburgh, Pennsylvania

Bruno Maranda, MD, MSc
Investigator
Mother and Child Axis
Centre de recherche de CHUS
Medical Geneticist
Centre Hospitalier Universitaire de Sherbrooke
Director of Department of Genetics
Assistant Professor
Department of Pediatrics
Division of Genetics
Faculty of Medicine and Health Sciences
Universite de Sherbrooke
Sherbrooke, Quebec, Canada

Bradley S. Marino, MD, MPP, MSCE
Staff Cardiac Intensivist
Cardiac Intensive Care Unit
Cincinnati Children's Hospital Medical Center
Cincinnati, Ohio

M. Michele Mariscalco, MD
Professor
Department of Pediatrics
Regional Dean
College of Medicine at Urbana–Champaign
Urbana, Illinois

Dolly Martin, AS
Data Coordinator and Analyst
Department of Transplantation Surgery
Children's Hospital of Pittsburgh/Thomas E. Starzl Transplantation Institute
UPMC Liver Cancer Center
Pittsburgh, Pennsylvania

Mudit Mathur, MD, FAAP, FCCP
Associate Professor of Pediatrics
Division of Pediatric Critical Care
Loma Linda University Children's Hospital
Loma Linda, California

Riza C. Mauricio, MD
Pediatric ICU Nurse Practitioner
Department of Pediatrics
Children's Hospital of MD Anderson Cancer Center
Houston, Texas

Patrick O'Neal Maynord, MD
Assistant Professor
Division of Critical Care Medicine
Department of Pediatrics
Vanderbilt University School of Medicine
Monroe Carell Jr Children's Hospital at Vanderbilt
Nashville, Tennessee

George V. Mazariegos, MD
Professor
Department of Surgery and Critical Care Medicine
University of Pittsburgh School of Medicine
Chief
Department of Pediatric Transplantation
Department of Surgery
Children's Hospital of Pittsburgh of UPMC
Pittsburgh, Pennsylvania

Jennifer A. McArthur, DO
Associate Professor
Division of Critical Care Medicine
Department of Pediatrics
Medical College of Wisconsin
Milwaukee, Wisconsin

Mary E. McBride, MD
Assistant Professor
Department of Pediatrics
Northwestern University Feinberg School of Medicine
Attending Physician
Division of Cardiology
Ann and Robert H. Lurie Children's Hospital of Chicago
Chicago, Illinois

Craig D. McClain, MD, MPH
Senior Associate in Perioperative Anesthesia
Boston Children's Hospital
Assistant Professor of Anaesthesia
Harvard Medical School
Boston, Massachusetts

Michael C. McCrory, MD, MS
Assistant Professor
Departments of Anesthesiology and Pediatrics
Wake Forest University School of Medicine
Winston-Salem, North Carolina

John K. McGuire, MD
Associate Professor
Department of Pediatrics
Associate Division Chief
Pediatric Critical Care Medicine
University of Washington School of Medicine
Seattle Children's Hospital
Seattle, Washington

Michael L. McManus, MD, MPH
Senior Associate
Department of Anesthesiology, Perioperative, and Pain Medicine
Division of Critical Care
Boston Children's Hospital and Harvard Medical School
Boston, Massachusetts

Nilesh M. Mehta, MD
Associate Professor of Anaesthesia
Harvard Medical School
Director
Critical Care Nutrition
Associate Medical Director
Critical Care Medicine
Department of Anesthesiology, Perioperative, and Pain Medicine
Boston Children's Hospital
Boston, Massachusetts

Rodrigo Mejia, MD, FCCM
Professor
Deputy Division Head
Director
Pediatric Critical Care
Division of Pediatrics
University of Texas MD Anderson Cancer Center
Houston, Texas

David J. Michelson, MD
Assistant Professor
Department of Pediatrics and Neurology
Loma Linda University School of Medicine
Loma Linda, California

Sabina Mir, MD
Assistant Professor
Division of Gastroenterology
Department of Pediatrics
University of North Carolina School of Medicine
Chapel Hill, North Carolina

Katsuyuki Miyasaka, MD, PhD, FAAP
Professor of Perianesthesia Nursing and Perioperative Center
St. Luke's International University and Hospital
Tokyo, Japan

Vinai Modem, MBBS, MS
Assistant Professor
Divisions of Critical Care and Nephrology
Department of Pediatrics
University of Texas Southwestern Medical Center
Dallas, Texas

Wynne Morrison, MD, MBE
Critical Care and Palliative Care
Director
Pediatric Advanced Care Team
The Children's Hospital of Philadelphia
Associate Professor
Department of Anesthesiology and Critical Care
Perelman School of Medicine
University of Pennsylvania
Philadelphia, Pennsylvania

Jennifer A. Muszynski, MD
Assistant Professor
Division of Critical Care Medicine
Department of Pediatrics
The Ohio State University College of Medicine
Nationwide Children's Hospital
Columbus, Ohio

Simon Nadel, FRCP
Adjunct Professor of Paediatric Intensive Care
St. Mary's Hospital and Imperial College Healthcare NHS Trust
London, United Kingdom

Vinay M. Nadkarni, MD, MS
Endowed Chair
Pediatric Critical Care Medicine
Departments of Anesthesia, Critical Care, and Pediatrics
Perelman School of Medicine
University of Pennsylvania
Department of Anesthesia and Critical Care
The Children's Hospital of Philadelphia
Philadelphia, Pennsylvania

Thomas A. Nakagawa, MD, FAAP, FCCM
Professor
Anesthesiology of Pediatrics
Department of Anesthesiology
Wake Forest University School of Medicine
Section Head
Pediatric Critical Care
Director
Pediatric Critical Care and Respiratory Care
Wake Forest Baptist Health
Brenner Children's Hospital
Winston-Salem, North Carolina

Michael A. Nares, MD
Assistant Professor
Department of Pediatrics
Miller School of Medicine
University of Miami
Pediatric Critical Care
Holtz Children's Hospital
Miami, Florida

David P. Nelson, MD
Professor
Department of Pediatrics
Director
Cardiac Intensive Care
The Heart Institute at Cincinnati Children's Hospital
Cincinnati, Ohio

Kristen Nelson McMillan, MD
Assistant Professor
Pediatric Critical Care
Departments of Anesthesiology and Critical Care Medicine and Pediatrics
Division of Pediatric Anesthesia and Critical Care Medicine
Director of Pediatric Cardiac Critical Care
Medical Director of Pediatric Ventricular Assist Device Program
Johns Hopkins University School of Medicine
Baltimore, Maryland

David G. Nichols, MD, MBA
Professor
Department of Anesthesiology and Critical Care Medicine and Pediatrics
Johns Hopkins University School of Medicine (on leave)
Baltimore, Maryland
President and CEO
The American Board of Pediatrics
Chapel Hill, North Carolina

Samuel Nurko, MD
Director
Center for Motility and Functional Gastrointestinal Disorders
Boston Children's Hospital
Boston, Massachusetts

Sharon E. Oberfield, MD
Professor
Department of Pediatrics
Columbia University
Director
Division of Pediatric Endocrinology, Diabetes, and Metabolism
Columbia University Medical Center
New York, New York

George Ofori-Amanfo, MD, ChB, FACC
Associate Professor
Department of Pediatrics
Duke University
Durham, North Carolina

Peter E. Oishi, MD
Associate Professor of Pediatrics
Pediatric Critical Care Medicine
University of California
UCSF Benioff Children's Hospital
San Francisco, California

Regina Okhuysen, MD
Associate Professor
Department of Pediatrics
University of Texas MD Anderson Cancer Center
Attending Physician
PICU
Pediatric Critical Care Medicine
MD Anderson's Children's Cancer Hospital
Houston, Texas

Richard A. Orr, MD, FCCM
Professor
Critical Care Medicine and Pediatrics
University of Pittsburgh School of Medicine
Children's Hospital of Pittsburgh
Pittsburgh, Pennsylvania

John Pappachan, MD
Senior Lecturer in Paediatric Intensive Care
University Hospital Southampton
NHS Foundation Trust
NIHR Southampton Respiratory Biomedical Research Unit
Southampton, United Kingdom

Robert I. Parker, MD
Professor
Pediatric Hematology/Oncology
Department of Pediatrics
Stony Brook University School of Medicine
Stony Brook, New York

Christopher S. Parshuram, MD
Physician Critical Care Program
Senior Scientist Child Health Evaluative Sciences
The Research Institute
Department of Critical Care Medicine
Hospital for Sick Children
Associate Professor
Department of Paediatrics, Critical Care, Health Policy, Management and Evaluation Faculty
Center for Patient Safety
University of Toronto
Toronto, Canada

Mark J. Peters, MD
Professor of Paediatric Intensive Care
UCL Institute of Child Health and Honorary Consultant Intensivist
Great Ormond Street Hospital
NHS Trust Foundation
London, United Kingdom

Matthew Pitt, MD, FRCP
Consultant Clinical Neurophysiologist
Department of Clinical Neurophysiology
Great Ormond Street Hospital
NHS Foundation Trust
London, United Kingdom

Renee M. Potera, MD
Instructor
Department of Pediatrics
University of Texas Southwestern Medical Center
Dallas, Texas

Frank L. Powell, PhD
Chief
Division of Physiology
Professor
Department of Medicine
University of California
La Jolla
San Diego, California

Jack F. Price, MD
Pediatric Cardiology
Department of Pediatrics
Baylor College of Medicine
Texas Children's Hospital
Houston, Texas

Elizabeth L. Raab, MD, MPH
Attending Neonatologist
Pediatrix Medical Group, Inc
Huntington Memorial Hospital
Pasadena, California

Surender Rajasekaran, MD, MPH
Pediatric Intensivist
Helen DeVos Children's Hospital
Grand Rapids, Michigan

Rangasamy Ramanathan, MBBS, MD
Professor of Pediatrics
Division Chief
Division of Neonatal Medicine
LAC + USC Medical Center
Director
NPM Fellowship Program and NICU
Associate Center Director
Center for Neonatal Medicine–CHLA
Keck School of Medicine of USC
Los Angeles, California

Courtney D. Ranallo, MD
Pediatric Critical Care-PICU
Oklahoma University Medicine
Oklahoma City, Oklahoma

Suchitra Ranjit, MD
Senior Consultant
Pediatric Intensive Care
Apollo Hospitals
Chennai, India

Chitra Ravishankar, MD
Attending Cardiologist
Staff Cardiologist
Cardiac Intensive Care Unit
Associate Director
Cardiology Fellowship Training Program
The Children's Hospital of Philadelphia
Assistant Professor of Pediatrics
Perelman School of Medicine
University of Pennsylvania
Philadelphia, Pennsylvania

Nidra I. Rodriguez, MD
Associate Professor
Department of Pediatrics
University of Texas Health Science Center
MD Anderson Cancer Center and Children's Memorial Hermann Hospital
Gulf States Hemophilia Treatment Center
Houston, Texas

Antonio Rodríguez-Núñez, MD, PhD
Pediatric Emergency and Critical Care Division
Hospital Clinico Universitario de Santiago de Compostela
Unidad de Cuidados Intensivos Pediatricos
Santiago de Compostela, Spain

Susan R. Rose, MD, Med
Professor
Department of Pediatrics and Endocrinology
Cincinnati Children's Hospital Medical Center and University of Cincinnati School of Medicine
Cincinnati, Ohio

Joseph W. Rossano, MD
Pediatric Cardiology
Department of Pediatrics
The Children's Hospital of Philadelphia
Perelman School of Medicine
University of Pennsylvania
Philadelphia, Pennsylvania

Eitan Rubinstein, MD
Center for Motility and Functional Gastrointestinal Disorders
Children's Hospital Boston
Boston, Massachusetts

Jeffrey A. Rudolph, MD
Assistant Professor
Department of Pediatrics
University of Pittsburgh
Director
Intestinal Care and Rehabilitation
Department of Pediatrics
Children's Hospital of Pittsburgh of UPMC
Pittsburgh, Pennsylvania

Ricardo D. Russo, MD
Chief of Pediatric Surgery
Co-Director of Fetal Surgery Program
Department of Pediatrics
Hospital Universitario Austral Pilar
Buenos Aires, Argentina

Monique M. Ryan, MD
Paediatric Neurologist
Children's Neuroscience Centre
Research Fellow
Murdoch Children's Research Institute
Royal Children's Hospital
Parkville, Victoria, Australia

Sanju S. Samuel, MD
Assistant Professor
Department of Pediatrics
University of Texas MD Anderson Cancer Center
Pediatric Intensive Care Physician
Pediatric Intensive Care Unit
MD Anderson Children's Cancer Hospital
Houston, Texas

Naveen Sankhyan, MD, DM
Pediatric Neurology Unit
Department of Pediatrics
Advanced Pediatrics Centre
Postgraduate Institute of Medical Education and Research
Chandigarh, India

Smarika Sapkota, MD
Resident Physician
Department of Internal Medicine
Marcy Catholic Medical Center
Aldan, Pennsylvania

Cheryl L. Sargel, PharmD
Clinical Pharmacy Specialist
Critical Care Medicine
Department of Pharmacy
Nationwide Children's Hospital
Columbus, Ohio

Stephen M. Schexnayder, MD, FAAP, FACP, FCCM
Professor and Vice Chairman
Department of Pediatrics College of Medicine
University of Arkansas for Medical Sciences
Arkansas Children's Hospital
Little Rock, Arkansas

Charles L. Schleien, MD, MBA
Philip Lanzkowsky Chairman of Pediatrics
Hofstra North Shore-LIJ School of Medicine
Cohen Children's Medical Center
New Hyde Park, New York

James Schneider, MD
Assistant Professor
Department of Pediatrics
Hofstra North Shore-LIJ School of Medicine
Cohen Children's Medical Center
New Hyde Park, New York

Eduardo J. Schnitzler, MD
Associate Professor
Department of Pediatrics
Hospital Universitario Austral Pilar
Buenos Aires, Argentina

Jennifer J. Schuette, MD, MS
Attending Physician
Cardiac Intensive Care Unit
Fellowship Director
Pediatric Critical Care Medicine
Children's National Health System
Assistant Professor of Pediatrics
George Washington University School of Medicine and Health Sciences
Washington, District of Columbia

Steven M. Schwartz, MD, FRCPC, FAHA
Professor of Paediatrics
Senior Associate Scientist
Head
Division of Cardiac Critical Care Medicine
Norine Rose Chair in Cardiovascular Sciences
The Labatt Family Heart Centre
Departments of Critical Care Medicine and Paediatrics
University of Toronto
Toronto, Canada

Istvan Seri, MD, PhD, HonD
Professor of Pediatrics
Weill Cornell Medical College
Professor of Pediatrics (Adjunct)
Keck School of Medicine of USC
Director
Sidra Neonatalogy Center of Excellence
Chief
Division of Neonatology
Vice Chair of Faculty Development
Department of Pediatrics
Sidra Medical and Research Center
Doha, Qatar

Christine B. Sethna, MD, EdM
Division Director
Pediatric Nephrology
Cohen Children's Medical Center
Assistant Professor
Hofstra North Shore-LIJ School of Medicine
New Hyde Park, New York

Donald H. Shaffner, MD
Associate Professor
Departments of Anesthesiology and Critical Care Medicine and Pediatrics
Division of Pediatric Anesthesiology and Critical Care Medicine
Johns Hopkins University School of Medicine
Baltimore, Maryland

Lara S. Shekerdemian, MB ChB, MD, MHA, FRACP
Professor and Vice Chair of Clinical Affairs
Diagnostic Imaging of the
Baylor College of Medicine
Chief of Critical Care
Texas Children's Hospital
Houston, Texas

Naoki Shimizu, MD, PhD
Chief
Department of Paediatric Emergency and Critical Care Medicine
Tokyo Metropolitan Children's Medical Centre
Tokyo, Japan

Peter Silver MD, MBA, FCCM
Chief
Pediatric Critical Care Medicine
Steven and Alexandra Cohen Children's Medical Center
Hofstra North Shore-LIJ School of Medicine
New Hyde Park, New York

Dennis W. Simon, MD
Assistant Professor of Critical Care Medicine and Pediatrics
Children's Hospital of Pittsburgh of UPMC
University of Pittsburgh School of Medicine
Pittsburgh, Pennsylvania

Rakesh Sindhi, MD
Professor
Department of Surgery
University of Pittsburgh
Surgeon
Department of Pediatric Abdominal Transplant
Children's Hospital of Pittsburgh of UPMC
Pittsburgh, Pennsylvania

Pratibha D. Singhi, MD, FIAP, FAMS
Chief
Pediatric Neurology and Neuro Development
Advanced Pediatrics Centre
Post Graduate Institute of Medical Education and Research
Chandigarh, India

Sunit C. Singhi, MBBS, MD, FIAP, FAMS, FISCCM, FICCM, FCCM
Head
Department of Pediatrics and Advanced Pediatrics Centre
Postgraduate Institute of Medical Education and Research
Chandigarh, India

Ruchi Sinha, MBChB, MRCPCH
Consultant Paediatric Intensivist
Paediatric Intensive Care
St. Mary's Hospital
Imperial College Healthcare NHS Trust
London, United Kingdom

Peter W. Skippen, MBBS, JFICM
Clinical investigator
Division of Pediatric Critical Care
Department of Pediatrics
BC Children's Hospital
Vancouver, British Columbia, Canada

Zdenek Slavik, MD, FRCPCH
Royal Brompton and Harefield NHS Trust
Royal Brompton Hospital
London, United Kingdom

Arthur J. Smerling, MD
Medical Director Cardiac Critical Care
Department of Pediatrics and Anesthesiology
Columbia University
New York, New York

Kyle A. Soltys, MD
Assistant Professor of Surgery
Department of Surgery
University of Pittsburgh
Surgeon
Pediatric Abdominal Transplant
Children's Hospital of Pittsburgh of UPMC
Pittsburgh, Pennsylvania

F. Meridith Sonnett, MD, FAAP, FACEP
Chief
Division of Pediatric Emergency Medicine
New York Presbyterian Morgan Stanley Children's Hospital
Associate Professor of Pediatrics
Columbia University Medical Center
Columbia College of Physicians and Surgeons
New York, New York

David S. Spar, MD
Assistant Professor
Department of Pediatrics
Pediatric cardiologist
The Heart Center
Division of Pediatric Cardiology
Cincinnati Children's Hospital Medical Center
Cincinnati, Ohio

Neil C. Spenceley, MB, ChB, MRCPCH
Lead Clinician/Patient Safety Fellow
Paediatric Critical Care
Royal Hospital for Sick Children
Glasgow, Scotland

Kevin B. Spicer, MD, PhD, MPH
Paediatric Consultant (Infectious Diseases)
Pietermaritzburg Metropolitan Hospitals Complex
Department of Health: KwaZulu-Natal
Pietermaritzburg, South Africa

Philip C. Spinella, MD, FCCM
Associate Professor
Division of Critical Care Medicine
Department of Pediatrics
Director
Critical Care Translational Research Program
Washington University School of Medicine
St. Louis, Missouri

Kurt R. Stenmark, MD
Professor of Pediatrics and Medicine
Division Head
Pediatric Critical Care Medicine
Director
Developmental Lung Biology and Cardiovascular Pulmonary Research Laboratories
University of Colorado Denver
Aurora, Colorado

John P. Straumanis, MD, FAAP, FCCM
Chief Medical Officer
Vice President of Medical Affairs
University of Maryland Rehabilitation and Orthopaedic Institute
Clinical Assistant Professor
University of Maryland Medical School
Baltimore, Maryland

Kevin J. Sullivan, MD
Assistant Professor
Department of Anesthesiology and Critical Care
Nemours Children's Specialty Care/Mayo School of Medicine
Jacksonville, Florida

Bo Sun, MD, PhD
Departments of Pediatrics and Neonatology
Children's Hospital of Fudan University
Shanghai, China

Clifford M. Takemoto, MD
Associate Professor
Division of Pediatric Hematology
Johns Hopkins School of Medicine
Baltimore, Maryland

Robert F. Tamburro, MD
Penn State Hershey Pediatric Critical Care Medicine
Hershey, Pennsylvania

Robert C. Tasker, MA, MD (Cantab), MBBS (Lond), DCH, FRCPCH, FRCP, FHEA (UK), AM (Harvard), MD (MA)
Professor of Neurology
Professor of Anaesthesia (Pediatrics)
Harvard Medical School
Chair in Neurocritical Care
Senior Associate Staff Physician
Department of Neurology
Department of Anesthesiology, Perioperative, and Pain Medicine
Division of Critical Care Medicine
Boston Children's Hospital
Boston, Massachusetts

Neal J. Thomas, MS, MSc
Professor of Pediatrics and Public Health Sciences
Division of Pediatric Critical Care Medicine
Penn State Hershey Children's Hospital
The Pennsylvania State University College of Medicine
Hershey, Pennsylvania

Jill S. Thomas, MSN, CRNP
Pediatric Critical Care Nurse Practitioner
Division of Pediatric Critical Care Medicine
Baltimore, Maryland

James Tibballs, MBBS, MD, FANZCA, FCICM, FACLM
Associate Professor
Departments of Paediatrics and Pharmacology
University of Melbourne
Deputy Director
Paediatric Intensive Care Unit
Royal Children's Hospital
Melbourne, Australia

Pierre Tissieres, MD, PhD
Director
Pediatric Intensive Care and Neonatal Medicine
Paris South University Hospitals
Le Kremlin Bicetre
Paris, France

Joseph D. Tobias, MD
Chairman
Department of Anesthesiology and Pain Medicine
Nationwide Children's Hospital
Professor of Anesthesiology and Pediatrics
The Ohio State University
Columbus, Ohio

Colin B. Van Orman, MD
Professor (Clinical) of Pediatrics and Neurology
University of Utah
Salt Lake City, Utah

Shekhar T. Venkataraman, MD
Professor
Department of Critical Care Medicine and Pediatrics
University of Pittsburgh School of Medicine
Pittsburgh, Pennsylvania

Kathleen M. Ventre, MD
Assistant Professor
Department of Pediatrics/Critical Care Medicine
University of Colorado
Attending Physician
Department of Pediatrics/Critical Care Medicine
Children's Hospital of Colorado
Aurora, Colorado

Hans-Dieter Volk, MD
Head
BCRT and IMI
Charité – University Medicine
Belrin
Germany

Steven A. Webber, MBChB (Hons), MRCP
James C. Overall Professor and Chair
Department of Pediatrics
Vanderbilt University School of Medicine
Monroe Carell Jr. Children's Hospital at Vanderbilt
Nashville, Tennessee

Stuart A. Weinzimer, MD
Associate Professor
Department of Pediatrics
Yale University School of Medicine
New Haven, Connecticut

Richard S. Weisman, PharmD
Associate Dean for Admissions and Professor of Pediatrics
University of Miami Miller School of Medicine
Director
Florida Poison Control'Miami
Miami, Florida

Scott L. Weiss, MD, MSCE
Assistant Professor of Anesthesia, Critical Care, and Pediatrics
Department of Anesthesiology and Critical Care Medicine
The Children's Hospital of Philadelphia
Philadelphia, Pennsylvania

David L. Wessel, MD
Executive Vice President
Chief Medical Officer for Hospital and Specialty Services
Ikaria Distinguished Professor of Critical Care Medicine
Division of Critical Care Medicine
Children's National Medical Center
Children's National Health System
Professor of Anesthesiology and Critical Care Medicine and Pediatrics
George Washington University School of Medicine and Health Sciences
Washington, District of Columbia

Derek S. Wheeler, MD, MMM
Associate Professor of Clinical Pediatrics
Associate Chair
Clinical Affairs
University of Cincinnati College of Medicine
Associate Chief of Staff
Division of Critical Care Medicine
Cincinnati Children's Hospital Medical Center
Cincinnati, Ohio

Michael Wilhelm, MD
Assistant Professor
Department of Pediatrics
Division of Critical Care
University of Wisconsin
Madison, Wisconsin

Kenneth D. Winkel, MBBS, BMedSci, PhD
Senior Research Fellow
Department of Pharmacology and Therapeutics
University of Melbourne
Victoria, Australia

Gerhard K. Wolf, MD
Associate in Critical Care Medicine
Pediatric Medical Director
Boston MedFlight
Assistant Professor of Anaesthesia
Division of Critical Care
Boston Children's Hospital
Boston, Massachusetts

Jennifer E. Wolford, DO, MPH
Assistant Professor
Department of Pediatrics
University of Pittsburgh School of Medicine
Pittsburgh, Pennsylvania

Edward C. C. Wong, MD
Director of Hematology
Associate Director of Transfusion Medicine
Center for Cancer and Blood Disorders
Division of Laboratory Medicine
Children's National Medical Center
Children's National Health System
Sheikh Zayed Campus for Advanced Children's Medicine
Associate Professor of Pediatrics and Pathology
George Washington University School of Medicine and Health Sciences
Washington, District of Columbia

Robert P. Woroniecki, MD, MS
Chief
Division of Pediatric Nephrology and Hypertension
Associate Professor of Clinical Pediatrics
Director
Pediatric Residency Scholarly Activity Program
SUNY School of Medicine
Stony Brook Children's Hospital
Stony Brook, New York

Angela T. Wratney, MD, MHSc
Attending Physician
Pediatric Critical Care
Children's National Medical Center
Assistant Professor
Department of Pediatrics
George Washington University School of Medicine and Health Sciences
Washington, District of Columbia

Roger W. Yurt, MD
Johnson & Johnson Professor and Vice Chairman
Department of Surgery
Chief
Division of Burns, Critical Care, and Trauma
New York Presbyterian Weill Medical Center
New York, New York

David A. Zideman, LVO, QHP(C), BSc, MBBS, FRCA, FRCP, FIMC, FERC
Consultant
Department of Anaesthetics
Hammersmith Hospital
Imperial College Healthcare NHS Trust
London, United Kingdom

PREFACE

This fifth edition of the *Rogers' Handbook of Pediatric Intensive Care* contains key clinical information from the *Rogers' Textbook of Pediatric Intensive Care* in a condensed version that is more portable and affordable. This edition of the Handbook also provides a bundled eBook that enhances its portability and availability. Chapters from the Rogers' Textbook with administrative and research focus have been omitted and the 96 most clinically relevant chapters included. The readers are urged to refer to the textbook for the references and for more detailed explanations of the subject matter.

The editors appreciate the original work of the chapter authors and section editors that went into the very comprehensive Rogers' Textbook. We also appreciate the work of the senior chapter authors who reviewed our condensed versions of their previous work for this Handbook. We are grateful for the editorial assistance provided by Nicole Dernoski and Franny Murphy. Our best wishes go to David Nichols and Mark Helfaer, who are friends, colleagues, and mentors, and who handed over to us the editorial work of this Handbook. It is our hope that this compilation of the clinical essence of the Rogers' Textbook facilitates the readers' practice of care for critically ill children.

Wynne Morrison
Kristen Nelson McMillan
Donald H. Shaffner

PREFACE TO PREVIOUS EDITION

The purpose of the *Rogers' Handbook of Pediatric Critical Care* is to be a companion to, not a replacement for, the *Rogers' Textbook of Pediatric Critical Care*. It is designed to be smaller and more economical than the *Textbook*, and in making it so, only essential information for the treatment of patients has been included in the *Handbook*. In addition to the references, we have omitted the first section of the *Textbook*, which contained chapters on the larger context of critical care medicine. The remaining chapters have been distilled to include the vital information needed for bedside care. It is the sound *practice of pediatric critical care* that is captured in the *Handbook*. Readers are encouraged to refer to the *Textbook* for a more comprehensive review of the material, as well as the references.

We thank the authors and section editors who submitted the full chapters for the *Textbook*. A special thanks also goes to Ms. Tzipora Sofare for her invaluable editorial assistance. As always, we are also indebted to the international patients, families, doctors, nurses, respiratory therapists, social workers, pharmacists, case managers, child-life specialists, nutritionists, and other members of the team who ensure the highest level of care for critically ill children. In addition, we thank our wives and children, who are always near and dear to our hearts.

M. A. Helfaer
D. G. Nichols

CONTENTS

SECTION VI ■ INFECTIOUS DISEASES

SECTION VII ■ NUTRITIONAL AND GASTROINTESTINAL DISORDERS

SECTION VIII ■ RENAL, ENDOCRINE, AND METABOLIC DISORDERS

SECTION IX ■ ONCOLOGIC AND HEMATOLOGIC DISORDERS

CHAPTER 1 ■ AIRWAY MANAGEMENT

DOMINIC CAVE, JONATHAN P. DUFF, ALLAN DE CAEN, AND MARY F. HAZINSKI

ANATOMY AND AIRWAY DEVELOPMENT

The Anatomy of the Airway

The pediatric airway can be divided into supraglottic, glottic, and subglottic structures. The *supraglottis*, or upper airway, includes the tongue, palate, posterior pharyngeal space, and epiglottis. The *glottis* includes the cartilages and muscular structures of the larynx. The larynx consists of nine cartilages, including the unpaired thyroid, cricoid, and epiglottis and the paired corniculate, cuneiform, and arytenoid cartilages. The *subglottis* or *infraglottis* includes the trachea (cricoid cartilage, tracheal rings, and mucosal surfaces) and the initial branches of the bronchial tree. The epiglottis is also proportionally larger and more "floppy." Because of the smaller diameter, a small change in tracheal radius can significantly increase resistance to airflow. Resistance to tracheal airflow is inversely related to the *fourth* power of the radius during quiet breathing (laminar airflow) but becomes inversely related to the *fifth* power of the radius when airflow is turbulent. The pediatric glottis is more *superior* (i.e., more cephalad) and more *anterior* than found in the adult airway (**Fig. 1.1**). The larynx has more angulation of the superior portion toward the provider, and can cause the tongue to obstruct the view of the airway. The rigid cricoid ring is the smallest functional part of the infant airway. In the adult, the larynx is more cylindrical in shape, with the narrowest segment at the level of the vocal cords.

Oral intubation with direct laryngoscopy requires the establishment of a line of vision from the mouth and teeth to the vocal cords. This line of vision requires the alignment of three axes (oral, pharyngeal, and laryngeal). Normally, the laryngeal axis is perpendicular to the oral axis and forms a 45-degree angle with the pharyngeal axis. The provider aligns the three axes in an older child or adult by placing a towel or other support beneath the occiput to flex the neck forward (at the shoulders) and lifts the chin to extend the neck (at the occiput) to achieve the *sniffing position* (**Fig. 1.2**). Because children <2 years have a relatively large occiput, it may only be necessary to lift the chin to produce extension of the neck and align the axes. For small infants, it may be necessary to place a support under the shoulders to achieve sniffing position.

INITIAL AIRWAY ASSESSMENT

Before performing an airway procedure, the provider must assess for a potentially difficult airway. The degree of mouth opening enables assessment of the palate, range of motion of the temporomandibular joint, and size of the tongue relative to the oral cavity. The *Mallampati assessment* relates visualization of the tonsillar pillars, soft palate, and uvula with the degree of difficulty of laryngoscopy. With a Class I airway, all three pharyngeal structures are visualized, and laryngoscopy yields adequate exposure in >99% of adult patients. With a Class II airway, uvula and soft palate are visible. With a Class III airway, only the soft palate and base of uvula are visible. With a Class IV airway, none of these structures can be seen, and laryngoscopy is adequate in 7% of adult patients. Reduced range of neck motion (*atlantooccipital joint extension*) may preclude successful alignment of the airway and visualization of the glottic opening. Mandibular hypoplasia can lead to difficulties and is assessed by evaluating the *thyromental distance* (from the upper aspect of the thyroid cartilage to the tip of the mandible); 1.5 cm in an infant or 3 cm in an adult is reassuring.

IDENTIFYING THE DIFFICULT AIRWAY

Definition and Priorities

A difficult airway is present if the provider has trouble providing bag-mask ventilation or intubating the trachea. The difficult pediatric airway is best managed by anticipation and careful planning. A history of stridor, snoring, or sleep apnea suggests a potentially difficult airway. A history of obesity, limited jaw or neck movement, craniofacial anomalies, facial trauma, or laryngeal abnormalities may lead to problems with intubation. Many patients who are labeled as having a difficult airway are actually difficult to intubate but easy to mask ventilate. The most concerning patients are difficult both to mask ventilate and to intubate (i.e., can lead to loss of the airway with administration of sedatives or paralytics). Having information displayed that explains

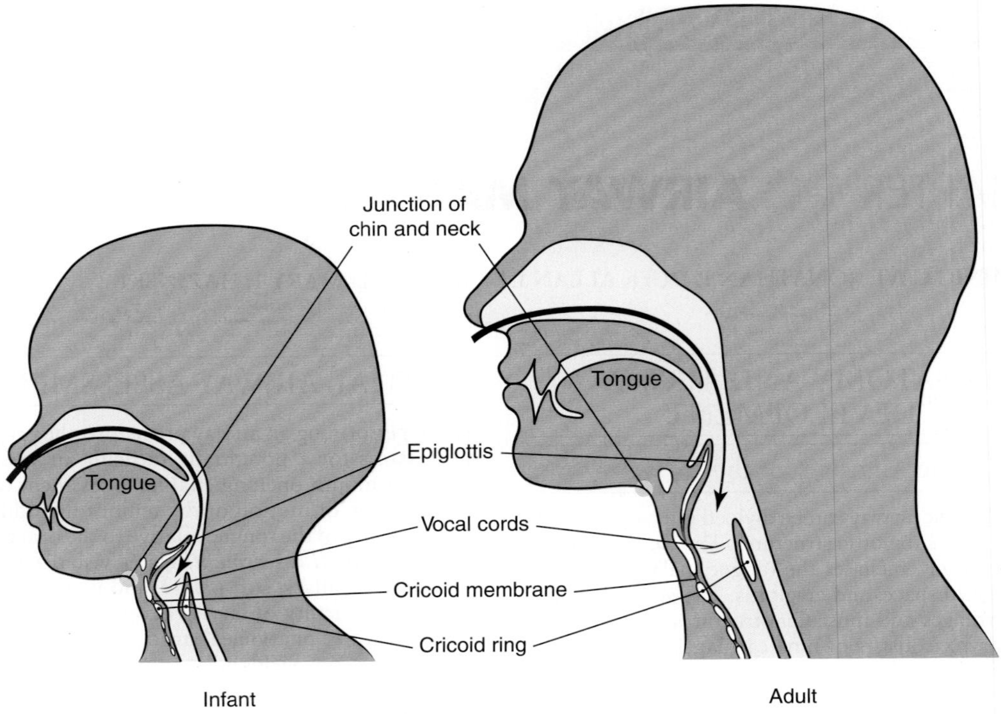

FIGURE 1.1. Children have (1) higher, more anterior position of the glottic opening (note the relationship of the vocal cords to the chin/neck junction); (2) relatively larger tongue in the infant, which lies between the mouth and glottic opening; (3) relatively larger and more floppy epiglottis in the child; (4) the cricoid ring is the narrowest portion of the pediatric airway versus the vocal cords in the adult; (5) position and size of the cricothyroid membrane in the infant; (6) sharper, more difficult angle for blind nasotracheal intubation; and (7) larger relative size of the occiput in the infant. (From Luten RC, Kissoon NJ. In: Walls R, Murphy MF, Luten LC, et al, eds. *Manual of Emergency Airway Management*. 2nd ed. Philadelphia, PA: Lippincott Williams & Wilkins, 2004:217, with permission.)

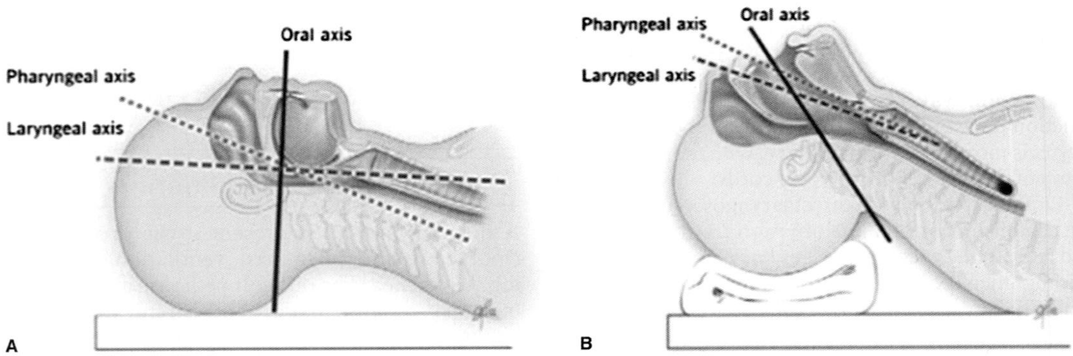

FIGURE 1.2. Correct positioning of the child over 2 years of age for ventilation and tracheal intubation. The oral, pharyngeal, and laryngeal/tracheal axes are optimally aligned for intubation when the child is placed in the "sniffing" position. A small towel is placed under the head (to extend the head forward at C1 and flex the neck slightly at C7). The opening of the ear canal should be above or just anterior to the front of the child's shoulder. **A:** Resting position. **B:** Proper positioning with both head position and neck extension (at C1) and flexion (at C7) for intubation. (From Mace SE. Challenges and advances in intubation: airway evaluation and controversies with intubation. *Emerg Med Clin North Am*. 2008;26(4):977–1000, ix.)

the patient's airway concerns and previously useful interventions can be lifesaving.

BASIC AIRWAY MANAGEMENT

Initial Maneuvers to Open the Airway

Often, airway obstruction can be relieved with a jaw-thrust maneuver. In cases with no suspected cervical spine injury, a head-tilt–chin-lift may also be successful. Both of these maneuvers are intended to create a patent airway for spontaneous ventilation and oxygenation without intubation. A jaw thrust can also be useful with bag-mask ventilation. Anterior displacement of the mandible (and indirectly the tongue) can be accomplished with pressure on the mentum (chin lift) or rami of the mandible (jaw lift). The combination of a bilateral jaw lift and caudad pressure on the chin to open the mouth is a jaw thrust. A one-handed jaw lift is used initially with mask ventilation by using anterior (lifting) pressure on the mandibular ramus with the fifth finger. Extension of the cranium at the junction with the cervical spine is a head tilt.

The *oropharyngeal airway* (OPA) consists of a flange, a short bite-block segment, and a curved plastic body. It provides an airway and suction channel through the mouth to the pharynx. It is designed to relieve airway obstruction by holding the tongue and the soft hypopharyngeal structures away from the posterior wall of the pharynx. Use of an OPA is not recommended in patients with intact cough or gag reflexes because it may stimulate gagging and vomiting. A correctly sized OPA approximates the distance from the corner of the mouth to the angle of the jaw. A tongue depressor may be used to insert the OPA, or it may be inserted sideways and then rotated (90 degrees) into position. Upside-down insertion with 180-degree rotation is not recommended because it may injure tissues or push the tongue posteriorly.

A *nasopharyngeal airway* (NPA) is a soft rubber or plastic tube (e.g., an endotracheal tube [ETT]) that provides an airway and channel for suctioning from the nares to the pharynx. NPAs may be used in patients with or without intact cough and gag reflexes. The NPA should be smaller than the inner aperture of the nares, and its length should approximate the distance from the tip of the nose to the tragus of the ear. If the NPA is too long, it may cause vagal stimulation and bradycardia, or injure the epiglottis or vocal cords. If the airway is too large, it will cause sustained blanching of the nostrils after insertion. It should be lubricated before inserting.

Bag-Mask Ventilation

If spontaneous respiratory effort is absent or insufficient to provide adequate ventilation or oxygenation, bag-mask ventilation is required. The most common technique for single-rescuer bag-mask ventilation involves the "E-C clamp" technique. The rescuer tilts the child's head and uses the last three fingers of one hand (forming a capital letter "E") to lift the jaw while pressing the mask against the face with the thumb and forefinger of the same hand (creating a "C"). The second hand squeezes the bag to produce visible chest rise. The jaw should be lifted to create the mask seal without pressing the mask down on the face. For larger patients, those with a difficult airway, or those with reduced lung compliance, a two-person bag-mask technique may be necessary. The first rescuer uses both hands to lift the jaw and open the airway while holding the mask to the face; the second rescuer squeezes the bag. In the out-of-hospital setting, bag-mask ventilation can be as effective as endotracheal intubation (ETI).

ADVANCED AIRWAY MANAGEMENT

Choice of Advanced Airway

Advanced airways can be divided into supraglottic, transglottic, or subglottic airways. The laryngeal mask airway (LMA) is a supraglottic airway. The LMA can bridge to a transglottic airway by guiding blind advancement or fiber-optic placement of an ETT. The ETT is the optimal advanced airway in most situations. The final option for difficult airway algorithms is the subglottic surgical airway (percutaneous cricothyrotomy or surgical tracheostomy).

Endotracheal Intubation

Preparation for laryngoscopy and intubation is essential; many airways assessed as difficult are simple airways that are inadequately supported. While providing effective oxygenation and ventilation, the provider should assure the necessary equipment and personnel are assembled (**Table 1.1**). Age-based formulas (**Table 1.2**) for ETT size are more reliable than estimates based on the size of the fifth finger, but are less accurate than length-based tapes. Providers generally use smaller-than-predicted ETTs in the setting of upper airway obstruction. Curved laryngoscope blades are often more effective for the child >2 years, while straight blades are used for children <2 years and those with a difficult airway.

After pharmacologic preparation of the patient (if appropriate), bag-mask ventilation should be interrupted to insert the ETT under direct visualization. The laryngoscope blade is used to deflect the tongue and lift the supraglottic structures (or tent the epiglottis) to visualize the glottis. The ETT is inserted through the vocal cords. Children have higher oxygen consumption (per kilogram body weight) than do adults and rapidly become hypoxemic during intubation. It is important to resume bag-mask ventilation if the patient's heart rate, oxygenation, or clinical appearance deteriorates.

TABLE 1.1

Equipment for Endotracheal Intubation

Monitoring Equipment (Apply before Intubation, if at All Possible)
Cardiorespiratory monitor (including monitoring of blood pressure, if possible)
Pulse oximeter
Length-based tape to estimate tube and equipment sizes
Confirmation Devices
Continuous waveform capnography preferred. In absence of continuous waveform capnography, the following may be used:
• Exhaled CO_2 colorimetric detector (pediatric size for patients <15 kg; adult size for patients >15 kg)
• Esophageal detector device (for children >20 kg with a perfusing rhythm) may be used.
Suction Equipment
Tonsil suction or large-bore suction device to suction pharynx
Suction catheter of appropriate size (to suction endotracheal tube)
Suction canister and device capable of generating suction of 280–2120 mm Hg (a wall-suction device capable of generating 2300 mm Hg is preferred)
Bag and Mask
Check size and oxygen connections
Connected to high-flow oxygen source with reservoir (capable of providing ~100% oxygen)
Medications
Anticholinergics (atropine)
Sedatives
Paralytics
Appropriate IV equipment and syringes for administration of medications
Intubation Equipment
Stylet
Cuffed or uncuffed tubes of estimated size and cuffed or uncuffed tubes that are 0.5 mm larger and smaller than estimated sizes
Laryngoscope blades (curved and straight) and handle with working light (keep extra batteries and bulb ready)
Water-soluble lubricant
Syringe to inflate tube cuff (if appropriate)
Towel or pad to place under patient (if appropriate)
Tape/Device to Secure Tube
Tape and tincture of benzoin or commercial device

External laryngeal manipulation (*b*ackward—posterior, *u*pward—cephalad, and *r*ightward *p*ush [BURP]) may help bring the glottis into view. If the provider can only visualize the posterior aspects of

TABLE 1.2

Formulas for Estimation of Endotracheal Tube Size and Depth of Insertion

Size
Uncuffed tube for infant: 3.0–3.5 mm ID
Uncuffed tube for child 1–2 y: 3.5–4.5 mm ID
Uncuffed tubes for children >2 y: size can be estimated with the following formula[a]:
$\text{Endotracheal tube (ID in mm)} = \frac{\text{Age(y)}}{4} + 4$
Cuffed tube for infant ≥ 3.5 kg and >1 y: 3.0 mm ID
Cuffed tube for child 1–2 y: 3.5 mm ID
Cuffed tubes for children >2 y: size can be estimated with the following formula:
$\text{Endotracheal tube (ID in mm)} = \frac{\text{Age(y)}}{3} + 3$
Depth of Insertion
$\text{Depth of insertion (cm)} = \frac{\text{Age(y)}}{2} + 12$
Depth of insertion = (ETT internal diameter) × 3

ID, internal diameter.

the glottis, successful intubation may be facilitated by using a stylet to create a bend ("hockey stick") in the end of the tracheal tube, taking care that the tip of the stylet does not protrude beyond the end of the tracheal tube.

Many uncuffed ETTs have depth indicators that should be positioned at or slightly distal to the vocal cords. Using the depth indicator helps ensure adequate depth while minimizing the risk of mainstem bronchus intubation. Cuffed tubes should be placed so that the cuff is positioned immediately below the level of the cords. Correct depth of insertion can be estimated from formulas using the child's age or the ETT size (see **Table 1.2**).

Nasotracheal Intubation

Nasotracheal intubation is sometimes used for patient comfort or ease of tube stabilization. Relative contraindications to nasotracheal intubation include coagulopathy, maxillofacial injury, or basilar skull fracture. A lubricated ETT is passed through one nare and guided through the larynx with McGill forceps during oral laryngoscopy (taking care to avoid rupturing the cuff with the forceps). If an orotracheal tube is in place, an assistant can remove it when the nasotracheal tube is in position and the glottis is well visualized. Blind nasotracheal intubation, sometimes used in awake adults, is generally difficult to perform in children. Complications of nasotracheal intubation include nosebleed, pressure-induced ischemic tissue injury to the rim of the nares, and nasal deformity due to nasal septal pressure necrosis. In older children, nasal intubation may be associated with a greater risk of sinusitis or otitis media.

Rapid Sequence Intubation

Rapid sequence intubation (RSI) is a technique used to secure the airway in the patient with a full (or presumed full) stomach when gastric insufflation may risk pulmonary aspiration. Medications are administered without awaiting the full effect of the preceding drug, and intubation occurs after a minimal delay based on the expected onset of action of the paralytic agent used. Bag-mask ventilation is classically avoided. Children become hypoxemic more rapidly, and those with intracranial or pulmonary hypertension may be intolerant of even brief periods of hypoxia or hypercapnia associated with apnea. For these reasons, a modified RSI technique with brief bag-mask ventilation may be used in the intubation of critically ill children.

Medications

No perfect combination of drugs exists for intubation of all patients, and so providers must select drugs based on the patient's condition and the provider's expertise. Some providers may choose to use atropine with intubation to prevent bradycardia, particularly in young infants, or with succinylcholine. The choice of sedative or anesthetic for intubation (**Table 1.3**) must be tailored to the patient and the clinical scenario. Hemodynamically unstable children who require intubation are likely to develop hypotension with the use of anesthetics that have significant vasodilatory properties (e.g., propofol or thiopental), but might well tolerate other anesthetic agents, such as ketamine or etomidate. Ketamine's bronchodilator properties are helpful when intubating children with asthma or other reactive airways disease.

Neuromuscular blocking (NMB) agents are used to facilitate the visualization and intubation of the airway. *Depolarizing neuromuscular blockers* bind the postsynaptic receptor of the neuromuscular junction, causing transient muscular fasciculation (seen less commonly in smaller infants) and then paralysis as the receptors remain occupied. Succinylcholine is the only agent in this group. Its advantages include rapid onset and relatively short duration of action. Complications include malignant hyperthermia, masseter spasm with subsequent airway obstruction, and a modest rise in serum potassium (typically, 0.5–1 mEq/L). Dangerous hyperkalemia is possible in patients with burns, myopathy (especially muscular dystrophy), peripheral nerve injury, renal failure, neuromuscular disease, or trauma with rhabdomyolysis.

Nondepolarizing neuromuscular blockers (e.g., rocuronium and vecuronium) bind the postsynaptic receptors of the neuromuscular junction, without causing postsynaptic depolarization and neuromuscular transmission. These agents have significantly longer duration than succinylcholine, and they are not reversible in time to allow spontaneous ventilation if the patient cannot be intubated or ventilated. Their use must be considered carefully in a patient with a potential difficult airway.

Airway Exchange Catheter

The *airway exchange catheter* is designed to be placed through an existing ETT to allow exchange with a new one. The airway exchange catheter often has a central lumen to allow oxygenation or placement over a guide wire during retrograde intubation.

Lighted Intubation Stylet

The *lighted intubation stylet*, also known as the light wand, is a rigid stylet with a fiber-optic light at the end. It can be used as a traditional stylet with direct laryngoscopy or blindly if direct laryngoscopy is impossible. It is contraindicated in conditions where there is laryngeal pathology. Any condition limiting transmission of light through the anterior neck (e.g., mass lesions, scarring, massive edema, or obesity) can interfere with its use.

Flexible Bronchoscopy

ETI over a flexible fiber-optic bronchoscope can be done directly or through an LMA. Once the fiber-optic bronchoscope is inserted into the trachea, a guidewire can be passed through the suction port or preferably a preloaded ETT can be passed over the scope into the trachea.

Videolaryngoscopy

Videolaryngoscopes are intubation devices with a camera on the distal end of the blade. They provide a more anterior laryngeal view and improve the view of the glottis when compared with direct laryngoscopy alone. They require less extension of the patient's head to provide a view of the glottis and may minimize the need to move the neck of a patient with cervical instability.

Laryngeal Mask Airway

The LMA consists of a small mask with an inflatable cuff that is connected to a plastic tube with a universal (15 mm) adaptor. It is placed in the oropharynx with its tip in the hypopharynx and the base of the mask above the epiglottis. When the cuff of the mask is inflated, it creates a seal with the supraglottic area, allowing air flow between the tube and the trachea. If the LMA is too large, it will be difficult to place, and if it is too small, it will not maintain an adequate seal to deliver effective positive pressure ventilation (PPV). The LMA can be inserted with the cuff fully or partially deflated; it is lubricated and then inserted

TABLE 1.3

Intubation Drugs and Doses

DRUG	ROUTE/DOSE	DURATION	COMMENTS
Anticholinergics			
Atropine	IV: 0.01–0.02 mg/kg (max: 1 mg)	>30 min	Both anticholinergics help prevent bradycardic response to vagal stimulation or succinylcholine. They may cause tachycardia and pupil dilation.
Glycopyrrolate	IV: 0.005–0.01 mg/kg (max: 0.2 mg)	>30 min	
Amnestic, Sedative Hypnotic, and Dissociative Agents			
Diazepam	IV: 0.1–0.2 mg/kg (max: 4 mg)	30–90 min	These 3 benzodiazepines are potent amnestic sedatives. They may cause respiratory depression or potentiate depressant effects of narcotics and barbiturates. They may cause hypotension and cardiac depression. They have no analgesic properties.
Lorazepam	IV: 0.05–0.1 mg/kg (max: 4 mg)	4–6 h	
Midazolam	IV: 0.1–0.3 mg/kg (max: 4 mg)	1–2 h	
Thiopental	IV: 2–5 mg/kg	5–10 min	Negative inotropic effects and systemic vasodilation often cause hypotension. Decreases cerebral metabolic rate and ICP. Potentiates respiratory depressive effects of narcotics and benzodiazepines. No analgesic properties.
Etomidate	IV: 0.2–0.4 mg/kg	5–15 min	Minimal cardiovascular effects. Decreases cerebral metabolic rate and ICP. May cause respiratory depression. Causes cortisol suppression; maybe contraindicated in patients dependent on endogenous cortisol response. No analgesic properties.
Propofol	IV: 2 mg/kg (up to 3 mg/kg in young children)	3–5 min	May cause hypotension, especially in hypovolemic patients. May cause pain on injection. Highly lipid soluble. No analgesic properties.
Ketamine	IV: 1–2 mg/kg, IM: 3–5 mg/kg	30–60 min	May increase blood pressure, heart rate, and cardiac output. May increase secretions. Bronchodilator. May cause hallucinations and emergence reactions. Has analgesic properties.
Analgesic Agents			
Lidocaine	IV: 1–2 mg/kg	~30 min	Causes myocardial and CNS toxicity with high doses. May decrease ICP during RSI. Hypotension occurs infrequently.
Fentanyl citrate	IV, IM: 2–45 mg/kg	IV: 30–60 min; IM: 1–2 h	May cause respiratory depression, hypotension, chest wall rigidity (usually with high dose, >5 μg/kg). May elevate ICP secondary to CO_2 retention.
Neuromuscular Blocking Agents			
Succinylcholine	Infant IV: 2 mg/kg, child IV: 1–1.5 mg/kg, IM: double the IV dose	3–5 min	Depolarizing muscle relaxant causes muscle fasciculation. May cause rise in intracranial, intraocular, and intragastric pressures. May cause rise in serum potassium. May cause bradycardia or ventricular arrhythmias. Avoid in renal failure, burns, crush injuries, or hyperkalemia.
cis-Atracurium	IV: 0.1 mg/kg, then 1–5 mg/kg/min	20–35 min	Metabolized by plasma hydrolysis. May cause mild histamine release.
Rocuronium	IV: 0.6–1.2 mg/kg	30–60 min	Few cardiovascular effects.
Vecuronium	IV: 0.1–0.2 mg/kg	30–60 min	Few cardiovascular effects.

Adapted from Hazinski M, Zaritsky A, Nadkarni V, et al. Rapid sequence intubation. In: *PALS Provider Manual*. Dallas, TX: American Heart Association, 2002; Venkataraman ST, Khan N, Brown A. Validation of predictors of extubation success and failure in mechanically ventilated infants and children. *Crit Care Med* 2000;28(8):2991–6.

and advanced with the aperture of the mask facing the tongue until the rescuer feels resistance, and the cuff is then inflated. Cuff inflation may push the LMA slightly out of the mouth, which may indicate that it is fully seated. See http://www.lmana.com/files/flexiblequick-reference-card.pdf for a size selection table.

Techniques Used to Verify Placement of Advanced Airway

Both clinical assessment (chest rise, auscultation, and vapor in the tube) and a device should be used to confirm airway placement. Detection of exhaled CO_2 after ETT insertion is a gold standard. When time permits, a chest radiograph should be obtained to confirm the proper depth of tube insertion. The tip of the ETT should be in midtrachea (approximately the level of the second to fourth thoracic vertebrae). The ETT will move further into the trachea when the neck is flexed and will move out of the trachea when the neck is extended.

Complications of ETI

Procedure Complications

Immediate complications of intubation can result from the medications administered, trauma to airway structures, injury to the cervical spine, or physiologic effects of laryngoscopy and PPV. Laryngoscopy can increase intracranial and intraocular pressures, coughing, regurgitation, aspiration, and laryngospasm (especially with inadequate sedation). Dental injury is common in school-aged children with loose deciduous teeth. A misplaced tube can be detected immediately with careful clinical assessment and evaluation of exhaled CO_2. Mainstem bronchus intubation (more commonly to the right side) can result in atelectasis, hypoxemia, and pneumothorax.

Late Complications

While the ETT is in place, the nares, lip, gum, and tongue should be assessed for signs of pressure injury. Ventilator-associated pneumonia and sinusitis can also occur in intubated patients. Subglottic fibrosis may develop and result in granuloma formation, especially posteriorly. Late complications including laryngeal and tracheal granulomas and vocal cord paralysis can develop up to 6 weeks after extubation.

MANAGEMENT OF THE DIFFICULT AIRWAY

General Principles of Difficult Airway Management

The American Society of Anesthesiologists has developed an algorithm for the approach to the difficult airway (www.asahq.org/~/media/sites/asahq/files/public/resources/standards-guidelines/practice-guidelines-for-management-of-the-difficult-airway.pdf). If time permits, the child should be moved to an environment where specialized equipment and personnel are available. Adequate preoxygenation with 100% oxygen can delay the onset of hypoxemia and bradycardia if intubation requires longer than anticipated. If initial tracheal intubation fails, it is important to make some change in technique or personnel before another attempt. The same careful preparations are required for extubation as for intubation because reintubation may be required and edema may make the reintubation even more difficult.

Surgical Airways: Percutaneous Needle Cricothyrotomy/Tracheostomy

Needle cricothyrotomy and tracheostomy are lifesaving procedures in patients who cannot be safely managed otherwise. They can be used in patients with obstruction proximal to the glottic opening or with abnormal anatomy that precludes laryngoscopic visualization of the glottic opening. Other clinical indications include facial trauma and angioedema.

MANAGEMENT OF SPECIFIC PROBLEMS

Cervical Spine Abnormalities and Injuries

Cervical spine anomalies, trauma, and conditions that limit neck movement interfere with visualization of the larynx. Movement of the neck for laryngoscopy in patients with an unstable cervical spine could result in spinal cord injury. Atlantoaxial instability is present in 10%–30% of patients with Down syndrome. In patients with presumed or diagnosed cervical spine instability, one provider must be assigned to stabilize the neck during airway manipulation until the airway is secured and immobilization devices can be applied. Although it is important to minimize neck movement in these patients, establishment of an adequate airway is the priority.

Intracranial Hypertension

Successful airway management for a patient with increased intracranial pressure (ICP) includes both advanced airway placement and prevention of secondary neurologic injury. Laryngoscopy and intubation can trigger spikes in ICP. Adequate anesthesia may blunt this rise in ICP, but hypotension from sedating agents should also be avoided. Lidocaine administration prior to intubation may help prevent an ICP spike; this is extrapolated from the use of lidocaine with tracheal suctioning. Because patients with increased ICP may not tolerate the hypoxemia or hypercapnia that can develop with a traditional RSI, a modified RSI technique is typically used.

Shock

When intubating a child in shock, sedatives/anesthetics should be selected with careful consideration of their associated hemodynamic effects. Drugs that are potent vasodilators (e.g., propofol and thiopental) should be used with extreme caution. Ketamine can be a useful drug in the hemodynamically unstable patient, but even it can have negative inotropic effects. Fentanyl at low doses is commonly used but may reduce sympathetic stimulation from pain. Etomidate maintains blood pressure but can cause adrenal suppression, especially in sepsis.

Facial or Laryngotracheal Injury

Facial injuries may be associated with profuse bleeding, fractures, and aspiration of blood, gastric contents, or teeth. If injury or uncontrolled bleeding obstructs the view of the larynx, fiber-optic or surgical techniques may be needed. Nasotracheal intubation is contraindicated until basilar skull fracture is ruled out because the ETT can migrate intracranially. Laryngeal injuries should be suspected in any patient with anterior neck trauma and hoarseness, stridor, subcutaneous emphysema, pneumomediastinum, or pneumothorax, and airway expertise sought. Inhalation injury should be anticipated in any burn patient with facial burns, singed nasal hairs, carbonaceous debris in the airway, or a history of closed-space exposure. Caustic ingestion can have a similar effect on airway structures. Anaphylaxis and hereditary angioedema are abrupt reactions that can result in severe airway edema.

Mediastinal Mass

The anterior mediastinal space can occasionally be occupied by masses, most commonly neoplasms. High-risk patients often present with positional symptoms. Changes in airway tone or chest wall compliance that result from anesthesia or neuromuscular blockade can lead to collapse or compression of the airway and nearby vascular structures, with consequent cardiorespiratory collapse. An ETT may not be able to bypass the area of the trachea compressed by the mass. The best plan is to keep the patient breathing spontaneously. Lateral or prone positioning may minimize airway compression. Because the transition from spontaneous breathing to PPV is a high-risk moment, it is prudent to briefly (and gently) assist spontaneous respiratory efforts with PPV to assess tolerance of PPV. Airway obstruction should be anticipated and equipment and personnel prepared in advance.

Acute Infectious Airway Obstruction

Infections of the deep neck space, including parapharyngeal, retropharyngeal, and peritonsillar infections, can lead to airway compromise. A protruding tongue can suggest infection in the submandibular or sublingual space (Ludwig angina). These conditions can rapidly progress to airway compromise. Therapy includes early antibiotics and surgical evaluation. *Laryngotracheobronchitis* (croup) presents with hoarseness, barky cough, and stridor and is almost always viral in origin. Only the most severe cases are not responsive to steroids or nebulized racemic epinephrine and require intubation. Subglottic narrowing may necessitate use of a much smaller diameter ETT than predicted. Bacterial laryngotracheobronchitis (bacterial tracheitis) is most commonly caused by *Staphylococcus aureus*. It often begins with a viral prodrome similar to croup but progresses rapidly with high fever, severe stridor, and respiratory distress. *Acute epiglottitis* is an airway emergency characterized by acute inflammation of the supraglottic region. Fortunately, this problem has almost vanished with the introduction of the *Haemophilus influenzae* type B vaccine. Epiglottitis is marked by sudden onset of fever, dysphagia, drooling, a “hot potato” voice, and toxemia. Unlike croup and bacterial tracheitis, cough is rarely present. Older patients often present in the “tripod” position (sitting and leaning forward braced on both arms) to maximize air entry. Antibiotic therapy is a priority. It is imperative to keep the child calm and allow a position of comfort; placing the child supine or performing unnecessary procedures, such as venipuncture, can trigger laryngospasm and irreversible airway obstruction. Intubation in the operating suite using an inhalational anesthetic is preferred.

CHAPTER 2 ■ CARDIOPULMONARY RESUSCITATION

ROBERT A. BERG, KATSUYUKI MIYASAKA, ANTONIO RODRÍGUEZ-NÚÑEZ, MARY F. HAZINSKI, DAVID A. ZIDEMAN, AND VINAY M. NADKARNI

Interventions to improve outcome from pediatric cardiac arrest should optimize therapies according to the etiology, timing, duration, intensity, and "phase" of resuscitation, as suggested in **Table 2.1**.

EPIDEMIOLOGY

Pediatric In-Hospital Cardiac Arrest

Survival to hospital discharge occurs in 25%–60% of children with in-hospital cardiopulmonary resuscitation (CPR) and aggressive postresuscitative care (70%–90% of survivors have favorable neurologic outcomes). Almost one-half of children have severe bradycardia and poor perfusion rather than a pulseless cardiac arrest when chest compressions are initiated. Children who received chest compressions initiated for bradycardia with pulses present have a much higher survival to hospital discharge rate (41%) than those whose chest compressions are initiated for nonshockable *pulseless* cardiac arrest (25%, $p < 0.001$).

Pediatric Out-of-Hospital Cardiac Arrest

The American Heart Association's (AHA) Chain of Survival highlights Prevention, Early CPR, Call for Help, Rapid Implementation of Advanced Life Support, and Aggressive Postresuscitation Care. *Bystander CPR* is key to increasing survival from out-of-hospital cardiac arrest (OHCA), yet only one-third to one-half of children receive bystander CPR (similar to adults). For children with sudden collapse (presumed arrest of cardiac etiology), hands-only bystander CPR is as effective as chest compression plus rescue breathing because the reservoir of air in the lungs oxygenates blood, perfusing the lungs during the low-flow state of CPR for 5–15 minutes; some gas exchange occurs with patient gasping; and some gas enters the lungs during the relaxation phase of compressions because of negative pressure generated with chest recoil. For pediatric OHCA from noncardiac causes, CPR with rescue breathing is preferred. The AHA recommends a C–A–B (compressions–airway–breathing) rather than the A–B–C (airway–breathing–compressions) approach because there is no flow until chest compressions are initiated and providing rescue breathing is complex and time-consuming and delays restarting circulation to vital organs.

Outcome from pediatric OHCA is worse than pediatric IHCA. Infants have both a higher incidence and mortality rate. The most common infant diagnosis of OHCA is sudden infant death syndrome (SIDS). The recent data suggest that the survival to discharge following pediatric OHCA is 3%–10%. The infant survival rate is only 3%–5%, and most surviving infants are severely neurologically impaired. The survival rate from a shockable rhythm (pulseless VT or VF) is ~20%, with >70% favorable neurologic outcome.

PEDIATRIC VENTRICULAR FIBRILLATION

Ventricular fibrillation (VF) is the *initial* rhythm in 19%–24% of pediatric OHCA. Conditions that increase the likelihood of VF in children include tricyclic antidepressant overdose, cardiomyopathy, renal failure with hyperkalemia, post–cardiac surgery, and prolonged QT syndromes. Mechanically initiated VF from *commotio cordis* (a low-energy chest-wall impact during repolarization, 10–30 milliseconds before the T wave peak) is seen in children 4–16 years old. The shockable rhythms of VF and pulseless ventricular tachycardia (VT) occur in 27% of pediatric in-hospital cardiac arrest (IHCA) at some point in time during the arrest and resuscitation (the most common initial rhythms during IHCA in children and adults are asystole and pulseless electrical activity [PEA]). Traditionally, VF and VT have been associated with better outcome than asystole and PEA. However, while outcome after *initial* VF/VT is good, outcome after *subsequent* VF/VT is worse, even when compared with asystole and PEA.

Termination of VF: Defibrillation

Defibrillation (defined as termination of VF) is necessary for the successful resuscitation from VF cardiac arrest. Defibrillation can result in asystole, PEA, or a perfusing rhythm. When an automated external defibrillator (AED) is used within 3 minutes

TABLE 2.1

Phases of Cardiac Arrest and Resuscitation

PHASE	INTERVENTIONS
Prearrest phase (protect)	Optimize community education regarding child safety
	Optimize patient monitoring and rapid emergency response
	Recognize and treat respiratory failure and/or shock to prevent cardiac arrest
Arrest (no-flow) phase (preserve)	Minimize interval to BLS and ALS (organized response)
	Minimize interval to defibrillation, when indicated
Low-flow (CPR) phase (resuscitate)	"Push hard, push fast"
	Allow full-chest recoil
	Minimize interruptions in compressions
	Avoid overventilation
	Titrate CPR to optimize myocardial blood flow (coronary perfusion pressures and exhaled CO_2)
	Consider adjuncts to improve vital organ perfusion during CPR
	Consider ECMO if standard CPR/ALS not promptly successful
Postresuscitation phase: short-term rehabilitation	Optimize cardiac output and cerebral perfusion
	Treat arrhythmias, if indicated
	Avoid hyperglycemia, hyperthermia, hyperventilation
	Consider mild postresuscitation systemic hypothermia
	Debrief to improve future responses to emergencies
Postresuscitation phase: longer-term rehabilitation (regenerate)	Early intervention with occupational and physical therapy
	Bioengineering and technology interface
	Possible future role for stem cell transplantation

BLS, basic life support; ALS, advanced life support; ECMO, extracorporeal membrane oxygenation; CPR, cardiopulmonary resuscitation.

of adult-witnessed VF, long-term survival is >70%. Mortality increases by 7%–10% per minute of delay to defibrillation.

Successful defibrillation requires an adequate current flow to depolarize a critical mass of myocardium. Current flow (amperes) is determined by the shock energy (joules) and the transthoracic impedance (ohms). Factors that affect transthoracic impedance include paddle size, thoracic gas volume, electrode/paddle contact, and conducting paste. Small paddle size increases resistance, which decreases current through the myocardium. Paddles/pads larger than the heart result in current flow through extramyocardial pathways and less current through the heart. Pediatric ("small") paddles are only used in infants (≤10 kg). Poor paddle contact and large lung volumes increase impedance, and conducting paste and increased pressure at the paddle–skin contact decrease impedance.

Defibrillation using biphasic defibrillators or the 150-J or 200-J biphasic AED dosage is nearly 90% successful for prolonged VF (compared with ~60% for 200-J monophasic defibrillation). The pediatric VF dose of 2 J/kg (monophasic or biphasic) is safe, but data are limited regarding effectiveness for prolonged VF. VF is usually prolonged in children with VF OHCA by the time a defibrillator is available. Mechanisms have been developed to attenuate the adult AED to deliver a dose to 50–86 J biphasic for children. However, use of an adult defibrillation dose is preferable to no defibrillation if a pediatric attenuator is not available.

INTERVENTIONS DURING THE PREARREST PHASE

Early warning scores and medical emergency teams (rapid response teams) are being implemented to recognize and intervene when cardiac arrest is impending. Their implementation has decreased the incidence of CPR on wards and is associated with improving survival rates.

INTERVENTIONS DURING THE CARDIAC ARREST (NO-FLOW) PHASE AND CARDIOPULMONARY (LOW-FLOW) PHASE

C–A–B Instead of A–B–C. First responders call for help and immediately start chest compressions while second and subsequent responders address the airway/breathing and rhythm issues. For shockable rhythms (VF/VT), chest compressions and defibrillation are the mainstays of treatment. For noncardiac causes (more common, asphyxia or hypotension) chest compressions are inadequate and rescue breathing is necessary. In sudden VF cardiac arrest, acceptable Pa_{O_2} and Pa_{CO_2} persist for 4–8 minutes during chest compressions without rescue breathing. In contrast, asphyxia results in significant arterial hypoxemia and acidemia prior to resuscitation. In this circumstance, rescue breathing can be lifesaving.

The Immediate Goal of Chest Compressions. CPR results in successful resuscitation only if it maintains adequate coronary perfusion pressure, the primary determinant of myocardial blood flow. A coronary perfusion pressure >20 mm Hg or arterial "diastolic/relaxation" pressure >30 mm Hg is associated with successful resuscitation. Titration of CPR efforts to adequate arterial diastolic/relaxation pressures is often feasible as many arrests occur in the intensive care unit (ICU) in patients with arterial catheter in place. End tidal carbon dioxide ($ETCO_2$) represents lung perfusion and is a surrogate for blood flow produced by CPR. Attaining $ETCO_2 > 15$ mm Hg is associated with survival and is recommended for monitoring during pediatric CPR.

Circumferential versus Focal Sternal Compressions. Circumferential chest compression provides better CPR hemodynamics than point compressions. This technique is recommended for smaller infants in whom it is often possible to encircle the chest with both hands and depress the sternum with the thumbs, while compressing the thorax circumferentially.

Open-Chest Compressions. Open-chest compressions are generally more effective than closed-chest compressions during CPR at generating myocardial and cerebral blood flow. They should be considered for children who have a chest that is open (recent cardiac surgery) or needs to be opened (penetrating chest injury).

Airway and Breathing. The most common precipitating events for pediatric cardiac arrest involve respiratory insufficiency. During CPR, cardiac output and pulmonary blood flow are ~10%–25% of normal. Consequently, less ventilation is necessary for adequate gas exchange from the pulmonary circulation during CPR. *Overventilation during CPR* is an important concern, it is both common and can compromise venous return and cardiac output. Overventilation can be due to frequent breaths (hyperventilation), which can interfere with the generation of negative intrathoracic pressure during the relaxation phase of chest compression or it can be due to too large breaths (overdistension) that may excessively increase intrathoracic pressure, pulmonary vascular resistance, and inhibit venous return. An additional concern in nonintubated patients is that delaying compressions to interpose ventilations increases the number of pauses in chest compression delivery and can contribute to worse survival outcomes. The final concern is that continued overventilation during into postresuscitation care may cause alkalosis, cerebral vasoconstriction, and limit cerebral blood flow.

Intraosseous Vascular Access. Intraosseous (IO) access provides access to a noncollapsible marrow venous plexus, which serves as a rapid, safe, and reliable route for the administration of drugs, crystalloids, colloids, and blood. Intraosseous vascular access can be achieved in 30–60 seconds. The onset of action and drug levels achieved with IO infusion during CPR are comparable to those following central vascular administration. Complications have been reported in <1% of patients following IO infusion (tibial fracture, lower extremity compartment syndrome, severe extravasation of drugs, and osteomyelitis).

Endotracheal Drug Administration. Epinephrine, atropine, naloxone, and lidocaine may be administered via the endotracheal route. Absorption into the circulation after endotracheal administration depends on dispersion over the respiratory mucosa, pulmonary blood flow, and matching of the ventilation (drug dispersal) to perfusion.

Medication Use during Cardiac Arrest

Vasopressors. During CPR, epinephrine's α-adrenergic effect on vascular tone increases systemic vascular resistance, diastolic blood pressure, coronary perfusion pressure and blood flow, and the likelihood of return of spontaneous circulation (ROSC). Epinephrine increases the vigor and intensity of VF, increasing the likelihood of successful defibrillation, presumably by increasing coronary perfusion. Epinephrine also increases cerebral blood flow during CPR because peripheral vasoconstriction directs flow to the cerebral circulation. However, epinephrine's β-adrenergic effect can increase myocardial oxygen consumption and worsen oxygen demand during CPR. Epinephrine administration during CPR can also worsen postresuscitation myocardial function and diminish microcirculatory flow in the organs through its α-adrenergic-mediated vasoconstriction. The use of *high-dose epinephrine* does not improve survival, may be associated with a worse neurologic outcome, and is not recommended for initial or rescue therapy.

Vasopressin is a long-acting endogenous hormone that mediates systemic vasoconstriction (V_1 receptor) and reabsorption of water in the renal tubule (V_2 receptor). Vasopressin increases blood flow to the heart and brain during CPR. It may decrease splanchnic blood flow during and following CPR. The increased afterload with this long-acting agent may exacerbate postresuscitation myocardial dysfunction. Vasopressin has comparable efficacy, but has not improved outcome compared with epinephrine.

Calcium. Calcium administration is only recommended during cardiac arrest for hypocalcemia, hyperkalemia, hypermagnesemia, and calcium-channel-blocker overdose. Calcium administration has not improved outcome in cardiac arrest and may worsen reperfusion injury. It may be useful for pediatric IHCA following cardiac surgery.

Buffer Solutions. Cardiac arrest results in lactic acidosis from inadequate organ blood flow and oxygen delivery. Acidosis depresses myocardial function, reduces systemic vascular resistance, and inhibits defibrillation. Sodium bicarbonate is indicated for arrest from hyperkalemia, tricyclic antidepressant overdose, or sodium-channel-blocker poisoning. Like calcium, bicarbonate administration during pediatric IHCA may be associated with worse outcomes. Side effects include hypernatremia, hyperosmolarity, metabolic alkalosis and hypercarbia. THAM is a non–carbon-dioxide-generating buffer that can be used during cardiac arrest.

Antiarrhythmic Medications. In children and adults, after an unsuccessful defibrillation attempt, epinephrine (with or without vasopressin) is administered before a subsequent attempt to defibrillate. If this fails, the antiarrhythmics *amiodarone* and *lidocaine* are considered. Amiodarone improves survival to hospital admission in the setting of shock-resistant VF.

POSTRESUSCITATION INTERVENTIONS

Targeted Temperature Management. Comatose adults, after resuscitation from witnessed VF OHCA, have improved outcome with induced hypothermia (32°–34°C). Targeted temperature management with close attention to postresuscitation supportive care may be equally effective at 32°C as at 36.5°C. Fever following cardiac arrest, brain trauma, stroke, and ischemia is associated with poor neurologic outcome. Hyperthermia following cardiac arrest is common in children. Until the benefit of postresuscitation hypothermia is determined for children, at least avoiding or actively treating hyperthermia following CPR is indicated.

Myocardial Support and Blood Pressure Management. Postarrest myocardial stunning occurs commonly and is pathophysiologically similar to sepsis-related or postcardiopulmonary bypass myocardial dysfunction (increases in inflammatory mediator and nitric oxide production). A significant proportion of children have hypotensive events following ROSC and require treatment with vasoactive medications.

Glucose Control. Hyperglycemia following adult cardiac arrest is associated with worse neurologic outcome after controlling for duration of arrest and presence of cardiogenic shock. Postresuscitation hyperglycemia is usually transient and children may be at increased risk for hypoglycemia after treatment. Care must be taken when hyperglycemia is treated and frequent monitoring used.

Post–Cardiac Arrest Seizures. Seizures after pediatric cardiac arrest are common. Continuous and reactive background patterns on electroencephalogram (EEG) are associated with good outcome, whereas burst-suppression and discontinuous backgrounds are associated with poor outcome. Continuous EEG monitoring can provide useful information to help minimize brain injury and enhance prognostication.

Postresuscitation Hyperoxia. The administration of 100% oxygen after ROSC is associated with worse neurologic outcome in animal models (thought due to free radical injury and oxidative stress). It is prudent to wean children from 100% oxygen post-ROSC while maintaining adequate oxygen saturations in vital organs.

Extracorporeal Membrane Oxygenation—Cardiopulmonary Resuscitation. Extracorporeal membrane oxygenation (ECMO) is a technology that can be used to control postresuscitation temperature and hemodynamic parameters. ECMO is also used as a rescue therapy for pediatric cardiac arrest (E-CPR).

POST–CARDIAC ARREST EVALUATION OF SUDDEN DEATH

Autopsy and genetic testing are important in the evaluation of an unexpected sudden death. The results may affect other members (or future members) of the victim's family.

Channelopathies. Genetic mutations that lead to channelopathies are common in infants and children with OHCAs (25%–53% of first- and second-degree relatives have these inherited arrhythmogenic diseases).

Hypertrophic Cardiomyopathy. Hypertrophic cardiomyopathy occurs among 1 in 500 in the general population with an annual risk of death of 1%, often caused by ventricular arrhythmias. It is the most common cause of sudden cardiac death among young athletes and often has no preceding symptoms.

Coronary Artery Abnormalities. Coronary artery abnormalities (generally aberrant coronary arteries with extrinsic obstruction) are the second leading cause of sudden death in athletes. Up to 17% of sudden deaths among young athletes have been attributed to anomalous coronary arteries.

CHAPTER 3 ■ STABILIZATION AND TRANSPORT

MONICA E. KLEINMAN, AARON J. DONOGHUE, RICHARD A. ORR,
AND NIRANJAN "TEX" KISSOON

ORGANIZATION OF PEDIATRIC TRANSPORT SYSTEMS

Essential components of a transport program include (a) online medical control by qualified physicians, (b) ground and air ambulance capabilities, (c) a coordinated communications system, (d) written clinical and operational guidelines, (e) a comprehensive quality and performance improvement program, (f) a database to track activity and facilitate patient follow-up, (g) medical and nursing leadership, (h) administrative resources, and (i) institutional endorsement and financial support.

Training, Certification, and Licensure

Most transport teams are multidisciplinary with highly trained hospital-based providers and include members with expertise in communications and out-of-hospital care. No uniform national curriculum exists for critical care transport clinicians, either adult or pediatric.

Finances and Reimbursement

A transport team's response to a request for emergent interfacility transfer should not depend on a patient's insurance status or ability to pay. Administrators must understand that transport teams facilitate patient entry into the hospital's system and are unlikely to be independently profitable. Reimbursement for critical care transport varies among states and insurance providers. If the transport team includes an attending physician, billing codes exist for face-to-face care of a child during transport, for telephone consultation with the referring physician prior to the transport team's arrival, and for non–face-to-face medical direction by the medical control physician.

Legal Considerations

In the United States, interfacility patient transfer is regulated by federal laws that protect patients with emergent conditions who present to Medicare-participating hospitals. The Consolidated Omnibus Budget Reconciliation Act (COBRA) was passed in 1986; one component of this legislation was the Emergency Medical Transportation and Labor Act (EMTALA). EMTALA was created to prevent "patient dumping", the transfer of an individual presenting for emergency care without assessment or stabilizing treatment (**Table 3.1**).

Risk Management and Insurance

Collisions and crashes involving pediatric or neonatal teams are uncommon, with one collision or crash for every 1000 patient transports. Collisions or crashes resulting in serious injuries or death are less common, with a rate of 0.55 injuries or deaths per 1000 transports. Disability coverage is important to provide financial security following an accident or work-related injury.

Transfer Agreements

Transfer agreements define administrative procedures and the roles and responsibilities of the referring and receiving facilities. The EMS for Children (EMSC) program has published sample pediatric transfer guidelines for adoption by states or programs (http://www.emscnrc.org).

TABLE 3.1

Requirements of the Emergency Medical Transportation and Labor Act

1. The transferring hospital provides medical treatment to the best of its ability, based on available resources.
2. The transferring physician contacts the receiving facility to determine that qualified personnel and space are available for treatment and to identify a receiving physician who will accept the patient.
3. The transferring hospital sends copies of all available medical records related to the patient's emergency medical condition.
4. The transfer is affected through qualified personnel and transportation equipment, including the use of advanced life support, if appropriate.

Quality Improvement and Accreditation

A written quality improvement (QI) plan is essential and should begin with an explanation of the mission of the transport service and the goals for the QI program. The medical director should oversee the posttransport case review process, including audits of charts, recorded audiotapes, and morbidity and mortality conferences. The Commission on Accreditation of Medical Transport Systems (CAMTS) aims to improve the quality of patient care and safety of the transport environment through its voluntary accreditation process. Accreditation standards are revised every 2–3 years.

THE TRANSPORT ENVIRONMENT

Prehospital Care versus Critical Care Transport

Most pediatric critical care transport programs provide interfacility transport but do not respond to the scene of an accident or emergency (unless a crash is encountered during travel or if a multicasualty incident or disaster occurs). Less than 10% of ambulance calls nationwide are for infants and children; few involve advanced life support, and even less can be classified as critical care. This frequency translates into three pediatric encounters per month for ~60% of the nation's paramedics, with <3% of the nation's paramedics providing emergency care for ≥15 children per month. Limited EMS provider exposure to critically ill children presents a challenge to maintaining pediatric assessment and treatment skills. This fact should be considered when selecting the appropriate mode of interfacility transport for an ill or injured child.

Mobile Intensive Care

Both ground and air transports result in noise levels that can prohibit auscultation of lung and heart sounds. Vehicular motion and vibration can result in artifacts in pulse oximetry, electrocardiography, and oscillometric blood pressure monitoring. Handheld and portable devices that enable point-of-care testing permit the analysis of whole-blood chemistries and blood gases. Most therapies available in the intensive care unit (ICU) can be employed during critical care transport.

Ground Transport Considerations

Transport by ground is the most common modality of interfacility and prehospital transport. The advantages of ground transport include virtually ubiquitous access, low cost, and ability to respond in most weather conditions. The disadvantages of ground transport include the impact of severe winter weather, traffic congestion, and road and highway conditions.

Aeromedical Transport

Both rotor-wing (helicopter) and fixed-wing (airplane) aircraft can be adapted for critical care transport vehicles. Barometric pressure is the sum of the partial pressures of each component gas in the atmosphere. Barometric pressure at sea level is 760 mm Hg. Total barometric pressure decreases with increasing altitude and the partial pressure of each gas is reduced. The *alveolar gas equation* defines the relationship between the alveolar partial pressure of oxygen (PAO_2), barometric pressure (PB), partial pressure of water vapor (PH_2O), fraction of oxygen in (FIO_2), alveolar partial pressure of carbon dioxide ($PACO_2$), and the respiratory quotient (R), as follows:

$$PAO_2 = (PB - PH_2O) \times FIO_2 - (PACO_2/R)$$

Assuming that R is 0.8, $PACO_2$ is normal (i.e., ~40 mm Hg), and the PH_2O at body temperature (37°C) is 47 mm Hg, the PAO_2 while breathing room air at sea level is calculated as follows:

$$PAO_2 = (760 \text{ mm Hg} - 47 \text{ mm Hg}) \times 0.21 - (40/0.8) = 99 \text{ mm Hg}$$

Thus, with increasing altitude and decreasing PB, the resultant PAO_2 will decrease. PAO_2 can be restored to baseline values by increasing the FIO_2. If other factors remain constant, the FIO_2 required to maintain the same PAO_2 at a lower barometric pressure can be calculated as follows:

$$FIO_{2(1)} \times PB_{(1)} = FIO_{2(2)} \times PB_{(2)}$$

The maintenance of a specific barometric pressure in the cabin of an aircraft (i.e., cabin pressurization) ameliorates this effect, but is only possible in fixed-wing aircraft and not in helicopters. For the patient with severe cardiac or pulmonary disease who is already requiring a FIO_2 of 1.0 at ground level, the effects of altitude can worsen the hypoxemia. An infant with cyanotic heart disease is similarly vulnerable to developing a critical level of tissue hypoxia.

A decrease in the ambient barometric pressure also has the potential to affect gas-filled compartments in the body. *Boyle's law* states an inverse relationship between volume and pressure of a gas; therefore, a decrease in pressure results in an increase in volume. Most medical helicopters travel 1500 and 5000 feet above ground level. If ground level represents sea level, then barometric pressure will decrease by 20% at 5000 feet, with a consequent 20% increase in gas volume. Most commercial aircraft maintain a cabin pressure equivalent to ~8000 feet above sea level, producing a 30% decrease in barometric pressure and a 30% increase in the volume of air-filled spaces. It is essential to anticipate and address the potential for gas expansion by such interventions as gastric drainage, pleural decompression, and replacement of air in an endotracheal tube cuff (using saline) prior to transport.

Rotor-Wing (Helicopter) Transport

Helicopter transport is generally faster than ground transport for patients >45 miles from the receiving facility. Hypothermia is a major risk for infants during helicopter transport if an Isolette is not used. In the unpressurized cabin, ambient air has less moisture, leading to increased risk of airway plugging. Humidified gases should be used as early as possible.

Fixed-Wing (Airplane) Transport

Fixed-wing transport is typically reserved for travel over long distances or open water. It has the fastest speed of the three commonly used transport modalities. Additional advantages include cabin pressurization, which minimizes the adverse physiologic effects of altitude, and the ability to fly in weather conditions that may not be favorable for helicopter transport.

Safety Considerations

Ground transport providers should be familiar with state and local regulations regarding child restraint, which often do not exempt emergency vehicles.

PATIENT CARE DURING TRANSPORT

Resuscitation, Stabilization, and Preparation for Transport

Length of stabilization time prior to transport does not appear to have an impact on early ICU mortality for critically ill children transported to receive intensive care. The transport team should know the patient's ongoing medical issues to be able to devise a plan in case of deterioration or complications; in some instances, this may involve consultation with the medical command physician and/or relevant specialists during stabilization and transport.

Communication

Initial communication should include a conversation between the referring and receiving physicians. The receiving physician may be asked for medical advice regarding patient management. Such advice should be clearly documented. The risks and benefits of interfacility transfer must be explained to family members and consent obtained, either in person or by phone.

Family and Ethical Considerations

Do-Not-Attempt-Resuscitation Orders

Transport team members should inquire about the presence of advanced directives and do-not-attempt-resuscitation (DNAR) orders and should not assume that such inquiries have been made by the providers at the referring facility. They should obtain specific details about the terms of an advanced directive. When ambiguity exists or family members appear uncertain, it is preferable for them to accompany the patient on the transport if possible (see Family Presence section).

Death on Transport

It is unusual for children to die during interfacility transport. Pediatric transport teams may arrive at a referring facility to find that a patient has failed to respond to resuscitative measures but the resuscitation team chose to continue efforts until arrival of the team. Transport team members should review the patient's status for potentially reversible causes of arrest and, in consultation with the medical control physician, use usual and customary criteria to discontinue resuscitation.

Transport team members should be familiar with state regulations regarding notification of the regional organ procurement organization and medical examiner's office following the death of a child. In most of the United States, it is illegal for anyone other than authorized funeral homes and the medical examiner's office staff to transport a patient who has been pronounced dead. In general, if cardiac arrest occurs after the team departs from the referring facility, the team should continue resuscitative efforts until arrival at the receiving facility.

Family Presence

Policy statements that encourage family presence in these situations now exist, but to date, no such formal recommendations have been formulated with respect to family presence during critical care transport. Data on the effect of parental presence during transport is limited but, for the most part, report its safety without impedance of care.

TRANSPORT CONSIDERATIONS FOR SPECIFIC POPULATIONS

Pediatric Emergency Department Considerations

It is estimated that <10% of hospitals in the United States have dedicated pediatric emergency departments (EDs). While physically separate care areas for children are ideal, they are not mandatory for the provision of quality pediatric emergency care.

Trauma Centers

Trauma is the leading cause of death for children 6 months to 14 years of age. Most pediatric trauma patients suffer blunt injuries that are managed nonoperatively. A small percentage of injured children (e.g., patients with expanding epidural hematomas) will require immediate surgery on arrival to the trauma center. Components of a "direct-to-the-OR" protocol include a communication system to notify the appropriate surgical service(s) and other essential personnel (e.g., anesthesia, operating room nursing, blood bank, radiology).

Burn Centers

Transfer to a pediatric burn center is often a secondary or tertiary transport following resuscitation and/or stabilization at a community hospital or trauma center without a burn unit. The American Burn Association (http://www.ameriburn.org) has developed guidelines for the transfer of children to a pediatric burn center (**Table 3.2**).

Extracorporeal Membrane Oxygenation and Inhaled Nitric Oxide

In general, the Extracorporeal Life Support Organization recommends that a neonate whose condition is deteriorating be transferred at a time when the conversion to conventional ventilation can still be tolerated and suggests that an infant who has not improved after 6 hours of high-frequency oscillatory ventilation (HFOV) be considered a candidate for expedient transfer. Individual institutions may use the alveolar–arterial oxygen difference, the oxygenation index, or the persistence of a PaO_2 of <50 torr as predictors of the need for extracorporeal membrane oxygenation (ECMO). The transport team must have the capability of providing inhaled nitric oxide (iNO) during transport if the patient is already receiving this therapy, because abrupt discontinuation may result in serious deleterious effects. If the patient is too unstable for transfer, a few select programs have the capability to respond to requests for transport by mobilizing an ECMO team that is capable of cannulating the patient at the referring facility, then transporting while on ECMO to the base institution.

TABLE 3.2

American Burn Association Burn Unit Referral Criteria

1. Partial thickness burns >10% total body surface area
2. Burns that involve the face, hands, feet, genitalia, perineum, or major joints
3. Third-degree burns in any age group
4. Electrical burns, including lightning injuries
5. Chemical burns
6. Inhalation injury
7. Burn injury in patients with preexisting medical disorders that could complicate management, prolong recovery, or affect mortality
8. Any patients with burns and concomitant trauma (e.g., fractures) in which the burn injury poses the greatest risk of morbidity or mortality. In such cases, the patient may be initially stabilized in a trauma center before being transferred to a burn unit. Physician judgment will be necessary in such situations and should be in concert with the regional medical control plan and triage protocols.
9. Burned children in hospitals without qualified personnel or equipment for the care of children
10. Burn injury in patients who will require special social, emotional, or long-term rehabilitative intervention

Resident Education in Transport Medicine

The Residency Review Committee of the Accreditation Council for Graduate Medical Education refers to pediatric resident involvement in critical care transport as follows: (a) participation in decision making in admitting, discharging, and transferring of patients to the ICU; and (b) resuscitation, stabilization, and transportation of patients to the ICU and within the hospital (http://www.acgme.org).

OUTCOMES

Transport Scoring Systems

Several scoring systems have been developed based on pretransport data, but their utility is limited by the subjective nature and variable accuracy of referring physicians' assessments. The Transport Risk Assessment in Pediatrics (TRAP) score uses physiologic variables to predict need for pediatric intensive care unit (PICU) admission and may support triage decision making.

Team Composition

Pediatric critical care transport teams may be staffed with a variety of personnel combinations including registered nurses or nurse practitioners, physicians, respiratory therapists, and paramedics. No studies have evaluated the effect of physician-versus-nonphysician team composition on the outcome of transported children.

Specialty Pediatric Teams versus General Teams

In a study involving 17,649 patients, the use of a pediatric specialty transport team was associated with improved survival. In addition to outcome, transport by specialty teams decreases costs through decreased adverse events as compared to nonspecialty teams.

Telemedicine

New technology makes it possible for patient assessment or test interpretation to be performed remotely, potentially improving pretransport care or, at the other extreme, obviating the need for patient transfer. *Tele-echocardiography* in particular has been used successfully to evaluate newborns with suspected congenital heart disease, preventing unnecessary transport for diagnostic testing for those infants who are clinically well.

CHAPTER 4 ■ INVASIVE PROCEDURES

STEPHEN M. SCHEXNAYDER, PRAVEEN KHILNANI, AND NAOKI SHIMIZU

Invasive procedures are necessary for the care of many critically ill children. Complications can be life-threatening and require careful assessment of risk and benefit.

CENTRAL VENOUS CATHETERIZATION

The indications for central venous catheter (CVC) placement include access for medication administration, monitoring of central venous pressure and central venous oxygen saturation, parenteral nutrition, frequent blood sampling, hemodialysis, hemofiltration, or apheresis. Bleeding complications may be the most common immediate adverse associated events. Subclavian catheters may carry the highest risk in very young or coagulopathic patients because of inability to effectively compress the subclavian vessels. Other complications can include infection, thrombosis, embolus (air or clot), vessel puncture or injury, nerve injury, lymphatic injury, catheter malfunction, wire-induced arrhythmia, or catheter displacement. Catheter-related bloodstream infection (CRBSI) can be reduced by using a "bundle" of practices during insertion and care of CVCs.

Three sites commonly used for CVCs in children are femoral, subclavian, and internal jugular. Peripherally inserted central catheters (PICCs) are an alternative for central access. Adult data indicate a lower risk of infection from subclavian sites; pediatric data are inconclusive. Recommended insertion techniques include strict hand washing prior to placement, skin antisepsis with chlorhexidine, and full barrier precautions (operator wearing hair covering, mask, sterile gown, and gloves, and use of a large sterile-field drape), but with ability to visualize the airway and peripheral vascular access site where medications are being administered. Sedation, analgesia, and local anesthesia facilitate placement.

Most CVCs are placed using the wire-guided (Seldinger) technique. A dilator is typically passed over the guide wire after the needle has been removed. Catheters should be flushed prior to insertion, and then clamped or capped to reduce the chance of air embolism. In hypovolemic patients, volume resuscitation prior to attempted CVC placement may facilitate cannulation.

Confirmation of venous placement can be by fluid-column drop test, the use of a pressure transducer, and blood gas analysis of a sample from the line. The recommended placement of the tip of the catheter is at or just above the junction of the superior vena cava and right atrium for upper body catheters to minimize risk of cardiac perforation or arrhythmia.

Femoral Venous Catheterization

For femoral venous cannulation, the lower extremity should be positioned with slight external rotation at the hip and flexion at the knee (frog-leg appearance). A rolled towel under the buttock may be useful. The femoral artery should be located by palpation and/or ultrasound or, in the pulseless patient, assumed to be at the midpoint between the pubic symphysis and anterior superior iliac spine. During cardiopulmonary resuscitation, pulsations may be felt in the femoral vein or artery; therefore, if cannulation is not successful medially, one should aim for the pulsation. The needle should be inserted 1–2 cm below the inguinal ligament, just medial to the artery, and slowly advanced while negative pressure is applied to a syringe attached to the introducer needle (**Fig. 4.1**).

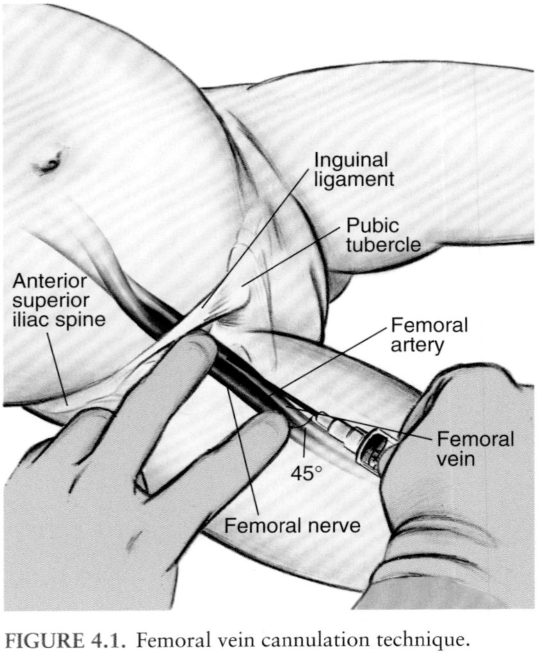

FIGURE 4.1. Femoral vein cannulation technique.

The needle should be directed at a 15–60-degree angle toward the umbilicus, with a flatter approach used in infants. Once venous blood is obtained, the syringe should be removed while the needle is stabilized and the guide wire is introduced gently. The guide wire should never be forced.

Subclavian Venous Catheterization

For cannulation of the subclavian vein, position the patient 30 degrees head-down (Trendelenburg) to distend the central veins and minimize the risk of air embolism. Extend the patient's neck, turn the patient's head away from the site of cannulation, and place a rolled towel beneath the patient's shoulder blades, along the axis of the thoracic spine. Keeping the head closer to midline may increase the diameter of the vein. The patient should be on an electrocardiogram (ECG) monitor.

The *infraclavicular approach* is most commonly used and will be described here. The needle should be introduced just under the clavicle at the junction of the middle and medial thirds and slowly advanced (**Fig. 4.2**). The needle should be inserted parallel with the frontal plane and directed medially and slightly cephalad, under the clavicle toward the lower end of the fingertip in the sternal notch. In ventilated patients, an expiratory hold while the needle is advanced may minimize the risk of pneumothorax. A fingertip should be placed over the needle hub as soon as the syringe is removed to prevent air entrainment. The guide wire should be introduced during inspiration in a patient on positive-pressure ventilation or during exhalation in a spontaneously breathing patient. An observer watches the ECG for arrhythmia. A chest X-ray should be obtained to verify position prior to use and to rule out pneumothorax or hemothorax.

Internal Jugular Catheterization

Internal jugular catheterization can be achieved via multiple approaches. When available, ultrasound guidance is preferable. Right-sided approaches are preferred as the thoracic duct is on the left side. The carotid artery should be palpated, as it lies medial to the internal jugular vein within the carotid sheath. For all approaches, the patient should be positioned supine and in a slight (15–30 degree) Trendelenburg position, with a shoulder roll and the head turned away from the site and ECG monitoring.

In the *anterior approach*, the needle is introduced along the anterior margin of the sternocleidomastoid muscle, halfway between the mastoid process and sternum (**Fig. 4.3A**). In the *middle approach*, the needle enters the apex of a triangle formed by the clavicle and the heads of the sternocleidomastoid muscle (**Fig. 4.3B**). The skin should be punctured with the needle at a 30–60-degree angle while the needle is directed toward the ipsilateral nipple. For the *posterior approach*, the needle should be introduced along the posterior border of the sternocleidomastoid cephalad to its bifurcation into the sternal and clavicular heads (**Fig. 4.3C**) and aimed toward the suprasternal notch. In all approaches, the needle should be advanced during exhalation to minimize the chance of pneumothorax. Monitor for arrhythmias during guide wire introduction. A chest X-ray should be obtained to verify position prior to use and to rule out pneumothorax or hemothorax.

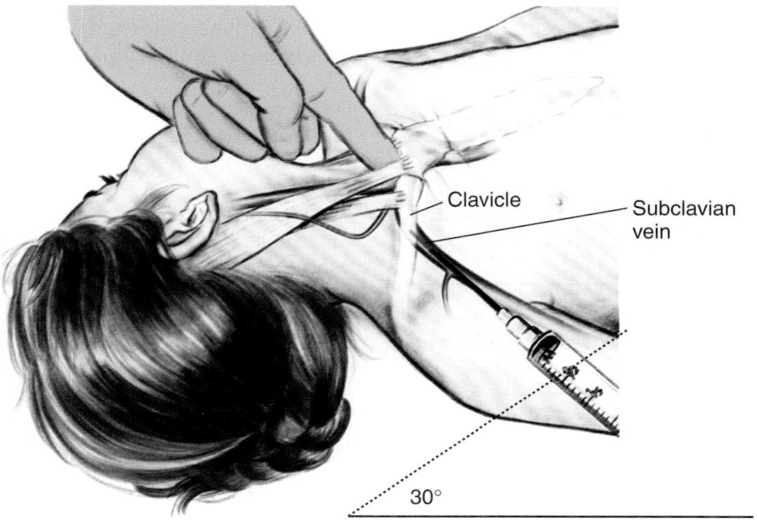

FIGURE 4.2. Cannulation of the subclavian vein.

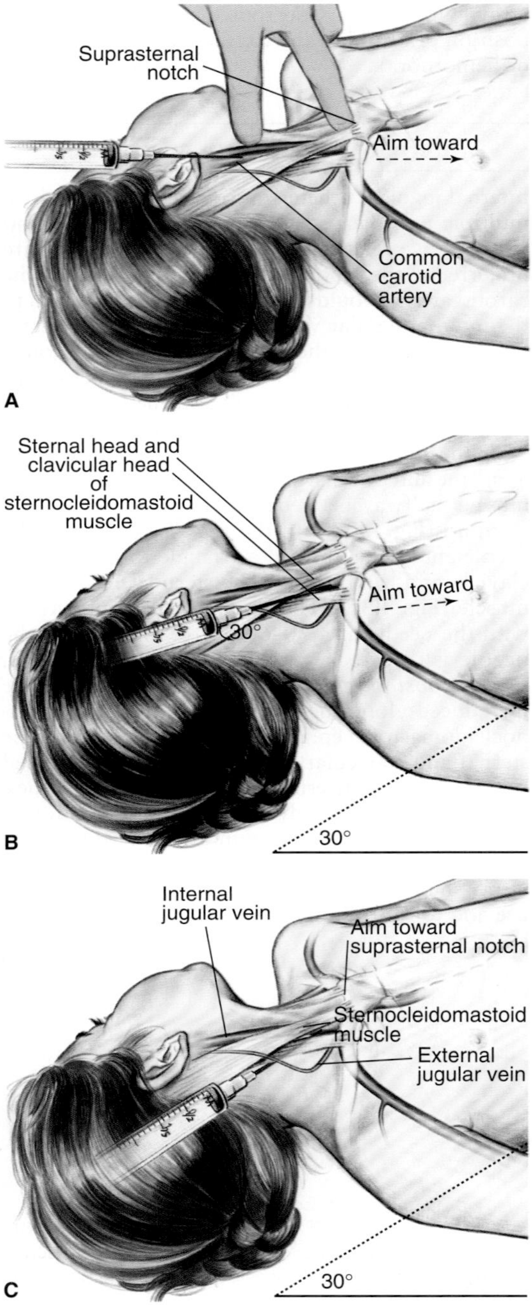

FIGURE 4.3. Technique for catheterization of the internal jugular vein. **A:** Anterior route. **B:** Middle route. **C:** Posterior route.

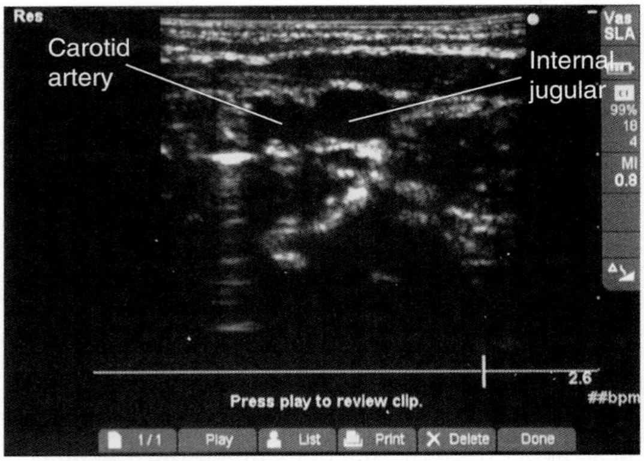

FIGURE 4.4. Anatomy seen during an ultrasound-assisted placement of a central venous line. The vein is often larger, more irregular, less pulsatile and more compressible than the artery.

Complications

Early complications of CVC placement include perforation of vessels or other structures by the needle, guide wire, dilator, or catheter. Hemothorax, hydrothorax, and pericardial tamponade may occur. The risk of catheter-induced erosion increases with catheter stiffness, catheter tip placement against a vessel bifurcation or the thin right atrium, or a catheter that remains in place for a long time. Pneumothoraces may occur with subclavian and internal jugular approaches and retroperitoneal hemorrhage with the femoral approach. Coagulopathy should be corrected prior to CVC attempts. Catheter or wire fracture may require retrieval under fluoroscopy.

CRBSI can be reduced by employing strict attention to the insertion technique, ongoing maintenance for the duration of its placement, minimizing entry into the catheter, daily assessment of the continued need for the catheter, and employing chlorhexidine skin prep during dressing changes. Both antibiotic- and antiseptic-impregnated catheters have been shown to reduce CRBSI. Deep venous thrombosis is found with all catheters sites and is associated with diabetic ketoacidosis and oncologic conditions.

Ultrasound Assistance in Central Venous Catheter Placement

Ultrasound guidance reduces complications of CVC placement (**Fig. 4.4**). To maintain strict antisepsis, use a long, sterile, ultrasound sheath. Ultrasonic gel is also required inside the sheath.

INTRAOSSEOUS INFUSION

Intraosseous (IO) needle placement is recommended as an emergency vascular access technique for all ages. It can be used for all medications that can be given IV. The IO route is preferred over endotracheal administration for drug delivery during cardiopulmonary resuscitation.

The most common site for IO placement is the proximal tibia. The distal tibia, distal femur, calcaneus, and anterior superior iliac spine are alternate lower body sites and the humerus and radius are alternative upper body sites. A sternal IO catheter placement system exists as does a drill for tibia or humerus placement. It is also possible to use a bone marrow aspiration or biopsy needle (use a stylet during advancement). A fracture or prior IO attempt at the same location are contraindications (medications and fluid may extravasate).

The skin should be prepared with chlorhexidine or povidone–iodine. The operator's hand should not be placed behind the extremity. The needle should be directed slightly away from the joint. When the needle reaches the periosteum, a firm twisting motion should be used to advance the needle through the cortical bone into the marrow cavity. Once a decrease in resistance is felt, the needle should be advanced no further. The cap should then be unscrewed and the stylet removed. If no marrow can be aspirated, infusion of a small amount of saline should be attempted. Infusion with little resistance indicates successful placement. Complications of IOs include fluid or drug extravasation, infection, compartment syndrome, and, potentially, growth failure if the IO is placed in the epiphysis. The area should be frequently assessed during IO infusion to detect infiltration early.

ARTERIAL CATHETERIZATION

Arterial access is indicated for arterial blood gas or other blood sampling and continuous blood pressure monitoring. Sterile technique should be employed and ultrasound may be useful.

Radial artery catheterization is frequently used but can be difficult in patients with shock. Some authorities recommend assessing collateral circulation using the modified Allen test, where both the ulnar and radial arteries are compressed, and after the hand becomes pale, the pressure on the ulnar artery is released. Perfusion should improve immediately if collateral circulation is adequate. The wrist should be placed on an appropriately sized arm board with a small roll under the dorsal surface. Skin antisepsis with chlorhexidine is then performed. Catheter-over-the-needle or Seldinger techniques may be used. For catheter-over-the-needle systems, some operators prefer to pass the needle completely through the artery to transfix the vessel, after which the needle is removed, the catheter withdrawn slowly, and the catheter advanced once blood flow returns. Other techniques include inserting a catheter over the needle through the skin until blood flow is noted. At that point, the catheter is slowly advanced while the needle is kept immobile. The catheter should advance easily. Pressure monitoring should be instituted quickly so that a disconnection will be rapidly recognized to avoid exsanguination. *Femoral artery catheterization* is used when other access sites are difficult but has a risk of causing lower extremity ischemia. The dorsalis pedis and posterior tibial arteries in the foot are alternative sites. The axillary artery is rarely used in children (complication is carotid emboli with fast flushes of catheter). Owing to the absence of collateral circulation, use of the brachial artery is not recommended.

THORACENTESIS/TUBE THORACOSTOMY

Tube thoracostomy or thoracentesis may be required to drain air (pneumothorax), blood (hemothorax), fluids (hydrothorax), or pus (empyema). Any abnormal collection in the pleural space may interfere with respiratory function and, in severe cases, impair cardiovascular function. Small pneumothoraces in spontaneously breathing patients may not require evacuation.

Needle Thoracostomy

Emergent decompression is indicated prior to chest X-ray for a suspected tension pneumothorax in a deteriorating patient. A needle or catheter-over-the-needle unit is inserted perpendicular to the chest wall and advanced along the superior border of the third rib (i.e., second intercostal space) in the midclavicular line until a rush of air is obtained. When spontaneous respirations are present, a one-way valve or stopcock should be attached to prevent air entry into the chest. Repeated aspiration of air may be required until a tube thoracostomy can be performed.

Thoracentesis

Thoracentesis may be used to symptomatically relieve respiratory distress in patients with large effusions and to obtain pleural fluid for diagnostic studies. The risks are increased if volume of fluid is small, if the patient is coagulopathic or if the patient is ventilated with positive pressure. Local anesthetics and sedation are often required for children. Larger patients may be positioned in a seated, upright position over a padded tray table. A young child may be held in an upright position or a partial lateral decubitus position. For simple aspiration of air, the supine position can be used. The usual site to obtain fluid is the posterior axillary line near the tip of the scapula, which represents the seventh intercostal space during full inspiration. Bedside ultrasound may be very helpful in localizing the best location for aspiration or tube placement. Pneumothorax and hemothorax are complications.

Tube Thoracostomy

Tube thoracostomy is performed for the ongoing drainage of air or fluid. Coagulopathy should be corrected when feasible. A hemothorax may tamponade ongoing bleeding so the need for rapid blood transfusion should be anticipated before drainage. The usual site of entry is into the fourth or fifth intercostal space in the anterior or midaxillary line. Ultrasound guidance can be helpful. In the prepubertal child, the nipple usually overlies the fourth intercostal space. The skin should be prepared with an antiseptic solution. For classical chest tube placement, a skin incision in an axis parallel to the rib is made and blunt dissection is performed using a curved hemostat or Kelly clamp through the incision and directed up to the superior intercostal space that has been chosen for chest wall entry. The clamp should be inserted with the tip closed; the tip is then spread to dissect the tissues. The clamp should be pushed firmly through the pleura while control is maintained so that the chest wall is not penetrated too deeply. Once the tube tip is within the thorax, the tube is advanced sufficiently so that all side holes are within the thoracic cavity. The drainage system should be connected and the tube sutured in place or secured with a device. An X-ray should be taken to verify the tube position and observe resolution of the pneumothorax or effusion. A number of percutaneous Seldinger technique chest-drainage systems are available, including pigtail catheters and tube-over-obturator systems. The dilator should only be inserted to the depth needed to penetrate the chest wall.

PERICARDIOCENTESIS

Pericardiocentesis is required for life-threatening cardiac tamponade or to obtain fluid for diagnostic purposes. Immediate complications include puncture or laceration of the ventricular epicardium or myocardium, laceration of a coronary artery or vein, hemopericardium, lethal arrhythmias, and pneumothorax. Delayed complications include slowly developing pneumothorax, pneumopericardium, diaphragm perforation, peritoneal puncture, esophageal puncture, pericardial leakage, fistula development, and infection.

The vital signs and ECG should be monitored. The xiphoid and subxiphoid areas and thorax should be disinfected. The child should be placed in a head-up position, if possible, to promote anterior pooling of the effusion. The overlying skin should be infiltrated with lidocaine, and a small stab incision should be made with a blade just below and to the left of tip of the xiphoid process. An 18- or 20-gauge pericardiocentesis needle is recommended. The needle should be inserted into the skin incision site at a 45-degree angle to the skin and directed toward the left nipple or the tip of the left scapula. The needle is advanced slowly, aspirating until pericardial fluid is aspirated. If an ECG lead is attached to the needle, contact with the ventricular wall is indicated by ECG changes. Once the needle tip is in the correct position, a J-tipped guide wire is introduced. A dilator is then inserted over the wire, a pigtail pericardial catheter is advanced over the guide wire, and the guide wire is removed. Draining a pericardial effusion with a needle alone risks laceration of the myocardium or coronary vessels. Echocardiography should be performed following placement to document evacuation of the fluid and catheter position.

TRANSPYLORIC FEEDING TUBE PLACEMENT

Nasogastric tube feeding is the first choice for enteral nutrition, but it may be poorly tolerated in critically ill children as a result of gastroparesis. Blind insertion of a transpyloric tube is usually performed at bedside. Right lateral decubitus positioning is often used. Even if postpyloric position is not achieved soon after the insertion, the tube may migrate through the pylorus over time. The use of pH assistance, magnet guidance, and motility (prokinetic) agents has been suggested as alternative techniques. Complications during insertion include perforation and tube misplacement. Tracheal or bronchial placement can occur, particularly in patients who are receiving sedation and neuromuscular blockade. Endoscopic tube placement may be needed.

ABDOMINAL PARACENTESIS

Abdominal paracentesis is performed for sampling and drainage in patients with ascites, peritonitis, or blunt abdominal trauma. Bleeding risk is fairly low even in coagulopathic patients, so platelets and fresh frozen plasma are not always given. Special caution is necessary in patients with severe bowel distension, history of previous abdominal or pelvic surgery, or distended bladder. Insertion sites where abdominal scar or cellulitis is apparent should be avoided. While rare, perforations of bowel or bladder, persistent leakage of fluid, intra-abdominal bleeding, infection, and hypovolemic shock may occur. Abdominal ultrasound should be used to aid in diagnosis and to perform ultrasound-guided aspiration. Sedation is usually required. A comparison of ascitic fluid composition by etiology is show in **Table 4.1**.

The area of needle insertion should be dependent and lateral, although some authorities prefer the midline 2 cm below the umbilicus. The patient should be in a supine position, with head elevated and the bladder empty. The insertion site is prepared with chlorhexidine or povidone–iodine and local anesthetic administered. A Z-track method minimizes the risk of fluid leak, compared with a direct linear-track insertion. The Z-track can be applied by placing caudal traction on the skin after the needle has been inserted perpendicular to the abdominal wall. The needle is advanced with constant negative pressure until a pop is felt as the needle enters the peritoneal cavity and fluid is aspirated. If a catheter-over-the-needle system is used, the catheter is advanced over the needle into the peritoneal cavity and the needle removed. Approximately 20–30 mL of fluid is usually enough for diagnostic studies, but for therapeutic drainage, more fluid may be required. A large volume drained quickly can result in hypotension; therefore, no more than 15–20 mL/kg should be drained at one time. Positional change may be necessary to facilitate drainage. A pigtail catheter may be used if longer-term drainage is required.

TABLE 4.1

Comparison of Ascitic Fluid by Etiology

ETIOLOGY	CELLS/APPEARANCE/ OTHER	TOTAL PROTEIN	LDH	GLUCOSE	PH	CULTURE/ GRAM STAIN	SERUM/ASCITES ALBUMIN
Spontaneous bacterial peritonitis	>250/mL	>1 g/dL	Normal	Normal	Low or normal	May be negative	>1.1 g/dL
Secondary bacterial peritonitis	>500/mL, polymorphonuclear predominance	<3 g/dL	> serum LDH	<50 mg/dL	Not reliable	Positive	<1.1 g/dL
Chylous ascites	1000–5000, lymphocytic predominance/milky or yellow/triglyceride level >> serum (>1500 g/dL)	<3 g/dL					
Pancreatic ascites	Increased/turbid, tea-colored, or bloody/amylase and lipase > serum levels	Increased					
Tuberculous ascites	>1000, predominant lymphocytes/ Bloody or yellow/firm clots	>2.5 g/dL		<30 mg/dL			
Urine ascites	Potassium and creatinine > serum	<1 g/dL					
Malignant ascites	Bloody fluid	Increased	Increased	Decreased			<1.1 g/dL
Nephrotic syndrome		<2.5 g/dL					
Biliary ascites	Bile-stained, Bilirubin >> serum bilirubin (100–400 mg/dL)						

LDH, lactate dehydrogenase.

CHAPTER 5 ■ RECOGNITION AND INITIAL MANAGEMENT OF SHOCK

RUCHI SINHA, SIMON NADEL, NIRANJAN "TEX" KISSOON, AND SUCHITRA RANJIT

Shock is a complex clinical syndrome characterized by an acute failure of the cardiovascular system to adequately deliver substrate or remove metabolic waste from tissues that results in anaerobic metabolism and acidosis. Shock progresses through three stages: the *compensated* stage, in which neurohumoral mechanisms maintain blood pressure (BP) and tissue perfusion and during which shock can be reversed with appropriate therapy; the *progressive* stage, which follows when compensatory mechanisms are exhausted and during which pathophysiologic derangements worsen; and finally, the *refractory* stage, which is due to the patient, without aggressive support, developing severe organ and tissue injury, which culminates in multiple organ failure and death.

CLASSIFICATION OF SHOCK

Shock is often classified based on five mechanisms that have important therapeutic implications:

- *Hypovolemic shock* includes hemorrhagic and nonhemorrhagic causes of fluid depletion.
- *Cardiogenic shock* occurs when cardiac compensatory mechanisms fail and may occur in children and infants with preexisting myocardial disease or injury.
- *Obstructive shock* is due to increased afterload of the right or left ventricle; examples include cardiac tamponade, pulmonary embolism, and tension pneumothorax.
- *Distributive shock*, such as septic and anaphylactic shock, is often associated with peripheral vasodilatation, pooling of venous blood, and decreased venous return to the heart (e.g., septic, neurogenic, and anaphylactic shock).
- *Dissociative shock* occurs as a result of inadequate oxygen-releasing capacity; examples include profound anemia, carbon monoxide poisoning, and methemoglobinemia.

PATHOPHYSIOLOGY

Oxygen Delivery

Circulatory failure results in a decrease in oxygen delivery (Do_2) to the tissues and is associated with a decrease in cellular partial pressure of oxygen (Po_2). Do_2 depends on two variables: the arterial oxygen content (Cao_2) and the cardiac output (CO). Oxygen uptake or consumption ($\dot{V}o_2$) and oxygen delivery (Do_2) can be quantified and are linked by the relationship:

$$\dot{V}o_2 = Do_2 \times O_2ER$$

where O_2ER = oxygen extraction ratio (O_2ER in %, $\dot{V}o_2$ and Do_2 in mL O_2/kg/min) and Do_2 = total flow of oxygen in arterial blood (related to CO and arterial oxygen content). Under normal conditions, oxygen demand equals $\dot{V}o_2$ (roughly equivalent to 2.4 mL O_2/kg/min when Do_2 is 12 mL O_2/kg/min, corresponding to an O_2ER of 20%). During circulatory shock or hypoxemia, as Do_2 declines, $\dot{V}o_2$ is maintained and O_2ER increases. However, if Do_2 falls further, a critical point is reached (Do_2crit) when O_2ER no longer increases and $\dot{V}o_2$ becomes dependent on Do_2 (**Fig. 5.1**).

Mixed Venous Oxygen Saturation

According to the Fick equation, tissue $\dot{V}o_2$ is proportional to CO:

$$\dot{V}o_2 = CO \times (Cao_2 - C\bar{v}o_2)$$

where Cvo_2 = mixed venous blood oxygen content. $\dot{V}o_2$ is proportional to CO × ($Sao_2 - Svo_2$) × Hb × 1.39. Therefore, it becomes apparent that Svo_2 is proportional to $Sao_2 - \dot{V}o_2/(CO \times Hb \times 1.39)$. Four conditions may cause Svo_2 to decrease: hypoxemia (decrease in Sao_2), increase in $\dot{V}o_2$, reduction in CO, and decrease in Hb concentration so that if Sao_2, Hb, and metabolism are stable, then Svo_2 changes reflect CO.

Decreased Oxygen Delivery (Quantitative Shock)

Decreased Flow (e.g., Hypovolemic, Cardiogenic Shock)

Decreased flow may be the consequence of either decreased circulating volume (absolute or relative hypovolemia) or failure of the cardiac pump for a variety of reasons.

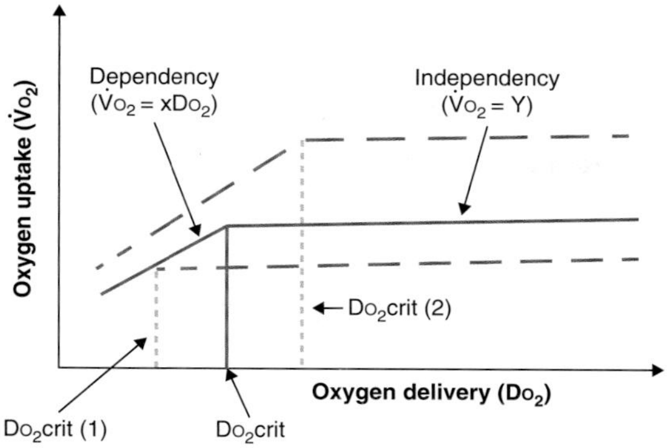

FIGURE 5.1. Relationship of oxygen uptake ($\dot{V}O_2$) to oxygen delivery (DO_2) (*solid line*): When $\dot{V}O_2$ is supply independent (independency), whole-body O_2 needs are met. When $\dot{V}O_2$ becomes dependent on DO_2 (dependency), $\dot{V}O_2$ becomes linearly dependent on DO_2 at the critical DO_2 (DO_2crit), which corresponds to the definition of "dysoxia." DO_2crit is influenced by global oxygen requirements: When $\dot{V}O_2$ is decreased (i.e., during sedation and hypothermia—*lower dotted line*), the DO_2crit is also decreased [DO_2crit (1)]. When $\dot{V}O_2$ is increased (i.e., agitation, hyperthermia, sepsis—*upper dotted line*), DO_2crit is increased [DO_2crit (2)].

Decreased Oxygen Content (e.g., Hemorrhagic Shock, Acute Hypoxemic Respiratory Failure, Poisoning)

Hemorrhagic shock is usually a result of hypovolemia and anemia. Decreased oxygen-carrying capacity of Hb, and therefore inadequate DO_2, may result in shock. With carbon monoxide poisoning, a decrease in DO_2 results from competitive binding of carbon monoxide in preference to O_2, resulting in shock that is both quantitative and distributive. In any respiratory cause of acute hypoxia, decreased SaO_2 leads to a decrease in DO_2 as soon as CO is unable to compensate for metabolic needs.

Decreased Oxygen Extraction (Distributive Shock)

Distributive shock often coexists with hypovolemic and/or cardiogenic shock. Spinal cord injury is a specific form of distributive shock that leads to loss of sympathetic outflow from the spinal cord, resulting in a sudden decrease in SVR and CO, while central venous pressure (CVP) remains unchanged.

ASSESSMENT

History and Physical Examination

Shock in children is characterized by tachycardia (may be absent in hypothermia) with signs of decreased organ or peripheral perfusion (e.g., decreased peripheral compared with central pulses, altered alertness, flash capillary refill or capillary refill >2 seconds, mottled or cool extremities, or decreased urine output).

Laboratory Markers of Shock

Serial blood gas and arterial lactate evaluations are used to complement the clinical assessment of systemic perfusion. Mixed venous O_2 saturation (SvO_2) can be used to assess whole-body $\dot{V}O_2$–DO_2 relationships, with continuous monitoring offering the advantage of real-time assessment.

Assessment of Global Blood Flow

Global blood flow is dependent on preload, myocardial function, afterload, and HR. Regional flow distribution is not homogeneous and is dependent on central and peripheral vascular tones, which determine SVR. Flow (Q) varies directly with perfusion pressure (dP) and inversely with resistance (R), mathematically represented by:

$$Q = dP/R$$

For the whole body, this relationship is represented by:

$$CO = MAP - CVP/SVR$$

This relationship also holds for individual organ perfusion. Some organs, including the kidney and brain, have vasomotor autoregulation that maintains flow in low-pressure states. However, at the lower limit of pressure autoregulation, perfusion pressure is reduced below the ability to maintain blood flow.

Pulmonary Artery Catheter Thermodilution

A pulmonary artery catheter (PAC) and pulmonary artery thermodilution (PATD) can be used to clarify cardiopulmonary physiology in children with refractory shock. However, evidence is not available to support the use of PAC in children, and catheter placement and interpretation of the hemodynamic data require experienced healthcare providers to avoid complications and misguided decision making.

Doppler Ultrasound

Doppler ultrasound cardiac monitors provide a rapid, noninvasive measure of cardiac function and can be used as trend monitors and for rapid detection of changes in CO, making them useful for monitoring therapeutic interventions, such as fluid administration.

Pulse Contour Analysis

Pulse contour analysis, like the PAC, can be used to estimate global blood flow as well as other hemodynamic variables such as end-diastolic volume (EDV). Stroke volume variability (SVV), derived from pulse contour analysis, has been suggested as a better determinant of preload compared with cardiac filling pressure (CVP or pulmonary capillary wedge pressure), volumetric parameters (right ventricular end-diastolic volume), and left ventricular end-diastolic area (echocardiography). Pulse oximetry uses photoelectric plethysmography to detect changes in blood volume at the site of measurement. It has been shown that pulse pressure variation by plethysmography is a reliable indicator of fluid responsiveness only when tidal volume is at least 8–12 mL/kg.

Echocardiography

Doppler echocardiography can be used to measure CO and superior vena cava (SVC) flow. Echocardiography can be used to rule out the presence of pericardial effusion, evaluate contractility, and check ventricular filling.

Assessment of Regional Blood Flow

Skin Temperature Gradient

Temperature gradients, peripheral-to-ambient (dTp-a) and central-to-peripheral (dTc-p), better reflect cutaneous blood flow than skin temperature itself. A gradient of 3°C–7°C indicates normal hemodynamic stability.

Peripheral Perfusion (Flow) Index

The peripheral perfusion (flow) index (PFI) is derived from the photoelectric plethysmographic signal of pulse oximetry and is the ratio of the light from the pulsatile component (arterial compartment) and the nonpulsatile component (other tissues).

Near-Infrared Spectroscopy

Near-infrared spectroscopy (NIRS) has a greater tissue penetration than pulse oximetry and provides a global assessment of oxygenation in all vascular compartments (arterial, venous, and capillary).

Orthogonal Polarization Spectral Imaging

Orthogonal polarization spectral (OPS) imaging is a noninvasive technique that uses reflected light to produce real-time images of the microcirculation, most readily by placement of the probe under the tongue.

Transcutaneous Oxygen and Carbon Dioxide Measurements

Transcutaneous sensors enable the estimation of arterial oxygen pressure (Pao_2) and arterial carbon dioxide pressure ($Paco_2$). When blood flow is adequate, transcutaneous oxygen ($P_{Tc}O_2$) and Pao_2 values are almost equal and the tc-index (changes in $P_{Tc}O_2$ relative to changes in Pao_2) is close to 1. A tc-index below 0.7 has been associated with hemodynamic instability. Differences between $Paco_2$ and transcutaneous carbon dioxide ($P_{Tc}CO_2$) have been explained by accumulation of CO_2 in the skin because of hypoperfusion; however, this technology has not gained widespread acceptance.

MANAGEMENT

Monitoring

In addition to repeated clinical examinations, monitoring for patients who are in either incipient or actual shock includes continuous electrocardiography, pulse oximetry, urine output, and either continuous invasive or rapid and regular noninvasive measurements of BP. A central venous catheter allows CVP monitoring, but is not essential in the early stages of management. In the sedated, ventilated patient, recordings of systolic pressure variation and/or pulse pressure variation may be helpful. The heart remains preload dependent until systolic pressure variation is <10 mm Hg, and/or pulse pressure variation is <10%. Blood gas analysis for metabolic acidosis and lactate concentration give an indication of global oxygenation, which reflects the adequacy of CO and oxygen delivery. The American College of Critical Care Medicine (ACCM) guidelines recommend the use of pulmonary artery thermodilution (PATD), pulse contour analysis, or Doppler ultrasound for monitoring CO in patients with septic shock.

General Supportive Measures

"Early goal-directed therapy" for shock includes prompt fluid resuscitation, targeted vasoactive therapy, early empiric antimicrobial therapy, and continuous monitoring of hemodynamic status. The ACCM guidelines for shock advocate peripheral inotropes until central venous access is established and encourage the use of noninvasive CO monitoring to direct therapies to achieve a CI of 3.3–6.0 L/min/m^2. To maximize Do_2, supplemental oxygen should be delivered to all patients with signs of shock and early tracheal intubation may be necessary. Acute circulatory failure should be initially treated by fluid challenge. Suggested protocols for management in the emergency department and after transition to the ICU are outlined in **Figures 5.2** and **5.3**.

Fluid Resuscitation

The goal of fluid administration is to optimize left ventricular preload and improve Do_2 by increasing CO via the Frank–Starling mechanism. Up to 60 mL/kg fluid may be given in the first hour of therapy to children with septic shock, without increasing the risk of pulmonary edema. The "surviving sepsis" and ACCM guidelines suggest initial resuscitation with infusion of crystalloid, with boluses of 20 mL/kg, over 5–10 minutes, titrated to clinical estimation of

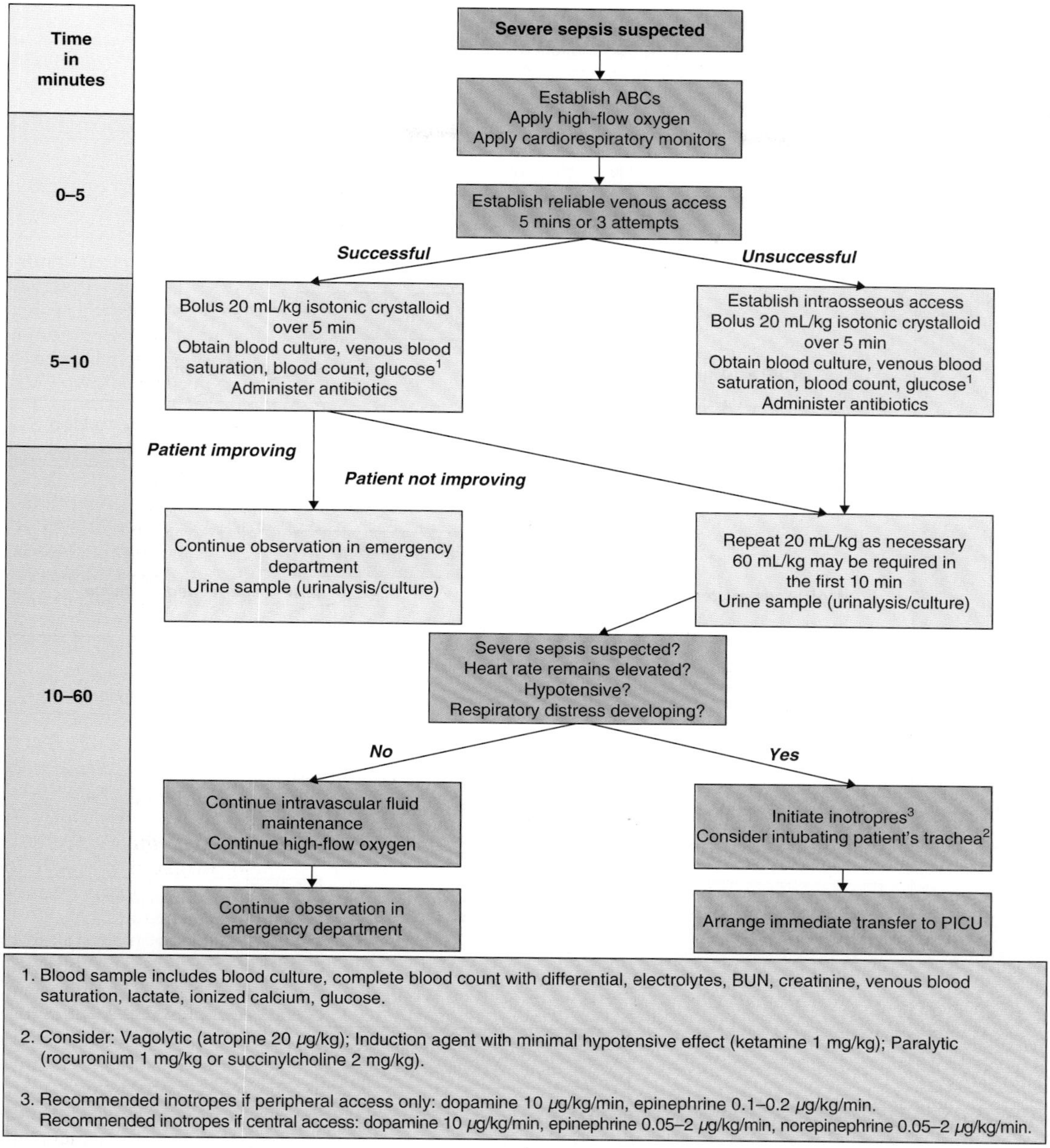

FIGURE 5.2. Suggested emergency department sepsis protocol.

CO. The ACCM guidelines recommend fluid removal using diuretics, peritoneal dialysis, or continuous renal replacement therapy (CRRT) in patients who have been adequately fluid resuscitated, but cannot subsequently maintain an even fluid balance via their native urine output in the ICU. Fluid-refractory shock is defined as the persistence of shock after the administration of sufficient fluids to achieve a CVP of 8–12 mm Hg and/or signs of fluid overload (hepatic congestion, pulmonary edema). Additional therapy, such as vasopressors/inotropes, should be administered.

Choice of Fluids

Either crystalloid or colloid may be used for early resuscitation of patients with sepsis. The choice of fluid may influence outcome in different populations of patients. For example, colloids should not be used in trauma and hydroxyethyl starch has been shown

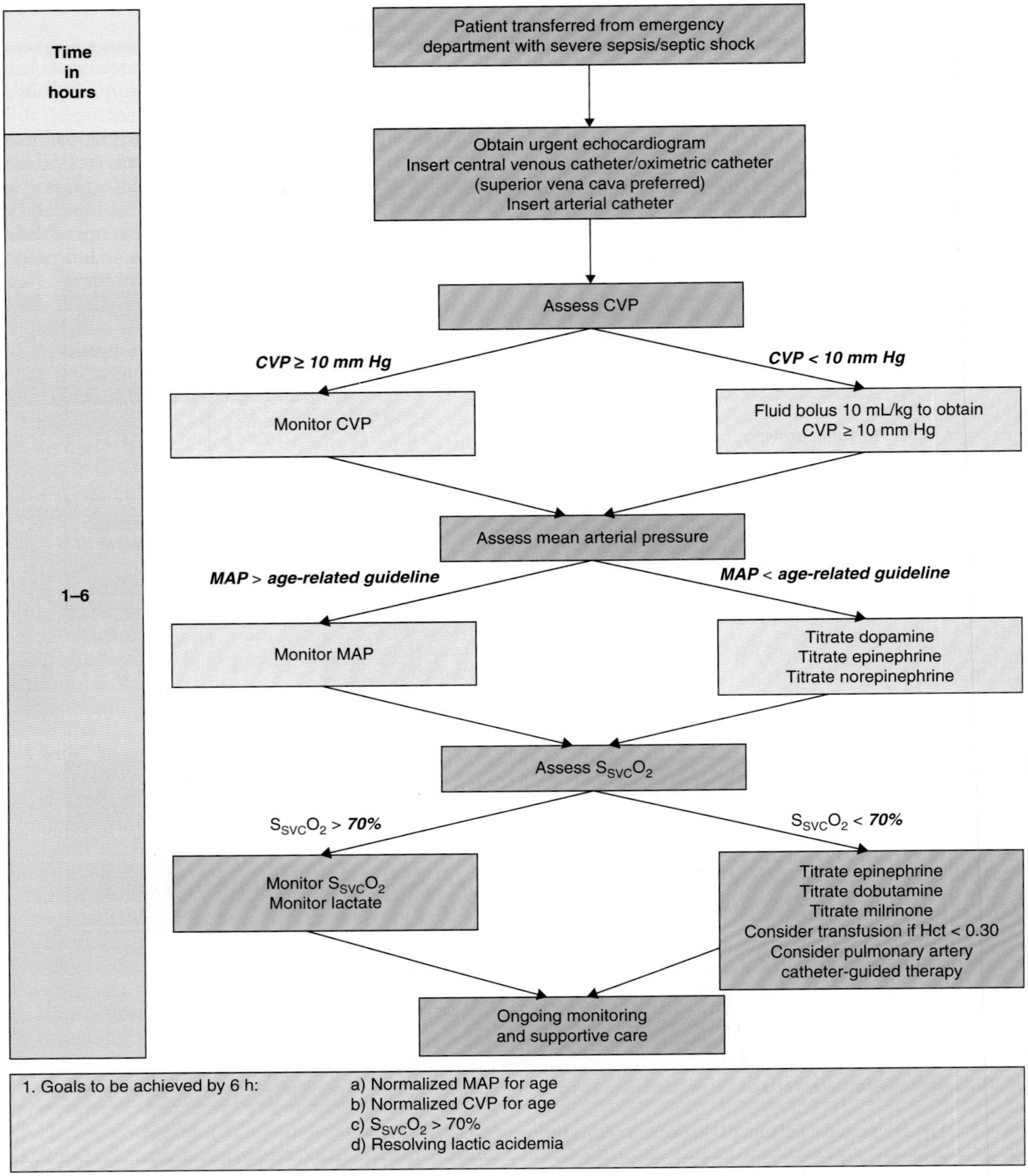

FIGURE 5.3. Suggested PICU sepsis protocol.

to increase the risk of death and the need for CRRT in septic patients.

Blood Replacement

Usually, blood replacement is not required unless shock is due to acute hemorrhage or anemia. However, an Hb of >8–10 g/dL is thought to be beneficial in patients with severe sepsis and/or decreased cardiac contractility.

Vasoactive Agents

Vasoactive agents have three main actions: effect on SVR (vasodilators and vasoconstrictors), effect on cardiac contractility (inotropes), and effect on HR (chronotropes). Inotropic agents can be subclassified as *inodilators* when they combine inotropic properties with vasodilation (e.g., dobutamine and milrinone) to increase blood flow, or *inoconstrictors* when they combine inotropic properties with vasoconstriction (e.g., dopamine, adrenaline, and noradrenaline) to increase perfusion pressure. Potent vasoconstrictors, such as vasopressin, its derivatives, and inhibitors of nitric oxide synthase, may also be used to treat shock. In vasodilated ("warm") shock (bounding pulses, warm extremities, normal capillary refill time [CRT]), the use of vasoconstrictor agents (e.g., noradrenaline) appears beneficial. Dopamine remains the first-line vasopressor for fluid-refractory hypotensive shock with low SVR in children while noradrenaline is now recommended as the first-line agent in adults with fluid-refractory shock. A predominantly poor CO state referred to as "cold shock," clinically manifested by weak pulses, cool extremities, and prolonged CRT, is associated with vasoconstriction and consequent increase in afterload. Using inotropic agents, such as dobutamine, adrenaline, or milrinone, would appear to be most beneficial. Rescue from refractory shock has been described using two other drugs: enoximone, which has type III phosphodiesterase activity; and levosimendan, which is a calcium-sensitizing agent that enhances myocardial contractility and vasodilation.

Antibiotic Therapy

Antibiotics should be administered within 1 hour of recognition of sepsis. The choice of antibiotics is vital and should be guided by the susceptibility of likely pathogens in the community and the hospital, specific knowledge about the patient, the underlying disease, and the clinical syndrome (**Table 5.1**).

Other Therapeutic Interventions

The importance of correcting metabolic abnormalities has been emphasized in treatment guidelines for children with meningococcal shock. However, the use of bicarbonate therapy to correct shock-induced metabolic acidosis failed to show any improvement in CO or reduction in inotrope requirement. Replacement low-dose steroid therapy has been shown to be beneficial in patients with septic shock and evidence of adrenal hyporesponsiveness, especially in those with high or increasing requirements for inotropes.

TABLE 5.1

Pediatric Antimicrobial Treatment Guide

<table>
<tr><th></th><th>NEONATE (<1 mo)</th><th>INFANT (1–3 mo)</th><th>PEDIATRIC (>3 mo)</th></tr>
<tr><td>Sepsis unknown source</td><td rowspan="3">Ampicillin + (gentamicin or cefotaxime)
<u>Ampicillin</u> 50 mg/kg/dose IV q6h (q8h if <1 wk old) plus
<u>Gentamicin</u> 2.5 mg/kg/dose IV q8h (q12h if <1 wk old) and Acyclovir 20 mg/kg/dose IV q8h
OR
<u>Ampicillin</u> 50 mg/kg/dose IV q6h (q8h if <1 wk old) plus
<u>Cefotaxime</u> 50 mg/kg/dose IV q8h (q12h if <1 wk old)</td><td rowspan="2">Ampicillin + cefotaxime
<u>Ampicillin</u> 50 mg/kg/dose IV q6h plus
<u>Cefotaxime</u> 50 mg/kg/dose IV q6h</td><td>Cloxacillin + cefotaxime
<u>Cloxacillin</u> 50 mg/kg/dose IV q6h (max 2 g/dose) plus
<u>Cefotaxime</u> 50 mg/kg/dose IV q6h (max 2 g/dose)</td></tr>
<tr><td rowspan="2">CNS suspected source</td><td>Cefotaxime ± vancomycin
<u>Cefotaxime</u> 75 mg/kg/dose IV q6h (max 2 g/dose) plus
Vancomycin 20 mg/kg IV × 1 dose, then 15 mg/kg/dose IV q6h</td></tr>
<tr><td colspan="2">Shunt/EVD
<u>Meropenem</u> 40 mg/kg dose IV q8h (max 2 g/dose) plus
<u>Vancomycin</u> 20 mg/kg IV × 1 dose, then 15 mg/kg/dose IV q6h</td></tr>
<tr><td>Pneumonia suspected source</td><td></td><td>Cloxacillin + cefotaxime
<u>Cloxacillin</u> 50 mg/kg/dose IV q6h (max 2 g/dose) plus
<u>Cefotaxime</u> 50 mg/kg/dose IV q6h (max 2 g/dose)</td><td>Cloxacillin + cefotaxime +/− azithromycin
<u>Cloxacillin</u> 50 mg/kg/dose IV q6h (max 2 g/dose) plus
<u>Cefotaxime</u> 50 mg/kg/dose IV q6h (max 2 g/dose) plus
<u>Azithromycin</u> 10 mg/kg/dose PO/IV × 1 dose (max 500 mg), then 5 mg/kg/dose PO/IV q24h (max 250 mg/dose) × 5 d</td></tr>
</table>

(continued)

TABLE 5.1

Pediatric Antimicrobial Treatment Guide (*continued*)

	■ NEONATE (<1 mo)	■ INFANT (1–3 mo) ■ PEDIATRIC (>3 mo)
GU suspected source	No known anatomic abnormalities or first presentation: Ampicillin + gentamicin *Ampicillin* 50 mg/kg/dose IV q6h (q8h if <1 wk old) **plus** *Gentamicin* 2.5 mg/kg/dose IV q8h (q12h if <1 wk old)	>1 mo old: No known anatomic abnormalities or first presentation: Ampicillin + gentamicin *Ampicillin* 50 mg/kg/dose IV q6h (max 3 g/dose) **plus** *Gentamicin* 7 mg/kg/dose IV q24h
	Known abnormality of GU tract: Piperacillin + gentamicin *Piperacillin* 75 mg/kg/dose IV q6h (q8h if <1 wk old) **plus** *Gentamicin* 2.5 mg/kg/dose IV q8h (q12h if <1 wk old)	Known abnormality of GU tract: Piperacillin/tazobactam + gentamicin *Piperacillin/tazobactam* 75 mg/kg/dose piperacillin component IV q6h (max 4 g/dose) **plus** *Gentamicin* 7 mg/kg/dose IV q24h
Skin/Soft tissue suspected source	Clindamycin + penicillin + gentamicin **OR** Clindamycin + cefotaxime *Clindamycin* 5 mg/kg/dose IV q6h (q8h if <1 wk old) **plus** *Penicillin* 50,000 units/kg/dose IV q6h (q8h if <1wk old) **plus** *Gentamicin* 2.5 mg/kg/dose IV q8h (q12h if <1wk old) **OR** *Clindamycin* 5 mg/kg/dose IV q6h (q8h if <1wk old) **plus** *Cefotaxime* 50 mg/kg/dose IV q8h (q12h if <1 wk old)	**>1 mo old:** Clindamycin + penicillin + gentamicin **OR** Clindamycin + cefotaxime *Clindamycin* 13 mg/kg/dose IV q8h (max 900 mg/dose) **plus** *Penicillin* 65,000 units/kg/dose IV q4h (max 4 million units/dose) **plus** *Gentamicin* 7 mg/kg/dose IV q24h **OR** *Clindamycin* 13 mg/kg/dose IV q8h (max 900 mg/dose) **plus** *Cefotaxime* 50 mg/kg/dose IV q6h (max 2 g/dose) if Group A Strep suspected Add IV immunoglobulin (IVIG) 1 g/kg/dose IV q24h × 2 doses Ordered from blood bank
Immunocompromised/Febrile neutropenic patient		>1 mo old: Piperacillin/tazobactam + gentamicin *Piperacillin/tazobactam* 75 mg/kg/dose piperacillin component IV q6h (max 4 g/dose) **plus** *Gentamicin* 7 mg/kg/dose IV q24h

IV, intravenous; CNS, central nervous system; EVD, external ventricular drain; PO, orally.

CHAPTER 6 ■ RAPID RESPONSE SYSTEMS

CHRISTOPHER P. BONAFIDE, RICHARD J. BRILLI, JAMES TIBBALLS,
CHRISTOPHER S. PARSHURAM, PATRICK W. BRADY, AND DEREK S. WHEELER

The hallmark of rapid response systems (RRSs) is their focus on identifying and mitigating reversible early signs of clinical deterioration in ward settings to prevent respiratory and cardiac arrest. They operate on the assumptions that (a) early, reversible clinical deterioration can be identified using tools that facilitate detection and standardize escalation of care on the wards, and (b) consulting a multidisciplinary team of critical care experts with the capability to rapidly intervene at the bedside can improve patients' outcomes. The organizational structure of RRSs should include two clinical components (afferent and efferent limbs) and two organizational components (process improvement and administrative limbs).

THE AFFERENT LIMB

The role of the afferent limb of RRSs is to identify or track patients at risk of deterioration and trigger an appropriate response based on the level of risk. Systems for prediction of deterioration are distinguished from systems for detection of deterioration. *Predictive tools* focus on "traits" rather than "states" and do not require continuous data collection. *Detective tools* focus on identifying critical illness by recognizing deterioration using highly time-varying data like vital signs. Detective systems require either frequent intermittent measurements or continuous data collection to identify early clinical instability and prevent progressive deterioration.

Predicting Deterioration

In comparison with detective tools, little work has been done to develop tools that predict clinical deterioration in hospitalized children using patient characteristics. A predictive model for clinical deterioration using non–vital sign patient characteristics was recently developed using a case-control design. The predictive model resulted in a 7-item weighted score that included age under 1 year, epilepsy, congenital/genetic conditions, history of transplant, presence of an enteral tube, hemoglobin less than 10 g/dL, and blood culture drawn in the preceding 72 hours. Predictive tools have the potential to identify and triage high-risk children who need intensive monitoring at the time of admission.

Detecting Deterioration

Single-Parameter Calling Criteria

The simplest and most widely used detective tool is a set of single-parameter calling criteria. They are easy for bedside use; if any criterion is met, the efferent limb should be activated. While the parameters are commonly objective clinical findings such as vital signs, they can also include diagnoses (such as suspected shock), events (such as seizures), subjective observations (such as increased work of breathing), and intuitive concerns (such as worried about the patient).

Multiparameter Early Warning Scores

Multiparameter tools combine several of the core components of single-parameter calling criteria. The scores may be weighted or unweighted. Weighted scores allocate points based on the degree to which patients' vital signs deviate from a (usually arbitrarily developed) "normal" or "expected" range. The scores are periodically calculated (manually or electronically), and the sum total score is used to trigger the efferent limb. The pediatric early warning score (PEWS) developed in England and the bedside pediatric early warning system score (Bedside PEWS) developed in Canada are the most rigorously evaluated.

Pediatric Early Warning Score. The PEWS, described in 2005, was developed using adult system concepts and includes three components: behavior, cardiovascular, and respiratory (**Table 6.1**). The total PEWS corresponded with a color, which was then used to indicate a suggested staff response, including, at the highest scores, calling the critical care outreach team.

Being the first early warning score (EWS) for children, the PEWS was widely disseminated and evaluated. The PEWS performed well in an analysis that used transfer to the intensive care unit (ICU) as the outcome and the highest score a patient had during hospitalization as the exposure. However, use of transfer alone as an outcome in a study in which the score was calculated as part of clinical care (and as such may have directly influenced decision making about transfer) introduces substantial limitations, as does using the highest score occurring during a hospitalization without regard to the timing of that

TABLE 6.1

The PEWS Tool

COMPONENT	POINTS FOR SUBSCORES 0	1	2	3
Behavior	Playing/appropriate	Sleeping	Irritable	Lethargic/confused. Reduced response to pain
Cardiovascular	Pink or capillary refill 1–2 s	Pale or capillary refill 3 s	Gray or capillary refill 4 s. Tachycardia of 20 above normal rate	Gray and mottled or capillary refill ≥ 5 s. Tachycardia of 30 above normal rate or bradycardia
Respiratory	Within normal parameters, no recession or tracheal tug	Rate > 10 above normal parameters, using accessory muscles $FIO_2 \geq 30\%$ or 4 L/min	Rate > 20 above normal parameters, recessing, tracheal tug $FIO_2 \geq 40\%$ or 6 L/min	Rate 5 below parameters with sternal recession, tracheal tug, or grunting $FIO_2 \geq 50\%$ or 8 L/min

Score 2 extra points for ¼ hourly nebulizers or persistent vomiting following surgery.
The total score is calculated as the sum of the subscores from each of the three components.
Adapted from Monaghan A. Detecting and managing deterioration in children. *Paediatr Nurs* 2005;17(1):32–5.

score in relationship to the transfer. Nevertheless, the score is widely used on pediatric wards.

Bedside PEWS. The initial Bedside PEWS was developed using expert opinion and consensus and refined using statistical methods. The 7-item score includes heart rate, systolic blood pressure, capillary refill time, respiratory rate, respiratory effort, oxygen therapy, and oxygen saturation (**Table 6.2**). Bedside PEWS has performed well in multiple retrospective evaluations, including a multicenter validation study.

The Bedside PEWS is being evaluated in the Evaluating Processes of Care and the Outcomes of Children in Hospital (EPOCH) study to determine the effect of its implementation on mortality, cardiac arrest rates, and processes of care among children hospitalized outside ICUs.

Family Concern as an Afferent Trigger

Data are scant regarding the effectiveness and unintended consequences of the use of family concern as a trigger. It appears that families infrequently activate these systems and that, when activated, the calls for assistance rarely represent urgent critical care needs.

Technologic Advancements

Intermittently Assessed Deterioration Surveillance

EWSs have been integrated into the electronic health records, leveraging the benefits of discrete vital sign data and subjective observations manually entered into electronic flow sheets with the ability to perform calculations and provide immediate clinical decision support to frontline staff. The Pediatric Rothman Index is an example of a commercially available score that integrates with existing electronic health records.

Continuous Deterioration Surveillance

Continuous multiparameter monitoring for early signs of deterioration offers the potential benefit of detecting critical illness earlier, without requiring manual measurement of vital signs or frequent calculation of complex scores. While there have been no reports of integrated systems for children hospitalized on wards, there have been reports of integrated systems developed for adult patients. Visensia is a commercially available system that integrates four continuously measured physiologic parameters (heart rate, respiration rate, oxygen saturation, and skin temperature) with one intermittently measured parameter (blood pressure) to generate a numerical patient status index. The index represents the amount of deviation of the patient's combined vital signs from a model of physiologic normality derived from a training data set of hospitalized adult patients.

THE EFFERENT LIMB

The role of the efferent limb of RRSs is to provide quickly dispatched teams of skilled personnel to address urgent care needs in patients on general medical and surgical wards. Teams may be reactive or proactive. The composition of these teams varies,

TABLE 6.2

The Bedside PEWS Tool

ITEM	AGE GROUP	ITEM SUBSCORE 0	1	2	4
Heart rate	0 to <3 mo	>110 and <150	≥150 or ≤110	≥180 or ≤90	≥190 or ≤80
	3 to <12 mo	>100 and <150	≥150 or ≤100	≥170 or ≤80	≥180 or ≤70
	1 to <4 y	>90 and <120	≥120 or ≤90	≥150 or ≤70	≥170 or ≤60
	4 to 12 y	>70 and <110	≥110 or ≤70	≥130 or ≤60	≥150 or ≤50
	>12 y	>60 and <100	≥100 or ≤60	≥120 or ≤50	≥140 or ≤40
Systolic blood pressure	0 to <3 mo	>60 and <80	≥80 or ≤60	≥100 or ≤50	≥130 or ≤45
	3 to <12 mo	>80 and <100	≥100 or ≤80	≥120 or ≤70	≥150 or ≤60
	1 to <4 y	>90 and <110	≥110 or ≤90	≥125 or ≤75	≥160 or ≤65
	4 to 12 y	>90 and <120	≥120 or ≤90	≥140 or ≤80	≥170 or ≤70
	>12 y	>100 and <130	≥130 or ≤100	≥150 or ≤85	≥190 or ≤75
Capillary refill time		<3 s			≥3 s
Respiratory rate	0 to <3 mo	>29 and <61	≥61 or ≤29	≥81 or ≤19	≥91 or ≤15
	3 to <12 mo	>24 or <51	≥51 or ≤24	≥71 or ≤19	≥81 or ≤15
	1 to <4 y	>19 or <41	≥41 or ≤19	≥61 or ≤15	≥71 or ≤12
	4 to 12 y	>19 or <31	≥31 or ≤19	≥41 or ≤14	≥51 or ≤10
	>12 y	>11 or <17	≥ 17 or ≤11	≥23 or ≤10	≥30 or ≤9
Respiratory effort		Normal	Mild increase	Moderate increase	Severe increase/ any apnea
Saturation (%)		>94	91–94	≤90	
Oxygen therapy		Room air		Any to <4 L/ min or <50%	≥4 L/min or ≥50%

The total score is calculated as the sum of the subscores from each of the items.
Reprinted from Parshuram CS, Duncan HP, Joffe AR, et al. Multi-centre validation of the Bedside Paediatric Early Warning System score: A severity of illness score to detect evolving critical illness in hospitalized children. *Crit Care* 2011;15(4):R184, an open access article.

but typically includes at least one critical care attending physician or fellow, at least one nurse, and often a respiratory therapist. A *medical emergency team* (MET) is defined as a physician-led team with full critical care capabilities, including (a) the ability to prescribe therapy, (b) advanced airway skills, (c) central venous access skills, and (d) the ability to initiate intensive care at the bedside. *Rapid response team* (RRT) refers to a team that does not necessarily have all of these capabilities, and may include only nonphysician responders with rapid access to physician assistance if needed. *Rover team* or *critical care outreach team* refers to a team structured like an RRT, with the addition of providing proactive outreach for patients at high risk of deterioration (e.g., those recently discharged from an ICU). Some teams exist with the primary goal of responding to the concerns of families. Each of these teams may function independently with distinct members, or they may comprise overlapping members who respond to different needs throughout the hospital.

Medical Emergency Teams

The most widely researched aspect of RRSs has been METs. MET implementation studies show a 34% reduction in cardiopulmonary arrest outside the ICU but no reduction in hospital mortality in adults, and a 38% reduction in cardiopulmonary arrest outside the ICU and a 21% reduction in hospital mortality in children. The findings from key pediatric MET studies generally support implementation. The variability in findings and the limitations of design lead make it unclear if MET implementation has a direct effect on mortality and arrest rates in children's hospitals, or if the improvements are due to other patient safety initiatives.

Proactive Rover and Outreach Teams

Rover and critical care outreach teams are structured like an MET, with the addition of providing proactive outreach for patients at high risk of deterioration. The Duke University's Children's Center proactive rover team comprises the same members as the MET, including a pediatric critical care nurse practitioner or fellow, the pediatric intensive care unit (PICU) charge nurse, and a PICU respiratory therapist. The team makes scheduled rounds to each inpatient care area and discusses at-risk patients identified by the ward's charge nurse and senior resident. The team also evaluates children discharged from the PICU in the preceding 12 hours and new admissions to the progressive care unit.

Family Concern Teams

Teams also exist to respond to the family member's concern about their child's condition. The Condition HELP team, implemented at Children's Hospital of Pittsburgh, comprises a physician, a nursing supervisor, and a patient advocate. On admission, families receive a verbal explanation of the program from their nurse, receive a brochure, and view a video presentation.

PROCESS IMPROVEMENT LIMB

This limb works with the administrative limb and should include membership/oversight from clinicians (including each discipline on team and members of activating and responding teams) as well as improvement science experts with experience in time series data analysis and improvement interventions. This limb addresses three categories of measures: (1) Do we see signs of improvement in patient outcomes (outcome measures)? (2) Is the RRS working as planned (process measures)? (3) What are the unintended consequences (balancing measures)?

Outcome Measures

The most frequent outcome measures have been rates of hospital-wide mortality, cardiac arrests, and respiratory arrests outside the ICU. Identifying deaths that were potentially preventable by an RRS versus those that occurred following a complex ICU course can be difficult and requires expertise. The rate of cardiopulmonary arrests occurring outside the ICU may be a better outcome measure for improvement work, in that the events are discrete and measurable.

Critical deterioration events are defined as ICU transfers with noninvasive ventilation, intubation, or vasopressor infusion initiated in the 12 hours following arrival in the ICU. This measure was associated with a >13-fold risk of mortality and occurred more than eight times more commonly than arrests outside the ICU. It was also used as the primary outcome measure in a recent quasi-experimental study of the impacts of RRS implementation. Unrecognized situation awareness failure events (UNSAFE transfers) are another proximate outcome measure for RRS effectiveness. These are defined as ward-to-ICU transfers where patients are intubated, placed on vasopressors, or receive three or more fluid boluses within the first 1 hour after transfer.

Process Measures

The most commonly used process measure is the number of MET calls, expressed as a rate per admission, patient-day, or non-ICU patient-day. There is uncertainty regarding the optimal rate. A complementary measure to this is the percentage of MET calls that result in transfer to the ICU. Although the optimal percentage is not known, 100% of MET calls resulting in ICU transfer reflect underuse. The time between initial physiologic abnormality and admission to ICU, or "score to door time," is a measure reflecting RRS efficiency, and may be helpful in setting expectations among activating teams and determining when more responding team resources may be needed.

Balancing Measures

Qualitative research on pediatric RRSs has revealed several important themes. First, team-based care on the wards that empowers nurses and families and supports a culture of teamwork, accountability, and safety is highly valued. Second, tools for displaying and monitoring data trends (including vital signs and EWSs) are desirable. Third, standardized processes and procedures at the organizational level including proper education and training on recognizing critical illness, a shared language around at-risk patients, and a structure to proactively support risk identification support a culture of reducing deterioration events. Barriers to seeking MET assistance include low perceived self-efficacy, both in terms of (a) recognizing deterioration and (b) activating the MET and intraprofessional and interprofessional hierarchies. In addition, expectations of adverse interpersonal interactions with sometimes brusque MET staff, or perceived suboptimal clinical outcomes from ICU transfers could lead to a reluctance among physicians to transfer patients to the ICU for fear of inappropriate (or at least different) management.

ADMINISTRATIVE LIMB

The role of the administrative limb of RRSs is to implement the system, manage each of its components, and support its ongoing operation. This requires a committee structure, which may be combined with the hospital's resuscitation/code blue committee.

Membership should include nurses, physicians, and respiratory therapists in frontline clinical roles as well as leadership roles in ICU and ward settings. In addition, at least one participant should be experienced in patient safety and quality improvement methodology.

Implementing a Rapid Response System and Operating Costs

The Ontario Pediatric Critical Care Response Team Collaborative recently published a detailed RRS implementation strategy, which is broadly generalizable. One study has examined the balance of costs and benefits of a pediatric MET. A research team at the Children's Hospital of Philadelphia found that critical deterioration events cost almost $100,000 in each instance and that an MET comprising a nurse, respiratory therapist, and ICU fellow with concurrent responsibilities would need to prevent only 3.5 critical deterioration events per year to recoup its cost.

CHAPTER 7 ■ MULTIPLE TRAUMA

JOHN S. BAIRD AND ARTHUR COOPER

EPIDEMIOLOGY OF PEDIATRIC TRAUMA

Trauma is the leading cause of death in children and young adults in developed countries. It comprises unintentional and intentional injuries. Most pediatric deaths from trauma are associated with motor vehicles and occur prior to hospital admission. Functional limitations frequently follow major traumatic injury. Injury rates have responded to community-based harm-reduction strategies.

PEDIATRIC INJURY: MECHANISMS AND PATTERNS

Intracranial injuries are the cause of most pediatric trauma. Blunt injuries outnumber penetrating injuries in children 12:1, a ratio that is decreasing. Injury mechanism is the main predictor of injury pattern. Pedestrian motor vehicle trauma injuries involve the head, torso, and lower extremities (*Waddell triad*). Occupant injuries involve the head, face, and neck in unrestrained passengers, and cervical spine injuries, bowel disruption or hematoma, and *Chance fractures* of the spine (flexion injury with anterior compression and posterior distraction) in restrained passengers. Bicycle trauma results in head (unhelmeted riders), upper extremity, and upper abdominal (from contact with the handlebar) injuries. Low falls, the most common cause of childhood injury, rarely produce significant trauma, but high falls (second story or higher) produce serious head, long-bone, intrathoracic, and intra-abdominal injuries.

INITIAL ASSESSMENT AND STABILIZATION

Emergency Medical Services

Prehospital transport of critically injured children presents a difficult decision between "scoop and run" or "stay and play," and delay should be avoided whenever possible. Interhospital transport should be conducted by physicians, nurses, and staff with special pediatric training.

Trauma Centers and Field Triage Recommendations

Trauma centers are hospitals with special expertise in trauma care. They are classified by the American College of Surgeons as Level One, Level Two (most but not all of the specialists and services of Level One), and Level Three (only core specialists and services available). Hospitals and clinics without trauma center designation should still be capable of routine resuscitation and stabilization of injured patients. In some states, pediatric trauma centers have been designated.

Severely injured children cared for in hospitals with a pediatric intensive care unit (PICU) or in pediatric trauma centers have an improved outcome. Referral of critically ill and injured children to qualified centers is a well-established practice. Abnormal vital signs and Glasgow Coma Scale (GCS) scores may be used in referral criteria, though, "when in doubt, transfer to a trauma center."

Scoring

Current trauma scoring systems include the *Injury Severity Score* and the *Revised Trauma Score*, although neither specifically addresses children. The GCS is used to assess gross neurologic status following injury and can be modified for infants and small children. The *Pediatric Risk of Mortality III* and *Pediatric Index of Mortality II* are focused on the outcome of patients admitted to a PICU. A Pediatric Trauma Score of <9 is consistent with significant risk of mortality.

Primary Survey

The body regions most frequently injured in major pediatric trauma are the head, neck, abdomen, and lower extremities; in minor pediatric injury, the soft tissue and upper extremity injuries predominate. Most pediatric trauma is blunt trauma involving the head and is primarily a disease of airway and breathing rather than circulation, bleeding, or shock. The primary survey (A, airway; B, breathing; C, circulation; D, disability/neurologic impairment; and E, exposure/environment) is vitally important in pediatric victims of multiple or severe trauma, and repeated evaluations are recommended. The primary survey requires full exposure (i.e., undressing) to assess injury, but hypothermia should be avoided. Children rapidly cool due to their large body surface area, increased minute ventilation, and decreased subcutaneous tissue.

Airway (and Cervical Spine Stabilization)

All patients undergoing a primary survey should receive supplemental oxygen (FIO_2 1.0). An airway obstructed by soft tissues or secretions is opened (utilizing the modified jaw-thrust maneuver with or without an oropharyngeal airway) while proper cervical spine precautions are taken. A head tilt is avoided in patients with possible cervical spine injury.

When tracheal intubation is required, rapid-sequence, oral–tracheal intubation using cervical spine protection is recommended (assume that patient has a full stomach and unstable neck). Nasal intubation is contraindicated in patients with severe facial or head trauma. Trauma patients should be considered to have a full stomach, independent of their last documented meal, as their gastric emptying may be delayed. Children are more likely to develop respiratory failure than adults with equivalent injury. A cuffed endotracheal tube may reduce the need for tube changes due to size issues. Infants may become hypoxemic after 30 seconds of apnea because their functional residual capacity is relatively smaller while oxygen consumption is increased. When endotracheal intubation is unsuccessful, the laryngeal mask airway may provide a temporary rescue until an alternative method of tracheal intubation is accomplished. Fiberoptic–assisted intubation may help in patients with injury to the upper airway.

Surgical approaches to establish an airway include needle and surgical cricothyroidotomy. A needle cricothyroidotomy can bypass upper airway obstruction but is contraindicated in the presence of laryngotracheal injury as it may exacerbate the injury. An emergent surgical cricothyroidotomy or tracheostomy may be needed.

Breathing

If ventilation is inadequate, positive-pressure ventilation (PPV) should be provided. Hypercarbia may occur rapidly, and decreased responsiveness may be the only sign. Hypoxia prevention should include titration of the FIO_2 to maintain saturation of ~95%. A chest radiograph or even an arterial blood gas level may be helpful. The decision to intubate is based on the patient's ability to adequately exchange gas and to maintain and protect the airway.

Circulation

The maintenance of adequate circulation may help attenuate the stress response and prevent delayed inflammatory complications of major trauma. The basic steps in the management of hemorrhagic shock are control of active hemorrhage, placement of intravascular access, and appropriate volume replacement or resuscitation. Most children in hypotensive shock following traumatic injury are victims of uncontrolled hemorrhage. Sites of unrecognized hemorrhage include body cavities large enough to sequester significant blood volume (hemithorax, retroperitoneum, and pelvis and thigh compartments). The first and most important step is direct pressure over actively bleeding wounds. Current military experience suggests that tourniquets used to control exsanguinating hemorrhage are associated with decreased mortality and no increase in limb amputations. Their use after the onset of shock was less helpful, and as a result, prehospital use only is recommended. Military antishock trousers are unlikely to be useful.

Coagulopathy in injured children is related to the dilution of platelets and coagulation factors during massive transfusion. Hypothermia and acidosis may also contribute. Massive transfusion protocols (MTPs) organize blood bank resources and balance the provision of packed red blood cells (PRBCs), fresh frozen plasma (FFP), and platelets in an attempt to avoid worsening coagulopathy. Military experience suggests providing blood components in a ratio of ~1:1:1 (PRBC:FFP:platelets), but appropriately powered studies in children are lacking. Laboratory tests of the coagulation system (prothrombin time, partial thromboplastin time, and platelet count) are used to guide replacement therapy, but blood product administration should not be delayed in the massively bleeding, unstable patient. The thromboelastogram or rotational thromboelastometry is a point-of-care assay that graphically represents the entire hemostatic system and may allow timely, goal-directed treatment of trauma-associated coagulopathy.

Aminocaproic acid has been used successfully in injured children to control hemorrhage associated with severe head injury or extracorporeal membrane oxygenation (ECMO). Recombinant factor VII use in adults with severe traumatic hemorrhage produced a significant reduction in red blood cell transfusions. No equivalent trial in children is available, and concern exists about thromboembolic events associated with the use of activated recombinant factor VII.

Placement of Intravascular Access. The child with major trauma and signs of hypovolemic shock requires volume resuscitation. Children maintain systemic vascular resistance (and systemic blood pressure) longer than do similarly injured adults. Hypotension is a late sign of pediatric shock, developing after 30%–35% of circulating blood volume is lost.

Resuscitation is best carried out by large-bore peripheral catheters placed in antecubital (elbow) or saphenous (ankle) veins. In the event that access cannot be rapidly established, intraosseous access should be utilized. Access by central venous catheter in the femoral, internal jugular, or subclavian veins or by cutdown in the ankle or groin is helpful during resuscitation if experienced operators are available and other means of vascular access are inadequate. Upper body sites are preferred in patients with abdominal trauma.

Volume Replacement. Hypovolemia usually responds to 20–40 mL/kg of warmed isotonic solution, but frank hypotension may require an additional 10–20 mL/kg of warmed PRBC. Continued instability suggests internal bleeding requiring emergency operation to control hemorrhage. In children in shock with no intrathoracic, intra-abdominal, or intrapelvic bleeding and who fail to improve despite volume resuscitation, other forms of shock (obstructive, cardiogenic, and neurogenic) should be considered. It is necessary to assess these children for tension pneumothorax, cardiac tamponade, myocardial contusion, or spinal cord injury.

The controversy regarding colloid versus crystalloid resuscitation persists, but meta-analyses show no additional benefit of colloid. Crystalloid solutions are less expensive and immediately available. The isotonic crystalloid solutions commonly utilized for resuscitations include normal saline and lactated Ringer solution. Excessive use of normal saline may lead to a hyperchloremic metabolic acidosis that obscures the metabolic acidosis from hypoperfusion. The lactate in lactated Ringer solution is metabolized by the liver to bicarbonate, which provides a buffer, if hepatic function remains intact.

In some patients with multiple trauma, including neurologic injury, the judicious use of hypertonic (3%) saline may be appropriate (data from clinical trials are not yet available, and appropriate limits for extracellular osmolality are still controversial). Both 5% and 25% (or "salt-poor") albumin have been used in the resuscitation of pediatric trauma patients; 5% albumin is preferred for acute resuscitation. Other colloid solutions include 6% hydroxyethyl starch and low-molecular-weight dextran, but there are serious concerns about adverse effects on platelet and renal function with both these agents.

The treatment of hemorrhagic shock must include transfusion of blood products. Time may not allow a full type and cross-match before transfusion. When possible, type-specific, uncross-matched blood is still preferable to type O, Rh-negative, uncross-matched blood. Blood warmers should be used when possible. The use of blood replacement products, such as stroma-free hemoglobin and human polymerized hemoglobin, is investigational.

Disability (Abbreviated Neurologic Exam)

Assessment of disability and the neurologic status includes ascertainment of the GCS (to assess level of consciousness), the pupillary responses (to exclude mass lesions), and evidence of an altered mental status. Traumatic coma (GCS $\leq$ 8) and pupillary asymmetry mandate immediate involvement of neurosurgical consultants. It is important to perform a rapid assessment of neurologic status while the severely injured patient is being prepared for endotracheal intubation.

Monitoring Resuscitation

Resuscitation proceeds concurrently with continuous reevaluation. The most sensitive monitor of cardiac output and volume status in children is heart rate. The perfusion of distal extremities is monitored by assessing capillary refill and skin turgor and by looking for cyanosis or other signs of circulatory embarrassment. The central venous pressure may be a helpful marker of intravascular volume, particularly in patients with extensive fluid resuscitation. Urinary output is an indicator of renal perfusion. Hourly output should be at least 1–2 mL/kg/h in infants and younger children and at least 0.5–1 mL/kg/h in children and adolescents. Placement of a urinary catheter should be deferred in patients with urethral injury, pelvic fractures, or gross hematuria. Additional helpful markers of adequate resuscitation include mixed venous oxygen saturation, arterial lactate concentration, and the base deficit.

SECONDARY SURVEY

Complete History and Physical Examination

Once the primary survey is complete, resuscitation is ongoing, and shock is being effectively treated, then a secondary survey is undertaken for definitive evaluation. The secondary survey consists of a "SAMPLE" history (*s*ymptoms, *a*llergies, *m*edications, *p*ast illnesses, *l*ast meal, *e*vents and environment), history of the injury, and a complete head-to-toe examination addressing all body regions and organ systems. The first priority is to identify life-threatening injuries that may have been overlooked during the primary survey.

Drainage from the nose or ears, evidence of mid-face instability, *hemotympanum*, or *Battle sign* (postauricular ecchymosis) suggests a basilar skull fracture. Following the lateral cervical spine radiograph, the neck is examined for tenderness, swelling, torticollis, or spasm (suggesting a cervical spine fracture). Cervical spine injuries may not be detected on lateral cervical spine films (i.e., *spinal cord injury without radiologic abnormality [SCIWORA]*). The trachea should be midline and the large vessels of the neck examined. Chest point tenderness, palpable bony deformity, crepitus, subcutaneous emphysema, or asymmetry in excursion suggests the presence of a rib fracture or air or blood in the thorax. Muffled or distant heart sounds with jugular venous distention may suggest cardiac tamponade. A distended abdomen following gastric decompression suggests intra-abdominal bleeding or a disrupted hollow viscus.

All skeletal components should be palpated for evidence of instability or discontinuity. Pelvic fractures should be suspected with an unstable pelvic girdle or perineal swelling or discoloration. Most long-bone fractures are self-evident but may be missed during the secondary survey. Reexamination of all injured extremities for pain, pallor, pulselessness, paresthesias, and paralysis (classical signs of associated vascular trauma, or, when advanced, compartmental hypertension) is necessary. The back should be completely examined.

Laboratory and Radiologic Evaluation

Serial hematocrits and a type and cross-match are essential. Elevations in serum transaminases, amylase, and lipase suggest injury to the liver or pancreas. Coagulopathy is common in children with extensive resuscitation or traumatic brain injury. Urinalysis should be performed with suspected abdominal injury. A pregnancy test is advisable for injured adolescent females.

Imaging studies should not take precedence over resuscitation from life-threatening injuries. CT scans of the head should be obtained for loss of consciousness or neurologic injury. CT scans of the abdomen should be obtained for abdominal tenderness, distention, bruising, gross hematuria, or penetrating injury. Children with severe, multiple trauma that prevents a complete physical examination benefit from routine CT of the head, thorax, abdomen, and pelvis. Angiography is appropriate for further study of injuries to large vessels in selected patients. MRI is necessary when SCIWORA is suspected but is not normally performed acutely. Focused assessment by sonography in trauma (*FAST*) may be useful in detecting intra-abdominal blood and assessments can be performed serially at the bedside. The role of FAST in the diagnosis of abdominal injury is increasing and diagnostic peritoneal lavage decreasing. However, FAST is not yet sufficiently reliable to exclude abdominal injury.

MANAGEMENT

With few exceptions, hypotensive pediatric trauma patients require immediate operation, Nonoperative management of blunt visceral trauma is often successful. Penetrating injuries of the head, neck, and abdomen also require surgical intervention, but most intrathoracic injuries, whether blunt or penetrating, require only tube thoracostomy. Emergency thoracotomy is rarely performed in children. Laparotomy is required for gunshot wounds to the abdomen, as well as for penetrating abdominal injury associated with hemorrhagic shock, peritonitis, or evisceration. Thoracoabdominal injury should be suspected (a) whenever the torso is penetrated between the nipple line and the umbilicus (anteriorly) or the costal margin (posteriorly), (b) if peritoneal irritation develops following thoracic penetration, (c) if food or chyme is recovered from the chest tube, or (d) if injury trajectory imaging suggests diaphragmatic penetration. If one or more of these signs is present, tube thoracostomy should be performed expeditiously, followed by laparotomy or laparoscopy for repair of the diaphragm and damaged organs. Skeletal injuries constitute the majority of cases in which surgical intervention is necessary. All penetrating wounds are contaminated, must be treated as infected, and accessible missile fragments removed.

Nutritional support with protein (even more than calories) and prophylaxis to prevent gastric stress ulcer bleeding is required for the care of children with major traumatic injury. Glucose supplementation is unnecessary in most noninfant trauma victims, unless hypoglycemia or underlying disease is noted. Close attention to avoid hypoglycemia is essential. Tetanus-prone wounds require tetanus toxoid, with or without tetanus-immune globulin, depending on immunization status and degree of contamination.

Social services, psychiatric support, pastoral care, and, when appropriate, law enforcement and child protective agencies should be involved. The emotional needs of the child and family, especially for those families who suffer the death of a child, should be addressed. Parents may feel loss of control over their child's destiny or enormous guilt, whether or not these feelings are warranted.

Definitive Management of Non-Neurologic Injuries

Chest Trauma

Intrathoracic injuries occur in 6% of pediatric trauma, 86% are due to blunt injury, and 74% are automobile related. The thoracic injury pattern includes lung contusion or laceration (48%), pneumothorax or hemothorax (41%), and rib or sternal fractures (32%). The heart, diaphragm, great vessels, bronchi, and esophagus are infrequently injured. A chest CT scan is useful with severe thoracic injuries and may help to grade the severity of lung injury. The chest wall of the child often escapes major harm. The pliable cartilaginous ribs permit compression without radiographic fractures but results in pulmonary contusions. Pneumothorax and hemothorax are uncommon but still risk ventilatory and circulatory compromise as the mediastinum shifts.

Pulmonary Contusion, Laceration, and Hematoma. Pulmonary parenchymal injury due to blunt trauma is characterized by alveolar hemorrhage, consolidation, and edema, leading to decreased gas exchange and pulmonary compliance. It may manifest as hemoptysis, subcutaneous emphysema, hypoxemia and respiratory distress. Secondary complications of pulmonary contusion include aspiration, infection, and ARDS (20% of children with pulmonary contusion). Pulmonary contusions uncomplicated by aspiration, overhydration, or infection resolve in 7–10 days. Fluid and blood in lung parenchyma provide an excellent "culture medium" for bacterial infection.

Hemopneumothorax. Penetrating trauma is associated with a higher incidence of hemopneumothorax than blunt trauma. Initial therapy includes a sterile, occlusive dressing to convert the open chest to a closed injury. A tube thoracostomy inserted via the fifth intercostal space in the mid-axillary line via open or Seldinger technique is then placed. Video-assisted thoracoscopy may be helpful when residual collections of blood persist. Definitive management of an open chest wound requires surgical intervention following stabilization.

Rib Fractures and Flail Chest. Rib fractures occur in one-third of children with blunt thoracic trauma, and their occurrence suggests a mechanism of injury with significant energy transfer. Rib fractures in infants and young children are frequently associated with child abuse in the absence of a history of major blunt trauma. Fracture of a first rib may be a marker of major vascular injury in children. A *flail chest* is characterized by a chest wall segment that has lost continuity with the thorax and moves paradoxically with changes in intrathoracic pressure and is rare in children. Diagnosis is made by the visual inspection of paradoxical movement of the chest wall. Definitive management includes controlled mechanical ventilation. Continued therapy is directed at the underlying pulmonary contusion.

Myocardial Contusion. Myocardial contusion is rare in children. Signs and symptoms include tachycardia, dysrhythmia, gallop rhythm, chest pain, myocardial dysfunction, and cardiogenic pulmonary edema. Myocardial enzymes are elevated. Treatment is supportive. Sudden death that occurs with relatively minor blunt trauma to the chest is known as *commotio cordis*. The mechanism of injury appears to be ventricular dysrhythmia. Survival is low but would likely improve with more community access to defibrillation.

Cardiac Tamponade. Pericardial contusions and lacerations may lead to hemopericardium and subsequent cardiac tamponade. Rising pericardial pressure obstructs venous return and cardiac output, leading to *Beck triad* (pulsus paradoxus, a quiet precordium, and distended neck veins). Unexplained tachycardia may be an early sign. FAST examination in selected patients may be diagnostic. Expansion of intravascular volume is useful to temporize as the patient is prepared for a pericardiocentesis or operative pericardial window. Sedation and PPV may worsen hemodynamic function.

Rupture of the Diaphragm. Traumatic rupture of the diaphragm results from severe compression forces over the lower chest and upper abdomen. Rupture is far more common on the left side. The diagnosis should be suspected when the left diaphragm is not clearly visualized or is abnormally elevated, abdominal visceral shadows are abnormally located on chest radiograph, or a nasogastric tube terminates in the hemithorax. Treatment is operative repair.

Aortic Disruption. Injury to the aorta is uncommon in children and usually occurs from a severe deceleration injury or fall from extreme heights. Most children with this injury die at the scene. Clinical symptoms and signs include back pain, a machinery-type heart murmur that radiates to the back, and hemorrhagic shock. Radiographic findings include widened mediastinum, loss of the aortic knob, rightward tracheal deviation, first or second rib fractures, or apical capping. Treatment is emergent surgical repair, usually with cardiopulmonary bypass.

Tracheobronchial Tears. Rupture of the tracheobronchial tree leads to symptoms and signs of airway obstruction (dyspnea and stridor), pneumothorax, pneumomediastinum, or subcutaneous emphysema. A persistent, large air leak following tube thoracostomy suggests the possibility of a tracheobronchial tear. PPV may exacerbate the leak. Some patients require multiple tube thoracostomies or emergent operative intervention. One-lung ventilation or ECMO may be lifesaving.

Abdominal Trauma

Serious intra-abdominal injuries occur in 8% of pediatric trauma victims and include injuries to the liver (27%), spleen (27%), kidneys (25%), and gastrointestinal tract (21%). Injuries to the genitourinary tract, pancreas, abdominal blood vessels, and pelvis are infrequent. Penetrating abdominal injury is less common than blunt trauma, and requires surgical exploration. Physical signs of significant abdominal injury in children include diminished bowel sounds, tenderness to palpation, guarding, rebound tenderness, and peritoneal irritation.

Abdominal radiographs should be assessed for free air. In patients with a concerning history or exam, CT scanning is the study of choice for both blunt and penetrating injury. Abdominal CT may reveal vascular blush or signs of contrast extravasation (evidence of extravasation does not mandate emergency laparotomy). A FAST examination may be useful to confirm abnormalities but is less helpful when negative.

Nonoperative treatment is successful for most solid visceral injuries, especially kidneys (98%), spleen (95%), and liver (90%). Bleeding from renal, splenic, or hepatic injuries is usually self-limited and resolves spontaneously. Operative intervention for bleeding is unnecessary unless the patient has hypotensive shock or the transfusion requirements exceed 40 mL/kg within 24 hours of injury. There is little role of peritoneal lavage to diagnose intra-abdominal hemorrhage due to reliance on imaging and nonoperative management. The indications for immediate surgery include ongoing intra-abdominal hemorrhage (shock), hollow viscus perforation (peritonitis), or evisceration.

Liver and Spleen. A grading system for anatomic findings in splenic and hepatic injury has been developed (**Table 7.1**) and helps in predicting outcome. An evidence-based guideline utilizing CT scan for the treatment of pediatric liver and spleen injuries below grade V includes ICU admission for patients with grade IV injury, activity restriction based on grade of injury, and no need for routine follow-up imaging. Angiographic control of bleeding may be helpful.

TABLE 7.1

Grading System[a] for Hepatic and Splenic Injuries

INJURY	GRADE I	GRADE II	GRADE III	GRADE IV	GRADE V	GRADE VI
Hematoma: liver, spleen	Subcapsular, <10% surface area	Subcapsular, 10%–50% surface area; intraparenchymal diameter <10 cm (liver) vs. <5 cm (spleen)	Subcapsular, >50% surface area or expanding; ruptured subcapsular or parenchymal hematoma; intraparenchymal hematoma >10 cm (liver) vs. >5 cm (spleen) or expanding			
Laceration: liver	Capsular tear <1 cm parenchymal depth	1–3 cm parenchymal depth, <10 cm in length (liver) vs. not involving a trabecular vessel (spleen)	>3 cm parenchymal depth or involving trabecular vessels (spleen)	Parenchymal disruption of 25%–75% of hepatic lobe, or 1–3 segments within a lobe	Parenchymal disruption >75% of hepatic lobe, or >3 segments within a lobe	
Laceration: spleen			Involvement of hilar vessels with >25% devascularization	Shattered spleen		
Vascular injury: liver					Juxtahepatic venous injuries	Hepatic avulsion
Vascular injury: spleen					Hilar injury with devascularization	

[a]Advance one grade for multiple injuries, up to grade III.
Adapted from Moore EE, Cogbill TH, Jurkovich GJ, et al. Organ injury scaling: Spleen and liver (1994 revision). *J Trauma* 1995;38:323–4.

Kidneys and Urinary Tract. Children are more susceptible to renal trauma than adults. Blunt trauma is more frequent and usually leads to a hematoma. Renal lacerations result from crush injuries against the ribs or spine. Gross hematuria is more sensitive than microscopic hematuria in detecting serious urologic injury. Rhabdomyolysis from crush injury may cause pigmented urine and a heme positive urinalysis. An abdominal CT scan with intravenous contrast is the most appropriate initial test for hemodynamically stable children with suspected renal trauma. A renal injury grading system is shown in **Table 7.2**. An IV urogram in the OR for patients requiring emergent surgical exploration provides information about renal function. The conservative management of renal injury in grades I to III is routine. In grades IV and V renal injury, indications for surgical exploration include persistent hemorrhage, expanding or uncontained retroperitoneal hematoma, or suspected renal pedicle avulsion. In addition, children with substantial devitalized renal parenchyma or urinary extravasation may also be candidates. Occasionally angiographic control of renal hemorrhage is feasible.

The ureters are protected by muscle and soft tissue and rarely injured. Ureteropelvic junction disruption may occur following severe abdominal trauma. The bladder is less protected in children. The approach for surgical repair of a ruptured bladder depends on the site of the leak; a cystostomy is often helpful. Pelvic fractures are associated with urethral injury, particularly in males, and blood is generally present at the urethral meatus. Diagnosis mandates retrograde urethrography. Management depends on the severity and site of urethral injury.

Gastrointestinal Tract. The esophagus is rarely injured by blunt thoracic trauma. Blunt injuries to the remainder of the gastrointestinal tract follow several patterns, including crush injury, burst injury, and shear injury. Subsequent damage includes hematoma, laceration, perforation, or transection of the gastrointestinal tract. Blunt stomach injury is more frequent in children and results in a perforation (*blowout injury*) along the greater curvature. Duodenal injuries are infrequent. CT scans (preferably with double contrast) differentiate between duodenal hematoma and perforation. Hematomas and perforations of the remainder of the small bowel may be difficult to diagnose early, as peritoneal signs may take several hours to develop.

The management of gastrointestinal tract perforation in children is surgical (nonoperative management of duodenal hematomas is possible). A colostomy may be necessary for extensive large bowel injury with perforation and fecal contamination. Primary repair is often feasible in an otherwise healthy child without shock or the need for multiple blood transfusions.

Pancreas. Pancreatic injury is infrequent in children, and diagnosis is often delayed. Diagnosis depends mainly on CT scan, although clinical and laboratory data may be useful. Routine surgical intervention is not recommended. Endoscopic retrograde cholangiopancreatography with stenting or distal pancreatectomy may have a role. Pseudocyst formation

TABLE 7.2

Grading System[a] for Renal Injury

INJURY	GRADE I	GRADE II	GRADE III	GRADE IV	GRADE V
Contusion	Microscopic or gross hematuria, normal urologic studies				
Hematoma	Subcapsular, nonexpanding	Nonexpanding perirenal hematoma confined to renal retroperitoneum			
Laceration		<1 cm parenchymal depth (renal cortex) without urinary extravasation	>1 cm parenchymal depth (renal cortex) without urinary extravasation	Extending through renal cortex, medulla, and collecting system	Shattered kidney
Vascular injury				Main renal artery or vein injury with contained hemorrhage	Avulsion of renal hilum

[a]Advance one grade for multiple injuries to the same organ.
Adapted from Moore EE, Shackford SR, Pachter HL, et al. Organ injury scaling: Spleen, liver, and kidney. *J Trauma* 1989;29:1664–6.

occurs in approximately one-third of children with pancreatic injuries.

Abdominal Compartment Syndrome. Trauma-associated abdominal compartment syndrome (ACS) is not common but may occur in pediatric blunt trauma or burn injury. Massive fluid resuscitation may be associated with the development of ACS. Increasing abdominal pressure decreases abdominal organ perfusion and venous return from the lower half of the body. Hypoperfusion injury worsens tissue edema, perfusion, and abdominal distention and results in organ dysfunction. Oliguria and respiratory insufficiency are common. Abdominal pressures can be measured via a bladder catheter. Treatment is with decompressive laparotomy.

Skeletal Trauma

Fractures in children are often incomplete or nondisplaced. They are also unique because of growth plates, rapid healing, a tendency to remodel in the plane of the fracture, and a high incidence of ischemic vascular injuries. Long-term growth disturbances may complicate childhood fractures. Joint dislocations and ligamentous injury are less common in children. The most common long-bone fractures from childhood pedestrian motor vehicle crashes involve the femur and tibia. Falls from significant height are associated with both upper and lower extremity fractures. Diagnosis of fractures is often delayed in multiply injured children.

Early stabilization decreases patient discomfort and limits blood loss. Closed treatment predominates for fractures of the clavicle, upper extremity, and tibia. Fractures of the femur increasingly involve internal fixation. An open fracture may have an innocuous-appearing puncture wound but requires antibiotics. Operative treatment is required for complex open fractures (for debridement and irrigation), displaced supracondylar fractures (association with ischemic vascular injury), and major or displaced physeal fractures (must be reduced anatomically). Frequent neurovascular checks are essential to assess for arterial insufficiency and compartment syndrome. Traumatic fat embolism (long-bone fractures) and rhabdomyolysis (severe crush injuries) are rare complications.

Compartment Syndrome. Fracture-associated arterial insufficiency is recognized by the presence of a pulse deficit and measurement of compartment pressures. Elevated compartment pressures impair capillary perfusion, and ischemia develops rapidly. Symptoms include the 5 Ps: pallor, pulselessness, paresthesia, paralysis, and pain. Pain is usually the earliest sign. Fasciotomy is indicated for a compartment pressure >40 cm H_2O. Lower pressures may mandate treatment if the child is symptomatic or if capillary perfusion pressure is reduced.

CHILD ABUSE

Child abuse is the presumed cause of 3% of major traumatic injuries in children. Child abuse should be suspected when there is an unexplained delay in obtaining treatment, the history is vague or incompatible with physical findings, the caretaker blames siblings, playmates, or other parties, or the caretaker protects other adults rather than the child. Every state requires reports of suspected child abuse be filed with local child protective services. The medical team should focus on the care of the child rather than attempts to determine perpetrators or accusations. Suspected abuse should be investigated expeditiously to protect siblings still in the home.

Victims of child abuse are younger, more severely injured, and more likely to die from their injuries than other pediatric trauma patients. The "shaken baby syndrome" or "whiplash shaken infant syndrome" comprises unique symptoms and signs peculiar to nonaccidental trauma. These patients have intracranial and intraocular hemorrhages in the absence of external head trauma or fracture of the calvaria. The "shaking" injuries result from bleeding of the easily torn bridging veins during rapid acceleration and deceleration forces (worsened if concomitant impact). Ophthalmologic examination often reveals retinal hemorrhages of varying severity, occasionally with retinal detachment. The prognosis is poor for many affected infants. Additional patterns of injury secondary to physical abuse include burns (shape often suggests mechanism, e.g. cigarette or hot iron), bruising (e.g., fingerprint contusions), asphyxiation, blunt abdominal injury, multiple fractures of various ages, and sexual abuse.

Findings on physical examination include signs of general neglect (poor skin hygiene, malnutrition, failure to thrive), hematomas and petechiae of various ages and distribution (the color of cutaneous contusions is not a sensitive nor specific indicator of contusion age), bite marks, burn injuries, abrasions, strap or belt injuries, and soft-tissue swelling. An ophthalmologic examination is mandatory in infants who are possible abuse victims. Infant victims require an examination for skeletal injury; either a skeletal survey with chest radiograph or a bone scan. Radiographic manifestations of child abuse include new and old injuries, subperiosteal hemorrhages, epiphyseal separations, periosteal shearing, metaphyseal fragmentations, previously healed periosteal calcifications, and shearing of the metaphysis.

CHAPTER 8 ■ DROWNING

KATHERINE V. BIAGAS AND LINDA APONTE-PATEL

The World Health Organization (WHO) estimates that nearly 400,000 persons die from drowning annually. In many countries, drowning is the second or third most frequent cause of childhood death. Despite recent prevention efforts and advances in medical care, the outcome remains quite poor.

EPIDEMIOLOGY

The majority of drowning events occur in freshwater; only 4% occur in salt water. (This incidence is higher in coastal communities.) The three pediatric groups at particular risk include the very young, adolescent males, and African-American children. Drowning events that involve infants and toddlers commonly occur in water in the home and have poor outcomes. Infants and toddlers are likely to have an unwitnessed event and a longer drowning time. Events in teenage boys are generally related to recreational water activities. Adolescent males have the highest rate of drowning while swimming, boating, or driving a car.

Drowning risk is elevated in children with epilepsy and neurologic disorders (especially autism and mental retardation). A prior history of seizure occurs in 7% of pediatric drowning victims. Hyperventilation due to swimming exertion may predispose a child with epilepsy to have a seizure. Long QT syndrome (LQTS) or other cardiac "channelopathies" increase the risk of ventricular tachyarrhythmias exacerbated by swimming. Swimming is an arrhythmogenic trigger with activation of the "diving reflex," which alters autonomic stability. Swimming also involves physical exertion, which is also a syncopal trigger. Screening of relatives is recommended for anyone suspected of having swimming-related arrhythmias. Counseling regarding safe water-related activities and β-blockade therapy are recommended. Other medical conditions that less frequently predispose to drowning include depression, coronary artery disease, cardiomyopathy, hypoglycemia, and hypothermia.

Thirty to seventy percent of boating and swimming fatalities in the adolescent and adult age groups have measurable blood alcohol levels. Cervical spine injury accompanies 0.5%–5.0% of drowning injuries in older children and adolescents. The mechanism of injury is a blow that hyperextends the cervical spine from diving or falling into a body of water. Immobilization of the cervical spine at the scene is important. Radiographs of the cervical spine may be normal despite cord injury.

PATHOPHYSIOLOGY

The sequence of events in drowning consists of an initial struggle, sometimes with a surprise inhalation, suspension of movement, and exhalation of a little air frequently followed by swallowing, violent struggle, convulsions with spasmodic respiratory efforts through an open mouth, loss of reflexes, and death. During the initial seconds of drowning, small amounts of aspirated fluid often cause laryngospasm. Victims who are resuscitated at this phase will have little water aspiration, but ventilation by rescue breathing may be difficult because of glottic closure. If the victim loses muscle tone while submerged, larger quantities of fluid may be aspirated. In addition, a victim may swallow a large amount of fluid, vomit, and aspirate gastric contents.

The development of hypothermia is common with drowning and is usually secondary to rapid radiant heat losses in tepid water. As core temperature drops below 32°–35°C, unconsciousness and muscular weakness develop and the risk of aspiration is increased. Atrial fibrillation occurs with core temperatures in the low 30°C range and ventricular fibrillation or asystole with severe hypothermia at a core temperature less than 28°C.

Respiratory and Cardiovascular Dysfunction

In patients with long hypoxic episodes and alveolar aspiration, surfactant washout, lung collapse, alveolar derecruitment, intrapulmonary shunting, raised pulmonary vascular resistance, and ventilation–perfusion mismatching occur. These processes create the clinical syndromes of acute lung injury (ALI) and acute respiratory distress syndrome (ARDS). Aspiration of gastric contents may add caustic injury. Neurogenic pulmonary edema can also occur.

The hallmark of cardiovascular dysfunction associated with drowning is decreased myocardial contractility with hypoxemia. Ventricular end-diastolic and atrial pressures are high with resultant congestion of central and pulmonary veins. Poor myocardial contractility, in combination with raised systemic vascular resistance, results in lower cardiac output.

Brain Injury

Metabolically active areas of the brain, such as subcortical tissues, and regions with so-called "watershed" perfusion are the most vulnerable to hypoxic injury. Global brain involvement is seen in the most severe cases.

Drowning in Ice-Cold Water

Brain function may be preserved in "ice-cold water drowning" with good (or even normal) neurologic outcome despite extensive submersion times. There are numerous reports of dramatic cases of intact neurologic recovery in children who drowned in ice-cold water. Patients who drown in more temperate water but become hypothermic should be considered to have hypothermia from prolonged submersion. Secondary hypothermia is often a poor prognostic sign. Arrhythmia is an important complication of ice-cold water drowning.

MANAGEMENT

Prehospital Management

The three most active areas of acute management of drowning patients are outlined in **Table 8.1.** Management at the scene should focus on rapid restoration of oxygenation and spontaneous circulation with basic life support. In patients who suffer respiratory arrest and continue to have spontaneous circulation, reestablishing ventilation often results in recovery with no serious morbidity. Time should not be wasted by attempting to drain water from the lungs before rescue breathing. Trained rescuers, equipped with buoyant rescue aids, should attempt in-water rescue breathing for victims found in deep water. Once on solid ground, chest compressions should be initiated unless signs of life are present. Cervical spine immobilization should be performed in cases with a history of diving, or when the cause of drowning is not known. Advanced life support (endotracheal intubation, manual ventilation, administration of fluid boluses, defibrillation, and administration of vasoactive medications) should be initiated for victims who do not regain spontaneous breathing and consciousness.

TABLE 8.1

Important Principles in the Management of Children with Drowning Events Arranged by Phase of Care

PHASE OF CARE	FOCUS OF THERAPY	SPECIFIC MEASURES
Prehospital	Initial rescue	Removal from water Activate EMS system
	Resuscitation	Rescue breathing Rescue breathing + chest compressions if "lifeless" Consider cervical collar for diving accidents
Emergency department	Oxygenation and ventilation	Supply supplemental oxygen Intubation if unable to protect airway Ventilation to provide normocarbia
	Brain resuscitation	Temperature monitoring to maintain body cooling Rewarming for persistent nonperfusing rhythms
	Circulation	Vasoactive agents for hypotension
	Disposition	Transfer victims not fully alert for definitive care
PICU	Brain resuscitation	Consider therapeutic hypothermia (32–34°C for 12–72 h) Control of fevers and seizures
	Respiratory management	"Lung protective" strategy ventilation for ALI/ARDS unless contributes to increased ICP
	Treatment of hypotension/shock	Vasoactive infusions
	Restore homeostatic systems	Control of dysglycemia Measurement and monitoring of electrolytes and fluid
	Assessment of prognosis	Repeated neurologic exams CT if concern for trauma MRI/MRS Electrophysiologic studies Measurement of biomarkers—future measure

EMS, emergency medical services; ALI, acute lung injury; ARDS, acute respiratory distress syndrome; ICP, intracranial pressure; CT, computerized tomography; MRI, magnetic resonance imaging; MRS, magnetic resonance spectroscopy.

Management in the Emergency Department

Advanced life support should focus on the establishment of adequate oxygenation, ventilation, and circulation and the determination of neurologic function. Intubation and positive pressure ventilation is required for patients who cannot protect their airway or who remain unconscious. Noninvasive ventilation may be sufficient support for those who are partially or fully conscious. Continuous infusions of vasopressor or inotropic agents should be administered to maintain a normal blood pressure. Initial neurologic status is approximated using the Glasgow Coma Score (GCS) with a more thorough neurologic examination performed later.

Temperature management is a key component of brain resuscitation. Aggressive rewarming should be avoided. In adults with cardiac arrest (CA), brain cooling may be neuroprotective and better-than-expected neurologic outcomes are possible. However, for victims with sustained ventricular fibrillation, rewarming may be necessary to establish a perfusing rhythm. Simple warming techniques include the use of warmed intravenous fluids, external radiant heat, and ventilation with heated gas. More aggressive efforts include warmed peritoneal lavage, dialysis fluids, or bladder washes. With severe hypothermia and absence of a perfusing rhythm, rewarming on cardiopulmonary bypass or extracorporeal cardiopulmonary resuscitation should be considered. Rewarming can induce peripheral vasodilatation and impaired cardiac output. Rewarming efforts should be employed solely to reestablish a perfusing rhythm and stopped as early as possible to prevent overshoot with hyperthermia.

Management in the Pediatric Intensive Care

Children who do not regain full consciousness should be transferred to a pediatric intensive care (PICU) facility. Ongoing efforts should be directed to aggressively treat any organ dysfunction. Neuronal injury cannot be reversed. Neurologic critical care is largely supportive. Hypermetabolic states of the brain (e.g., seizures and fevers) should be aggressively treated. Electroencephalography (EEG) may be needed to detect subclinical seizures and to titrate antiepileptic therapy.

In the 1970s, therapy included moderate dehydration, controlled hyperventilation, deep hypothermia (30°C), barbiturate coma, corticosteroids, and continuous muscular paralysis for 48–72 hours. Studies of children who received deep hypothermia for pulseless victims resulted in an increase in the number of survivors who suffered a persistent vegetative state and increased infectious complications. The promising results of moderate hypothermia in adults following witnessed out-of-hospital CA and in asphyxiated newborns and animal models of asphyxic CA suggest possible usefulness of this therapy. Targeted temperature management in the normothermic range and prevention of hyperthermia may be a reasonable alternative.

For patients with ALI or ARDS, an "open-lung strategy" should be employed. Usual ventilator management includes limiting peak pressures to 25 torr, tidal volumes to 6–8 mL/kg, and increasing positive end-expiratory pressure (PEEP) until fraction of inspired oxygen is <0.6. Permissive hypercapnia, a commonly used lung protective strategy, may adversely affect intracranial pressure (ICP) due to the elevation in P_{CO_2}. Moreover, the increase in intrathoracic pressure associated with high levels of PEEP may be transmitted to the intracranial space and further increase ICP as well as diminish cerebral venous return.

Lung injury following drowning is partly related to surfactant washout. The efficacy of surfactant administration has only been shown in case reports. Other extraordinary methods of lung support, including extracorporeal membrane oxygenation, inhaled nitric oxide, and prone positioning, may be considered.

Continuous vasoactive infusions may be required to treat myocardial dysfunction and to correct abnormal peripheral vascular resistance. Treatment should concentrate on normalizing blood pressure, organ perfusion, and gas exchange for as long as needed.

Postmortem examinations demonstrate mild to moderate hyponatremia and hypotonic hemolysis in victims who drowned in freshwater and moderate hypernatremia and hyperchloremia after salt water drowning. However, clinically important abnormalities in serum electrolyte concentrations are not usually found. Exceptions to this generality are found in drowning that occurs in high-salinity water (e.g., the Dead Sea). Hemodilution and hypervolemia may be found with fresh-water-associated drowning but these are generally mild as the absorbed fluid is readily excreted in survivors.

PREVENTION

Prevention strategies should focus on the supervision of young children around any water, the risks of recreation-related incidents, the need for CPR training of parents and caretakers, and the use of effective pool and water hazard barriers. Supervision of young children around water sources is paramount. Parents and caretakers need to be knowledgeable about the risks of all water hazards, including wading pools, spas, drainage ditches, toilets, buckets, and moderate-sized containers. A water-filled 5-gallon bucket has sufficient depth to cause a toddler to drown. The absence of proper fencing increases pool-related drowning by three to fivefold.

The American Academy of Pediatrics (AAP) recommendations for anticipatory guidance can be found at http://www.aap.org/en-us/about-the-aap/aap-press-room/Pages/AAP-Gives-Updated-Advice-on-Drowning-Prevention.aspx. Additional prevention tips and information on safety barriers can be found on the Consumer Product Safety Commission website http://www.cpsc.gov/en/Safety-Education/

Neighborhood-Safety-Network/Toolkits/Drowning-Prevention/. Such educational strategies have been met with demonstrable success.

OUTCOMES

Outcome from drowning is often related to the extent of neurologic injury. Poor prognostic signs include an unwitnessed event, prolonged time to resuscitation, the need for CPR at the scene, the need for continued CPR in the ED, and prolonged coma. The best independent predictor of survival is drowning time; however, accurate data are not known for many patients. Predictors of outcomes at the time of PICU admission are of mixed certainty. Drowning victims who are awake on admission have generally good outcomes, yet those who remain nonresponsive at 24 hours after admission do not necessarily have poor outcomes.

Adjunct radiographic studies can aid in the determination of the extent of the initial injury and contribute to the understanding of ongoing disease. Brain CT is often used in the initial assessment, especially in patients with a possible associated traumatic injury. Magnetic resonance imaging (MRI) and MR spectroscopy (MRS) scans detect subtle injury. Diffusion-weighted imaging detects early (minutes to hours) injury after CA and may provide information about prognosis. Repeat MR scans (4–7 days after injury) may be the most predictive and MRS may aid in this determination.

Electrophysiologic studies may provide additional information. Brain stem auditory-evoked responses (BSAER) have been used to evaluate prolonged functional outcome with some success. A combination of electrophysiologic modalities, including sleep recordings, BSAER, somatosensory evoked potentials, and polysomnography may give better prediction over the use of EEG alone; however, cost issues and availability of resources may make this impractical.

CHAPTER 9 ■ BURNS AND SMOKE INHALATION

ROGER W. YURT, JAMES J. GALLAGHER, JOY D. HOWELL, AND BRUCE M. GREENWALD

After a major burn injury, wounds provide a portal for loss of fluid and body heat, systemic responses stress the homeostatic mechanisms, and the loss of skin integrity exposes the child to bacterial, fungal, and viral pathogens.

EVALUATION OF THE PATIENT

Initial evaluation of the burn patient is the same as for any injury. The adequacy of airway, breathing, and circulation are assessed followed by a rapid overall evaluation simultaneous with resuscitation. The possibility of coexisting trauma should be considered.

Extent of Burn Injury

The extent of a burn injury is quantified by surface area (SA) and depth of the injury. This determination guides fluid resuscitation and informs prognosis. A Lund & Browder chart or Berkow's formula can estimate burn SA percentage. The "rule of nines" calculations are less accurate in children <15 years of age. The distribution of SA by age is shown in **Table 9.1**.

A first-degree burn is characterized as erythematous, painful, and dry, whereas a third-degree burn (also known as a full-thickness burn) is leathery, dry, and insensate. Burn injuries at an intermediate depth of partial thickness are more difficult to assess. They are divided into superficial and deep partial-thickness wounds and may appear very similar on physical examination. They are erythematous, moist, and painful. Evaluation of wounds is complicated by the fact that they evolve over time. The importance of differentiating depth of injury is that a superficial partial-thickness burn will reepithelialize in 2 weeks, whereas deeper wounds need skin grafting to avoid scarring. Except for small SA wounds, full-thickness wounds should be either excised and closed primarily or grafted with the patient's skin.

TABLE 9.1

Distribution of Body Surface Area by Age as Percentage of Total Body Surface Area

■ AREA	■ AGE IN YEARS 0–1	1–4	5–9	10–14	15
Head	19	17	13	11	9
Neck	2	2	2	2	2
Anterior trunk	13	13	13	13	13
Posterior trunk	13	13	13	13	13
Each buttock	2.5	2.5	2.5	2.5	2.5
Genitalia	1	1	1	1	1
Each upper arm	4	4	4	4	4
Each lower arm	3	3	3	3	3
Each hand	2.5	2.5	2.5	2.5	2.5
Each thigh	5.5	6.5	8	8.5	9
Each leg	5	5	5.5	6	6.5
Each foot	3.5	3.5	3.5	3.5	3.5

Types of Injury

The depth of the injury in burns caused by scalding, flame, or contact with a hot object is directly related to the temperature, duration of exposure, and thickness of the tissue. Three zones of injury have been identified in burn-injured skin. The outer *zone of coagulative necrosis* includes necrotic tissue that is irreversibly damaged by heat or chemical. Below that is the *zone of stasis* in which some viable tissue remains if it is protected from ongoing damage. Care must be taken to avoid aggressive debridement and harsh cleansing agents. Compromised cardiac output due to inadequate resuscitation can increase depth of injury. The third zone is the *zone of hyperemia*, characterized by increased blood flow and local inflammatory response to the injury.

Chemical burns cause denaturation of proteins and disruption of cellular integrity. The degree of injury is dependent on the time of exposure, the strength of the agent, and the solubility of the agent in tissue. Alkaline agents penetrate deeper into tissues than do acids (an exception is hydrofluoric acid, which readily penetrates lipid membranes).

Electrical injury accounts for 2%–3% of pediatric burns seen in the emergency department. Electrical injury can occur from direct contact or by an arc (e.g., lightning strike). Direct contact causes damage at the entry, exit, and along the path of the current. Arcs associated with high voltage can be extremely hot and cause deep thermal burns at the entrance site as well as current injury along the path. Electricity occurs in two forms: alternating current (AC), where the current flows back and forth, and direct current (DC), where flow is in one direction. Battery power and lightning are examples of DC. AC is more dangerous at a given voltage because tetanic muscular contraction prevents the victim from letting go and prolongs contact.

Tissue necrosis caused by electrical injury comes from the conversion of current to thermal energy as it passes through tissues. Indirect injury occurs if muscle contractions cause the victim to suffer a fall, arrhythmia, asphyxia, or spinal cord injury. When resistance is high, there is greater tissue damage. The resistance of wet skin is almost zero, and more damage occurs to internal organs and less to the skin. Bone and tendon have high resistance and can lead to more injury at joints. Current passing in the region of the heart, even at low voltage, can cause arrhythmia and death. In high-voltage injury, aggressive evaluation for rhabdomyolysis or compartment syndromes due to muscle necrosis is necessary to avoid additional tissue loss. Excision of dead muscle or early surgical decompression may be needed.

Lightning has an extremely high DC current (more than 1 million volts). This energy is transformed into an arc of current, releasing light and extreme heat. Eyes and ears may be points of entry or damaged by blast effect, with frequent ruptured tympanic membranes. Transient autonomic disturbances may cause fixed and dilated pupils and unconsciousness or even asystole. Late sequelae of electrical injury include the development of cataracts and transverse myelitis of the spinal cord.

In any electrical injury, the surface injury is often not indicative of the extent of injury to subcutaneous tissues, muscle, and bone. If current passes through the torso, visceral organ injury may result, including the pancreas and gastrointestinal tract. Patients who contact a low-voltage (<1000 V) source may be cared for as an outpatient if they have no electrocardiographic abnormalities and no loss of consciousness. Patients who contact high-voltage sources should be admitted and placed on cardiac monitoring. Creatine kinase levels, including the MB subunit, do not reliably indicate the extent of myocardial injury.

RESUSCITATION

General Principles

Peripheral venous cannulation is preferred over central access and may be performed through burn-injured tissue if access through noninjured sites is not available. Children with >10% total body surface area (TBSA) injury require IV fluid resuscitation and should have a urinary catheter. During transport and resuscitation, body temperature should be maintained. Patients should be wrapped in clean sheets or blankets and the room and resuscitation fluids warmed.

Fluid Resuscitation

Burn injury leads to intravascular volume depletion because fluid is lost into burn-injured tissue, through the wound, and into noninjured tissue. Formulas have been developed to provide an estimate of crystalloid requirement. Myocardial depression also occurs in the first 24–36 hours after injury. Assessment of the patient's response to resuscitation should be used (not the formula) to determine fluid administration. The adequacy of resuscitation in burn injury is based on urine output as a marker of tissue perfusion. Fluids are titrated to maintain hourly urine output of 1 mL/kg/hour in the infant and young child and 0.5 mL/kg/hour in the child >12 years of age or >50 kg in weight. Urine output above these goals should motivate the clinician to decrease resuscitation fluid volumes. The crystalloid-based Parkland formula is most commonly used to estimate initial fluid requirements. This formula calls for the initiation of resuscitation with lactated Ringer solution at a rate based on the BSA of burn injury and the patient's body weight. The resuscitation volume for the first 24 hours is

$$\text{Resuscitation } (4 \text{ mL} \times \text{weight in kg} \times \%\text{BSA burn}) + \text{Maintenance}$$

Maintenance fluid for children who weigh <40 kg is 5% dextrose in lactated Ringer solution and should be estimated as daily requirements of 100 mL/kg for the first 10 kg, plus 50 mL/kg for the second 10 kg, and plus 20 mL/kg above 20-kg body weight (hourly fluid requirements of 4 mL/kg/h for 0–10 kg, plus 2 mL/kg/h for the next 10kg, and plus 1mL/kg/h for >20kg). For children who weigh >40 kg and adults, maintenance fluids are not included in the estimate of fluid requirements. Half of the resuscitation volume is given in the first 8 hours after injury, and the other half is given in the following 16 hours. Excessive volume resuscitation has been associated with pulmonary edema in patients with inhalation injury and increased subeschar pressures in the extremities and the abdomen that can lead to compartment syndrome.

After the first 24 hours, fluids are given to meet maintenance requirements and to replace ongoing losses. The hourly evaporative fluid loss from the patient's wounds can be estimated as:

$$(25 \text{ mL} + \% \text{ BSA burn}) \times \text{total BSA}$$

Evaporative losses are primarily free water. However, to avoid rapid changes in sodium concentration in children, this loss is replaced with a salt-containing solution, such as 5% dextrose in 0.2% normal saline. Protein replacement with 5% albumin may also be necessary if a burn injury exceeds 40% BSA.

Inhalation Injury

Inhalation injury can cause upper airway direct thermal burn, chemical pneumonitis from products of combustion, and systemic poisoning from inhalation of cyanide and carbon monoxide. The decision to intubate a burn victim is straightforward if the victim is unconscious or has stridor. More commonly, a stable patient presents with soot on the face and in the mouth. In this case, a history of having been trapped in a space with smoke, and findings such as a change in voice, hoarseness, or increased work of breathing suggest that the airway may become compromised.

Pulmonary parenchymal pathology evolves following inhalation injury with a peak at 3–5 days. Timing depends upon the combustibles present in the fire. Burning plastics produce cyanide gas and carbon monoxide, leading to systemic poisoning. Pneumonitis is caused by inhaled chemicals deposited in the airways. Bronchoscopy may reveal erythema and edema of the airway, blistering, ulceration, erosions, and sloughing of the mucosa. Casts can form, leading to obstruction of terminal bronchioles. Increases in pulmonary lymph flow and microvascular permeability lead to pulmonary edema. Mucociliary dysfunction impairs airway clearance. Patients may deteriorate days after the injury and require intubation and mechanical ventilation. The incidence of pneumonia after inhalation injury is as high as 70% within a week of injury.

Management of Inhalation Injury

Therapy for inhalation injury consists of aggressive pulmonary toilet, mucolytics, early detection and treatment of infection, and supportive care. *N*-acetylcysteine and nebulized heparin have been used for smoke inhalation treatment in adults. Antibiotic prophylaxis and corticosteroids are not indicated. Frequent therapeutic bronchoscopy may facilitate removal of bronchial casts.

Approximately 12% of pediatric burn center patients require intubation, with the majority having sustained inhalation injury. Cuffed endotracheal tubes and lung-protective ventilator strategies should be employed in patients at risk for acute lung injury. High-frequency oscillatory ventilation has been used as a rescue therapy, and high-frequency percussive ventilation has been used for secretion clearance in adult case series. Early tracheostomy should be considered in children with severe burns for whom a prolonged course of mechanical ventilation is anticipated.

Blood sampling for carbon monoxide (CO) should be performed on admission. Treatment for CO poisoning begins with the administration of 100% oxygen. The existing evidence is insufficient to mandate the use of hyperbaric oxygen (HBO) for CO poisoning, although suggested indications for HBO include loss of consciousness, ischemic cardiac changes, neurologic deficits, significant metabolic acidosis, or COHb level >25%. In situations when the patient must be transferred to receive HBO therapy, the risk to an unstable patient needs to be considered. The goal of treatment is to minimize neurologic deficits from CO poisoning.

Cyanide poisoning can occur with inhalation of toxins from burning plastics. Cyanide gas can be rapidly fatal so first responders now carry cyanide antidote kits. Cyanide causes metabolic acidosis with high central venous oxygen saturation. Hydroxocobalamin (a precursor to vitamin B_{12}) is administered IV. Cyanide has a greater affinity for cobalamin than cytochrome oxidase, and cyanocobalamin is eliminated in the urine (which becomes dark purple or red). Cyanide antidotes that produce methemoglobin (amyl nitrite or sodium nitrite) may increase CO toxicity and should be avoided until it is determined that CO is not present in the blood.

Patients with burns >30% of their BSA, with injury of critical body parts, or with significant preexisting disease should be cared for in a burn center. A great strength of specialized burn centers is the significant nursing expertise in wound care. A collaborative decision should be made regarding the best location for the care of young children if advanced pediatric expertise is not available at the same center. Active participation by child life therapists as well as child psychiatrists often helps patients cope with their injuries and treatments and should yield the best psychological outcome.

Neglect and Abuse

The incidence of child abuse is as high as 16% of children admitted to burn centers. Most nonaccidental injuries occur between 2 and 4 years of age. A history that is inconsistent with the physical exam or conflicting histories are sufficient reasons to launch a deeper investigation. Well-defined lines of demarcation between burned and unburned skin in a scald burn and the absence of splash burns are suggestive of intentional injury. However, splash burns can also be seen in intentional scald-burning cases. In addition, sparing of areas of skin may be suggestive of an intentional injury, particularly when the extremity is held in flexion and the area around the joint is protected and spared. Contact burns present with well-defined margins; the object that caused the injury can be determined by the outline of the wound. All states require the reporting of suspected neglect and/or abuse of children.

WOUND CARE

General Principles

The objective of wound care is to avoid infection and protect from further injury. Small (<2 cm) blisters are left intact, whereas larger blisters and full-thickness wounds are debrided and covered with a topical agent. Debridement is painful and may require deep sedation or general anesthesia. Even without debridement, burns are painful, and patients usually require opioid analgesia.

Sterile gloves should be worn at all times when the wound is manipulated. Chemical injury of tissue is treated with irrigation with copious amounts of either normal saline or tap water for as long as 6 hours. Neutralizing agents are not used because they can lead to additional tissue damage from heat generated in an exothermic reaction. Hydrofluoric acid injuries can lead to systemic hypocalcemia and be rapidly fatal; topical calcium gluconate gel can be used.

Prophylaxis against Wound Infection

Systemic antimicrobials are not used unless wound infection is apparent. Topical antimicrobial agents have substantially reduced the mortality associated with burn-wound infection. Common topical agents are listed in **Table 9.2**. Silver sulfadiazine is the agent most commonly used. Mafenide acetate penetrates the wound well and is used for therapy of burn-wound infection. Silver-containing dressings can decrease the frequency of dressing changes. Silver sulfadiazine is not used in infants <2 months of age or pregnant patients, due to an association with kernicterus.

Surgical Care

First-degree burns heal without a scar. Third-degree burns require surgery for wound closure unless they are very small. Second-degree burns include deep and superficial burns with varying degrees of healing potential. The closure of the wound, function, and cosmetic result are considered in the decision regarding surgery. Therapy for closure of a significant excised wound requires the use of an autograft. The preferred skin graft in children is a split-thickness autograft. A full-thickness graft is preferred for cosmetic reconstruction and areas where scarring leads to functional compromise, but may require that the donor site be grafted. Autograft can be enlarged up to four to six times the SA of the original donor skin by passing it through a meshing device.

Allograft may also be used as a test graft in areas where infection is of concern or when the adequacy of the excised wound bed is suspect. Skin substitutes have been developed that replace the function of some or all layers of the skin. Immediate application of other products (pigskin or a commercially available synthetic membrane) on a partial-thickness wound moderates pain and eliminates the need to change dressings.

Circumferential burns can compromise blood flow to other viable tissue. The threshold for performing an escharotomy to release subeschar pressure should be low. A "compartment syndrome" can occur in the chest or abdomen in patients with circumferential full-thickness burns in these areas. Escharotomy of the chest will often decrease the inspiratory pressures required to maintain tidal volume. Abdominal compartment syndrome may be relieved by escharotomy, drainage of peritoneal fluid, or decompressive laparotomy.

TABLE 9.2

Topical Antimicrobial Agents for Treatment of Burn Injury by Type

TYPE	APPLICATION	ADVANTAGES	DISADVANTAGES
Ointment			
Bacitracin	Second-degree burns, small areas	Not water soluble, good on face	Not indicated for large surface area
Cream			
Silver sulfadiazine	Second- and third-degree burns	Soothing, good for range of motion	Possible neutropenia; little penetration
Mafenide acetate	Second- and third-degree burns	Penetrates eschar	Painful, metabolic acidosis
Solution			
Aqueous silver nitrate (0.5%)	Second- and third-degree burns	Good antimicrobial	Hyponatremia, stains wound, little penetration
Mafenide acetate (5%)	Graft dressing, open wound soak	Broad activity, moist dressing	Not used for unexcised wound
Impregnated Dressing			
Acticoat	Second-degree burns	Dressing change every 3 days	Only second-degree burns
Aquacel Ag	Second-degree burns	Leave on for 21 days	Less flexibility and ease of motion; only second-degree burns

INFECTION

The systemic inflammatory response associated with major burns can be difficult to distinguish from infection. Yet, the incidence of actual infection is higher in burn-injured children compared to other critically ill children. Four categories of wound-related infection have been proposed. *Impetigo* "involves the loss of epithelium from a previously reepithelialized surface such as a grafted burn, a partial-thickness burn allowed to heal by secondary intention, or a healed donor site". Also called "melting graft syndrome," it is not necessarily associated with systemic signs of infection, fever, or an elevated white blood cell count. The cause is usually streptococcal or staphylococcal. Treatment consists of local care and systemic antibiotics. *Open surgical wound infections* are associated with a surgical intervention that has not healed. These infections usually require the addition of a topical antimicrobial agent, more frequent dressing changes, and the administration of systemic antibiotics. Burn-associated *cellulitis* presents as erythema and edema. It must be differentiated from the normal local inflammatory response. The definition requires at least one of the following: (a) localized pain, tenderness, swelling, or warmth; (b) systemic signs of infection, such as hyperemia, leukocytosis, or septicemia; (c) progression of erythema and swelling; or (d) signs of lymphangitis, lymphadenitis, or both. Systemic antibiotics are required. The diagnosis of *invasive infection* of a burn wound rests on the recognition of changes in the wound (black, purple, or reddish discoloration; maceration; or early separation of eschar) and systemic manifestations of infection. Biopsy may be performed for quantitative culture or histologic evaluation. Invasive wound infection requires surgical excision of the wound to the level of viable tissue and administration of systemic antibiotics. Non–wound-related infections seen in burn patients include pneumonia, suppurative thrombophlebitis, chondritis (e.g., the cartilage of the ear), sinusitis, urinary tract infections, sinusitis, bacteremia, and endocarditis.

HYPERMETABOLISM AND NUTRITION

The classical metabolic response to injury includes an early ebb phase characterized by low cardiac output and decreased metabolic rate followed by a hypermetabolic phase that begins 24–36 hours later. This increased catabolic state can persist for 9–12 months. Early and aggressive nutritional support reduces the elevated resting energy expenditure (REE) in burn victims. Measurement of REE by indirect calorimetry is the best way to estimate caloric needs in children during the hypermetabolic phase.

The enteral route is the preferred route for nutrition. In addition to vitamin A, other vitamins, minerals, and trace elements may be required in excess of recommended daily allowances, including calcium, magnesium, vitamin D, zinc, copper, and other micronutrients. Attempts have been made to pharmacologically mitigate the persistent hypermetabolic state that follows burn injury. The hypermetabolism can be blunted by β-blockade, leading to the use of propranolol in children. Muscle wasting, decreased bone mineralization, and retarded linear growth can be profound. Recombinant human growth hormone and testosterone are treatments with little benefit demonstrated and concern about side effects. A synthetic testosterone analog, oxandrolone, may show some benefits but is not yet considered to be standard care.

Hypoalbuminemia is associated with edema, particularly of the pulmonary interstitium and bowel wall. Albumin is often administered to avoid exacerbating acute lung injury, diarrhea, feeding intolerance, and impaired wound healing. The use of albumin in burn patients and in those with critical illness has been extensively studied, with great variability in results.

OUTCOME

Patient age and extent of injury are the two most powerful predictors of outcome. The mortality for a severe burn injury of 60%–69.9% TBSA is 50% in the newborn to 1.9-year-old group, 22.6% in those between 2 and 4.9 years of age, and 18.3% in those between 5 and 19.9 years of age. Mortality rate increases as much as 20% when inhalation injury accompanies thermal injury.

Improvement in medical care resulting in increased survival has led to a renewed emphasis on quality of life after thermal injuries. Splinting of injured extremities begins as soon as the patient is stabilized, and range-of-motion exercises begin within the first 24 hours. As soon as wounds have a stable epidermal closure, attention is turned to wound and scar management. Garments that apply pressure to the wounds are tailor-made for the patient and worn 24 hours per day. The development of cicatrix can best be modulated when the wound is immature and actively remodeling. This period may extend up to a year postinjury, but mechanical intervention is of little benefit beyond that time. Surgical intervention for cosmetic deformity is usually delayed until the wound is mature, as is intervention for functional restriction, unless necessary to allow for physical therapy.

CHAPTER 10 ■ INJURY FROM CHEMICAL, BIOLOGIC, RADIOLOGIC, AND NUCLEAR AGENTS

PETER SILVER, F. MERIDITH SONNETT, AND GEORGE L. FOLTIN

The use of chemical, biologic, radiologic, or nuclear (CBRN) agents to deliberately harm civilians can challenge healthcare systems beyond their capacity to provide treatment.

CHEMICAL AGENTS

Chemical agents include nerve agents, asphyxiants, choking (pulmonary) agents, and vesicant (blistering) agents. These chemical terrorism agents often originate from military, industrial, or medical sources.

Initial Approach to Chemical Attack

The single most important step for treating chemical exposures is decontamination. Rapid removal of patient clothing can eliminate ~90% of contaminants. After the clothing is put in sealed bags, the patient's skin and eyes may require decontamination. In most cases, decontamination of skin can be achieved by washing with water and soap, ideally at the scene.

Nerve Agents

Pathophysiology

The nerve agents include Sarin, Soman, Tabun, and Venom X (VX). They are organophosphate compounds that inhibit acetylcholinesterase and cause cholinergic crisis. These agents are usually colorless, odorless, tasteless, and nonirritating to the skin. Nerve agent vapors are denser than air and accumulate in low-lying areas, putting children at risk for higher exposure. Exposure can result from inhalational, dermal, or gastrointestinal absorption.

Clinical Signs and Symptoms

Symptoms include muscarinic and nicotinic effects. Muscarinic effects involve multiple organ systems, respiratory (shortness of breath, rhinorrhea, bronchorrhea, bronchospasm), cardiovascular (bradycardia, arrhythmias), gastrointestinal (salivation, nausea, vomiting, diarrhea, abdominal cramping), ophthalmologic (miosis, lacrimation), and genitourinary (incontinence). Nicotinic effects involve muscle fasciculations progressing to weakness or flaccid paralysis. Sympathetic effects include tachycardia and hypertension. Central nervous system (CNS) symptoms include altered consciousness ranging from agitation or lethargy to coma and seizures. Severe exposure produces unconsciousness, convulsions, apnea, or flaccid paralysis.

Management

Emergent treatment of nerve agent toxicity is described in **Table 10.1**. Initial treatment includes administration of atropine followed by *pralidoxime* (2-PAM, 2-pyridine aldoxime methyl chloride) and benzodiazepines. The first dose of atropine should be given IM to delay peak blood level in hypoxic patients because ventricular fibrillation is seen with IV administration in animal models. Adult nerve gas survivors have required up to 20 mg of atropine in the first 24 hours, along with frequent doses or a continuous infusion of pralidoxime. Survivors may need atropine for several days. Benzodiazepines are effective for nerve agent–induced seizure activity. Topical cycloplegics may reduce nerve agent–induced ocular pain.

Asphyxiants

Pathophysiology

Asphyxiants are toxic compounds that inhibit cytochrome oxidase and mitochondrial oxidative metabolism, which causes cellular anoxia and lactic acidosis. Hydrogen cyanide is the most common toxin in this class. Cyanide is a colorless liquid or gas that smells like bitter almonds. Cyanide is also a direct neurotoxin contributing to excitatory brain injury. Cyanide's efficacy as a weapon of chemical terrorism is limited by its volatility in open air and lower lethality than nerve agents. If released in closed, crowded quarters, the effects would be severe.

Clinical Signs and Symptoms

Early findings include tachypnea, hyperpnea, tachycardia, flushing, dizziness, headache, and diaphoresis. Symptoms associated with exposures to high concentrations include rapid onset of tachypnea and hyperpnea (15 seconds), followed by seizures (30 seconds), coma and apnea (2–4 minutes), and cardiac arrest (4–8 minutes). Classical signs of cyanide poisoning include severe dyspnea without cyanosis (cherry-red skin from a lack of peripheral oxygen use), and a bitter almond odor to the breath and body fluids. Laboratory findings include an anion-gap acidosis, increased lactate, and high mixed venous oxygen saturation. Blood cyanide levels can be determined but usually not on an emergent basis.

Management

Initial management includes removal of the victim from the contaminated environment, administration of 100% oxygen, correction of acidosis with sodium bicarbonate, and seizure control with benzodiazepines. Antidotal therapy is a multiple-step process (**Table 10.1**). First, inhaled amyl nitrite and IV sodium nitrite are given to form methemoglobin. Methemoglobin has a high affinity for cyanide, and forms cyanomethemoglobin, which helps restore cellular respiration. The second step is to administer IV sodium thiosulfate, which provides substrate for conversion of cyanide to thiocyanate, which is eliminated in the urine. Nitrite administration should be done carefully, as it may cause hypotension or produce excess methemoglobin that may compromise oxygen-carrying capacity. IV hydroxocobalamin is an alternative antidote. It should not be given in the same IV line as thiosulfate.

TABLE 10.1

Findings and Management of Specific Chemical Agents

AGENT	FINDINGS	TREATMENT
Nerve agents Sarin Soman Tabun VX	Rhinorrhea Bronchorrhea Eye pain Bronchospasm Apnea Respiratory muscle paralysis Unconsciousness Convulsions	Airway, breathing, circulation support, 100% oxygen Atropine IM (autoinjector) or IV, every 2–5 min for secretions and respiratory symptoms Then Pralidoxime (2-PAM) IM (autoinjector) or IV Diazepam or midazolam for seizures or if seriously ill[a]
Asphyxiant Cyanide	Cherry-red skin Tachypnea Seizures	Airway, breathing, circulation support, 100% oxygen If conscious No antidote If unconscious Sodium nitrite 3%: 0.12–0.33 mL/kg (max 10 mL) slow IV (minimum 5 min); causes orthostatic hypotension Sodium thiosulfate 25%: 1.65 mL/kg (max 50 mL) IV over 10–20 min Sodium bicarbonate for acidosis after above if unresponsive
Choking agents Chlorine Phosgene	Ear, nose, throat irritation Stridor Bronchospasm Pulmonary edema (esp. phosgene)	Symptomatic care Possible bronchoscopy Aggressive management of pulmonary edema
Blistering/vesicants Sulfur mustard Lewisite	Skin erythema Bullae, ulcers Skin sloughing Ocular inflammation Respiratory tract inflammation Hyperexcitability, seizures	Symptomatic care Burn care Cycloplegics for eyes Possible use of hematopoietic growth factors BAL (dimercaprol, if available) 3 mg/kg IM q4–6h for systemic effects in severe cases

[a]Some authorities recommend seizure prophylaxis with benzodiazepines, while others suggest that use be reserved for treatment of seizures.

IM, intramuscular; IV, intravenous; VX, Venom X; BAL, British anti-Lewisite.

Choking (Pulmonary) Agents

Pathophysiology

Choking agents include chlorine and phosgene, which are gases at room temperature. Millions of tons of these chemicals are produced each year for the textile, paint, and dye industries. These agents may be released during terrorist acts or industrial accidents. Chlorine has a strong, characteristic odor. It acts primarily on the epithelium of the bronchi and larger bronchioles, resulting in necrosis, denudation, and the formation of pseudomembranes. Phosgene has a characteristic odor of "freshly mown hay." Phosgene harms the gas-exchange regions of the respiratory system (bronchioles, alveolar ducts, and alveoli), causing pulmonary edema. Both gases are heavier than air and settle close to the ground, which is significant for small children.

Clinical Signs and Symptoms

Initial symptoms of chlorine poisoning include mucosal irritation of the eyes, nose, and upper airways and a sensation of choking. Greater exposure leads to hoarseness, aphonia, stridor, and bronchospasm. Phosgene toxicity typically presents with coughing and sneezing. Dyspnea and respiratory distress due to pulmonary edema occurs late, after a several-hour period of latency.

Management

After decontamination with copious water irrigation of the eyes and mucosal membranes, management is largely supportive (**Table 10.1**). Corticosteroids may be helpful in patients with bronchospasm or history of asthma. Bronchoscopy may be needed to remove pseudomembranes. Secondary bacterial infection often occurs, but prophylactic antibiotics are not helpful.

Vesicant (Blistering) Agents

Pathophysiology

Vesicants are chemical agents that cause blistering of the skin; they include sulfur mustard and Lewisite. Vesicant exposure is associated with significant and prolonged morbidity. Sulfur mustard is an alkylating agent, highly toxic to rapidly reproducing and poorly differentiated cells (e.g., skin, pulmonary parenchyma, and bone marrow). Its odor resembles garlic or mustard. It is rapidly absorbed by tissue surfaces, and damages cells within minutes. Lewisite is an arsenical compound that affects skin and eyes immediately upon exposure.

Clinical Signs and Symptoms

Skin findings progress from erythema resembling sunburn to yellow blisters, which coalesce into bullae and then ulcers, which may take months to heal (**Table 10.1**). Victims may present with full-thickness skin sloughing. Ocular symptoms include conjunctivitis, corneal ulceration, and globe perforation. Respiratory symptoms range from hoarseness and cough to respiratory failure due to epithelial necrosis and airway obstruction from pseudomembranes. Secondary bacterial pneumonia may occur. All cellular elements of the bone marrow can be affected. Gastrointestinal involvement produces cholinergic activity, mucosal injury, abdominal pain, vomiting, and diarrhea. CNS manifestations include hyperexcitability, convulsions, and coma.

Management

There is no specific antidote for mustard exposure. The most effective treatment is prompt decontamination. Anyone assisting must take proper precautions. Eye treatment includes copious irrigation, cycloplegics for comfort and prevention of synechiae, and topical antibiotics with lubricating agents to prevent adhesions and scarring. Lung involvement often requires positive-pressure ventilation and frequent bronchoscopy. Hematopoietic growth factors may shorten the bone marrow suppression. Treatment for Lewisite is also supportive but includes the specific antidote *British anti-Lewisite* (BAL), also called *Dimercaprol*. This chelating agent should only be administered to victims with shock or significant pulmonary injury.

BIOLOGIC AGENTS (BIOTERRORISM)

Bioterrorism involves the intentional release of bacteria, viruses, or other infectious agents that result in morbidity, mortality, or physical damage to humans, livestock, or crops. Agents include bacteria, *Bacillus anthracis* (anthrax), *Yersinia pestis* (plague), and *Francisella tularensis* (tularemia); viruses, variola (smallpox) and hemorrhagic fevers (Ebola virus and Marburg hemorrhagic fever); and toxins, botulism from *Clostridium botulinum*. Lower mortality agents include brucellosis, *Salmonella*, *Shigella*, ricin toxin, and *Vibrio cholerae*. The ability to differentiate an attack from a natural outbreak can be difficult as symptoms may be delayed for days after exposure. A sudden outbreak of an unusual illness is likely to be the first indication.

Terror-Related Bacterial Agents

Bacillus anthracis (Anthrax)

Pathophysiology. Anthrax is caused by spores from *B. anthracis*, an aerobic gram-positive rod-shaped bacterium. It occurs naturally in soil and often affects domestic and wild animals in developing countries. Spores are easily found in nature, can be produced in the laboratory, are durable, and easily dispersed in powders, sprays, food, or water. *Cutaneous anthrax* occurs after a spore enters the skin through an open laceration or abrasion, and accounts for 95% of anthrax disease in the United States. *Gastrointestinal anthrax* occurs after consumption of food (usually the meat of an animal that died of the disease) contaminated with *B. anthracis* bacilli or spores. *Inhalation anthrax* occurs by breathing airborne spores. Infection in both cutaneous and gastrointestinal anthrax is typically at a low level, with local edema and necrosis. In inhalation anthrax, and advanced cutaneous or gastrointestinal anthrax, spores are phagocytosed by macrophages, transported to regional lymph nodes, and germinate into toxin-producing bacteria causing hemorrhagic lymphadenitis and septicemia. Severe edema, bacteremia, and toxemia can occur.

Clinical Signs and Symptoms. The skin lesions progress from pruritic papules or vesicles into painless, depressed black eschars (necrosis) surrounded by moderate to severe edema. The common symptoms of gastrointestinal anthrax in children are fever, abdominal pain, vomiting, diarrhea, and bloody stools. Inhalational illness is biphasic, an initial nonspecific period involving fever, fatigue, cough, and myalgia followed by a brief improvement, then a fulminant phase with high fever, respiratory failure (pleural effusions, pulmonary hemorrhage), and bacteremia that results in severe edema and shock. Chest radiographs may be notable for pleural effusion (69%) and widened mediastinum (52%). Meningoencephalitis occurs in ~50% of adult cases. Mortality from inhalation anthrax is 40% with treatment (nearly 100% without).

Management. Antimicrobial treatment is with ciprofloxacin or doxycycline. Drainage of pleural effusions and ascites is often indicated. Corticosteroids are used for suspected or confirmed adrenal failure, and may have a role in anthrax meningoencephalitis. Two antitoxin products *raxibacumab* (a humanized monoclonal antibody) and *anthrax immune globulin* (a polyclonal human immunoglobulin) are used in conjunction with antibiotics.

Yersinia pestis (Plague)

Pathophysiology. Plague is caused by the bacterium *Yersinia pestis*. It occurs in three forms. *Bubonic plague* occurs following a bite from a rodent flea or by handling an infected animal with plague. *Septicemic plague* occurs either as the spread of bubonic plague or as the first symptom of plague. *Pneumonic plague* is the most serious form of the disease; it can be the result of hematogenous spread or be caused by aerosolized *Y. pestis* delivery in bioterrorism. It causes a multilobar hemorrhagic and necrotizing bronchopneumonia.

Clinical Signs and Symptoms. In bubonic plague, patients develop fever, headache, weakness, and swollen, tender lymph nodes near a bite from an infected flea. Septicemic plague involves fever, chills, extreme weakness, hemorrhage (including into the skin), and shock. Pneumonic plague presents with fever, cough, purulent sputum, hemoptysis, and desaturation.

Management. *Y. pestis* can be isolated from lymph node aspiration, blood culture, sputum culture, or bronchial washing. Polymerase chain reaction (PCR) testing is available. Treatment should not be delayed for testing. Gentamicin or streptomycin is equally effective. Alternatives are tetracycline, doxycycline, chloramphenicol, and ciprofloxacin.

Francisella tularensis (Tularemia)

Pathophysiology. *F. tularensis* is a highly virulent, small, nonmotile, aerobic, gram-negative bacillus. It multiplies within macrophages, allowing it to invade the lymph nodes, lungs, pleura, spleen, and liver. Humans are infected via tick bite, deer fly bite, skin contact with infected animals (rodents, rabbits), or inhalation of contaminated dusts or aerosols. The forms of tularemia include ulceroglandular (most common), glandular, oculoglandular, oropharyngeal, and pneumonic. *Pneumonic tularemia* is the most severe and results either from direct inhalation or from hematogenous spread from other sites.

Clinical Signs and Symptoms. Patients develop fever, chills, headache, and atypical pneumonia 1 to 14 days postexposure and hilar adenopathy on chest radiograph. In *ulceroglandular tularemia*, there is a skin ulcer at the point of contact, with swelling of regional lymph nodes. After inhalational exposure, hemorrhagic airway inflammation develops and progresses to necrotizing pneumonia. Pleural disease is common. Bacteremia is also common, particularly early.

Management. Streptomycin or gentamicin is recommended, and doxycycline is an alternative. Isolation is not required.

Terror-Related Viral Agents

Variola Virus (Smallpox)

Pathophysiology. Smallpox is caused by Variola virus. The last natural case occurred in 1977 and routine vaccination is no longer performed. Smallpox still exists in laboratory stockpiles, and is a potential bioterrorism agent. Smallpox is spread by contact with infected body fluids, respiratory secretions, contaminated objects, or face-to-face contact with an infected individual. Macrophages are infected first; the virus then migrates along the lymphatics and multiplies in lymph nodes. Infected macrophages migrate into the epidermis, with subsequent edema and necrosis. Polymorphonuclear leukocytes migrate into these areas, forming pustules.

Clinical Signs and Symptoms. Historically, mortality rates in unimmunized patients were as high as 30%, and occurred from multiorgan failure secondary to overwhelming viremia.

Management. Care is generally supportive. Dehydration and electrolyte abnormalities may occur. Bacterial superinfections should be treated with antibiotics. The antiviral agents ribavirin and cidofovir experimentally inhibit viral replication, but their effect in humans is unknown. Vaccination within 72–96 hours of exposure provides protection against fatal disease. Patients with smallpox should be cared for in a negative-pressure environment, utilizing both airborne and contact precautions. Ideally, only staff previously vaccinated should care for victims.

Viral Hemorrhagic Fevers

Pathophysiology. Viral hemorrhagic fevers are caused by a variety of agents, most notably Ebola and Marburg viruses, both members of the filovirus family. Spread occurs rapidly, through direct contact with blood, body fluids, and contaminated objects.

Clinical Signs and Symptoms. After an incubation of 2–21 days (shorter for Marburg virus), patients develop fever, severe headache, and muscle ache. Gastrointestinal symptoms include abdominal pain, vomiting, and voluminous diarrhea. The clinical course can progress to massive hemorrhage, shock, and multiorgan dysfunction. Diagnosis can be made by antigen-capture enzyme-linked immunosorbent assay (ELISA), PCR, or IgM-capture ELISA.

Management. Treatment includes aggressive rehydration, replacement of potassium and calcium from gastrointestinal loss, and administration of blood products as needed. An experimental monoclonal antibody (ZMapp, Mapp Pharmaceutical, San Diego, CA) has been used for Ebola. Disease can spread quickly within a healthcare setting. The care for these patients should include the use of dedicated medical equipment (disposable), proper sterilization of nondisposable equipment, personal protective equipment, and isolation. Mortality is 40%–90%. Aggressive fluid and electrolyte replacement is associated with a better outcome.

Terror-Related Toxin-Mediated Disease

Pathophysiology

Botulism is a neuroparalytic illness caused by the toxin produced by *Clostridium botulinum* (found ubiquitously in soil and water). Natural forms of botulism include foodborne, infantile, and wound botulism. *Inhalational botulism* does not occur naturally. Botulinum toxin inhibits acetylcholine release, leading to weakness, aspiration, respiratory failure, and death.

Clinical Signs and Symptoms

Patients present with symmetrical cranial neuropathy, and progress to descending weakness, respiratory failure, and flaccid paralysis. Inhibition of acetylcholine release at parasympathetic terminals leads to autonomic signs and symptoms. Mental status and sensation remain intact.

Management

Therapy is supportive. Bedside pulmonary function testing is used to assess the need for mechanical ventilation. Botulinum antitoxin can arrest the progression of paralysis, but it is best used early as it neutralizes only molecules still unbound to nerve endings. Antitoxin is an equine product and has a risk of serum sickness; skin testing and possible desensitization are necessary. Complete recovery of muscle function may take as long as 3–6 months.

RADIOLOGIC AND NUCLEAR AGENTS

Radiologic terrorism could include detonation of nuclear weapons, conventional explosives to deploy radioactive materials (dirty bomb), or placement of a radioactive source (nuclear waste material) in a public location. Immediate morbidity and mortality result from explosive force. *Acute radiation syndrome*, or *radiation sickness*, can occur in survivors. Nuclear power reactors cannot detonate like a nuclear bomb (reactor fuel does not contain the highly enriched uranium needed for detonation), and so the primary hazard of a nuclear power plant attack would be downwind exposure of radioactive iodine gas.

Decontamination

Unlike scenarios described previously, decontamination of radiologic victims is less time sensitive. Life-threatening conditions should be treated before decontamination. Also, a patient exposed to radioactive material and alive upon arrival at the hospital is unlikely to be sufficiently contaminated to harm healthcare workers. After stabilization, the patient can be disrobed and washed with soap and water; runoff and the discarded clothes should be contained and disposed of following hazardous waste guidelines. The eyes may then be flushed. Care should be taken not to irritate or abrade the skin. Washings should continue until the patient's radiation level is no more than twice the background level. Standard precautions are the only measures required for healthcare workers who do not come into direct contact with radioactive dust or debris.

Pathophysiology

Acute radiation syndrome is most likely to occur in those who were exposed to a nuclear detonation but were far enough away to survive the blast. A radiologic dispersal device is much less likely to cause acute radiation syndrome. Military, industrial, and medical exposures can also lead to acute radiation syndrome. Cells with active mitoses are very radiosensitive and include spermatogonia, lymphocytes, erythroblasts, other hematopoietic cells, and cells of the gastrointestinal tract. Muscle, bone, and collagen-producing cells are less sensitive.

Clinical Signs and Symptoms

Victims of radiation exposure follow a course with four clinical stages: prodromal, latent, manifest illness, and recovery. In the *prodromal stage*, nausea and vomiting predominate, with the nonspecific signs and symptoms of fever, headache, abdominal cramping, and skin erythema. In the *latent stage*, the patient experiences apparent improvement (hours to weeks). During the *manifest illness stage*, patients suffer hematopoietic system loss that causes hemorrhage and sepsis. Gastrointestinal effects include mucosal sloughing, hemorrhage, obstruction, and sepsis. Radiation pneumonitis can occur. High doses of radiation cause microvascular injury of the CNS leading to cerebral edema, increased intracranial pressure, and intractable seizures. The fourth stage is the *recovery stage*, which can last weeks to years.

Treatment

Life-threatening injuries should be treated before decontamination occurs. Removal of external contamination, dose estimation, supportive care, symptomatic treatment, and replacement of fluid and electrolytes should be the goals of early medical management. As patients become neutropenic, hematopoietic growth factors should be administered. Health physicists and/or nuclear medicine physicians may help to determine the specific exposure and prognosis. Specific antidotes are unlikely to be helpful in the critical care environment (some victims will have been given potassium iodide to avoid the carcinogenic effects of radioactive iodine, which could be released in a nuclear power plant incident).

CHAPTER 11 ■ MASS CASUALTY EVENTS

MARIA C. ESPERANZA

Globally, natural disasters affected 211 million people and there were 54,000 terrorist-related casualties in 2008. During mass casualty events (MCEs), local health systems may be overwhelmed, requiring redistribution of casualties and request for external assistance. The best response is provided by a collaboration and resource sharing among hospitals.

BACKGROUND

MCEs affect at least 10 patients and 3–4 severely wounded patients can arrive at the same hospital, exceeding therapeutic capacity and requiring external assistance. Local infrastructure such as roads or hospitals may be destroyed. Events may cause large population movements and overwhelm healthcare resources. Much of the emergency response to MCEs is directed toward the management of trauma-related injuries, but providers must also be ready to deal with environmental effects (hypothermia, heat stroke, electrolyte imbalance, dehydration, and infections) and psychological stress. Pediatrics has not been viewed as a separate population but does require separate study and planning (**Table 11.1**).

THE STATE OF PEDIATRIC EMERGENCY PREPAREDNESS

Children (<17 years) represent 8%–30% of MCE victims. The distribution of knowledge, logistics, and infrastructure support for pediatric healthcare

TABLE 11.1

Pediatric-Specific Vulnerabilities during Mass Casualty Events

Increased susceptibility to effects of exposure to terrorism-related agents	Increased respiratory exposure	Higher minute ventilation Located closer to the ground
	Increased dermal exposure	Thinner, more permeable skin, less fat Larger BSA/mass ratio
	More virulent disease manifestations from infectious agents	Immature immune system
	Less capable of escaping attack and taking appropriate protective actions	Motor and cognitive immaturity Dependence on caregivers
More susceptible to development of secondary medical problems	Increased risk of dehydration due to toxin-induced vomiting and diarrhea	Decreased intravascular volume Larger BSA/mass ratio May be dependent on caregivers for access to fluids
	Increased risk of hypothermia	Larger BSA/mass ratio Immature temperature regulation in infants
	Increased incidence of multiple organ injury	Thoracic cage less developed Small size with more force applied per unit body area Less fat protecting internal organs
	Increased incidence of head injury	Larger head-to-body ratio Thinner calvarium
	Increased fractures	Incomplete ossification of skeletal system Smaller body mass
	Increased mental health needs	Separation from primary caregiver (need for reunification) Developmental immaturity

Adapted from Henretig FM, Ciesiak TJ, Eitzen EM Jr. Biologic and chemical terrorism. *J Pediatr* 2002;141:311–26.

delivery is highly variable. In 2012, only 17 states had plans for four key components of the pediatric disaster response: evacuation/relocation, family and child reunification, children with special needs, and a K-12 multiple-disaster plan. Five states had not met any of the standards. Only 19% of emergency medical service (EMS) agencies utilize pediatric triage protocols, and the majority do not address MCEs at schools or have accommodations for people with special healthcare needs. Availability of pediatric equipment on ambulances is also poor. Most hospitals do not have a pediatric intensive care unit (PICU) or pediatric trauma service, opting instead to transfer patients requiring specialized care. Only 5% of emergency departments (EDs) have all recommended pediatric supplies. In an MCE, all hospitals must be prepared to receive and stabilize critically injured children before a secondary interfacility transport for definitive care. Many hospitals will need to provide a level of care beyond what they would normally provide.

PEDIATRIC DISASTER TRIAGE

A finite amount of resources dictates that care is provided to patients with survivable injuries. A high rate of *undertriage* (underestimation of the severity of injuries) will lead to missed injuries and avoidable deaths. MCE response favors *overtriage* (overestimation of the severity of injuries) in order not to miss potentially salvageable patients. However, high overtriage rates will flood hospitals with patients who could have received delayed care. Acceptable undertriage and overtriage rates by the American College of Surgeons are 5%–10% and 30%–50%, respectively.

The Simple Treatment and Rapid Transport (START) protocol is a commonly used triage tool and includes an assessment of mobility, frequency of respirations, presence of a palpable pulse, and the ability to follow commands. Patients are classified into four categories on the basis of their needs for advanced care: deceased or expected to die from incident (black), immediate (red), delayed (yellow), or ambulatory (green). The Sacco triage method (a computer model) orders patients on the basis of their probability of survival, potential for deterioration, and available resources. When applied to pediatric data, it shows high reliability in predicting mortality. No evidence supports the use of any one triage tool.

The performance of secondary triage in the field through the Secondary Assessment of Victim Endpoint (SAVE) methodology establishes the order with which patients receive care at the hospital, or in the setting of delayed transport, at the scene. It is most effective in MCEs where treatment occurs under less than ideal conditions. Pediatric-specific triage tools such as JumpSTART (for 1–8 years of age) and Pediatric Triage Tape (PTT) are modifications to adult triage tools using pediatric vital sign ranges. The Care Flight triage tool uses qualitative observations with no vital sign measurements rendering it amenable to pediatric use. None of the tools have been field-tested, and all show poor sensitivity for detecting critically ill children.

HOSPITAL RESPONSE TO MASS CASUALTY EVENTS

The type and magnitude of MCE response are affected by the nature of the precipitating event; location, date, and time of event; weather patterns; and population density. Disaster plans must address the aspects of response that are common to all types of MCEs (e.g., evacuation plans, allocation of supplies and personnel, etc.).

Surge Response

MCEs can be "big bang" events that occur suddenly (e.g., earthquakes, transport accidents, or terrorist bombing) or "rising tide" events that develop slowly (e.g., pandemics or flooding). In "big bang" MCEs, most casualties occur at the time of the event and the number remains relatively constant. In rising tide events, the number of victims gradually increases at an unknown rate and for an undetermined duration. Big bang events immediately overwhelm health systems, and disaster planning involves this type of scenario. The first wave is a sudden influx (50% within the first hour) of patients who self-triage and have minor injuries. The second wave is more critically injured patients. They arrive within 15 minutes of the beginning of the event, and within 90 minutes, 80% of casualties will arrive. The final phase consists of patients with minor injuries and emotional stress and may last days.

Pediatric victims from MCEs have a high overtriage rate, with 4% requiring PICU admission. Mechanical ventilation is needed for 75% of the PICU admissions. The high acuity of admitted survivors makes PICU surge capacity an integral part of MCE response. Upon notification of an MCE, the PICU should plan for a 300% increase in bed capacity. Satellite critical care units may be established in postanesthesia care units, intermediate care units, large procedure suites, telemetry units, or hospital wards. Some hospitals may have to increase critical care surge capacity above 300% if ICU beds for their catchment area are inadequate at baseline. Interfacility transfer and sharing healthcare resources may be necessary.

Maintenance of normal staffing patterns may be difficult. Hospital personnel or their families may be affected, and staff may be reluctant to report to work. Altered staffing patterns may have to be adopted and responsibilities delegated. Existing policies and procedure should be followed to minimize variability and iatrogenic complications.

Alternate Levels of Care and Allocation of Scarce Resources

Existing standards of care should be maintained during an MCE. Stepwise changes in resource utilization are

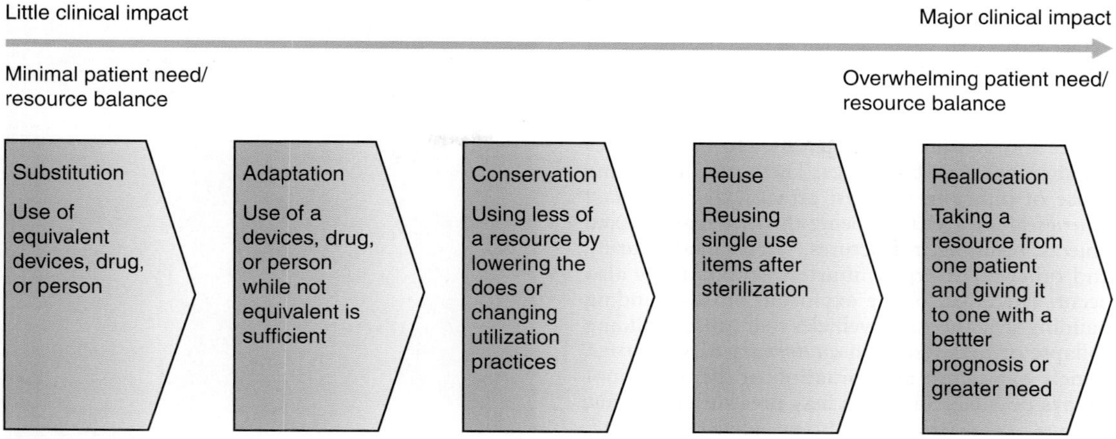
Little clinical impact
Major clinical impact
Minimal patient need/ resource balance
Overwhelming patient need/ resource balance
Substitution
Use of equivalent devices, drug, or person
Adaptation
Use of a devices, drug, or person while not equivalent is sufficient
Conservation
Using less of a resource by lowering the does or changing utilization practices
Reuse
Reusing single use items after sterilization
Reallocation
Taking a resource from one patient and giving it to one with a bettter prognosis or greater need

FIGURE 11.1. Stepwise approach to altered resource utilization and standard of care. (Adapted from Christian MD, Deveraux AV, Dichter JR, et al. Definitive care for the critically ill during a disaster: Current capabilities and limitations from a Task Force for Mass Critical Care Summit meeting, January 26–27, 2007, Chicago, IL. *Chest* 2008;133(5 suppl):8S–17S.)

recommended until reallocation is the only feasible option (**Fig. 11.1**). Explicit policies and procedures should detail how to proceed if hospitals change standards of care.

Children with Special Needs and the Technology-Dependent Child

There are 200 million children worldwide who have disabilities, and they represent a significant at-risk population. The Federal Emergency Management Agency helps support state's efforts to increase preparedness for disabled individuals. Loss of electricity and consumption of resources (medications, formula, or oxygen) may require these patients to present to a hospital.

BOMBINGS AND BLAST INJURIES

Background

Explosives remain the most common cause of MCEs. In addition to casualties from the immediate area, first responders and onlookers may be injured by subsequent blasts, fire, or building collapse. Terrorists use this *second-hit principle* to maximize damage and casualties. Containment of the scene and ensuring the safety of responders is part of on-scene management. Protection of medical assets by keeping them away from the explosion and areas with a high probability of attack is essential.

Blast injuries present in a number of patterns that include burn, blunt, penetrating, inhalational, and crush injuries. Incidents with structural collapse have higher immediate mortality (87%–100%). Most survivors have noncritical injuries (soft tissue and bone injuries). Critically injured patients comprise 8%–34% of survivors. Head injuries are most common followed by pulmonary, abdominal, and chest injuries. Most head injuries are noncritical. MCE victims are often more severely injured than the typical pediatric trauma population and require more operative interventions, ICU admissions, and longer hospitalization. Pediatric MCE survivors appear to be less debilitated than adults, with fewer discharges to rehabilitation centers.

Mechanisms, Manifestations, and Management of Blast Injuries

Explosions generate a blast wave (a high-pressure *shock wave*) that travels at the speed of sound away from the detonation center. As the wave travels, it rapidly loses pressure and velocity. If reflected off solid surfaces, it may multiply eight to nine times and lead to greater injury. The magnitude and duration of the blast wave depend on the type of explosive and the medium (air or water) through which it travels. As the blast wave displaces surrounding air, it propels individuals and bomb fragments, causing additional injury.

Explosion-related injuries are classified by mechanism into four categories. *Primary blast injuries* are due to barotrauma from the blast wave, and are most severe when they occur in a confined space. As the blast wave enters the body, it creates stress, shock, and shear waves. *Stress waves* are longitudinal pressure forces that create a spalling effect (breaking into small pieces) at air–fluid interfaces that result in microvascular damage and tissue disruption. Gas-filled organs (e.g., middle ear, lung, and gastrointestinal tract) are commonly affected. *Shear waves* are transverse waves that cause asynchronous movement of tissue, tissue disruption, and traumatic amputation. *Secondary blast injuries* involve penetrating injuries caused by projectile particles from the explosive device and surrounding materials. The highest rates occur in open-air bombings. These are the leading cause of injury in terrorist attacks. *Tertiary blast injuries* involve victims being thrown against fixed objects, resulting in fractures, intracranial injuries, and other solid organ injuries. Amputations also occur. The effect of the explosion on surrounding building structures and vehicles that causes building collapse or fires results in *quaternary blast injuries*. Timely extraction and initiation of therapy is not always possible. Survivors may present with burns, fractures, compartment syndrome, inhalational, head, and crush injuries. Late complications include acute respiratory distress syndrome, acute kidney injury, chemical and radiation exposure, and exacerbation of preexisting conditions.

Aural Injuries

With blast injuries, perforation of the tympanic membrane (TM) is common. Patients may present with deafness, tinnitus, or vertigo. The ossicles of the middle ear can be dislocated. Traumatic disruption of the oval or round window may lead to permanent hearing loss.

Blast Lung Injury

Pulmonary injuries are often the most common critical injury. The pressure differential across the alveolar–capillary barrier causes disruption of alveolar septa and capillaries, leading to acute pulmonary hemorrhage, pulmonary edema, and hypoxic respiratory failure. Pneumothorax, hemothorax, pneumomediastinum, and subcutaneous emphysema have all been described. Acute gas embolism from pulmonary disruption can cause sudden death. Blast lung injury should be suspected in patients presenting with apnea, bradycardia, dyspnea, hypoxemia, or hypotension. Chest X-ray shows the characteristic butterfly or batwing infiltrates (**Fig. 11.2**) caused by reflection of the blast wave off mediastinal structures. Patients are at high risk for pneumothoraces and positive-pressure ventilation should therefore be avoided if possible. With severe pulmonary hemorrhage and hypoxemia, endotracheal intubation and mechanical ventilation are necessary. The use of lung protective strategies is recommended. Providers must be cautious and avoid worsening pulmonary edema from fluid overload. There is no evidence to support the routine use of corticosteroids or antibiotics.

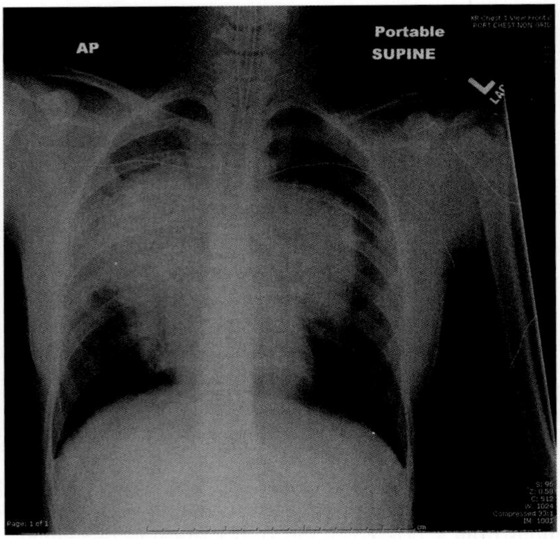

FIGURE 11.2. Pediatric blast lung injury with typical butterfly pattern. (From Ratto J, Johnson BK, Condra CS, et al. Pediatric blast lung injury from a fireworks-related explosion. *Pediatr Emerg Care* 2012;28(6):573–6.)

Gastrointestinal Blast Injury

Gastrointestinal (GI) blast injuries are rare. The rapid compression and expansion of air in gas-filled organs result in contusions, intramural hemorrhage, and perforation. Tearing of mesenteric vessels leads to mesenteric ischemia or infarction. Rupture of solid organs (liver, spleen, or kidney) with resulting hemorrhage can occur. GI injuries usually present 8–36 hours postevent. Signs and symptoms include abdominal pain, nausea, vomiting, hematemesis, melena, rebound tenderness, and abdominal rigidity. Hemodynamic instability may be seen with mesenteric vessel and solid organ injury. Pneumoperitoneum, free fluid, and a sentinel clot adjacent to bowel wall or mesentery may be seen on abdominal CT scan. Patient deterioration requires a laparotomy to control hemorrhage or GI contamination of the peritoneal cavity.

Cardiovascular Effects of Blast Injury

Cardiac contusion or air embolization to the coronaries may occur from blast waves. Cardiac index can be low with normal systemic vascular resistance. Apnea is brief and followed by tachypnea. Bradycardia has a rapid onset, is severe, and is typically protracted. Blast survivors may lose the tachycardic response to hemorrhage. Atropine may be used for bradycardia.

Traumatic Amputations

A traumatic amputation is an indicator of the severity of the blast wave. The transmission of energy through the extremities causes fracture through the shaft rather than the joint. Secondary and tertiary soft tissue injury results from shrapnel and debris from structural collapse. Open wounds, lacerations, and crush injuries should be managed using general trauma principles.

Neurologic Injuries

Primary blast injury from the blast wave can cause neurologic injury. Fractures around sinuses, air embolism in cerebral vessels, cerebral contusion, and intracranial hemorrhage have been described. Shearing and diffuse axonal injuries with activation of inflammatory mechanisms produce both immediate and delayed symptoms. Children are more likely to demonstrate persistent functional deficits in neuropsychological, behavioral, adaptive, and academic outcomes, but improvement over time does occur.

SCHOOL MASS SHOOTINGS

High-profile cases (e.g., Columbine, Virginia Tech, and Sandy Hook) have drawn attention to public mass shootings at academic institutions. It is estimated that 15% of public mass shootings occur in academic institutions. While many schools have disaster plans, a significant number do not address children with special healthcare needs or postdisaster counseling. Shooting events have a high immediate mortality rate (77%). While 60% of bombing victims are at the hospital within 30 minutes, only 22% of shooting victims arrive during that time frame. MCE-related shooting patients had higher mortality (2.75 times) than for non-MCE shooting casualties.

CHEMICAL AND RADIOLOGIC MASS CASUALTY EVENTS

Chemical Mass Casualty Events

Chemical agents are more prevalent than radiologic agents due to their application in many sectors of society. Most enter the body through inhalation, ingestion, absorption, or inoculation. With their rapid minute ventilation and large body surface area, children are at increased risk for serious toxicity. The chemical agents are often classified as (a) nerve agents, (b) vesicants, (c) choking agents, or (d) asphyxiants.

Duration of contact with the agent increases the likelihood of severe illness. Rapid decontamination of the victim is the first step in management. Patient stabilization may need to be delayed until after decontamination. This delay should not put the patient at additional risk. Decontamination procedures need to be flexible and consider severity of illness, physical nature of the agent, and weather conditions. Important principles include the following: (1) decontaminate as soon as possible, (2) decontaminate by priority of patients needing stabilization, (3) decontaminate only what is necessary, and (4) decontaminate as far away from the hot zone as possible. Effective decontamination reduces the risk of secondary contamination of healthcare workers. The use of a heated room, water warmed to 37.8°C, and the availability of new clothing may help prevent hypothermia. Family presence may minimize fear and decrease psychological trauma. Presentation and management of patients exposed to specific nerve agents, vesicants, and asphyxiants are discussed in Chapter 10.

Radiologic/Nuclear Mass Casualty Events

The full effects of a nuclear MCE may not be immediately evident. Acute radiation syndrome (toxicity may occur within minutes and usually in <24 hours) will develop in individuals exposed to a nuclear detonation who are close enough to sustain blast injuries. Decontamination (which can usually be deferred for stabilization) and the time course of symptom development are outlined in Chapter 10. Treatment is supportive. Fluids, antibiotics, hematopoietic growth factors, nutrition, and skin care are provided when indicated. Potassium iodide administration within 8 hours prevents incorporation of inhaled or ingested radioiodines, thus reducing the possibility of thyroid cancer. Other antidotes include Prussian blue for exposure to cesium-137 and thallium. For plutonium, curium, and americium exposures, treatment is through chelation with pentetate calcium trisodium, pentetate zinc trisodium, or 2,3-dimercaptopropane-1-sulfonic acid, which bind radioactive elements/heavy metals and remove them through the urine.

CHAPTER 12 ■ POISONING

MICHAEL A. NARES, G. PATRICIA CANTWELL, AND RICHARD S. WEISMAN

More than 2 million childhood poisonings are reported yearly in the United States and most cause minimal harm. Poisoning in children <5 years of age is usually accidental and accounts for ~85%–90% of pediatric cases. Poisoning in a child >5 years is often intentional. Unintentional overdose occasionally occurs in teenagers who take alcohol and street drugs. Teenage exposures may also be due to suicide gestures or attempts.

EPIDEMIOLOGY

The majority of poison control center calls involve cosmetics, personal care products, cleaning substances, analgesics, foreign bodies, topical agents, and plants. Fatalities most often involve analgesics, hydrocarbons, antidepressants, gases, fumes, stimulants, street drugs, cardiovascular drugs, anticonvulsants, sedative/hypnotics, antipsychotics, and chemicals.

CLINICAL APPROACH TO THE POISONED CHILD

Initial evaluation includes triage and determination of the appropriate decontamination and treatment regimens. The primary survey involves evaluation of airway, breathing, and circulation. Toxins may depress respiratory drive, impair the central nervous system (CNS), inhibit airway reflexes, or cause direct pulmonary toxicity. Airway management requires a low threshold for intubation and presumption of a full stomach, with risk of aspiration. Monitoring is necessary for dysrhythmias and hypotension. Consideration of decontamination and personal protective equipment (PPE) is important to ensure safety of personnel.

Patient History

A comprehensive history for toxic exposure may be obtained from witnesses, family members, friends, and emergency medical services personnel. It is important to obtain a list of available toxins (including over-the-counter medications and nonpharmaceutical agents such as plants and cleaning agents), information about the environment, circumstances surrounding a toxic exposure, smells, unusual items, occupations of those in the home, and the presence of a suicide note. Additionally, determine the maximum amount of toxin available and the minimum amount per kilogram to produce symptoms. Product containers and medication labels identify specific toxic contents. The extremely dangerous single agents are camphor, chloroquine, hydroxychloroquine, imipramine, desipramine, quinine, methyl salicylate, theophylline, thioridazine, and chlorpromazine. Inhaled toxins to evaluate for include carbon monoxide, cyanide, ozone, smoke, volatile hydrocarbons, and mercury vapor. The *regional poison control center (1-800-222-1222)* provides rapid access to a toxicology consultant.

Physical Examination

Signs and symptoms that suggest specific classes of poisoning are referred to as toxidromes. The four classical toxidromes are discussed later. The aberrations of various organ systems caused by toxins are outlined in **Table 12.1**. Symmetric pupillary changes are typical of toxic exposures. Asymmetric pupils suggest a neurologic abnormality such as traumatic brain injury. Drug withdrawal may be heralded by agitation, abnormal vital signs, irritability, and an altered sensorium. Nystagmus, tinnitus, and visual disturbances are common in specific intoxications. Inhalant abuse may lead to skin rashes around the nose and the mouth. Needle tracks or characteristic tattooing suggest IV drug use. Alopecia or jaundice can suggest specific toxic exposures. Odors may suggest specific exposures.

Laboratory Evaluation

Laboratory evaluation is essential in intoxications with acetaminophen, ethanol, methanol, ethylene glycol, lithium, salicylates, iron, lead, mercury, arsenic, phenobarbital, carbon monoxide, methemoglobin, and theophylline. A negative toxicology screen does not exclude a toxic exposure. It is helpful to inform laboratory personnel of suspected toxins. Some toxins are better detected in urine than in blood. Urine screens may detect drugs or metabolites for days after exposure, and symptoms may not be due to the drug detected. Acetaminophen levels are important in any poisoned patient to ensure that urgent treatment is addressed. Comprehensive drug screens and levels are rarely available at the time of initial intervention. Blood glucose level should be assessed in any patient with an altered sensorium. Urine pregnancy tests are

TABLE 12.1

Clinical Manifestations of Poisoning

Skin	
Cyanosis (unresponsive to oxygen, methemoglobinemia)	Nitrates, nitrites, phenacetin, benzocaine
Red flush	Carbon monoxide, cyanide, boric acid, anticholinergics
Sweating	Amphetamines, LSD, organophosphates, cocaine, barbiturates
Dry	Anticholinergics
Bullae	Barbiturates, carbon monoxide
Jaundice	Acetaminophen, mushrooms, carbon tetrachloride, iron, phosphorus
Purpura	Aspirin, warfarin, snakebite
Temperature	
Hypothermia	Sedative hypnotics, ethanol, carbon monoxide, phenothiazines, TCAs, clonidine
Hyperthermia	Anticholinergics, salicylates, phenothiazines, TCAs, cocaine, amphetamines, theophylline
Blood Pressure	
Hypertension	Sympathomimetics (especially phenylpropanolamine in over-the-counter cold remedies) organophosphates, amphetamines, PCP
Hypotension	Narcotics, sedative hypnotics, TCAs, phenothiazines, clonidine, β-blockers, calcium channel blockers
Pulse Rate	
Bradycardia	Digitalis, sedative hypnotics, β-blockers, ethchlorvynol, calcium channel blockers
Tachycardia	Anticholinergics, sympathomimetics, amphetamines, alcohol, aspirin, theophylline, cocaine, TCAs
Arrhythmias	Anticholinergics, TCAs, organophosphates, phenothiazines, digoxin, β-blockers, carbon monoxide, cyanide, theophylline
Mucous Membranes	
Dry	Anticholinergics
Salivation	Organophosphates, carbamates
Oral lesions	Corrosives, paraquat
Lacrimation	Caustics, organophosphates, irritant gases
Respiration	
Depressed	Alcohol, narcotics, barbiturates, sedative/hypnotics
Tachypnea	Salicylates, amphetamines, carbon monoxide
Kussmaul	Methanol, ethylene glycol, salicylates
Wheezing	Organophosphates
Pneumonia	Hydrocarbons
Pulmonary edema	Aspiration, salicylates, narcotics, sympathomimetics
CNS	
Seizures	TCAs, cocaine, phenothiazines, amphetamines, camphor, lead, salicylates, isoniazid, organophosphates, antihistamines, propoxyphene, strychnine
Pupils, miosis	Narcotics (except Demerol and Lomotil), phenothiazines, organophosphates, diazepam, barbiturates, mushrooms (muscarine types)
Mydriasis	Anticholinergics, sympathomimetics, cocaine, TCAs, methanol, glutethimide, LSD
Blindness, optic atrophy	Methanol
Fasciculation	Organophosphates
Nystagmus	Diphenylhydantoin, barbiturates, carbamazepine, PCP, carbon monoxide, glutethimide, ethanol
Hypertonus	Anticholinergics, strychnine, phenothiazines
Myoclonus, rigidity	Anticholinergics, phenothiazines, haloperidol
Delirium/psychosis	Anticholinergics, sympathomimetics, alcohol, phenothiazines, PCP, LSD, marijuana, cocaine, heroin, methaqualone, heavy metals
Coma	Alcohols, anticholinergics, sedative hypnotics, narcotics, carbon monoxide, TCAs, salicylates, organophosphates, barbiturates
Weakness, paralysis	Organophosphates, carbamates, heavy metals

(continued)

TABLE 12.1

Clinical Manifestations of Poisoning (*continued*)

Gastrointestinal System	
Vomiting, diarrhea, abdominal pain	Iron, phosphorus, heavy metals, lithium, mushrooms, fluoride, organophosphates, arsenic

LSD, lysergic acid diethylamide; PCP, phencyclidine; TCA, tricyclic antidepressants.
Adapted from Guzzardi L, Bayer MJ. Emergency management of the poisoned patient. In: Bayer M, Rumack BH, Wanke LA, eds. *Toxicologic Emergencies*. Bowie, MD: Robert J. Brady, 1984.

important for adolescent girls. Urinalysis may reveal specific crystals or myoglobinuria.

Electrolytes, blood urea nitrogen (BUN), and creatinine levels assess anion-gap acidosis, basic electrolytes, and renal function. The *anion-gap* calculation is:

$$Na\ (mEq/L) - [Cl\ (mEq/L) + HCO_3\ (mEq/L)]$$

The normal anion gap is 3–16 mEq/L. Agents that cause anion-gap acidosis are listed in **Table 12.2**. Arterial blood gas analysis is useful for the evaluation of acid–base status. The addition of co-oximetry can identify carboxyhemoglobin, methemoglobin, and sulfhemoglobin.

Calculated serum osmolality is determined using:

$$2 \times Na\ (mEq/L) + BUN\ (g/L)/2.8 + glucose\ (mg/dL)/18$$

The *osmolal gap* is evaluated by subtracting the calculated osmolality from the measured osmolality. The normal range is -3 to $+6$ mOsm/kg H_2O. An increased osmolal gap (>10 mOsm/kg) indicates the presence of abnormal osmotically active substances (e.g., methanol, ethanol, ethylene glycol, acetone, or isopropanol). Calculation of the osmolal gap may be confounded by lipemia or osmotic agents (mannitol or radiologic contrast).

Electrocardiogram

The 12-lead electrocardiogram can detect dysrhythmias and conduction abnormalities (e.g., wide QRS complex or prolonged QT interval). Findings may suggest specific toxins or indicate a risk of serious hemodynamic compromise.

TABLE 12.2

Anion-Gap Acidosis (Mudpiles)

Methanol
Uremia
Diabetic ketoacidosis
Paraldehyde and phenformin
Isoniazid and iron
Lactic acidosis
Ethanol and ethylene glycol
Salicylates

Radiologic Imaging

Imaging can reveal foreign bodies, radiopaque drugs, metals, and chemicals. Disc battery ingestion can be a medical emergency. Radiopaque compounds may be grouped by the mnemonic "COINS": chloral hydrate and cocaine (packets), opiate (packets), iron and heavy metals (lead, arsenic, and mercury), neuroleptics, and sustained-release or enteric-coated tablets.

MANAGEMENT

Regional poison control hotlines have extensive information regarding drug identification, pharmacokinetics, drug interactions, and precautions. Also helpful are the Poisindex computer database (Micromedex Corporation, Greenwood Village, CO) and Drug Information Centers in large medical centers.

Toxicokinetics

Limiting the time of exposure to a toxin may dramatically reduce toxicity (i.e., washing a toxin from the skin or removing a patient from an environment with a toxic gas). Preventing absorption from the gastrointestinal (GI) tract is more complex, as factors such as pH, pKa of the toxin, and lipid solubility may alter absorption. Activated charcoal may provide adsorption of the toxin within the GI lumen. Enteric-coated tablets and sustained-release formulations may have a delayed time to peak serum concentrations. Whole-bowel irrigation may force transit of enteric-coated tablets or sustained-release formulations before absorption begins.

Decontamination

Aggressive gastric decontamination and syrup of *ipecac* (to induce vomiting) were standard management.

Ipecac is no longer recommended because of a brief time window for efficacy and the risk of airway compromise from vomiting. *Gastric lavage* is also used less frequently, and contraindications include inadequate upper airway protection, ingestion of corrosive substances or hydrocarbons, and risk for GI perforation or hemorrhage. *Activated charcoal* may be efficacious but not for iron, alcohols, cyanide, pesticides, and lithium. It is not as useful beyond >1 hour after ingestion. If activated charcoal is indicated in a patient with poor airway protection, the patient should first undergo intubation. Multiple doses may be used for substances with prolonged half-lives and small volumes of distribution such as carbamazepine, dapsone, phenytoin, phenobarbital, quinine, salicylates, and theophylline. *Whole-bowel irrigation* utilizes polyethylene glycol electrolyte solutions (PEG-ES) to enhance the elimination of toxins prior to absorption, and may be useful with ingestions of heavy metals, iron, sustained-release or enteric-coated tablets, and illegal drug packets. It should not be used in patients with an unprotected airway, hemodynamic compromise, intractable vomiting, GI hemorrhage, ileus, perforation, or obstruction. *Surgical decontamination* may prove useful in rare cases, such as in bowel obstruction due to heroin or cocaine packets or in massive iron ingestion.

Antidotes

Specific antidotes as well as modes of enhancing elimination are listed in **Table 12.3**. In some cases, supportive care is safer than antidotes. *Flumazenil* is a benzodiazepine antagonist that can be useful in isolated benzodiazepine overdose, but may precipitate difficult-to-control seizures. It should be avoided in unknown overdoses or in mixed ingestions. *Lipid emulsion infusions* (LEIs) are increasingly used to reverse cardiotoxicity from lipophilic drugs. First described to treat arrhythmias secondary to local anesthetic toxicity in the operating room, LEI therapy use includes intoxication by calcium channel blockers, β-blockers, and psychiatric medications.

Extracorporeal Elimination

Hemodialysis may be effective for the removal of small compounds concentrated in the intravascular compartment with low protein binding. Its use includes severe salicylate and lithium exposures, methanol and ethylene glycol, and when hydrophilic drugs with a low volume of distribution and low protein binding result in severe or life-threatening symptoms. *Charcoal hemoperfusion* is preferred in the instance of toxicity with larger, lipid-soluble compounds with greater affinity for plasma proteins, such as theophylline.

Diuresis and Urine pH Management

Elimination of some drugs (salicylates, phenobarbital, chlorpropamide, and the chlorophenoxy herbicides) may be facilitated by ensuring adequate urine output and using intravenous sodium bicarbonate to alter the urinary pH and prevent reabsorption across the renal tubular epithelium.

TOXIDROMES

Sympathomimetic/Adrenergic Agents

Cocaine is the classical sympathomimetic drug of abuse. Sympathomimetics cause agitation, tachycardia, hypertension, diaphoresis, fever, and seizures. Rhabdomyolysis, myocardial ischemia, or stroke is possible. Caffeine and theophylline are not sympathomimetics but result in similar symptomatology. Benzodiazepines may be effective in controlling hypertension, tachycardia, agitation, and extreme muscle activity. β-Blockers may result in unopposed α-receptor stimulation and are best avoided. Hypoglycemia may be present. Short-acting antihypertensive agents are preferred for treating these overdoses. The sympathomimetic toxidrome is not seen with centrally acting α-agonists (e.g., clonidine) which decrease sympathetic outflow and cause bradycardia, hypotension, and CNS and respiratory depression.

Cholinergic Agents

Cholinergic agonists include muscarinic agents, nicotinic agents, and cholinesterase inhibitors. Signs and symptoms are listed in **Table 12.4.** This toxidrome is effectively managed with atropine and supportive care. Organophosphate pesticides and nerve agents are examples of cholinesterase inhibitors. Dermal exposure results in local hyperhidrosis, followed by systemic involvement as the drug is absorbed. Topical decontamination with utilization of PPE is essential. Inhalational exposure is marked by upper airway involvement and subsequent respiratory distress. Vomiting and drooling are most commonly seen following ingestion. Fatality is usually attributed to respiratory failure that results from bronchorrhea, bronchospasm, diminished respiratory drive, and neuromuscular blockade. Seizures and severe CNS toxicity occur following large exposures to household products or small exposures to industrial pesticides and "nerve agents." Management includes atropine to reverse the muscarinic effects, an oxime (Pralidoxime) to facilitate reactivation of acetylcholinesterase and reverse the neuromuscular blockade, and benzodiazepines to control seizures. There is a potential for prolonged paralysis with succinylcholine, because its half-life is prolonged by the organophosphate-induced inhibition of cholinesterase production.

TABLE 12.3

Selected Antidotes and Methods of Enhancing Toxin Elimination

ANTIDOTE	TOXIN
Antivenoms	
Crotalidae	North American Pit Viper envenomation
Polyvalent	
Polyvalent immune Fab	
Micrurus sp.	Eastern or Texas coral snake envenomation
Latrodectus mactans	Black widow spider envenomation
Atropine	Organophosphate, carbamate poisoning, bradydysrhythmias, Centruroides (scorpion) envenomation
Calcium (chloride or gluconate)	Calcium channel blocker overdose, hydrofluoric acid ingestion/exposure
Cyanide antidote package	Cyanide, acetonitrile (artificial nail remover), amygdalin (peach, apricot pits), nitroprusside (thiosulfate only)
Amyl nitrite	
Sodium nitrite	
Sodium thiosulfate	
Deferoxamine	Iron
Digoxin-specific antibody fragments	Digoxin, digitoxin, natural cardiac glycosides (e.g., oleander, red squill, Bufo toad venom)
Flumazenil	Benzodiazepines
Fomepizole	Toxic alcohols (ethylene glycol, methanol)
Glucagon	Calcium channel blocker, β-blocker toxicity
Glucose (dextrose)	Sulfonylureas, insulin, hypoglycemia (multiple toxins)
Hydroxocobalamin (vitamin B_{12})[a]	Cyanide, acetonitrile, amygdalin, nitroprusside
Insulin (high dose)/euglycemia[b]	Calcium channel blocker, β-blocker toxicity
Lipid emulsion, 20%	Lipophilic drugs, local anesthetics, calcium channel blocker, β-blocker toxicity
Methylene blue	Methemoglobinemia
N-acetylcysteine	Acetaminophen, pennyroyal oil, carbon tetrachloride
Naloxone	Opioid toxicity
Octreotide	Sulfonylurea toxicity
Physostigmine	Antimuscarinic delirium (as a diagnostic tool only)
Pralidoxime	Organophosphate poisoning (insecticides, nerve agents)
Protamine sulfate	Heparins
Pyridoxine	Isoniazid, monomethylhydrazine (rocket fuel), Gyromitra mushrooms
Thiamine	Deficiency states (e.g., alcoholism, anorexia nervosa)
Sodium bicarbonate	Sodium channel blocking cardiotoxins, salicylates
METHOD OF REMOVAL	**INDICATION**
Dialysis	Toxic alcohols, salicylates, lithium, theophylline, valproic acid, atenolol, sotalol, others
Urinary alkalinization with sodium bicarbonate	Salicylates, phenobarbital, chlorpropamide, chlorophenoxy herbicides, methotrexate

[a]Not FDA approved for this use.
[b]Anecdotal experience.
From Barry JD. Diagnosis and management of the poisoned child. *Pediatr Ann* 2005;34:937–46, with permission.

TABLE 12.4

Cholinergic Toxidrome Features

Muscarinic Effects (DUMBBELLS)
Diarrhea/defecation
Urinary incontinence
Miosis
Bradycardia
Bronchorrhea/bronchospasm
Emesis
Lacrimation
Lethargy
Salivation/sweating
Nicotinic Effects
Fasciculations
Weakness
Paralysis
Tachycardia
Hypertension
Agitation
Central Effects
Lethargy
Coma
Agitation
Seizures

TABLE 12.5

Anticholinergic Agents

Antihistamines—diphenhydramine, hydroxyzine
Atropine
Benztropine mesylate
Carbamazepine
Cyclic antidepressants
Cyclobenzaprine
Hyoscyamine
Jimsonweed
Oxybutynin
Phenothiazines
Scopolamine
Trihexyphenidyl

TABLE 12.6

Anticholinergic Toxidrome

Agitation
Delirium
Coma
Mydriasis
Dry mouth
Warm, dry, flushed skin
Tachycardia
Hypertension
Fever
Urinary retention
Decreased bowel sounds

Anticholinergic Agents

Agents that produce antimuscarinic properties (**Table 12.5**) result in symptoms and signs referred to as the anticholinergic toxidrome (**Table 12.6**). It is similar to the sympathomimetic toxidrome, but sympathomimetic toxicity results in diaphoresis and cool skin, whereas anticholinergic toxicity is marked by impaired sweating and warm, dry skin. Sympathomimetics result in hyperactive bowel sounds, whereas anticholinergics cause diminished bowel sounds or ileus. Management focuses on controlling agitation to minimize hyperthermia in the face of impaired sweating mechanisms. Benzodiazepines may be extremely helpful. Physostigmine may reverse central and peripheral manifestations; however, it is not recommended for management of tricyclic antidepressant toxicity because of reported convulsions and asystole.

Opioid Agents

Opioids typically cause a triad of respiratory depression, coma, and miosis. An exception is meperidine, which manifests as respiratory depression, coma, *mydriasis*, and *seizures*. Physical findings often include bradycardia, hypotension, and decreased GI motility. Naloxone, an opiate-receptor antagonist, rapidly reverses toxicity. Naloxone may precipitate acute withdrawal in opiate-dependent patients or severe symptoms in patients with a source of pain (e.g., the postoperative setting) so initial doses should be low and titrated to effect. The duration of action of naloxone is shorter than that of many opioids; repeat dosing or an infusion may be needed. Clonidine is a centrally acting α-agonist that is often included in the opiate toxidrome owing to the diminished sympathetic tone, its ability to cause miosis, and CNS and respiratory depression. There may be some response to naloxone, but its use is controversial. In the event of respiratory failure, airway management takes precedence over naloxone. Many opiates are formulated in combination with acetaminophen or aspirin, so it is important to maintain a high index of suspicion for combined toxicity. Fentanyl patches contain a high concentration of drug, and significant toxicity can result from ingestion.

FOCUSED REVIEW OF COMMON TOXINS

Acetaminophen

Acetaminophen is the most common intentional overdose. Toxicity results in fulminant hepatic failure. Acetaminophen is metabolized in the liver by glucuronidation and sulfation to form nontoxic metabolites that are renally excreted. Glutathione is depleted by significant overdose, which allows the toxic intermediate *N*-acetyl-p-benzoquinone-imine (NAPQI) to bind to the hepatocytes and cause cell death. Early clinical signs (if symptomatic) are nausea and vomiting. Acidosis occurs in extreme overdoses. Transaminases increase (by 24 hours after ingestion) while symptoms abate. Liver function abnormalities peak at 48–72 hours, and symptoms return with nausea, vomiting, and anorexia. The clinical course varies from complete recovery to fulminant hepatic failure. Therapy involves the administration of *N-acetylcysteine* (NAC), which can replenish glutathione and detoxify NAPQI. Initiation of NAC within 10 hours of ingestion is recommended, but it may be beneficial up to 24 hours. The *Rumack–Matthew nomogram* helps predict toxicity when the time since ingestion is known. NAC therapy should continue until all doses are administered, even if the acetaminophen plasma level drops below the toxic range.

Salicylates

Acetylsalicylic acid (aspirin) is the most commonly encountered salicylate ingestion. Methyl salicylate (oil of wintergreen) is especially dangerous. Topical aspirin-containing compounds may be absorbed cutaneously. Respiratory alkalosis from hyperventilation is often the first sign of salicylate intoxication. Nausea, vomiting, dehydration, and tinnitus are common. CNS manifestations include lethargy, coma, and seizures. Uncoupling of oxidative phosphorylation results in hyperpyrexia and metabolic acidosis. Salicylate intoxication may mimic diabetes mellitus with hyperglycemia and glycosuria. Chronic salicylate toxicity can be fatal with pulmonary and cerebral edema. Plasma salicylate levels should be monitored for at least 24 hours after ingestion of sustained-release or enteric-coated capsules. Therapy includes activated charcoal to prevent absorption and alkalinization of the urine to enhance elimination. Hemodialysis is recommended for extreme salicylate levels (>100 mg/dL), renal insufficiency, significant volume overload, pulmonary edema, or severe electrolyte aberrations.

Alcohols

Ethanol is the most commonly ingested alcohol and can pose a hazard in beverage form, mouthwash, perfume, cologne, or topical antiseptic. Children may present with nausea, vomiting, stupor, and ataxia. Infants and toddlers may develop coma, hypothermia, and hypoglycemia. Metabolic acidosis is typical. Management of respiratory compromise and blood glucose determination are priorities. Ethanol is rapidly absorbed, so GI decontamination is rarely useful. Hemodialysis increases the rate of elimination, but is rarely necessary.

Isopropyl alcohol is found in rubbing alcohol, aftershave lotions, perfumes, skin lotions, and antifreeze. Toxicity manifests as vomiting, abdominal pain, and hematemesis (due to gastritis). CNS manifestations include lethargy, dizziness, ataxia, and coma. Patients may have ketosis and ketonemia without acidemia. Children are at extreme risk for hypoglycemia.

Methanol and *ethylene glycol* (commonly found in antifreeze) are metabolized by alcohol dehydrogenase to toxic metabolites. Methanol is metabolized to formic acid, which causes severe metabolic acidosis and retinal toxicity. Ethylene glycol is metabolized to oxalate, causing severe anion-gap metabolic acidosis, hypocalcemia, and renal failure. *Fomepizole* treatment blocks this metabolism. Hemodialysis is recommended for very high levels.

Caustics

Alkaline ingestion causes deep tissue injury, usually with liquefaction necrosis, in the oropharynx and proximal esophagus. Perforation occurs in severe exposure. Automatic dishwasher detergents have extremely high alkalinity. *Acid ingestion* causes a superficial coagulation necrosis, with heat production and eschar formation. Absorption may result in metabolic acidosis, hemolysis, and renal failure. Management involves aggressive decontamination, with washing and diluting of dermal or ocular exposures, fresh air and oxygen for inhalational injury, and removal of any oral matter if ingested. Eye exposure requires urgent ophthalmologic consult. Neutralization is contraindicated, as an exothermic reaction can yield more extensive tissue destruction. Ipecac, gastric lavage, and activated charcoal are not indicated. Endoscopy is recommended within the first 24 hours. The use of steroids is controversial.

Iron

The first 30 minutes after iron intoxication is marked by vomiting, diarrhea, hematemesis, or hematochezia followed by malaise and metabolic acidosis. Hemodynamic instability and shock may occur after 12 hours. Late sequelae include liver failure and GI tract scarring or strictures. GI lavage or whole-bowel irrigation may be used. *Deferoxamine* chelation is indicated for serum iron levels >500 mcg/dL or hemodynamic collapse. Brisk urine output is essential for the excretion of the iron–deferoxamine complex.

Calcium Channel Blockers

Calcium channel antagonists cause negative inotropic, chronotropic, and dromotropic effects. Vasodilation from effects on arteriolar smooth muscle results in hypotension. Bradydysrhythmias are common and electrocardiographic changes include prolonged PR interval, inverted P waves, AV dissociation, AV block,

ST-segment changes, sinus arrest, and asystole. Patients may have altered mental status, seizures, coma, and poor GI motility. Fluid resuscitation, atropine, IV calcium, *glucagon*, and vasopressors may be needed. Activated charcoal should be administered and repeated if the ingestion was a sustained-release formulation. Whole-bowel irrigation should be considered. Hyperinsulinemia/euglycemia therapy may reverse cardiogenic shock. Severe cases may require transvenous pacing, ventricular assist device, or extracorporeal life support. Lipid emulsion therapy may be useful.

β-Blockers

β-Adrenergic antagonists competitively inhibit sympathetic neurotransmission at a variety of sites. β-Blocker toxicity results in bradycardia, hypotension, conduction delay, bronchospasm, and hypoglycemia. Severe toxicity may result in torsades de pointes, ventricular fibrillation, or asystole. Propranolol intoxication can result in coma and seizures. Atropine is helpful to reverse symptomatic bradycardia. Therapy with mixed β-agonists may result in an exacerbation of hypotension owing to β_2-receptor-mediated vasodilatation. Epinephrine infusions have been efficacious. Milrinone may enhance cardiac contractility. Severe toxicity may be managed with glucagon, transvenous pacing, and extracorporeal life support.

Digoxin

Digoxin toxicity produces increased sympathetic tone and cardiac automaticity. Manifestations include nausea, vomiting, altered sensorium, and dysrhythmias. The most typical dysrhythmias are bidirectional ventricular tachycardia and atrial tachycardia with AV block. Serum drug levels are available. Heart block or sinus bradycardia may be managed with atropine. For serious dysrhythmias, therapy is digoxin-specific Fab fragments (Digibind, DigiFab). Hypokalemia exacerbates digitalis-associated dysrhythmias. Intracellular calcium is increased, so additional calcium should be avoided. Cardiac pacing may be used to treat heart block or other life-threatening bradydysrhythmias. Amiodarone, magnesium sulfate, and phenytoin have been used for recurrent life-threatening tachydysrhythmias.

Tricyclic Antidepressants

Tricyclic antidepressants (TCAs) have anticholinergic properties, inhibit α-adrenergic receptors, and cause sedation and hypotension. Blockade of cardiac sodium channels decreases myocardial contractility, delays conduction, and widens QRS complexes. Blockade of potassium channels results in prolonged QT intervals. Effects on GABA and the reuptake of biogenic amines in the CNS cause seizures, which can be controlled with benzodiazepines (flumazenil should be avoided). Alkalinization increases protein binding of the drug and may restore normal cardiac conduction. TCA-induced hemodynamic compromise refractory to alkalinization therapy may benefit from vasopressors or lipid emulsion therapy. Flecanide, procainamide, amiodarone, or physostigmine may cause severe cardiac deterioration in the setting of TCA ingestion.

CLUB DRUGS

The increased popularity of club drugs emerged with the rave scene. Substances frequently ingested are ecstasy, amphetamines, marijuana, cocaine, inhalants, ketamine, and γ-hydroxybutyrate (GHB). Inhaled drugs of abuse include hydrocarbons (aliphatic and halogenated hydrocarbons and solvents), nitrous oxide, and nitrites. Clinical effects usually occur within seconds to minutes. These compounds can cause significant organ damage. Inhalation of volatile compounds may result in chemical pneumonitis. CNS depression may also occur.

Ecstasy (X, E, XTC, Adam, Molly)

Ecstasy, 3,4-methylenedioxymethylamphetamine (MDMA), is a selective serotoninergic neurotoxin that is utilized to foster a sense of enhanced empathy, relaxation, and closeness. Dehydration is a frequent manifestation of intoxication. Mild cases present with anxiety attacks, muscle cramping, trismus, or urinary retention due to urethral sphincter spasm. More severe symptoms include hyperthermia, malignant hyperthermia, rhabdomyolysis, disseminated intravascular coagulation, renal failure, seizures, dysrhythmias, intracranial hemorrhage, brain infarction, or death. Hyponatremia secondary to excessive water consumption is common.

γ-Hydroxybutyrate (G, Liquid Ecstasy, Liquid E)

GHB is a CNS depressant that results in euphoria, disinhibition, and heightened sexuality, making it a "date-rape drug." Effects include drowsiness, dizziness, nausea, vomiting, amnesia, hallucinations, convulsions, respiratory failure, coma, and death. Aggressive supportive care is the mainstay of management, and patients tend to have a sudden reversal of loss of consciousness. Emergence may be marked by myoclonic jerking, confusion, or combativeness.

Methamphetamines (Tina, Ice, Crystal Meth, Tweak, Crank, Glass)

Methamphetamine may be taken orally, rectally, IV, smoked, or snorted intranasally and is extremely addictive. Symptoms are sympathomimetic. Manifestations include headache, pallor, tachycardia, hypertension, chest pain, palpitations, arrhythmias, hyperthermia, rhabdomyolysis, convulsions, and death. Patients are agitated, anxious, flushed, and diaphoretic and have mydriasis. Management includes fluid and electrolyte replacement, as well as benzodiazepines.

Cocaine

Cocaine toxicity presents with the sympathomimetic toxidrome. It may be inhaled (cocaine alkaloid, or "crack"), or taken in by nasal insufflation, IV, or GI route. Crack cocaine is considered the most potent and addictive form. Manifestations include extreme CNS stimulation, seizures, hypertension, CNS bleeding and infarction, hemodynamic collapse, coma, and death. An acute coronary syndrome can result from increased myocardial oxygen demand in the setting of coronary artery constriction. Tachydysrhythmias and rhabdomyolysis also occur. Management includes benzodiazepines to control seizure activity and to help tachycardia and hypertension. Vasoconstriction of the coronary arteries may be managed with morphine, oxygen, nitroglycerin, aspirin, and phentolamine (an α-adrenergic antagonist). β-Blockers are contraindicated.

CHAPTER 13 THERMOREGULATION

ADNAN M. BAKAR AND CHARLES L. SCHLEIEN

PHYSIOLOGY OF THERMOREGULATION

Normal body temperature is maintained via thermoregulatory mechanisms that balance heat loss and heat gain. Extreme environmental temperatures can overcome thermoregulatory function and cause heat- or cold-related illnesses. Thermoreceptors exist in the cortex, hypothalamus, midbrain, medulla, spinal cord, deep abdominal structures, and the skin. Thermoregulation is initiated when sensed temperature differs from the hypothalamic set point.

Heat Gain

Warm-blooded animals have the capacity to raise their body temperature above environmental temperature. Heat is generated from basal metabolism, physical activity, food consumption, metabolic activity, emotional change, hormonal effects, and medications that increase metabolism. The body also acquires heat when the environmental temperature exceeds body temperature.

Heat Loss

Heat is lost from the body via *conduction*, *convection*, *radiation*, and *evaporation*. *Conduction* is heat loss by transfer from a warmer to a cooler object via direct contact. Approximately 3% of body heat is lost by conduction; it may cause major heat loss in wet clothing or immersion incidents. *Convection* is heat loss by the circulation of air or fluid around the skin. Windy conditions increase heat loss by removing the insulating warm air layer that surrounds the body. Approximately 12%–15% of heat is lost by convection. *Radiation* is heat loss due to infrared heat emission to surrounding air. Heat loss occurs primarily from the head and noninsulated areas of the body and can occur rapidly. Approximately 55%–65% of heat is lost by radiation. *Evaporation* is heat loss by the conversion of water from a liquid (sweat) to a gas via the skin or respiration. Approximately 25% of heat is lost by evaporation, depending on surface area, temperature difference, and humidity.

HYPERTHERMIA

Hyperthermia is a body temperature elevation beyond the hypothalamic set point. Antipyretics (aspirin, acetaminophen, and nonsteroidal anti-inflammatories) lower the set point; they have no effect in environmental hyperthermia. *Fever* is a regulated temperature elevation (>38.5°C) to a new, higher, hypothalamic set point. Fever is due to cytokine release and rarely exceeds 41°C.

Classification of Hyperthermia Syndromes

Hyperthermia syndromes may be classified as environmental (or exertional), drug (or toxin) induced, or of genetic/unknown origin. The severity of heat-related injury depends on the extent of core temperature elevation and its duration, and so early identification and treatment are important.

Heat Stroke (Environmental/Exertional Heat-Related Illness)

Heat-related illnesses range from *heat stress* (benign) to *heat stroke* (potentially fatal). Heat-related deaths in the United States with respect to the victim's age are approximately 6% for those <15 years of age, 50% for those between 15 and 64 years old, and 44% for those >65 years old. Heat stroke is characterized by an elevation of core temperature above 40°C, often with nervous system dysfunction manifesting in delirium, convulsions, or coma. Mortality is up to 50%, and survivors may sustain neurologic damage. Heat stroke is subdivided into environmental or exertional. *Environmental heat stroke* is more common in young children. *Exertional heat stroke* is most likely to occur when an individual engages in heavy exercise in hot, humid conditions. Individuals genetically predisposed to exertional heat stroke have a predominance of type II muscle fibers and lower exercise capacity and more easily develop lactatemia and rhabdomyolysis.

Prevention

Multiple factors may increase the risk of heat-related illness (**Table 13.1**). Recent illness increases the risk through effects on hydration status and regulation of body temperature. Chronic conditions such as diabetes insipidus, diabetes mellitus, obesity, hyperthyroidism, and cystic fibrosis may also affect thermoregulation. Acclimatization can be protective. Preventive measures include drinking adequate quantities of fluids before and during physical activity.

Core Pathophysiology

Most heat loss in these situations occurs from the skin through perspiration-induced evaporation. Cutaneous vasodilation brings skin temperature nearer to core temperature. The sympathetic nervous system controls skin blood flow through modulation of adrenergic vasoconstriction and vasodilation. Heat stress–induced vasodilatation can increase cutaneous blood flow to 60% of cardiac output. *Acclimatization* is an adaptation response that occurs over weeks in a hot environment. Adaptive responses include increase in plasma volume, enhancement of cardiovascular performance, activation of renin–angiotensin–aldosterone axis, ability to increase sweating, salt retention by sweat glands and kidneys, rise of the glomerular filtration rate, and inhibition of rhabdomyolysis. The cytokine response to temperature elevation may help prevent multi-organ dysfunction. Heat stress induces transcription of heat shock proteins, which improve the cell's ability to survive injury. Advanced age, failure to acclimatize, and genetic factors are associated with inadequate heat shock protein release.

TABLE 13.1

Risk Factors for Heat-Related Illness

FACTORS	DESCRIPTION
Socioeconomic factors	Lack of access to air conditioners; living on upper floors of buildings especially with flat roof tops; social isolation; closed doors and windows during hot weather conditions
Weather conditions	Factors that prevent heat loss from the body: reduced wind, elevated barometric pressure, high humidity, high environmental temperature at or above body temperature for prolonged periods of time
Drugs	Alcohol, amphetamines, anticholinergics, anti-Parkinson medications, β-blockers, cocaine, diuretics, ecstasy, ephedra-containing diet supplements, neuroleptics, phenothiazines, tricyclic antidepressants
Body habitus	Obesity (BMI > 85th percentile for age)
Clothing	Thick, nonabsorbable clothing
Illnesses	Mental handicap; febrile illnesses; dehydrating illnesses (diabetes insipidus, diabetes mellitus, diarrhea, and vomiting); skin diseases (anhidrosis); heat-producing illnesses (thyrotoxicosis); lack of sleep, food, or water; diminished sweating (cystic fibrosis); lack of acclimatization; previous heat stroke
Exertional heat illness	Athletes, military personnel, manual laborers, multiple same day sessions, insufficient rest/recovery between sessions, excessive physical exertion, poor acclimatization

Decompensated Response

Body temperature of 41°C–42°C leads to tissue injury within 1–8 hours and >49°C within 5 minutes. Hypovolemia follows, with a resultant decrease in skin blood flow and compromised thermoregulation. Sweating is decreased, and vasoconstriction secondary to hypovolemia further compromises heat loss. Cutaneous vasodilatation results in reduced blood flow to the gastrointestinal tract, leading to translocation of endotoxin and release of proinflammatory cytokines. The coagulation cascade is activated by heat injury, with the development of thrombin–antithrombin complexes, decreased anticoagulant protein production, and enhanced expression of adhesion molecules.

Clinical Features

Individuals who suffer from heat exposure can present with delirium, seizures, lethargy, or coma due to metabolic disturbances, cerebral edema, or infarcts. Intracranial bleeding, central pontine myelinolysis, disruption of the blood–brain barrier, and demyelination can also occur. Guillain–Barré syndrome may develop 7–10 days later.

Translocation of blood from the central circulation to the periphery can lead to hypotension, especially with hypovolemia. Conduction defects and changes in the QT interval or the ST segment can occur. Sinus tachycardia, supraventricular tachycardia, and atrial fibrillation may be observed. Tachycardia, hypotension, and increased tissue oxygen demand lead to a risk of myocardial infarction. Acute respiratory distress syndrome may develop after heat stroke, with unpredictable timing. Disseminated intravascular coagulation (DIC) may be a risk factor.

Acute tubular necrosis may result from hypovolemia, rhabdomyolysis, DIC, and direct effects of thermal injury. Lactic acidosis occurs in exertional heat stroke. Hyponatremia, hypokalemia, hypomagnesemia, and hypophosphatemia may be present initially, with eventual hyperkalemia and hyperuricemia possible from tissue damage in the setting of renal dysfunction. Hypoglycemia occurs due to rapid depletion of glycogen, rapid utilization of glucose, and liver dysfunction from splanchnic ischemia.

Liver damage from direct heat injury or hypoxemia secondary to splanchnic ischemia results in elevated transaminases, bilirubin, γ-glutamyl transpeptidase, and lactic dehydrogenase that peak at 72 hours after injury. Fulminant liver failure is uncommon. DIC may be worsened by liver dysfunction. Splanchnic ischemia leads to translocation of bacteria and endotoxin production, with subsequent release of proinflammatory mediators, leading to multisystem organ dysfunction.

Rhabdomyolysis occurs more commonly in exertional than in environmental heat stroke. It results in hyperkalemia leading to cardiotoxicity, myoglobinuria resulting in renal failure, shock or compartment syndrome from sequestration of fluid into injured muscle, and muscle necrosis of the diaphragm leading to respiratory failure.

Treatment

Emergency cooling should be undertaken without delay. The victim should be moved, sprinkled with water, and fanned constantly. Tight clothing should be removed. Cooling victims to <39°C in <30 minutes greatly improves outcome. Core temperature should be monitored. Methods of cooling and their advantages are listed in **Table 13.2**. Shivering increases body temperature and can be prevented with diazepam. Ringer lactate or normal saline is used for hydration. Seizures are treated with a benzodiazepine.

Therapy at the Tertiary Center

Body cooling should be continued until core temperature is below 39°C. Overhydration should be avoided to minimize the development of pulmonary and cerebral edema. Low cardiac output, elevated central venous pressure, mild right heart failure, and low systemic vascular resistance are seen in most victims until cooling results in vasoconstriction and increased blood pressure. Avoidance of α-adrenergic agents (vasoconstriction prevents heat loss from the skin) and anticholinergic agents (prevent sweating and increase body temperature) is important.

Hypocalcemia should be corrected cautiously due to the risk of deposition of calcium carbonate and calcium phosphate in injured skeletal muscles.

TABLE 13.2

Methods of Cooling

COOLING METHOD	DESCRIPTION	ADVANTAGES	DISADVANTAGES
External Cooling			
Immersion	Immersion of body in ice water	Faster cooling, greater temperature gradient between core and periphery	Vasoconstriction impedes heat loss; shivering; makes resuscitative measures difficult
Body-cooling unit	Spraying finely atomized water mixed with warm air to keep body temperature above 32°C–33°C	Faster cooling (mean cooling rate of 0.31°C/min or 0.56°F/min); comfortable to the patient; heat is lost by evaporation and convection	Sophisticated unit that requires maintenance and storage
Wet sheet and fan	Patients are covered with a sheet, water is sprayed over the sheet, and fans are used to blow over the wet sheet	Heat lost by evaporation; heat loss is comparable to body-cooling unit; easy maintenance	
Ice packs	Ice packs are placed over the groin, axillae, and neck	Simple and readily available; inexpensive; shorter cooling time when combined with evaporative technique	Longer cooling time compared to evaporative technique
Core Cooling			
Cold water irrigation	Gastric, bladder, peritoneal lavage, extracorporeal technique	Not well studied	Invasive, especially peritoneal and extracorporeal techniques
IV fluids	Cold IV fluid administration	Not studied	Invasive

Rhabdomyolysis, identified by elevated creatine kinase and myoglobinuria, requires aggressive hydration in order to increase urine output to >3 mL/kg/h. Alkalinization may be no better than early, aggressive hydration for treatment of rhabdomyolysis. Acute renal failure occurs in 30% of patients with exertional heat stroke and in 5% with environmental heat stroke. The most important aspect in the prevention of renal failure is to maintain adequate hydration. Shock requires fluid resuscitation, which can increase edema in injured muscles. Compartment syndrome may occur 3–4 days following injury, and fasciotomy may be required. Coagulation abnormalities peak at 24–36 hours. DIC is treated with fresh frozen plasma or cryoprecipitate if hypofibrinogenemia is also present.

HYPERTHERMIA SYNDROMES

Malignant Hyperthermia

Malignant hyperthermia (MH) occurs in genetically predisposed individuals following exposure to inhaled general anesthetics (halothane, isoflurane, sevoflurane) or succinylcholine. It is most often caused by a point mutation in the gene encoding the ryanodine receptor RYR1 leading to sustained $Ca^{2}+$ release from the sarcoplasmic reticulum on exposure to a triggering agent. Patients suspected of having MH should undergo testing at an MH testing center and wear a "Medic Alert" bracelet. Up-to-date information from the Malignant Hyperthermia Association is available at http://www.mhaus.org. The cardinal features of MH include muscle rigidity (sustained contracture), increased carbon dioxide production, acidosis, tachypnea, and tachycardia. The body temperature often exceeds 41°C. Rhabdomyolysis, hyperkalemia, ventricular tachycardia, myoglobinuric renal failure, and cardiac arrest may occur. Therapy consists of immediate discontinuation of the trigger agent. The muscle relaxant dantrolene is given as rapidly as possible and may be repeated.

Malignant Hyperthermia-Like Syndrome is a hyperglycemic, hyperosmolar nonketotic state with diabetic coma that usually occurs in obese teenage boys. Severe hyperthermia may occur after the administration of insulin. Rhabdomyolysis, hemodynamic instability, and organ failure occur with a mortality rate as high as 50%. The insulin preservative *m*-creosol, underlying fatty acid oxidation defects, and infection have been proposed as potential causes. Case reports suggest that dantrolene may be effective. Hypertonic saline may be required simultaneously since dantrolene is diluted in sterile water.

Neuroleptic Malignant Syndrome

Neuroleptic malignant syndrome (NMS) is a rare clinical syndrome associated with the use of antipsychotic drugs and characterized classically by four cardinal signs: muscle rigidity, mental status changes (confusion, agitation, catatonia, bradykinesia, encephalopathy, coma), hyperthermia, and autonomic instability (tachycardia, labile hypertension, diaphoresis). Every type of neuroleptic agent that antagonizes dopamine D_2 receptors has been associated with NMS, including haloperidol, chlorpromazine, fluphenazine, risperidone, clozapine, and olanzapine. Promethazine and metoclopramide have also been implicated. Therapy has been reported with dantrolene, bromocriptine, and amantadine. Triggering agents must be discontinued emergently.

Serotonin Syndrome

Serotonin syndrome (SS) is due to excess postsynaptic serotonergic neurotransmission, and the classical triad includes abnormalities of mental status (agitation, delirium, hypervigilance), neuromuscular function (hyperreflexia, clonus, hypertonicity, tremor, hyperkinesia), and autonomic function (hyperthermia, tachycardia, hypertension, diaphoresis, vomiting, diarrhea). A variety of psychiatric medications, herbal medications, illicit drugs, and antiemetics can predispose to SS. The management of SS relies on immediate discontinuation of the serotonergic drug and supportive care. Agitated patients should receive benzodiazepines. If the triggering agent is a monoamine oxidase inhibitor (MAOI), it is prudent to avoid inotropes (e.g., dopamine) that are metabolized by monoamine oxidase inhibitors. Severely hyperthermic patients should undergo endotracheal intubation and neuromuscular blockade to eliminate motor activity until hyperthermia resolves. An antidote is cyproheptadine, a histamine-1 (H_1) receptor antagonist with nonspecific serotonergic ($5\text{-}HT_{1A}$ and $5\text{-}HT_{2A}$) antagonistic properties, although its efficacy has not been rigorously studied.

HYPOTHERMIA

Cold-induced injuries range from frostnip and frostbite to severe hypothermia. Although hypothermia is most common during exposure to cold environments, it can also develop secondary to toxin exposure, metabolic derangement, infection, and central nervous system (CNS) or endocrine system dysfunction. *Frostnip* (also known as first-degree frostbite) is a nonfreezing injury of skin tissues, usually of the face, fingertips, or toes, following exposure to cold. Superficial ice crystals may form, but no tissue destruction occurs. Pallor and numbness or tingling of the affected skin are seen until warming occurs. Treatment is with simple rewarming. *Frostbite* is the destruction of skin or other tissues caused by freezing. It is classified as superficial (affecting skin and subcutaneous tissues) or deep (affecting bones, joints, and tendons). Reduced blood flow from vasoconstriction exacerbates the cooling process. Increased blood viscosity leads to worse microvascular damage and tissue edema.

Vasoconstriction may be followed by vasodilation as a protective response, but this shift can further decrease core body temperature.

Below-freezing temperatures, low wind-chill, high humidity, and prolonged exposure to cold are risk factors for frostbite. Superficial frostbite leads to pallor, edema, blistering, and desquamation. Deep frostbite can lead to hemorrhagic blisters, anesthesia, hyperesthesia, ulceration, and gangrene. Treatment involves removal of nonadherent wet clothing, rapid rewarming, and avoidance of rubbing damaged tissue. Preparation and protection from the effects of cold weather is the best prevention for frostbite.

When adaptive thermoregulation is overwhelmed, the body cannot generate sufficient heat and hypothermia occurs. *Hypothermia* is classified based on core body temperature as mild (35°C–32°C), moderate (<32°C–28°C), or severe (<28°C). Measurements made with infrared thermometers are often inaccurate in patients with hypothermia.

Mechanisms of Disease

Thermoregulatory response to cold requires input from peripheral skin receptors and core thermoreceptors (distributed along the internal carotid arteries and the posterior hypothalamus). Thermosensitive neurons are located throughout the CNS in close proximity to arteries so that blood and brain temperatures are closely coupled. Normal *thermogenesis*, or heat production, occurs through basal metabolism and exercise. *Facultative (adaptive) thermogenesis* occurs via voluntary physical activity, shivering, or humoral response. Shivering is the production of heat generation by muscle tremor and produces a fivefold increase in metabolic rate. Humoral thermogenesis involves release of norepinephrine leading to the production of heat by uncoupling of the metabolic chain from oxidative phosphorylation in the mitochondria. Cutaneous vasoconstriction conserves heat, and skin blood flow can be downregulated to nearly zero in extreme cold. Heat may also be conserved with insulation secondary to subcutaneous fat and by normal behavioral responses to cold exposure, both of which are less effective at the extremes of age.

Organ System Response to Hypothermia

CNS responses are slowed, and severe mental status changes and unconsciousness occur below 32°C. Myocardial irritability develops and may lead to atrial and ventricular arrhythmias, including ventricular fibrillation. J (Osborn) waves may be seen on electrocardiogram, represented by an elevation at the QRS–ST junction in the inferior and lateral precordial leads. A cold-induced diuresis occurs from increased renal blood flow, eventual loss of distal tubular reabsorption of water and sodium, and a resistance to the action of antidiuretic hormones.

The heat loss by conduction in cold water is ~20 times greater than in air and leads to very rapid cooling and decrease in organ blood flow. Conditions that involve total immersion (including the head) initiate a "diving reflex" that consists of apnea, marked bradycardia, increased peripheral vascular resistance, and increased blood supply to the brain and heart. The early shunting of oxygen to essential vascular beds and overall decrease in metabolic rate due to rapid cooling may explain survival after prolonged immersion reported in some patients.

Etiology of Hypothermia

Common Causes

Primary hypothermia occurs in otherwise healthy individuals whose ability to produce heat is overcome by excessive cold. Secondary hypothermia occurs due to an underlying condition, and death in patients with secondary hypothermia is usually due to the underlying condition.

Predisposing Factors

The high body surface area to mass ratio in infants and children results in faster rates of cooling. Low body fat decreases tissue insulation and small muscle mass lowers metabolic heat production. Neonates and the elderly can be dysthermic at seasonal temperature extremes. Alcohol and sedative drugs cause cutaneous vasodilation, inhibit the shivering response to cold, impair awareness of the cold, and impair judgment to seek shelter and warm clothing.

Clinical Presentation and Diagnosis

Even with no history of cold exposure, hypothermia must be considered in patients with typical clinical features. Pulses may be difficult to palpate due to profound bradycardia and frozen extremities. Clinical features of mild, moderate, and severe hypothermia are listed in **Table 13.3**.

Laboratory Data

Hypothermia leads to acidosis, altered blood clotting, and decreased renal function. Hypokalemia or hyperkalemia can occur. Liver function tests are abnormal secondary to reduced cardiac output. Hyperglycemia occurs acutely, but hypoglycemia may predominate later. It is important to know whether blood gas results are temperature corrected.

Clinical Management

All patients should be removed from the cold environment, wet clothing removed, and rewarmed. Evidence is lacking to support the benefit of one method of rewarming, but slow rewarming may be safer than rapid rewarming.

TABLE 13.3

Clinical Features of Hypothermia

	MILD HYPOTHERMIA (35°C–32°C)	MODERATE HYPOTHERMIA (<32°C–28°C)	SEVERE HYPOTHERMIA (<28°C)
Thermoregulatory	Shivering	Extinction of shivering	No shivering
Respiratory	Tachypnea	Hypoventilation, respiratory acidosis, hypoxemia, aspiration pneumonia, atelectasis	Apnea, pulmonary edema, acute respiratory distress syndrome
Cardiovascular	Tachycardia, hypertension	Bradycardia, hypotension, prolonged QT interval, J wave, atrial arrhythmias	Pulseless electrical activity, atrial and ventricular fibrillation, asystole
Gastrointestinal	Ileus, nausea, vomiting	Pancreatitis, gastric erosions	Pancreatitis, gastric erosions
Renal/fluid/ electrolyte	Cold diuresis, hypokalemia, alkalosis	Hyperkalemia, hyperglycemia, lactic acidosis	Hyperkalemia, hyperglycemia, lactic acidosis
Muscular	Hypertonia	Rigidity	Rhabdomyolysis
Hematologic		Hemoconcentratio, hypercoagulability	Thrombocytopeni, disseminated intravascular coagulation, bleeding
Neurologic	Disorientation, impaired judgment, dysarthria, ataxia, hyperreflexia	Agitation, hallucination, unconsciousness, dilated pupils, diminished gag reflex, hyporeflexia	Coma, nonreactive pupils, areflexia, brain-dead-like state

Passive External Rewarming

Passive rewarming (covering the head, neck, and body with blankets) reduces evaporative heat loss and allows rewarming at a rate of 0.5°C–4°C per hour. This method will be unsuccessful if shivering or other thermoregulatory mechanisms are absent, but may be adequate for patients with mild hypothermia.

Active External Rewarming

Active external warming—the application of heat directly to the skin—is only effective if the patient has an intact circulation that can return peripherally rewarmed blood to the core. Caution is necessary to prevent skin burns. Convective, forced-heated-air devices can rewarm at a rate of 1°C–2.5°C per hour. Warm water immersion is not recommended. External methods of rewarming are usually effective for mild-to-moderate hypothermia. Complications include *afterdrop*, a decrease in core temperature secondary to the rapid return of cold peripheral blood to the heart. Acidosis due to return of pooled lactic acid to the central circulation may be seen.

Active Internal Rewarming

Active internal warming methods include heated (42°C), humidified air via an endotracheal tube and heated (42°C) IV fluids via rapid infusion. Together, these methods can warm at a rate of 1°C–2°C per hour. More invasive techniques include body cavity lavage (gastric, bladder, colon, pleural, peritoneal) with warmed saline, which can warm at a rate of 1°C–4°C per hour. The most invasive methods of active internal rewarming are extracorporeal and include continuous arteriovenous or venovenous warming, hemodialysis, and cardiopulmonary bypass. Cardiopulmonary bypass is highly effective and can increase the core temperature by 1°C–2°C every 3–5 minutes and provides the benefit of full circulatory support.

Management of Patients with Arrhythmias and Cardiac Arrest

Most arrhythmias caused by hypothermia correct with rewarming alone. CPR (cardiopulmonary resuscitation) should be administered without delay in hypothermic patients with cardiac arrest. Resuscitative efforts may be prolonged, especially if extracorporeal warming is not immediately available. Resuscitative efforts should continue until the patient has been rewarmed to ~34°C, spontaneous circulation has been restored, or clearly lethal injuries are identified.

Outcomes

There are approximately 750 deaths annually in the United States due to hypothermia. The outcome of hypothermia depends on cause and comorbid conditions. The lowest initial temperatures recorded in survivors were 14.2°C in a child and 13.7°C in an adult. In patients with multisystem trauma, uncorrectable spontaneous hypothermia is associated with poor outcome.

CHAPTER 14 ENVENOMATION SYNDROMES

JAMES TIBBALLS AND KENNETH D. WINKEL

SNAKEBITE

Worldwide, there are an estimated 2 million snakebites annually, with 5%–10% mortality. The four families of venomous snakes include two major families—the Elapidae and Viperidae. Elapids include dangerous snakes from Australia (taipan, brown, death adder, tiger, and black snakes), Asia and Africa (cobras, mambas, and kraits), and Americas (coral snakes). Elapid venoms are highly neurotoxic. Vipers include the rattlesnakes of the Americas, and the old and new world vipers. Their venom causes bite site swelling and tissue destruction.

Diagnosis of Envenomation

Signs of snakebite include puncture marks (usually on a limb) accompanied by bruising, bleeding, blistering, or regional tender lymphadenopathy. If envenomation occurs, signs and symptoms (**Table 14.1**) develop, often in a predictable sequence. A more rapid illness is seen with multiple bites or in a small child.

Treatment of Venomous Snakebite

First Aid

It is prudent to treat all snakebites as serious since the degree of envenomation is not predictable. Little venom is removed by incision or excision, and so these practices are not recommended. Tourniquets are also not recommended. The pressure-immobilization technique retards the movement of venom from the bite site into the circulation, gaining time for the victim to reach medical care. A continuous bandage (as tight as when binding a sprain, 40–70 mm Hg) is applied to the whole limb with a splint (to further prevent movement). The patient is kept still. Bandages and splints should not be left in place for prolonged periods. Immobilization without pressure may be preferred for viper bites due to concerns about potentiating tissue damage by trapping venom locally.

Medical Treatment of Envenomation

If the patient has not developed symptoms or signs of envenomation within 4–6 hours of a bite, significant envenomation is unlikely. The onset of neurotoxicity and rhabdomyolysis can be delayed, and so observation should occur for at least 24 hours, particularly if the patient is a small child.

Local Effects. Viper venom causes local effects (skin blistering, limb swelling, and tissue necrosis). Fasciotomy is not helpful when crotaline antivenom has been administered. Blistering may progress to full-thickness skin necrosis over 3–7 days, and bites are prone to infection.

Coagulopathy. Australian elapid venom causes consumption of coagulation factors with thrombosis

TABLE 14.1

Expected Sequence of Symptoms and Signs after Envenomation by Elapid Snakes

<1 Hour after Bite
Headache
Nausea, vomiting, abdominal pain
Transient hypotension associated with confusion or loss of consciousness
Coagulopathy (laboratory testing or whole blood clotting time)
Regional lymphadenitis
1–3 Hours after Bite
Paresis/paralysis of cranial nerves (e.g., ptosis, double vision, external ophthalmoplegia, dysphonia, dysphagia, and myopathic facies)
Hemorrhage from mucosal surfaces and needle punctures secondary to disseminated intravascular coagulation (DIC)
Tachycardia, hypotension
Tachypnea, shallow tidal volume
>3 Hours after Bite
Paresis/paralysis of truncal and limb muscles
Paresis/paralysis of respiratory muscles (respiratory failure)
Peripheral circulatory failure (shock), hypoxemia, cyanosis
Rhabdomyolysis
Dark urine (due to myoglobinuria or hemoglobin)
Renal failure secondary to combinations of shock, hypoxemia, DIC, rhabdomyolysis, and hemolysis
Coma secondary to cerebral hypoxemia or ischemia, occasionally due to hemorrhage

and microangiopathy. Platelet consumption and fibrinolysis may occur. Fresh frozen plasma (FFP) may exacerbate these effects and is withheld unless active bleeding occurs.

Neurotoxicity. Descending paralysis, starting with ptosis and external ophthalmoplegia and progressing to respiratory failure, is typical of bites by Elapidae and a few species of Viperidae. If antivenom is delayed or inadequate doses are given, recovery may be prolonged (days to weeks).

Rhabdomyolysis and Renal Failure. Many factors may contribute to renal failure including shock, a direct toxic effect of venom, rhabdomyolysis, and disseminated intravascular coagulation (DIC). Hemodialysis is occasionally required, and long-term renal morbidity may occur.

Shock and Cardiotoxicity. Shock may be caused by fluid sequestration into necrotic tissue, altered vascular permeability, autopharmacologic phenomena, acute reactions to venom or antivenom, or cardiotoxicity (either primary or secondary to hypoxemia or ischemia). Procoagulopathy may contribute to myocardial ischemia and pulmonary hypertension.

Other. Spitting cobras of Asia and Africa and the rinkhals of South Africa spray venom from their fangs into a victim's eyes, causing blindness and painful chemical conjunctivitis. The eyes should be irrigated immediately followed by cycloplegics, topical antibiotics, and analgesia. Victims should receive tetanus prophylaxis, but antibiotic prophylaxis is only warranted for contaminated wounds.

Antivenom

Antivenom should be administered for systemic envenomation, progressive limb swelling, or limb necrosis. Symptoms or signs could include headache, nausea or vomiting, irritability, confusion, collapse, hypotension, neurologic impairment, abnormal bleeding, hematuria, or myoglobinuria. Laboratory abnormalities include a disordered coagulation profile, low or undetectable levels of fibrinogen, raised levels of fibrin degradation products, elevated serum creatine kinase level, hemoglobinuria, or myoglobinuria. Antivenom is not indicated for puncture marks and lymphadenopathy.

The correct antivenom may be selected on the basis of unequivocal morphologic identification of the snake, venom testing, or genus-specific clinical scenarios. Local poison information centers may be able to source appropriate antivenom. If a reliable identification of the snake cannot be made, then polyvalent antivenom or a selection of monovalent antivenoms, covering likely species, is used. Snake antivenoms are given intravenously. Skin testing only delays urgent therapy. Initial administration should be slow while observing for allergic reaction. Adverse reactions are common and are divided into early hypersensitivity (usually anaphylactoid), pyrogenic, and late allergic (serum sickness). Prior allergy to antivenom is not an absolute contraindication to subsequent administration. Larger initial doses should be considered if there is evidence of severe envenomation (multiple bites, rapidly progressive symptoms, or large snakes). The dose of antivenom for children should not be reduced according to weight, since the amount of venom injected is independent of victim's size. Severely envenomated patients may require multiple doses.

Premedication to reduce adverse antivenom reactions is endorsed. Subcutaneous epinephrine is recommended for polyvalent antivenom in a low-resource setting and for higher-risk patients, such as those with equine allergy and asthma. Antihistamines are not recommended on the basis of ineffectiveness. Serum sickness, due to the deposition of immune complexes, is a recognized complication of the administration of foreign protein solutions such as antivenoms. Symptoms include fever, rash, arthralgia, lymphadenopathy, and a flu-like illness occurring 7–10 days after antivenom administration. Corticosteroids should be considered if a large volume of antivenom (polyvalent antivenom or multiple ampules of monovalent antivenom) has been administered, or if the patient had a previous exposure to equine protein.

SPIDERBITE

Most spiderbites result in transient local (or radiating) pain, erythema, swelling, and itchiness. Spiders with the greatest potential to harm include funnel-web (*Atrax* or *Hadronyche* species), comb-footed (*Latrodectus* species), and recluse or violin spiders (*Loxosceles* species).

Funnel-Web Spiders

Funnel-web spiders are found on the eastern seaboard of Australia. Most funnel-web spider bites are asymptomatic, but they can cause death within 2 hours. The venom triggers the release of excessive catecholamines, eventual exhaustion of sympathetic neurotransmitters, and a characteristic biphasic syndrome. Acetylcholine is also released at neuromuscular junctions. Early symptoms are characterized by bite site pain, local swelling, erythema, numbness around the mouth, spasms or fasciculation of the tongue, nausea, vomiting, abdominal pain, sweating, salivation, lacrimation, piloerection, and severe dyspnea. Confusion can progress to coma. Initial symptoms include hypertension and tachycardia; late symptoms include hypotension, hypoventilation, apnea, acute noncardiogenic pulmonary edema, coma, and cardiac arrest. Treatment includes pressure-immobilization and antivenom. Supportive care includes atropine to reduce salivation and bronchorrhea, nasogastric aspiration to relieve gastric distension, sympathetic blockade for hypertension and severe tachycardia, and fluid resuscitation for hypotension. Tetanus prophylaxis is provided when indicated.

Comb-Footed (Widow) Spiders

The "comb-footed" spiders of the family Theridiidae are ubiquitous throughout the world. Mortality from envenomation is rare. The key toxin, *a*-Latrotoxin, forms Ca^{++} permeable pores in presynaptic membranes and stimulates the release of catecholamines from sympathetic nerves and acetylcholine from motor nerve endings. Envenomation may progress and persist for days to months. Usually the bite is painful but it may go unnoticed. Progression of illness is slow. Signs and symptoms include local pain that may last >24 hours, localized redness, piloerection, painful regional lymphadenopathy, and sweating. Systemic features include fever, hypertension, tachycardia, nausea, vomiting, abdominal pain, headache, lethargy, and insomnia. Myalgia or neck spasms may be a prominent feature in children >4 years of age. Migratory arthralgia and paresthesias can be seen. Rare complications include neurologic symptoms associated with the neuromuscular blockade and excessive catecholamine release. Antivenom is administered for pain unrelieved by simple analgesia or systemic signs of envenomation. Several vials may be required, especially if the victim sustains more than one bite or presents late. The dose should not be reduced for children. Acute reaction to redback antivenom is unusual, as is the incidence of serum sickness, and corticosteroids are not routinely recommended.

Recluse or Violin Spiders

The venom from *Loxosceles* species has variable toxicity; some species' venom causes relatively mild skin lesions and others' systemic illness. The venoms contain multiple enzymes and Sphingomyelinase D which cause dermonecrosis, myolysis, and hemolysis. The characteristic necrotic skin lesions result from the direct effect on cellular and basal membrane components and the extracellular matrix. *Cutaneous Loxoscelism* is characterized by a dermonecrotic lesion at the bite site taking weeks to heal. A perimeter of blanched skin due to venom-induced vasoconstriction surrounds lesions. A larger area of erythema may evolve in reaction to the chemical mediators leaching into surrounding tissue. A fine, macular eruption over the entire body may occur. By the third or fourth day, the hemorrhagic area degrades into a central area of blue necrosis, eventually forming an eschar and sinking below the surface of the skin. This common pattern is referred to as the "red, white, and blue sign." Eschars eventually dehisce, usually with scar formation. Venom-induced lymphangitis can be confused with a secondary infection. Transient constitutional signs and symptoms such as myalgia, malaise, fever, chills, nausea, vomiting, generalized rashes, and headache may occur. *Viscerocutaneous Loxoscelism* is more severe, consisting of low-grade fever, arthralgia, diarrhea, vomiting, coagulopathy, DIC, hemolysis, petechiae, thrombocytopenia, urticaria, and sometimes rhabdomyolysis. It occurs more frequently in children.

No definitive therapy exists. Dapsone, which inhibits polymorphonuclear cell degranulation, for loxoscelism, has inconclusive results, and side effects can be severe. Surgical debridement and skin grafting was an initial intervention for cutaneous loxoscelism, but increased acute-phase reactant release secondary to surgery may exacerbate venom effects and prolong tissue injury. Delaying surgical excision for 2–8 weeks allows dissipation of venom and acute-phase reactants. Systemic corticosteroids are not recommended for isolated cutaneous disease, but may have a role for viscerocutaneous loxoscelism. Necrotic lesions are often treated with oral antibiotics to prevent infection, but this may not be necessary. Hyperbaric oxygen treatment has been used for cutaneous loxoscelism, but there is no conclusive evidence to support its use. Antivenom is not widely available and is usually reserved for systemic loxoscelism. Regional sympathetic blockade is a potential adjunct to treat neuropathic pain, improve blood supply, and to promote healing.

SCORPION STINGS

Scorpion stings are estimated to exceed 1.2 million worldwide with 3,250 deaths annually. Scorpions are nocturnally active and inhabit hot, dry climates. Scorpion venom is a complex mixture of mucopolysaccharides, hyaluronidase, serotonin, histamine, protease inhibitors, histamine releasers, protein neurotoxins, and channel inhibitors. Life-threatening cardiovascular and neurotoxic effects are caused by most species. Pain is a universal feature of envenomation. Other neurologic symptoms include coma, convulsions, cerebral edema, external ophthalmoplegia, mydriasis, meiosis, agitation, rigidity, tremor, twitching, tongue and muscle fasciculation, respiratory failure, gastric and pancreatic hypersecretion, bradycardia, tachycardia, salivation, sweating, abdominal pain, vomiting, and priapism. Myocardial ischemia or myocarditis with raised CPK-MB isoenzymes and troponin I levels may occur in children. Direct cardiotoxicity and release of endogenous catecholamines are responsible for high systemic and pulmonary vascular resistance, low cardiac output, elevated left atrial pressure, and pulmonary edema. While antivenom reduces circulating venom antigens, the clinical relevance is questionable. The incidence of acute and delayed adverse reactions to antivenom may be significant. Supportive care is essential. In early envenomation, catecholamine release causes hypertension but later culminates in cardiac failure and hypotension. The use of hydrocortisone has not influenced outcome.

BEE, WASP, AND ANT (HYMENOPTERA) STINGS

Most stings by Hymenoptera are mild and self-limiting. Life-threatening immediate hypersensitivity reactions (anaphylaxis) can occur and cause death in minutes in hypersensitive patients. Severe systemic reactions are less common in children than adults. The risk of recurrence can persist for decades with a 30% chance of a similar reaction even 20 years later. The effects of multiple bee, wasp, or ant stings are dramatically amplified, and systemic effects include headache, vomiting, thirst, pain, edema, discolored urine (hematuria and/or myoglobinuria), jaundice, and confusion. Rhabdomyolysis may cause acute renal failure. Intravascular hemolysis, coagulopathy, thrombocytopenia, metabolic disturbances, encephalopathy, liver dysfunction, and myocardial damage may occur. The inflammatory response may precipitate an acute coronary syndrome. Treatment involves removing the stinger as soon as possible (the method is unimportant) to limit the amount of venom injected. Cold packs and oral analgesia are valuable. Large local reactions usually respond well to symptomatic treatment with nonsteroidal anti-inflammatory agents and topical steroid creams. Oral steroids and antihistamines are often used. Treatment of anaphylaxis is with epinephrine and supportive therapy with oxygen, and β-agonists for bronchoconstriction, steroids, and intravenous fluid. Individuals at risk of anaphylaxis from insect stings should carry IM epinephrine autoinjectors. Maintenance immunotherapy (with small quantities of bee or wasp venom) may be valuable.

TICK BITE

Tick bites can cause paralysis, allergic reactions, infection (zoonoses), secondary infection, and foreign body granulomas. *Tick paralysis* occurs from bites of females in a variety of *Ixodes* species. The tick may be hidden above the hairline, in a skin fold, or in any body orifice. Regional lymphadenopathy may be present. Intoxication occurs after the tick has been feeding for >3 days. Progressive weakness and ataxia develop. The paralysis commences as ascending, symmetric, lower motor neuron weakness progressing to the upper limbs and, terminally, the muscles of swallowing and breathing. Reflexes are diminished or absent. Double vision, photophobia, nystagmus, or pupillary dilation may be present. Prompt and careful removal of the offending tick(s) is essential. Failure to recover should prompt a search for additional ticks.

Zoonoses include rickettsial diseases (Q fever, tick typhus, and spotted fevers such as Rocky Mountain spotted fever), Lyme disease, and viral encephalitis. Other bacterial zoonoses include tick-borne relapsing fever caused by *Borrelia persica* and infections by *Babesia*, *Ehrlichia/Anaplasma,* and *Francisella* species. Tick-borne encephalitis, Omsk hemorrhagic fever, louping ill, and Crimean-Congo hemorrhagic fever have mortality rates of a few percent.

JELLYFISH STINGS

Jellyfish and hydroids of the Phylum Cnidaria are characterized by possession of nematocysts (stinging cells) and cause human envenomation. Tentacles are covered with millions of nematocysts ("spring loaded syringes"), which discharge toxins via a penetrating everting thread or tube upon contact. Pain increases in mounting waves, despite removal of the tentacles. The victim may scream and become irrational. The lesions resemble marks made by a whip 8–10 mm wide with a "frosted ladder pattern." Whealing is prompt and massive. Edema, erythema, and vesiculation soon follow, and when these subside (after days), patches of full-thickness necrosis leave permanent scars. Most stings are minor, although some deaths are reported. *Chironex fleckeri* antivenom is the only jellyfish antivenom manufactured. Vinegar (4%–6% acetic acid) inactivates undischarged nematocysts, and pouring it over adhering tentacles for 30 seconds prevents further envenomation. Alcohol, in any form, discharges nematocysts and must not be used for this purpose. Treatment with verapamil has been proposed to counteract the elevation of cytosolic calcium, but little evidence supports its use, and it may be harmful. Magnesium is a potential adjunct to improve antivenom effectiveness, but more studies are needed.

Irukandji syndrome is caused by small Carybdeid jellyfish. Sodium channel modulation by toxin increases catecholamines levels, causing tachycardia, increased cardiac output, and systemic and pulmonary hypertension. Severe low back pain, cramping muscle pains, nausea, vomiting, profuse sweating, headache, restlessness, and agitation occur, sometimes with hypertension. Cerebral edema and heart failure can occur. "Jellyfish" of the genus *Physalia* (Portuguese Man-o'-War, Bluebottle) are the most frequent cause of significantly painful stings. Physalitoxin is a glycoprotein with cardiovascular toxicity, leading to occasional deaths. Upon contact, contracted tentacles produce a linear lesion, like a row of beans or buttons, while uncontracted tentacles cause fine linear stings. Most stings are minor. Immersion of a stung limb in hot water provides pain relief.

OTHER STINGS

Numerous fish have dorsal or pectoral spines, which may inflict a traumatic wound made worse by deposition of venom. *Stonefish* venom depresses the cardiovascular and neuromuscular systems and has a direct effect on muscle. Less-dangerous effects are hemolysis, an increase in vascular permeability, and effects due to a variety of enzymes including hyaluronidase. Local swelling, pain, muscle weakness, and paralysis may develop in the affected limb, and shock may occur. Antivenom is recommended for all cases, except those involving only a single puncture wound with moderate discomfort. Administration of an antibiotic active against pathogens found in salt or brackish water is recommended. Tetanus prophylaxis should be given if appropriate. Severe injuries may require surgical debridement and skin grafting.

Stingrays have barbed tails, which may inflict serious leg, abdominal, or chest wounds. Direct damage by penetration of the stinging barb is of greater importance than the introduction of venom. Penetrating wounds to the chest or abdomen, however minor, should be imaged or explored, because of likely damage to internal organs. Tetanus and introduction of marine bacterial infection is possible.

Octopus bites can be highly venomous. The toxin (tetrodotoxin) causes flaccid paralysis by reversibly blocking neuronal sodium channels. Vomiting often occurs. In severe cases, complete flaccid paralysis and apnea may progress rapidly.

Cone snails fire a venom-laden miniature harpoon to rapidly paralyze prey. Conotoxins cause rapid disruption of neuronal transmission, neurotransmitter release (particularly acetylcholine), and neuroreceptor activation. A sharp stinging pain is followed by local numbness or paresthesia. In serious envenomation, weakness and incoordination of voluntary muscles occur. Recovery of full neuromuscular function may take days to weeks.

CHAPTER 15 ■ MECHANICAL VENTILATION

MARK J. HEULITT, COURTNEY D. RANALLO, GERHARD K. WOLF, AND JOHN H. ARNOLD

PHYSIOLOGY OF MECHANICAL VENTILATION

Positive-pressure mechanical ventilation requires a pressure necessary to cause a flow of gas to enter the airway and increase the volume of gas in the lungs. The volume of gas (ΔV) and the gas flow ($\dot{V}$) entering any lung unit are related to the applied pressure (ΔP) by

$$\Delta P = \Delta V/C + \dot{V} \cdot R + k$$

where R is the airway resistance, C is the lung compliance, and k is a constant that defines end-expiratory pressure.

The above equation is the *equation of motion* for the respiratory system. The applied pressure to the respiratory system is the sum of the muscle and the ventilator pressures. Pressure and flow can be measured by transducers in the ventilator. Volume is derived mathematically from the integration of the flow waveform.

To generate a volume displacement, the total forces have to overcome elastic and resistive elements of the lung and airway/chest wall. Elastic force depends on both the volume insufflated in excess of resting volume and respiratory system compliance. To generate a flow of gas, the total forces must overcome the resistive forces of the airway and the endotracheal tube (ETT) against the driving pressure gradients. We commonly measure the result of these forces as the airway pressure (P_{AWO}). In conventional ventilation, the airway pressure can be calculated as:

$$P_{AWO} = \frac{\text{Volume}}{\text{Compliance}} + \text{Resistance} \times \text{Flow}$$

The quotient of volume displacement over compliance of the respiratory system represents the pressure needed to overcome the elastic forces above the resting lung volume (i.e., the functional residual capacity, FRC). Pressure, volume, and flow are all measured relative to baseline values. Thus, the pressure necessary to cause inspiration is the change in airway pressure above positive end-expiratory pressure (PEEP), representing the change from baseline pressure to peak inspiratory pressure. The same principle applies to the volume generated during inspiration (the tidal volume, V_T), the change in lung volume during inspiration above FRC. The pressure necessary to overcome the resistive forces of the respiratory tract is the product of the maximum airway resistance (R_{max}) and the inspiratory flow. Flow is measured relative to its end-expiratory value and is usually zero at the beginning of an inspiratory effort, unless *intrinsic PEEP* ($PEEP_i$) is present. In this circumstance, flow may still be occurring within the lung as alveoli attempt to achieve their baseline state (i.e., due to time-constant differences, overfilled alveoli may be emptying into underfilled alveoli to help both to achieve their "best" resting volume), an effect known as *pendelluft*. When $PEEP_i$ is present, it takes greater "effort" from the patient and the ventilator to generate sufficient flow to move gas into the lung. Pressure, volume, and flow are clinician-controlled variables, while resistance and compliance depend on the resistive and elastic properties of the respiratory system and cannot be directly controlled.

VENTILATOR CONTROLLERS

The *mode of ventilation* determines how the ventilator delivers the mechanical breath. Any of the three variables (pressure, volume, or flow expressed as functions of time) can be predetermined. This principle is the basis for classifying ventilators as *pressure, volume,* or *flow* controllers. The ventilator controls the airway pressure waveform, the inspired volume waveform, or the inspiratory flow waveform. In this context, pressure, volume, and flow are the *control variables*. The determinants of how a mechanical breath is delivered include not only control variables, but also phase and conditional variables. *Conditional* variables are determinants of a response to a preset threshold, which are clinician set and influenced by dependent and independent variables. *Phase variables* are those that are used to start, sustain, and end the phase.

Control Variables

Compliance relates to the change in volume in the lung as a result of a change in pressure. Thus, pressure is related to volume and to the patient's compliance.

$$\text{Pressure} = \frac{\text{Volume}}{\text{Compliance}}$$

If the clinician sets pressure as the control variable, volume varies directly with the compliance of the respiratory system. During expiration, the elastic and resistive elements of the respiratory system are passive, and expiratory waveforms are not directly affected by the modes of ventilation or the controller. For the resistive components of the equation of motion,

$$\text{Pressure} = \text{Resistance} \times \text{Flow}$$

When a ventilator operates as a constant-pressure controller, the set pressure is delivered and maintained constant throughout inspiration, independent of the resistive or elastic forces of the respiratory system. Even though pressure is constant, the delivered V_T will vary as a function of compliance and resistance, and the flow will also vary with time. When a ventilator operates as a constant-flow controller, pressure and V_T vary with time, depending on the compliance and resistance. Modern ventilators can operate as a *flow controller* or *pressure controller*.

In pressure control (PC) ventilation, the pressure pattern is "square," but flow increases rapidly at the beginning of the inspiratory phase to generate the set pressure limit, and then decays exponentially over the inspiratory time. This flow pattern is described as *decelerating flow*. In PC mode, the initial "snap" of high flow may be beneficial in opening stiff alveoli in conditions such as acute respiratory distress syndrome (ARDS) or surfactant deficiency. Decelerating flow may improve gas exchange and distribution of ventilation among lung units with heterogeneous time constants. For this reason, clinicians often choose PC ventilation in patients with poor compliance, although the benefit of PC has not been well established in animal or clinical studies.

If the clinician sets volume as a function of time, then pressure varies with compliance. Volume is the independent variable and pressure the dependent variable. Most ventilators cannot directly measure volume; rather, they calculate volume delivered from flow over a period of time. The ventilator is referred to as *volume cycled*, but it is really acting as a flow controller.

Volume Measurement

The goals of modern mechanical ventilation in infants and children have focused on preventing overdistension of alveoli by limiting V_T, thus reducing volutrauma. During the inflation phase of mechanical ventilation, pressure rises within the ventilator circuit, causing elongation and distension of the tubing. The volume compressed within the ventilator tubing that never reaches the patient is termed the *compressible volume of the circuit*. When compression volume is accounted for in determining V_T, the resultant volume is termed the *effective tidal volume* (eV_T), which means that this is the V_T that reaches the patient's lungs.

The optimal site for monitoring volumes in infants and children is unclear. The inability to accurately measure V_T is caused by difficulty compensating for volume loss in the ventilator circuit or humidifier and changes in temperature, humidification, and secretions that influence the amount of gas delivered. Air leaks around the ETT are another source of volume measurement error. Measuring V_T at the proximal airway eliminates most circuit compliance and other dead-space factors, but requires placing a pneumotachograph at the patient's airway opening or ETT, which creates dead space and makes suctioning more difficult. Secretions can distort measurements, and increased weight on the ETT may increase the risk of extubation.

When examining volume inaccuracies, the first source of error would be loss within the ventilator circuit resulting from compression volume. The volume loss can be affected by temperature and humidity of the circuit and changes in the patient's compliance and resistance. Manufacturers have attempted to compensate for volume losses within the ventilator by measuring compression volume loss in the system. Generally, the ventilator-displayed V_T is overestimated without software compensation for circuit compliance and underestimated when the circuit-compliance compensation is on.

Phase Variables

Phase variables control the ventilator during the period between the beginning of one breath and the initiation of the next breath. Expiration is passive and not described in this terminology. In each phase, a particular variable is measured and used to initiate, sustain, or end the phase. The phase variables include trigger variable (determines initiation of inspiration), limit variable (determines what sustains inspiration), and cycle variable (determines termination of inspiration).

Trigger Variables

A ventilator breath can be initiated in two ways; a controlled breath is delivered independent of the patient's desire or coordinated with the patient's effort. Inspiration is initiated when one of the variables (pressure, volume, flow, or time) reaches a preset value. A *patient-triggered* breath provides patients with some autonomy to alter breathing patterns. Such systems must sense a signal from the patient, recognize the beginning of inspiration, and then begin a breath. Finally, the system must recognize the end of inspiration and termination of the breath. If this interaction is optimized, patient comfort could be improved. Recognition of the signal from the patient to begin inspiration is *triggering*. The most common trigger variables are time and flow.

In *time-triggering*, the ventilator initiates a breath according to a set frequency independent of the patient's efforts. In *flow-triggering*, the ventilator senses the patient's inspiratory effort as a change in flow from baseline. Ventilator features that affect the trigger phase include the response time of the ventilator and the presence of bias flow. *Bias flow* is a continuous delivery of fresh gas circulating through the inspiratory and expiratory limbs of the circuit. Theoretically, bias flow reduces the work of breathing (WOB) by making flow available to satisfy the earliest demand of the patient during inspiration. Flow-triggering allows the patient to trigger the ventilator with less effort and a faster response time. *Pressure-triggering* requires a negative pressure to be created, which can be difficult when the patient has a small ETT or if intrinsic PEEP is present.

Neurally adjusted ventilatory assist (NAVA) involves acquisition of the patient's neural respiratory transmission through the phrenic nerve to the diaphragm. An esophageal catheter with imbedded electrodes captures the electrical signal of the diaphragm, and NAVA provides the requested level of ventilatory support. NAVA is being investigated in clinical trials in Europe.

Work of Breathing

The forces encountered while breathing include the elastic forces of the chest wall and lungs, the viscous and turbulent resistance of air, the nonelastic tissue impedance, and inertia. Work is performed to expand and contract the lungs by pressures applied from the ventilator, respiratory muscles, or both. During normal ventilation, WOB overcomes the elastic and frictional resistance of the lungs and chest wall. Resistive WOB is also imposed by the breathing apparatus (e.g., ETT, breathing circuit, and ventilator demand-flow system) and the airway physiology. WOB increases during weaning from prolonged mechanical ventilation. Equipment factors affect the ability of the mechanical ventilator to meet the needs of the patient and have increased significance in patients with poor pulmonary reserve or high airway resistance.

Limit Variable

The limit variable is the modality that sustains inspiration. Inspiration time is the time interval from the beginning of inspiratory flow to the beginning of expiratory flow. During inspiration, pressure, volume, and flow increase above their end-expiratory values. If one of these variables increases to a preset value, it becomes a *limit variable*. The limit variable determines what *sustains* inspiration and differs from the *cycle variable*, which determines the *end* of inspiration.

Cycle Variable

The cycle variable terminates inspiration, and varies according to the mode of ventilation. In *pressure-support ventilation* (PSV), the termination of inspiration is triggered by reaching either an absolute level or fixed percentage of peak inspiratory flow. In a patient with increased airway resistance and dynamic hyperinflation, a short inspiratory phase and prolonged expiratory phase may be desirable. The opposite may be true for patients with decreased pulmonary compliance.

PATIENT–VENTILATOR ASYNCHRONY

Patient–ventilator asynchrony is failure of two controllers to act in harmony (the clinician-controlled ventilator and the patient's respiratory muscles). Asynchrony can occur through several different mechanisms.

Trigger Asynchrony

Trigger asynchrony occurs when muscular effort fails to trigger a breath. It can occur in almost any ventilator mode. Trigger asynchrony is also associated with the development of auto-PEEP. To trigger the ventilator, patients with obstructive lung disease who develop $PEEP_i$ must generate enough negative intrapleural pressure to match the value of $PEEP_i$ plus the sensitivity threshold. Dynamic hyperinflation ($PEEP_i$) in patients with obstructive lung disease results in frequent nontriggering of breaths, wasted breathing effort, and patient distress. In patients in whom $PEEP_i$ is present, application of external PEEP may reduce nontriggered breaths by narrowing the difference between mouth pressure and alveolar pressure at end expiration. Similarly, in patients with high resistance to airflow from airway edema or constriction (such as asthma), external PEEP can help to "stent open" airways and improve flow during expiration.

Flow Asynchrony

Flow asynchrony occurs when the ventilator flow does not match the patient's flow need. Flow from the ventilator can be delivered in a fixed (VC ventilation) or variable flow pattern (PC or PRVC). During ventilation with variable flow, the peak flow depends on set target pressure, patient effort, and the compliance and resistance of the respiratory system. In PC mode, the clinician can set target pressure and rate of flow acceleration (rise time). Patients may require a rapid rise time to match demand. While adequate flow is necessary, too much flow in children with small ETTs may lead to increased turbulence of gas and increased asynchrony.

Termination Asynchrony

Termination asynchrony occurs when patient inspiratory time and ventilator inspiratory time differ. The most common cause is delayed termination, but it can also be premature termination. Delayed termination can result in dynamic hyperinflation and missed trigger attempts if the patient cannot overcome the effects of $PEEP_i$. Patients with high airway resistance (e.g., bronchopulmonary dysplasia or chronic obstructive pulmonary disease) may have prolonged inspiratory time if using a ventilator mode that allows the patient to trigger spontaneous breaths. This situation can occur in PSV and result in early activation of expiratory muscles with premature termination of the ventilator breath.

Expiratory Asynchrony

Expiratory asynchrony occurs due to a shortened expiratory time, a prolonged expiratory time, or patient efforts during expiration when the ventilator is unresponsive. Shortened expiratory time creates the potential for hyperinflation secondary to air trapping. Current active exhalation valves sense patient effort even during exhalation. This mechanism contrasts with systems that require the patient to wait for expiration to terminate before another ventilator breath can be triggered.

DETERMINING INITIAL SETTINGS FOR MECHANICAL VENTILATION

The clinician must recognize that the goal of ventilatory support is not to achieve a normal blood gas at the cost of ventilator-induced lung injury. Lung protective strategies for obstructive lung disease (e.g., asthma) avoid high airway pressures and hyperinflation-associated complications by using lower V_Ts and prolonged exhalation times. Spontaneous breathing in a support mode provides more patient control over exhalation time. Previously, minimal levels of PEEP were used in patients with obstructive disease; however, levels of PEEP that match the level of auto-PEEP can splint airways open, ensure adequate oxygenation, and improve exhalation. Patients with poor lung compliance require settings that provide lung recruitment. Lung protection in this situation is accomplished by limiting excessive distension and changes in alveoli distending pressure and providing adequate PEEP to maintain alveolar recruitment during expiration.

LUNG RECRUITMENT

Lung recruitment is a strategy to re-expand collapsed lung and maintain adequate PEEP to prevent "derecruitment." The benefits of optimal lung recruitment are (a) reduced intrapulmonary shunt fraction with improved arterial oxygenation, (b) improved pulmonary compliance by shifting the compliance curve to the point where less pressure is required for the same change in volume, and (c) prevention of a cyclic opening and collapse of alveolar units. The use of a recruitment maneuver may provide a long-term improvement in oxygenation.

Ideal patients for recruitment maneuvers are those with early ARDS (before the onset of fibroproliferation). Preexisting focal lung disease that predisposes to barotrauma (e.g., extensive apical bullous lung disease) is a relative contraindication. Patients with "secondary" ARDS (e.g., following abdominal sepsis) are more likely to respond favorably to recruitment maneuvers than patients with "primary" lung disease. Several methods are used clinically for recruitment. Most apply an intermittent increased positive pressure to the lung for a limited time.

POSITIVE END-EXPIRATORY PRESSURE

PEEP can be added to any mode of mechanical ventilation. PEEP delivers a distending pressure to increase FRC. Maintaining PEEP above closing pressure minimizes alveolar collapse, which decreases intrapulmonary shunting of blood and improves arterial oxygenation. PEEP increases intrathoracic pressure with potential hemodynamic consequences for both the right and left heart. The most dramatic effect is decreased venous return to the right heart. In children with normal cardiac function, increasing intravascular volume with administration of isotonic crystalloids or colloids can overcome this problem.

PEEP Titration

Although many methods have been used to identify the "best" PEEP in patients with lung disease, none conclusively improves survival. Most methods use an analysis of flow, volume, and pressure at varying PEEPs to determine a point of optimal recruitment (**Fig. 15.1**). As the lung is inflated from zero end-expiratory pressure, the point at which the compliance and hence volume abruptly increase is the *lower inflection point* (LIP), the point at which alveolar recruitment occurs. As the lung is further inflated, another point is reached where the pressure–volume slope (i.e., compliance) abruptly decreases, the *upper inflection point* (UIP). Ultimately, volume no longer changes with each change in pressure and represents overdistension of the lung. Ideal PEEP is thought to be 2–3 cm H_2O greater than the LIP and less than the UIP. Other studies have suggested titrating the PEEP to just above the critical *closing* pressure (deflection point) measured during expiration. Titrating PEEP to maximize O_2 delivery is another method to achieve lung recruitment, avoid overdistension, and maintain hemodynamic stability at lower FIO_2, especially when P–V measurement is impractical.

MODES OF VENTILATION

Intermittent Mandatory Ventilation

During intermittent mandatory ventilation (IMV), a preset number of positive-pressure (mandatory)

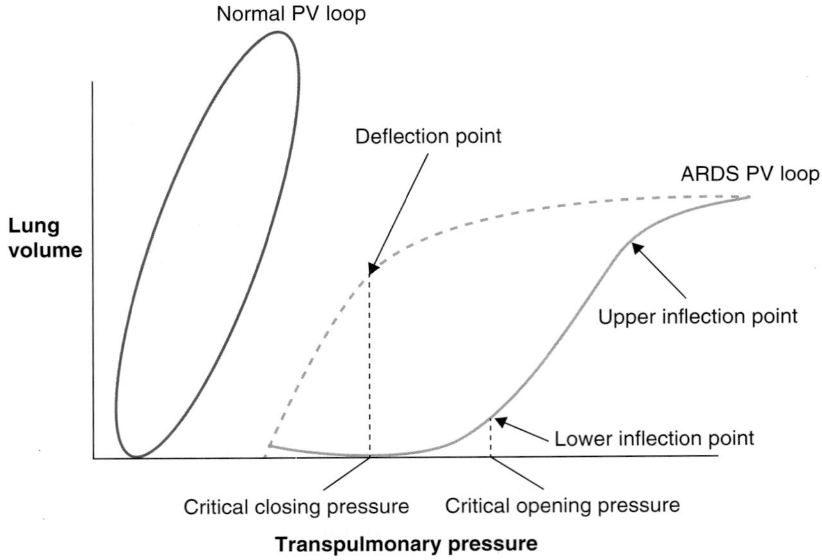

FIGURE 15.1. Pressure–volume (P–V) loop of the normal lung (blue) and the acute respiratory distress syndrome (ARDS) lung (red) with inspiratory limb (solid) and expiratory limb (dashed). Note that the lung volumes and compliance (slope of inspiratory P–V limb) are reduced in ARDS. During inflation of the ARDS lung, the lower inflection point is reached where lung units open and compliance increases until overdistension decreases compliance at the upper inflection point. During deflation, a point is reached (deflection point) where lung volume suddenly decreases as lung units close.

breaths are delivered between which the patient can breathe spontaneously. The variables of volume or pressure can control the mandatory breaths. IMV contrasts with single-control modes (assist control, PC, VC) because the patient is allowed to breathe spontaneously between mandatory breaths. The most common mode of IMV is SIMV, in which mandatory (machine) breaths are synchronized via a timing window to the patient's effort (**Fig. 15.2**). This mode is commonly combined with PS (to provide support for nonmandatory breaths).

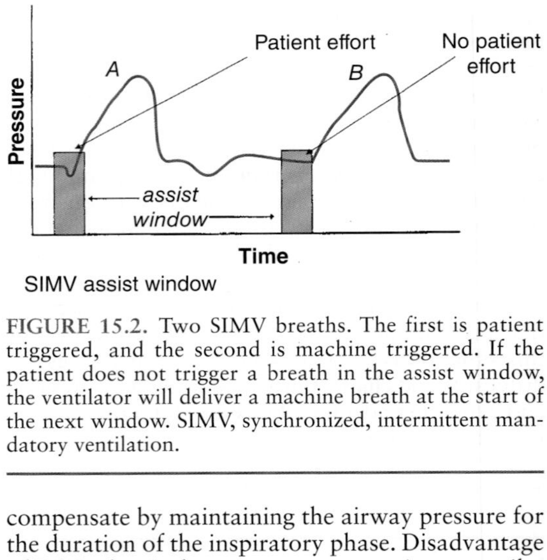

FIGURE 15.2. Two SIMV breaths. The first is patient triggered, and the second is machine triggered. If the patient does not trigger a breath in the assist window, the ventilator will deliver a machine breath at the start of the next window. SIMV, synchronized, intermittent mandatory ventilation.

Pressure-Controlled Ventilation

During PC ventilation, a pressure-limited breath is delivered during a preset inspiratory time at a preset respiratory rate (**Fig. 15.3**). The V_T is determined by the preset pressure limit and the respiratory compliance and resistance. The flow waveform is decelerating. As the alveolar pressure rises with increasing alveolar volume, the rate of flow drops off. The set pressure is maintained for the duration of inspiration. The high initial flow with PC ventilation easily meets the patient's flow demands, especially in patients with "stiff" lungs. The peak inspiratory pressure during PC ventilation is usually lower than VC ventilation for the same V_T. During PC breaths, the distribution of ventilation may be more even in a lung with heterogeneous mechanical properties. PC is also useful in the patient with an air leak. Although volume is lost through the leak, the ventilator will attempt to compensate by maintaining the airway pressure for the duration of the inspiratory phase. Disadvantage of PC is that it does not guarantee minute ventilation, and therefore requires close observation if compliance is changing. Worsening compliance may result in hypoventilation and hypoxia, and improved compliance may lead to volutrauma.

Volume-Controlled Ventilation

In the VC mode, the ventilator delivers a set V_T with a constant flow during a set inspiratory time at a

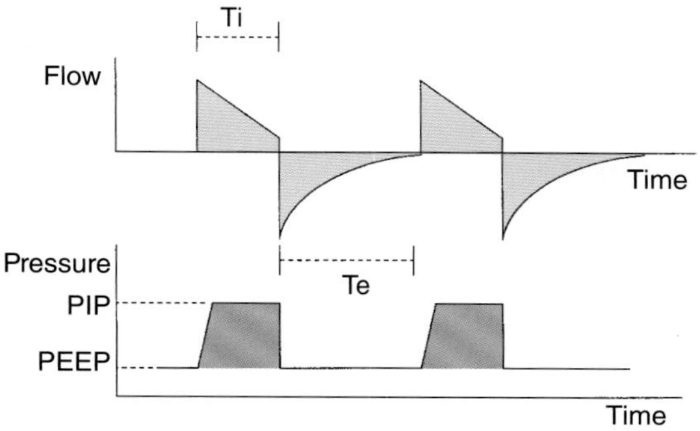

FIGURE 15.3. Pressure-controlled breath. Note that the flow pattern is rapidly decelerating from high initial flow to baseline. Ti, inspiratory time; Te, expiratory time.

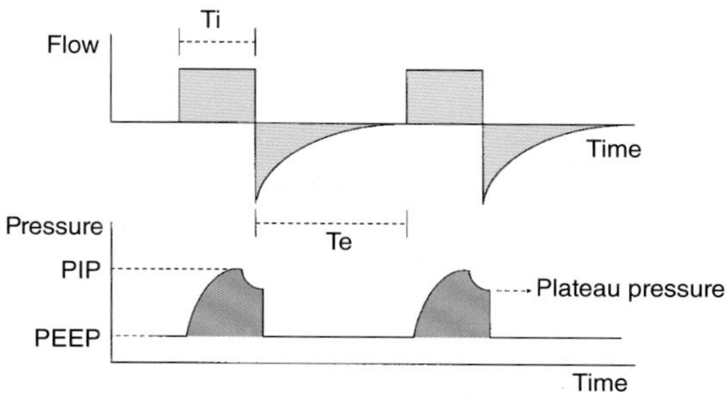

FIGURE 15.4. Volume-controlled breath. Note that the flow pattern is square with an initial high flow that is maintained during inspiration and then quickly terminated at expiration. Ti, inspiratory time; Te, expiratory time.

set respiratory rate (**Fig. 15.4**). Airway and alveolar pressures are dependent variables and will rise or fall depending upon changes in lung mechanics or patient effort. There is control of the patient's minute ventilation, if only a small leak is present around the ETT. The constant-flow delivery in VC may not meet patient demands and the peak inspiratory pressure is higher.

Proportional-Assist Ventilation

Proportional-assist ventilation (PAV) amplifies airway pressure proportional to inspiratory flow and volume. In PAV, the level of support is determined in an interaction between the patient and the ventilator. Despite some potential advantages, no studies have demonstrated outcome benefits. PAV is currently not available in the United States.

Airway-Pressure-Release Ventilation

Airway-pressure-release ventilation (APRV) is a high-level CPAP mode with intermittent brief terminations. The elevated mean helps oxygenation, and the releases assist CO_2 removal. Spontaneous breathing is allowed during all phases of the cycle (**Fig. 15.5**). In addition to FIO_2, the set parameters in APRV mode are P_{high}, T_{high}, P_{low}, and T_{low}, where P and T equate to pressure and time. P_{high} should be set at a level equivalent to the plateau pressure being used in a conventional mode when transitioning to APRV. If APRV is the first mode to be used, P_{high} is set at ~20–30 cm H_2O, P_{low} at zero, T_{high} at ~4–6 seconds, and T_{low} initially at ~0.2–0.6 seconds. T_{low} should then be adjusted based on the expiratory gas flow waveform so that the expiratory flow falls to ~25%–75% of peak expiratory flow. Generally, T_{low} will be shortened in restrictive disease and lengthened in obstructive disease. The P_{high} and T_{high} control oxygenation and alveolar ventilation. Counterintuitive to conventional concepts of ventilation, the extension of T_{high} can be associated with a decrease in $PaCO_2$ as machine frequency decreases. To minimize derecruitment, the time (T_{low}) at P_{low} is brief. Partial assistance (tube compensation) can be added to the spontaneous breaths. After the patient improves, APRV can gradually be weaned by lowering the P_{high} and extending the T_{high}. The goal is to arrive at straight CPAP. The ability to breathe spontaneously may decrease the need for sedation or neuromuscular blockade. Disadvantages are that V_T varies and spontaneous breaths may increase end-inspiratory lung volume beyond that set by the inflation pressure. APRV has not been compared to other forms of ventilation in a controlled fashion.

Hybrid Techniques

Pressure-regulated volume control (PRVC, adaptive pressure ventilation, variable PC, autoflow, or volume control plus) is a dual-control (pressure and volume regulated), breath-to-breath mode. PRVC has a variable decelerating flow pattern with time-cycled breaths. All breaths are volume targeted, with pressure adjusted to reach that volume target. Minute ventilation is assured, pressure-induced lung damage is minimized, and automatic weaning of pressure occurs as the patient's compliance improves.

Support Modes of Ventilation

PSV delivers a clinician-selected amount of positive pressure to assist a spontaneous inspiratory effort. PSV can be used to overcome the work associated with ETT resistance or, at higher levels, as a standalone support mode. Changes in resistance and compliance will affect the V_T delivered. Sedation can decrease respiratory drive and require a back-up rate. *Volume-support ventilation* is essentially PS with a V_T target. Most hybrid modes will automatically

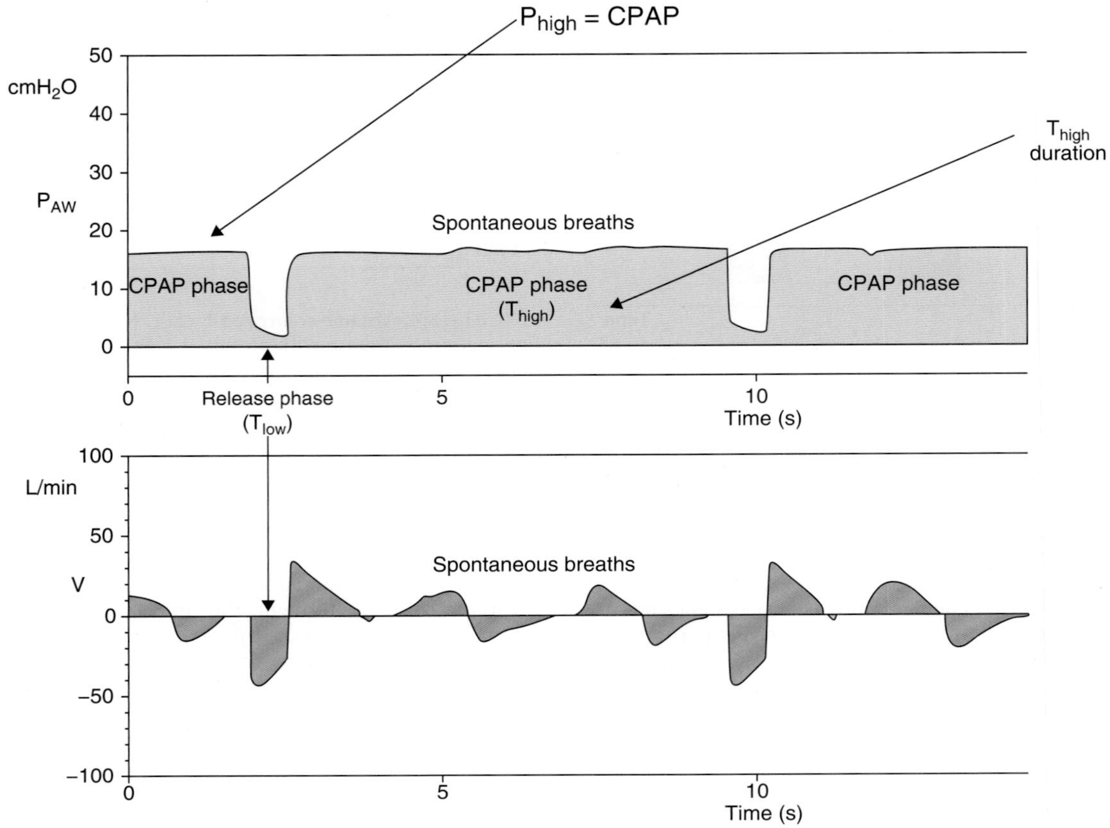

FIGURE 15.5. APRV: The CPAP phase (P_{high}) is intermittently released to a P_{low} for a brief duration (T_{low}) reestablishing the CPAP level after a set time. Spontaneous breathing may be superimposed at both pressure levels and is independent of time-cycling. (Adapted from Slonim AD, Pollack MM. Mechanical ventilation. In: Slonim AD, Pollack MM, Bell MJ, et al. eds. *Pediatric Critical Care Medicine*. Philadelphia, PA: Lippincott Williams & Wilkins, 2006.)

alarm and switch to an assist-control or SIMV mode if the patient's respiratory rate becomes inadequate.

HIGH-FREQUENCY VENTILATION

High-frequency ventilation (HFV) delivers minimal V_Ts that approximate the anatomic dead space at respiratory rates that greatly exceed normal. The strategy is to limit the delivered V_Ts and optimize recruitment to minimize atelectrauma and volutrauma.

In *high-frequency oscillation ventilation* (HFOV), a nearly square waveform is generated either by a diaphragm or piston. Inspiration and expiration are both active. Fresh gas flow pressurizes the system to the required MAP. The magnitude of the oscillations (often referred to as ΔP) is controlled by the distance traveled by the piston or the diaphragm. The inspiratory time is set as a percentage of the respiratory cycle. Inspiratory times of 33% or 50% (I:E ratio of 1:2 or 1:1) are frequently used. Frequencies range from 3 to 15 Hz (180–900 breaths/min). MAPs for neonates and infants range from 3 to 45 cm H_2O. Adults and children >35 kg usually require an oscillator model with a more powerful diaphragm and can require MAPs up to 55 cm H_2O.

In *high-frequency jet ventilation*, a jet ventilator is combined with a conventional ventilator. The jet ventilator is the source of small delivered V_Ts and the conventional ventilator provides the bias flow. The V_T of the jet ventilator is a result of the driving pressure of the jet, resistance of the ETT, and the set inspiratory time. *High-frequency flow interrupters* involve the use of a valve mechanism in the ventilator's expiratory limb that rapidly alters flow and causes a pulsating gas flow. Due to their limited bias flow, they are usually limited to neonates.

Mechanisms of Gas Exchange

Despite V_Ts that approach anatomic dead space, adequate gas exchange is maintained. Gas exchange

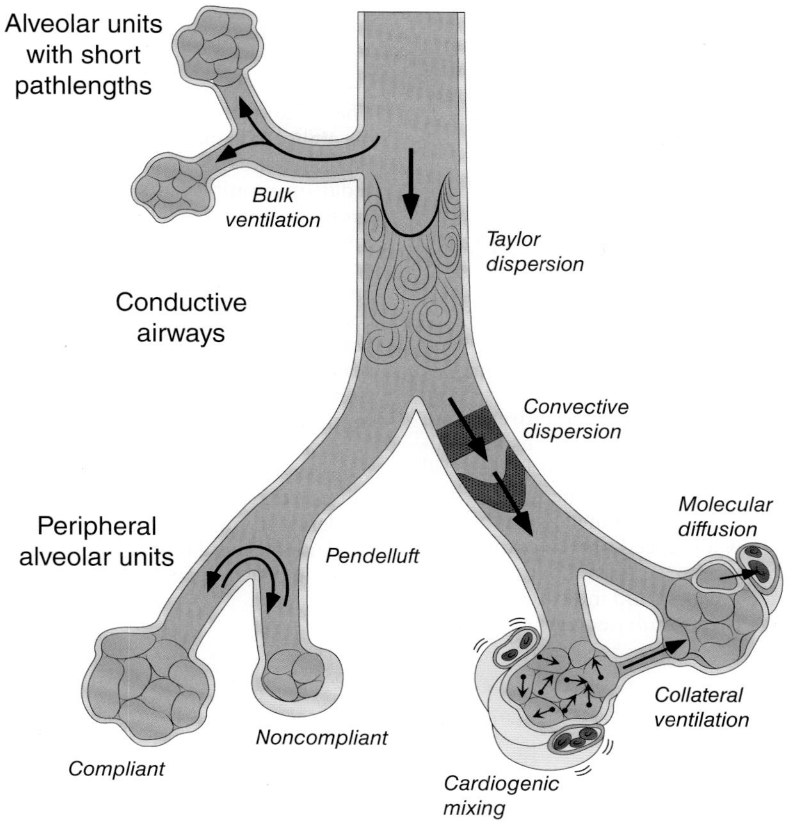

FIGURE 15.6. Mechanisms of gas exchange during high-frequency ventilation.

is achieved by a complex interplay of different mechanisms (**Fig. 15.6**). A small V_T may reach proximal alveoli with short path lengths by *bulk ventilation*. *Taylor Dispersion* occurs when the initial planar surface of a gas column transforms into a parabolic surface, allowing longitudinal mixing and dispersion. Turbulence further contributes to gas exchange. *Convective dispersion* occurs when air molecules undergo mixing as molecules in the center of the gas column move distally and the molecules near the wall stay behind. *Pendelluft* refers to the equilibration of gas between lung units with different time constants and regional mixing contributes to gas exchange. *Collateral ventilation* occurs between neighboring alveoli through collateral channels such as the *interalveolar pores of Kohn*. *Molecular diffusion* is the passive diffusion of gas molecules through the alveolocapillary membrane that occurs in peripheral lung units. *Cardiogenic mixing* occurs when cardiac-induced pressure changes in the vascular bed add to gas mixing on the alveolar level.

Technical Description of High-Frequency Ventilation

Alveolar Recruitment

Mean Airway Pressure. Optimal lung volume during HFV is the lowest MAP that achieves oxygenating efficiency and maintains lung volume. The diameter and length of the ETT affect both MAP and pressure amplitude. Air trapping occurs if the inspiratory time is increased at the expense of the expiratory time, and I:E ratios are typically limited to 1:2.

Carbon Dioxide Elimination

Alveolar Ventilation. Alveolar ventilation is a function of the rate of oscillations and the squared V_T ($V_{CO_2} = f \times V_T^2$). V_T contributes more to CO_2 elimination than frequency. Increasing the amplitude leads to increasing V_Ts and improves CO_2 elimination. Conversely, decreasing the amplitude decreases the delivered V_T and CO_2 elimination. The frequency has a significant effect on delivered V_T. As V_Ts are more important than rate for CO_2 elimination, decreasing the rate results in more efficient oscillations, larger V_Ts, and improved CO_2 clearance. An ETT cuff leak can enhance CO_2 clearance in HFV. The leak allows a path of CO_2 egress around the ETT.

WEANING FROM MECHANICAL VENTILATORY SUPPORT

Predictive Indices for Discontinuation from Mechanical Ventilatory Support

Predicting the success of weaning children from mechanical ventilation has been defined using clinical signs and symptoms, yet extubation failure still occurs in 24% of cases. Respiratory therapist-driven weaning protocols are being examined and adult and pediatric studies show a reduced time to extubation. It is not reasonable to expect an extubation failure rate to be 0% because this would indicate that some patients could have been extubated earlier.

Noninvasive Mechanical Ventilatory Support

The advantages of NIV over invasive ventilation are the ability to maintain speech, cough, and gag reflexes, flexibility in the suspension of the therapy, lower sedation requirements (especially older children), avoidance of laryngeal damage/tracheal stenosis, and lower secondary pneumonia rates. Complications of NIV include skin breakdown, gastric distention, and interface discomfort. While NIV should not be considered in pending respiratory arrest or shock, patients with acute or chronic respiratory failure may benefit from NIV (especially those in whom intubation has high complication rates, such as asthma or immunocompromised patients).

A well-fitted interface is key to the success of NIV; whether that can be accomplished with a nasal or full face mask depends on the patient facial structure, tendency to mouth breathe, and patient size. High-flow nasal cannula therapy appears to improve WOB in some disease processes.

CHAPTER 16 ■ INHALED GASES AND NONINVASIVE VENTILATION

ANGELA T. WRATNEY, DONNA S. HAMEL, IRA M. CHEIFETZ, AND DAVID G. NICHOLS

The use of inhaled gases and of noninvasive respiratory support provides therapeutic resources fundamental to the management of critical care illness.

HUMIDIFICATION

Providing inhaled gas therapy that bypasses the upper airway, or is administered with high pressure or flow, requires careful attention to temperature, humidification, and infection. The risks include hypothermia, inspissated secretions, airway injury, and the development of ventilator-associated pneumonia.

OXYGEN

O_2 is provided to patients with impaired respiratory function to improve arterial O_2 saturation, to vasodilate the pulmonary capillary bed, and to enhance systemic oxygen delivery. Arterial O_2 tension may fail to rise despite supplemental O_2 for the following reasons: 1) hypoventilation (e.g., oversedation); 2) decreased ventilation -perfusion ($\dot{V}/\dot{Q}$) matching in the lung (e.g., pneumonia, atelectasis). Low mixed venous O_2 saturation magnifies hypoxemia from decreased $\dot{V}/\dot{Q}$ ratios. The mixed venous O_2 saturation is reduced when systemic O_2 demand exceeds O_2 supply (e.g., shock, anemia); and 3) anatomic right-to-left shunt (e.g., cyanotic congenital heart disease).

Oxygen Delivery Systems

Depending on the desired F_{IO_2}, a variety of devices exist for administering supplemental O_2 (**Table 16.1**).

Nasal Cannulae

Although highly variable in practice, a general "rule of thumb" states that for each liter of supplemental O_2 flow, the inspired O_2 concentration increases by −4%. Rapid respiratory rates, large tidal volumes, and short inspiratory times increase air dilution and reduce F_{IO_2}. High flow (e.g., >2 L) may provide significant positive end-expiratory pressure (PEEP) to infants, and heating and humidification are necessary to prevent nasal drying, irritation, and heat loss.

Face Masks

A *non-rebreathing face mask* has one-way valves to ensure that each inspiration consists of fresh gas without entrainment of room air and that exhaled gas is eliminated into the environment rather than the reservoir bag. A *partial rebreathing mask* has an attached reservoir bag and an inflow gas source, but lacks unidirectional valves. To avoid rebreathing exhaled CO_2, the inspired gas flow rate should be maintained at or above 6 L/min. *Venturi masks* are high-flow systems that provide fixed concentrations of O_2. Dependable O_2 concentrations are administered as long as total gas flow exceeds the patient's peak inspiratory flow rate.

Risks

Oxygen Toxicity

O_2-mediated pulmonary toxicity pathologically resembles acute respiratory distress syndrome (ARDS). The patient may complain of chest pain, cough, and tracheal inflammation. Decreased pulmonary

TABLE 16.1

Fraction of Inspired Oxygen Provided by Various Delivery

DELIVERY SYSTEM	F_{IO_2} DELIVERY (%)	FLOW REQUIRED (L)
Nasal cannula	24–50	<6
Face mask	<60	6–10
Venturi mask	<60	Variable
Partial rebreather	<60	15
Non-rebreather	~100	15

compliance and abnormal gas exchange result from impaired surfactant activity. Inflammatory cell infiltrates contribute to proteolytic damage, loss of the alveolar–capillary membrane integrity, and pulmonary edema. Although an FIO_2 of 0.50 is commonly regarded as safe, toxicity may be seen with even brief periods of exposure to lower levels of O_2. The mechanism underlying oxygen toxicity involves the creation of reactive oxygen species, which results in oxidative injury in organs rich in lipids and proteins, such as the pulmonary and central nervous system.

Hypercapnia

Administering oxygen to patients with a chronically compensated respiratory acidosis may induce an increase in $PaCO_2$. Hypercarbia may occur secondary to (a) loss of hypoxic pulmonary vasoconstriction, (b) decreased stimulation of peripheral chemoreceptors resulting in reduced ventilatory drive, and (c) the decreased CO_2-binding affinity of oxyhemoglobin (i.e., the Haldane effect).

INHALED NITRIC OXIDE

Inhaled NO (iNO) is used as a selective pulmonary vasodilator to reduce pulmonary vascular resistance and treat pulmonary arteriolar hypertension. Endogenous NO is synthesized within most cells of the human body from arginine and O_2 by one of three isoforms of NO synthase (NOS): neural, inducible, and endothelial. Constitutive NO production is found in the vascular endothelium, neurons, platelets, adrenal medulla, and macula densa of the kidney. NO induces upregulation of cytosolic guanylyl cyclase, triggering the activation of cyclic guanosine 3′,5′-monophosphate (cGMP)–dependent protein kinases (**Fig. 16.1**) and resulting in smooth muscle cell relaxation and pulmonary arteriolar vasodilation due to decreased intracellular calcium levels. Phosphodiesterase enzymes cause cGMP levels within the smooth muscle cell to fall. Phosphodiesterase enzyme inhibitors (e.g., sildenafil, zaprinast, and dipyridamole) preserve the cGMP-dependent cascade and may provide a synergistic increase in the vasodilatory effects of iNO. iNO provides a selective pulmonary vasodilator due to rapid inactivation of iNO to nitrosylmethemoglobin before it enters the systemic circulation.

Nitric Oxide Delivery Systems

iNO is generally delivered during mechanical ventilation, but can also be delivered to nonintubated patients via a tight-fitting face mask, transtracheal O_2 catheter, or nasal cannula. During mechanical ventilation, iNO is injected into the inspiratory limb of the ventilator circuit in synchrony with each inspiratory breath. iNO has an effective half-life of 15–30 seconds.

NO Metabolite Monitoring

During iNO administration, the measurements of NO_2 and methemoglobin levels are necessary to prevent NO-induced toxicity. Toxic levels of NO_2 (>2 ppm) are rare when administering iNO at doses <40 ppm. Blood methemoglobin levels should be monitored within 4 hours of initiating iNO and after every 24 hours of continued treatment.

NO Dosing and Weaning

iNO doses 5–20 ppm should produce a clinical response in oxygenation and/or pulmonary vascular resistance. Continuous iNO >40 ppm does not produce greater benefit and results in increased methemoglobin and nitrogen dioxide levels. Abrupt discontinuation of iNO may precipitate $\dot{V}/\dot{Q}$ mismatch, pulmonary hypertension, and hemodynamic compromise. The addition of enteral pulmonary vasodilators (e.g., sildenafil and bosentan) may facilitate weaning from iNO and help to prevent rebound pulmonary hypertension.

HELIUM–OXYGEN MIXTURES (HELIOX)

Helium is administered clinically as a helium–oxygen mixture, referred to as *heliox*. Owing to its low density, heliox can improve respiratory distress, work of breathing, and deposition of bronchodilator therapy to obstructed lower airways. Heliox therapy in *viral croup* appears to benefit children short term while awaiting the onset of the effects of dexamethasone. The National Asthma Education and Prevention Program (NAEPP) indicates that heliox may be added to inhaled β-agonists for impending respiratory refractory to other therapies.

Helium is an odorless, tasteless, and noncombustible gas. Premixed heliox provides 20% O_2 (80:20 mixture), 30% O_2 (70:30 mixture), or 40% O_2 (60:40 mixture). As gas flow becomes less turbulent in the affected airways, flow velocity is reduced, and the flow pattern may transition from turbulent to more laminar. This transitional zone is represented by the Reynolds number (Re). A lower Re indicates gas flow with greater laminar flow characteristics.

$$Re = 2Vr\rho/\eta$$

where V = gas velocity, r = airway radius, ρ = gas density, and η = gas viscosity.

Heliox Delivery Systems

Heliox is normally administered to nonventilated patients in respiratory distress via a face mask with a reservoir bag or non-rebreather mask. Heliox delivery through mechanical ventilators may also be effective to reduce air trapping and airways resistance

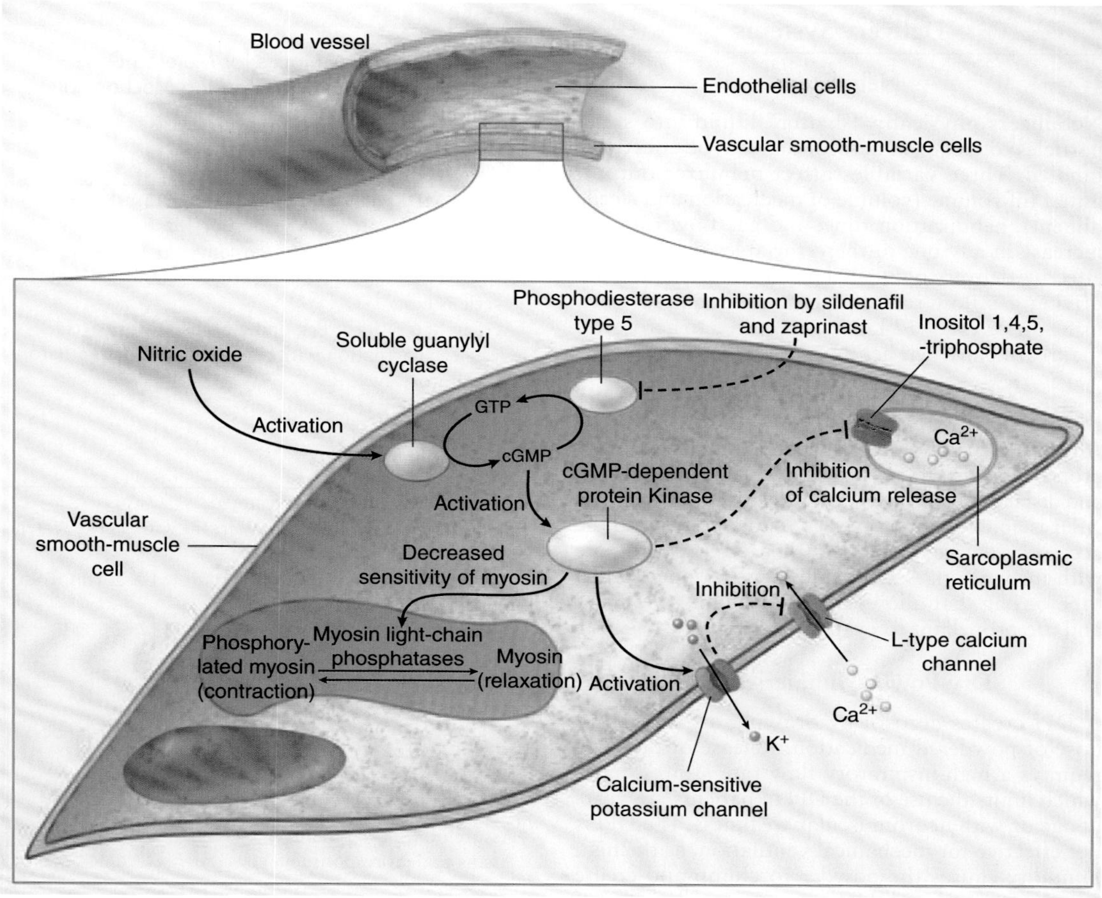

FIGURE 16.1. iNO causes pulmonary vascular endothelial smooth muscle cell relaxation, induces pulmonary capillary smooth muscle cell relaxation, and induces upregulation of guanylyl cyclase, resulting in cytosolic increase of cyclic guanosine 3′,5′-monophosphate (cGMP). cGMP-dependent protein kinase (cGKI) ultimately lowers the intracellular calcium concentration and decreases the sensitivity of myosin to calcium-induced contraction. (Adapted from Griffiths MJD, TW Evans. Drug therapy: Inhaled nitric oxide therapy in adults. *N Engl J Med* 2005;353:2683–95.)

in partially obstructed airways. Most mechanical ventilators can be adapted to administer heliox, but calibration is required. One must also account for the greater flow rate delivery when heliox is used.

Safety Considerations

When heliox is in use, air flow turbulence is minimized and coughing efficacy may be reduced. Removing the face mask briefly to wash out the heliox gas effects allows the patient to generate an effective cough.

INHALED BRONCHODILATOR THERAPY

Inhaled bronchodilator therapy is provided to relieve lower airway bronchoconstriction, reduce airway resistance, and improve $\dot{V}/\dot{Q}$ matching. The inhaled β-agonists (e.g., albuterol, metaproterenol, pirbuterol, levalbuterol, fenoterol, and salbutamol) interact with type 2 β-receptors (β_2) on the luminal surface of bronchial smooth muscle cells. The inhaled anticholinergic agent ipratropium bromide competitively inhibits acetylcholine binding at the M_3 muscarinic receptor located on bronchial smooth muscle cells to decrease intracellular cyclic AMP (cAMP) and cause bronchodilation.

Adverse effects of β_2 agents include vasodilation, decreased systemic vascular resistance, tremors, and hypoinsulinemia, which may result in a widened pulse pressure, hyperglycemia, and hypokalemia. β-Adrenergic type 1 receptor binding causes tachycardia, palpitations, and arrhythmias. Albuterol is a 1:1 racemic mixture of the R- and S-isomers. The R-isomer, levalbuterol, is responsible for bronchodilation while the S-isomer contributes to side effects, toxicity, and tolerance (observed with chronic use).

Delivery Systems

Nebulizers

Nebulizers physically "shatter" liquid into small particles to create an aerosol that can be effectively inhaled. Three variables affect nebulizer output: initial fill volume (volume of medication and sterile diluent), nebulization time, and gas flow rate. An increase in any one of these variables increases the effective delivery of inhaled medication. A minimum driving gas flow rate of 8 L/min is required when using air or O_2; >12 L/min is required to aerosolize the treatment when heliox is used.

Metered-Dose Inhaler (MDI)

An MDI consists of drug suspended in a mixture of propellants, surfactants, preservatives, flavoring agents, and dispersal agents within a pressurized canister. The MDI is actuated once every 15–20 seconds into the accessory device, to reduce the need to coordinate with inspiration. A spacer device is an open-ended tube or bag that allows the MDI plume to expand and the propellant to evaporate.

Dry-Powder Inhalers (DPI)

A DPI creates aerosol by drawing air through a dose of powdered medication. Release of the drug requires a high-inspiratory flow rate (>50 L/min), which limits the use of the DPI in patients <6 years of age or with neuromuscular weakness. The DPI is not effective for mechanical ventilation, as the high humidity causes the powder to clump and create large particles that do not aerosolize well.

Mechanically Ventilated Patients

Inhaled bronchodilators may be effectively administered and equally therapeutic in the mechanically ventilated patient using a nebulizer or MDI. Humidity within the circuit significantly decreases aerosol deposition. Positioning the delivery device so that it bypasses the humidifier increases medication delivery by a factor of 4 (**Table 16.2**).

TABLE 16.2

Recommended Techniques for Metered-Dose Inhaler and Nebulizer Use during Mechanical Ventilation

Metered-Dose Inhaler
Agitate MDI and warm to hand temperature
Place MDI adaptor into inspiratory limb of circuit (18–30 cm from the Y-piece connector)
Attach MDI to adaptor in ventilator circuit (chamber-style is best)
Actuate ≥6 puffs at beginning of inspiratory cycle
Cycle each actuation with a spontaneous or ventilator inspiratory cycle
Wait ≥5 s between actuations
Assess patient response
Nebulizer
Establish dose to be administered
Place drug in nebulizer reservoir; fill with sterile water to ≥4 mL
Place nebulizer in inspiratory circuit ≥18–30 cm from the patient Y-piece connector
Initiate driving gas flow of oxygen ≥6 L/min; ≥12 L/min when heliox is used
Turn off flow by or continuous flow during nebulization
Continue nebulization treatment until sputtering occurs, indicating end of treatment
Remove nebulizer and return ventilator to previous settings
Assure no leak in circuit
Assess patient response

Adapted from Fink JB. Metered-dose inhalers, dry powdered inhalers, and transitions. *Respi Care*. 2000;45(6);623–35.

INHALATIONAL ANESTHETICS

Inhalational anesthetics have been administered in the intensive care unit (ICU) to treat medically refractory bronchospasm (isoflurane, desflurane), refractory pain (isoflurane, N_2O), refractory status epilepticus (isoflurane), and for sedation (isoflurane, desflurane, sevoflurane). Inhaled anesthetics should be used only under the supervision of an anesthesiologist.

General Principles

To reach peak sedative effect, the inspired concentration must reach equilibrium within the pulmonary alveolar capillary and subsequently with brain tissue. The end-tidal alveolar gas concentration is continuously monitored to determine the number of minimum alveolar concentration (MAC) of the volatile agent administered to the patient. For each inhaled anesthetic agent, 1 MAC refers to the concentration required to prevent movement in 50% of patients in response to surgical stimuli.

Isoflurane

Isoflurane (1-chloro-2,2,2-trifluoroethyl difluoromethyl ether) is a fluorinated, nonflammable ether that is volatile at room temperature. In the ICU, isoflurane has been used to treat severe bronchospasm in cases refractory to conventional medical therapies. Isoflurane may affect multiple pathways involved in the relief of bronchospasm, and antagonize the actions of both histamine and acetylcholine. It is postulated that isoflurane activates the sympathetic system to cause elevated endogenous catecholamine levels, leading to bronchodilation. Isoflurane is eliminated almost completely from the lungs.

Isoflurane dosing in the ICU setting is initiated at 0.5% and titrated to clinical effect up to 2%. Dose-dependent side effects include systemic vasodilation and increased sympathetic stimuli, which result in increased cardiac output, skin flushing, and tachycardia. Isoflurane increases cerebral blood flow, may increase intracranial pressure, but reduces cerebral O_2 consumption. It is a potent coronary vasodilator, which improves coronary blood flow and decreases myocardial O_2 consumption. The bronchodilator effect is immediate and sustained. For patients who do not respond within 4–6 hours of maximal anesthetic support, consideration for extracorporeal support is warranted. Slow weaning of isoflurane 0.1%–0.2% on average every 30 minutes to 1 hour is recommended.

Delivery Systems

The ICU ventilator is usually adapted for use with inhaled anesthetics and an active scavenging system added. Active scavenging systems and appropriate turnover of ambient air are required to protect patients and staff from inadvertent exposure. Continuous infrared monitoring equipment for both the inspired and the expired concentrations of O_2, CO_2, and the inhalational agent is necessary.

Safety Considerations

The safety of prolonged inhaled anesthetic administration, particularly in the critically ill, has not been established. Abstinence syndrome has been reported. Fluoride ion nephrotoxicity is associated with prolonged isoflurane exposure. Nephrotoxicity has been reported with serum fluoride levels ≥50 μM/L, resulting in decreased glomerular filtration rate and nephrogenic diabetes insipidus. Acute concerns during use of inhalational anesthetics include the rare, but treatable, onset of malignant hyperthermia. Continuous temperature monitoring is necessary, and dantrolene sodium should be readily available for any patient receiving an inhaled volatile anesthetic.

NONINVASIVE VENTILATION

Noninvasive Positive-Pressure Ventilation (CPAP and BiPAP)

The noninvasive positive-pressure ventilation (NIPPV) interface may be nasal prongs, a nasal or full face mask, or helmet. Exhalation ports exist on the mask or within a separate attachment in the circuit (non-rebreathing valves or exhalation ports) to introduce an intentional leak and prevent rebreathing of exhaled carbon dioxide. A soft adhesive gelatin patch is often used to protect the nasal bridge. NIPPV may be applied in the mode of CPAP or BiPAP. BiPAP permits the clinician to set the inspiratory positive airway pressure (IPAP) and expiratory positive airway pressure (EPAP) separately. The difference between the IPAP and EPAP is known as the pressure support, and should be at least 4 cm H_2O. CPAP delivers a continuous level of positive airway pressure.

NIPPV is indicated in patients with acute respiratory failure, dynamic upper airway obstruction, alveolar hypoventilation syndromes, and chronic respiratory failure. Other indications include the following:

1. Infants and children with poor systolic ventricular function after open-heart surgery. These patients are very sensitive to increased afterload to the heart, which is reflected by the left ventricular transmural pressure (LV_{TM}), where
   LV_{TM} = aortic pressure − pleural pressure
   Infants with cardiac disease and respiratory distress develop very negative pleural pressures, which lead to increased LV_{TM} and increased LV afterload.
2. After extubation from mechanical ventilation. The elective application of NIPPV immediately after extubation appears to be more effective than rescue NIPPV.
3. To support patients with chronic neuromuscular disease at baseline, during respiratory illness, for postoperative recovery, and in settings of acute illness. The IPAP is often increased to 12–24 cm H_2O and EPAP to 3–8 cm H_2O. Clinicians should attempt to wean FIO_2 as tolerated. An increasing supplemental oxygen requirement may mask atelectasis owing to retained secretions in these patients.

Safety Considerations

NIV allows enteral nutrition in most patients, although there are no guidelines to favor a specific mode of enteral feeding (continuous vs. intermittent, gastric vs. postpyloric). However, a recent meta-analysis revealed that jejunal feedings were associated with a lower relative risk of pneumonia (but no difference in vomiting or aspiration) compared with gastric feedings.

High-Flow Nasal Cannula

High-flow nasal cannula (HFNC) systems offer independent adjustment of FIO_2 and humidified, warmed, gas flow to match the inspiratory flow demands of tachypneic patients. Recommended flow rates are ≤2 L/min for premature or term infants, up to 12 L/min for older infants to toddlers, up to 30 L/min for children, and up to 40 L/min for adults.

Safety Considerations

We generally recommend postpyloric feeds when older infants receive HFNC ≥ 8–10 L and in patients of any age who have reflux or a history of aspiration, or require the higher HFNC flows for age.

CHAPTER 17 ■ EXTRACORPOREAL LIFE SUPPORT

GRAEME MACLAREN, STEVEN A. CONRAD, AND HEIDI J. DALTON

Extracorporeal life support (ECLS) or extracorporeal membrane oxygenation (ECMO) is the use of a modified cardiopulmonary bypass (CPB) circuit to support children with refractory respiratory and/or circulatory failure.

CIRCUIT COMPONENTS

The components of an ECLS circuit, while based on the CPB circuit, have been developed or adapted for long-term support (**Fig. 17.1**).

Oxygenator

The latest generation of artificial lungs is hollow-fiber oxygenators. Many are coated with heparin to decrease the risk of clotting. Blood flows over the hollow fibers while fresh gas (100% oxygen or an air–oxygen mixture) runs through them, facilitating gas exchange. The rate of fresh gas flow ("sweep") is the principal determinant of carbon dioxide clearance.

Blood Pump

Two types of blood pumps are being used for ECMO. The roller pump is a positive-displacement pump in which a rotating roller head squeezes a length of blood-filled tubing against a backing plate as the roller head rotates. This pump is used with gravity drainage and requires an assist reservoir (bladder) at the pump inlet to maintain a continuous supply of blood. The centrifugal pump is a nonocclusive pump that generates flow via a rotating impeller. These pumps have extremely low incidence of mechanical failure. The main risk with their use is hemolysis, which manifests as increased plasma hemoglobin levels.

Vascular Cannulas

Traditional cannulation involves separate single-lumen cannulas for venous drainage and for return to the circulation. Double-lumen cannulas have been developed specifically for venovenous (VV) ECLS. Placed through the internal jugular vein, these VV

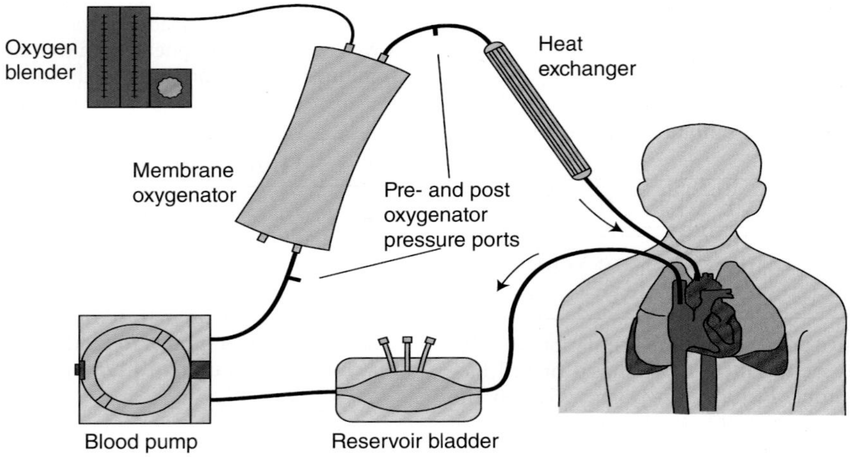

FIGURE 17.1. Components of a typical extracorporeal circuit. The circuit consists of a drainage reservoir (bladder), blood pump, membrane lung, heater–cooler, and connecting tubing. In many modern centrifugal pump circuits, the heater–cooler is integrated into the oxygenator and no reservoir is used.

cannulas have drainage ports located near both atriocaval junctions and a reinfusion port located between and directed toward the tricuspid valve. Most centers have a cannulation chart for bedside use that compares cannula size, expected blood flow rate, and patient weight.

Other Components

The heater–cooler unit is essential in children on ECLS, especially infants. Pressure monitors are used to monitor the development of excessive pressures across the membrane oxygenator, providing an indication of the development of clotting and impairment of blood flow.

PATIENT SELECTION

Indications

Hypoxemic Respiratory Failure

The most common causes of hypoxemic respiratory failure in children that lead to ECLS are viral pneumonia (19%), bacterial pneumonia (11%), and acute respiratory distress syndrome (ARDS) (10%). The selection criteria for ECLS are reviewed in **Table 17.1**.

Hypercapnic Respiratory Failure

Severe hypercapnia with respiratory acidosis, in particular severe asthma, is effectively managed by VV extracorporeal support. Low-flow extracorporeal CO_2 removal ($ECCO_2R$) can be delivered with blood flow of ≤20% of the cardiac output.

TABLE 17.1

Criteria Used in Selection of Patients for ECLS for Pulmonary Support in Hypoxemic Respiratory Failure

Severe, potentially reversible acute respiratory failure
Lack of response to conventional support measures[a]
Severe hypoxemia
$PaO_2/FIO_2 < 80$
Oxygenation index > 40
Qs/Qt > 0.5
Elevated inflation pressures
MAP > 20 on conventional ventilation, >30 on HFOV
Persistent air leak or interstitial air
Cardiovascular depression with shock (pH < 7.25)
Lack of irreversible ventilator-induced lung injury
Duration of mechanical ventilation <14 d

[a]Conventional support may include measures such as high-frequency oscillation, inhaled nitric oxide, prone positioning, surfactant, or others.
Qs/Qt, intrapulmonary shunt; MAP, mean airway pressure; HFOV, high-frequency oscillatory ventilation.

Circulatory Failure

Circulatory failure refractory to conventional treatment accounts for >50% of pediatric ECLS beyond the neonatal period. Venoarterial (VA) support is the mode of choice, as it provides CPB and maintains systemic circulatory flow at normal levels. In cases of severe myocardial dysfunction, the ventricle cannot empty against the afterload associated with ECLS-maintained arterial pressure. Persistent elevation of end-diastolic pressure can result in pulmonary hypertension, pulmonary edema, pulmonary hemorrhage, and impairment of myocardial recovery. When required, the left heart can be decompressed via atrial septostomy, performed in the cardiac catheterization suite or at the bedside. If this is not possible, the systemic ventricle can be vented by surgical insertion of an atrial or ventricular drainage cannula, which is then incorporated into the venous drainage of the ECLS circuit by means of a Y connector. VA ECLS can be used as a bridge to transplantation, but long-term outcomes may be better with a ventricular assist device (VAD) rather than ECMO.

Newer Indications

The American College of Critical Care Medicine provides an algorithm of recommendations prior to instituting ECLS in refractory pediatric septic shock. Patients with septic shock may require high circuit flows to meet increased metabolic demand while preventing differential cyanosis (see below). Central cannulation (right atrium and aorta) may be helpful in shock states to provide higher flows. Another evolving use of ECLS is extracorporeal cardiopulmonary resuscitation (ECPR), involving the rapid institution of ECLS during cardiac arrest.

Contraindications

Contraindications to ECLS are shown in **Table 17.2**, which should not be offered if likely to be futile.

TABLE 17.2

Potential Contraindications to ECLS

Absolute Contraindications
Extremes of prematurity or low birth weight (<32 wk gestational age or <1.5 kg)
Lethal chromosomal abnormalities (e.g., Trisomy 13 or 18)
Uncontrollable hemorrhage
Irreversible brain damage
Relative Contraindications
Intracranial hemorrhage
Less extreme prematurity or low birth weight in neonates (<34 wk gestational age or <2.0 kg)
Irreversible organ failure in a patient ineligible for transplantation
Prolonged intubation and mechanical ventilation (>2 wk) prior to ECLS

TABLE 17.3

Comparison of Cardiopulmonary Bypass and Different Modes of ECLS

	CPB	VA ECMO	VV ECMO	VAV ECMO	$AVCO_2R$
Setting	Cardiac surgery	Prolonged support	Prolonged support	Prolonged support	ED or ICU support
Support	Total cardiac and pulmonary	Cardiac and pulmonary	Pulmonary	Cardiac and pulmonary	Pulmonary
Cannulation	Intrathoracic (surgical)	Extrathoracic (surgical)	Extrathoracic (percutaneous)	Extrathoracic (percutaneous)	Extrathoracic (percutaneous)
Blood pump	Roller or centrifugal	Roller or centrifugal	Roller or centrifugal	Roller or centrifugal	None (pumpless)
ECMO blood flow (fraction of CO)	Total (100%)	Subtotal (70%–90%)	Subtotal	Subtotal (1/3–2/3 arterial, remainder venous)	Low (10%–20%)
Pulmonary flow	None	Low	Unchanged	Moderate decrease	Unchanged
Length of support	Hours	Days to weeks	Days to weeks	Days to weeks	Days
Anticoagulation	ACT > 400	ACT 180–200	ACT 180–200	ACT 180–200	ACT 200–220
Reservoir	Large	Small or none[a]	Small or none[a]	Small or none[a]	None

[a]Reservoir used for roller pump, optional for centrifugal pump.
CPB, cardiopulmonary bypass; VA, venoarterial; ECMO, extracorporeal membrane oxygenation; VV, venovenous; VAV, venoarteriovenous; $AVCO_2R$, arteriovenous carbon dioxide removal; ED, emergency department; ICU, intensive care unit; CO, cardiac output; ACT, activated coagulation time.

MODES

ECLS modes have advantages and disadvantages for different clinical situations (**Table 17.3**).

Venovenous

VV ECLS is the preferred mode for management of severe respiratory failure in children. No direct cardiac support is delivered, and myocardial function commonly improves with increased myocardial oxygenation and reduced intrathoracic pressures.

Venoarterial

VA support is based on CPB; blood is drained from the right atrium and returned to the proximal arterial system, bypassing the ventricles and the pulmonary system. There is a higher potential for complications (e.g., cerebral embolism, reduced pulmonary blood flow, increased ventricular afterload, and loss of right carotid circulation from ligation).

Venoarteriovenous

The venoarteriovenous (VAV, also venovenoarterial) mode is a hybrid, combining VV support for pulmonary failure with partial VA support, and it has the advantage of percutaneous cannulation.

Arteriovenous

The application of AV CO_2 removal ($AVCO_2R$) is identical to $ECCO_2R$, without the need for a pump. It reduces mechanical ventilatory support and controls hypercapnia.

CANNULATION

Patients placed on ECLS in the operating room may be centrally cannulated. The cervical approach (carotid and internal jugular cannulation) is common in children not yet able to walk. In older children (>15 kg), percutaneous femoral approach may be adequate but limb ischemia is a potential hazard (risk reduced by a surgically placed anterograde perfusion cannula).

Percutaneous Cannulation

VV support is almost exclusively approached percutaneously. Dual-lumen catheters are available in sizes from 13 to 31 Fr, suitable for neonates to adults. The catheter is placed by percutaneous puncture of the right internal jugular using the Seldinger technique, and the tip is maneuvered into the inferior vena cava under ultrasound or fluoroscopic guidance. Percutaneous arterial cannulation is limited to the femoral artery in larger children who require VA ECLS.

Peripheral Surgical Cannulation

The open surgical technique is preferred for VA support through the common carotid artery and internal jugular (IJ) vein. Femoral cannulation is an additional option for VA support. Surgical placement of a dual-lumen venous cannula into the IJ for VV bypass can also be performed.

Central Cannulation

ECLS following failure to wean from CPB or sternotomy for resuscitation uses the same cannulas placed for intraoperative support. The chest is incompletely closed and dressed, usually with a silastic membrane sutured over the defect.

PHYSIOLOGY OF EXTRACORPOREAL CIRCULATION

Venovenous

The aims of VV ECLS for isolated respiratory failure are oxygenation, CO_2 clearance, and lung rest. Less blood flow (e.g., 10–15 mL/kg/min) is needed to remove CO_2 than to oxygenate blood (generally >40–50 mL/kg/min). The goal is to place the catheter with the largest diameter and shortest length as allowed by the venous anatomy to maximize blood flow.

Venoarterial

Venoarterial ECLS provides circulatory support by returning oxygenated blood under pressure into the arterial circulation, with circuit blood flow rates set to arbitrary norms based on the child's weight. In septic shock (higher flows may be needed), it is appropriate to use the same time-critical, goal-directed principles as for patients not receiving ECLS.

Adverse Effects

Nonpulsatile Flow

Stroke volume diminishes as ECLS flow increases and is recognized as a diminishing pulse pressure on the arterial waveform. When cardiac contractility is sufficiently impaired and unable to eject blood against the afterload provided by the circuit, distension of the left ventricle may result and may require the left-heart decompression as previously discussed.

Blood Component Damage

High shear rates applied to erythrocytes induce membrane changes (altered deformability) or disruption (hemolysis). Injury to plasma proteins, platelets, and white blood cells contributes to activation of coagulation and inflammation.

Activation of Coagulation and Systemic Inflammation

The ECLS circuit is a large, nonendothelial contact surface that activates the coagulation system. Systemic anticoagulation is mandatory (usually with heparin which accelerates the action of antithrombin III but does not inhibit thrombin formation). Activation of macrophages and other immune cells produces pro-inflammatory mediators (e.g., tumor necrosis factor [TNF], interleukin-1 [IL-1], and IL-6) and results in systemic inflammation.

CIRCUIT MANAGEMENT

Priming and Initiation of Support

The ECLS circuit volume is substantial relative to patient blood volume, mandating that the circuit prime consist of a solution that has normal electrolyte concentrations. A blood prime is necessary in smaller children, especially neonates. Cannulation takes place at the bedside under local or general anesthesia, or in a nearby procedure suite if fluoroscopy is used. An initial bolus of heparin (50–100 U/kg) is administered just prior to cannulation.

Anticoagulation and Hematologic Management

The procoagulant ECLS circuit requires continuous administration of a systemic anticoagulant. The goal activated clotting time (ACT) is usually between 180 and 200 seconds. Multiple factors influence ACTs and other coagulation tests may be needed. Platelet dysfunction is common during ECLS support (possibly an acquired von Willebrand syndrome). A platelet count of 80,000–100,000 is maintained initially and during bleeding complications, lower values may be accepted once transfusion requirements bleeding have stabilized.

Troubleshooting

Thrombi (*clots*) forming postoxygenator on VA ECLS have the potential to cause systemic embolization to the patient. Thrombi detection should prompt a review of anticoagulation strategies, an evaluation for hemolysis, and discussion of when to change the circuit.

Air embolism is a rare but serious complication of ECLS. The oxygenator acts as a bubble trap to minimize this risk. Bubble detectors can inform of the problem and stop circuit flow.

Differential cyanosis may occur on VA ECLS and is most commonly seen with femoral cannulation when there is a combination of significant ventricular ejection and profound lung disease. Pulse oximetry on the right hand should be monitored as a surrogate for right coronary and carotid oxygenation. A right radial arterial line and cerebral near-infrared spectroscopy (NIRS) are additional monitoring options. If blood passing through the lungs cannot be adequately oxygenated by modest increases in positive end-expiratory pressure (PEEP) and FIO_2, then consideration should be given to changing to VV, VAV, or central VA ECLS.

Weaning

For weaning from VV ECLS, the ventilator is set for moderate support (e.g., PIP $\leq$ 30 cm H_2O, $FIO_2 \leq$ 50%, PEEP $\leq$ 10 cm H_2O, and rate < 20–30) and the fresh gas flow to the oxygenator is turned off. For weaning from VA ECLS, the patient is fully ventilated and ECLS flow is reduced at discrete intervals over a period of 4–8 hours, with serial assessment of perfusion, myocardial function, and blood gases until a terminal flow of 25% of full support is achieved.

PATIENT MANAGEMENT

Ventilator Management

The goal is to maintain alveolar recruitment, avoid overdistension, minimize shear stress associated with tidal ventilation, and avoid O_2 toxicity. Use of pressure-limited ventilation, elevated levels of PEEP (10–12 cm H_2O), low ventilator rates (6–10/min), and small tidal volumes (<6 mL/kg) usually meet these goals. PEEP is usually lower (5–10 cm H_2O) in patients with heart disease on VA ECLS. Spontaneous breathing with coughing better clears lower airway secretions. Early tracheostomy or extubation while on ECLS allows mobility of patients and facilitates spontaneous breathing and may be desirable in specific scenarios.

Hemodynamic Management

After the initiation of ECLS support, vasoactive agents can often be weaned off. In patients on VA ECLS with severe cardiac dysfunction, it is common to enhance contractility with low-dose inotropes (e.g., ≤0.05 mcg/kg/min epinephrine or ≤5 mcg/kg/min dobutamine) to facilitate aortic valve opening and prevent stasis of blood in the systemic ventricle and aortic root.

Sedation and Analgesia

Increased dosing may be required for sedation and analgesia due to medications being adsorbed by the circuit, tolerance developing, and hemofiltration removing drugs. To minimize sedation, allow spontaneous breathing, and improve interaction, atypical antipsychotic agents may be effective in reducing agitation and delirium without sedation. Dexmedetomidine provides sedation from which the patient can be easily aroused.

Fluids and Renal Replacement Therapy

Maintenance of normal intravascular volume is necessary to maintain pump flow. To reduce edema, diuretics are the first choice, but hemofiltration can be incorporated into the circuit. Plasmapheresis can be performed in the management of sepsis, immunologic disorders, and hepatic failure through the ECLS circuit without the need for additional vascular access.

Nutritional Support

Initiation of enteral nutrition can begin after resuscitation is complete and perfusion is restored, usually in 12–24 hours. The absence of bowel sounds does not predict intolerance. Postpyloric feeding may be better tolerated than gastric feeding. Promotility agents (e.g., erythromycin) allow successful gastric feeding in most patients. IV nutritional support is used when enteral is contraindicated or to supplement it when full support is not achieved by enteral alone.

Duration of Support and Withdrawal of Care

The average duration of support is 3–5 days for postoperative cardiac dysfunction and 7–9 days for myocarditis and nonoperative cardiomyopathy. Support duration is longer for pulmonary dysfunction (11–13 days); however, lung function can take several months to recover. For the terminal withdrawal of VA support in patients with residual cardiac function, two short clamps are placed on each cannula and cut in between them to avoid an intravascular shunt.

COMPLICATIONS

Bleeding

If no surgical cause for bleeding is found, the platelet count is increased and the anticoagulation decreased. An ACT of 160–180 or 140–160 seconds may be required for a short time. If bleeding continues, aminocaproic acid can be used as an antifibrinolytic, and an IV loading dose (100 mg/kg) is followed by an infusion of 25–50 mg/kg. Tranexamic acid is another option. Recombinant factor VII has been used for severe bleeding but is not recommended as standard rescue therapy.

Heparin-induced thrombocytopenia (*HIT*) due to heparin-associated antibodies is uncommon but a potentially life-threatening complication of heparin use. Direct thrombin inhibitors are the first alternative to heparin in cases of HIT.

Neurologic Injury

Neurologic injury can occur with either respiratory or cardiac ECLS. In children with an anterior fontanelle, it is usual to perform daily or second daily cranial ultrasounds to monitor for cerebral thromboembolism, bleeding, or edema. Continuous EEG monitoring detects seizures in high-risk patients. Prevention of neurologic injury involves strict control of anticoagulation and the prompt institution of ECLS in severely hypoxic or hypotensive patients.

Vascular Injury

Vascular injury can present as posterior perforation with extravascular placement, subintimal placement, or vessel transection. Failure to complete cannulation may result from using a cannula larger than the vein can accommodate or from placement of the guidewire in a tributary instead of the major vessel. These usually require surgical exploration and management.

Infection

The most important risk factor for nosocomial infection is the duration of support. Infection can result in longer durations of ECMO and mechanical ventilation time and increased mortality.

OUTCOMES FROM ECLS

Survival in pediatric ECLS for respiratory failure is 65% with 56% surviving to hospital discharge. Survival for cardiac support is also 65% surviving ECLS but with 49% surviving to discharge. ECPR has the lowest survival (40% to discharge), but this level of survival is remarkable given the patient condition at time of cannulation.

Long-Term Outcomes

Neurologic impairment on ECLS may manifest as brain death, seizures, and CNS infarction or hemorrhage. Long-term outcomes have reported severe disability rates of at least 4%. It is likely that many long-term effects are due to the underlying illness rather than ECLS.

CHAPTER 18 ■ EXTRACORPOREAL ORGAN SUPPORT THERAPY

WARWICK W. BUTT, PETER W. SKIPPEN, PHILIPPE JOUVET, AND JIM FORTENBERRY

Extracorporeal *organ* support therapy (ECOST) encompasses various renal replacement therapies (RRTs), liver support therapies, and total plasma exchange.

GENERAL CONCEPTS

The ECOST Circuit Components

The basic ECOST filter circuit is shown in **Figure 18.1**.

Catheters: There is a large range of double-lumen, variable-length catheters. These catheters contain a proximal withdrawal lumen that has multiple side holes and a distal, single-end lumen for reinfusion to the patient. They are firm so that they will not collapse with suction applied by the system. Recommended sizes for hemofiltration/plasmafiltration catheters for children are listed in **Table 18.1**. The largest percutaneously accessible vessel is the subclavian vein, followed by the internal jugular and femoral vein. The closer the tip of the vascular catheter is to the right atrium, the better the flow obtained, although placing the catheter deep in the right atrium increases the risk of perforation. At high blood flow rates, high negative pressure can be generated in the dialysis circuit. Both blood drainage and blood return can be impaired. In situations in which drainage is inadequate, the filter connections can be reversed so that the inflow (blood drainage) cannula is the single-end hole and the blood-return lumen is the side hole.

Hemofilters: Filter function is determined by size and type of membrane. The larger surface area filter allows more effective filtration (a higher filtration fraction [FF]) and less hemoconcentration within the filter. However, larger filters require larger priming volumes (potential for hemodilution) and slower blood flow within the filter. The membrane may be either microtubules or a plate membrane.

Pumps: Almost all circuits use roller pumps to accurately control blood flow, ultrafiltrate flow, and replacement fluid.

Heater: The use of extracorporeal circulation (ECC) and the infusion of solute with high flow rates can create substantial heat loss, and so heating systems are recommended.

Circuit Priming

In children who weigh >10 kg, circuit priming often uses 0.9% saline or albumin with 5 U/mL of heparin. In children who weigh <10 kg, in children in whom the priming volume is >10% –15% of estimated patient blood volume, or in patients who are hemodynamically compromised, it is a common practice to use a blood prime. Hematocrit of the priming fluid should be >40%. The amount of albumin and packed red blood cells to be added to the circuit can be calculated as

$$(V_{\text{prbc}} \times \text{Hct}_{\text{prbc}}/P_{\text{hct}})\ V_{\text{prbc}} = V_{\text{alb}}$$

where V_{prbc} = the volume of packed red blood cells for the prime, Hct_{prbc} = the hematocrit of the prime red blood cells, P_{hct} = the desired hematocrit of the prime, and V_{alb} = the volume of 5% albumin to be

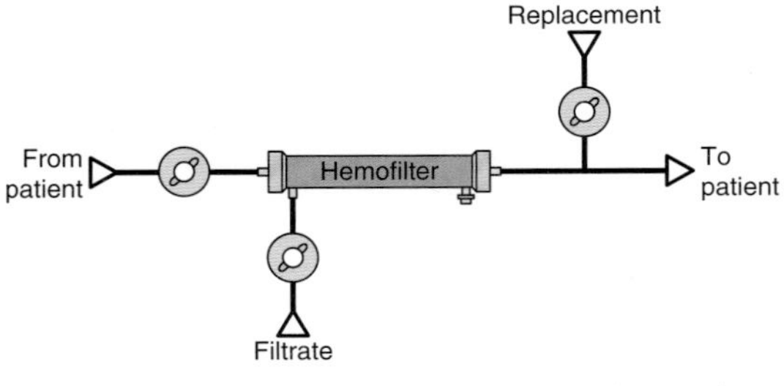

FIGURE 18.1. Basic ECOST circuit with catheters (from and to patient), hemofilter, filtrate, and replacement fluids. Roller pumps control flow rates for hemofilter blood, (ultra) filtrate, and replacement fluid.

TABLE 18.1

Suggested Sizes of Catheters for Use in CVVH/CVVP

■ PATIENT AGE (y)	■ CATHETER SIZE (French)	■ FLOW (mL/min)
Neonate	Single-lumen 5 or Dual-lumen 6.5–7	25–40
1–4	Dual-lumen 7.0–8.5	40–80
5–10	Dual-lumen 8.5–11.5	50–100
>10	Dual-lumen 11.5–14	80–150

added to the prime solution. Small infants are prone to hypotension when filtration is started, and the child's blood ionized calcium levels and hemodynamic parameters should be carefully monitored.

Complications of Extracorporeal Therapy

Access: Large veins are needed for the large catheters, and the risk of complications of insertion is inevitable but may be minimized by use of an ultrasound-guided insertion by an experienced person.

Infection: Prevention of catheter-related infection requires aseptic technique during insertion and access of circuit.

Technical: Equipment malfunction is always possible, and so trained staff must be available.

Clotting of blood vessel or membrane filter: Clotting of vessels is often related to catheter dysfunction (size of the catheter close to the size of the vessel). Clotting may also be increased by infection. Despite the use of heparin, clots in the blood vessel used for cannulation occur in 30%–50% of patients with large filtration catheters. Clotting of the filter is increased if there is a high FF (which causes hemoconcentration in the distal end of the filter), in instances of slow blood flow in large surface area filters, or if long microtubules with high resistance are used.

Bleeding: Platelet dysfunction or disseminated intravascular coagulation is much more likely to cause patient bleeding than the anticoagulants used for ECOST.

Embolism: Although uncommon, embolization of air, clots, or debris returning from the circuit can occur.

Anticoagulation Use

The factors that affect the decision to anticoagulate a patient for continuous RRT (CRRT) include patient age, underlying condition, medications (coexisting heparin therapy), and platelet counts. Many factors lead to clotting within the circuit including kinking of catheters; high circuit resistance; obstruction to inflow (blood drainage from patient); obstruction of catheter (often by side-hole occlusion by the vessel wall); slow blood flow or stasis; high blood viscosity due to high hematocrit, high plasma proteins, or from hemoconcentration due to excess fluid filtration; fibrin-strand formation from binding to the plastic surface of tubing or the filter; circulating procoagulants (particularly in sepsis or systemic inflammatory response syndrome); and inadequate anticoagulation. Most pediatric filtration is performed with anticoagulation. In patients with coagulopathy, such as sepsis, severe brain injury, trauma, liver failure, or active bleeding, it is logical to use regional anticoagulation, whereby the circuit is anticoagulated but the effect is reversed prior to blood return to the patient. Most pediatric intensive care units (PICUs) follow one of the following schemes:

Infusion of heparin: About 10–20 U/kg/h heparin prefilter and 1–2 U/kg/h heparin postfilter and maintenance of activated clotting time (ACT) at 1.5–2 times normal (to limit clots on the return line and tip of vascular-access catheter). This method is usually considered the easiest.

Regional anticoagulation with citrate: Trisodium citrate (0.5%) is infused prefilter, with the goal of maintaining a postfilter ionized Ca^{2+} (iCa^{2+}) of 0.3–0.4 mmol/L. (The prefilter citrate infusion is *increased* if the postfilter iCa^{2+} is >0.4 mmol/L and *decreased* if the iCa^{2+} is <0.3 mmol/L.) A *systemic calcium* infusion maintains the patient's iCa^{2+} of 1–1.2 mmol/L.

Regional anticoagulation with heparin: Heparin is infused prefilter 10–20 U/kg/h and reversed postfilter with *protamine* (1 mg for every 100 U of heparin given prefilter).

Anticoagulation Monitoring

The tests used to monitor heparin anticoagulation include (1) bedside tests such as ACT with a goal level 1.5–2 times normal (the thromboelastogram (TEG) is more informative and used instead of, or in addition to, the ACT) and (2) laboratory blood tests such as aPTT, D-dimers, or Anti-Xa (for fractionated or low molecular heparins) or antithrombin III (ATIII; the preferred aPTT is 1.5–2 times normal).

The key to safe citrate anticoagulation is similarly a systematic approach and adequate monitoring of (1) postfilter iCa^{2+} to maintain levels 0.3–0.4 mmol/L, (2) patient systemic iCa^{2+} levels 1–1.2 mmol/L, (3) daily total calcium levels to monitor for citrate toxicity, and (4) avoiding excessive blood flow to minimize citrate flows and hence minimize risks of citrate toxicity.

RENAL REPLACEMENT THERAPIES

There are renal and nonrenal therapy indications for RRT; a guide to determine the type of RRT most appropriate appears in **Table 18.2**. The *renal indications for RRT* include oliguria (unresponsive to diuretics and/or fluid challenge), anuria (nonobstructive), metabolic acidosis, hyperkalemia, azotemia, uremia symptoms (encephalopathy, myopathy, pericarditis, bleeding), and hyperphosphatemia. *The nonrenal indications for RRT* include fluid overload, anticipated large transfusion in trauma or coagulopathy, inborn errors of metabolism, sepsis, post-CPB systemic inflammatory response syndrome, pancreatitis, and drug overdose. RRT is used in a variety of clinical situations to remove endogenous or exogenous toxins and to restore water, acid–base, or electrolyte balance. Very few absolute contraindications to CRRT exist.

TABLE 18.2

Specifics of the Three Techniques of RRT in the PICU

	PD	iHD	CRRT
Method Specificities			
Vascular access (ECC)	No	Yes	Yes
Complex method with specific expertise	Low	High	Moderate
Systemic or regional anticoagulation	No	Frequent	Frequent
Dialysis Dose			
Efficacy to remove a toxin	Moderate	High	High
Efficacy to remove fluid	Moderate	Moderate	High
Clinical Situation Indication			
Hemodynamic instability	Yes	No	Yes
Intracranial hypertension	Yes	±	Yes
ARDS	±	Yes	Yes
Abdominal surgery	±	Yes	Yes

PD, peritoneal dialysis; iHD, intermittent hemodialysis; CRRT, continuous renal replacement therapy; ECC, extracorporeal circulation; ARDS, acute respiratory distress syndrome.

Even in the presence of intracranial hemorrhage or systemic bleeding, CRRT can be safely performed by using no anticoagulation, using small doses of heparin with close serial monitoring by ACT, or using regional anticoagulation provided by citrate/calcium.

PERITONEAL DIALYSIS

Peritoneal dialysis (PD) is the oldest, simplest, and still the most commonly used form of RRT in children. PD requires the bidirectional exchange of fluid and solute between dialysis fluid and blood across the peritoneal membrane. The other major mechanism involved in fluid and solute clearance is peritoneal lymph drainage. Up to 50% of capillary ultrafiltrate can be reabsorbed via the lymphatics, which can limit fluid removal.

Physiology of Peritoneal Dialysis

The surface area of the peritoneal cavity is directly proportional to the patient's body surface area (~0.6 m^2/m^2 of body surface area), and peritoneal permeability is similar in all patients from 2 years to adulthood. The peritoneal membrane is relatively impermeable to protein, unless diseases such as sepsis, systemic inflammatory response syndrome, cardiopulmonary bypass (CPB), pancreatitis, or shock have caused a marked increase in capillary permeability. Clearance achieved by PD depends on the following factors: (1) size of the molecule (smaller molecules are cleared more quickly); (2) dialysis fluid osmolality (the higher the glucose concentration, the more rapid the fluid removal); (3) dwell time (most fluid removal occurs within the first 30 minutes, because the concentration gradients change the most during this period); and (4) volume of dialysis fluid (the larger the dialysate volume, the greater the clearance because more fluid is in contact with the peritoneal membrane and its large surface area).

Indications for Peritoneal Dialysis

The standard indications for RRT also apply to PD. The absolute and relative contraindications to PD include a defect in the peritoneal membrane or cavity, such as diaphragmatic hernia, gastroschisis, omphalocele, or postsurgical thoracoabdominal communication (absolute); abdominal sepsis with adhesions (absolute); fulminant necrotizing enterocolitis with perforation (absolute); ventriculo-peritoneal shunt (relative); profound shock or cardiac failure (relative); and massive rapid clearance required (relative).

Catheters Used for Peritoneal Dialysis

The Tenckhoff catheter is most commonly used for PD; it is available as either a straight or a curled catheter. It can be inserted by a surgeon in the operating theater (after CPB) or in the PICU. Administration of a single dose of prophylactic antibiotics at the time of insertion is recommended.

Complications of Peritoneal Dialysis

PD can be associated with fluid and electrolyte abnormalities, in particular, potassium, sodium, and, in small infants, lactate (if lactate dialysate solute is used). *Peritonitis* is an uncommon complication that is mainly related to poor aseptic insertion or handling of the circuit. Diagnosis of peritonitis is confirmed if the dialysate fluid is cloudy, if the white blood cell count is >100/mm^3, and if >50% of the cells are polymorphonuclear cells. Early empiric therapy with intraperitoneal cefazolin and gentamicin is commenced. A single IV dose of vancomycin may also be given if the patient is clinically unstable. Evidence of a *pneumoperitoneum* is also found in some patients with PD. Pneumoperitoneum usually results from air entrainment in the dialysis fluid, rather than from bowel perforation, although making the distinction between the two is obviously important. *Catheter-related problems* with PD can occur frequently. Poor flow into the peritoneum can occur from kinking of the catheter, crystallization around the catheter instillation/drainage holes, or infection. Poor drainage can occur with kinking, malposition of the catheter, or from omentum wrapped around catheter drainage holes. Leakage at the site of entry can also occur from excessive dwell volumes with a newly placed catheter, local irritation of the site of entry, or initial poor surgical technique. *Inguinal hernias* can occur because of increased intra-abdominal pressure, and the development of scrotal fluid (hydrocele) is common in the neonate.

Peritoneal Dialysis Fluid Composition

The choice of PD solution depends on the amount of fluid to be removed, the age of the patient, and whether metabolic acidosis is present. Instillation of 10–20 mL/kg normally provides good clearance and minimal risk of intra-abdominal hypertension. Increased volume of dialysate to 30–40 mL/kg gives a better clearance of solutes, but an increased likelihood of intra-abdominal hypertension, respiratory embarrassment, or leakage from the insertion site of a newly placed catheter. Usually, a total time of 30–240 minutes (depending on diagnosis and clearance required) is provided for instillation, dwell time, and drainage, with dwell time providing 66%–85% of the total cycle time.

Cardiopulmonary Interactions

Increased PD volumes and abdominal muscle tone increases may impair ventilation, gas exchange, and cardiac performance.

HEMODIALYSIS

Hemodialysis (HD) is the extracorporeal exchange of fluid and solute that occurs across an artificial, semipermeable membrane between blood and dialysis fluid moving in opposite (countercurrent) directions. HD uses dialyzers with larger filter surface area, higher blood flow rates, and higher dialysis flow rates than CRRT. Thus, HD is much more efficient at removing solute than CRRT. The intermittent nature of the technique (sessions usually last 4–6 hours and are repeated three times per week) lends itself to being used in stable children with chronic renal failure or acute renal failure (ARF) due to renal disease (such as hemolytic uremic syndrome [HUS] or glomerulonephritis), as well as patients with hyperammonemia, inborn errors of metabolism, and drug overdoses in which rapid substance removal may be desirable.

Physiology of Hemodialysis

Fluid removal is accomplished via the ultrafiltration along a transmembrane pressure (TMP) gradient, which is determined by the hydrostatic pressure difference across the semipermeable membrane minus the plasma oncotic pressure (which tends to retain fluid in the blood) and is of the order of 20–30 mm Hg. *Solute removal* in HD occurs by diffusive transport along a concentration gradient; the larger the concentration gradient, the faster the removal (clearance) of solute or waste products. Solute removal also depends on the time allowed for dialysis, as well as the volume of distribution for the particular solute. Countercurrent flow is important to improve the efficiency of solute removal because it maintains a continuous concentration gradient along the entire length of the dialyzer fibers. The size of the solute molecule is important; transfer across the dialysis membrane depends on blood flow rates for small molecules and membrane characteristics for large molecules. Small molecules (<300 Da) move easily across the membrane. Increasing blood flow rate increases solute transfer by maintaining a concentrated solute, and increased dialysate flow maintains low solute levels on the dialysate side, thereby maintaining the concentration gradient; thus, small-molecule clearance is flow dependent. Large molecules do not diffuse as easily and, therefore, are not flow dependent, but they are dependent on physical characteristics (thickness, surface area, and type) of the plastic that constitutes the membrane dialyzer.

Catheters

In general, similar catheters are used in acute HD and in CRRT. A large range of catheters for acute HD are available—from 6.5 to 7 French in the newborn, to 14 French in the large adolescent (**Table 18.1**). Most centers use double-lumen catheters for acute HD and they must be large enough to obtain blood flow rates of 3–5 mL/kg/min to achieve adequate solute clearance.

Dialyzer Membrane

A large range of dialyzer membranes are used, and they have a number of features in common: small priming volume, biocompatibility (with minimal cytokine release), known sieving and filtration coefficients, known and consistent relationships between solute clearance and blood and dialysate flows, and low pressure drop across the membrane. Most centers use hollow-fiber (capillary) membranes. It is prudent to choose a membrane size that has a surface area that is less than the surface area of the patient and a priming volume that is less than 10% of the patient's circulating blood volume.

Choice of Dialysis Solution

Normalization of electrolytes focuses on key electrolytes of plasma, including sodium, potassium, calcium, magnesium, and chloride. Buffering of the dialysate is usually accomplished by the addition of bicarbonate in concentrations of 30–35 mmol/L to the dialysis fluid.

Complications of Hemodialysis

Vascular-access risks include problems related to insertion, infection, thrombosis, embolism, and hemorrhage. Longer-term complications include vascular stenosis and vessel occlusion with clot. *Disequilibrium syndrome* occurs when the patients' plasma becomes hypotonic relative to their brain cells and water enters the brain. Initial symptoms include nausea, headache, dizziness, and vomiting but can rapidly progress to seizures or coma. Children most at risk are those with high serum sodium or urea and those in whom very rapid HD is performed. When disequilibrium syndrome is recognized or anticipated, an attempt should be made to have slow changes of solute occur by using low blood flow rates to decrease the rate of clearance. Mannitol at doses of 0.25–1.0 g/kg may also be helpful. *Hemolysis* can occur from the use of a dialysate solution that is hypo-osmolar; hyperthermic; hyponatremic; or contaminated with formaldehyde, bleach, copper, or nitrates. Other causes of hemolysis include use of faulty blood pumps, which cause trauma to blood cells; inadequate anticoagulation leading to clot formation; and excess suction in the venous drainage line due to hypovolemia or kinking/obstruction of the dialysis catheter. The main danger that results from hemolysis is acute hyperkalemia (arrhythmia) and high plasma-free hemoglobin. *Anaphylaxis reactions* still occur, albeit much less frequently than with cellulose/cuprophane membranes. *Bacteremia/infection* can occur with poor aseptic technique. *Air embolism* is also possible, as is a blood or dialysate leak. *Hypothermia/hyperthermia* can occur if heaters or temperature baths malfunction. Dosage adjustment of drugs, due to both renal failure and removal of drug by HD, is essential.

Recirculation can occur because of high blood flows and, especially in small children, the proximity of the two ends (the drainage and reinfusion holes) of the catheters. The percentage of recirculation can be calculated as

$$\% \text{ recirculation} \times 100 = (U_{\text{systemic}} - U_{\text{arterial line}})/(U_{\text{systemic}} - U_{\text{venous return line}})$$

where U_{systemic} = urea concentration in peripheral blood, $U_{\text{arterial line}}$ = urea concentration in the predialyzer arterial line, and $U_{\text{venous return line}}$ = urea concentration in the postdialyzer venous return line. No recirculation occurs when $U_{\text{arterial}} = U_{\text{systemic.}}$ Some recirculation is occurring if $U_{\text{arterial}} < U_{\text{systemic}}$. If recirculation is greater than 20%, the efficiency of HD is diminished and should be corrected.

CONTINUOUS RENAL REPLACEMENT THERAPY

CRRT is a "gentler" form of removal of fluid and solute than intermittent hemodialysis (iHD). It can be equivalent in efficiency to iHD and has the benefit of more hemodynamic stability. The amount of fluid overload present at initiation CRRT may be related to outcome, suggesting that earlier use of CRRT to control fluid balance may improve outcome.

Physiology of Continuous Renal Replacement Therapy

The filtration of blood during CRRT is analogous to native glomerular filtration and is determined by fluid movement across a semipermeable membrane down a pressure gradient. Bulk flow of solute (convection) also occurs concurrently. Simply stated, the filter acts as a sieve, allowing molecules dissolved in water to be carried along to the other side. Each filter is composed of many microtubules that act independently of each other but function with the same principles. The process of convective ultrafiltration is driven by three key factors: filter blood flow, TMP, and FF.

Filter Blood Flow

Poiseuille's law governs laminar flow through a tube and is defined by the following parameters:

$$Qb = \Delta p - \pi r^4/8L\mu$$

where Qb = blood flow, Δp = change in pressure across the tube, r = radius of the tube, L = length of the tube, and μ = viscosity of the blood. Δp is the difference between the filter inlet and filter outlet pressure. The desired blood flow is set on the machine. Lower blood flow across the filter can result in a higher tendency for clotting to occur. As the filter clots, resistance to flow will increase, and filter pressure will increase as well.

Transmembrane Pressure

Transmembrane pressure (TMP) is the major force that acts on water and solute clearance outside the microtubule. Fluid moves through the microtubule into the external chamber of the filter, where it is removed as ultrafiltrate. The amount of ultrafiltrate obtained varies with the surface area, length and type of material from which the filter is made, and the patient's blood viscosity. In continuous arteriovenous hemofiltration (CAVH), the TMP is usually determined by the height difference between the filter and the continuous column of ultrafiltrate as it enters the collecting bag. All other forms of CRRT utilize a pump on the ultrafiltrate line to apply a precise amount of suction (negative pressure) to the ultrafiltrate line, thereby allowing precise determination of TMP to yield a controlled ultrafiltrate production.

Filtration Fraction

Filtration fraction (FF) represents the efficiency of plasma water removal through filtration and is the ratio of ultrafiltration rate (UFR) to the plasma flow rate (Q_P) through the filter. The FF depends on TMP, surface area of the filter, permeability of the membrane, plasma oncotic pressure, and hematocrit. An FF greater than 30% increases the risk of filter clotting. The clearance of a substance in CRRT modes can be increased with higher blood flow, higher TMPs, and higher FFs. Thus, larger surface area and increased filter permeability will increase the efficiency of filtration, whereas higher hematocrit and high plasma protein concentration will decrease efficiency of filtration. It is important to note that use of postfilter fluid replacement provides more efficient clearance than prefilter replacement.

Sieving Coefficient and Solute Removal

CRRT removes solute from the blood via filtration and adsorption (to the surfaces of the circuit tubing and filter). The efficiency of solute transfer from the blood side of the membrane to the ultrafiltrate side is expressed by the sieving coefficient (SC), which is the concentration of a solute in the ultrafiltrate ($[\text{solute}]_{UF}$) divided by the concentration of the same solute in the plasma ($[\text{solute}]_{plasma}$). Many small molecules have an SC of ~1, indicating free convective movement from plasma to ultrafiltrate. CRRT may clear a variety of "middle" molecules, including cytokines, complement, tumor necrosis factor (TNF), interleukins (IL-1, IL-6, and IL-8), prostaglandin, myocardial depressant factor, interferon, and even gram-positive bacterial exotoxins. Drug clearance is also affected by the size, charge, and protein binding of the drug.

Pre- or Postfilter Infusion of Replacement Fluids

The advantages of replacement fluid placement prior to the filter (predilution) are increased urea clearance as diffusion of red blood cell urea into the plasma occurs, and increase in filter survival due to hemodilution of blood and clotting factors. Thus, predilution placement is preferred in some PICUs. However, predilution placement decreases the SC of most solutes by lowering the filter inlet concentration of these substances.

Modes of Continuous Renal Replacement Therapy

Continuous Arteriovenous Hemofiltration

In CAVH mode, the drainage catheter is placed in an artery, and the return catheter in a vein (either peripheral or central). CAVH provides a potential volume load to the heart in small infants that may not be well tolerated. In this mode, blood flows from artery to vein, and filtrate production depends on the patient's blood pressure, the filter surface area, and the height of the collecting system below the filter.

Slow Continuous Ultrafiltration

Slow continuous ultrafiltration (SCUF) uses a low volume of filtrate with no replacement solution and is useful in removing small amounts of fluid. The SCUF circuit design is analogous to CAVH except that the driving pressure in SCUF comes from the blood pump, whereas in CAVH it comes from the patient's heart creating an arterial pressure.

Continuous Venovenous Hemofiltration

Continuous venovenous hemofiltration (CVVH) is the most common form of CRRT. The critical difference between SCUF and CVVH is the addition of replacement fluid (**Fig. 18.1**), which drives convection (solute drag). Hence, CVVH allows solute removal in addition to fluid removal. When a net fluid loss is desired in the fluid-overloaded patient, the replacement fluid rate (RFR) is set such that the sum of all outputs (ultrafiltrate, urine, chest tubes, etc.) exceeds the sum of all inputs (replacement fluid, IV fluids, nutrition, etc.) by a defined amount every hour. The typical range of ultrafiltration rates for PICU patients is 10–50 mL/kg/h (10–20 mL/min/1.73 m^2). Blood flow through the filter is maintained at a level that is at least three times the UFR. Inadequate blood flow risks clotting the filter, whereas excessive flow produces hemolysis. The faster the replacement fluid infusion rate, the greater the convective solute clearance.

Continuous Venovenous Hemodialysis

Continuous venovenous hemodialysis (CVVHD) removes solute through diffusion rather than the convection mechanism seen in CVVH. CVVHD is more efficient than CVVH at removing small molecules such as urea, whereas CVVH can remove both small and larger molecules. Dialysate is infused into the filter of the CVVHD circuit, but replacement fluid is not used. Dialysate (countercurrent) flow removes solute through diffusion. The greater hydrostatic pressure in the filter compared with the filtrate drainage bag results in fluid removal.

Continuous Venovenous Hemodiafiltration

Continuous venovenous hemodiafiltration (CVVHDF) combines hemofiltration (through convection) and dialysis (through diffusion). Both dialysis and replacement fluids are infused into (and removed from) the filter. Increased clearance of small molecules is obtained by increasing dialysis flow (and ultrafiltrate flow in an equal amount). Clearance of middle molecules requires an increase in the percentage of ultrafiltrate flow from hemofiltration and convection by increasing the filter blood flow rate and/or the RFR.

Complications of Continuous Renal Replacement Therapy

Filter clotting: Although common, effective anticoagulation strategies can increase filter survival. An increased TMP or a large rate of change of TMP substantially contributes to filter clotting.

Fluid imbalance: Hypo- or hypervolemia may occur from imbalances in fluid intake and filtration flow. Obtaining patient weights (if the patient's condition allows) is very important in the assessment of fluid balance.

Electrolyte abnormalities: Phosphate losses can be expected and require replacement. Some units add 1 mmol/L Na- or K-phosphate to replacement and dialysis solutions. A systemic calcium infusion is required to prevent systemic hypocalcemia when using citrate anticoagulation. Magnesium losses can also be expected when using citrate anticoagulation and should be replaced.

Metabolic acidosis or alkalosis: Either acidosis or alkalosis may occur during CRRT. Alkalosis is more common with citrate anticoagulation as citrate metabolism creates a large alkali load (see under Citrate Toxicity). High blood flow rates require increased citrate flow rates and increase the alkalosis. This often requires the replacement of chloride through manipulation of the dialysate solution. Use of dialysis or replacement solutions that contain lactate can lead to metabolic acidosis from hyperlactatemia.

Citrate toxicity: High blood flow rates require increased citrate flow rates. Citrate toxicity should be suspected with rising systemic calcium infusion requirements, falling systemic *ionized* Ca levels, rising *total* serum calcium levels, and a total:ionized calcium ratio > 2.25. It can be managed by reducing the blood flow rate (and therefore citrate flow rate) and increasing clearance of the citrate load through increasing replacement fluid flow rates.

Hypothermia: Hypothermia occurs often from extracorporeal blood cooling and the infusion of large volumes of dialysate or replacement fluids at room temperature. Several complications are associated with hypothermia, including altered immune function, glucose and electrolyte imbalance, and prolonged clotting times.

Thrombocytopenia: It is not uncommon to see a decrement in platelet count of up to 50% of baseline values every time a patient is placed on a new filter. The exposure to a new filter does not seem to affect white blood cell count or cause a rise in cytokines or inflammatory mediators.

Hypotension upon initiation of CRRT: Hemodynamically unstable patients receiving vasopressors may experience hypotension and circulatory collapse upon initiation of CRRT, likely due to dilution and binding of catecholamine to the plastic of the circuit. Thus, in patients on large doses of vasoconstrictors and inotropic drugs, an effective strategy may be to double drug infusion rates before starting CVVH and to begin with a slow blood flow that is gradually increased over 5–10 minutes to the desired rate.

Hypoxemia: Neonates with severe lung disease who begin CRRT with a "blood-primed" circuit may experience hypoxemia from initial exposure to venous blood in the priming volume. This may be avoided by increasing the FIO_2 up to 100% before beginning CRRT in such patients.

How to Choose the Type of Renal Replacement Therapy

The main types of RRT (PD, iHD, and CRRT) are available at most PICUs. PD is often used in infants (<10 kg) after cardiac surgery and in patients with early-onset chronic renal failure, CRRT in the very sick or unstable patient with multiorgan failure, and iHD in hemodynamically stable patients with acute or chronic renal failure.

Extracorporeal Membrane Oxygenation and CRRT

Fluid overload or ARF often develops in patients with sepsis or cardiogenic shock receiving ECMO for hemodynamic support. These patients are on extracorporeal therapy and are anticoagulated so there is no additional access or bleeding risk with adding CVVH, CVVH DF, or CVVHD to the ECMO circuit. The CVVH circuit runs from the higher- to the lower-pressure end of the oxygenator and represents a small shunt.

Cardiopulmonary Bypass and CRRT

The *CPB-based inflammatory response* may be limited by prebypass corticosteroids, heparin-bonded circuits, albumin priming of circuits, and modified ultrafiltration on CPB. It appears that modified ultrafiltration and early use of PD after pediatric cardiac surgery may decrease length of intubation and bleeding.

THERAPEUTIC PLASMA EXCHANGE

Therapeutic plasma exchange (TPE), also known as plasmapheresis, is a technique for removing potentially harmful large molecules such as autoantibodies, immune complexes, or endotoxin from the circulation.

Background

Two methods are used to separate plasma from the blood. *Centrifugation with* a centrifugal pump has been the conventional method to separate the blood into cellular and noncellular elements for apheresis. The noncellular plasma is removed and replaced with an albumin/saline solution. *Filtration* is a newer method for separation of blood components. This approach (also known as "membrane plasma separation") replaces the hemofilter of a CVVH circuit with one containing larger pore sizes to filter (protein) molecules, up to 2 million Daltons. The filtered plasma containing unwanted proteins is replaced with albumin or fresh frozen plasma.

Continuous Venovenous Plasmafiltration

The basic principles of continuous venovenous plasmafiltration (CVVP) are similar to CVVH with a few important differences: (1) The replacement fluid in CVVP must contain protein because large protein molecules have been removed. The typical choices are 5% albumin, an albumin/saline mixture, or fresh frozen plasma (FFP). Prolonged CVVP or large volume of CVVP will filter immunoglobulins and clotting factors, which may require specific replacement. Replacement with FFP is indicated for thrombotic thrombocytopenic purpura and HUS. (2) Even small imbalances in CVVP intake and output will affect intravascular volume and risk of hypo- or hypertension. (3) Protein-bound drugs are removed, and drug levels should be measured and dosing adjusted. (4) Heparin and citrate have unique disadvantages in CVVP. An increasing proportion of protein-bound heparin is removed at lower hematocrits, necessitating increased heparin administration in the anemic patient. Citrate anticoagulation combined with FFP replacement may lead to citrate toxicity because FFP consists of 14% citrate by volume.

Indications for Therapeutic Plasma Exchange

The American Society for Apheresis (ASFA) divides the indications for TPE into four categories based on the evidence for clinical efficacy. The following lists some of the more common PICU indications in each category.

Category I (TPE accepted as first-line therapy). Guillain–Barrè syndrome (GBS), thrombotic thrombocytopenic purpura, HUS (atypical HUS due to autoantibody to factor H), antibody-mediated transplantation rejection, myasthenia gravis, and Wilson disease (fulminant).

Category II (TPE accepted as second-line therapy). Acute disseminated encephalomyelitis, mushroom poisoning, severe systemic lupus erythematosus (e.g., diffuse alveolar hemorrhage, cerebritis), atypical HUS (due to complement factor gene mutation), and humoral renal transplant rejection.

Category III (optimum TPE role not established). Dilated cardiomyopathy, Henoch–Schonlein purpura (severe extrarenal disease), acute liver failure, sepsis with multiorgan failure, envenomation, refractory stem cell transplantation-associated thrombotic microangiopathy, and refractory toxic epidermal necrolysis.

Category IV (TPE ineffective or harmful). Dermatomyositis, polymyositis, shiga-toxin HUS, and refractory immune thrombocytopenia.

Guillain–Barrè Syndrome

Despite physiologic changes in patients with GBS, patient outcomes are excellent. Treatment with immunoglobulin (IVIG) is equally efficacious. IVIG is often used for children admitted to the ward, but TPE (plus IVIG immediately following TPE) is used if children develop respiratory failure.

Drug Overdose

TPE may be useful in overdose or poisoning with drugs/toxins that are highly protein bound with a low volume of distribution. It is effective for theophylline, vancomycin, colchicines, neonatal lead poisoning in combination with chelation, and isobutyl nitrate–induced methemoglobinemia.

Sepsis with or without Thrombocytopenia-Associated Multiple Organ Failure

Interest in the use of TPE in sepsis has focused on a subset of children with thrombocytopenia-associated multiple organ failure (TAMOF). Some patients with TAMOF have reduced or absent von Willebrand factor cleaving protease activity, now known as ADAMTS-13 (A Disintegrin And Metalloprotease with Thrombo-Spondin motifs), similar to TTP phenotypes that demonstrate excellent response to plasma exchange.

CHAPTER 19 ■ BLOOD PRODUCTS AND TRANSFUSION THERAPY

OLIVER KARAM, PHILIP C. SPINELLA, EDWARD C.C. WONG, AND NAOMI L.C. LUBAN

RED BLOOD CELL TRANSFUSION

Scientific Foundation of Red Blood Cell Transfusion

Oxygen Transport

Oxygen delivery (Do_2, in mL O_2/min) is described by:

$$Do_2 = \text{cardiac output} \times \text{arterial } O_2 \text{ content}$$

Arterial O_2 content (Cao_2) is:

$$Cao_2 = (Sao_2 \times Hb \times 1.34) + (0.003 \times Pao_2)$$

where Cao_2 and Pao_2 are expressed in mm Hg, arterial saturation in oxygen (Sao_2) is expressed as a fraction, and hemoglobin (Hb) concentration is expressed in g/dL. The amount of oxygen utilized by the cells can be calculated by the oxygen consumption ($\dot{V}o_2$) equation:

$$\dot{V}o_2 = \text{cardiac output} \times 1.34 \times Hb \times (Sao_2 - Svo_2)$$

where arterial and venous saturations in oxygen (Sao_2 and Svo_2) are expressed as a fraction, and hemoglobin (Hb) concentration is expressed in g/dL. Under normal circumstances, Do_2 exceeds $\dot{V}o_2$. If Do_2 decreases beyond a threshold, the physiologic Do_2 reserve is exhausted, and thereafter $\dot{V}o_2$ decreases linearly with further decreases in Do_2. This point in the $Do_2/\dot{V}o_2$ relationship is the "critical threshold" and indicates that $\dot{V}o_2$ is no longer governed by the metabolic need of the tissues but becomes limited by O_2 supply (Do_2). Tissue hypoxia from low Do_2 may be due to a low Hb concentration (anemic hypoxia), low cardiac output (stagnant hypoxia), or low Hb saturation (hypoxic hypoxia). This is illustrated in **Figure 19.1**.

Adaptation to Anemia. The physiologic adaptation to anemia is an increase in the other Do_2 variables or a decrease in $\dot{V}o_2$. Examples include increased extraction of O_2, increased heart rate and stroke volume (i.e., cardiac output), redistribution of blood flow from nonvital organs to the heart and brain (at the expense of the splanchnic vascular bed), and a left shift in the oxyhemoglobin dissociation curve (i.e., decreased O_2 affinity).

Impairment in Adaptive Mechanisms. Diseases can impair the adaptive mechanisms to anemia (e.g., increased metabolic rate and decreased Do_2 reserve from sepsis). Host characteristics specific to children and infants can impair adaptive mechanisms (e.g., physiologic anemia in the first months of life, lower myocardial compliance in the neonate that limits increases in stroke volume, or elevated heart rate in neonates that limits additional heart rate contribution to increase cardiac output).

Microcirculatory Effects of Transfused Red Blood Cells

During red blood cell (RBC) storage, 2,3-DPG is diminished, nitric oxide (NO) bioavailability is reduced, the membranes lose deformability, adhesion and aggregation increase, and membrane microparticles are generated, resulting in reduced perfusion and oxygen delivery. Microparticles have immune suppressive and procoagulant properties. Free intravascular Hb (from hemolysis) as well as Hb within RBC membrane microvesicles binds NO and causes vasoconstriction.

Immunologic Effects of Allogeneic Red Blood Cell Transfusions

The proinflammatory molecules detected in RBC units include cytokines, complement activators, O_2 free radicals, histamine, lysophosphatidylcholine species, and other bioreactive substances such as RBC membrane microparticles that may initiate, maintain, or enhance an inflammatory process. Transfusion can cause immunosuppression, increase the risk of nosocomial infections, and reinforce systemic inflammatory response syndrome (SIRS) that progresses to multiple organ dysfunction syndrome (MODS).

Transfusion of Red Blood Cells: Application to the PICU

Hemorrhagic Shock. Pediatric advanced life support (PALS) and advanced trauma life support (ATLS) guidelines recommend initiating volume resuscitation with 40–60 mL/kg of crystalloid solutions (normal saline or Ringer lactate) before transfusing RBC units based on animal data and very small human studies. Recent large observational studies of massive transfusion for hemorrhagic shock dispute this.

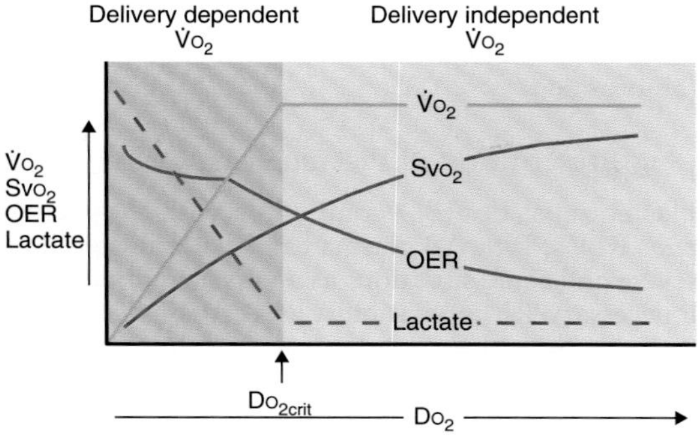

FIGURE 19.1. Effect of the oxygen delivery (DO_2) on the oxygen consumption ($\dot{V}O_2$), central venous oxygen saturation (SvO_2), oxygen extraction ratio (OER), and lactate levels.

Unstable Patients. It is reasonable to transfuse RBCs for a threshold of 7 g/dL in children who are unstable (in shock). It is possible that patients with severe sepsis have better outcome if the Hb threshold is 10 g/dL during the hours following diagnosis. There is insufficient evidence in children to standardize this approach.

Stabilized Patients. Once stabilized, critically ill children are able to tolerate Hb concentrations as low as 7 g/dL.

Cyanotic Congenital Heart Disease. Non–evidence-based thresholds as high as 13 g/dL are recommended. It might be reasonable to adopt a restrictive transfusion strategy (transfuse only when Hb is <9.0 g/dL) in non–stage 1 cyanotic congenital heart disease (results of a small RCT need to be confirmed in a larger trial).

Chronic Anemia. Patients with chronic anemia usually increase their cardiac output (to maintain DO_2) or decrease their $\dot{V}O_2$. Although a threshold for transfusion below Hb of 5 g/dL seems reasonable to many physicians, no recommendation can be made until a proper study is undertaken.

Red Blood Cell Products

RBCs adenine saline added are prepared by centrifuging whole blood to remove plasma and replace it with 100–110 mL of a solution that contains dextrose, adenine, sodium chloride, and either monobasic sodium phosphate (AS-3) or mannitol (AS-1 and AS-5). The hematocrit of these products varies between 55% and 65%. RBCs stored with an additive solution have an extended shelf life, dependent on the solution (42 days for RBCs in AS).

Leukocyte-reduced RBCs have the advantages of leukocyte reduction that include decreased transmission of infections carried by leukocytes (cytomegalovirus [CMV]), decreased febrile transfusion reactions, and decreased transfusion-related immune modulation (TRIM) caused by residual white blood cells. Leukocyte-reduced preparations still contain leukocytes and should not be given to patients at risk for transfusion-associated graft-versus-host disease (TA-GVHD). The intensivist should order leukocyte-reduced blood for transplant patients, children with a history of febrile nonhemolytic transfusion reactions, and CMV-seronegative patients for whom seronegative PRBC units are not available. *Washed RBCs* are RBC units in which the plasma is removed and replaced with either normal saline or plasma substitute. Washing removes 98% and 99% of plasma constituents. They are used for recurrent severe allergic reactions or to deplete potassium. *Frozen deglycerolized RBCs* may be indicated for patients with previous severe allergic transfusion reactions; the process efficiently removes plasma constituents. *Irradiated RBCs* are used to prevent TA-GVHD. GVHD is a rare but potentially fatal complication of RBC transfusion in an immunosuppressed or immunodeficient patient. It is caused by donor T lymphocytes in the RBC unit that proliferate in the transfusion recipient (host). Gamma irradiation of the PRBC unit inactivates T-lymphocyte proliferation and prevents TA-GVHD in the susceptible recipient. *Emergency-release (universal donor) blood* is type O un-crossmatched RBCs. Rh(D) negative is recommended for females and either Rh(D) negative or positive for males. Prior to administration of any blood, collect a blood sample from the patient for subsequent ABO testing.

PLASMA

Constitution of Plasma

Plasma units contain the acellular portion of blood (i.e., the supernatant after centrifugation of whole blood). The RBCs, WBCs, and platelets precipitate and are almost completely removed. One mL of plasma contains ~1 unit of each coagulation factor. Labile coagulation factors (factors V and VIII) are unstable in plasma stored at 1°C–6°C, and plasma is usually stored frozen at or below −18°C. Plasma also contains fibrin, immunoglobulins, antithrombin, protein C, protein S, allergens, and significant amounts of glucose (535 mg/dL or 30 mmol/L), sodium (172 mEq/L), potassium (15 mEq/L), and proteins (5.5 g/dL with 60% albumin).

Scientific Foundation of Transfusion of Plasma

Immunologic Effects of Plasma Transfusions

Plasma contains bioactive substances (cytokines, immunoglobulin, and coagulation factors) that can interact with the patient's immune system. The process of freezing and thawing plasma increases histamine and other bioactive products. Plasma transfusion induces the production of TNF-α and IL-10 and increases lymphocyte count.

Transfusion of Plasma: Application to PICU

Risk of Bleeding

Coagulation tests (e.g., prothrombin time [PT] or activated partial thromboplastin time [aPTT]) do not correlate with the risk of bleeding in patients without active bleeding. Thromboelastography (TEG)-based algorithms reduce transfusion requirements and blood loss in cardiac surgery, liver transplantation, and massive trauma.

Prophylactic. Current recommendations advise against the use of plasma for volume expansion and in nonbleeding patients, except in preparation for surgery or invasive procedures.

Therapeutic. In the massive bleeding patient at risk for exsanguination, plasma should be transfused before classical coagulation test results are available. In the nonmassive bleeding patient, plasma should be considered only if the PT or aPTT ratio is higher than 1.5, or the INR is above 2.0. Prothrombin complex concentrates are indicated for reversal of vitamin K antagonists. If they are not available, plasma is appropriate in the presence of major or intracranial hemorrhage or in preparation for emergent surgery. Plasma exchange therapy is indicated for treatment of thrombotic micro-angiopathies (e.g., thrombotic thrombocytopenic purpura, atypical hemolytic-uremic syndrome). Plasma is also indicated as reconstitution of whole blood for exchange transfusions, as well as for hereditary angioedema when C1-esterase inhibitor is not available.

Plasma Products

Fresh frozen plasma (FFP) is prepared from whole blood or apheresis collection and frozen at −18°C or colder temperature. Most units contain 200–250 mL, but apheresis-derived units may contain as much as 400–600 mL. FFP contains plasma proteins and all coagulation factors. *Frozen plasma* (plasma frozen within 24 hours after phlebotomy *[FP24]*) is prepared from a whole blood or apheresis collection. The product is stored at 1°C–6°C within 8 hours of collection and frozen at −18°C or below within 24 hours of collection. Most plasma proteins are at levels similar to FFP, except that levels of factor VIII and protein C are reduced and levels of factor V and other labile plasma proteins are variable compared with FFP. *Thawed plasma* is thawed at 30°C–37°C and maintained at 1°C–6°C for up to 5 days after the initial 24-hour postthaw period has elapsed. Thawed plasma contains stable coagulation factors of factor II and fibrinogen in concentrations clinically similar to those of FFP, but variably reduced amounts of other factors. It is often used in the setting of massive transfusion protocols, especially in adult trauma settings. *Solvent/detergent plasma* is used to reduce the risk of infectious transmission from pooled donors, and so multiple pathogen inactivation methods are used, such as solvent/detergent (S/D) treatment, methylene blue, ultraviolet light with riboflavin, and psoralens (amotosalen).

Prescription of Plasma Transfusions

Plasma must be ABO compatible with the recipient's RBCs. Type AB plasma can be administered in severe and acute situations as a universal donor type if necessary. Rh compatibility and crossmatching are not considered because there are virtually no RBCs in FFP. Plasma dosing is calculated at 10–20 mL/kg.

PLATELETS

Constitution of Platelets

Platelet concentrates are prepared within hours of collection from units of whole blood or through apheresis from a single donor. Platelets are stored between 20°C and 24°C to have superior survival.

Immunologic Effects of Platelet Transfusions

Platelet transfusions contain plasma or cellular elements (platelets and leukocytes) and can result in immunomodulation (via transfusion of cytokines or immunomodulatory proteins, such as IL-1, IL-6, and IL-8, or soluble CD40 ligand) or development of antibodies directed against histocompatibility (typically class I) antigens or specific platelet antigens.

Transfusion of Platelets: Application to the PICU

Prophylactic. Prophylactic platelet transfusion is considered if the platelet count is <5–10 × 10^9/L (<5000–10,000/mm^3). For intensive care unit (ICU) patients, the threshold is 50 × 10^9/L (50,000/mm^3) for surgical or invasive procedures, and 100 × 10^9/L (100,000/mm^3) for surgical interventions in critical sites (ocular or neurosurgery). Guidelines for oncology and hematopoietic stem cell transplant (HSCT) patients suggest that platelet counts greater than 10–20 × 10^9/L (10,000–20,000/mm^3) may be helpful in preventing life-threatening hemorrhage. Platelet transfusion should not be used for the treatment of immune thrombocytopenic purpura (ITP) except in the presence of intracranial or life-threatening bleeding. Platelets are also contraindicated in cases of thrombotic thrombocytopenic purpura (TTP) and heparin-induced thrombocytopenia (HIT) because of increased thrombotic risk. However, in the case of life-threatening bleeding, it is permissible to transfuse platelets in patients with TTP. Alternatives to platelet transfusion, such as DDAVP or antifibrinolytic agents, the use of steroids, plasmapheresis, and avoidance of heparin, should be considered as first-line therapies in patients with nonhypoproliferative thrombocytopenia.

Therapeutic. In general, bleeding patients should have their platelet counts maintained $>50 \times 10^9$/L (50,000/mm^3) depending on the clinical situation and the location of the bleeding. Patients on ventricular assist devices and extracorporeal membrane oxygenation (ECMO) should have platelet counts at least $>100 \times 10^9$/L (100,000/mm^3).

Platelet Products

Apheresis platelets contain $\geq 3.0 \times 10^{11}$ platelets, equivalent to 4–6 units of random donor platelets (RDPs) but are collected from a single donor. *Apheresis platelets leukocytes reduced* should contain $\geq 3.0 \times 10^{11}$ platelets and $<5.0 \times 10^6$ leukocytes. *Pooled platelets*, also called *random donor platelets*, are a concentrate of platelets, which have been separated from a single unit of whole blood. *Leukocyte-reduced* product is also available.

Prescription of Platelets Transfusions

It is prudent to use ABO-matched platelets. The use of ABO-incompatible platelets requires the removal of incompatible plasma, which decreases platelet content by 15%–20%, shortens the storage time to 4 hours, and delays platelet release by ~1 hour. Administering 10 mL/kg of platelet concentrate should increase the platelet count by 50×10^9/L (50,000/mm^3).

Preparation of volume-reduced platelets for volume-sensitive patients results in decreased storage life of platelets and decreases platelet content. An anti-D immunoglobulin preparation (WinRho SDR) may be given to avoid the development of anti-D if the patient is Rh negative, the donor is Rh positive, and RBC contamination of the platelet product is known or expected.

Irradiation is necessary to prevent T-lymphocyte proliferation and eliminate the risk of TA-GVHD. TA-GVHD is associated with a mortality of 90% despite treatment. TA-GVHD has been associated with most blood components, with the exceptions being FFP, frozen deglycerolized RBCs, and cryoprecipitate. Patients most at risk for TA-GVHD include patients with congenital cellular immunodeficiency, patients undergoing stem cell or solid organ transplantation or chemotherapy, and patients receiving HLA-matched products or directed donations from blood relatives.

GRANULOCYTES

Constitution of Granulocyte Concentrates

Granulocyte concentrates are collected using apheresis from donors who have undergone either steroid or growth factor (granulocyte colony-stimulating factor, G-CSF) stimulation. The product contains RBCs and must be crossmatched to the recipient.

Granulocyte Transfusion: Application to PICU

Indications

Therapeutic granulocyte transfusions are indicated for febrile neutropenic (absolute neutrophil count $< 0.5 \times 10^9$/L) patients who have a severe bacterial or fungal infection refractory to antimicrobials and in whom bone marrow recovery is expected to be delayed for as long as 2–3 weeks. These patients have usually failed to respond to a trial G-CSF therapy.

Prescription of Granulocyte Concentrates

A relative contraindication to granulocyte transfusions is if the recipient has anti-HLAs or antigranulocyte antibodies because of the possibility of developing transfusion-related acute lung injury (TRALI). Irradiation of the product is recommended to prevent the proliferation of T lymphocytes, given the immunocompromised state of the recipient and because of the possibility of HLA-matched (including related family member) donations that increases the risk of TA-GVHD. Granulocytes should be transfused over 1–2 hours and should be separated by as much time as possible (at least 4 hours) from amphotericin transfusion as severe pulmonary reactions have been associated with the simultaneous infusion of both products.

WHOLE BLOOD

Constitution of Whole Blood

Whole blood is stored after donation without separation into components. A whole blood unit is typically between 450 and 500 mL, with 63 mL of this volume containing citrate–phosphate–dextrose (CPD) solution, and can be stored at 4°C for up to 21 days.

Transfusion of Whole Blood: Application to PICU

Proposed benefits of whole blood for patients at risk for hemorrhagic shock or requiring massive transfusion include (a) increased concentration of hemoglobin, coagulation factors, and platelets relative to reconstitution with individual components; (b) limited impact of processing on function (with regard to both O_2 transport and coagulation); (c) avoidance of risk associated with extended storage duration; and (d) reduced donor exposure.

TABLE 19.1

Acute and Delayed Transfusion Reactions

Acute (<24 h): Immunologic	
Hemolytic	
ABO/Rh mismatched	1:40,000
Acute hemolytic transfusion reaction	1:76,000
Fatal	1:1.8 million
Febrile, nonhemolytic	0.1%–1% (universal leukoreduction)
Urticarial	1:100–1:33 (1%–3%)
Anaphylaxis	1:20,000–1:50,000
Transfusion-related acute lung injury (TRALI)	1:1200–1:190,000
Acute (<24 h): Nonimmunologic	
Transfusion-associated sepsis	~1:3000 (after implementation of platelet bacterial testing)
Hypotension associated with ACE inhibition	Depends on clinical situation
Transfusion-associated circulatory overload (TACO)	<1%
Nonimmunologic hemolysis	Rare
Air embolus	Rare
Hypocalcemia	Depends on clinical situation
Delayed (>24 h): Immunologic	
Alloimmunization, RBC antigens	1:100 (1%)
Alloimmunization, HLAs	1:10 (10%)
Hemolytic	1:2500–1:11,000
Graft-versus-host disease	Rare
Posttransfusion purpura	Rare
Delayed (>24 h): Nonimmunologic	
Iron overload	Typically after 100 RBC units
Viral and parasitic	See **Table 19.2**

ACE, angiotensin-converting enzyme.
Modified from Mazzei CA, Popovsky MA, Kopko PM. Noninfectious complications of blood transfusion. In: Grossman BJ, Harris T, Roback JD, et al., eds. *AAB Technical Manual.* Bethesda, MD: American Association of Blood Banks Press, 2011.

MASSIVE TRANSFUSIONS

The definition of massive transfusion in children ranges between 40 and 80 mL/kg of RBCs transfused in a 24-hour period. For children with life-threatening bleeding, the classical approach taught within ATLS courses is being replaced with damage control resuscitation (DCR). DCR principles support the use of permissive hypotension (except in patients with severe traumatic brain injury), the rapid surgical control of bleeding, avoidance of hypothermia and acidosis, minimal use of crystalloids, treatment of hypocalcemia, and the use of empiric high unit ratios of plasma and platelets to RBCs to provide a balanced treatment of both shock and coagulopathy for patients with immediate life-threatening hemorrhagic shock.

COMMON COMPLICATIONS OF BLOOD PRODUCT TRANSFUSIONS

Early Reactions

The most common early transfusion reactions include *mild allergic and febrile nonhemolytic reactions*, the latter of which is defined as an increase in temperature equal to or greater than 1°C that cannot be explained by the patient's clinical condition (i.e., other causes of fever must be ruled out) (**Table 19.1**). Febrile nonhemolytic transfusion reactions are typically caused by cytokines generated by leukocytes present within the blood product (most commonly in nonleukoreduced platelet products). *Hemolytic transfusion reaction* is

TABLE 19.2

Viral and Parasitic Infectious Risks

INFECTIOUS AGENT	INCIDENCE
HIV (with NAT)	1:1,467,000 (first-time donors)
HCV (with NAT)	1:1,149,000 (first-time donors)
HTLV	1:2,993,000
HBV	1:280,000
HAV	<1:1 million
Malaria	1:4 million
Chagas disease	Unknown (rare)
Cytomegalovirus	Unknown (presumed rare)
West Nile virus	Unknown (rare break-through despite NAT)
Epstein–Barr virus	Unknown (rare)

NAT, nucleic acid–based tests; HCV, hepatitis C virus; HIV, human immunodeficiency virus; HTLV, human T-lymphocyte viruses; HBV, hepatitis B virus; HAV, hepatitis A virus.
Based on Galel SA. Infectious disease screening. In: Roback JD, Grossman BJ, Harris T, et al., eds. *AABB Technical Manual*. Bethesda, MD: American Association of Blood Banks Press, 2011.

defined as hemoglobinuria or hemoglobinemia (measured as plasma-free hemoglobin above the normal range) with at least one of the following symptoms/signs: fever, dyspnea, hypotension and/or tachycardia, anxiety/agitation, and pain. *Major allergic and anaphylactic reaction*, which may be fatal, is defined as at least one of the following symptoms/signs: (a) cardiac arrest; (b) generalized allergic reaction or anaphylactic reaction; (c) angioedema (facial and/or laryngeal); (d) upper airway obstruction; (e) dyspnea, wheezing; (f) hypotension, shock; (g) precordial pain or chest tightness; (h) cardiac arrhythmia; and (i) loss of consciousness. Older units of RBCs, even more so if irradiated in order to avoid GVHD, are known to have elevated K^+ levels and hyperkalemia can also result from exchange transfusion and after massive transfusion in cardiopulmonary bypass.

Delayed Reactions

Delayed reactions may occur and include transfusion-transmitted viral and parasitic infectious disease; TA-GVHD; and alloimmunization to RBC, platelet-specific (or HLA), or granulocyte antigens. The incidence of viral and parasitic disease transmission is seen in **Table 19.2.**

LIMITING BLOOD PRODUCT UTILIZATION

Reduction in operative blood loss can be achieved by prescribing erythropoietin and iron supplements. The risk of prothrombotic events with erythropoietin must be taken into consideration prior to administration. In addition, the use of fibrin sealants, antifibrinolytics, and recombinant coagulation factor agents, and the judicious use of plasma and platelets instead of crystalloid-based resuscitation for patients with significant bleeding have the potential to reduce bleeding and the need for blood products.

CHAPTER 20 ■ RESPIRATORY PHYSIOLOGY

FRANK L. POWELL, GREGORY P. HELDT, AND GABRIEL G. HADDAD

PULMONARY GAS EXCHANGE

Pulmonary gas exchange describes the process of O_2 uptake and CO_2 elimination by the lungs to supply the metabolic demands of the body. The *oxygen cascade* represents the change in partial pressure of O_2 (Po_2) values measured in gas, blood, and tissue in a resting adult at sea level. The large drop in Po_2 between inspired and alveolar gas is a function of ventilation. Diffusion across the blood–gas barrier, such as shunts and mismatching of ventilation and pulmonary blood flow, explains the small decrease in Po_2 between alveolar gas and arterial blood. The O_2 diffusion from capillaries to tissues causes the large decreases in Po_2 between arterial and venous blood, and between blood and mitochondria in the tissues.

Oxygen in Blood

Hemoglobin

The normal O_2 concentration in arterial blood (Cao_2) is ~20 mL/dL, with only 0.3 mL/dL physically dissolved. Hemoglobin (Hb) is responsible for blood's O_2-carrying capacity. Hb consists of four polypeptide chains, each with a heme (iron-containing) protein that binds O_2 with iron in the ferrous (Fe^{2+}) form. Methemoglobin results when iron is in the ferric form (Fe^{3+}) and cannot bind O_2. Small amounts of methemoglobin normally occur. Methemoglobin reduces O_2 binding to Hb.

Blood–Oxygen Equilibrium Curves

Blood–O_2 equilibrium curves (O_2 dissociation curves) display O_2 carriage as concentration versus Po_2 (**Fig. 20.1**). The sigmoidal shape of the O_2–Hb equilibrium curve facilitates O_2 loading into blood in the lungs and O_2 unloading from blood in the tissues. Remembering four points on the curve allows one to solve many common problems of O_2 transport:

a. Po_2 = 0 mm Hg, So_2 = 0% (the origin of the curve)
b. Po_2 = 100 mm Hg, So_2 = 98% (normal arterial blood, which is almost fully saturated)
c. Po_2 = 40 mm Hg, So_2 = 75% (normal mixed-venous blood)
d. Po_2 = 26 mm Hg, So_2 = 50% (i.e., P_{50})

The P_{50} quantifies the affinity of Hb for O_2 as the Po_2 at 50% saturation under standard conditions of partial pressure of CO_2 (Pco_2) = 40 mm Hg, pH = 7.4, and 37°C. A decrease in P_{50} indicates an increase in O_2 affinity because So_2 or Co_2 is greater for a given Po_2.

Modulation of Blood–Oxygen Equilibrium Curves

The horizontal position of the Hb–O_2 equilibrium curves reflects the affinity of Hb for O_2. Changes in horizontal position are quantified as changes in P_{50} (**Fig. 20.2**). A decrease in P_{50} causes a *left shift* of the equilibrium curve and indicates increased Hb–O_2 affinity; So_2 or Cao_2 is increased for a given Po_2. Similarly, increased P_{50}, or a *right shift*, reflects decreased Hb–O_2 affinity. The three most important physiologic variables that can modulate P_{50} are pH,

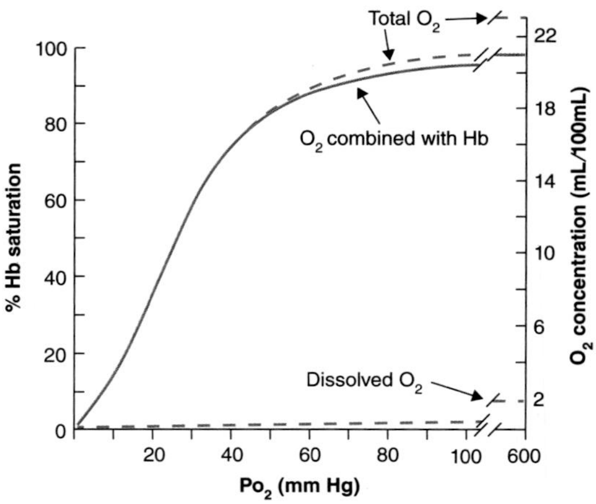

FIGURE 20.1. Standard human O_2–blood equilibrium (or dissociation) curve at pH = 7.4, Pco_2 = 40 mm Hg, and 37°C. Left ordinate shows O_2 saturation of hemoglobin (Hb) available for O_2 binding; right ordinate shows absolute O_2 concentration in blood. Most O_2 is bound to hemoglobin, and dissolved O_2 contributes very little to total O_2 concentration. (From Powell FL. Oxygen and CO_2 transport in the blood. In: Johnson LR, ed. *Essential Medical Physiology*. 3rd ed. Boston, MA: Elsevier/Academic Press, 2003, with permission.)

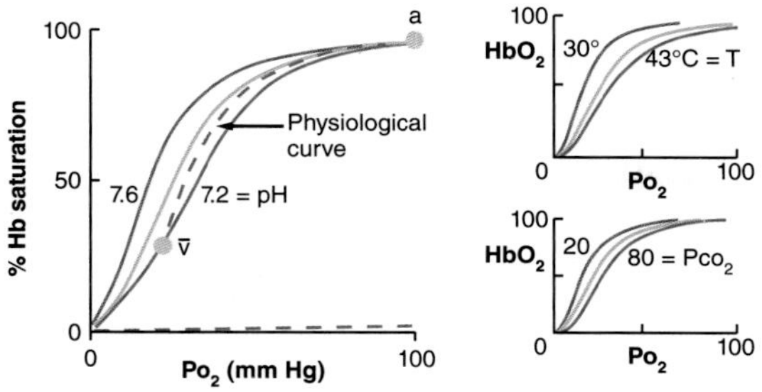

FIGURE 20.2. Effects of pH and P_{CO_2} (i.e., Bohr effect) and temperature on the position of the O_2–hemoglobin (HbO_2) equilibrium curve. The "physiologic" curve connects the arterial (a) and mixed-venous points ($\bar{v}$), so that the in vivo curve is steeper than the standard curve at pH = 7.4 (green). (From Powell FL. Oxygen and CO_2 transport in the blood. In: Johnson LR, ed. *Essential Medical Physiology*. 3rd ed. Boston, MA: Elsevier/Academic Press, 2003, with permission.)

P_{CO_2}, and temperature. The *Bohr effect* describes changes in P_{50} with changes in blood P_{CO_2} and pH. The physiologic advantage of the Bohr effect is facilitation of O_2 loading in the lungs, where CO_2 is low and pH is high. In the tissues, the increased CO_2 and decreased pH facilitate O_2 unloading from Hb to the tissues. The effect of temperature on Hb–O_2 affinity also has physiologic advantages.

Hb–O_2 affinity is also affected by *2,3-diphosphoglycerate* (2,3-DPG) levels. Physiologic stimuli that enhance O_2 delivery (e.g., chronic decreases in blood P_{O_2} levels) lead to increased concentration of 2,3-DPG and O_2 delivery to tissues. In stored blood, 2,3-DPG is decreased, which increases Hb–O_2 affinity and can lead to problems in O_2 delivery after blood transfusion.

The affinity of Hb for *carbon monoxide* (CO) is 240 times greater than for O_2, and so even small amounts of CO greatly reduce the capacity for Hb to bind O_2. CO also causes a left shift of the curve by altering the ability of the Hb molecule to bind O_2; therefore, blood O_2 concentration remains high until P_{O_2} decreases to very low levels, which impairs O_2 unloading from blood to tissues.

Oxygen Transport in Fetal Blood

Fetal Hb (HbF) P_{50} is 20 torr (adult P_{50} is 26 torr); this facilitates O_2 transfer from the placenta to the fetus. HbF is replaced by adult Hb in the first year. Both the left shift of the fetal (versus adult) O_2–Hb equilibrium curve and a high fetal O_2 capacity facilitate O_2 unloading from the mother to the fetus.

Carbon Dioxide in Blood

The CO_2–blood equilibrium curve is steeper than the O_2 curve, resulting in a smaller range of physiologic P_{CO_2} values. The difference between arterial and venous concentrations is similar for CO_2 and O_2 (~5 mL/dL).

Carbon Dioxide and Blood Acid–Base

Dissolved CO_2 contributes ~5% of total CO_2 concentration in arterial blood. *Carbamino compounds* also comprise 5% of arterial CO_2. *Bicarbonate ion* (HCO_3^-) is the most important form of CO_2 carriage in blood. The rapid conversion of CO_2 to bicarbonate results in ~90% of the CO_2 in arterial blood.

Modulation of Blood–Carbon Dioxide Equilibrium Curves

Increasing O_2 decreases the affinity of Hb for H^+ and blood CO_2 concentration (Haldane effect), and increased [H^+] decreases the affinity of Hb for O_2 (Bohr effect). The Haldane effect promotes unloading of CO_2 in the lungs when blood is oxygenated and CO_2 loading in the blood when O_2 is released to tissues.

Alveolar Ventilation and Alveolar P_{O_2}

The conducting zone includes the conducting airways from the trachea to the terminal bronchioles (the 16th order of bronchial branching). The gas volume of the conducting zone equals the *anatomic dead space.* The respiratory zone comprises the rest of the lung (the 17th to 23rd orders of bronchial branching—respiratory bronchioles to alveolar sacs—where all gas exchange occurs). Total cross-sectional area of the airways in distal parts of the lung is greatly increased; therefore, the respiratory zone comprises most of the lung volume.

Alveolar Ventilation Equation Predicts Alveolar P_{CO_2}

Alveolar ventilation $\dot{V}_A$ is the difference between total ventilation ($\dot{V}_T$) and dead space ventilation ($\dot{V}_{DS}$), and it is the effective conductance for pulmonary gas exchange. Although anatomic dead space can be measured, it is more relevant to estimate physiologic dead space (also called *Bohr dead space*). Physiologic dead space includes all "wasted ventilation" and can exceed anatomic dead space. Physiologic dead space can be calculated from rearrangement of the Fick principle applied to CO_2 elimination by the lungs as:

$$\dot{V}_{DS}/V_T = (P_{ACO_2} - P\bar{E}_{CO_2})/P_{ACO_2}$$

where $P\bar{E}_{CO_2}$ = *mixed-expired* P_{CO_2} that is measured by collecting all expired gas and includes gas exhaled from the alveoli *and* dead space. In practice, arterial P_{CO_2} is easier to measure and substituted for alveolar P_{CO_2}.

Alveolar Gas Equation Predicts Alveolar P_{O_2}

Alveolar P_{O_2} (P_{AO_2}) can be predicted from the *alveolar gas equation* that models an "ideal lung" with only physiologic dead space:

$$P_{AO_2} = P_{IO_2} - (P_{ACO_2}/R) + F$$

where P_{IO_2} is inspired P_{O_2}, P_{ACO_2} is alveolar P_{CO_2}, R is the respiratory exchange ratio, and F is a constant that is ignored under normal conditions. Arterial P_{CO_2} is substituted for alveolar P_{CO_2}. The *respiratory exchange ratio* (R) is the ratio of uptake to CO_2 elimination by the lungs:

$$R = \dot{V}_{CO_2}/\dot{V}_{O_2}.$$

Under steady-state conditions, R equals the *respiratory quotient* (RQ), which is the ratio of CO_2 production to O_2 consumption in metabolizing tissues. RQ averages 0.8 on a normal, mixed, adult diet, but it can range from 0.67 to 1, depending on the relative amounts of fat, protein, and carbohydrate being metabolized.

Diffusion

Diffusion of O_2 from alveoli to pulmonary capillary blood is the next step in the O_2 cascade after alveolar ventilation. O_2 moves from the alveoli to pulmonary capillary blood barrier according to Fick's first law of diffusion:

$$\dot{V}_{O_2} = \Delta P_{O_2} \times D_{O_2}$$

where ΔP_{O_2} is the average P_{O_2} gradient across the blood–gas barrier and D_{O_2} is a diffusing capacity.

Blood–Gas Barrier

The pathway of an O_2 molecule diffusing from alveolar gas to Hb inside a red blood cell is the anatomic basis for D_{O_2}. The blood–gas barrier consists of three different layers. The "thin" side of a pulmonary capillary (0.3 µm) separates gas from plasma with (a) thin cytoplasmic extensions from type I alveolar epithelial cells, (b) a thin basement membrane, and (c) thin cytoplasmic extensions from capillary endothelial cells. The thicker side of a capillary has collagen in the interstitial space to provide mechanical strength in the alveoli. Finally, O_2 must diffuse through plasma and across the red blood cell membrane before it can combine with Hb. The diffusing capacity for O_2 between the alveolar gas and Hb is called the *membrane diffusing capacity for* O_2, or D_{MO_2}. After O_2 diffuses into red blood cells, the finite *rate of reaction between* O_2 *and Hb* (abbreviated with the symbol θ) offers an additional "resistance" to O_2 uptake. The magnitude of this chemical resistance depends on θ and the total amount of Hb, which is a physiologic function of pulmonary capillary volume (V_C). The total resistance to O_2 diffusion in the lung can be defined as:

$$1/D_{LO_2} = 1/D_{MO_2} + 1/(\theta V_C)$$

where D_{LO_2} *is the lung diffusing capacity for* O_2. (D_{LO_2} is a conductance; recall that conductance is the inverse of resistance, and resistors in series are additive.)

P_{O_2} Changes along the Pulmonary Capillary

Normally, P_{O_2} changes along the capillary in adult lungs and the P_{O_2} in capillary blood increases from mixed-venous levels at the beginning to arterial levels at the end of the capillary. Two conditions cause diffusion limitation for O_2 in healthy adults. Elite athletes with abnormally high cardiac outputs move blood through capillaries in less than 0.25 seconds and diffusion limitation results. Second, normal adults exercising at altitude may not achieve diffusion equilibrium because transit time and P_{AO_2} decrease. Both of these types of diffusion limitation are different than hypoxemia in the intensive care unit (ICU) where metabolic rate and cardiac output may be depressed. Hypoxemia from a decrease in lung diffusing capacity (e.g., thickening of the blood–gas barrier from edema) may be corrected by increasing inspired O_2 levels.

Diffusion-Limited and Perfusion-Limited Gases

The anesthetic gas nitrous oxide (N_2O) achieves equilibrium rapidly, whereas CO never comes close to diffusion equilibrium. N_2O is a *perfusion-limited gas*. Changes in the diffusing capacity have no effect on the uptake of a perfusion-limited gas or its partial pressure in the blood. All anesthetic and "inert" gases that do not react chemically with blood are perfusion-limited. The uptake of a gas that does not achieve diffusion equilibrium could obviously increase if the diffusing capacity increased. CO is an example of such a *diffusion-limited gas*. As Hb has a very high affinity for CO, the effective solubility of CO in blood is large. Therefore, increases in the CO concentration in blood are not effective at increasing partial pressure of carbon monoxide (P_{CO}), which keeps blood P_{CO} lower than alveolar P_{CO} and results in a large disequilibrium and diffusion limitation. In practice, the only diffusion-limited gases are CO and O_2 under hypoxic conditions. All other gases are perfusion-limited, including O_2 under normoxic conditions in healthy lungs.

Four Causes of Hypoxemia

Arterial hypoxemia (decreased P_{aO_2}) indicates a limitation of pulmonary gas exchange. Gas-exchange limitations in the lungs can reduce P_{O_2} throughout the O_2 cascade but they do not decrease resting oxygen consumption. The four kinds of pulmonary gas-exchange limitations are (a) hypoventilation, (b) diffusion limitation, (c) pulmonary blood-flow shunt, and (d) mismatching of ventilation and blood flow in the lung.

Hypoventilation

Hypoventilation is the only gas-exchange limitation that does not increase the alveolar–arterial PO_2 difference. The magnitude of hypoxemia caused by hypoventilation is predicted by the alveolar gas equation. If R = 1, then PAO_2 decreases 1 mm Hg for every 1 mm Hg increase in $PACO_2$. However, a normal value for R is 0.8, and this magnifies the effects of hypoventilation and increased $PaCO_2$ on hypoxemia. Two primary classes of problems that cause hypoventilation are (a) mechanical limitations and (b) ventilatory control abnormalities.

Diffusion Limitation

Pulmonary diffusion limitation decreases PaO_2 by increasing the alveolar–arterial PO_2 difference, which occurs with (a) decreases in the partial pressure driving O_2 across the blood–gas barrier (PAO_2), or (b) low diffusing capacity for O_2 (DLO_2). With lung disease, the measured DLCO can decrease with destruction of surface area and capillary volume (e.g., emphysema) or thickening of the blood–gas barrier (e.g., edema). However, DLCO must decrease to <50% of normal before arterial hypoxemia is observed in resting patients. Arterial hypoxemia caused by a diffusion limitation can be relieved rapidly by increasing inspired O_2 (within several breaths).

Shunt

Shunt flow is defined as deoxygenated venous blood flow that enters the arterial circulation without going through ventilated alveoli in the pulmonary circulation. This kind of shunt is also called *right-to-left shunt.* Alveolar and end-capillary PaO_2 are predicted to be >600 mm Hg during pure O_2 breathing. However, shunt significantly decreases PaO_2 because of the shape of the O_2–blood equilibrium curve. Persistent hypoxemia during 100% O_2 breathing indicates a shunt. Normally, shunt during O_2 breathing averages <5% of cardiac output. It includes (a) venous blood from the bronchial circulation that drains directly into the pulmonary veins, and (b) venous blood from the coronary circulation that enters the left ventricle through the Thebesian veins. If shunt is calculated during room air breathing, it is called *venous admixture,* which occurs in healthy lungs because of ventilation–perfusion mismatching. Shunts in the newborn are common, especially during transition to air breathing. Most newborns with pulmonary hypertension have a PDA if pulmonary arterial pressure exceeds systemic arterial pressure. Measuring PaO_2 simultaneously from the preductal area (upper right chest or right radial artery) and the postductal area (umbilical artery, left radial artery, or legs) can measure this shunt.

Ventilation–Perfusion Mismatching

Mismatching of ventilation and blood flow in different parts of the lung is the most common cause of hypoxemia and increased alveolar–arterial PO_2 differences in health and disease. It is also the most complicated mechanism of hypoxemia and will be approached in two steps.

The $\dot{V}A/\dot{Q}$ Ratio. PAO_2 increases with $\dot{V}A$ according to the alveolar ventilation and alveolar gas equations. $\dot{V}A/\dot{Q}$ adds the concept of blood flow ($\dot{Q}$). If $\dot{Q}$ suddenly increases and removes more O_2 from the alveoli (recall that O_2 is normally a perfusion-limited gas), then PAO_2 will decrease. However, if $\dot{V}A$ increases O_2 delivery to match increased O_2 removal (returning the $\dot{V}A/\dot{Q}$ ratio to normal), then PAO_2 will return to normal. When $\dot{V}A/\dot{Q} = 0$, a shunt is indicated. Dead space is indicated when $\dot{V}A/\dot{Q}$ is infinite. As dead space receives no blood flow, this alveolus equilibrates with inspired gas.

$\dot{V}A/\dot{Q}$ Mismatching Between Different Lung Regions. Regional differences in alveolar ventilation occur because of the mechanical properties of the lung. In upright adults, gravity tends to distort the lung, and alveoli in the apex are more expanded than in the base of the lung, resulting in basal alveoli operating on a steeper part of the lung's compliance curve, so that $\dot{V}A$ is greater at the bottom than at the top of the lung. $\dot{V}A/\dot{Q}$ heterogeneity occurs in healthy lungs and explains the small but measurable alveolar–arterial PO_2 in young adults. $\dot{V}A/\dot{Q}$ heterogeneity can be diagnosed clinically by eliminating other causes of hypoxemia. Hypoventilation is ruled out if arterial PCO_2 is normal. Diffusion limitation can be ruled out if the measured DLCO is at least 50% of normal or if breathing high inspired O_2 relieves hypoxemia and decreases the alveolar–arterial PO_2 difference. O_2 breathing improves hypoxemia from $\dot{V}A/\dot{Q}$ heterogeneity but not as quickly as with a pure diffusion limitation (which requires <1 minute). If shunt is present, 100% O_2 breathing will never resolve hypoxemia or decrease the alveolar–arterial PO_2 difference.

Carbon Dioxide Exchange

The Fick principle can also be used to calculate the normal arterial–venous CO_2 concentration difference:

$$\dot{V}CO_2 = \dot{Q}\ (CaCO_2 - C\bar{v}\text{–}CO_2)$$

For normal values of $\dot{V}CO_2$ = 240 mL of CO_2/min and $\dot{Q}$= 6 L/min, the arterial–venous CO_2 concentration difference is 4 mL/dL. $PaCO_2$ is the most important value in determining resting ventilation, and ventilatory reflexes tend to increase $\dot{V}A$ as much as necessary to restore normal $PaCO_2$ when gas exchange is altered.

Cardiovascular and Tissue Oxygen Transport

The mitochondria are the ultimate site of O_2 consumption and CO_2 production. The magnitude of the PO_2

decrease between arterial and venous blood depends on both the cardiovascular O_2 delivery and tissue O_2 demand. O_2 delivery is the product of cardiac output and arterial O_2 concentration ($\dot{Q}Ca_{O_2}$). The tissues will extract enough O_2 to meet their needs as long as O_2 supply is sufficient. Hence, O_2 supply and demand determine venous O_2 levels. These factors are related by the Fick principle, which describes O_2 transport by the cardiovascular system as:

$$\dot{V}o_2 = \dot{Q}\,(Cao_2 - C\bar{v}o_2)$$

where $\dot{V}o_2$ is O_2 consumption, $\dot{Q}$ is cardiac output, and the last term is the arterial–venous O_2 concentration difference. Changes in $\dot{V}o_2$ can be achieved by increasing cardiac output ("flow reserve") or increasing the arterial–venous O_2 difference. Increasing $\dot{V}o_2$ by increasing venous O_2 extraction represents the "extraction reserve." Changes in $P\bar{v}o_2$ are minimized with large decreases in venous O_2 concentration by the shape of the O_2–blood equilibrium curve. A right shift of the curve can increase $P\bar{v}o_2$ for a given $C\bar{v}o_2$ ("O_2-dissociation reserve"). Maintaining a high $P\bar{v}o_2$ is important for tissue gas exchange and the "microcirculatory and tissue reserve." All these reserves are important mechanisms for meeting increased O_2 demands during exercise.

Increases in O_2 delivery are achieved primarily through increases in cardiac output in normoxic conditions. Increasing alveolar and arterial Po_2 is not effective at increasing Cao_2 in normoxic conditions because the slope of the O_2–blood equilibrium curve is flat at normal Pao_2 values ("ventilatory reserve"). Changes in Pao_2 are much more effective at changing O_2 delivery when Po_2 is low and O_2 exchange occurs on a steep part of the O_2–blood equilibrium curve. Changes in Hct and Hb concentration, which occur with chronic hypoxia, can increase O_2 delivery by increasing total O_2 concentration for any given Po_2 ("erythropoietic reserve").

Tissue Gas Exchange

Tissue gas exchange describes the process of O_2 moving out of systemic capillaries to the mitochondria by diffusion. The difference between O_2 diffusion in tissue and the lung is that diffusion pathways are longer in tissue. Additional capillaries are recruited during exercise, maintaining adequate O_2 supply by decreasing diffusion distances. Myoglobin facilitates O_2 diffusion in muscle by shuttling O_2 to sites far from a capillary.

LUNG MECHANICS, RESPIRATORY, AND AIRWAY MUSCLES

Pressure–Flow Relationships in the Respiratory System

The mammalian lung has a natural tendency to collapse. The respiratory muscles and the chest wall oppose this tendency and apply a continuous tension to the structure of the lungs to maintain lung volume at end-expiration. The sum of the forces that make the lungs collapse is referred to as the *elastic recoil*.

Developmental Aspects of the Lung as They Affect Elastic Recoil

Lung development begins with the formation of the respiratory diverticulum from the ventral foregut. Differentiation of the lungs is under the control of the extracellular matrix that is laid down in the mesenchyme, into which the developing lung bud grows. Much of the early branching is controlled by the presence of syndecan, a proteoglycan that is abundant in the mesenchyme and is critical to the formation of epithelial tubes. The main elastic elements of the lung are collagen and elastin. The central airways have two collagen/elastin layers: one longitudinal and one circumferential. These grow out past the respiratory and terminal bronchioles and become thin fibers that spiral into the alveolar ducts. These fibers are continuous with the fibers of the blood vessels, airways, and the pleura. Inflammation in the developing lung dramatically affects normal lung development and is thought to be a major mechanism in the development of BPD in low–birth weight infants.

Surface Tension and Elastic Recoil

The elastic skeleton of the lung predicts a simple, linear relationship between the volume of the lung and the pressure applied across it. It has long been observed that pulmonary surfactant contributes greatly to the pressure–volume characteristics of the lungs. When lungs are washed of surfactant, the alveolar ducts increase in size, which suggests that alveolar collapse redistributes stress to the more proximal airway. At 23–30 weeks gestation, when many premature infants are born, the elastic fibers are not yet developed and cannot bear the stress imposed by alveolar collapse. This effect is greater during mechanical ventilation. Rupture of the airways and the capillaries causes the formation of edema and hyaline membranes, the pathologic precursor of BPD.

Flow Limitation

The second element in the mechanics of breathing involves where and how airflow limitation occurs. Airway resistance is usually modeled by the aerodynamics of flow through tubes. Flow through the airways is driven by a pressure drop between the alveoli and the atmosphere or the endotracheal tube. Laminar flow (described by Poiseuille) has the least possible pressure drop or energy dissipation for a given flow and tube diameter:

$$\text{Resistance} = (8 \times \text{viscosity} \times \text{length}) / (\pi \times \text{radius}^4)$$

The resistance is dependent on the viscosity of the gas and is inversely proportional to the fourth power of the radius. The Reynolds number is a dimensionless number proportional to the product of the gas density, the flow rate, and the diameter of the tube. When the Reynolds number is greater than ~2300, the inertial forces are greater than the viscous forces, and laminar flow cannot be established. Rather than moving in smooth lines straight down the tube, the gas is turbulent. From estimates of the Reynolds number and dimensions of the airways obtained from anatomic casts, flow in the large airways is turbulent. Laminar flow becomes established between the 4th and 15th generation of airways. In cases of extreme large-airway obstruction, the resistance can be decreased by reducing the density of the gas with a mixture of helium and O_2 (Heliox).

The airways are flexible tubes and will collapse if the transmural pressure becomes negative. The peribronchial pressure approximates the pleural pressure. Applying additional pressure upstream, such as during active expiration, does not allow transmission of the pressure or flow downstream because the transmural pressure in the large airways becomes negative (**Fig. 20.3**). The transmural pressure reflects the elastic recoil pressure of the lung, because the lung parenchyma is closely linked mechanically to the peribronchiolar space. Thus, at high lung volume, when recoil pressure is greatest, the flow limitation is in the 2nd and 3rd generation of bronchi. At lower lung volumes, flow decreases and the sites of flow limitation move peripherally.

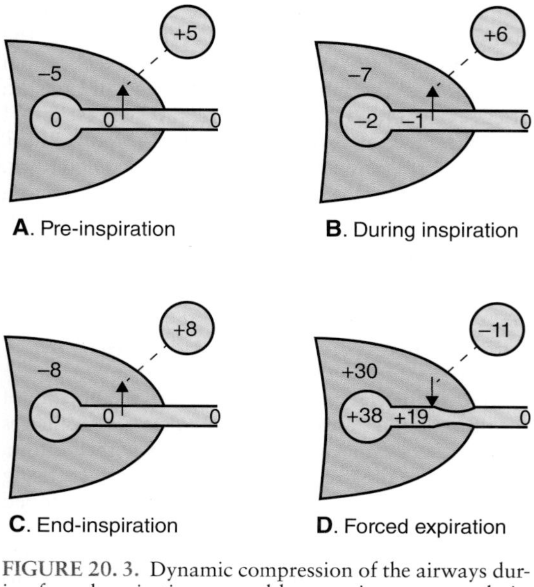

FIGURE 20. 3. Dynamic compression of the airways during forced expiration, caused by negative transmural airway pressure (D) beyond the equal pressure point. (From Powell FL. Mechanics of breathing. In: Johnson LR, ed. *Essential Medical Physiology*. 3rd ed. London, England: Elsevier/Academic Press, 2003, with permission.)

PULMONARY CIRCULATION

The adult pulmonary circulation is unique because the lung is the only organ to receive the entire cardiac output. Low pulmonary vascular pressure is beneficial for reducing the stress on the extremely delicate pulmonary capillaries, which are as thin as possible to enhance diffusion of O_2 and CO_2.

Fetal and Perinatal Pulmonary Circulation

The pulmonary circulation in the fetus differs from the adult because the placenta is the gasexchange organ. Fetal blood flows into the placenta through the umbilical arteries. O_2 diffuses from the maternal circulation into the fetus. Diffusion is inefficient in the placenta compared to the lungs, but O_2 transfer is enhanced by the high O_2 affinity of fetal Hb. The result is a maximum Po_2 of 30 torr in the fetal circulation in blood leaving the placenta and entering the inferior vena cava. Blood is pumped from the right ventricle into the pulmonary artery, 10% flows into the lungs and the remainder goes to the aorta via the ductus arteriosus. Some pulmonary blood flow is important for development of the lungs and the surfactant system. The ductus arteriosus joins the aorta distal to the carotid and coronary arteries. This anatomy maximizes the Po_2 in blood that perfuses the brain and heart because Po_2 is greater in the left ventricle than in the right ventricle. It is important to note that the output of the left ventricle is approximately half that of the right ventricle in the fetus, in contrast to being equal in adults, because the ductus arteriosus shunts blood from the pulmonary to systemic circulations.

Fetal transition takes place in three stages. The first stage reduces the PVR to ~50% of the fetal level, and occurs with the first few effective breaths. The second stage takes up to 1 hour, during which time the ductus arteriosus constricts, and relief of the hypoxic pulmonary vasoconstriction is stabilized. During this stage, the PVR is reduced by ~75% of the fetal level. This third stage takes several hours to days, during which complete relaxation of the hypoxic vasoconstriction and remodeling of the vascular smooth muscle occur.

Pulmonary Vascular Pressures

The pressure drop from artery to vein is more uniform in the adult pulmonary circulation than in the systemic circulation, and this is the same for newborns. Capillaries are more important determinants of total resistance in the pulmonary than systemic circulation. During positive-pressure ventilation, alveolar and intrapleural pressures may increase considerably during inflation, leading to large increases in pulmonary circulatory pressures. However, PVR can increase also, which may limit pulmonary blood flow and cardiac output.

Pulmonary Vascular Resistance

PVR is low compared to systemic vascular resistance. PVR is the resistance for both lungs; in adults ~1.7 (mm Hg × minute)/L for a normal cardiac output of 6 L/min, with an average pressure drop of 10 mm Hg from the pulmonary artery to left atrium. The resistance to flow through a vessel depends on its dimensions. Because the pulmonary capillaries are surrounded by open air spaces rather than solid tissue the primary determinant of vessel size in the lungs is the *transmural pressure*, the pressure difference between inside and outside the vessel. Increasing pulmonary arterial pressure increases flow by increasing the pressure gradient and increasing the transmural pressure, which increases vessel size and decreases PVR. Increasing pulmonary venous pressure also decreases PVR by dilating capillaries.

Alveolar pressure is the outside pressure for calculating transmural pressure. Alveolar pressure varies with the ventilatory cycle, but it is generally near zero (i.e., atmospheric pressure). Therefore, vascular pressure is the primary determinant of transmural pressure. Large positive alveolar pressures from artificial ventilation or PEEP can collapse pulmonary capillaries. Increased pulmonary arterial or venous pressures do not necessarily decrease vascular resistance unless they increase transmural pressure. Increasing transmural pressure can affect capillary dimensions by recruitment and distention. At very low pressures, some capillaries may be closed, and increasing pressure opens them by recruitment. At higher pressures, capillaries are open, but they may be distended or stretched by increased transmural pressure. Together, recruitment and distention increase the effective size of the pulmonary capillaries and reduce PVR. Another important determinant of pulmonary vessel size is lung volume. This effect differs for different types of vessels. Extra-alveolar vessels are surrounded by lung parenchyma, which acts as a tether or support structure to hold the vessels open. At high lung volumes, above functional residual capacity (FRC), the extra-alveolar vessels are pulled open by tissues outside the vessels. At low lung volumes, below FRC, this tethering effect is reduced and the extra-alveolar vessels narrow. The effects of lung volume on alveolar vessels are generally opposite to those on extra-alveolar vessels. These factors account for why PVR is at its lowest at FRC—the lung volume at which normal tidal ventilation occurs. When end-expiratory lung volume is greater or less than physiologic FRC, PVR is increased.

Hypoxic Pulmonary Vasoconstriction

Hypoxic pulmonary vasoconstriction is an important physiologic mechanism that actively controls PVR and blood flow in the lungs and is critical to the transition to neonatal circulation. Currently, the bulk of evidence suggests that the primary sensor is mitochondria in pulmonary artery smooth muscle cells. **Figure 20.4** shows the effect of Po_2 on PVR in the newborn; the main effect of Po_2 occurs at very low levels, which are found in the fetus. However, blood pH has an effect even at high Po_2; therefore, the increase in pH with the onset of air breathing will also reduce PVR as Po_2 increases with air breathing in the newborn. Other physiologic factors capable of influencing the adult pulmonary circulation include a weak vasoconstrictor effect from the sympathetic nervous system and potent vasoconstriction by endothelins.

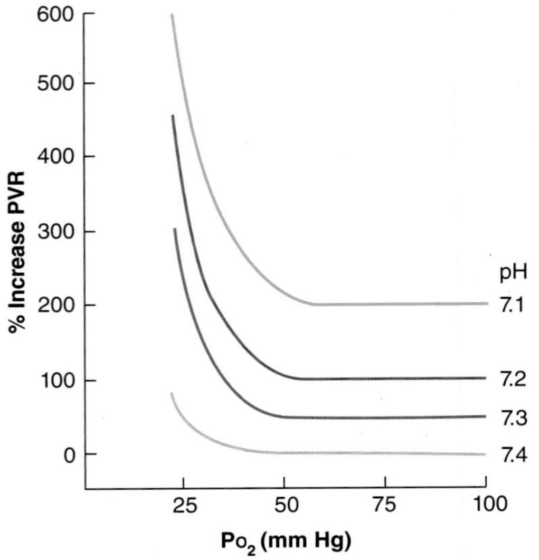

FIGURE 20.4. Decreasing O_2 in inspired gas (Po_2) causes hypoxic vasoconstriction and increases pulmonary vascular resistance (PVR). Arterial acidosis exaggerates this effect in newborns and may be important in helping to establish the adult pattern of circulation. (From Powell FL. Pulmonary gas exchange. In: Johnson LR, ed. *Essential Medical Physiology*. 3rd ed. Boston, MA: Elsevier Academic Press, 2003, with permission.)

Distribution of Pulmonary Blood Flow

Gravity increases vascular pressures in the bottom of the upright lung. This recruits and distends capillaries to decrease resistance and increase flow in the bottom, compared to the top, of the lung. These effects using the zone model for pulmonary blood flow developed by West are illustrated in **Figure 20.5**. Zone 1 occurs at the top of the lung, where the pulmonary arterial pressure is not sufficient to pump blood to the top. Zone 1 does not occur in the normal adult lung because the normal pulmonary arterial pressure (30 cm H_2O) is greater than the height of a water column between the heart and top of the lung (~15 cm). Zone 2 describes the flow in most of the lung. In this

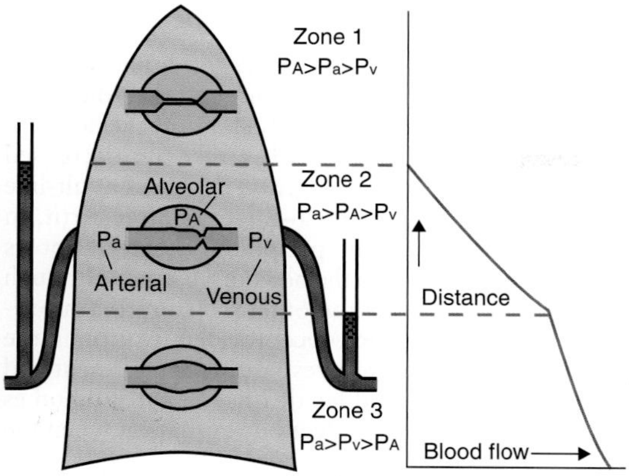

FIGURE 20.5. West's zone model for pulmonary blood flow predicts increasing blood flow down the lung because of the effects of gravity on pressures. PA, arterial pressure; PA, alveolar pressure; Pv, venous pressure. (From Powell FL. Structure and function of the respiratory system. In: Johnson LR, ed. *Essential Medical Physiology*. 3rd ed. London, England: Elsevier/Academic Press, 2003, with permission.)

zone, which occurs near the bottom of the lung, the relevant pressure gradient driving blood flow is the arterial–alveolar difference. Elevating alveolar pressure with mechanical ventilation converts some zone 2 lung to zone 1 (more alveolar dead space) and some zone 3 lung to zone 2 (improves V/Q mismatch).

Bronchial Circulation

The bronchial circulation is part of the systemic circulation and serves the metabolic needs of the large airways and blood vessels. Bronchial arteries arise from the aorta and intercostal arteries, and the bronchial circulation returns blood to the heart by two pathways. Bronchial veins from large airways return approximately half of the bronchial blood flow to the right heart via the azygos vein. The other half of the bronchial circulation drains directly into the pulmonary circulation, which constitutes an anatomic shunt. The bronchial circulation is only 1%–2% of cardiac output in normal adults and this anatomic shunt has a small effect on arterial O_2 levels.

Lung Fluid Balance

The pulmonary capillaries are extremely thin and contain pores that allow fluid to move across their walls. Starling's law states that the net fluid flux across the capillary depends on a balance of hydrostatic forces (P) and colloid osmotic (or oncotic) forces (π):

$$\text{Net fluid flux} = K_{fc}\,[(Pc - Pi) - \sigma\,(\pi c - \pi i)]$$

where K_{fc} is a filtration coefficient that depends on the total surface area of the capillary and the number and size of pores in the capillary. Hydrostatic pressure in the capillary (Pc) tends to move fluid out, and interstitial pressure (Pi) tends to move fluid into the capillary. Conversely, capillary osmotic pressure (πc) tends to hold fluid in the capillary, and interstitial osmotic pressure (πi) tends to draw fluid out of the capillary. Normally, the balance of forces results in net filtration, or the movement of a few milliliters per hour of fluid out of the capillaries in adults. The osmotic forces promote absorption. When this balance of forces is disturbed, filtration can exceed reabsorption and lymphatic drainage and fluid accumulates in the interstitium. Pulmonary edema fluid accumulates first in the peribronchiolar and perivascular spaces; this is called *interstitial edema*. Interstitial edema can alter local ventilation and perfusion and make gas exchange inefficient by decreasing compliance, increasing the work of breathing, and loss of lung volume. Only in severe pathology does fluid cross directly from capillary lumen into alveolus because the basement membrane between the endothelial and epithelial cells is quite impervious to water.

RESPIRATORY CONTROL

General Concepts

Respiratory Control Concepts

Respiration is controlled via α negative feedback system, using α controller in the CNS. The carotid bodies inform the central controller of the O_2 level. The external intercostal and diaphragm muscles are the major muscles of respiration.

Central neuronal processing and integration in the brainstem is hierarchical. Respiratory muscles are recruited to perform different tasks at different times, such as for respiration, jumping, splinting the abdomen, and Valsalva maneuvers. In other conditions, respiratory muscles can be totally inhibited. An example relevant to infants is bottle- or breast-feeding, which can be associated with a reduction in ventilation and Po_2 because respiratory muscles and breathing efforts are inhibited. Brainstem neurons have cellular and membrane properties that allow them to beat (cycle) spontaneously. The respiratory rhythm is generated by an oscillating neuronal network in the ventrolateral formation of the medulla.

Afferent information is not essential for generation of breathing, but modulates respiration. Chemoreceptors and mechanoreceptors in the larynx and upper airways sense stretch, temperature, and chemical changes over the mucosa and relay this information to the brainstem. Afferent impulses from these areas travel through the superior laryngeal nerve and vagus. Changes in O_2 or CO_2 tensions are sensed at the carotid and aortic bodies, and afferent impulses travel through the carotid and aortic sinus nerves. Thermal or metabolic changes are sensed by skin or mucosal receptors or by hypothalamic neurons and carried through spinal tracts to the brainstem.

In the absence of afferent information, the inherent rhythm of the central generator (indexed by respiratory frequency) is slowed. Chemoreceptor afferents modulate respiration and rhythmic behavior.

Developmental Aspects of Respiratory Control

Central Aspects of Respiratory Control

The discharge of central neurons in the adult or neonate is affected by peripheral input, including input from the vagus nerve, and the respiratory feedback system can operate on a breath-by-breath basis.

Peripheral Sensory Aspects

The primary O_2 sensors in the carotids show major differences between the newborn and the adult. The increase in $Pa{O_2}$ at birth virtually shuts off chemoreceptor activity in the newborn. However, this decreased sensitivity does not last long, and a normal adult-like sensitivity takes place by 1–2 weeks after birth. In comparison to the adult, peripheral chemoreceptors assume a greater role in the newborn period. Although not essential for initiation of fetal respiratory movements, peripheral chemoreceptor denervation in the newborn results in severe respiratory impairment and high probability of sudden death. The carotid bodies discharge and have an effect on ventilation when the $Pa{O_2}$ reaches below 55–60 torr.

CHAPTER 21 ■ THE MOLECULAR BIOLOGY OF ACUTE LUNG INJURY

TODD CARPENTER AND KURT R. STENMARK

The central derangement in acute respiratory distress syndrome (ARDS) is the disruption of the alveolar–capillary barrier, which allows protein-rich plasma components to cross into the airspaces. Once alveoli are flooded, surfactant is inactivated and a cycle of inflammation and local hypoxia leads to injury progression, which is worsened by the mechanical forces of artificial ventilation and oxidant stress from high inspired O_2 concentrations. This early phase of ARDS is characterized by pulmonary edema, hypoxemic respiratory failure, poor lung compliance, and pulmonary hypertension (**Fig. 21.1**). The illness progresses to a fibroproliferative phase with progressive scarring and thickening of the lung interstitium. Many survivors have long-lasting pulmonary function deficits.

INJURY, INFLAMMATION, AND EDEMA FORMATION

Toll-like Receptors/Mitochondrial DNA/ Danger-Associated Molecular Patterns and Pathogen-Associated Molecular Patterns

ARDS is initiated by either direct injury to the lung (respiratory infections, acid aspiration, or pulmonary contusion) or distant tissue injuries (sepsis or trauma). The innate immune system then triggers and amplifies inflammatory responses to the injury. Initial recognition of tissue injury occurs through pattern recognition receptors (PRRs), which include the Toll-like receptors (TLRs), NOD-like receptors (NLRs), and RIG-like receptors (RLRs). PRRs bind specific molecular patterns, which can be typical of pathogens (pathogen-associated molecular patterns [PAMPs]) or damaged cells and tissues (danger-associated molecular patterns [DAMPs]), and initiate signaling cascades that activate proinflammatory transcription factors, most prominently nuclear factor-κB (NF-κB). TLR signaling activates both inflammation and protective responses (i.e., there is reduced survival in some models of impaired TLR signaling).

Mitochondrial DNA, which shares evolutionary origins with bacterial DNA, when released from damaged cells activates TLR9, leading to inflammation and neutrophil activation. Other DAMPs contributing to lung injury include nucleic acids (DNA, RNA, microRNAs), extracellular matrix proteins (fibronectin, hyaluronin), and metabolic products (uric acid). Nuclear histone proteins are also highly toxic to cells when released into the extracellular space.

Inflammatory Mediators in Lung Injury

A multitude of inflammatory mediators are responsible for the physiologic derangements in ARDS (e.g., disrupted endothelial and epithelial barriers, alveolar flooding, and intense inflammation). While these cascades of mediators explain the difficulty encountered in devising targeted therapies, they also provide opportunities for the development of specific interventions.

Signaling and Transcriptional Mediators

The protein kinase C (PKC) family of serine/threonine kinases is among the best-described intracellular signaling pathways implicated in the development of ARDS. These molecules contribute to the control of endothelial permeability in the injured lung. Many transcription factors are involved in ARDS, including hypoxia-inducible factor (HIF) 1, NF-κB, and SMAD transcription factors. HIF-1 is ubiquitously expressed and is a critical regulator of cellular responses to hypoxia. NF-κB is the most prominent transcriptional regulator of inflammatory responses and cytokine production and in the control of inflammation in injured lung. SMAD transcription factors act downstream of TGF-β and control endothelial and epithelial permeability and the fibrotic response.

Cytokine Mediators

Activation of transcriptional regulators produces a number of cytokine and chemokine mediators, which recruit inflammatory cells to injured lung and amplify the inflammatory and reparative responses. Transforming growth factor (TGF)-β is ubiquitously expressed, secreted by most cells, and stored in latent form in the extracellular matrix. It is linked to activation of the coagulation system (in the form of thrombin). It contributes to lung injury in high tidal volume ventilation and in lung injury models.

Many cytokines involved in systemic inflammatory responses to sepsis are implicated in ARDS (e.g.,

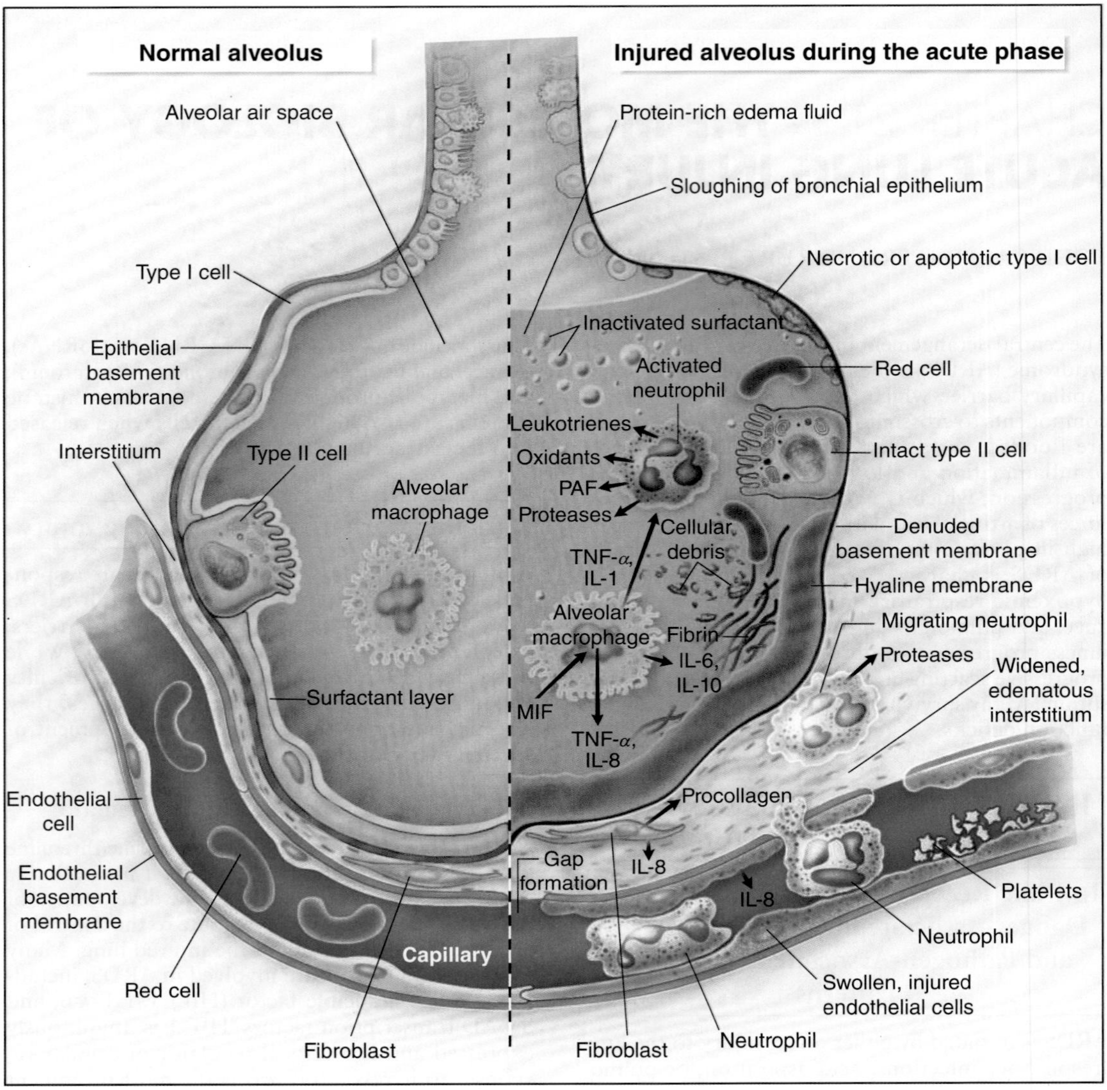

FIGURE 21.1. Cellular and molecular mechanisms of acute lung injury. Changes that occur as part of the early acute phase of lung injury are visible on the *right half* of the diagram in comparison to the *left*, including disruption of the endothelial and epithelial barriers, alveolar flooding, and influx of activated inflammatory cells into the alveolus and interstitium of the lung. PAF, platelet activating factor; TNF, tumor necrosis factor; IL, interleukin; MIF, macrophage migration inhibitory factor.

TNF-α and IL-1β). TNF-α stimulation upregulates adhesion molecules in lung endothelium, which increases PMN attachment, cytoskeletal changes, and endothelial barrier dysfunction. IL-1β increases endothelial cell permeability and stimulates a variety of chemotactic cytokines. Strong correlations exist between measures of IL-1β activity and clinical lung injury severity. IL-6 and IL-10 have also been implicated, IL-6 increases endothelial permeability through activation of PKC, and IL-10 (a potent anti-inflammatory cytokine) inhibits cytokine production by macrophages.

Macrophage migration inhibitory factor (MIF) is produced by alveolar macrophages and bronchial epithelial cells. MIF and TNF-α promote each other's production. MIF potentiates endotoxin and regulates macrophage responses through TLR4 expression.

Inflammatory Cells and Chemokines

Neutrophils are abundant in airspaces in ARDS. Neutrophil numbers and neutrophil persistence after the first week of ARDS are associated with mortality. Lung cellular injury and ARDS can occur in neutropenic patients. Lung dysfunction also worsens during resolution of neutropenia, as PMNs are recruited to injured lungs. PMNs are likely neither necessary nor sufficient to cause lung injury. The most important neutrophil chemoattractants in the injured lung are produced by human alveolar macrophages and include the CXC family of chemokines, IL-8, epithelial-derived neutrophil-activating peptide-78 (ENA-78), growth-related oncogene (GRO), and granulocyte chemotactic peptide (GCP)-2. IL-8 is the dominant PMN chemoattractant.

Thrombin

Important links exist between the coagulation system and lung injury. Proinflammatory cytokines activate the coagulation system (upregulation of tissue factor expression and subsequent activation of the extrinsic clotting cascade). The generation of thrombin leads to increased inflammation and cytokine release. Thrombin has potent permeability-inducing effects.

Angiogenic Mediators

Mediators involved in the formation of new blood vessels (angiogenesis) are activated by tissue injury and many increase vascular permeability in the lung and other vascular beds. Three major families control angiogenesis: the VEGFs, the angiopoietins, and the ephrins. The *VEGF family* of receptors and ligands are potent regulators of blood vessel formation and vascular permeability and play key roles in lung development and repair. VEGF is produced and secreted by many lung and inflammatory cells. VEGF alveolar levels in normal lung far exceed plasma. This alveolar reservoir promotes epithelial integrity. VEGF expression is strongly upregulated by hypoxia, cytokines, and inflammatory mediators. VEGF increases endothelial permeability in vascular beds through increased nitric oxide (NO) production and increased cellular cGMP. Overexpression of VEGF leads to pulmonary edema, and VEGF antagonists reduce lung injury and edema formation in lung injury models of viral infection, high tidal volume ventilation, and LPS instillation. VEGF may also be required for healing of epithelial injury.

The angiopoietin family includes the important ligands angiopoietins-1 (Ang1) and -2 (Ang2) and transmembrane receptor tyrosine kinases TIE-1 and TIE-2. The balance between Ang1 and Ang2 expression regulates endothelial barrier properties. The signaling mechanisms involve Rho family GTPases.

Ephrin family ligands and receptors regulate cell–cell interactions including nervous system and vascular development, tissue morphogenesis, and cancer growth and metastasis. Ephrin signaling activates pathways through the Rho family GTPases and guanine nuclear exchange factors to exert effects. Ephrins regulate vascular permeability and inflammation.

Barrier-Protective Mediators

Lung mediators that can stabilize barriers and reduce permeability include Ang1 and Sphingosine-1-phosphate (S1P), a lipid mediator released from activated platelets. S1P receptor ligands reduce endothelial chemokine generation in experimental pandemic influenza infection, suggesting a possible therapeutic role. S1P effects on other cell types may limit its application. The Slit–Robo system has also been implicated in barrier regulation. Slit ligands are a family of neural guidance molecules released by epithelial and endothelial cells that promote barrier stabilization. In sepsis and influenza models, administration of Slit2 reduces vascular leak and mortality without altering cytokine levels.

REGULATION OF THE ALVEOLAR–CAPILLARY BARRIER

Mechanisms of Increased Endothelial Permeability

Molecular strategies aimed at improving barrier function may improve outcomes from lung injury. The permeability of endothelial layers is determined by the intercellular junctions between endothelial cells and by the cytoskeleton of endothelial cells. Loosening of the intercellular junctions or contraction of the cytoskeleton opens paracellular gaps for fluid movement. Several types of junctions regulate the endothelial barrier: tight junctions, adherens junctions, and focal adhesions. *Tight junctions* include occludens, claudins, and zonula occludens (ZO) proteins and are the major permeability-regulating element of the blood–brain barrier. Their role in lung vascular and epithelial permeability remains uncertain. *Adherens junctions* may be more important in controlling lung vascular permeability. In the pulmonary endothelium, adherens junctions are composed of vascular/endothelial-cadherin (VE-cadherin) and catenin proteins. The adherens junctions connect to neighboring cells and intracellularly to the actin cytoskeleton. Adherens junctions break down in response to permeability-increasing stimuli (e.g., thrombin and oxidant stress) and VE-cadherin function-blocking antibodies. *Focal adhesions* connect endothelial cells to the extracellular matrix via integrin receptors and cytoplasmic focal adhesion proteins.

Connected to these junctional complexes is the endothelial cytoskeleton with its principal components: actin fibers, microtubules, and intermediate filaments. The actin cytoskeleton appears to be most important in controlling lung endothelial barrier function. Stress fiber formation and actin–myosin interactions result from phosphorylation of the myosin light chain (MLC) molecule. MLC phosphorylation is regulated by a balance in activity of MLC kinase (MLCK) and myosin phosphatase (MYPT). Many mediators that effect endothelial barrier function modulate these enzymes.

Calcium handling is key in the control of the endothelial cytoskeleton. MLCK activation is calcium-dependent and increased intracellular calcium increases endothelial permeability. In nonexcitable cells like endothelial cells, calcium entry is mediated by store-operated calcium (SOC) channels. Their role in acute lung injury remains uncertain.

Rho family GTPases regulate actin cytoskeleton and endothelial permeability. They function as switches and their activation increases MLC phosphorylation, actin–myosin interaction, and endothelial cell gap formation. This mechanism is important in permeability changes induced by thrombin, TNF-*α*, lysophosphatidic acid, and LPS.

Epithelial Barrier Integrity and Function in the Injured Lung

Once plasma fluids have breached the endothelial barrier, they must cross the epithelial barrier to reach the alveolar airspace. The permeability of the epithelial barrier is ~10-fold lower than the endothelial barrier (i.e., the epithelium is the greater barrier to edema). Tight junctions also exist in the alveolar epithelium and contain claudins, occludens, and ZO proteins. Adherens junctions are also important in the epithelial barrier. The predominant cadherin protein is E-cadherin, rather than VE-cadherin as in the endothelium. Changes in epithelial permeability are associated with actin cytoskeleton rearrangements, although MLCK and Rho kinase activity is uncertain.

Epithelial cell death from bacteria, viruses, inhaled toxins, or ventilator mechanical injury can alter permeability. LPS and cytokines increase epithelial monolayer permeability. Hypoxia increases epithelial permeability and breaks down epithelial tight junctions.

For edema to result in alveolar flooding, the movement of fluid must overwhelm alveolar fluid clearance mechanisms. Alveolar liquid clearance is the result of active sodium transport. Both type 1 and type 2 alveolar epithelial cells express Na/K-ATPases on their basolateral membranes. These enzymes pump sodium out of the epithelial cell and into the interstitium. The epithelial cell also expresses sodium channels that allow sodium to move passively down the concentration gradient created by the basolateral pumps, out of airspaces and into the epithelial cell. Water moves out of the alveolus via specific water channels (aquaporins) and paracellular routes.

Both inflammation and infection impair liquid clearance by altering sodium channel expression or activity. Hypoxia also impairs epithelial sodium transport. Thrombin reduces liquid clearance by promoting endocytosis of Na/K-ATPases. *β*-Adrenergic agents, corticosteroids, and aldosterone interact with these pathways. Using *β*-agonists to increase alveolar liquid clearance in adult ARDS patients showed no benefit.

CONTROL OF PULMONARY VASCULAR TONE

The regulation of pulmonary vascular tone is important to the pathophysiology and treatment of ARDS. Ventilation–perfusion matching is impaired in ARDS, and the maldistribution in pulmonary blood flow and increased intrapulmonary shunting contribute to hypoxemia. Increased pulmonary arterial pressure is common and correlates with worse outcome. While elevated vascular pressures severe enough to cause right heart failure are rare, changes in vascular tone may contribute to pulmonary edema in many patients.

At the molecular level, the key cell is the vascular smooth muscle cell. In contrast to endothelial cells, smooth muscle cells express voltage-gated ion channels. When the intracellular calcium concentration reaches a threshold level, the cell depolarizes and opens voltage-gated calcium channels, flooding the cell with calcium. Calmodulin is then activated and activates MLCK, which phosphorylates MLCs, enabling the interaction of myosin with actin and cell contraction. Some agonists also stimulate Rho/Rho kinase signaling, which reduces MYPT activity, leading to "calcium sensitization," in which contractile tone is increased independently of increased intracellular calcium.

Pulmonary vascular tone results from a balance between endogenous vasoconstrictors and vasodilators. Endothelin (ET) is one of the most important endogenous vasoconstrictors. This small peptide is produced by many cells in the lung. Binding to its receptor on smooth muscle cells leads to intense constriction of either the airway or blood vessel. In addition to vascular effects, ET is a potent cytokine and contributes to inflammation and fibrosis. ET expression in the lung is upregulated by hypoxia and inflammatory cytokines. The ET system has been clearly implicated in lung injury.

The roles of NO in the lung include immune modulation, epithelial function, and control of endothelial permeability. NO acts in vascular smooth muscle by stimulating soluble guanylate cyclase to produce cyclic guanosine monophosphate (cGMP). cGMP activates cGMP-dependent protein kinases that reduce intracellular calcium levels via an effect on calcium flux out of the sarcoplasmic reticulum and reduce calcium sensitization by activating MYPT. The net effect reduces vascular smooth muscle contraction. NO can also increase or decrease lung microvascular permeability. NO is produced by NO synthases (NOS). eNOS is constitutively expressed by endothelial cells, and neuronal NOS (nNOS) is expressed in neurons. Inducible NOS (iNOS) can be expressed, as a response to inflammation or injury, by lung macrophages and neutrophils in the setting of lung injury.

In ARDS, hypoxia upregulates many of the transcriptional and signaling mechanisms and contributes to lung injury. The increased pulmonary vascular resistance is predominantly attributable to the effects of vasoactive mediators rather than to the O_2 tension.

Surfactant Biochemistry in the Injured Lung

A major consequence of alveolar flooding and epithelial cell dysfunction is inactivation and loss of surfactant. Pulmonary surfactant reduces surface tension, facilitates the stability of the expanded alveolus, and is essential for normal lung function.

When surfactant activity is lost, the alveolus becomes prone to collapse. Surfactant also contributes to the innate defense system and possesses anti-inflammatory properties. Surfactant proteins (SP-A, SP-B, SP-C, and SP-D) play an important role in these processes, especially the small, hydrophobic proteins SP-B and SP-C. Deficiencies of either surfactant phospholipids or surfactant proteins can lead to impaired lung function, including poor compliance, atelectasis, inflammation, infection, and hypoxemia.

FIBROPROLIFERATION AND REPAIR IN THE INJURED LUNG

The pathophysiology of ARDS consists of overlapping acute inflammatory and delayed "repair/fibrotic" phases. Overlapping with the acute exudative phase of ARDS (rather than following it, as was previously thought) is a process of repair. Markers of the repair process occur as early as a few hours into the course of disease. This process is characterized by intra-alveolar mesenchymal cells/fibroblasts, type II cell hyperproliferation, and extracellular matrix turnover. In many cases, repair proceeds normally but in some cases results in a restrictive ventilatory defect and evidence of impaired alveolar membrane function, characterized by a prolonged reduction in the diffusing capacity for carbon monoxide.

Alveolar Epithelial Repair

Restoration of the airspace architecture requires reconstitution of the denuded type I alveolar epithelial cells. Regeneration of type II epithelial cells, in coordination with extracellular matrix turnover, is important in reestablishing surfactant production and ion transport, functions essential for maintaining open and dry alveoli. Efficient restoration of the alveolar epithelium in the early phase of ARDS may speed recovery by enhancing alveolar liquid clearance and preventing the development of pulmonary fibrosis. EGF, TGF-α, and their common receptor, EGF receptor (EGFR) participate in epithelial repair following injury. Keratinocyte growth factor (KGF) and hepatocyte growth factor (HGF) play a role in lung repair. It is not determined if alveolar epithelial repair processes can be manipulated as a therapeutic strategy.

Mechanisms of Fibroproliferation

Either during or after the acute inflammatory response, interstitial fibroblasts migrate into the alveolar space, marking the fibroproliferative phase of ARDS (**Fig. 21.2**). These interstitial fibroblasts differentiate into myofibroblasts. Fibroproliferation is also seen in the microcirculation of the lung. In the airspace,

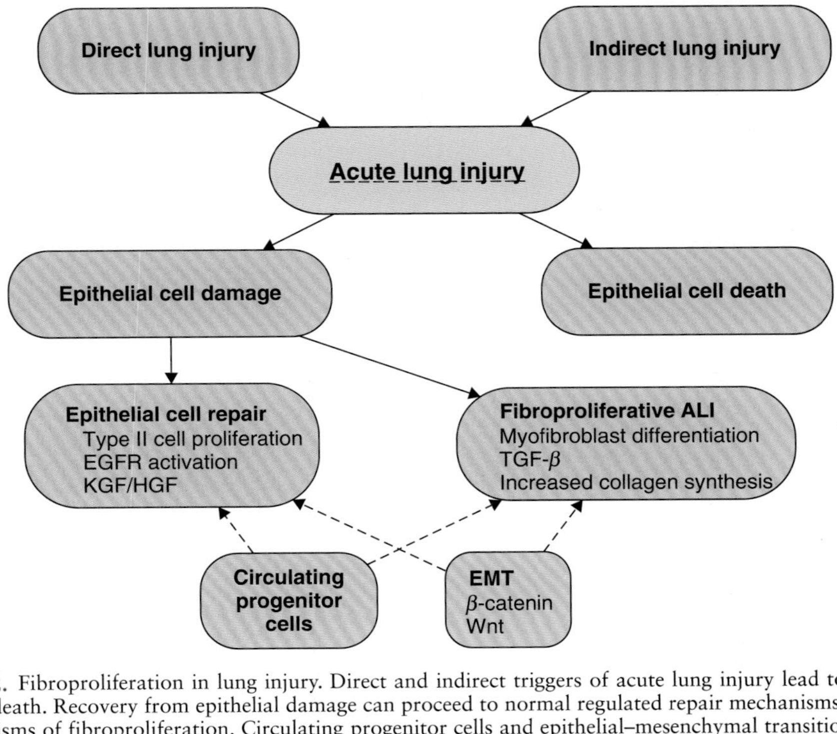

FIGURE 21.2. Fibroproliferation in lung injury. Direct and indirect triggers of acute lung injury lead to epithelial cell damage and death. Recovery from epithelial damage can proceed to normal regulated repair mechanisms or to dysregulated mechanisms of fibroproliferation. Circulating progenitor cells and epithelial–mesenchymal transitions (EMT) may contribute to both repair and fibroproliferation. ALI, acute lung injury; EGFR, epidermal growth factor receptor; TGF-β, transforming growth factor-β; KGF, keratinocyte growth factor; HGF, hepatocyte growth factor.

fibroproliferation leads to shunt; in the microcirculation, it contributes to pulmonary hypertension.

TGF-β is a major regulator of gene expression of extracellular matrix molecules in mesenchymal cells and lung fibroblasts. It induces collagen synthesis and the differentiation of fibroblasts into myofibroblasts, but inhibits collagenase production. During the resolution of the fibrotic phase, apoptosis of mesenchymal cells may be an essential component of normal repair and resolution, and dysregulation of this process may lead to persistent or nonresolving ARDS.

Stem Cells in the Injured Lung

Research suggests that when the lung is damaged by a variety of causes (chemicals, infection, or radiation), progenitor cells released from the bone marrow are attracted to the damaged lung. These cells repair the lung. Progenitor cells could also, under certain circumstances, contribute to ongoing fibroproliferative responses. The most promising stem cell work involves mesenchymal stem cells (MSCs). The beneficial actions of MSCs encompass antiapoptotic and cytoprotective effects in the promotion of angiogenesis and are powerful modulators of the immune response. Preclinical studies demonstrate that MSCs can reduce lung injury caused by endotoxin, pneumonia, and systemic sepsis. Safety concerns represent a significant barrier to the translation of MSCs into clinical therapeutic intervention.

CHAPTER 22 ■ RESPIRATORY MONITORING

IRA M. CHEIFETZ, JAN H. LEE, AND SHEKHAR T. VENKATARAMAN

PHYSICAL ASSESSMENT

Respiratory Rate and Pattern

Physical assessment and observation should always be used to complement electronic surveillance. Physical examination remains the primary method to measure respiratory rate. Impedance pneumography is most often used to measure respiratory movements in spontaneously breathing children. Variable impedance to current flow through the electrodes on the chest is converted into a waveform and displayed on a monitor. *Respiratory pauses* last <5 seconds and usually occur in children <3 months of age. Pauses occur in groups of three or more, are separated by <20 seconds, and generally resolve by 6 months of age without medical intervention. *Apnea* is cessation of breathing for >20 seconds or any respiratory pause associated with bradycardia, pallor, or cyanosis. The relationship between infantile apnea and sudden infant death syndrome (SIDS) remains controversial.

GUIDELINES AND PRINCIPLES

Assessment of the Lung as an Oxygenator

Indices that assess the lung as an oxygenator are (a) arterial oxygen tension (Pao_2), (b) arterial blood oxygen saturation (Sao_2), (c) intrapulmonary shunt fraction (Qs/Qt), (d) alveolar-to-arterial oxygen tension difference ($P_A\text{-}ao_2$), (e) arterial-to-alveolar oxygen tension ratio (Pao_2/P_{AO_2}), and (f) arterial-to-fraction of inspired oxygen ratio (Pao_2/F_{IO_2}). Pao_2 represents the net effect of oxygen exchange in the lung. At sea level, the normal Pao_2 in a newborn infant is 40–70 mm Hg when breathing room air. Pao_2 increases with age until it reaches the adult value of 90–120 mm Hg. *Hypoxemia* is defined as a Pao_2 lower than the acceptable range for age, whereas hypoxia is inadequate tissue oxygenation. For a child, a Pao_2 of <60 mm Hg is defined as hypoxemia, although that may be an acceptable level for a newborn. The *intrapulmonary shunt fraction*, Qs/Qt, is defined as the fraction of right ventricular output that enters the left ventricle without oxygen transfer. In the absence of intracardiac shunts, Qs/Qt is calculated by the formula

$$Qs/Qt = (Cc'O_2 - Cao_2)/(Cc'O_2 - C\bar{v}o_2)$$

where $Cc'O_2$ is the oxygen content of the pulmonary venous blood (assumes the lung is a perfect oxygenator), Cao_2 is the arterial oxygen content, and $C\bar{v}o_2$ is the mixed venous oxygen content. *Oxygen content* is the amount of O_2 carried by a unit volume of blood and is equal to the amount bound to hemoglobin (Hb) and dissolved in plasma. The oxygen content of whole blood is calculated as $(Hb \times 1.34 \times So_2/100) + (0.003 \times Po_2)$. Intrapulmonary shunt may consist of three components: anatomic shunt, capillary shunt, and venous admixture. $Cc'O_2$ is most affected by F_{IO_2}, Cao_2 is affected mostly by intrapulmonary shunting, and $C\bar{v}o_2$ is affected mostly by cardiac output and O_2 consumption.

$P_A\text{-}ao_2$, Pao_2/P_{AO_2}, and Pao_2/F_{IO_2}

P_{AO_2} is calculated from the simplified alveolar gas equation

$$P_{AO_2} = (P_B - P_{H_2O}) \times F_{IO_2} - Paco_2/RQ$$

where P_B is the barometric pressure, P_{H_2O} is the partial pressure of water vapor (47 mm Hg when fully saturated with H_2O), and RQ is the respiratory quotient (CO_2 production/O_2 consumption). With intrapulmonary shunting, Pao_2 is less than P_{AO_2}. The normal alveolar-arterial (Aa) oxygen gradient ($P_A\text{-}ao_2$) is <20 mm Hg in a child and <50 mm Hg in a newborn. $P_A\text{-}ao_2$ is affected not only by intrapulmonary shunting, but also by mixed venous oxygen saturation (Svo_2). Pao_2/F_{IO_2} ratio is the easiest index to calculate and does not require calculation of P_{AO_2}. The normal Pao_2/F_{IO_2} in a child breathing room air at sea level is >400 mm Hg.

Oxygen Delivery

Oxygen delivery (Do_2) is the amount of O_2 delivered to the tissues every minute. It is calculated as: $Do_2 = Cao_2 \times CO$, where CO is the cardiac output in mL/min. The oxygen delivery index (Do_2I) uses cardiac index in place of cardiac output; a normal Do_2I in a child is ~650–750 mL/min. The major determinants of Do_2 are Hb and CO. Mild hypoxemia can be compensated by increasing Hb and/or CO.

Assessment of Oxygen Utilization

Oxygen consumption ($\dot{V}o_2$) is the amount of O_2 utilized by the body in a minute, and it can be measured as: $\dot{V}O_2 = CO\ (CaO_2 - C\bar{v}O_2)$. Fever, thyrotoxicosis, and increased catecholamine release or administration increase $\dot{V}O_2$. Hypothermia and hypothyroidism tend to decrease $\dot{V}O_2$.

Mixed Venous Oxygen Saturation

A low $S\bar{v}O_2$ usually signifies that DO_2 is decreased and commonly occurs with hypovolemic and cardiogenic shock. In sepsis (maldistribution of blood flow is present) and in inborn errors of metabolism (where O_2 utilization can be abnormal), $S\bar{v}O_2$ may be normal or increased despite O_2 deficits in the tissues. A high $S\bar{v}O_2$ is seen in hypothermia (decreased O_2 demand) and in brain death (the brain is a major site of O_2 consumption). The normal saturation of Hb in the pulmonary artery is ~78% (range, 73%–85%).

PULSE OXIMETRY

Pulse oximetry (SpO_2) provides a continuous, noninvasive measure of the percent O_2 saturation of arterial Hb.

Oxygen-Dissociation Curve

The arterial O_2 saturation of Hb (SaO_2) is the percent oxyhemoglobin in the arterial blood. The O_2-dissociation curve describes the avidity with which O_2 binds to Hb. Acidemia, hypercarbia, increased temperature, and increased red-cell 2,3-diphosphoglycerate (2,3-DPG) level shift the curve to the right (decrease affinity).

Beer–Lambert Law

The Beer–Lambert law states that the concentration of a solute in a solvent can be determined by light absorption. Pulse oximetry estimates SaO_2 by measuring the absorption of light in tissues. Wavelengths of 660 nm (red) and 940 nm (infrared) are used because the absorption characteristics of oxygenated and deoxygenated Hbs are significantly different at these two wavelengths (**Fig. 22.1**). By using the two wavelengths of light, the pulse oximeter determines *functional saturation*. Functional $SpO_2 = HbO_2/(HbO_2 + Hb)$, where HbO_2 is the oxygenated Hb and Hb is the nonoxygenated Hb. Functional SpO_2 is contrasted with *fractional saturation* measured by co-oximetry on most blood gas analyzers. Fractional SpO_2 provides the ratio of oxygenated Hb to the sum of *all Hb types*, including carboxyhemoglobin (COHb) and methemoglobin (MetHb), which do not carry O_2: Fractional $SpO_2 = HbO_2/(HbO_2 + Hb + COHb + MetHb)$.

Factors That Affect the Performance of Pulse Oximeters

The factors that contribute to potential inaccuracy of pulse oximetry include poor cardiac output/low-perfusion states, motion artifact, increased venous pulsations, optical interference from the environment,

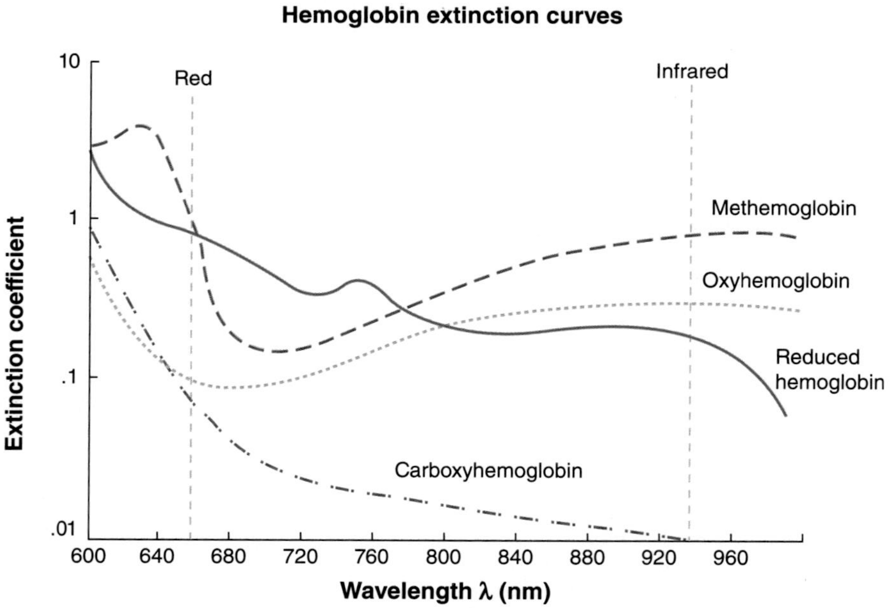

FIGURE 22.1. Hemoglobin extinction curves. The extinction curves of four hemoglobin species (oxyhemoglobin, reduced hemoglobin, methemoglobin, and carboxyhemoglobin) are displayed from red (660 nm) to infrared (940 nm). (From Tremper KK, Barker SJ. Pulse oximetry. *Anesthesiology* 1989;70:98–108, with permission.)

dyshemoglobinemias (carboxyhemoglobin, methemoglobin, fetal hemoglobin), and dyes and pigments (methylene blue, indocyanine green).

Carboxyhemoglobin

Carboxyhemoglobin is interpreted as oxyhemoglobin by the pulse oximeter, as both carboxy- and oxy-hemoglobin absorb similar amounts of light at 660 nm (**Fig. 22.1**). Thus, functional Spo_2 overestimates HbO_2, but fractional Spo_2 is dramatically decreased with carboxyhemoglobin. In patients with smoke inhalation or coma of uncertain cause (i.e., carbon monoxide poisoning), it is necessary to use co-oximetry to determine Sao_2.

Methemoglobin

MetHb absorbs significant light at both 660- and 940-nm wavelengths, thus causing the oximeter to register that both HbO_2 and reduced Hb are increased, resulting in a Spo_2 of ~85%.

Methylene Blue

Methylene blue has a maximum absorbance at 668 nm. The oximeter interprets this extra absorbance as reduced Hb and, therefore, a lower Spo_2. Clinically, this is seen as a sudden (<30 seconds) and limited (~2 minutes) drop in saturation when methylene blue is injected for therapeutic or diagnostic purposes.

Low-Perfusion States

Pulse oximetry depends on optical plethysmography (i.e., a pulsatile change in arterial blood). Shock states, high vasopressor doses, severe edema, hypothermia, and peripheral vascular disease interfere with interpreting signal versus background. Recent improvement enables saturation monitoring despite decreased perfusion.

TRANSCUTANEOUS MEASUREMENT OF GAS TENSION

The transcutaneous measurement of gas tensions (oxygen, $P_{Tc}O_2$, and carbon dioxide, $P_{Tc}CO_2$) involves warming the skin to cause hyperperfusion and diffusion of gases through the dermis and epidermis. Electrodes are attached to the skin, by adhesive patches, to well-perfused, nonbony surfaces (i.e., abdomen, inner thigh, lower back, and chest in neonates; chest, abdomen, and lower back in larger children and adults). O_2 tension decreases linearly along the skin capillaries due to O_2 consumption in the dermis, which results in an arteriovenous difference in Po_2, with the Po_2 in the capillary dome being intermediate. The correlation between $P_{Tc}O_2$ and Pao_2 is excellent only when the blood pressure and peripheral circulation are normal. When the peripheral circulation is affected by hypotension, acidosis (pH < 7.1), hypothermia (<35°C), cyanosis (Pao_2 < 30 mm Hg), or drugs, the correlation becomes less reliable. $P_{Tc}O_2$ correlates with Pao_2 in the range of 30–200 mm Hg but underestimates O_2 tensions >200 mm Hg and overestimates Po_2 < 30 mm Hg.

CAPNOGRAPHY

Capnography is the graphic waveform produced by variations in CO_2 concentration through the respiratory cycle as a function of time.

Sampling Techniques

Capnometers use two sampling techniques, sidestream and mainstream. Sidestream sampling aspirates a small quantity of gas continuously from the ventilator circuit, or at the nares in spontaneously breathing patients (i.e., via a nasal cannula). Mainstream capnography incorporates a light-emitting source and detector on opposite sides of an airway adaptor. The *end-tidal carbon dioxide* level ($ETCO_2$) is defined as the peak CO_2 value during expiration and depends on adequate pulmonary capillary blood flow and right and left heart function. The normal $ETCO_2$ in healthy subjects is generally <5 mm Hg lower than the $Paco_2$, representing normal anatomic dead space of the upper airway. Clinical conditions associated with alterations in $ETCO_2$ are shown in **Table 22.1.** Of note, changes in capnography tend to occur more rapidly than changes in pulse oximetry.

TABLE 22.1

Clinical Conditions Associated with Alterations in $ETCO_2$

Increases in $ETCO_2$
Increased pulmonary capillary blood flow
Increased cardiac output
Hypoventilation
Increased CO_2 production
Sudden release of a tourniquet
Sodium bicarbonate administration
Decreases in $ETCO_2$
Decreased pulmonary capillary blood flow
Pulmonary hypertension
Pulmonary embolus (thrombus or air)
Decreased cardiac output
Hyperventilation
Ventilator circuit leak
Obstructed endotracheal tube
Decreased CO_2 production
Absent $ETCO_2$
Esophageal intubation
Ventilator disconnect

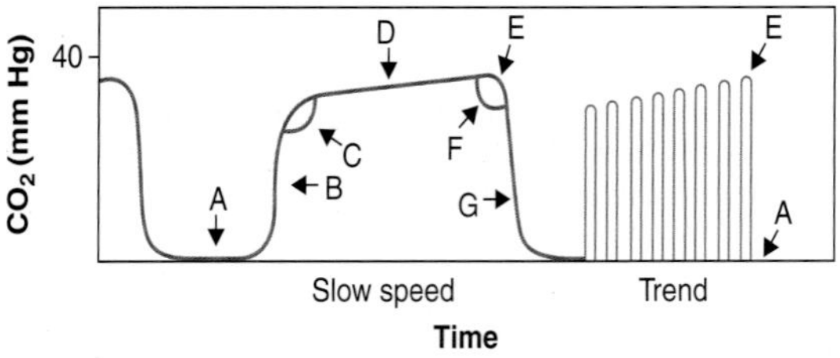

FIGURE 22.2. Normal features of a capnogram. *A*, baseline, represents the beginning of expiration and should start at zero. *B*, the transitional part of the curve, represents mixing of dead space and alveolar gas. *C*, the α angle, represents the change to alveolar gas. *D*, the alveolar part of the curve, represents the plateau average alveolar gas concentration. *E* is the end-tidal CO_2 value. *F*, the β angle, represents the change to the inspiratory part of the cycle. *G*, the inspiration part of the curve, shows a rapid decrease in CO_2 concentration. (From Thompson JE, Jaffe MB. Capnographic waveforms in the mechanically ventilated patient. *Respir Care* 2005;50(1):100–9, with permission.)

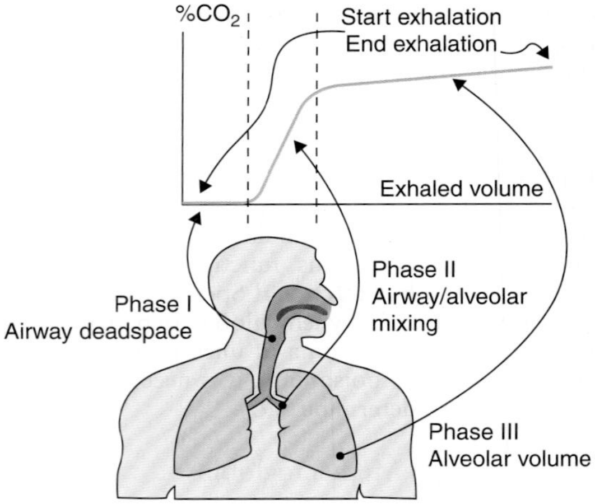

FIGURE 22.3. Volumetric capnogram. The initial portion of the volumetric capnogram (phase I) represents the quantity of CO_2 eliminated from the large airways. Phase II is the transitional zone, which represents ventilation from both small and large airways. The third phase of the capnogram represents CO_2 elimination from the alveoli and, thus, the quantity of gas involved with alveolar ventilation. (Courtesy of Respironics, Inc., and its affiliates, Wallingford, Connecticut.)

Evaluation of Respiratory Pattern

The phasic changes in CO_2 concentration that occur during the respiratory cycle are shown in **Figure 22.2.**

Clinical Applications

False-positive $ETCO_2$ values may occur when the ETT is in the esophagus (following mouth-to-mouth ventilation or ingestion of antacids or carbonated beverages) or when the tip of the ETT is in the pharynx. False-negative $ETCO_2$ readings (no $ETCO_2$ when the ETT is in trachea) may occur with severe airway obstruction, poor cardiac output, pulmonary emboli, or pulmonary hypertension. During cardiopulmonary resuscitation, capnography can be utilized to assess the quality of chest compressions and provide an early indication of return of spontaneous circulation. Effective chest compression should produce enough pulmonary blood flow to generate an exhaled CO_2 value of >10 mm Hg.

Time-Based versus Volumetric Capnography

Time-based capnography is limited to the measurement and display of the respiratory waveform and $ETCO_2$ value (**Fig. 22.2**). $ETCO_2$ can be used to trend changes in $Paco_2$ for patients in whom physiologic dead space is not significantly elevated or changing. The integration of flow and volume graphically displayed (**Fig. 22.3**) is the basis of volumetric capnography. Volumetric capnography provides a measurement of CO_2 production (Vco_2) and enables calculation of alveolar minute ventilation and the ratio of volume of dead space (Vd) to tidal volume (V_T), Vd/V_T. Although there are no absolute cutoff values, Vd/V_T values of <0.5–0.55 and >0.65 have been proposed as predictive of extubation success and failure, respectively.

MONITORING RESPIRATORY MECHANICS

Respiratory Inductive Plethysmography

Respiratory inductive plethysmography uses two coils of insulated wires sewn in a sinusoidal pattern in elastic-fabricated bands. One band encircles the chest, with the upper level of the band just under the axillae, and the other encircles the abdomen, with the band located midway between the lower ribs and the upper edge of the iliac crests. Movement causes voltage changes, which can be interpolated to indicate changes in thoracic volume.

Application in Critically Ill Patients

Minute ventilation is the product of V_T and respiratory frequency (*f*) or:

$$V = V_T/T_i \times T_i/T_{tot} \times 60$$

where *V* is the minute ventilation (L/min), T_i is the inspiratory time (seconds), and T_{tot} is the total respiratory cycle (seconds). The parameter V_T/T_i is the *mean inspiratory flow*, and T_i/T_{tot} is the *fractional inspiratory time*. V_T/T_i is a measure of respiratory drive and correlates well with other indices of respiratory drive such as $P_{0.1}$ and the ventilatory response to hypercapnia. $P_{0.1}$ is the pressure generated in the first 100 milliseconds after the onset of inspiratory effort against an occluded airway.

Monitoring of Respiratory Muscle Function

Maximal inspiratory pressure (P_{Imax}), often called *negative inspiratory force* (NIF), is the maximal static pressure that can be generated with forceful efforts against an occluded airway and provides a noninvasive index of global muscle strength in both nonintubated and intubated patients. In normal infants, P_{Imax} during crying is -118 ± 21 cm H_2O. In children 6–17 years of age, the P_{Imax} is -70 to -110 cm H_2O, and pubertal children are capable of generating P_{Imax} of -80 to -120 cm H_2O. In adults, a P_{Imax} more negative than -30 cm H_2O has been reported to be associated with extubation success, and a value less negative than -20 cm H_2O has been associated with extubation failure. In children, P_{Imax} is poorly discriminative between extubation success and failure. The clinician should use additional assessments of muscle strength such as hip flexion in the infant and head lift >5 seconds in the adolescent as well as careful observation of spontaneous breathing without distress, hypoxemia, or hypercapnia before deciding on readiness for extubation.

Monitoring Respiratory Mechanics in Ventilated Patients

Compliance and Elastance

Lung compliance is the change in lung volume divided by the transalveolar pressure, which is equal to the difference between the alveolar pressure (P_{alv}) at the end of inflation and the pleural pressure (P_{pl} or P_{es}). At the bedside, the P_{plat} can be substituted for P_{alv} and tidal volume can be substituted for a change in lung volume, such that $C_{lung} = V_T/(P_{plat} - P_{es})$. C_{lung} is also called *static lung compliance* (C_{stat}). Since esophageal pressure is often not measured in children, C_{lung} can be calculated by $C_{lung} = V_{T(effective)}/(P_{plat} - PEEP)$, where $V_{T(effective)}$ is the tidal volume delivered to the patient. *Chest-wall compliance* is the change in thoracic volume divided by the transthoracic pressure (atmospheric pressure (P_{atm}) $-$ P_{es}). To compare among patients, compliance values should be indexed to body weight. *Elastance* is the reciprocal of compliance.

Dynamic Compliance

Dynamic compliance (C_{dyn}) is defined as the change in volume divided by the change in airway pressure from end expiration to end inspiration during a mechanical breath: $C_{dyn} = V_T/(P_{max} - PEEP)$.

Tidal Volume Measurement

In adults, the inspiratory V_T displayed by the ventilator can generally be used for compliance calculations and for most aspects of mechanical ventilation. In children, the fraction of the V_{Tdel} that is distributed to the ventilator circuit is substantially higher than in adults and can be as much as 70% in critically ill infants. To determine the actual V_T delivered to the lungs without requiring additional equipment (i.e., a pneumotachometer), a mathematical formula can be used to correct for the compliance of the ventilator circuit: $V_{Teff} = V_{Tdel} - C_{vent}$ (PIP $-$ PEEP), where V_{Teff} is the effective tidal volume that reaches the ETT, PIP is the peak inspiratory pressure, and C_{vent} is the compliance of the ventilator circuit.

Intrinsic PEEP

The static recoil pressure of the respiratory system at end expiration may be elevated in patients who receive mechanical ventilation, especially in those who have lower-airway disease and obstruction. Inspiration that begins before exhalation is complete results in an end-expiratory alveolar pressure that remains elevated above the proximal airway pressure. This positive recoil pressure, or static $PEEP_i$, can be quantified in relaxed patients by using an end-expiratory hold maneuver on a mechanical ventilator immediately before the onset of the next breath. Spontaneously breathing patient have to overcome $PEEP_i$ to trigger a ventilator and develop muscle fatigue. Excessive $PEEP_i$ may also result in poor triggering because the patient is unable to generate the necessary negative pressure in the central airway. This problem can be largely overcome by flow triggering.

Static Pressure–Volume Curves

The inspiratory phase of the PV curve consists of three sections. As the lung is inflated from low lung volumes, the initial lung compliance is low (**Fig. 22.4**).

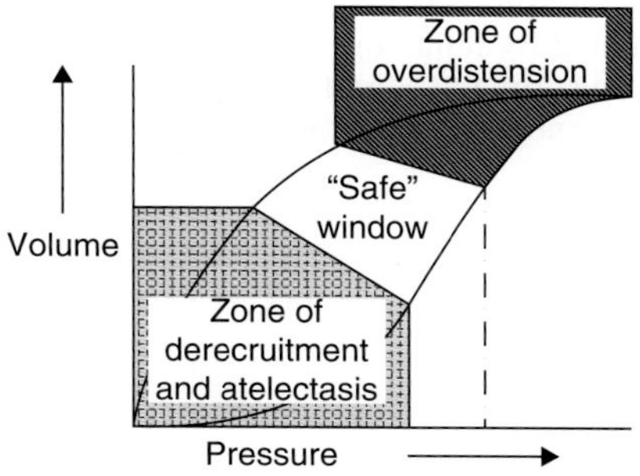

FIGURE 22.4. Pressure–volume curve. The inspiratory phase of the pressure–volume curve consists of three sections. As the lung is inflated from an initial low lung volume, the lung compliance is low. As airway pressure is increased, lung compliance improves, which continues until the lung is fully inflated. Inflating the lung further results in a reduction in the lung compliance at the end of inflation as the lung overdistends. The goal is to ventilate in the "safe window." (From Froese AB. High-frequency oscillatory ventilation for adult respiratory distress syndrome: Let's get it right this time! *Crit Care Med* 1997;25(6):906–8, with permission.)

The junction between the first and second portions of the curve is called the *lower inflection point* (LIP). The junction of the second and third portions of the curve is called the *upper inflection point* (UIP). The LIP is thought to represent the point of alveolar recruitment, and the UIP is thought to represent overdistension. In patients with acute lung injury, some investigators recommend that PEEP is set at a pressure slightly above the LIP on a static PV curve.

Mechanical Ventilators and Airway Graphics Monitoring

Airway Scalars

Airway scalars, the most commonly reported waveforms, comprise three distinct waveforms (flow, pressure, and volume) plotted against time. Conventionally, positive values correspond to inspiration events and negative values correspond to expiration. Volume is generally measured by integrating the flow signal over time. The upward deflection of the graphic represents the volume delivered to the patient, while the downward deflection represents the total expiratory volume. Inspiratory and expiratory volumes should be equal. However, patients with uncuffed ETTs or inadequate cuff inflation may have expiratory volume less than the inspiratory volume.

Scalar Display of Volume-Limited Ventilation

A typical airway graphic during time-cycled, volume-limited ventilation is displayed in **Figure 22.5**. The top graphic displays flow on the vertical axis and time on the horizontal axis. The bottom graphic displays airway pressure versus time. During volume-limited ventilation, the V_T is set, and the PIP is determined by lung compliance, airway resistance, inspiratory time (T_i), and flow characteristics. This mode of ventilation is characterized by a square-wave, constant-flow inspiratory flow pattern. When an unacceptable PIP occurs during volume-limited ventilation, consideration of increasing Ti, decreasing V_T (allowing permissive hypercapnia), or changing the ventilation mode to a variable, decelerating inspiratory flow pattern (e.g. pressure-regulated volume control) will decrease the PIP.

Scalar Display of Pressure-Limited Ventilation

A typical airway graphic during pressure-limited ventilation with a variable, decelerating inspiratory flow pattern (i.e., pressure-control ventilation) is displayed in **Figure 22.6**. During pressure-limited ventilation, the PIP is set, and the V_T is determined by lung compliance, airway resistance, and delivered flow rate. During pressure-limited ventilation, if V_T decreases, increasing the PIP limit, increasing the T_i, or optimizing the PEEP should be considered.

Pressure–Volume and Flow–Volume Loops

The first portion of inspiratory curve in the pressure-volume loop in **Figure 22.4** shows a significant increase in pressure with little increase in volume (low compliance). The following rapid upsloping, an increase in volume per pressure delivered (high compliance), is the previously described *LIP* that is created by a sudden opening of alveoli. The flow–volume loop depicts flow on the vertical axis and volume on the horizontal axis. Inspiration is seen on the upper portion of the loop, with exhalation depicted on the lower portion.

Pressure–Volume and Flow–Volume Loops in Volume-Limited Ventilation

The typical PV and flow–volume loops during volume-limited ventilation are displayed in **Figure 22.7**. As the ventilator delivers gas to the patient, airway pressure increases from the set PEEP level until the set V_T is reached and inspiration is terminated. Dynamic

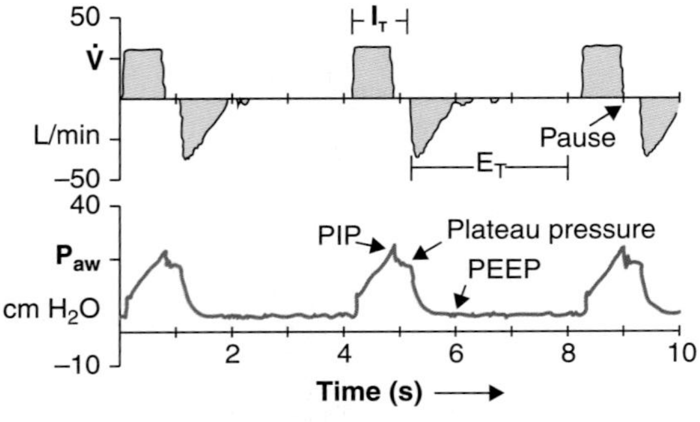

FIGURE 22.5. Normal scalar display of flow versus time and airway pressure versus time for volume-limited ventilation. P_{aw}, airway pressure; PIP, peak inspiratory pressure; PEEP, positive end-expiratory pressure. (Courtesy of VIASYS Healthcare Inc., Yorba Linda, CA.)

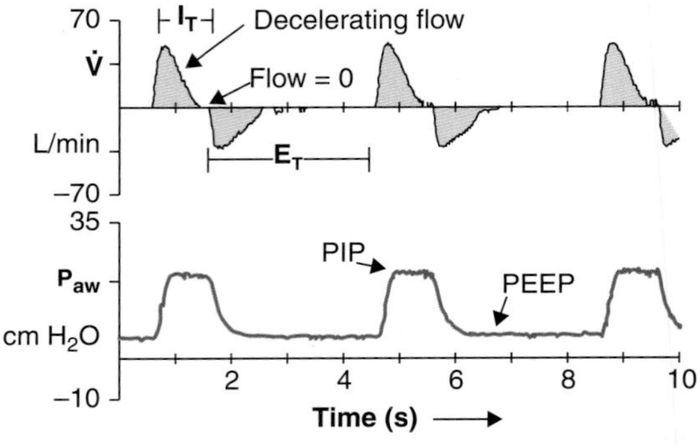

FIGURE 22.6. Normal scalar display of flow versus time and airway pressure versus time for pressure-limited ventilation. (Courtesy of VIASYS Healthcare, Inc., Yorba Linda, CA.)

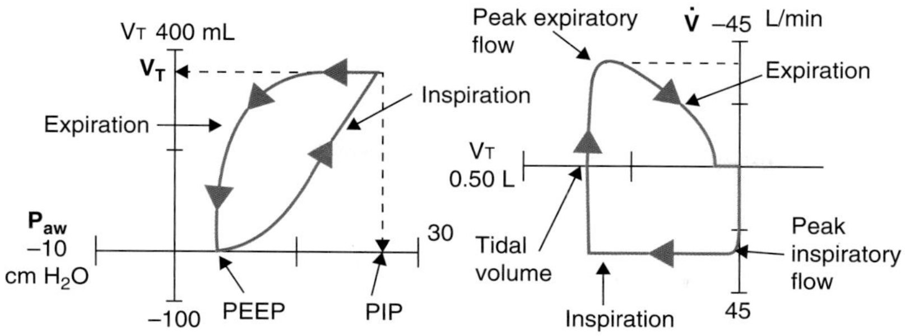

FIGURE 22.7. The pressure–volume graphic displays tidal volume on the vertical axis and airway pressure on the horizontal axis. The flow–volume graphic displays flow on the vertical axis and tidal volume on the horizontal axis. Note that in this flow–volume loop, the delivered inspiratory flow is represented during volume-limited ventilation below the baseline as a square wave. (Courtesy of VIASYS Healthcare, Inc., Yorba Linda, CA.)

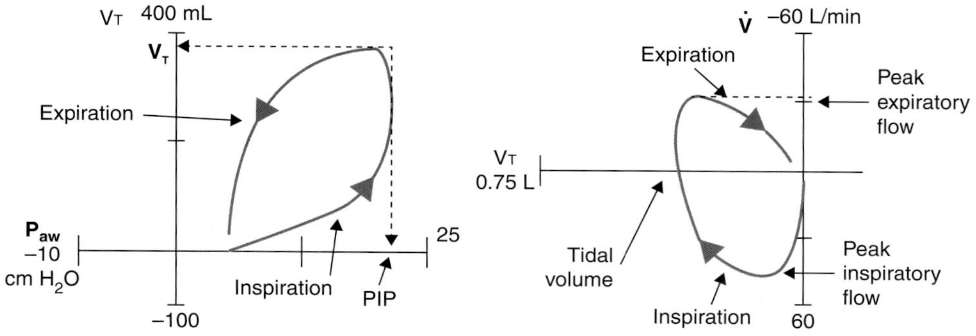

FIGURE 22.8. Normal pressure–volume and flow–volume loops for pressure-limited ventilation. V_T, tidal volume. (Figure courtesy of VIASYS Healthcare, Inc., Yorba Linda, CA.)

compliance, which is the slope of the line connecting the PEEP with the PIP, is calculated as V_{Tdel}/(PIP − PEEP). Hysteresis, which is a nonlinear change in the PV relationship over time, is present during both inspiration and expiration. A decrease in compliance results in higher airway pressures being required to achieve a similar V_T. As a result, the PV loop flattens, and the curvature of the inspiratory and expiratory limbs decreases (decreased hysteresis).

Pressure–Volume and Flow–Volume Loops in Pressure-Limited Ventilation

The decelerating flow pattern of pressure-control ventilation results in a more rapid rise in airway pressure during the initial phase of inspiration, versus a volume-limited breath. The corresponding PV loop is demonstrated in **Figure 22.8**. During the initial phase of inspiration, the airway pressures are higher for a given V_T, and the PV loop demonstrates an initial "scooping." Although the initial airway pressures are higher for a given V_T, the V_T is delivered at a lower PIP, and dynamic compliance is improved. This increase in dynamic compliance is demonstrated by the increased slope of the inspiratory loop (line connecting PEEP with PIP).

Detection of Overdistension Using Pressure–Volume Loops

Pulmonary overdistension is an abrupt decrease in compliance at the end of inspiration and occurs when the volume limit of the lung is approached. Dynamic compliance is decreased and the inspiratory loop has a reduced slope and terminal "beaking." Overdistension increases dead space, leads to volutrauma, and increases pulmonary vascular resistance. To eliminate overdistension, the set PIP or V_T should be decreased. Excessive PEEP leads to overdistension of compliant regions of lung and should be titrated carefully.

Flow–Volume Loops Demonstrating Airway Obstruction

In **Figure 22.9A**, the delivered inspiratory flow is represented below the baseline as a decelerating wave. During early exhalation, near-complete obstruction to flow results in a high expiratory resistance. In

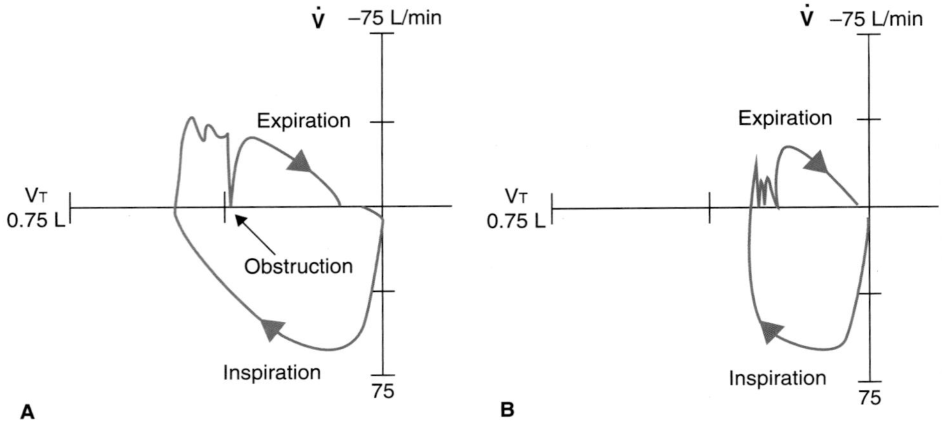

FIGURE 22.9. Flow–volume loops demonstrating airway obstruction. **A:** Mild airway obstruction, resulting in a high expiratory resistance. **B:** Severe airway obstruction that involves increased inspiratory and expiratory resistance. (Courtesy of VIASYS Healthcare, Inc., Yorba Linda, CA.)

Figure 22.9B, the airway obstruction is more severe; in the inspiratory phase, the decelerating wave form is blunted and approaches a square wave, while in the expiratory phase, the peak flow is limited. Both inspiratory resistance and expiratory resistance are elevated, indicating a fixed airway obstruction.

Optimizing Positive End-Expiratory Pressure during Acute Respiratory Distress Syndrome

Acute respiratory distress syndrome (ARDS) causes a loss of alveolar stability and diffuse atelectasis. As lung volume is restored toward functional residual capacity by optimizing PEEP, the PIP required to deliver the V_T may decrease. As a result, the lung is more compliant, and the V_T can be delivered with a smaller change in airway pressure. Excessive levels of PEEP cause detrimental cardiorespiratory effects including (a) a reduction of venous return and cardiac output secondary to increased mean intrathoracic pressure and (b) overdistension of compliant lung units with redistribution of blood flow to the less-compliant lung units.

Dynamic Hyperexpansion/Intrinsic Positive End-Expiratory Pressure

Prolongation of the T_i may be beneficial in ARDS by decreasing PIP and increasing mean airway pressure, which should improve oxygenation. If exhalation time before the next breath is initiated is inadequate, dynamic hyperexpansion or "gas trapping" occurs. Dynamic hyperexpansion may result in $PEEP_i$, which elevates the baseline airway pressure (externally applied PEEP + $PEEP_i$). The increase in the baseline airway pressure secondary to $PEEP_i$ results in an increase in PIP that is required to maintain the set V_T during volume-limited ventilation or results in a decrease in V_T during pressure-limited ventilation (i.e., set total PIP). The combination of an increased PIP and development of $PEEP_i$ will cause the mean airway pressure to rise. $PEEP_i$ may be desirable in the management of ARDS, as it results in improved oxygenation. However, careful monitoring of the amount of $PEEP_i$ is required to limit the development of secondary lung injury and hemodynamic compromise due to the increased mean intrathoracic pressure.

Patient–Ventilator Asynchrony: Inaccurate Sensing of Patient Effort

With inadequate trigger sensitivity, the ventilator is unable to detect that patient effort has occurred. Inadequate detection of patient effort leads to tachypnea, increased effort, patient–ventilator asynchrony, and patient discomfort ("fighting the ventilator"). Trigger sensitivity must be improved to correct this situation. Asynchrony may also occur when an air leak leads to the loss of PEEP, resulting in excessive ventilator triggering. This reduction in airway pressure or flow may be misinterpreted by the ventilator as a patient effort and result in a mechanical breath being triggered (referred to as *autocycling*, frequent ventilator triggering without patient effort). In this case, the trigger sensitivity setting and the ETT air leak must be assessed.

Patient–Ventilator Asynchrony: Inadequate Ventilatory Support

Another cause of patient-ventilator asynchrony is inadequate ventilator support to meet the patient's inspiratory needs. Increasing the flow rate during patient-assisted, volume-limited ventilation (i.e., constant, square-wave inspiratory flow) may eliminate flow asynchrony. Additionally, decreasing the T_i or changing to another mode of ventilation with a variable, decelerating inspiratory flow is often beneficial, such as pressure-support ventilation, pressure-assist/control ventilation, and pressure-regulated volume control. When increasing the flow rate or changing the inspiratory flow pattern is unsuccessful, inadequate ventilatory support should be considered as the cause of the patient–ventilator asynchrony.

Esophageal and Gastric Manometry

Esophageal and gastric manometry are invasive methods to assess pressures generated during breathing. Esophageal pressure monitoring complements extubation readiness testing when patients are being weaned from mechanical ventilation.

Measurements of Diaphragmatic Function

Transdiaphragmatic Pressure

Transdiaphragmatic pressure (P_{di}) is the difference between intrathoracic and abdominal pressures. It is usually calculated as the difference between P_{es} and gastric pressure (P_{ga}). Measurement of P_{di} is useful in the diagnosis of diaphragmatic strength, weakness, and fatigability; data are lacking in critically ill children.

Diaphragmatic Ultrasonography and Fluoroscopy

Diaphragmatic paresis and paralysis can occur from injury to the phrenic nerve or diaphragm weakness. Diaphragmatic paresis is diagnosed by the reduction in diaphragm excursion during spontaneous breathing. Unilateral diaphragmatic paralysis can result in paradoxical movement of the paralyzed hemidiaphragm, during inspiration, the normal diaphragm moves downward and the paralyzed diaphragm moves upward. It is important that testing be performed without positive pressure applied to the airway.

Measures of Inspiratory Drive

The pressure generated after the onset of inspiratory effort against an occluded airway in the first 100 milliseconds ($P_{0.1}$) provides a measure of respiratory drive. In adults, $P_{0.1}$ can be used to predict weaning outcome. For extubated children, $P_{0.1}$ can be measured by placing a tight-fitting mask over the face and attaching a one-way valve that allows exhalation but not inspiration. In children who are mechanically ventilated, $P_{0.1}$ can be measured using either a one-way valve attached to the ETT, similar to that used to measure P_{Imax}, and the pressure can be recorded through a side port. It is important that there be no leak in the system. This maneuver cannot be performed with an uncuffed ETT. An easier index to measure is the *mean inspiratory flow* (derived by dividing the V_T by the T_i), which can be determined in intubated patients by measuring spontaneous V_T and T_i using a pneumotachometer attached to the ETT without applying positive pressure to the airway.

CHAPTER 23 ■ STATUS ASTHMATICUS

MICHAEL T. BIGHAM AND RICHARD J. BRILLI

Asthma is "a chronic inflammatory disorder that causes recurrent episodes of wheezing, breathlessness, chest tightness, and coughing associated with airflow obstruction that is often reversible." *Status asthmaticus* is a condition of progressively worsening bronchospasm and respiratory dysfunction unresponsive to standard therapy and may progress to respiratory failure.

EPIDEMIOLOGY

Asthma-related deaths in American children nearly doubled between 1980 and 1995, but recently stabilized or even decreased. Most deaths are associated with cardiac arrest prior to pediatric intensive care unit (PICU) admission. Risks for severe disease include a history of ICU admission, respiratory failure, or sudden, severe deterioration. Other risk factors include poor compliance with outpatient treatment, inner-city residence, and denial of disease severity. Fatal asthma exacerbations may occur in children with mild asthma.

MECHANISM OF DISEASE: CORE PATHOPHYSIOLOGY

Asthma is an inflammatory disease characterized by airflow obstruction due to airway hyperresponsiveness, bronchospasm, and airway inflammation with mucosal edema and mucous plugging of small airways. The cascade of inflammation begins with degranulation of mast cells, usually in response to allergen exposure. Submucosal infiltration by eosinophils, neutrophils, and activated lymphocytes is responsible for late or delayed bronchospasm. "Early" bronchospasm may be more sensitive to bronchodilating agents, whereas "late" bronchospasm is more sensitive to anti-inflammatory therapy. Parasympathetic activation also contributes to bronchospasm and mucous production.

Pulmonary Mechanics and Gas-Exchange Abnormalities

Pulmonary mechanical dysfunction results from bronchial smooth muscle contraction, mucosal edema, and increased mucous production that leads to decreased airway diameter and increased airflow resistance. During inspiration, negative pleural pressure causes physiologic intrathoracic airway dilation; however, during expiration, pleural pressure approaching zero causes airway narrowing. In status asthmaticus, these changes in airway diameter during expiration cause airflow obstruction, air trapping, and lung hyperinflation. Expiration becomes active, which results in increased work of breathing (WOB). Diaphragmatic flattening from hyperinflation causes additional mechanical disadvantages. Forced expiratory volume and forced vital capacity are decreased, and total lung volumes and functional residual capacity are increased.

Gas-exchange abnormalities in status asthmaticus are due to ventilation–perfusion (V/Q) mismatch, including increased intrapulmonary shunt (atelectasis) and increased dead space (airway overdistension) from small-airway obstruction. Atelectasis causes areas of decreased ventilation but adequate pulmonary blood flow (shunt) and arterial hypoxemia. As disease severity worsens, greater distal airway obstruction causes alveolar distension and increased pulmonary dead space. Tachypnea compensates for worsening V/Q mismatch. Despite increasing dead space–tidal volume ratio (V_d/V_T), hypocarbia is initially present because minute ventilation increases. Eventually, intercostal and diaphragmatic muscles fatigue and progressive hypoxemia and hypercarbia result.

Cardiopulmonary Interactions in Asthma

Dynamic hyperinflation in severe asthma can have significant cardiopulmonary consequences. High lung volumes stretch the pulmonary vasculature (i.e., increases pulmonary vascular resistance and right ventricular afterload) and compromise right ventricular function. The fluctuations in pleural pressures produce significant effects on the intrathoracic vessels and right atrial venous return. The large, negative intrathoracic pressure produced during inspiration increases left ventricular afterload and decreases systolic blood pressure. The exaggerated variation in blood pressure associated with intrathoracic pressure change is termed *pulsus paradoxus* (**Fig. 23.1**).

CLINICAL PRESENTATION

Entities that must be distinguished from asthma include pneumonia, foreign-body aspiration, and congestive heart failure. Upper airway obstruction

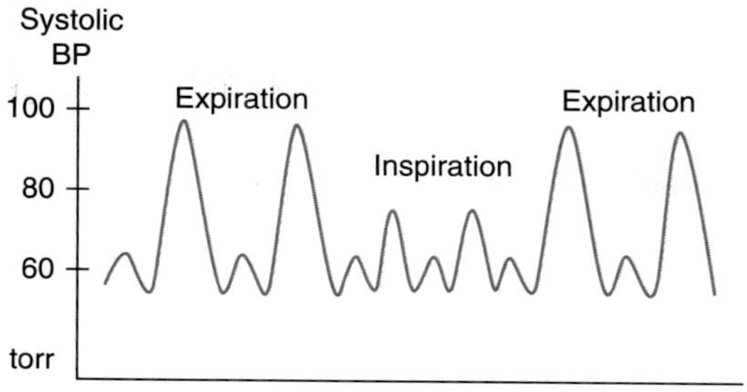

FIGURE 23.1. Pulsus paradoxus in status asthmaticus.

can also present with wheezing but usually presents with stridor. Diagnostic considerations include vocal cord paralysis, anatomic webs, airway hemangiomas, laryngomalacia, tracheomalacia, or bronchomalacia. Congenital anomalies, such as complete tracheal rings and bronchial slings, may also present with wheezing.

Children typically present with respiratory distress, cough, and wheezing that progresses over 1–2 days. Allergen exposure and upper respiratory tract infection can be triggers. In contrast, foreign-body aspiration presents with an abrupt onset of symptoms. The presence of fever suggests lower respiratory infection, though asthma and pneumonia can occur together. Children with severe status asthmaticus often appear lethargic and diaphoretic, cannot phonate, and have severe retractions and paradoxical thoracoabdominal breathing. Poor air movement on chest auscultation is an ominous sign of impending respiratory or cardiopulmonary failure.

Wheezing, which reflects turbulent airflow in obstructed airways, is usually equal bilaterally. Asymmetric wheezing may imply atelectasis, pneumothorax, or foreign body. Expiratory wheezing alone is found in mild-to-moderate illness, whereas expiratory plus inspiratory wheezing is present in moderate-to-severe status asthmaticus. The "silent chest" is an ominous sign and may indicate either pneumothorax or severe airway obstruction. Hypoxemia is another sign of severe asthma. Clinical asthma scores are valuable in research but are not in predicting progression of clinical illness. The peak expiratory flow rate (PEFR) is an excellent measure of airway narrowing, and can be less than 50% of normal values in severe exacerbations. PEFRs are often used to monitor response to therapy.

For spontaneously breathing children with status asthmaticus, clinical interventions should be based upon physical examination and not blood gas determinations. Normal $Paco_2$ in a tachypneic, hyperventilating child with status asthmaticus may be a sign of early respiratory muscle fatigue. Lactic acidosis is often present and reflects a combination of dehydration and overuse of the respiratory musculature. Hypokalemia may result from intracellular shifts from β-agonist therapy. Serum magnesium levels may be important because the correction of relative hypomagnesemia in status asthmaticus may improve outcome. Children with first-time wheezing or who require PICU admission should receive a chest X-ray to evaluate for an infectious infiltrate, pneumothorax, cardiomegaly, pulmonary edema, or unsuspected chest masses.

CLINICAL MANAGEMENT

Most children with asthma exacerbations do not require hospital admission. A small percentage will have a history of rapid clinical deterioration, limited air entry, air hunger, an inability to phonate despite bronchodilator therapy, or a Becker asthma score ≥ 7 and should be considered for PICU admission. Other indications for PICU admission include a sense of impending doom, altered mental status, respiratory arrest, or a rising $Paco_2$ coupled with clinical signs of fatigue.

Emergency-department management should provide supplemental O_2, continuous inhaled β-agonists, and IV methylprednisolone. Some suggest that IV magnesium and/or IV β-agonists should be administered to prevent progression to mechanical ventilation. Evidence-based clinical pathways are designed to reduce variation and standardize the delivery of high-quality care. PICU asthma pathway use can reduce ICU length of stay (LOS) and enhance adherence to national recommendations around asthma education and asthma specialist referral.

Children are often dehydrated as a result of decreased oral intake and increased insensible losses from increased minute ventilation. Providing appropriate fluid resuscitation is essential; however, overhydration should be avoided. Pulmonary edema is a risk due to microvascular permeability, increased left ventricular afterload, and alveolar fluid migration associated with the inflammatory lung process. In lung segments with atelectasis, compensatory hypoxic pulmonary vasoconstriction is often present. Treatment with inhaled β-agonists may induce generalized pulmonary vasodilatation, exacerbate mismatch, and worsen hypoxemia.

Corticosteroids

The overriding physiologic derangement in asthma is airway inflammation, and corticosteroids are a mainstay in the management of both acute and chronic asthma. Glucocorticosteroids suppress cytokine production, granulocyte-macrophage colony-stimulating factor production, and inducible nitric oxide synthase activation. They also impede recruitment and activation of inflammatory cells, decrease airway mucous production, and attenuate microvascular permeability. Systemic corticosteroids reduce hospitalization rates and LOS. Inhaled corticosteroids are of no benefit in status asthmaticus. While enteral and parenteral administration of corticosteroids may be of equal efficacy, the child in the PICU is less likely to tolerate oral medications, and IV methylprednisolone is preferred. Systemic corticosteroids begin to exert effect in 1–3 hours and reach maximal effect in 4–8 hours. Treatment continues until the exacerbation is resolved. Side effects observed in critically ill children include hyperglycemia, hypertension, and agitation related to steroid-induced psychosis. Prolonged steroid use may cause hypothalamic–pituitary–adrenal axis suppression, osteoporosis, myopathy, and weakness. The incidence of myopathy and weakness is increased when neuromuscular blocking agents are concomitantly administered.

Inhaled β-Agonists

Stimulation of the β_2-adrenergic receptor activates adenylate cyclase and increases cyclic AMP (cAMP) and cAMP-dependent protein kinase (protein kinase A, PKA) which inhibit Ca^+ influx in the sarcolemma and cause smooth muscle relaxation. Inhaled β-agonists are a bridge to support ventilation and oxygenation until the anti-inflammatory effects of corticosteroids take effect. Albuterol for inhalation is available in two forms: albuterol (salbutamol) and levalbuterol. Albuterol is a racemic mixture of equal parts of R- and S-enantiomers. The R-enantiomer is pharmacologically active, whereas the S-enantiomer is considered pharmacologically inactive and may contribute to airway irritation as a spasmogen. Levalbuterol consists solely of the R-enantiomer of albuterol, but has not proved superior to racemic albuterol in clinical trials. The two primary albuterol delivery mechanisms are nebulizer and metered-dose inhaler (MDI), usually with a vehicle-delivery device (i.e., spacer). Continuous albuterol nebulization may lead to a more rapid clinical improvement than intermittent administration. Some practitioners transition to MDI treatments when weaning.

Side effects of continuous albuterol are usually minor. Sinus tachycardia is common. Other cardiovascular effects include palpitations, hypertension, diastolic hypotension, and, rarely, ventricular dysrhythmias. Excessive central nervous system (CNS) stimulation occurs with hyperactivity, tremors, and nausea/vomiting. Hypokalemia and hyperglycemia are common but do not usually require treatment. Long-acting inhaled β-agonists (LABAs) are used predominately as controller medications for asthma and there are no data to support their use in pediatric status asthmaticus.

Intravenous and Subcutaneous β-Agonists

IV and subcutaneous administration of β-agonists may help children with severely limited airflow, when distribution of inhaled medications may be reduced. Nonselective β-agonists, such as ephedrine, epinephrine, and isoproterenol, are rarely used because of their high side-effect profile. Terbutaline, a relatively selective β_2-agonist, is available for IV or subcutaneous administration. The subcutaneous route is useful for children with no IV access. The side effects of subcutaneous or IV-administered terbutaline are similar to inhaled β-agonists. Elevation in troponin I levels occur in 10%–50% of pediatric asthmatics during IV terbutaline therapy. ST analysis on continuous electrocardiography and following creatine phosphokinase or troponin in children who are receiving IV β-agonists, including terbutaline, may be useful.

Methylxanthines

Methylxanthines promote relaxation of the bronchial smooth muscles; however, the exact mechanism of action remains controversial. Previously a mainstay in the treatment, recent data have made their use in the ICU controversial. They may have a role in critically ill children not responsive to steroids, inhaled and IV β-agonists, and O_2. Theophylline is administered by continuous IV infusion, and levels should be measured 1–2 hours after the loading dose is completed. Theophylline clearance is reduced in infants and adolescents. Serum levels >20 μg/mL are associated with adverse effects that include nausea, jitters or restlessness, tachycardia, and irritability. Serum levels >35 μg/mL have been associated with seizures and dysrhythmias.

Anticholinergics

Ipratropium bromide is the most frequently used anticholinergic agent in the treatment of status asthmaticus. Aerosolized ipratropium blocks acetylcholine interactions with the muscarinic receptor on bronchial smooth muscle cells, reducing intracellular cyclic guanosine monophosphate levels, and relaxing bronchial smooth muscle. Ipratropium promotes bronchodilation without inhibiting mucociliary clearance (unlike atropine). Although it has no proven benefit in moderately ill children with asthma, it may be prudent to add inhaled ipratropium therapy for these patients. Ipratropium has few adverse effects because of poor systemic absorption. The most common untoward effects are dry mouth, bitter taste, flushing, tachycardia, and dizziness. Tiotropium bromide, a long-acting selective anticholinergic compound with a higher affinity for the muscarinic receptors in the airway, has shown promising clinical benefits in chronic asthma management.

Magnesium Sulfate

Magnesium acts as a bronchodilator through its activity as a calcium channel blocker and in activating adenylate cyclase in smooth muscle cells. Magnesium given in the emergency department reduces hospitalization rates, improve short-term PFTs, and improve clinical asthma scores. No data are available regarding the efficacy of magnesium in the ICU. A target magnesium level of 4 mg/dL may achieve maximal effect. Side effects include hypotension, CNS depression, muscle weakness, and flushing. Severe complications, such as cardiac arrhythmia, respiratory failure due to severe muscle weakness, and sudden cardiopulmonary arrest, may occur in the setting of very high serum magnesium levels (usually >10–12 mg/dL).

Helium–Oxygen

Helium is a biologically inert, low-density gas that reduces airflow resistance in small airways by enhancing laminar gas flow. It may also enhance particle deposition of aerosolized medications in distal lung segments. A Cochrane review concluded that heliox was not beneficial in asthma (most of the studies cited were in adults). Pediatric studies are mixed. The use of heliox is sometimes limited by hypoxemia. If substantial supplemental O_2 is added to mixtures of helium/oxygen, the salutary effect of low-density gas administration on reducing turbulent gas flow is lost. Ventilator measurement of tidal volumes may be affected by its use.

Noninvasive Mechanical Ventilation

Noninvasive positive-pressure ventilation (NIPPV) is an alternative to conventional mechanical ventilation and is used in 3%–5% of critically ill asthmatic children. Small studies suggest benefit. It remains an unproven therapy for children with status asthmaticus; however, it is relatively easy to institute, and a trial may be warranted prior to tracheal intubation.

Mechanical Ventilation

Currently, <1% of children with status asthmaticus require mechanical ventilation. Children initially cared for at a community hospital were three times more likely to be intubated. Children who require mechanical ventilation are at increased risk for pulmonary barotrauma, nosocomial infection, pulmonary edema, circulatory dysfunction, steroid/muscle relaxant-associated myopathy, and death. In status asthmaticus, the indications for tracheal intubation for children include cardiorespiratory arrest, refractory hypoxemia, or significant respiratory acidosis unresponsive to pharmacotherapy. Tracheal intubation of the asthmatic child requires preparation. Hypotension should be anticipated secondary to hypovolemia exacerbated by reduced preload as positive-pressure ventilation is initiated and by vasodilation caused by sedative use for tracheal intubation. Histamine-producing agents, such as morphine or atracurium should be avoided. Ketamine is preferred for induction because of its relatively long half-life, bronchodilating properties, and preservation of hemodynamic stability. A large diameter, cuffed, endotracheal tube should be used, as high ventilatory pressures are often required.

Ventilatory support in status asthmaticus should maintain adequate oxygenation, allow for permissive hypercarbia, and adjust minute ventilation (peak pressure, tidal volume, and rate) to maintain an arterial pH of >7.2. Ventilator management strategies should attempt to minimize dynamic hyperinflation and air trapping. This can usually be accomplished by employing slow ventilator rates with prolonged expiratory phase and short inspiratory time.

Volume-control ventilation with constant or accelerating flow wave forms will provide stable tidal volumes but, in the setting of dynamic airway resistance, may result in high peak airway pressures, uneven distribution of tidal breaths, and increased risk for pulmonary barotrauma. Pressure-control ventilation with decelerating flow pattern results in lower peak pressure, higher mean airway pressure, and better distribution of gas into high-resistance, long time-constant airways. PEEP administration is controversial, reduced PEEP may help because patients with status asthmaticus already have increased functional residual capacity, or increased PEEP may stent small airways open at end of expiration and facilitate full expiration in patients that have dynamic collapse of small airways during forced exhalation. Review of graphically displayed flow–time curves will demonstrate whether expiratory flow is completed prior to the next breath. The use of high-frequency ventilation has been described and requires careful attention to the amplitude settings to avoid further hyperinflation. Tracheal gas insufflation has been used to facilitate expiratory gas flow and reduce severe hypercarbia. Pressure-support ventilation without any preset rate allows spontaneous breathing, avoids muscle relaxants, and allows forced exhalation.

Tracheal extubation should occur as soon as possible. The presence of the breathing tube, especially in awake children, may stimulate further bronchospasm. Decreasing peak inspiratory pressure, adequate air movement by auscultation, and graphic evidence of full expiration of are sufficient criteria for tracheal extubation, even if wheezing is still present.

Chest Physiotherapy

Chest physiotherapy (CPT) may augment airway clearance and encourage resolution of mucous plugging; but should only be considered in children with clear segmental or lobar atelectasis. In all other populations of children with status asthmaticus, CPT has no therapeutic benefit.

Antibiotics

Most asthma exacerbations are associated with viral infections and not bacterial infections, and empiric antibiotic treatment is not indicated. Isolated lower respiratory tract bacterial infections do occur. The most commonly identified organisms are *Mycoplasma pneumoniae* and *Chlamydia pneumoniae*. When findings on chest X-ray, leukocytosis, and fever suggest pneumonia, appropriate antibiotics should be administered. Sinusitis should also be considered in patients without evidence of bacterial pneumonia, but with high fever and peripheral blood leukocytosis.

Sedation, Analgesia, Muscle Relaxants, and Inhalational Anesthetics

Sedation of the unintubated asthmatic is generally not indicated. Mechanically ventilated children require sedation and may need muscle relaxation to prevent ventilator–patient asynchrony and reduce the risk of cough-induced barotrauma. Ketamine by continuous infusion is often chosen for sedation, usually combined with intermittent or continuous benzodiazepines. Increased respiratory secretions can occur with ketamine administration, but are usually manageable. When opiates are used, morphine is avoided as it causes histamine release and may exacerbate bronchospasm. Neuromuscular blocking agents should be titrated to train-of-four monitoring—usually one to two twitches. Drug holidays can be used to reduce the risk of overdose, prolonged paresis, and myopathy that are sometimes observed.

Inhaled volatile anesthetics have bronchodilating effects and have been used when other measures are failing. Several small pediatric studies describe the safe use of isoflurane in the management of refractory status asthmaticus. Appropriate expertise is needed for delivery and scavenging. Hypotension, impaired renal perfusion, and cardiac dysrhythmias are associated with their use and are more likely to occur in hypoxemic children.

Extracorporeal Membrane Oxygenation Support

When maximal medical therapy fails, ECMO should be considered. Numerous case reports demonstrate high survival rates (~90%), even in a gravely ill patient population.

OUTCOMES

Mortality rates for children with severe status asthmaticus who arrive at the hospital intact are nearly zero. Sophisticated ventilatory strategies, the availability of more selective, less toxic bronchodilating agents, and the selective use of ECMO have contributed to this good prognosis.

CHAPTER 24 ■ NEONATAL RESPIRATORY FAILURE

NARAYAN PRABHU IYER, PHILIPPE S. FRIEDLICH, ELIZABETH L. RAAB, RANGASAMY RAMANATHAN, AND ISTVAN SERI

DEVELOPMENTALLY REGULATED DISORDERS: RESPIRATORY CONDITIONS ASSOCIATED WITH PREMATURE LUNG

Respiratory Distress Syndrome

Respiratory distress syndrome (RDS) due to surfactant deficiency is a significant life-threatening condition that primarily occurs in preterm infants. The incidence and severity of RDS is inversely proportional to gestational age (GA). RDS occurs in about 50% of infants born at <29 weeks and in 25% of infants born at >29 weeks of gestation. The combination of prenatal steroid and postnatal surfactant therapy has significantly reduced mortality and morbidity from RDS.

Pathophysiology of Respiratory Distress Syndrome

Surfactant Synthesis, Metabolism, and Function. Surfactant coats the lung surface at the air–liquid interface in the alveoli and maintains a low surface tension that prevents collapse during expiration. Surfactant is primarily composed of phospholipids (80%–90%) and surfactant proteins (SP) SP-A, SP-B, SP-C, and SP-D. Dipalmitoyl phosphatidylcholine (DPPC) constitutes the major phospholipid. Type II pneumocytes that line alveoli synthesize surfactant. Surfactant equalizes surface tension forces across the lung, resulting in more uniform alveolar expansion. Infants with RDS have reduced available surfactant, which results in low pulmonary compliance and an inability to maintain functional residual capacity (FRC). Surfactant deficiency results in a heterogeneous distribution with underaerated alveoli emptying into adjacent overdistended alveoli. Pulmonary edema inactivates and dilutes the remaining surfactant, furthering injury.

Management of Respiratory Distress Syndrome

Surfactant Therapy for Respiratory Distress Syndrome. Surfactant therapy decreases mortality and the incidence of pneumothorax and is the standard of care for infants with RDS. Early use is better than delayed, but intubation solely for surfactant administration is controversial. Natural modified surfactants (derived from animal sources) and synthetic surfactants are available. Luminactant is the only synthetic surfactant currently in use. Natural surfactants that have been extensively studied include beractant (Survanta), calfactant (Infasurf), SF-RI 1 (Alveofact), and poractant alfa (Curosurf). They differ in composition, onset of response, duration of action, dosing volume, and the need for additional doses. Based on randomized controlled trials (RCTs) and large retrospective studies, treatment with poractant alfa is consistently associated with improved outcomes, likely due to the use of a higher initial dose.

Attempts have been made to apply less invasive techniques of surfactant delivery. The Intubate–Surfactant–Extubate (INSURE) technique involves a very brief period of intubation and positive-pressure ventilation for surfactant administration. Techniques for administration that avoid endotracheal intubation include surfactant aerosols and administration using catheters, feeding tubes, or a laryngeal mask airway (LMA). The impact of techniques that avoid intubation on the rate of bronchopulmonary dysplasia (BPD) is still being evaluated.

Noninvasive Respiratory Support in the Management of Respiratory Distress Syndrome. Modes of noninvasive respiratory support in newborn infants include nasal continuous positive airway pressure (NCPAP), synchronized inspiratory positive airway pressure (Si-PAP), noninvasive positive-pressure ventilation (NIPPV), heated humidified high-flow nasal cannula (HFNC), and nasal high-frequency oscillatory ventilation (HFOV) (**Table 24.1**). The use of noninvasive support can prevent lung collapse and decrease the need for invasive mechanical ventilation. Complications can include nasal trauma, pneumothorax, and feeding intolerance from gastric distention.

Oxygenation and Ventilation Targets in Preterm Infants with Respiratory Distress Syndrome

Exposure to hyperoxia is associated with retinopathy of prematurity (ROP) and possibly with BPD. Trials to identify the optimal oxygen saturation target for

TABLE 24.1

Different Modes of Noninvasive Respiratory Support

■ MODE	■ MECHANISM	■ TYPICAL SETTINGS
Nasal continuous positive airway pressure (NCPAP)	Provides continuous distending pressure, improves functional residual capacity (FRC), and stents open upper airway. By preventing alveolar collapse NCPAP also helps conserve surfactant.	4–8 cm H_2O
Synchronized inspiratory positive airway pressure (Si-PAP)	Provides "biphasic" CPAP, allowing infant to breathe at two levels of pressure, further augmenting the FRC. Synchronized Si-PAP (not available in the United States) can be used to synchronize the "high pressure" with inspiration.	Positive end-expiratory pressure (PEEP): 4–8 cm H_2O Peak inspiratory pressure (PIP): 8–15 cm H_2O
Nasal intermittent positive-pressure ventilation	Provides a peak inspiratory pressure in addition to CPAP, thereby augmenting ventilation.	PEEP: 4–8 cm H_2O PIP: 15–30 cm H_2O
Heated humidified high-flow nasal cannula (HFNC)	Reduces work of breathing by "washout" of nasopharyngeal dead space. Also produces distending pressure comparable to NCPAP.	2–8 L/min Pressure generated cannot be measured or controlled by the user.
Nasal high-frequency oscillatory ventilation (HFOV)	Augmentation of FRC. Theoretically, does not require synchronization.	Mean airway pressure (MAP): 8–14 cm H_2O (usually 1–3 cm H_2O above the MAP used during conventional ventilation) Amplitude: 20–40 cm H_2O; Frequency:10–15 Hz
Noninvasive neurally adjusted ventilator assist (NIV-NAVA)	Provides noninvasive ventilation proportional to and synchronized with diaphragmatic electric activity. Support is not affected by leak conditions at nasal interface.	PEEP: 4–8 cm H_2O NAVA level: 0.5–3 cm H_2O/mV; Electrical activity of the diaphragm (Edi) peak goal is 5–15 and Edi minimum is <3 cm H_2O

preterm infants have raised concerns for worsened mortality and necrotizing enterocolitis in the low-saturation target (85%–89%) groups and more ROP in the high-saturation target (91%–95%) groups. Another change is allowing Pa_{CO_2} levels above 40 mm Hg to reduce ventilator-induced barotrauma. Although practices differ, Pa_{CO_2} levels of 45–55 mm Hg are generally accepted. The long-term neurodevelopmental effects need to be investigated.

Bronchopulmonary Dysplasia

BPD (chronic lung disease of prematurity) is the most common chronic lung disease of childhood. The classic severe form of BPD is less frequent due to antenatal steroids, postnatal surfactant, and a shorter period of mechanical ventilation despite more severe immaturity. An increasing number of small preterm infants survive with more uniform lung inflation on X-ray and minimal evidence of fibrosis. Infants with BPD have alveoli that are *larger, more simplified, and fewer in number* as well as variable airway smooth muscle hyperplasia. An *arrest of vascular growth* contributes to ventilation–perfusion mismatch and pulmonary hypertension.

Etiology, Pathogenesis, and Prevention

Infants most commonly affected with BPD are usually born at <28 weeks of gestation. They may worsen after a period of initial apparent stability. In addition to prematurity, intrauterine growth retardation and prolonged mechanical ventilation increase the risk of BPD. Noninvasive respiratory support might reduce rates of BPD. A reduction in BPD has not been found when comparing HFOV with conventional ventilation. Results are conflicting regarding an association between chorioamnionitis and BPD.

Pharmacotherapy for Bronchopulmonary Dysplasia Prevention

Steroids for the Prevention of Bronchopulmonary Dysplasia. Dexamethasone was a key part of efforts to prevent or treat BPD. Recent concerns involve long-term neurodevelopmental outcome and the risk of spontaneous intestinal perforation (SIP). Dexamethasone is now reserved for patients with the most severe lung disease using lower doses and shorter courses. Trials using hydrocortisone to prevent BPD are currently recruiting patients.

Nonsteroidal Agents. Vitamin A, caffeine, inositol, and clarithromycin have shown promise for BPD prevention. A beneficial effect of caffeine was found as a secondary outcome in the Caffeine for Apnea of Prematurity trial. Inositol and clarithromycin have been studied in single-center randomized trials. Ibuprofen used to close a patent ductus arteriosus has been associated with an increased risk of BPD.

Management

The management of infants at risk for developing BPD should (a) minimize ventilatory support and alveolar overdistension, (b) maintain adequate FRC with optimal positive end expiratory pressure, (c) optimize growth, and (d) judiciously use of diuretics and bronchodilators. Inhaled β_2 adrenergic agonists improve airway resistance and ventilation. Inhaled corticosteroids can minimize the inflammatory process that exacerbates BPD. There is no evidence that inhaled corticosteroids improve pulmonary outcome.

Implications for Long-Term Outcome

Although alveolar growth accelerates in the first 2 years of life, infants with BPD have a reduced pulmonary diffusion capacity and persistent impairment of expiratory flow in small airways. Unfortunately, lung function can deteriorate in adults who once had BPD and infants with BPD need to be followed long into adulthood. BPD is associated with poor neurodevelopmental outcome, although it is not easy to separate the effects of BPD from the effects of immaturity and complications of premature birth.

DISORDERS OF TRANSITION

Transient Tachypnea of the Newborn

Transient tachypnea of the newborn (TTN) is a syndrome of early-onset respiratory distress, radiographic findings (increased pulmonary vascular markings, pulmonary edema, mild hyperexpansion, and mild cardiomegaly), and symptoms that resolved within 2–5 days. It is thought to be due to a delay in the cessation of production and clearance of fetal lung fluid. Infants born by elective cesarean section are at a significantly higher risk of developing TTN, most likely because they do not undergo the normal hormonal changes accompanying the transition to extrauterine life. The diagnosis of TTN is a diagnosis of exclusion. Treatment is supportive with oxygen, positive-pressure ventilation as needed, radiographs to rule out lung malformations, antibiotics during evaluation for sepsis, and an echocardiogram if indicated.

Persistent Pulmonary Hypertension of the Newborn

Persistent pulmonary hypertension of the newborn (PPHN) is characterized by failure of the normal pulmonary vascular transition to extrauterine life. It results in increased pulmonary pressures, hypoxemia, and respiratory distress and occurs in ~1–2/1000 live born births. In utero, the placenta serves as the organ of gas exchange, and pulmonary resistance is maintained at or above systemic levels. As the fetus approaches term, vasodilatory pathways (NO and prostacyclin) are upregulated. At birth, multiple factors dilate the pulmonary vasculature during the first few breaths. Significant derangements in metabolic homeostasis (i.e., acidosis, hypoxemia, or hypercarbia) prevent the coordinated transition from vasoconstriction to vasodilation, leading to the clinical syndrome of PPHN. The most common precipitating diseases of PPHN are meconium aspiration syndrome (MAS), sepsis/pneumonia, perinatal depression/acidosis, abnormal pulmonary vascular development, congenital diaphragmatic hernia/pulmonary hypoplasia, and idiopathic "black lung" PPHN.

Initial treatment includes correction of hypothermia, hypoglycemia, hypocalcemia, anemia, polycythemia, and hypovolemia. Induced alkalosis has been linked with adverse outcomes; however, correction of metabolic acidosis to physiologic pH is standard therapy. The practice of using vasopressors/inotropes to drive the blood pressure to supraphysiologic levels in order to "force" the blood through the lungs cannot be recommended as concomitant increases in PVR may occur. Oxygen is a pulmonary vasodilator, so normal oxygenation should be maintained. The goal of mechanical ventilation is to achieve "optimal" lung volume and recruitment, as both atelectasis and lung overdistension limit pulmonary blood flow. Inhaled NO (iNO) has been shown to improve oxygenation and decrease the need for extracorporeal membrane oxygenation (ECMO). Sildenafil has been used for the treatment of pulmonary hypertension in the setting of BPD and congenital diaphragmatic hernia (CDH), although there are concerns about possible increased mortality in children treated with high doses. Other off-label pulmonary vasodilators include prostanoids (PGI2, epoprostenol, treprostinil), milrinone (phosphodiesterase 3 inhibitor), and bosentan (endothelin receptor antagonist). ECMO remains the final rescue therapy for infants with PPHN.

CONGENITAL LUNG ANOMALIES

Congenital Diaphragmatic Hernia

CDH occurs due to a failure of closure of the pleuroperitoneal folds at around gestational week 5, resulting in a posterolateral diaphragmatic defect (Bochdalek hernia). The defect is most often on the left. CDH is almost universally associated with lung hypoplasia. In ~40% of cases, CDH is associated with another major anomaly or syndrome. Tracheal occlusion has been studied as a fetal intervention, as blocking fluid egress from the fetal lung increases lung growth.

Unfortunately, human studies using the tracheal occlusion strategy have failed to show benefit. Delivery room management of a neonate with known CDH focuses on immediate intubation and the avoidance of bag and mask ventilation in order to minimize distension of the stomach and the proximal intestine. The stomach should immediately be decompressed. Asymmetric breath sounds and a scaphoid abdomen at birth are clues to the diagnosis for infants not diagnosed prenatally. Current practice usually involves delaying surgery 1–2 weeks to allow PVR to fall prior to surgical repair. iNO and ECMO are frequently used to stabilize the infant during this time period.

Congenital Cystic Adenomatoid Malformation and Bronchopulmonary Sequestration

Congenital Pulmonary Airway (Cystic Adenomatoid) Malformation

Congenital pulmonary airway malformation (CPAM), previously known as congenital cystic adenomatoid malformation (CCAM), is a relatively rare developmental abnormality. It is believed to occur because of a failure of the normal bronchoalveolar development of the pulmonary mesenchyme between weeks 5 and 7 of gestation. The lesions are typically unilateral and isolated to one lobe (bilateral in <10%). The lesions typically grow significantly between 20 and 26 weeks of gestation and can lead to mediastinal shift and hydrops fetalis. Occasionally, the lesions regress as pregnancy develops. The severity of respiratory compromise cannot always be predicted antenatally. Timing of surgical resection depends on the severity of the symptoms and ranges from 1 to 2 days to 4 to 6 months of age. Eventual resection is recommended in all cases in view of the high likelihood of chronic infections within the lesion and the possibility of malignant transformation.

Pulmonary Sequestration

Pulmonary sequestration is a cystic lesion of the lung differentiated from CPAM by the origin of its blood supply (systemic rather than pulmonary). Sequestrations can be intrapulmonary or extrapulmonary. Sequestration is believed to occur due to development of an accessory lung bud. Many infants with sequestration are asymptomatic at birth, although they may be diagnosed early as part of an evaluation of other congenital anomalies. Sequestrations present a significant risk for recurrent infections. Resection is recommended in the first year of life.

Pulmonary Hypoplasia

Pulmonary hypoplasia represents a broad spectrum of anatomic malformations ranging from total bronchial agenesis to mild parenchymal hypoplasia and may be either primary or secondary to other lesions. It can be associated with CDH, skeletal or neuromuscular disease that decreases fetal movement, or the oligohydramnios sequence.

ACQUIRED DISEASE

Pulmonary Interstitial Emphysema

Pulmonary interstitial emphysema (PIE) is a consequence of the overdistension of distal airways and usually occurs in the most immature babies. Ruptured airways provide a pathway for leakage of air into the connective tissue sheets that results in the radiographic findings of PIE (linear and cyst-like radiolucencies that reflect the accumulation of interstitial air). Ventilatory techniques to minimize alveolar and airway distension are tried. When PIE is unilateral, it is often suggested that the infant be positioned with the affected side down. One can attempt to decompress the air leaks by using a short inspiratory time, low inflation pressures, and small tidal volumes. High-frequency ventilation may allow for adequate ventilation and oxygenation in infants with PIE at lower peak and mean airway pressures than with conventional ventilation.

Pneumomediastinum and Pneumothorax

About 3%–5% of normal term newborns may have asymptomatic, spontaneous, nontension pneumothoraces during the first few postnatal hours, likely from the large negative intrapleural pressure required to inflate the lungs immediately after delivery. In neonates with lung disease, it is believed that up to 10% develop an air leak syndrome as a result of poor lung compliance. When air is constrained to the mediastinum, it is unusual for the volume of air to cause circulatory compromise. Tension pneumothorax can result in high intrapleural pressures, collapse of the ipsilateral lung, hypoxia, hypercapnia, and mediastinal shift. The mediastinal shift can impede cardiac output and lead to cardiovascular collapse. Differential breath sounds are unreliable for the diagnosis of pneumothorax in infants, but transillumination of the chest may be helpful. Acute clinical deterioration in a mechanically ventilated infant should raise immediate concerns. Recent studies of infants with spontaneous pneumothorax did not show any difference in time to resolution between room air and a 100% oxygen washout, and the risk of oxygen toxicity may outweigh the benefit. Tube thoracotomy is indicated in neonates with cardiorespiratory compromise or those receiving mechanical ventilation.

CHAPTER 25 ■ PNEUMONIA AND BRONCHIOLITIS

WERTHER BRUNOW DE CARVALHO, MARCELO CUNIO MACHADO FONSECA, CINTIA JOHNSTON, AND DAVID G. NICHOLS

PNEUMONIA

Pneumonia is an inflammatory condition of the lung parenchyma, which distinguishes it from inflammatory conditions of the airways (bronchiolitis, bronchitis, or tracheitis). The etiology can be infection, aspiration, hypersensitivity to inhaled materials (hydrocarbon and lipoid pneumonia), and drug- or radiation-induced. Pneumonia usually presents with signs of alveolar compromise and radiographic opacification without lung volume loss. Recurrent pneumonia raises the possibility of an underlying disease (e.g., acquired or congenital lung anatomical abnormalities, immunodeficiency, prematurity, lung sequestration, tracheoesophageal fistula, foreign body, cystic fibrosis, heart failure, cleft palate, bronchiectasis, ciliary dyskinesia, neutropenia, or increased pulmonary blood flow). Other predisposing factors are lower socioeconomic status, parental smoking, and prolonged critical illness.

Pneumonia occurs either by colonization of the upper airway that spreads to the lower respiratory tract or, less commonly, through hematogenous spread to pulmonary parenchyma (e.g., *Streptococcus pneumoniae* and *Staphylococcus aureus*). The child may experience cough, coryza, or pharyngitis. Inflammatory responses lead to increased airway reactivity, transudation of plasma into the air spaces, and excess mucus production. The bronchiolar and alveolar epithelia become necrotic in severe cases. The accumulation of fluid and cellular debris in the alveoli may lead to decreased ventilation relative to perfusion and hypoxia. Viral pneumonia also affects the lung through direct invasion, and the resulting mucosal inflammation and cilial injury predispose to secondary bacterial infection.

Neonatal Pneumonia

Newborns with bacterial pneumonia present with tachypnea, grunting, nasal flaring, and chest wall retractions. Other nonspecific signs (poor feeding, vomiting, irritability, lethargy, and apnea) are also seen with bacteremia and meningitis, which makes diagnosing pneumonia difficult without a chest radiography. In preterm newborns, pneumonia may present as apnea without fever or tachycardia. Infants with *Chlamydia trachomatis* pneumonia present between 3 weeks and 3 months of age with staccato cough, tachypnea, and rales.

Group B Streptococcus (GBS) is the most common cause of early-onset pneumonia in developed countries. Vaginal colonization, prematurity, and premature or prolonged (>18 hours) rupture of membranes are risk factors. Severely affected infants may develop persistent pulmonary hypertension of the newborn. Maternal screening for GBS colonization and the use of intrapartum antibiotic prophylaxis have decreased the incidence and severity of GBS pneumonia. Among viral etiologies of neonatal pneumonia, herpes simplex virus (HSV) is most common and carries a high mortality rate. Ampicillin, gentamicin, and acyclovir are a useful antibiotic combination until cultures and polymerase chain reaction (PCR) studies are available to tailor therapy. *Meconium aspiration syndrome* (MAS) can also cause neonatal respiratory distress but is usually readily distinguished from infectious early-onset pneumonia based on clinical and radiographic criteria.

Prolonged mechanical ventilation is the greatest risk factor for pneumonia that presents after the first 48 hours of life. The usual pathogens for this neonatal ventilator-associated pneumonia (VAP) are *Pseudomonas aeruginosa* and *Staphylococcus*. Late-onset GBS usually presents as bacteremia or meningitis, not pneumonia. Respiratory syncytial virus (RSV) is the most common cause of late-onset neonatal viral pneumonia.

Community-Acquired Pneumonia

Community-acquired pneumonia (CAP) is a lung parenchymal infection acquired outside the hospital. Most children >6 months of age with CAP are managed as outpatients. For infants <2 months, the bacterial etiologies include *Streptococcus pneumoniae,* group B streptococci, gram-negative bacilli (from maternal genital tract or hospital flora), *Staphylococcus aureus*, and *C. trachomatis*. Young infants with bacterial pneumonia are usually highly febrile (>39°C) and tachypneic, and appear toxic. *C. trachomatis* (less commonly *Mycoplasma hominis* or *Ureaplasma urealyticum*) may cause an "afebrile pneumonia of infancy" in 2-week- to 4-month-olds.

Pertussis ("whooping cough") is making a resurgence worldwide. Young infants are at greatest risk for complications. The presentation is characteristic with prolonged staccato cough, sometimes followed by an inspiratory "whoop," and posttussive emesis. Extreme leukocytosis (lymphocytosis), pulmonary hypertension, hypoxia, apnea, and seizures can occur. Viruses are the main pathogens among infants 6–12 months old. RSV and influenza are most common, but parainfluenza, adenovirus, rhinovirus, coronavirus, measles, rubella, varicella, cytomegalovirus, or herpes may also cause pneumonia. Among children 1–5 years old, viruses remain the predominant cause, but *S. pneumonia* is a common bacterial pathogen. Methicillin-resistant *Staphylococcus aureus* (MRSA) is more commonly associated with necrotizing pneumonia and empyema than other organisms. Less common pathogens include helminths (*Ascaris lumbricoides*, *Strongyloides stercoralis*, *Toxocara kennels*), human metapneumovirus (hMPV), *B. pertussis*, *Mycobacterium tuberculosis*, *Listeria monocytogenes*, *Legionella pneumophila*, Hantavirus, *Coxiella burnetii*, protozoa (e.g., *Toxoplasma gondii*), fungi (including *Pneumocystis jiroveci*), and physical and chemical agents. The relative incidence of *Mycoplasma* pneumonia increases with age and is common in young adults.

The evidence-based recommendations for CAP antibiotic therapy depend on the child's immunization status. For patients with suspicion for *S. pneumoniae* pneumonia, IV ampicillin (ceftriaxone if suspected penicillin resistance) is used. Vancomycin should be added if MRSA is prevalent. When infection due to Hib is suspected (e.g., unimmunized child), ceftriaxone, cefotaxime, or ampicillin–sulbactam should be used because of β-lactamase–mediated resistance. Initial empiric therapy can be modified after the identification of the etiologic agent. A macrolide, doxycycline or levofloxacin, should be considered if atypical pneumonia is suspected.

Pneumonia in the Immunocompromised Host

Several chronic immune deficiency states are associated with characteristic pneumonia syndromes. The radiologic pattern may be characteristic, as with focal consolidation (*Streptococcus pneumoniae*, *H. influenzae*, *Legionella* sp., mycobacteria, and fungi), a micronodular pattern (viruses, mycobacteria, *Histoplasma*, *Candida* sp., and *Cryptococcus*), a nodular pattern (*Aspergillus* sp., other fungi, mucormycosis, *Nocardia* sp., and Epstein–Barr virus lymphoproliferative disease), or diffuse interstitial pattern (viruses, *M. pneumoniae*, Chlamydia, and *P. jiroveci*). Early, empiric therapy is very important and bronchopulmonary lavage or lung biopsy may be needed for a definitive diagnosis.

Nosocomial Pneumonia

Pneumonia acquired after 48 hours of hospitalization is considered nosocomial. Pneumonia associated with mechanical ventilation (*VAP*) is the second leading cause of nosocomial infection (20%). The most frequent microorganism recovered is *P. aeruginosa*, followed by *S. aureus* and then other gram-negative organisms such as *Klebsiella* spp., *Escherichia coli*, *Enterobacter* spp., *Serratia marcescens*, and *Acinetobacter*. Empiric treatment is usually combination therapy including an aminoglycoside due to the risk of gram-negative infections. Vancomycin is added if MRSA is a risk.

Aspiration Pneumonia

Aspiration pneumonia occurs when airway protective reflexes are inadequate or overwhelmed. The nature of the resulting pneumonia depends on whether the aspirate consists of gastric acid (chemical pneumonitis), upper airway flora (bacterial pneumonia), or particulate matter (airway obstruction). Prevention includes head of bed elevation to 30 degrees, endotracheal intubation for patients who lost protective airway reflexes, and good dental hygiene. Large particulate matter may require bronchoscopic removal. Corticosteroids do not improve outcome. Empiric coverage for aspiration of oral secretions includes ampicillin and clindamycin (for anaerobic coverage). Gastric acid aspiration alone does not require antibiotic coverage.

Diagnosis

Bacterial diagnosis from blood cultures is unusual (3%–11%) and rarely modifies management. The identification of a specific organism is especially useful in serious cases or with pleural effusions. Viral diagnosis is important in guiding therapy (especially for immunocompromised children) and for infection control precautions. PCR is useful for *Mycoplasma* and urinary antigen for *Legionella*. When chest X-ray or risk factors indicate tuberculosis, a skin test should be performed. Radiographic findings often lag behind clinical examination, especially in the presence of dehydration. Bacterial infection is likely with large pleural effusions, necrotizing pneumonia, and abscesses. High-resolution computed tomography (HRCT) shows anatomical structures and is more sensitive than chest X-ray for the detection of pneumonia. Lung ultrasound is potentially useful and avoids ionizing radiation.

Complications

Pneumonia complications include pleural effusions, empyema, extrapulmonary infection, sepsis, acute respiratory distress syndrome, shock, lung abscess, pneumothorax, atelectasis, and multiple organ system dysfunction. Pleural effusion and empyema are frequent acute complications and are referred to as parapneumonic effusions. Pleural effusion represents a fluid collection within the pleural cavity. Inflammation of the pleura results in leakage of plasma and

TABLE 25.1

Pleural Fluid Characteristics

	TRANSUDATE	EXUDATE
pH	>7.20	<7.20
Proteins (pleural fluid/serum level rate)	<0.5	≥0.5
LDH (pleural fluid/serum level)	<0.6	≥0.6
LDH (IU/L)	<200	≥200
Glucose (mg/dL)	>40	<40
Red cells (mm^3)	<5000	>5000
Leukocytes (mm^3)	<10,000 (PMN)	>10,000 (PMN)

LDH, lactate dehydrogenase; PMN, polymorphonuclear neutrophil.

white cells into the pleural cavity. Pleural effusions are classified as transudates or exudates depending on the laboratory analysis (**Table 25.1**). Additional data include a positive microbiologic study (Gram test, culture, or other diagnostic tests, such as PCR).

Conservative treatment of pleural infection consists of isolated antibiotic therapy or antibiotic therapy and simple drainage. Pleural effusions that increase in volume or compromise breathing must be drained. Insertion of a thoracostomy tube is preferable to repeated thoracentesis punctures.

Pneumonia with pleural fluid containing pus is termed empyema. Chronic complications include bronchial wall thickening, bronchiectasis, predisposition to asthma, constrictive bronchiolitis, fibrothorax, mediastinal fibrosis, constrictive pericarditis, and pleural thickening. Intrapleural fibrinolytics can be used for complicated parapneumonic effusions (loculated thick fluid) or empyema. Urokinase has been evaluated in pediatric trials. Surgical treatment is considered in patients who are septic from persistent pleural collection despite chest thoracostomy and antibiotic therapy. The surgical options are video-assisted thoracic surgery (VATS), minithoracotomy (similar to VATS but an open procedure), and decortication. Infants and children have a better ability than adults to resolve pleural thickening without detrimental effect on lung growth and function.

BRONCHIOLITIS

Acute bronchiolitis (AB) is a respiratory illness in infants and toddlers caused by viral infection that results in respiratory distress, wheezing, and crackles. The diagnosis is primarily clinical. Most AB cases are mild, self-limited, and symptoms last 3–7 days. Transmission of pathogens is likely for hospitalized patients; hence, selective control measures are needed. RSV is the main pathogen, although other viruses are involved. AB epidemics occur during the fall and winter. High-risk infants (premature, immunocompromised, or those with bronchopulmonary dysplasia or congenital heart disease) may have prolonged disease and higher mortality. More than half of AB patients have recurring episodes of wheezing until 7–11 years of age.

Pathogenesis

Viral infection of the distal bronchiolar epithelial cells leads to cell swelling, mucus production, cellular necrosis, and sloughing. Inflammation produces submucosal and adventitial edema. Goblet cells proliferate and produce excessive mucus that is poorly eliminated by the nonciliated (regenerating) epithelial cells. Plugs of mucus laden with cellular debris cause airway obstruction, hyperinflation, increased airway resistance, atelectasis, and ventilation–perfusion mismatch. Bronchial smooth muscle constriction appears to have little part in the disease course. Infants are particularly at risk because of their small airways, high closing volumes, insufficient collateral ventilation, increased airway smooth muscle reactivity, and absence of immunity against respiratory viruses. The ciliated epithelium takes 13–17 weeks to be restored. The inflammatory response is different from that in asthma and allergies; neutrophils rather than eosinophils predominate.

Specific Pathogens

Respiratory Syncytial Virus

RSV is a single-stranded RNA virus member of the Paramyxoviridae family. RSV may persist for several hours on surfaces, and careful hand-washing forms the main infection control measure. Prior infection generates serum antibodies but only offers partial protection. High maternal antibody levels are associated with lower infection rates in infants. Prophylactic administration of antibodies reduces but does not eliminate severe RSV disease.

Rhinovirus

The rhinovirus, usually associated with the common cold, is the second most common cause of bronchiolitis. The >100 serotypes of rhinovirus are single-stranded RNA and members of the Picornavirus family. Transmission occurs by self-inoculation into nasopharynx or conjunctiva and by aerosol droplets.

Influenza Virus

Influenza infection is usually self-limited but may cause complications (e.g., pneumonia, Reye syndrome, myositis, febrile convulsion, and acute encephalopathy). Hospitalization, increased severity, and complications are more frequent in children <2 years and those with risk factors (asthma, chronic pulmonary disease, severe heart disease, immunocompromise, hemoglobinopathies, and diabetes mellitus).

Human Metapneumovirus

Human Metapneumovirus (hMPV), described in 2001, has probably been infecting humans for 50 years. The clinical syndrome ranges from mild respiratory symptoms to AB and pneumonia. It mostly affects children <2 years of age (usually 3–5 months). Epidemics occur during fall and winter. Due to heterogeneity, multiple reinfections may occur in the same patient, particularly in the aged and immunocompromised.

Coronavirus

Manifestations of coronavirus infection include fever >38°C, dry cough, dyspnea, and hypoxemia are milder in young children than adolescents and adults. Laboratory changes include leukopenia or moderate lymphopenia with liver enzyme elevation. A coronavirus was identified as causing severe acute respiratory syndrome (SARS) in China in 2003. Infants and young children were not a risk group.

Adenovirus

Adenovirus is a DNA virus, has no lipid viral envelope, is highly stable outside of host cells, and stays infectious at room temperature for 2 weeks. It frequently causes acute respiratory infection and conjunctivitis, and may be latent with later relapse. Lower respiratory infections include pneumonia, AB, laryngotracheobronchitis, or pertussis-like cough. Gastrointestinal disease and aseptic meningitis can occur.

Parainfluenza

Every second year, type 1 parainfluenza virus causes an epidemic, with a larger number of croup cases than AB. Type 2 parainfluenza virus epidemic is erratic and comes just after a type 1 epidemic. A type 3 parainfluenza epidemic occurs yearly (spring and summer) and has a prolonged duration in relation to types 1 and 2. Parainfluenza viruses cause a disease similar to RSV with a lower hospitalization rate. Generally, these infections involve upper airways, frequently with acute otitis.

Diagnosis

Laboratory studies are not necessary to diagnose AB when history and physical examination are consistent, but may be useful in high-risk patients or those with severe disease. The indication for bacterial cultures and complete blood count (CBC) in febrile young infants with bronchiolitis has been controversial. Febrile (>38.3°C) infants <3 months old with presumed bronchiolitis can have a urinary tract infection rate of 3.3%, bacteremia rate from 0.2% to 1.4%. Neonates with fever require a full evaluation. Viruses may be detected from nasopharyngeal samples, bronchoalveolar lavage fluid, or lung tissue by direct immunofluorescent antibody staining, enzyme-linked immunosorbent assay (ELISA), PCR, or direct culture. Testing for influenza virus may guide treatment with oseltamivir. Diagnoses that mimic AB include congenital heart disease, gastroesophageal reflux, aspiration pneumonia, *Mycoplasma* pneumonia, other bacterial pneumonias, or foreign-body aspiration.

Supportive Therapy

Adequate monitoring, hydration, and oxygenation are the backbone of AB treatment. No specific therapy improves outcome for critically ill infants with bronchiolitis. Chest physiotherapy does not improve severity of illness, oxygen requirement, or outcome. β-Agonists (e.g., albuterol, salbutamol) do not improve oxygen saturation, reduce hospital admission, or shorten length of stay. Inhaled epinephrine decreases the need for hospital admission, but does not shorten the length of stay. Bronchodilator studies in bronchiolitis suffer from the limitation that it is clinically difficult to distinguish bronchiolitis from acute asthma triggered by a viral infection. Anticholinergics, corticosteroids (inhaled or systemic) and aerosolized recombinant human DNase have not been shown to have added benefit. Current evidence supports a trial of α- or β-adrenergic medication with subsequent discontinuation if a dose does not result in clinical improvement.

Nebulized hypertonic (3%) saline may improve mucociliary clearance of airway secretions by reducing viscosity, breaking ionic bonds within mucus, rehydrating mucus, absorbing water from the mucosa and submucosa, reducing wall edema, inducing sputum production and cough, and inducing cilial mobility by releasing prostaglandin E_2.

Ribavirin inhibits viral structural protein synthesis, reducing viral replication and immunoglobulin (Ig) E response. Problematic issues involve its high cost, logistic issues, possible teratogenicity, and low clinical efficacy. Ribavirin should be reserved for immunosuppressed patients with severe disease who are also under the care of infectious diseases specialists.

In infants with AB and fever, the risk of coexisting bacteremia is lower (0%–3.7%) than in a comparable population of febrile young infants without recognizable viral infection. Antibiotics are administered only if there are specific indications of a coexisting bacterial infection.

Supplementation with exogenous surfactant in infants requiring intensive care and mechanical ventilation has been associated with a shorter duration of mechanical ventilation and PICU length of stay, but evidence is insufficient to provide an estimate of its effectiveness.

Complications

Apnea

Apnea is linked to several different respiratory tract infections in infants exhibiting clinical syndromes analogous to AB. The mechanism of apnea in AB is uncertain, but may resemble that of prematurity and upper airway reflex apnea. There are reports suggesting that RSV has direct effect on CNS. Although bronchiolitis-related apnea usually resolves within 48 hours, recurrent apnea spells may occur. Caffeine may decrease the need for intubation in infants with bronchiolitis and apnea.

Respiratory Failure

High-flow nasal cannula (HFNC) may decrease the need for intubation and length of stay in children with bronchiolitis. Risk factors for respiratory failure include young age (<2 months), low birth weight (<2.26 kg), maternal smoking history, onset of respiratory symptoms <1 day before admission, presence of apnea, severe retractions, room air oxygen saturation <85%, and insufficient oral intake. There is no clear evidence on which ventilation mode to select. CPAP or BiPAP is often used as an alternative before invasive ventilation. Patients with refractory hypoxemia and hypercapnia will require intubation and mechanical ventilation. High-frequency oscillatory ventilation (HFOV) has been successful in infants with bronchiolitis and severe hypoxemia. As with other forms of life-threatening respiratory failures that are refractory to all other interventions, extracorporeal membrane oxygenation may be employed.

Immunoprophylaxis (Palivizumab)

Immunoprophylaxis for RSV has relied on two potential approaches: vaccines (active immunization) and monoclonal antibodies. Efforts to obtain an effective vaccine have been unsuccessful. Passive immunization against RSV uses humanized monoclonal antibodies (palivizumab). Palivizumab is administered intramuscularly to high-risk groups once per month for a maximum of 5 months (during the epidemic months). Among high-risk groups, hospitalization rates due to RSV are reduced by 39%–82%.

CHAPTER 26 ■ ACUTE LUNG INJURY AND ACUTE RESPIRATORY DISTRESS SYNDROME

KATHLEEN M. VENTRE AND JOHN H. ARNOLD

INTRODUCTION AND DEFINITIONS

In 1994, the American-European Consensus Conference defined "adult" or "acute" respiratory distress syndrome (ARDS) as a severe form of acute lung injury (ALI) characterized by acute, noncardiogenic pulmonary edema with bilateral pulmonary infiltrates on chest X-ray and a ratio of Pao_2 to Fio_2 of <200. The term *acute lung injury* was adopted to describe patients with Pao_2/Fio_2 <300 who otherwise meet the criteria for ARDS. Recent data indicate that ARDS occurs in 1%–4% of pediatric intensive care unit (PICU) admissions and 8%–10% of children requiring mechanical ventilation. Historically, mortality for pediatric ARDS has ranged between 20% and 75%, but data from contemporary epidemiologic studies and the control groups of recent multicenter trials indicate that mortality in pediatric ALI/ARDS now ranges between 8% and 36%. Among immunocompromised children with ALI/ARDS, mortality remains as high as 60%.

The ALI/ARDS continuum does not represent a single disease. These terms describe a diverse group of conditions for which the final common pathway involves the acute onset of permeability edema, parenchymal opacification, and marked oxygenation impairment. The ARDS Definition Task Force has proposed a revised definition (**Table 26.1**) that accounts for the effect of ventilator settings, accepts that ALI can coexist with hydrostatic pulmonary edema, and acknowledges that there can be variability in radiograph interpretation. The task force proposed eliminating the term *acute lung injury* in favor of simply classifying the degree of oxygenation impairment in ARDS patients as "mild," "moderate," or "severe."

TABLE 26.1

The Acute Respiratory Distress Syndrome (Berlin Definition)

Time	Onset within 1 wk of a known clinical trigger, or new/worsening respiratory symptoms
Imaging	Bilateral chest opacities not explained by effusion, regional atelectasis, or nodules
Origin	Respiratory failure not fully explained by cardiac failure or fluid overload. Echocardiography used to exclude hydrostatic edema in the absence of specific risk factors.
Oxygenation Impairment	
Mild ARDS	$200 < Pao_2/Fio_2 \leq 300$ with PEEP or CPAP ≥ 5 cm H_2O
Moderate ARDS	$100 < Pao_2/Fio_2 \leq 200$ with PEEP ≥ 5 cm H_2O
Severe ARDS	$Pao_2/Fio_2 \leq 100$ with PEEP ≥ 5 cm H_2O

Adapted from Ranieri VM, Rubenfeld GD, Thompson BT, et al. ARDS Definition Task Force. Acute respiratory distress syndrome: The Berlin Definition. *JAMA* 2012; 307(23):2526–33.

MECHANISM OF DISEASE: CORE PATHOPHYSIOLOGY

ARDS develops following either "direct" or "indirect" lung injury. Pneumonia and pulmonary aspiration, traumatic pulmonary contusion, fat embolism, submersion injury, and inhalational injury are causes of direct lung injury. The most common forms of indirect lung injury include systemic conditions such as sepsis, shock, cardiopulmonary bypass, or blood product transfusion. Direct injury is thought to cause regional consolidation from destruction of the alveolar architecture, while indirect injury is believed to be associated with pulmonary vascular congestion, interstitial edema, and less severe alveolar involvement.

Regardless of its inciting factors, ARDS commonly progresses through stages defined by distinct clinical, radiographic, and histopathologic features. The *exudative phase* is characterized by the acute development of decreased pulmonary compliance and arterial hypoxemia. The chest radiograph reveals diffuse alveolar infiltrates from pulmonary edema. In the *fibroproliferative stage*, increased alveolar dead-space fraction and refractory pulmonary hypertension may develop as a result of chronic inflammation and scarring of the alveolar–capillary unit. During the *recovery phase*, there is restoration of the alveolar epithelial barrier, gradual improvement in pulmonary compliance, resolution of hypoxemia, and eventual return to premorbid pulmonary function.

Edema in ARDS is not caused primarily by cardiac failure but rather by disruption of the structural components that regulate alveolar fluid balance. Normally, attachments between endothelial cells allow movement of fluid, but not proteins or solutes, into the interstitial space. The rate of fluid movement into the interstitium depends on net differences between hydrostatic and osmotic pressures in the pulmonary capillaries relative to the interstitial environment. Interstitial fluid clearance by the pulmonary lymphatic system is disrupted in ARDS by injury to the alveolar epithelium and/or pulmonary capillary endothelium. These events trigger the host immune response, causing neutrophil activation and elaboration of proinflammatory cytokines.

Surfactant is produced by alveolar epithelial type II cells and contains phospholipid and protein components. It promotes alveolar and small airway stability by lowering surface tension. Surfactant's principal protein constituents also facilitate clearance of infectious organisms. Following lung injury, surfactant production declines, and the activity of what remains is impaired due to alterations in phospholipids and inactivation by alveolar exudates. In the nondiseased state, the interaction of surfactant with the elastic properties of the lung and chest wall contributes to *pulmonary hysteresis*, a phenomenon allowing for the maintenance of lung volume at lower transpulmonary pressures during expiration than are required during inspiration. During inspiration, increasing transpulmonary pressure produces little change in lung volume until the patient reaches a lower inflection point on the inspiratory limb of the curve (lower Pflex) (**Fig. 26.1**). At that point, the change in lung volume produced by each upward increment of pressure (i.e., compliance) increases quickly, and then more slowly, until reaching an upper inflection point (upper Pflex) (**Fig. 26.1**) where compliance again decreases. In the injured lung, the entire curve

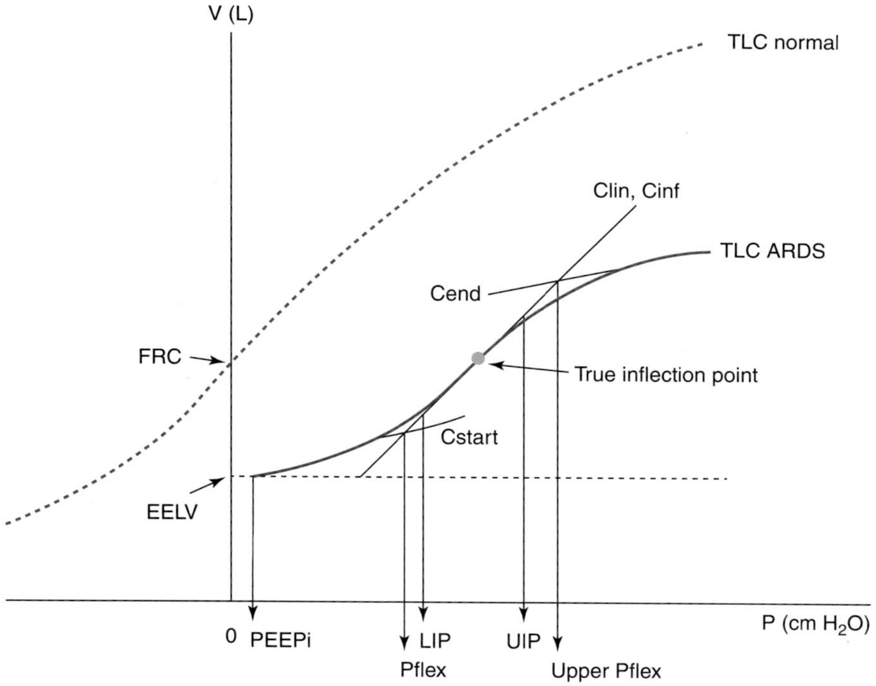

FIGURE 26.1. Volume–pressure curve in absence of disease (*dashed lines*) and in ARDS (*solid line*). Inspiratory curves are shown. Important transitions during lung inflation are indicated on the ARDS curve. Note that in ARDS, total lung capacity (TLC) is reduced, compared to TLC in the normal lung. In this example, a small amount of positive end-expiratory pressure (intrinsic PEEP [PEEPi]) is present at end-expiratory lung volume (EELV) in the ARDS lung. EELV in the ARDS lung is below functional residual capacity (FRC). Compliance is indicated at various points as the slope of the volume–pressure curve. Pflex is indicated on the curve as the intersection of the low-compliance portion of the curve obtained at low lung volume (Cstart). Upper Pflex is indicated at the transition between the nearly linear zone of maximal compliance (Clin) and the zone of low compliance at high lung volume (Cend). The lower inflection point (LIP) and upper inflection point (UIP) are points at which the volume pressure curve begins to depart from Clin at the extremes of lung volume. The "true inflection point" marks the actual change in concavity of the volume–pressure curve. (From Harris RS. Pressure-volume curves of the respiratory system. *Respir Care* 2005;50:78–98, with permission.)

is displaced downward and rightward, reflecting the higher pressures required to achieve and maintain lung recruitment, and a decrease in lung compliance throughout the respiratory cycle.

Mechanisms of Alveolar Fluid Clearance

Clearance of fluid accumulated in the alveolar space is regulated by ion channels in distal airway Clara cells and alveolar epithelial type I and type II cells. Type I cells make up about 95% of the alveolar epithelial lining and are highly permeable to water. Type II cells are responsible for producing pulmonary surfactant and for facilitating transepithelial ion transport. Once sodium enters through channels on the apical surface of type II cells, Na^+/K^+-ATPases located on the basolateral cell membrane actively transport sodium into the interstitial space, creating a gradient for the movement of water across the alveolar epithelium and back into the interstitium (**Fig. 26.2**). ALI undermines alveolar fluid clearance owing to at least two important reasons: epithelial damage compromises the membrane proteins that regulate alveolar fluid balance, and hypoxia inhibits transepithelial sodium transport. The permeability edema that is the defining feature of early ALI/ARDS sets the stage for decreased pulmonary compliance and a reduction in end-expiratory lung volume (EELV) to a level approaching closing volume, leading to regional atelectasis and widespread intrapulmonary shunt.

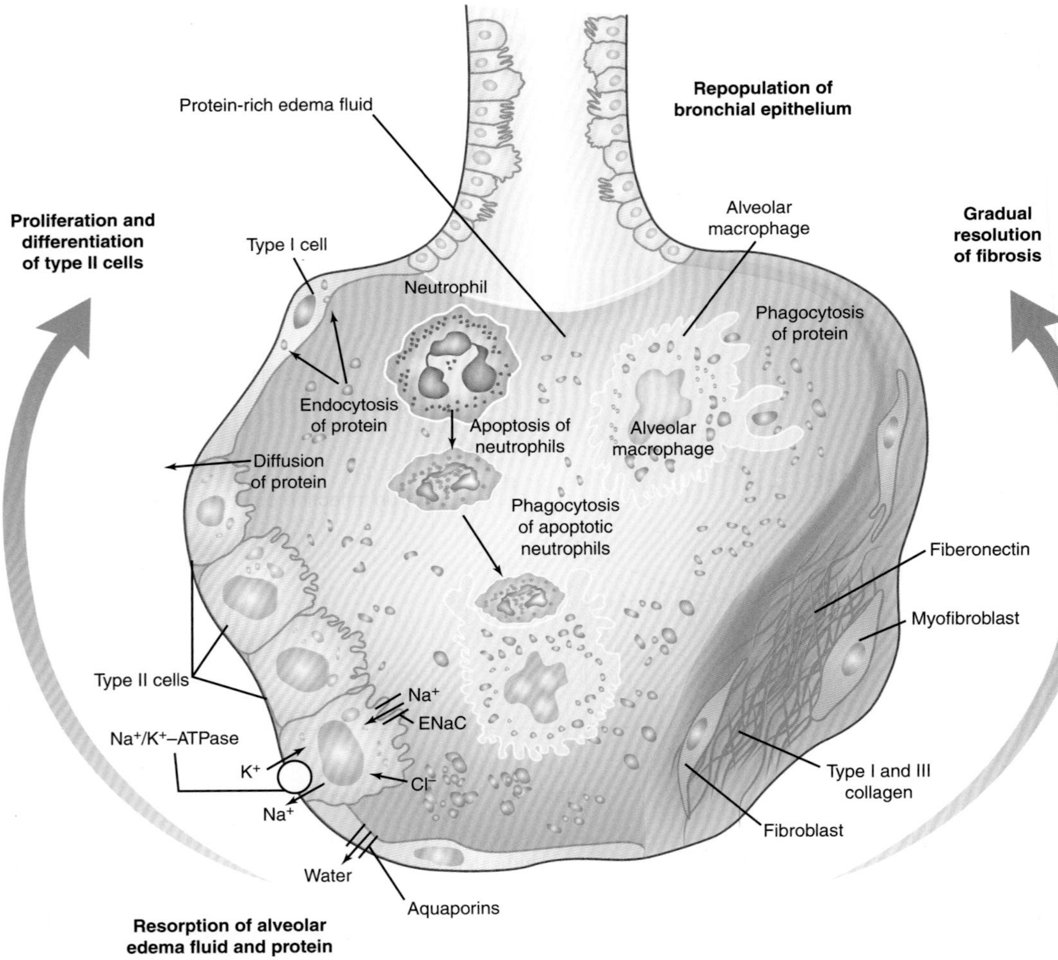

FIGURE 26.2. Cellular mechanisms of ARDS resolution. Repopulation of the alveolar epithelial barrier is shown on the left side of the figure. It is now believed this process may involve endogenous stem cell proliferation (see text). Within the alveolus, neutrophils are undergoing apoptosis and phagocytosis by alveolar macrophages. Structural elements governing fluid transport across the alveolar epithelium are illustrated. (From Ware LB, Matthay MA. The acute respiratory distress syndrome. *N Engl J Med* 2000;342(18):1334–49, with permission.)

Alteration of Gas Exchange in ALI and ARDS

There are many potential sources of hypoxia in ALI and ARDS. Edema in the interstitial compartment or in the alveoli inhibits gas exchange, and blood flowing past compromised or collapsed lung units is poorly oxygenated. Intrapulmonary shunt does not raise systemic $Pa{CO_2}$ because sensitive chemoreceptors stimulate respiratory drive. Intrapulmonary shunt is attenuated by pulmonary vasoconstriction, which redirects blood toward better-ventilated units. The pulmonary vasculature is unique in human physiology in that its smooth muscle *contracts* in response to hypoxia.

The relationship of alveolar ventilation ($\dot{V}$) to perfusion ($\dot{Q}$) is not anatomically fixed. In the upright, nondiseased human lung subjected to gravitational forces, spontaneous breathing creates a decreasing gradient of transpulmonary pressure from apex to base, creating a driving pressure for alveolar filling that is greater in the (nondependent) apex than at the (dependent) base. Dependent alveoli are positioned on a more compliant portion of the volume–pressure curve, compared to more distended nondependent alveoli, a phenomenon harmonizing with the fact that blood flow in the upright lung is greater in dependent regions than in nondependent regions. However, it is important to recognize that local variability in pulmonary blood flow distribution is not completely explained by gravity and is likely dictated to a large degree by the pulmonary vascular architecture. Large animal experimental models have demonstrated that in the supine position, pulmonary blood flow tends to be distributed preferentially to the dorsal (dependent) region, although marked heterogeneity of perfusion exists. In the prone position, pulmonary blood flow remains preferentially distributed to the dorsal (now nondependent) region.

"Physiologic shunt" fraction comprises about 10% of cardiac output and arises from baseline $\dot{V}/\dot{Q}$ inequality as well as blood from the bronchial, pleural, and thebesian veins, which returns to the systemic circulation without passing through the pulmonary vascular bed. In ARDS, fluid-filled alveoli act as low $\dot{V}/\dot{Q}$ lung units. Alveolar overdistension in other areas creates dead space. Distension from positive-pressure ventilation displaces local pulmonary blood flow, creating even more $\dot{V}/\dot{Q}$ inequality. Studies suggest that intrapulmonary shunt is the dominant cause of arterial hypoxemia in ARDS.

Host Immune Response: Role of Cytokines and Alteration of Hemostasis

Exposure to one or more inciting factors produces a swift and robust response from the host's innate immune system that upsets the precarious balances between proinflammation and anti-inflammation, and procoagulation and anticoagulation. Release of reactive oxygen species potentiates additional damage to alveolar epithelial cells, leading to their dysfunction and apoptosis. Products of cellular injury then serve to perpetuate the cycle of tissue injury by renewing the inflammatory response. TNF-α and IL-6 act in a complementary fashion on hemostasis, by either promoting coagulation or impairing fibrinolysis. Whether the individual patient with ARDS expresses a predominantly procoagulant or anticoagulant phenotype seems likely to be a function of the interaction between host genetics and the specific inciting factors that lead to disease.

Alteration of Cardiovascular Function: Effects on Pulmonary Hemodynamics

Lung injury has the potential to increase pulmonary vascular resistance (PVR), adding to right ventricular afterload and potentially compromising cardiac output. PVR is minimal (or "optimal") at the lung volume that corresponds to FRC. If EELV approaches total lung capacity or decreases toward residual volume, PVR increases exponentially. In addition, collapse of small airways as lung compliance falls results in alveolar hypoxia and reflex pulmonary vasoconstriction. Collectively, the effects of lung volume on PVR produce a parabolic curve whose nadir occurs at FRC (**Fig. 26.3**). Increases in right ventricular afterload can reduce systemic cardiac output, as increased end-diastolic volume in the highly compliant right ventricle (RV) shifts the interventricular septum toward the left, resulting in poor LV filling.

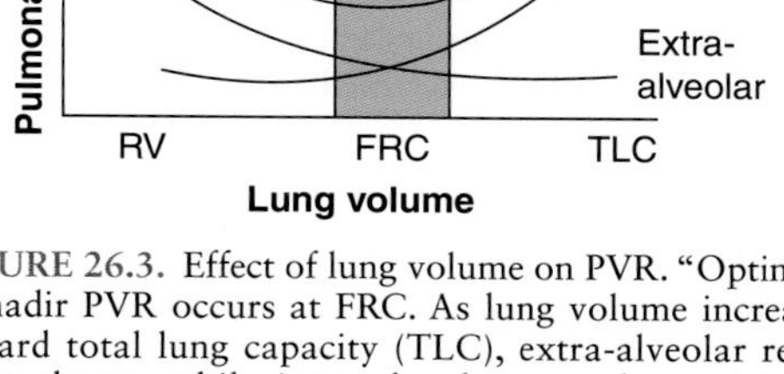

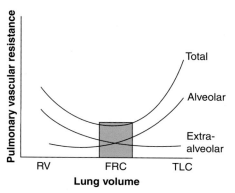

FIGURE 26.3. Effect of lung volume on PVR. "Optimal" or nadir PVR occurs at FRC. As lung volume increases toward total lung capacity (TLC), extra-alveolar resistance drops, while intra-alveolar vascular resistance escalates. As lung volume drops toward residual volume (RV), extra-alveolar vascular resistance increases as these vessels become tortuous, while alveolar hypoxia results in intra-alveolar vasoconstriction. The "total" or net effect of these findings on overall PVR is represented by the uppermost curve. (From Shekerdemian L, Bohn D. Cardiovascular effects of mechanical ventilation. *Arch Dis Child* 1999;80(5):475–80.)

CLINICAL PRESENTATION

Leakage of proteinaceous fluid into the alveolar spaces and regional atelectasis leads to rapidly worsening hypoxia and labored breathing from the transpulmonary pressures needed to maintain alveolar patency. Hypocarbia occurs early, when the patient first manifests tachypnea. The $PaCO_2$ subsequently rises as respiratory muscle fatigue ensues. The patient often presents râles over atelectasis-prone or congested lung units, decreased air entry over areas of consolidation, and wheezes over areas where small airways closure is occurring.

Imaging Studies

Among patients with ALI/ARDS, early findings on chest radiograph often include diffuse alveolar infiltrates, air bronchograms, effusions and atelectasis. Lung injury evolving into fibrosis appears as prominent reticular opacities. Computed tomography (CT) reveals that lung consolidation occurs along the gravitational axis. In later stages of the disease, fibrosis begins to be identifiable in nondependent areas. This pattern develops in lung areas subject to repetitive cycles of expansion and collapse.

PRINCIPLES OF CLINICAL MANAGEMENT

The mainstay of ALI/ARDS management remains supportive care, of which positive-pressure ventilation plays a critical role as both a necessary therapeutic strategy and as a potential trigger for further lung injury (**Table 26.2**). Positive-pressure ventilation is typically required to stabilize consolidated or

TABLE 26.2

Suggested Therapy Guidelines for ALI/ARDS

	■ PULMONARY	■ CARDIOVASCULAR	■ OTHER
Resuscitation	Supplemental O_2 Early arterial access for disease identification (PaO_2/FIO_2, OI) and early implementation of therapy Consider early NPPV for alveolar recruitment in alert, cooperative patient Endotracheal intubation and positive-pressure ventilation for respiratory failure failing noninvasive therapy Titrate PEEP to achieve $FIO_2 \leq$ 0.5–0.6/SpO_2 88%–95% Limit tidal volume (6 cc/kg *ideal* body weight) and alveolar plateau pressure (≤30 cm H_20)[a] Permissive hypercapnia unless contraindicated (e.g., coexisting increased intracranial pressure)	Crystalloid, colloid, or blood to optimize intravascular volume and support hemodynamics[b] Anticipate potentially adverse hemodynamic consequences of transition to positive-pressure ventilation in setting of intravascular volume depletion Titrate supportive therapy to correct perfusion abnormalities and optimize urine output	Cultures Broad-spectrum antimicrobial agents Consider antifungal, antiviral, atypical agent coverage in immunocompromised population Consider early bronchoalveolar lavage in immunocompromised population
Escalation	Titrate PEEP upward if ongoing hypoxemia in setting of alveolar derecruitment Early transition to HFOV if high inflation pressures are necessary Consider prone positioning in selected cases Short-term administration of neuromuscular blocking agents to facilitate mechanical ventilation may benefit patients with severe disease	Titrate fluid and vasoactive infusions to achieve age-appropriate blood pressure parameters and adequate end-organ function	Sedation/analgesia Neuromuscular blockade if necessary

TABLE 26.2

Suggested Therapy Guidelines for ALI/ARDS (*continued*)

	■ PULMONARY	■ CARDIOVASCULAR	■ OTHER
Maintenance	Follow OI to track response to therapy Wean ventilator as allowable	Monitoring: CVP, serial clinical examination, and review of organ function[c] Maintain euvolemia Diuretics	Nutrition: Implement enteral nutrition early. Avoid excess glucose administration. Careful attention to nitrogen balance Neuromuscular blockade: Interrupt infusion daily and discontinue as soon as feasible Sedation and analgesia: Interrupt infusion daily and wean during plateau phase of illness
Advanced therapy	OI not improving on optimal ventilator strategy/HFOV: Consider ECMO	Consider early RRT for persistent hypervolemia and oliguria despite diuretics	

[a]Optimal tidal volume and plateau pressure are not known, but high tidal volumes are associated with proinflammatory cytokine release. The use of 6 cc/kg has been associated with a 22% relative mortality benefit compared to 12 cc/kg.
[b]Optimal hemoglobin concentration is not known. In physiologically stable critically ill children, hemoglobin of 7 g/dL is probably adequate and may avert adverse effects of red cell transfusion.
[c]Pulmonary artery catheter use in ALI/ARDS is not associated with improved outcomes and may be associated with increased incidence of catheter-related complications. CVP must be interpreted in the context of surrounding compartment pressure (e.g., intrathoracic pressure for SVC lines) and/or myocardial compliance. In absence of coexisting intracardiac shunt, mixed venous oxygen saturation may clarify adequacy of cardiac output.
OI, oxygenation index [100 × mean airway pressure × FiO_2]/PaO_2; NPPV, noninvasive positive-pressure ventilation; PEEP, positive end-expiratory pressure; HFOV, high-frequency oscillatory ventilation; CVP, central venous pressure; ECMO, extracorporeal membrane oxygenation. RRT, renal replacement therapy.
Adapted from Fackler JC, Arnold JH, Nichols DG, et al. Acute respiratory distress syndrome. In: Rogers M, ed. *Textbook of Pediatric Intensive Care*. 3rd ed. Baltimore, MD: Williams and Wilkins, 1996:197–233.

collapsed alveoli to provide oxygenation without the use of high FiO_2. While the salutary effects of PEEP have been well established, PEEP can add to anatomical dead space by distending large airways and increasing alveolar dead space.

Although positive-pressure ventilation is required to restore lung volume toward FRC and achieve adequate gas exchange, it increases right atrial pressure, which decreases systemic venous return and right ventricular stroke volume. However, positive-pressure ventilation can enhance LV function because of favorable effects on LV afterload. Although cardiac filling can be affected by intravascular volume loading and the use of vasoactive infusions, the effects of positive-pressure ventilation on cardiac output have much to do with the relationship between alveolar volume and pulmonary blood flow. Titrating positive pressure (or PEEP) in a way that achieves alveolar recruitment, avoids alveolar overdistension, and optimizes the relationship of ventilation to perfusion will provide adequate gas exchange while limiting excess lung injury and adverse cardiovascular effects.

In heterogeneous conditions such as ARDS, it is difficult to know what level of PEEP will open enough alveoli to produce adequate oxygenation without creating conditions for ongoing stress-induced lung injury. Recognizing the prudence of limiting a patient's exposure to high concentrations of supplementary oxygen and high transpulmonary pressures, a logical strategy suggests stepwise escalation of PEEP in 3–5 cm H_2O increments, until arriving at the minimum PEEP that allows for a PaO_2 in the range of 55–80 mm Hg, with peripheral oxygen saturation (SpO_2) of 88%–95%, using an FiO_2 of $\leq$0.5–0.6.

Limiting phasic changes in lung volume and preventing alveolar overdistension at end-inspiration may reduce the risk of ventilator-associated lung injury. When the lung is heterogeneously inflated, some lung units remain collapsed throughout the respiratory cycle. This shifts stress and strain forces onto adjacent, more compliant lung units, making them vulnerable to structural deformations that are capable of provoking an inflammatory response. A landmark multicenter trial has shown that limiting tidal volumes to 6 cc/kg ideal body weight versus 12 cc/kg ideal body weight results in a significant mortality reduction among adults with ARDS. Subsequent trials examining the effects of applied PEEP and recruitment maneuvers have not demonstrated mortality benefit.

The use of high-frequency oscillatory ventilation (HFOV) as a supportive care strategy for patients with ALI/ARDS has intuitive appeal for potentially mitigating the risk of excess lung injury. Theoretically, HFOV provides the ultimate "open-lung" strategy by preserving EELV, minimizing cyclic stretch, and avoiding parenchymal overdistension at end-inspiration. One randomized controlled crossover trial has evaluated the effect of HFOV versus conventional ventilation in children with diffuse alveolar disease and/or airleak. While there was no difference in survival or duration of mechanical ventilation between children receiving HFOV versus conventional ventilation, fewer children randomized to HFOV remained dependent on supplemental oxygen at 30 days. Both pediatric and neonatal trials suggest that HFOV may be more successful if employed early in the course of disease. In a recent adult trial on the early use of HFOV versus conventional ventilation in adults with ARDS, the HFOV group had a higher in-hospital mortality rate. It is not clear whether this finding is related to the population studied, the HFOV strategy employed, or to the HFOV device itself. The generalizability of these data to the pediatric population is problematic and more data are needed to assess the efficacy of early HFOV use in children.

Fluid Management

Lower intravascular and cardiac filling pressures may limit extravascular lung water accumulation without impairing tissue oxygenation, yet lung-protective strategies using high levels of PEEP may lead to a need for intravascular volume supplementation to optimize $\dot{V}/\dot{Q}$ relations and improve cardiac output. An adult trial of conservative versus liberal administration of IV fluids in adult ARDS patients past their initial resuscitation phase showed mortality was similar between groups but the conservative strategy was associated with an improvement in oxygenation index and in ventilator-free days.

Adjuvant Therapies in ALI and ARDS

Prone Positioning

The physiologic rationale for prone positioning in ARDS patients is premised on the accompanying reduction in chest wall compliance, which allows for more efficient transmission of airway pressure to the alveoli. Theoretically this would result in a stabilization of alveolar volume and a more even distribution of stress and strain forces over a larger portion of previously nonaerated lung units. Multiple adult studies of prone positioning have shown an oxygenation benefit but no change in mortality, with one recent trial showing a dramatic mortality benefit in adult patients with severe ARDS. Taken together, the existing data do not support routine use of prone positioning for infants and young children with ALI/ARDS, but clinicians may choose to use it in individual patients with specific pathophysiologic features suggesting that their gas exchange efficiency may improve as a result.

Surfactant

Whether by aerosol or intratracheal instillation, surfactant administration has repeatedly been approached as an adjuvant therapy for ALI/ARDS. While no trial has demonstrated a survival benefit, post hoc analyses have suggested potential benefit in patients with direct lung injury. This observation was further evaluated in a pediatric trial that included immunocompromised patients. Importantly, the risk-adjusted analysis that accounted for the asymmetric randomization of immunocompromised patients eliminated the statistically significant mortality benefit attributed to surfactant administration. In general, outcome benefits associated with the use of surfactant have not come close to those reported in association with its use in surfactant-deficient neonates. Interpretation of the surfactant literature is complicated by the fact that the specific surfactant preparation, the dosing regimen, and the mechanical ventilation strategy vary across studies, and each of these factors can modify patient outcomes. Although the data have yet to identify a clear indication for the use of surfactant in ALI/ARDS, arriving at the "ideal" surfactant dose and composition, as well as the timing of its administration, will ultimately depend on understanding its interaction with the chosen mechanical ventilation strategy.

Corticosteroids

Corticosteroids are intuitively appealing as an adjunct therapy for ARDS but few data support their widespread use. Short courses of high-dose corticosteroids administered early in ARDS have not demonstrated an outcome benefit. A single study of methylprednisolone administration in 24 patients with persistent ARDS reported a decrease in mortality when the drug was initiated after 7 days. A multicenter, randomized controlled trial published 8 years later found no mortality benefit associated with the use of methylprednisolone as compared to placebo in 180 patients with persistent ARDS.

Inhaled Nitric Oxide

Nitric oxide (NO) mediates vasodilation through smooth muscle relaxation and also plays a role in modifying immune function and platelet aggregation. NO avidly binds hemoglobin, a phenomenon that leads to its rapid inactivation. Its short half-life enables NO to be a selective pulmonary vasodilator when administered by inhalation. It has been difficult to demonstrate a benefit in outcome from iNO in ARDS. The use of iNO in ARDS is associated with early, nonsustained increases in PaO_2 and decreases in oxygenation index that do not translate to a difference in mortality or ventilator-free days. Routine administration of iNO to nonseptic patients with

ALI/ARDS is not supported by existing data, but individuals suspected of having particularly reactive pulmonary vasculature may potentially benefit from this therapy.

Modifying Alveolar Fluid Clearance

Preclinical investigations suggest that β-agonists may affect alveolar ion and fluid transport and may inhibit proinflammatory cytokine release, coagulation, and neutrophil activation. A follow-up phase II trial demonstrated a reduction in extravascular lung water with treatment, but subsequent randomized trials involving adult ALI/ARDS patients showed no outcome improvement and one was stopped for higher mortality in those treated with IV β-agonists.

Nutritional Support in ALI and ARDS

Enteral, rather than parenteral, nutrition may preserve functional integrity of the gastrointestinal mucosal barrier and decrease intestinal bacterial translocation. Substantial practice variation exists regarding timing, volume, and composition of enteral feeding. One trial of trophic feedings versus full enteral feedings did not show a difference in outcome.

Fatty acid metabolism may be an important mediator of the inflammatory cascade. Administration of arachidonic acid precursors to patients with ALI and ARDS seems to increase thromboxane A_2 production, while inhibiting cyclooxygenase activity seems to improve gas exchange, relieve vasoconstriction, and decrease airways resistance. Experience with providing alternative ratios of fatty acids in an attempt to repopulate host cell membranes has demonstrated that feedings enriched with "omega-3" fatty acids, such as EPA and DHA, decrease proinflammatory cytokine concentrations in animal models. Such dietary manipulations result in favorable short-term improvements in relevant physiologic parameters, but a larger randomized trial ended early because of worsened outcomes (ventilator-free days) in the intervention group.

Extracorporeal Membrane Oxygenation

Current registry data indicate that overall survival for children who require extracorporeal membrane oxygenation (ECMO) for nonneonatal respiratory failure is 57%. An increasing proportion of children who receive ECMO for acute respiratory failure also have extrapulmonary organ failures, which reduces their prospects for survival. The best outcomes with ECMO can be expected from patients with reversible lung injury who fail conventional therapy before they develop nonpulmonary organ failures. Early recognition of the patient with hypoxic respiratory failure who is destined to fail even the most strategic mode of mechanical ventilation is difficult. The trend in oxygenation index is used to assess a response to mechanical ventilation and may assist in identifying patients who may benefit from ECMO.

OUTCOMES IN PEDIATRIC ALI AND ARDS

Mortality in pediatric ALI and ARDS seems to be decreasing from a high of 50%–75% 15–20 years ago to <10% more recently. Outcomes are improving, even for immunocompromised children. It is not clear whether lung-protective ventilation or supportive care advances are responsible for this encouraging trend. Among ARDS patients, death most often occurs in association with multiorgan dysfunction.

CHAPTER 27 ■ CHRONIC RESPIRATORY FAILURE

THOMAS G. KEENS, SHEILA S. KUN, AND SALLY L. DAVIDSON WARD

Neurologic control of breathing must ensure adequate ventilation to meet metabolic needs. Ventilation becomes less adequate during sleep. It is less responsive to modulation by chemoreceptor input during rapid eye movement (REM) or active sleep. Immaturity of the respiratory control systems in infants and young children predisposes them to apnea and hypoventilation. Inadequate gas exchange during sleep is part of chronic respiratory failure (CRF). The factors that predispose to ventilatory muscle fatigue include hypoxia, hypercapnia, acidosis, malnutrition, hyperinflation, changes in pulmonary mechanics that increase work of breathing, and disuse. The infant diaphragm has significantly less fatigue-resistant muscle fibers and is weaker than in older children and adults.

ACUTE RESPIRATORY FAILURE

Acute respiratory failure is most commonly seen in children who experience an abrupt onset of a severe respiratory disorder, such as severe pneumonia or acute respiratory distress syndrome (ARDS). The increase in respiratory load exceeds the ability to work at that level. Ventilatory muscle fatigue results in hypoxia, hypercapnia, and acidosis. In adults, this limit for diaphragmatic work is ~40% of maximal diaphragm strength and 60%–70% of combined inspiratory muscle strength. If the work of breathing associated with a respiratory illness remains below the fatigue threshold, the child continues to breathe spontaneously and acute respiratory failure may not occur.

CHRONIC RESPIRATORY FAILURE

CRF implies that a persistent, perhaps irreversible, disorder is causing inadequate ventilation or oxygenation. The diagnosis is often made when a patient is unable to wean from assisted ventilation for 1 month without superimposed acute respiratory disease. CRF is also diagnosed when there is no prospect of being weaned from the ventilator, such as high spinal cord injury.

Reduce the Respiratory Load

Reducing the respiratory load involves optimizing pulmonary mechanics. Infection is vigorously treated. Aggressive chest physiotherapy, inhaled bronchodilators, and anti-inflammatory agents reduce atelectasis and airway resistance by enhancing mucociliary activity and clearing secretions.

Increase Ventilatory Muscle Power

Hypoxia, hypercapnia, and acidosis decrease muscle energy production and predispose the muscle to fatigue. Malnutrition decreases oxidative energy-producing enzymes in muscle. Hyperinflation places the diaphragm at a mechanical disadvantage so that the same muscle tension develops less pressure. Infants have decreased strength and endurance of the ventilatory muscles. Prolonged assisted ventilation causes muscle change from disuse. Pharmacologic neuromuscular blockade, sedation, and pain medications decrease respiratory muscle function and should be weaned as tolerated. Weaning from the ventilator should be designed to improve ventilatory muscle power to raise the fatigue threshold (an approach similar to athletic training of skeletal muscles). "Sprint weaning" is analogous to this form of athletic training, and produces ventilatory muscle training. In children with prolonged respiratory failure (not yet met the definition of CRF), sprint weaning, or sprinting, is instituted in the following way. The ventilator is set to meet the child's ventilatory demands by the use of an appropriate rate for age and normal gas exchange by noninvasive monitoring ($Spo_2 \geq 95\%$ and end-tidal Pco_2 [$ETCO_2$] of 30–40 torr). The goal is to provide total ventilatory muscle rest. The patient is then removed from the ventilator for short periods of time during wakefulness, two to four times per day. In some cases, these initial sprints last only 1–2 minutes. The child is carefully monitored during sprints to detect hypoxia or hypercapnia. Increased supplemental oxygen may be required during sprinting. If the child develops signs of distress such as tachypnea, retractions, diaphoresis, tachycardia, hypoxia, or hypercapnia, the sprint should be stopped. The length of each sprint is increased daily as tolerated.

Usually a child is weaned off the ventilator completely during wakefulness, before attempting to reduce sleeping ventilatory support.

Improve Central Respiratory Drive

Chronic metabolic alkalosis decreases central respiratory drive. Thus, electrolyte balance should maintain serum chloride concentrations >95 mEq/dL and avoid alkalosis. Chronic hypoxia or hypercapnia may cause habituation of chemoreceptors, leading to a decrease in respiratory center stimulation, and decreased central respiratory drive.

This approach to reduce load, increase power, and improve drive in children with prolonged respiratory failure may result in successful weaning from assisted ventilation (**Table 27.1**). When children remain ventilator dependent for at least 1 month despite use of the above techniques, the cause of respiratory failure may be irreversible, or weaning from assisted ventilation may take months to years, the diagnosis of "CRF" is made, and chronic ventilatory support will be required.

DECISION TO INITIATE CHRONIC VENTILATORY SUPPORT

Increasingly, the decision to initiate chronic ventilatory support is being made electively to preserve physiologic function and improve the quality of life. Families need to be informed that home mechanical ventilation (HMV) does not guarantee survival. Children receiving HMV via tracheostomy face a 20% mortality rate in the first 5 years after discharge home.

CANDIDATES FOR HOME MECHANICAL VENTILATION

Children with CRF and relatively stable ventilator settings are candidates for HMV. Generally, the FIO_2 should be <40% and the peak inspiratory pressure (PIP) should be <40 cm H_2O. Children with CRF fall into three diagnostic categories: ventilatory muscle weakness and neuromuscular diseases, central

TABLE 27.1

Approaches to Weaning Children with Prolonged Respiratory Failure

Reduce the Respiratory Load	
Relieve bronchospasm	Aerosolized bronchodilator Aerosolized corticosteroids or other anti-inflammatory agents
Remove excessive pulmonary secretions	Chest physiotherapy If ventilatory muscle weakness, cough assist device
Reduce lung fluid and pulmonary edema	Diuretics with careful attention to electrolyte balance
Treat pulmonary infections	Antibiotics Consider aerosolized antibiotics for chronically colonized patients
Increase Ventilatory Muscle Power	
Increase ventilatory muscle strength	Eliminate or reduce hyperinflation
Increase ventilatory muscle endurance	Adequate oxygenation Avoid hypercapnia Avoid acidosis Optimize nutrition Reduce respiratory load (as above)
Train ventilatory muscles to improve strength and endurance	Sprint weaning
Improve Central Respiratory Drive	
Avoid hypochloremic alkalosis	Maintain serum $[Cl^-] \geq 95$ mEq/dL Avoid alkalosis
Reset chemoreceptors	Ventilate to adequate oxygenation ($Spo_2 \geq 95\%$) and ventilation ($ETCO_2 \leq 40$ torr)
Avoid respiratory depression	Reduce or avoid central nervous system–depressant medications

hypoventilation syndromes, and chronic pulmonary disease.

Ventilatory Muscle Weakness and Neuromuscular Diseases

Ventilatory muscle weakness has important physiologic consequences. Inspiratory muscle weakness prevents deep inspiration and results in atelectasis. Expiratory muscle weakness prevents effective coughing and results in decreased removal of pulmonary secretions and foreign material from the lungs. All of these increase the incidence and severity of pneumonia, which is the leading cause of morbidity and mortality in children with neuromuscular disease. Frequent or severe pneumonia is an indication of significant ventilatory muscle weakness, and should prompt investigation of the adequacy of spontaneous ventilation, especially during sleep.

Both progressive and nonprogressive ventilatory muscle weakness are seen in neuromuscular disease. In progressive neuromuscular disease (e.g., spinal muscular atrophy and Duchene muscular dystrophy), muscle weakness worsens with time and eventually results in the CRF. In nonprogressive neuromuscular diseases (e.g., congenital myopathy), muscle weakness does not progress but muscle strength does not increase to meet functional demands of somatic growth. Many children with static neuromuscular disorders become nonambulatory and ventilator dependent in association with the pubertal growth spurt. The development of neuromuscular scoliosis also contributes to respiratory failure.

Children with chronically hypercarbia ($Pco_2 >$ 55–60 torr) due to ventilatory muscle weakness can develop progressive pulmonary hypertension. While oxygen administration relieves their hypoxia, it is inadequate, and hypoventilation results in atelectasis, recurrent respiratory infections, and pulmonary hypertension. These children go on to require HMV.

Central Hypoventilation Syndromes

An inadequate central respiratory drive (congenital or acquired) is the cause of CRF in children with central hypoventilation syndrome. The congenital form may be idiopathic (congenital central hypoventilation syndrome [CCHS] or Ondine's curse) or due to an identifiable brainstem lesion (Chiari malformation type II in myelomeningocele). Causes of acquired central hypoventilation syndrome include brainstem trauma, tumor, hemorrhage, stroke, or infection. In children with respiratory control disorders, it is difficult to augment central respiratory drive. It can be further inhibited by metabolic imbalance, and so serum chloride concentrations should be maintained at >95 mmol/L, and alkalosis avoided. Sedatives and central nervous system depressants should be avoided. Children with respiratory control disorders are good candidates for chronic HMV. Typically, their lungs and ventilatory muscles are normal and reasonable ventilator settings achieve adequate gas exchange.

Chronic Pulmonary Disease

Chronic pulmonary disease may increase the work of breathing beyond a sustainable level. There is no consensus on the Pco_2 level at which a child with chronic lung disease progresses to CRF and requires chronic ventilatory support. Children with Pco_2 consistently ≥60 torr may have a better clinical outcome if chronic ventilatory support is used to keep Pco_2 ≤ 45–50 torr. If damaging ventilator settings are required, rather than risk of ventilator-induced lung injury, a higher level of Pco_2 is accepted. Many of the children requiring HMV because of chronic lung disease are able to wean from chronic ventilatory support with time.

PHILOSOPHY OF CHRONIC VENTILATORY SUPPORT

For most children on HMV, weaning is not realistic in the short term. Ventilators are adjusted to completely meet their ventilatory demands, leaving much of their energy available for other activities. For children without lung disease, ventilators are adjusted to provide an $ETCO_2$ of 30–35 torr and Spo_2 ≥ 95%. Children who can spontaneously ventilate when awake do better if ventilated to a $Pco_2 \leq 35$ torr during sleep. Optimal ventilation also avoids atelectasis and the development of lung disease. Even if a child cannot be completely weaned from assisted ventilation, nocturnal ventilation preserves quality of life when awake and allows the ventilatory muscles to recover during the time when the patient is at highest risk for hypoventilation. Weaning of daytime-assisted ventilation is best accomplished by sprint weaning.

MODALITIES OF HOME MECHANICAL VENTILATION

Portable Positive-Pressure Ventilator via Tracheostomy

Portable positive-pressure ventilation (PPV) via tracheostomy is the most common method of providing assisted ventilation at home. Small, uncuffed tracheostomy tubes are preferred for HMV. The work of breathing to overcome the increased resistance is performed by the ventilator, not the child. The rationale for the small uncuffed tube is to (a) minimize the risk of tracheomalacia and tracheal injury, (b) allow an expiratory leak for speech, and (c) increase safety by allowing ventilation around the tracheostomy tube.

Pressure ventilation is preferred for infants and smaller children as the tracheostomy leak can be large and variable and is unlikely to be compensated for by a volume setting. A backup ventilator is required if ventilatory support is required ≥20 h/day or there is a long distance from emergency service in the event of malfunction.

Tracheostomy

A tracheostomy is performed when CRF is established. The most common complication for a tracheostomy is mucous plugging. When in doubt, caregivers should suction and then change the entire tracheostomy tube if there is any concern. The weight of ventilator tubing pulling on the tracheostomy can cause erosion, laceration of the skin, and an exacerbation of granulation tissue. Bleeding from suctioning is another common problem that may lead to life-threatening bleeding in extreme situations. Granulation tissue forms from persistent irritation from suctioning and can obstruct the airway, compromising ventilation. Granulation tissue formation is an indication for bronchoscopy and possible laser removal. Tracheitis is also a common complaint. When systemic signs and symptoms of infection are not present, inhaled antibiotics are helpful to reduce upper respiratory infection and prevent pneumonia. If a tracheostomy tube is accidentally dislodged, an immediate replacement is recommended to ensure adequate ventilation and airway access. Tracheostomy stomas can constrict and close in a very short time. A spare tracheostomy tube is necessary as a backup at all times.

Some children may need cuffed tubes to decrease the leak and allow better ventilation during sleep, when upper airway resistance decreases. Cuffed tubes, which are inflated during sleep, can almost always be deflated during wakefulness, permitting speech. Auto-cycling is a sign that the leak has increased to the extent that the ventilator can no longer compensate by increasing flow to deliver the desired inspiratory pressure.

Ventilator Circuits

A circuit delivers humidified air from a positive-pressure ventilator to the patient. The desired temperature is 26°C–29°C (80°F–85°F). Dead space between the tracheostomy and exhalation valve should be minimized, to avoid hypercarbia. Two to three circuits should be available for home care. Circuits are changed each day.

Monitoring and Alarm Systems

Positive-pressure ventilators have a low-pressure alarm, which sounds when a minimally acceptable pressure level is not achieved. These alarms detect a sudden disconnect of the ventilator from the tracheostomy or large leaks in the circuit. They are usually set to alarm if the maximal airway pressure on a breath is 10 cm H_2O less than the desired PIP. High-pressure alarms sound if the pressure used to deliver a breath is too high. They are very useful to detect a plug or occlusion of the tracheostomy tube. The pulse oximeter alarm should be used at all times during sleep and when a ventilator-dependent patient is not being observed. Sophisticated home ventilators have low- and high-minute ventilation alarms. The low-minute ventilation alarm sounds for airway occlusion and the high-minute ventilation alarm sounds for a disconnection.

Noninvasive Positive-Pressure Ventilation by Mask or Nasal Prongs

Noninvasive intermittent positive-pressure ventilation (NIPPV) is delivered via a nasal mask, nasal prongs, or face mask using a noninvasive positive-pressure ventilator. It is most frequently used in children with neuromuscular disorders and central hypoventilation syndromes. NIPPV has also been used for children with chronic lung disease who require ventilatory muscle rest. Inspiratory positive airway pressure (I-PAP) and expiratory positive airway pressure (E-PAP) can be adjusted independently. When NIPPV ventilators are used for ventilatory assistance rather than for obstructive sleep apnea, a large I-PAP to E-PAP difference is desirable. Tidal volume increases linearly, with I-PAP to E-PAP difference up to ~14 cm H_2O. The lowest E-PAP that can be used without CO_2 accumulation at the interface is 4 cm H_2O. The highest I-PAP that can be used is usually 24 cm H_2O, but some NIPPV ventilators can go to an I-PAP of 30 cm H_2O. For infants with neuromuscular diseases, one can start with an I-PAP of ~15 cm H_2O, and increase as required. Humidification and supplemental oxygen can be added to the circuit, though they are not always necessary.

Four modes of NIPPV can be used: (a) continuous positive airway pressure, (b) spontaneous mode—only assists spontaneously generated breaths, (c) timed mode—controls ventilation at a set rate, and (d) spontaneous/timed mode—assists generated breaths when the patient breathes at least the backup rate and adds control breaths if the patient does not breathe the minimum backup rate. Only the timed mode guarantees breath delivery and should be used in children with respiratory control disorders. It is important to set the rate to at least that which is physiologic for the patient's age. Because of the risk of aspiration, children who are unable to remove their own masks should not have full-face masks unless they are closely observed.

Negative-Pressure Ventilation

Negative-pressure ventilators (NPVs) apply a negative pressure outside the chest and abdomen to generate inspiration. A chest NPV uses a shell over the anterior chest and abdomen. The negative-pressure wrap ventilator is a "jump suit" that fits snugly around the neck, wrists, and ankles to minimize leaks. A portable tank is a negative-pressure ventilator into which the child's torso is placed, with the head outside. These ventilators can provide effective ventilation in children and adolescents, sometimes without a tracheostomy. In order for negative-pressure shell ventilators to provide adequate ventilation, the shell must be closely fitted to the chest to avoid large leaks. Negative-pressure wrap ventilators or portable tanks need not exactly conform to the chest. They are better suited for children who are small, have scoliosis, or have chest wall deformities. The effectiveness of negative-pressure ventilation depends on the ability to move the chest wall. Children with marked restrictive disease from scoliosis or chest wall deformities are not good candidates for NPV. NPVs can be used to enhance airway clearance by high-frequency chest oscillation and compression, to simulate a cough.

Diaphragm Pacing

Diaphragm pacing uses the child's diaphragm as the respiratory pump. A phrenic nerve electrode is implanted thoracoscopically, and connected by a lead wire to a receiver in a subcutaneous pocket in the abdomen. The electrical stimulation of the phrenic nerve causes a diaphragmatic contraction, which generates the breath. The amount of electrical voltage is proportional to the diaphragmatic contraction, which generates tidal volume. In children, simultaneous bilateral diaphragm pacing is generally required to achieve optimal ventilation. In older children or adolescents who have a stable chest wall, adequate ventilation may be achieved by pacing only one side. Ventilatory muscle myopathy or phrenic neuropathy is a contraindication to pacer use. Obstructive apnea can be a complication of pacing during sleep, because synchronous upper airway skeletal muscle contraction does not occur with inspiration. This can often be overcome by adjusting settings on the pacers to lengthen inspiratory time and/or decrease the force of inspiration. In general, diaphragm pacers can be used only up to ~14 hours a day, and cannot be used for 24 hours continuously. This may provide benefit to select groups of children with central hypoventilation syndrome or high cervical spinal cord injury.

HOSPITAL MANAGEMENT PRIOR TO DISCHARGE

Nearly all infants and young children who receive HMV develop chronic lung disease with elements of bronchoconstriction, chronic inflammation of the airway, and impaired mucociliary clearance. These children usually benefit from aerosolized bronchodilators followed by intensive pulmonary physiotherapy on a routine basis. Patients should receive the routine immunizations and annual split virion influenza vaccine. The patient's respiratory status must be stable on the home ventilator for 1–2 weeks prior to discharge. Patients tolerate a $Paco_2$ slightly lower than physiologic (30–35 torr) which provides a margin of safety and eliminates subjective feelings of dyspnea.

There are many pieces of equipment essential for home care of the ventilator-assisted child. Prompt 24-hour emergency availability of the respiratory equipment vendor is essential in the event of equipment malfunction. A backup ventilator and other essential equipment should be provided to all families, but *must* be provided for children who are ventilator dependent ≥20 h/day or who live long distances from medical or technical assistance. A resuscitation bag is necessary for resuscitation and to permit manual ventilation in the event of power failure or ventilator malfunction. An appropriate-size mask made for the resuscitation bag is needed in the event the tracheostomy is decannulated and cannot be readily reinserted. The physical environment of the home should be evaluated for adequacy of space, grounded electrical outlets, and wiring.

Prior to discharge from the hospital, the family must demonstrate competency in equipment operation, tracheostomy care, ability to change the tracheostomy (both routinely and in emergencies), pulmonary physiotherapy, administration of medications (including aerosols), and cardiopulmonary resuscitation. Families must become adept at recognizing signs of respiratory compromise. Nurses with pediatric critical care expertise are helpful in assisting families for 8–24 h/day in the home care of their child, especially for infants and young children. Before a child is discharged from the hospital, each nurse who will care for the child at home should receive in-service training on the child's care, preferably from the child's primary nurse. Training for caregivers of children on HMV should focus on technical aspects of ventilator alarms and emergency responses.

Children who are ventilator assisted in the home must be closely linked to a medical center capable of providing the subspecialty care required. When possible, a local primary pediatrician should be recruited to provide routine pediatric care. The local emergency department or paramedics should be familiar with the child and be able to provide emergency care or transport to the medical center when necessary. The local telephone and utility companies must be notified in writing of the patient's location and condition. In the event of a power outage or interruption of service, the home ventilator patient should be given priority for restoration of service.

HOME MANAGEMENT OF THE VENTILATOR-ASSISTED CHILD

Routine evaluation of ventilator settings should be performed on a regular basis, so that ventilation meets the changing requirements of the growing child. These evaluations are usually performed by polysomnography. It is important to monitor $ETCO_2$ as an indication of the adequacy of ventilation. Sleep studies during daytime naps may also be adequate for the evaluation of ventilator settings if the child's clinical course is reasonably stable. Sleep studies may also be used to predict the success of sprint weaning during sleep when sprinting schedules are advancing in the home.

Because HMV may not completely meet the ventilatory requirements at all times, even the most successfully managed patients may be exposed to periods of alveolar hypoxia and hypoventilation. Thus, ventilator-assisted children are at risk for the development of pulmonary hypertension and cor pulmonale. The usual clinical findings of right heart failure may not be present until late in the course. Echocardiography may be a more sensitive method for following right heart function and should be obtained annually or more often if clinically indicated. When signs of pulmonary hypertension are discovered, it should be assumed that an inadequate level of mechanical ventilation is the cause until proven otherwise.

Growth failure can result from chronic hypoxemia and/or inadequate ventilation. Some patients, especially those with ventilatory muscle weakness, may have a decreased caloric expenditure due to decreased body movement. Monitoring for appropriate growth is important during HMV.

A number of normal host defenses against disease are either lost or impaired in chronically ventilated patients. Breathing via tracheostomy bypasses the humidifying and filtering functions of the upper airway, predisposing to inspissated secretions and tracheobronchitis. Ineffective cough leads to decreased clearance of pulmonary secretions. Because of changes in the ventilatory requirements during illness, hospitalization for blood gas monitoring and frequent ventilator changes may be required.

The first month after discharge is a critical time for unplanned readmission of children on HMV. A multidisciplinary action plan (MAP) should include the plans and management strategies post discharge. Fortunately, because many chronic lung diseases improve with age, half of children on HMV due to chronic lung disease were able to wean off ventilatory support by 5 years after discharge.

CHAPTER 28 ▪ SLEEP AND BREATHING

SALLY L. DAVIDSON WARD AND THOMAS G. KEENS

RESPIRATORY CONTROL AND SLEEP

Breathing is under both voluntary and involuntary control during wakefulness. Chemoreceptor activity matches minute ventilation to metabolic needs, while voluntary control of ventilation allows the integrated performance of complex behavioral activities. The muscles of the upper airway maintain sufficient tone for unobstructed breathing during wakefulness. Respiratory control and upper airway muscle tone change during sleep, predisposing to upper airway obstruction and instability. As sleep commences, $Paco_2$ normally rises by several mm Hg. The ventilatory responses to hypoxemia and hypercapnia, potent stimuli of chemoreceptor activity during wakefulness, are blunted during sleep. Important respiratory reflexes (e.g., cough and swallow) are inhibited. The respiratory pattern becomes irregular during rapid eye movement (REM) sleep with a variable rate and tidal volume and frequent pauses. Skeletal muscle atonia leads to collapsibility of the upper airway and a decrease in functional residual capacity. These changes predispose to obstructive sleep apnea (OSA) and impaired gas exchange.

OBSTRUCTIVE SLEEP APNEA SYNDROME

The most common sleep-related breathing disorder (SRBD) in childhood is obstructive sleep apnea syndrome (OSAS). OSA is defined as an absence of airflow at the nose and mouth despite continued respiratory efforts. Discrete events with reduced, but not absent, airflow are termed obstructive hypopneas. Apneas and hypopnea are often accompanied by hypoxemia, hypercapnia, and sleep disruption. Parents may describe snoring, gasping, choking, or apnea during their child's sleep and may reposition their children several times during the night. Nocturnal symptoms may be accompanied by excessive sleepiness and neurocognitive impairment during the day. The physical exam during wakefulness may not predict OSAS, and correction of anatomic defects by surgery may not relieve symptoms. The significant familial pattern to the risk of OSAS is likely related to both heritable anatomic and central nervous system (CNS) factors.

The most common conditions that predispose to OSAS are listed in **Table 28.1**. Obesity has increased the number of children and adolescents at risk for severe obesity-related OSAS. Obstructive apneas and hypopneas can result in continuous or episodic hypoxemia and hypoventilation during sleep, as well as repetitive arousals. These stimuli alter the function of the autonomic nervous system, and systemic hypertension and pulmonary hypertension are recognized complications of OSAS. Although children with OSAS may not have daytime sleepiness, they may suffer from other neurobehavioral complications, including school failure, hyperactivity, and mood or conduct disorders. A correlation exists between the severity of OSAS and the extent of these complications. A trial of early adenotonsillectomy (T&A) for mild-to-moderate pediatric OSA found that the surgical group had improvements in quality of life and measures of behavior, but not in neuropsychological estimates of attention and executive function. Other potential complications of OSA include failure to thrive, nocturnal enuresis, and worsening of parasomnias such as sleepwalking. Sleep disruption and hypoxemia also contribute to abnormalities of glucose homeostasis in obese children with SRBD.

A polysomnogram (PSG; sleep study) is required to reliably make the diagnosis of OSAS. Normal children have only one to two obstructive apneas or hypopneas per hour of sleep. Adults may have as many as five obstructive events per hour of sleep and be considered normal.

The first approach to therapy for OSAS is usually adenotonsillectomy (T&A). Complications of T&A include postoperative bleeding, upper airway obstruction secondary to airway edema, pulmonary edema,

TABLE 28.1

Conditions That Predispose to Obstructive Sleep Apnea Syndrome in Children

- Adenotonsillar hypertrophy
- Obesity
- Craniofacial abnormalities
- Down syndrome
- Sickle cell disease
- Cerebral palsy

TABLE 28.2

Conditions with a Higher Risk of Complications Following Adenotonsillectomy

- Age less than 3 y
- Severe OSAS (profound hypoxemia, AHI > 10, significant hypoventilation)
- Morbid obesity
- Neuromuscular disease
- Pulmonary hypertension
- Down syndrome
- Craniofacial anomalies

OSAS, obstructive sleep apnea syndrome; AHI, apnea hypopnea index.

or respiratory failure. Groups at the highest risk for postoperative complications are listed in **Table 28.2**. Retrospective pediatric studies have identified rates of postoperative respiratory compromise as high as 23% in children admitted following T&A, with young age, higher apnea hypopnea index (AHI) on preoperative PSG, laryngospasm in the operating room, hypoxemia in the postanesthesia care unit, underlying illness other than OSAS, and extremes of weight found to be risk factors.

Infants and children with craniofacial abnormalities (especially micrognathia or midfacial hypoplasia) can have severe OSAS. It is reported that surgery for OSAS in patients with craniofacial malformations is less likely to succeed in infants <12 months of age, results in long hospital stays, and presents more difficulty with extubation than in older children undergoing these procedures. Children with Down syndrome have multiple reasons for severe OSAS, including midface hypoplasia, relative macroglossia, hypotonia, obesity, and occasionally hypothyroidism.

In patients with postoperative difficulties, noninvasive ventilation, either continuous positive airway pressure (CPAP) or bilevel positive airway pressure (BiPAP), is attractive as it avoids intubation and can be performed on a pediatric unit after the patient is stable. Some practitioners question the safety of BiPAP in the immediate postoperative period with concerns regarding subcutaneous emphysema dissecting at the surgical site, bleeding, and drying of the upper airway. The surgical team should be involved in decisions to use CPAP or BiPAP.

Some children with OSAS will require uvulopalatopharyngoplasty, a more extensive procedure that includes removal of the tonsils, the tonsillar pillars, and the uvula. Mandibular distraction osteogenesis is being used with increasing frequency for infants and children with micrognathia. This procedure represents a considerable therapeutic advance, as previously many of these patients required tracheostomy. Treatment of OSAS in patients with Beckwith–Wiedemann or Down syndrome may require tongue reduction surgery. Despite surgical therapy, some will have only minimal improvement in OSAS and need long-term positive-pressure therapy or tracheostomy placement.

Unrecognized cases of OSAS can present to the pediatric intensive care unit (PICU) following other surgical procedures, trauma, or other medical illnesses. Unrecognized sleep apnea can adversely affect surgical outcomes. Changes in respiratory control following anesthesia can worsen symptoms of OSAS. Sleep fragmentation, inherent in hospitalization, may change upper airway neuromuscular function, favoring airway obstruction and apnea. Studies of adults with OSAS who underwent orthopedic procedures document cardiorespiratory complications in one-third of patients, including unplanned ICU transfers and reintubation. Careful screening of surgical patients for OSAS and its recognition in postoperative patients are essential.

The adult OSAS literature contains evidence that stabilization by positive airway pressure (CPAP or BiPAP) therapy prior to elective surgery reduces operative risk and improves postoperative course. Although patients with untreated OSAS may benefit from positive-pressure support after surgery, pressure titration and adaptation to the mask may be difficult in a child recovering from surgery. Judicious use of narcotics, avoiding or minimizing sedation, and careful respiratory monitoring with frequent assessment of airway status are required.

SUDDEN INFANT DEATH SYNDROME

Sudden infant death syndrome (SIDS) is the sudden unexpected death of an infant, under 1 year of age, with onset of the fatal episode apparently occurring during sleep, and that remains unexplained after a thorough investigation (complete autopsy and review of the clinical history and circumstances of death). SIDS is the most common cause of death in infants 1 month to 1 year of age, yet its cause remains unknown. The typical scenario is that caregivers place an apparently healthy baby for an overnight sleep or daytime nap and later find the baby lifeless. In some cases, the caregivers have been within hearing distance and have come back within 30 minutes, to find that the baby has died. That no sounds of struggling occur suggests that SIDS occurs swiftly and silently.

SIDS is most common between 2 and 4 months of age, and ~ 95% of SIDS deaths occur before 6 months of age. It is slightly more common in males. The risk of SIDS is higher in infants born prematurely or with low birth weight. Babies born to mothers who smoked cigarettes, drank alcohol, or used illicit drugs during pregnancy are at increased risk. African-American and Native American babies have increased risk. Although the cause of SIDS is unknown, most researchers believe that it results from an interaction of a developmental window of vulnerability (age 2–4 months), extrinsic environmental risks, and intrinsic infant vulnerability (infants have immature protective responses to environmental and physiologic challenges).

Sleeping in the prone position, on soft bedding, with soft items in the bed, overheating, and bed-sharing are associated with SIDS. The SIDS rate has fallen dramatically since 1992 owing to the "Back to Sleep" and "Safe to Sleep" campaigns, which educate parents to place their babies in a safe sleeping environment. However, even babies whose parents have followed these recommendations continue to die of SIDS.

Most SIDS infants are without vital signs when found. Many receive cardiopulmonary resuscitation by emergency responders and are often transported to a nearby hospital. In a small percentage of babies, resuscitation successfully restores a heartbeat but not respiratory effort. These cases are frequently referred to as "aborted" or "interrupted" SIDS. These babies usually develop signs of brain death by 24–48 hours. These infants should be evaluated for conditions such as sepsis, trauma (particularly head trauma), cardiac lesions (particularly serious arrhythmias or anomalous coronary arteries), metabolic disorders, and respiratory disorders (particularly pneumonia, or craniofacial abnormalities predisposing to OSAS). If child abuse or neglect is suspected, the intensivist should notify appropriate legal authorities. The United States and most Western countries require a thorough postmortem investigation for babies who die suddenly at home, in child care, or outside a hospital setting. An examination of the arrest scene by trained coroner's investigators and a complete autopsy by skilled pathologists should be performed.

Parent grief following an SIDS death is complicated by the fact that no one can tell parents why their baby died. SIDS parent support groups are the best source of support and information for them. SIDS parents from these groups are available 24 hours per day to speak with bereaved parents and to provide comfort and support. In the United States, the national SIDS parent support organization is First Candle/SIDS Alliance. In the United Kingdom, the national SIDS parent support organization is Foundation for the Study and Prevention of Infant Deaths.

APPARENT LIFE-THREATENING EVENTS

An apparent life-threatening event (ALTE) involves a witnessed color change (cyanosis or pallor), tone change (limpness or rarely stiffness), or apnea. Vigorous stimulation, mouth-to-mouth breathing, or resuscitation is required to revive the infant. In most cases, observers feared that the infant was dying. Some infants respond quickly and are normal on evaluation, while others require intensive intervention and may exhibit signs of a serious hypoxic event.

Initial Evaluation

There are no diagnostic tests that can be used to determine whether a child experienced an ALTE. However, laboratory evidence for severe hypoxia (acidosis, lactate, liver enzymes, or urinary hypoxanthines) can be used to assess the severity of the event. Infants with a concerning history or persistent signs and symptoms require a diagnostic evaluation to discover the etiology of the event. Infants presenting with an ALTE, who have recurrent events and are <1 month of age, are more likely to have subsequent events, require subsequent intervention, or have a diagnosis for which hospitalization is required. ALTEs often raise a concern for SIDS, yet there is no scientific evidence that ALTE confers an increased risk.

Diagnostic Evaluation

Arterial blood gas, blood sugar, and chest X-ray are first-line diagnostic procedures. If the infant appears septic, then evaluation for sepsis is necessary, including a lumbar puncture. Other diagnostic evaluations should be performed as indicated by the clinical history of the event and physical examination. A list of possible etiologies and appropriate diagnostic testing is shown in **Table 28.3**. Only those tests indicated by the history and physical examination should be performed. In a series of 243 infants presenting with ALTE, only 17% of the diagnostic tests were positive, and only 6% contributed to a diagnosis. Tests most likely to be positive include blood count, blood gases, chest X-ray, and evaluation for gastroesophageal reflux.

Etiology

A diagnosis is identified in 50%–70% of ALTE and up to 50% are caused by gastrointestinal disorders. Gastroesophageal reflux disease (GERD) is frequently found during diagnostic testing. ALTEs of gastrointestinal origin usually occur during or shortly after feeding, are likely to occur during wakefulness, and may be accompanied by choking, vomiting, or coughing. Neurologic problems, especially seizures, account for up to 30% of ALTEs. Electroencephalograms should be performed when seizures are suspected. Congenital brainstem anomalies, especially Arnold Chiari type I or II, may cause apnea, and a brainstem magnetic resonance imaging (MRI) may be helpful. Approximately 20% of ALTEs are due to respiratory disorders. Apnea can occur with viral infections (e.g., CMV, RSV, or influenza). Craniofacial anomalies predispose to obstructive apnea in infants. CNS-depressant medications enhance susceptibility to OSAS. OSAS can be idiopathic in infants, especially if premature and exacerbated by anemia. A history of noisy breathing, snoring, or excessive sweating during sleep should prompt a further evaluation for OSAS. Cardiovascular problems account for only ~5%

TABLE 28.3

Diagnostic Evaluation for Apparent Life-Threatening Event Infants

■ POTENTIAL DIAGNOSIS/ETIOLOGY	■ DIAGNOSTIC TESTS
Infection, sepsis	Complete blood count. Blood, urine, and cerebrospinal fluid cultures
Hypocalcemia	Serum calcium
Electrolyte imbalance	Serum electrolytes
Dehydration	BUN, creatinine
Hypoglycemia	Blood sugar
Asphyxia	Arterial blood gas (pH)
Pneumonia, chronic lung disease	Chest X-ray
Congenital heart disease, cardiomyopathy	Electrocardiogram, echocardiogram
Cardiac arrhythmia, prolonged QT interval syndrome	Electrocardiogram, 24-h Holter monitoring
Trauma, child abuse	Skeletal series, skull X-ray, head CT scan, retinal examination
Seizures	Electroencephalogram
GERD	Barium swallow, gastric scintiscan
Sleep-disordered breathing, OSA, central hypoventilation syndrome	Overnight polysomnography
Upper airway obstruction, craniofacial abnormality, congenital airway anomaly	Laryngoscopy, bronchoscopy
Inborn errors of metabolism	Serum ammonia level, urine organic acids, plasma amino acids
Drug ingestion, toxic exposure	Serum and urine toxicology

BUN, blood urea nitrogen; GERD, gastroesophageal reflux disease; OSA, obstructive sleep apnea.

of ALTEs. Inborn errors of metabolism account for 2%–5% of ALTEs. These are associated with fasting, fever, or vomiting. Inborn errors of β-oxidation of fatty acids have been described in ALTE babies with severe recurrent events, those that persist beyond a year of age, and in babies with a family history of previous infant deaths and/or severe apneas. Less than 3% of ALTEs appear to be due to child abuse. A family history of previous SIDS, infant deaths, or ALTE, especially if there are unusual associated circumstances, may increase suspicion for child abuse.

Management

Medical management of the ALTE infant in the ICU is primarily directed toward stabilizing the cardiorespiratory status. Treatment should be directed toward any underlying diagnosis; however, in 50% of ALTE infants, a specific etiology will not be determined. Home apnea–bradycardia monitoring has been used to manage infants with no identified etiology. However, few infants have recurrent events, and infants have died despite home apnea–bradycardia monitoring.

SLEEP IN THE INTENSIVE CARE UNIT

The purpose of sleep is not fully understood, but the consequences of sleep deprivation are well described. Sleep in critically ill patients is characterized by an abnormal distribution, with sleep periods scattered over 24 hours instead of being consolidated at night. Because of fragmentation, the restorative properties may be lacking. The organization, or architecture, of sleep stages is also affected with an increase in "light sleep" (stage N1) and decreased time in deeper sleep (stages N2, N3, and REM). Sleep deprivation results in neurologic and behavioral complications that include mood alterations (irritability), organic brain dysfunction (delusions and hallucinations), and delirium. Sleep deprivation is a physiologic stressor and affects autonomic, immunologic, metabolic, and hormonal functions. Both sleep deprivation and critical illness cause insulin resistance. Patients identify poor sleep as a great hardship during ICU stay.

Medications impact sleep, both during use and after discontinuation. Benzodiazepines and opioids cause REM suppression, and the *REM rebound effect* that follows discontinuation results in nightmares and disturbing dreams. The use and discontinuation of other medications also affects sleep (e.g., abrupt discontinuation of a β-blocker fragments sleep). Noise and light levels in the ICU are high and not conducive to sleep. It is important to engage ICU staff in efforts to reduce noise levels and limit care activities between midnight and 05:00 to provide consolidated sleep. Controlling light exposure with open blinds during the day and decreased light at night is also recommended. Melatonin therapy may entrain circadian rhythm–based results.

CHAPTER 29 ■ ELECTRODIAGNOSTIC TECHNIQUES IN NEUROMUSCULAR DISEASE

MATTHEW PITT

The peripheral nervous system (PNS) is defined as the motor nervous system from the anterior horn cell to the muscle and the sensory pathways up to and including the dorsal root ganglia. Electrodiagnostic techniques (nerve conduction studies [NCS] and needle electromyography [EMG]) are useful for the diagnosis of neuromuscular disorders and for unexplained weaknesses that develop during pediatric intensive care unit (PICU) admission.

Disorders of the PNS can be divided into those affecting the anterior horn cell, the peripheral nerves, neuromuscular junction (NMJ), and the muscle. ICU-pertinent *hereditary neuromuscular conditions* include the severe forms of spinal muscular atrophy, hypomyelinating and Dejerine Sottas neuropathies, congenital myasthenic syndromes, myotonic dystrophy, and nemaline and centronuclear myopathies. The relevant *acquired neuromuscular conditions* include poliomyelitis, acute inflammatory demyelinating polyneuropathy, infantile botulism, tick paralysis, autoimmune myasthenia gravis, and acute myositis. *Conditions acquired during ICU care* include critical care neuromyopathy and mononeuropathies from pressure or ischemic injury.

SIGNAL RECORDING

Electrodes

Surface electrodes, concentric needle electrodes, and single fiber needle electrodes are used in EMG and NCS. *Surface electrodes* are used to record compound muscle action potentials (CMAP). They are placed over the muscle of interest along with electrodes used to record nerve action potentials over the related nerve. *Concentric needle electrodes* have a recording surface at the tip. When placed into a muscle, they allow the recording of activity from fibers that lie within a radius of ~0.5 mm. *Single fiber needle electrodes* have recording surfaces on the side of the needle (behind the tip), and have a smaller range (1–3 muscle fibers, because of the arrangement of muscle fibers in the motor unit).

Definitions and Diagnostic Findings

Guidelines, consensus statements, and recommendations from the *American Association of Neuromuscular & Neurodiagnostic Medicine* are available at their website: http://www.aanem.org/.

Electromyography Patterns

At rest, muscle is electrically inactive. On piercing the muscle with a recording needle, brief bursts of activity are due to mechanical stimulation. At full contraction, there is a disorderly group of action potentials of varying rates and amplitudes. The EMG can be used to diagnose neuropathies, NMJ diseases, and myopathies (**Table 29.1**). Other phenomena recorded include muscle fibrillations, fasciculations, and jitter. *Fibrillations* are biphasic potentials regarded as the key feature of denervation when present at more than one site in a muscle. *Fasciculations* are variably shaped waveforms of high amplitude observed in lower motor neuron disease (poliomyelitis, spinal

TABLE 29.1

Typical EMG Findings in Neuropathic and Myopathic Disease

■ DISEASE	■ TYPICAL EMG FEATURES: ■ ACTION POTENTIAL AMPLITUDE	■ ACTION POTENTIAL DURATION	■ MOTOR UNIT NUMBER ESTIMATES
Neuropathic	Increased (×2) due to more fibers per motor unit	Increased	Decreased
Myopathic	Reduced area-to-amplitude ratio of the action potential	Reduced	Decreased in severe cases

muscular atrophy), medications (stimulants, succinylcholine), and hypomagnesemia. *Jitter* arises from small variations in the timing of action potentials when two muscle fiber action potentials are recorded from the same motor unit. *Blocking* occurs when neuromuscular transmission is sufficiently impaired such that an individual endplate potential does not reach threshold and a muscle fiber action potential is not generated. The decremental response recorded in patients with myasthenia gravis during repetitive motor nerve stimulation is related to blocking of individual muscle fiber action potentials.

Nerve Conduction Study Results

Nerve Conduction Velocity. Motor and sensory NCS data are obtained from electrical stimulation of appropriate nerves. *Latency* (milliseconds) is the time for the electrical impulse to travel from the stimulation to the recording site, *amplitude* (millivolts) is the height of the response, and *duration* (milliseconds) is the length of the response (**Fig. 29.1A** and **B**). Motor nerve conduction velocities (NCVs) require stimulation of two or more sites along the same nerve and calculation of the difference in latencies and distance between stimulating electrodes. Sensory NCVs are calculated using the latency and distance between stimulating and recording electrodes from a sensory portion of the nerve being stimulated. Sensory nerve amplitudes are much smaller than motor nerve amplitudes. **M-wave.** *The M-wave*, recorded in the muscle, represents the orthodromic response to a stimulus traveling from the motor neuron to the muscle. The M-wave amplitude increases with stimulus intensity (**Fig. 29.2**).

F-wave. The *F-wave study* involves a supramaximal stimulation of the motor nerve and recording of action potentials from the muscle supplied. In this recording, the action potential travels from the site of stimulation to the anterior horn (antidromic) and back to the limb (orthodromic) through that same nerve. The F-wave latency can be used to calculate the NCV of the nerve between the limb and spine.

H-reflex. The *H-reflex study* uses the stimulation of a sensory nerve and records the reflex muscle activity in the limb. This reflex also assesses conduction between the limb and the spinal cord, but in contrast to the F-wave, the afferent and efferent impulses are from sensory and motor nerves, respectively. Since the H-wave decreases with stimulus intensity and the F-wave increases with stimulus intensity, the H-wave can be readily identified at lower stimulus intensity.

PERFORMING ELECTROMYOGRAPHY AND NERVE CONDUCTION STUDIES IN THE PICU

Most children with disorders of the PNS have generalized abnormalities and an EMG protocol can be standardized. The first test is the sensory nerve action potential (SNAP) amplitude and velocity in the leg. In small babies, the medial plantar nerve is used, because greater distance between the stimulating and recording electrodes reduces stimulus artifact. In older children, either the superficial peroneal or the sural nerve is used. If results are normal, the arms do not need to be tested. Motor nerve stimulation, recording either the peroneal nerve from extensor digitorum brevis or the ulnar nerve from adductor pollicis, is the next test. In the presence of abnormalities of the sensory nerve, it may be possible to

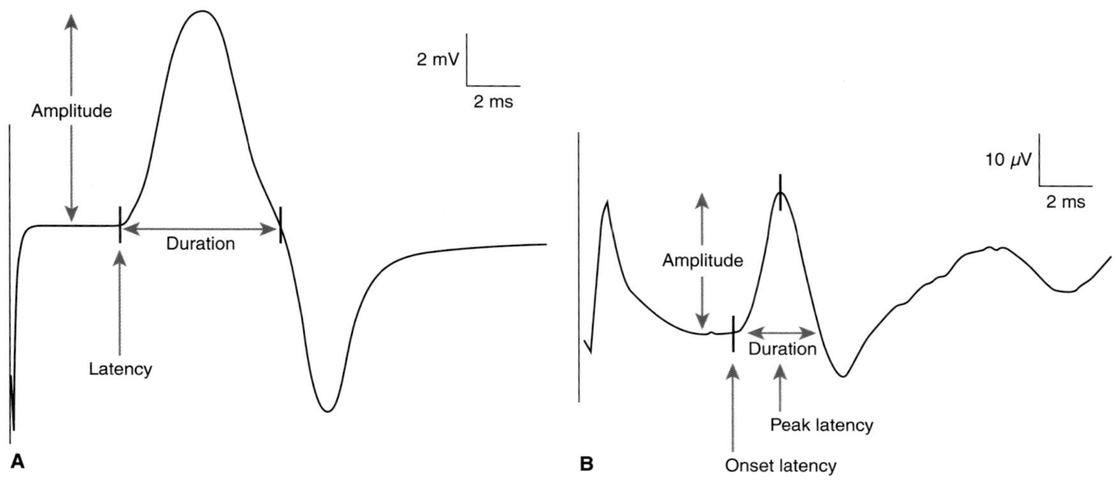

FIGURE 29.1. Basic nerve conduction studies. Components and shapes of (**A**) compound muscle action potential (CMAP) and (**B**) sensory nerve action potential (SNAP). (From Preston DC, Shapiro BE. *Electromyography and Neuromuscular Disorders: Clinical–Electrophysiologic Correlations*. 3rd ed. Philadelphia, PA: Elsevier, 2013.)

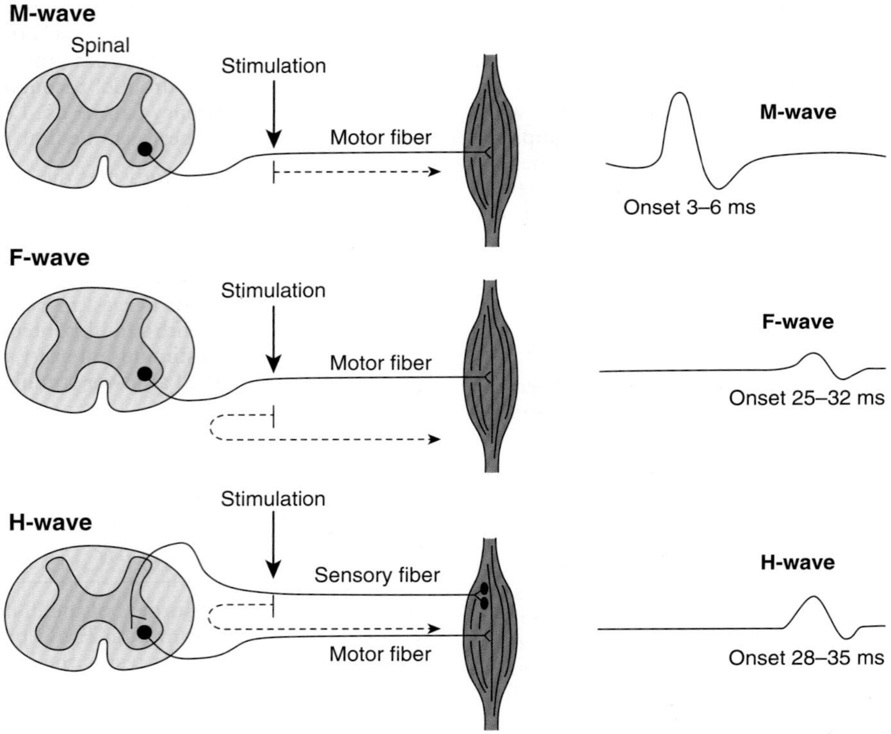

FIGURE 29.2. **M-wave:** Excitement is conducted along motor neuron from stimulus to recording at muscle fiber (orthodromic); M-wave increases as stimulus increases. **F-wave:** Excitement is conducted along motor neuron from stimulus to nerve body (antidromic) before returning along the motor neuron to the muscle fiber (orthodromic); F-wave increases slightly as stimulus increases. **H-wave:** Excitement is conducted along the sensory neuron to the motor neuron (antidromic), and then travels down motor neuron to muscle (orthodromic); H-wave decreases as stimulus increases. (Modified from Kai S, Nakabayashi K. Evoked EMG makes measurement of muscle tone possible by analysis of the H/M ratio. In: Turker H, ed. *New Frontiers of Clinical Research*. Croatia: Intech, 2013.)

document motor nerve involvement and indicate whether this might be due to demyelination or axonal degeneration. Since effective reinnervation may restore CMAP, EMG should be performed to look for signs of chronic denervation (**Table 29.1**). EMG is performed with small (30 g) needles placed in the tibialis anterior, which is easily activated by stimulating the sole of the foot. If abnormal, and motor neuropathy is suspected, the tongue should be sampled next by the submental route. Abnormal results will indicate that the motor neuronopathy is generalized rather than due to segmental spinal cord involvement. Depending on the findings, other muscles may be sampled.

This protocol will demonstrate abnormalities if a neuromuscular condition is present. If not, there are occasions (e.g., cervical segmental myelopathy) when examination of the arm is needed. However, if no abnormality is seen, it is very important to include single muscle fiber needle EMG (SFEMG) to rule out a myasthenic syndrome. Stimulation SFEMG (StimSFEMG) of the orbicularis oculi muscles may be the only test to show abnormality. Specific examination of the diaphragm or bulbar muscles may be requested. Undiagnosed bulbar palsies are increasingly common reasons for children to be admitted to the PICU (i.e., lack of airway protection).

PERIPHERAL NERVOUS SYSTEM DISORDERS

Hereditary Conditions

Anterior Horn Cell Disease

Spinal Muscular Atrophy. The most common anterior horn cell disease is spinal muscular atrophy (SMA) due to mutations on the 5q chromosome. SMA is the most common genetic neuromuscular disorder of childhood. It is classified according to severity, with SMA 0 the worst affected (present as a hypotonic neonate) and SMA 3 the least affected (often unrecognized until adulthood). Diagnosis with EMG and NCS of severe SMA in infancy is not straightforward. It is common for sensory nerve fibers to be affected due to associated dorsal root ganglionopathy, which makes distinction from early neuropathy difficult. Furthermore, while the reduction in the CMAP indicates a severe loss of muscle fibers, the EMG may not show classic neuropathic abnormalities (**Table 29.1**). Reinnervated motor units (an expected feature of anterior horn cell disease) may not have developed. Fibrillation potentials are regarded as an important sign, but can be seen in other conditions (e.g., acute myositis or severe myopathy) and their presence does not confirm SMA. The genetic test is globally available and is positive in severe cases.

Spinal Muscular Atrophy with Respiratory Distress. *Spinal muscular atrophy with respiratory distress* (SMARD) is another anterior horn cell condition, exceedingly rare, and associated with the immunoglobulin mu-binding protein 2 (IGHMBP2) gene abnormality. Affected babies usually have intrauterine growth retardation and present at 3 months of age with respiratory compromise. Investigation shows an abnormality of the diaphragm, often unilateral and suggestive of a diaphragmatic eventration. It is not unusual for the infant to have surgery that reveals a very thin diaphragm and then be unable to wean from the ventilator. The clinical neurophysiology often shows no sensory response in the legs. The motor fibers have strikingly slow NCVs similar to a demyelinating neuropathy. However, motor and sensory NCVs are typically normal in the upper limbs. The EMG shows the well-recognized chronic neuropathic change, most marked distally suggesting distal SMA. This combination of axonal degeneration by EMG but demyelination by NCS is unique. EMG of the diaphragm can be diagnostic. Widespread denervation in the diaphragm, often with no abnormality in the intercostal muscles (found during passage through the chest wall), is pathognomonic.

Disorders of the Nerve

Charcot–Marie–Tooth disease. The most common hereditary disorder of the nerve is *Charcot–Marie–tooth disease* (CMT) type I. Affected children rarely need intensive care unless exposure to neurotoxins (vincristine) causes profound weakness and unmasks undiagnosed CMT. The mutations that cause CMT are associated with more severe forms of hereditary neuropathy that can present with sufficient weakness in a newborn to require ventilation. Two conditions that cause this are *Dejerine Sottas disease* (DSD) and *congenital hypomyelinating neuropathy*. Affected children are born very hypotonic and require mechanical ventilation. A very increased stimulus may be needed to provoke a response from the nerve. Response may be missed because the recording is not long enough to allow the long distal motor latency to be captured. The EMG may show fibrillation potentials consistent with secondary axonal degeneration. Genetic confirmation follows.

Neuromuscular Junction Disorders

Congenital Myasthenic Syndromes. The *congenital myasthenic syndromes* (CMS) are hereditary disorders of the proteins in and around pre-and postsynaptic areas of the NMJ. They are rare, but may be treatable. StimSFEMG has revolutionized detection of this unusual condition. The most common cause of CMS is a mutation of the epsilon subunit of the acetylcholine receptor. Because affected patients continue to produce the fetal form of the acetylcholine receptor (containing a gamma subunit), the weakness is less profound. The particular conditions that should be considered include CMS with episodic apnea (CMS-EA, previously called infantile myasthenic syndrome), which is associated with a presynaptic abnormality of the choline acetyltransferase enzyme (CHAT). Rapsyn (receptor-associated proteins of the synapse) mutations may also be associated with apnea. Conditions that present with stridor and require ventilatory support can also be associated with Dok7 mutation (Dok7 CMS). Other (nonmyasthenic) conditions show abnormalities of StimSFEMG, such as central hypoventilation syndrome due to PHOX2B, Prader Willi syndrome, and some myopathies. If the StimSFEMG is normal, the likelihood of myasthenia is low, but not absent. Repetitive nerve stimulation is easy to perform, but not routine, as it has a significantly reduced sensitivity in comparison with StimSFEMG.

Muscle Disease

Myotonic Dystrophy. Babies with myotonic dystrophy inherit it from the mother (the mother may be undiagnosed until they have careful examination and EMG testing). EMG testing of the neonate is usually unnecessary, and examination of CTG trinucleotide (cytosine–thymine–guanine) repeats on the *DMPK* gene (code for myotonic dystrophy protein kinase) secures the diagnosis. EMG myotonic discharges, seen in older children and adults, may not be seen in babies.

Other Myopathies. Nemaline rod myopathy and minitubular (centronuclear) myopathy are among the few myopathies that are sufficiently devastating to require ventilatory support from birth. EMG is usually clearly abnormal, but further delineation of the exact condition requires muscle biopsy or genetic analysis.

Acquired Disorders of the PNS

Anterior Horn Cell Disease

Poliomyelitis. Historically, poliovirus was the most common infection causing anterior horn cell disease. Enteroviruses other than poliovirus have been implicated in a poliomyelitis-like *acute flaccid paralysis (AFP)*. Coxsackie or Echo viruses may exhibit anterior horn cell involvement. The most commonly implicated virus varies according to region. West Nile virus is seen in the United States. Other causes of AFP include the viruses causing Japanese B encephalitis, Murray Valley encephalitis, St Louis encephalitis, Russian Spring encephalitis, tick-borne viruses, and the herpes virus. AFP should be considered in the child who has respiratory illness and becomes overly weak, but does not have Guillain–Barré syndrome (GBS).

Disorders of the Peripheral Nerve

Guillain–Barré Syndrome. GBS is the most common cause of acute nontraumatic paralysis in children and is linked to antibodies that cross-react with neuronal gangliosides. These children present with gastrointestinal or respiratory illness preceding an ascending weakness and neuropathic pain. Children have most of the recognized changes of GBS such as increase in the distal motor latency, temporal dispersion, and slowing of the main nerve trunk velocity. Some changes are subtle and may only manifest as absent F-waves. Computed tomography (CT) scans or magnetic resonance imaging (MRI) show inflammation around nerve roots, and cerebrospinal fluid (CSF) shows elevated protein levels.

Neuromuscular Junction Abnormalities

Botulism. Botulinum toxin is one of the most potent poisons known. Infantile botulism is due to colonization of the intestine and production of toxin by *Clostridium botulinum*. Constipation is followed by paralysis that starts cranially and descends (contrasts the ascending paralysis in GBS). Infantile botulism is most common in specific regions possibly related to climatic environments that support spore development or construction work causing spores to be airborne. Children can have the organism in their bowels and be asymptomatic. The well-recognized finding of a small CMAP, with a significant increment on rapid repetitive nerve stimulation (up to a 200% increase at stimulation rates of 20 and above), occurs only at a particular level of NMJ involvement. When all NMJs are paralyzed, no responses are seen; if there is minimal infection, then only a small proportion will demonstrate abnormalities. It is unequivocal that NMJ function will be affected (demonstrated by StimSFEMG) and jitter reduced at faster rates of stimulation. Botulism immune globulin (BIG) neutralizes unbound toxin, has revolutionized treatment, and can reduce ICU stay.

Tick Paralysis. In areas where tick paralysis is seen, GBS should not be diagnosed without looking carefully for a tick. The removal of the tick immediately restores strength.

Autoimmune Myasthenia Gravis. In *congenital autoimmune myasthenia gravis* (AIMG), a mother with myasthenia gravis gives birth to a baby paralyzed by the transplacental diffusion of antibodies against the NMJ. After birth, the child recovers over a period of weeks. A confusing situation can occur when a child is born with arthrogryposis and the Pena–Shokeir phenotype that occurs from lack of in utero movement. They have antibodies against the adult form of the NMJ (against its alpha subunit). There is a further form of congenital AIMG in which the maternal antibodies are against the gamma subunit (seen only in the fetal NMJ and replaced by the epsilon subunit in the adult NMJ). These children may also be born with arthrogryposis, and the mother will have had a succession of miscarriages. The diagnosis is often delayed; this is a rare disorder and testing for acetylcholine receptor antibodies looks for those against the adult, not the fetal, form. All these children have abnormalities on StimSFEMG. Outside of the neonatal period, AIMG can be caused either by receptor antibodies or by antibodies against the muscle-specific kinase (MuSK) receptors.

Acute Muscle Disease

It is very rare that an acute muscle disease is sufficiently severe for a child to need intensive care. When it presents, an extremely elevated CPK and rhabdomyolysis with concomitant renal changes facilitate diagnosis. EMG and NCS usually have no role in their diagnosis.

CONDITIONS ACQUIRED IN THE PICU AFFECTING THE PERIPHERAL NERVOUS SYSTEM

Critical Illness Neuromyopathy

Weakness in the context of critical illness can occur from one of three causes: a critical illness neuropathy, a critical illness myopathy, or a combination of two (critical illness polyneuropathy and myopathy). The neuropathy is usually an axonal neuropathy, with the motor nerve affected more than the sensory. This assumption is based on a marked reduction in CMAP amplitude in the context of preserved or only slightly affected SNAPs (**Fig. 29.3**). If present, this indicates a slow and prolonged recovery. Reports vary regarding the prevalence of this condition in children.

Critical illness myopathy may be more common in adults and children. Studies of the nerves notice the differences in the evoked responses from the muscle according to whether you stimulate the nerve or the muscle itself. Other studies include those looking at muscle fiber conduction velocity or at muscle fiber excitability. The duration and the configuration of the CMAPs have a very close relationship to muscle conduction velocity.

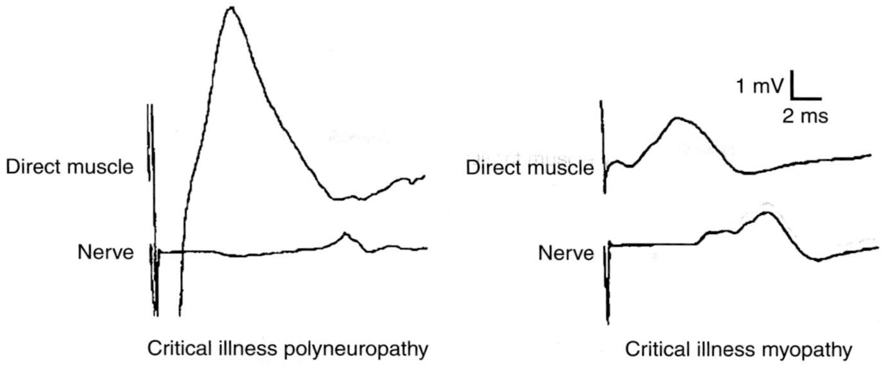

FIGURE 29.3. Studies showing critical illness polyneuropathy and critical illness myopathy. Compound muscle action potentials from the tibialis anterior muscle of a patient with critical illness neuropathy (**left**) and critical illness myopathy (**right**). Note the higher amplitude with direct muscle stimulation compared with nerve stimulation in the patient with critical illness neuropathy, whereas there is little difference in amplitude between direct muscle and nerve stimulation in the patient with critical illness myopathy. (From Preston DC, Shapiro BE. *Electromyography and Neuromuscular Disorders: Clinical–Electrophysiologic Correlations*. 3rd ed. Philadelphia, PA: Elsevier, 2013.)

Mononeuropathies That Develop in the PICU

The mononeuropathies that occur in the PICU are usually the result of pressure or inadvertent damage from resuscitation or monitoring procedures. The lower limb nerves seem more susceptible to injury, and in particular the sciatic nerve. Children with sciatic nerve injury often present with a foot drop. Cachectic children undergoing prolonged surgery are at particular risk. It is possible that there is a vascular element in addition to pressure. The sciatic nerve's blood supply comes from the femoral artery and can be compromised by femoral artery cannulation. The neurophysiologic findings of sciatic nerve palsy require the demonstration of abnormalities in the peroneal and the tibial elements of the nerve. Recovery from sciatic nerve palsies can be poor because of the long distance for the nerve to regrow.

CHAPTER 30 ■ ACUTE NEUROMUSCULAR DISEASE

SUNIT C. SINGHI, NAVEEN SANKHYAN, AND ARUN BANSAL

Children with acute neuromuscular disease (NMD) require critical care due to poor airway protection, respiratory failure, or autonomic nervous system involvement with cardiovascular instability. NMDs are classified according to the site of pathology: brain, spinal cord, peripheral nerve, neuromuscular junction, or the skeletal muscle (**Table 30.1**).

TABLE 30.1

Anatomic Classification and Examples of Conditions with Neuromuscular Weakness

Brain
Intracranial hemorrhage
Hypoxic ischemic encephalopathy
Meningoencephalitis
Acute demyelinating encephalomyelitis
Spinal Cord
Trauma
Epidural abscess
Myelitis
Acute poliomyelitis
Spinal muscular atrophy
Peripheral Nerve
Guillain–Barré syndrome
Critical illness polyneuropathy
Toxic (lead, arsenic) neuropathy
Drug-induced neuropathy, e.g., vincristine
Diphtheric polyneuropathy
Acute porphyria
Phrenic nerve injury—diaphragmatic paralysis
Neuromuscular Junction
Myasthenia gravis and congenital myasthenic syndromes
Prolonged neuromuscular blockade
Antibiotic (aminoglycoside, D-penicillamine) therapy
Snake bite and scorpion sting
Organophosphorus poisoning
Botulism
Tick paralysis
Hypermagnesemia
Muscle
Critical illness myopathy
Hypokalemia
Muscular dystrophies
Congenital myopathies
Acute rhabdomyolysis
Inflammatory myopathies, e.g., dermatomyositis

RESPIRATORY DYSFUNCTION IN A PATIENT WITH A NEUROMUSCULAR DISORDER

Brain and brainstem conditions that cause respiratory depression manifest as hyperventilation, irregular or ataxic (cluster) breathing, hiccups, hypopnea, and apnea, and if bulbar involvement, impaired secretion clearance and aspiration. Neuromuscular weakness manifests as rapid shallow breathing from decreased tidal volume and minute ventilation. An ineffective cough results in retention and aspiration of secretions and microatelectasis. Lack of muscle tone also results in unopposed recoil pressure of the lung that results in decreased functional residual capacity and impaired gas exchange. The development of respiratory symptoms may be insidious or sudden. Weakness of oropharyngeal muscles causes choking, slurred speech, dysphonia, difficulty clearing secretions, or aspiration. Patients may have shortness of breath at rest or on exertion, or nonspecific symptoms such as restlessness, difficulty sleeping, or fatigue. Early morning headache, daytime somnolence, and poor school performance suggest nocturnal hypoventilation. Weakness of the diaphragm results in daytime dependency on accessory muscles and can lead to nighttime hypoventilation (intercostal muscles become hypotonic during rapid eye movement sleep, REM atonia). Patients with diaphragmatic weakness may report distress when supine. Patients with an intact diaphragm but weak intercostal and abdominal muscles may develop respiratory distress while upright. *Paradoxical breathing* occurs when, during inspiration, the chest wall is pulled inward due to weak intercostal muscles while the abdomen expands outward as the diaphragm contracts downward (a rocking motion of chest and abdomen).

Spirometry

A single-breath counting test may be used to follow progression of weakness. Counting to 10 in one breath is associated with a forced vital capacity (FVC) at least 15–20 mL/kg and to 25 a FVC ~30–40 mL/kg. In children older than 5 years, spirometry is used to monitor progression of weakness. Vital capacity is measured from maximum inspiration to maximum expiration (normal is 55–80 mL/kg). Maximum inspiratory pressure is measured at residual volume, and maximum expiratory pressure is measured at total lung capacity. These values are sensitive indicators of respiratory muscle strength. In adults, a vital capacity of ~20 mL/kg, a maximum inspiratory pressure less negative than −30 cm H_2O, or a maximum expiratory pressure of <40 cm H_2O are minimal values that raise concern. Values that fall by 50% from baseline or >30% in a 24-hour period are of concern. Life-threatening respiratory failure occurs when vital capacity drops below 20 mL/kg or 30% of predicted values.

Tracheostomy

Advantages of early tracheostomy include increased comfort, airway safety, and easier weaning from ventilation. No guidelines exist for tracheostomy in children with these disorders. Some disease-specific data suggest that children are less likely to require tracheostomy than are adults.

General Supportive Care

General care should prevent complications from immobilization and includes physiotherapy, splints to prevent contractures, prevention of deep vein thrombosis, and careful positioning and repositioning. Enteral nutrition should begin as early as possible. Chest physiotherapy may help prevent mucus retention. In patients with facial nerve palsy, eye care prevents desiccation and corneal injury. Constipation from immobilization and opiate use should be prevented.

GUILLAIN–BARRÉ SYNDROME

Guillain–Barré syndrome (GBS) is an acute, autoimmune disorder of the peripheral nervous system characterized by areflexic weakness of limbs. GBS may encompass a group of acute peripheral-nerve disorders. GBS is the most common cause of acquired, nontraumatic paralysis. It can occur at any age (incidence increases with age), in any race, and in all climates. The incidence in children <9 years of age is 0.62 per 100,000, and the overall annual incidence is ~1.3 per 100,000. Males have a slight predilection. An infectious illness in the month preceding the onset of neurologic symptoms is present in 70% of cases.

The common variants include acute inflammatory demyelinating polyradiculopathy (AIDP), acute motor axonal neuropathy (AMAN), and acute motor and sensory axonal neuropathy (AMSAN). The Miller Fisher variant is characterized by a triad of ophthalmoplegia, ataxia, and areflexia. It is believed that GBS results from an antibody against an infecting organism that cross-reacts with the host's gangliosides. Molecular similarity of myelin and ganglioside antigens to constituents of the infecting organism results in a hyperimmune response. Demyelinating lesions occur along the entire peripheral nerve including the nerve roots. All nerve types are involved (e.g., autonomic, motor, and sensory), but motor nerve involvement predominates. Schwann-cell proliferation with imperfect remyelination is seen during recovery.

Clinical Features

Initial symptoms of GBS include paresthesias (toes and fingers) or limb pains followed by progressive weakness of the lower limbs and unsteady gait. Over hours to weeks, upper limb weakness and cranial nerve palsies develop. Ascending weakness is symmetrical. Pain may be an initial complaint. Urinary retention occurs in 10%–15% of children. Dysautonomia, including dizziness, hypertension, excessive sweating, and tachycardia, can occur. The symptoms progress for a median of 7 days and plateau for a variable period and then improvement begins.

The hallmark of GBS is an ascending motor weakness and areflexia that may ascend to involve respiratory muscles. Cranial nerve involvement (35%–50%), autonomic instability (26%–50%), ataxia (23%), or dysesthesia (20%) occur. The signs of autonomic dysfunction are sinus tachycardia, bradycardia, or hypertension. Severely affected patients have arrhythmias and changes in vasomotor tone that manifest as hypotension and blood pressure lability. Loss of vasoregulation is associated with exaggerated hemodynamic responses to drugs and anesthetics. Volume and electrolyte disturbances are common. Hyponatremia and excess antidiuretic hormone may be caused by hypovolemia, hypotension, or positive-pressure ventilation.

Variant clinical features include fever at onset, severe sensory loss with pain (myalgias, arthralgias, meningismus, and radicular and back pain), sphincter dysfunction (urinary retention), ileus, central nervous system (CNS) involvement (cerebellar ataxia, extensor planter response, absent pupillary response, and rarely, loss of all brainstem reflexes), and papilledema. Adults with GBS may experience an abnormal mental state, vivid dreams, hallucinations, delusions, and psychosis. Rare variants in children include descending GBS (facial or bulbar muscles involved first), Miller Fischer syndrome, polyneuritis cranialis, pharyngocervicobrachial syndrome, acute sensory neuropathy of childhood, and acute pandysautonomia (**Table 30.2**).

In evolving GBS, other causes of progressive symmetric weakness must be considered (e.g., transverse myelitis, toxins or heavy metal polyneuropathies, organophosphate poisoning, tick paralysis, acute porphyria, diphtheria polyneuropathy, myelopathies [polio or other viral infections of anterior horn cell], myasthenia gravis [MG], and hypokalemia). Evidence of neurotoxic conditions, persistent asymmetric involvement, preserved reflexes, severe sensory signs, or distinct sensory level should suggest a diagnosis other than GBS. MG presents with intact tendon reflexes, no dysautonomia, and normal cerebrospinal fluid (CSF). Enteroviral infections have CSF pleocytosis and motor neuronal injury on electromyogram (EMG). Transverse myelitis causes a sensory-deficit level, urinary incontinence, and CSF pleocytosis. Botulism may mimic GBS but has ophthalmoplegia, pupillary involvement, dry mouth, and ileus. Tick paralysis can cause acute ascending paralysis with areflexia, but patients have complete ophthalmoplegia and preserved sensation, and a tick is usually found on the scalp or behind the ear.

CSF findings in GBS reveal elevated protein (>45 mg/dL) without CSF pleocytosis (<10 cells/mm^3) (albuminocytologic dissociation). More than 50 cells/mm^3 should prompt a reconsideration of the diagnosis. Lumbar puncture can rule out infection. Imaging is used to exclude myelitis. In GBS, 2 weeks after the onset of symptoms, lumbosacral magnetic resonance imaging (MRI) with gadolinium contrast reveals enhancement of the cauda equina nerve roots.

Management

Rapid progression, bilateral facial nerve palsy, and autonomic dysfunction have been associated with need for intubation. Respiratory failure requiring

TABLE 30.2

Selected Subtypes of Guillain–Barré Syndrome

SUBTYPE	PATHOLOGIC AND IMMUNOLOGIC FEATURES	CLINICAL FEATURES
Guillain–Barré Syndrome		
AIDP	Multifocal demyelination, pathologic antibodies unknown	Progressive, ascending, symmetrical, areflexic or hyporeflexic weakness
Facial diplegia	Pathologic antibodies unknown	Bilateral facial weakness
AMAN	Antibodies against gangliosides GM1, GD1a, GNalNAc-GD1a, and GD1b affecting motor axons only	Acute motor neuropathy of variable severity, reflexes may be preserved in a few patients
Acute motor conduction blocks neuropathy	Antibodies against gangliosides GM1, GD1a, affecting motor axons only	Milder form of acute axonal neuropathy, does not progress to axonal degeneration
AMSAN	Above plus sensory axons affected	Sensory symptoms predominate
Pharyngo-cervico-brachial weakness	Antibodies against gangliosides GT1a, GQ1b, GD1a	Prominent pharyngeal, neck, and shoulder weakness
Miller Fisher Syndrome		
Miller Fisher syndrome	Demyelination, antibodies against gangliosides GQ1b, GT1a, GD3	Ophthalmoplegia, ataxia, Areflexia. Incomplete forms occur, can overlap with generalized weakness
Acute ataxic neuropathy	Antibodies against gangliosides GQ1b, GT1a, GD1b	Acute ataxia, no ophthalmoplegia, considered an incomplete form of Fisher syndrome
Acute oropharyngeal palsy	Antibodies against gangliosides GQ1b, GT1a	Acute oropharyngeal weakness
Others		
Acute autonomic neuropathy	Pathologic antibodies unknown	Acute autonomic failure due to cardiovascular involvement

AIDP, Acute inflammatory demyelinating polyneuropathy; AMAN, Acute motor axonal neuropathy; AMSAN, Acute motor sensory axonal neuropathy.
Adapted from Yuki N, Hartung HP. Guillain–Barré syndrome. *N Engl J Med* 2012;366:2294–304.

mechanical ventilation occurs in 15%–25% of children with GBS and is associated with rapid progression, upper limb weakness, autonomic dysfunction, and cranial nerve involvement. Dysautonomia exaggerates the hemodynamic response to drugs used for intubation. Patients without full stomachs or ileus may benefit from topical/local anesthetic administration to blunt airway response. The risk of hyperkalemia from succinylcholine use should be considered and weighed against alternatives.

Mechanical ventilation is indicated for ventilatory muscle insufficiency, increased O_2 requirement to maintain Spo_2 >92%, or alveolar hypoventilation (e.g., $Pco_2 > 50$ torr). Other indications are FVC <15 mL/kg, rapid decline in vital capacity by 50% from baseline, and inability to generate a maximum NIF more negative than −20 cm H_2O. Recovery from respiratory failure is expected though some motor weakness may remain. Early tracheostomy may benefit patients who have severe GBS, but it can be deferred a few weeks until the time course of recovery is more clear.

Fatal cardiovascular collapse from autonomic dysfunction occurs in 2%–10% of seriously ill patients, with the highest risk in patients with respiratory failure, quadriplegia, or bulbar involvement. A reduction of "beat to beat" variation in heart rate suggests vagal involvement and indicates a risk of arrhythmia. Transcutaneous pacing and volume repletion may be needed. For hypotension refractory to fluids, pure α-agonists (e.g., phenylephrine) avoid the arrhythmogenic effects from combined α- and β-agonists. Hypertension does not need specific treatment unless it is associated with signs of end-organ damage. Constipation is seen in more than 50% of patients, but prokinetic bowel motility drugs are contraindicated in patients with dysautonomia.

Immunomodulation

Corticosteroids. Corticosteroids do not hasten recovery or affect long-term outcome when used alone or in combination with intravenous immunoglobulin (IVIG).

Plasma Exchange. Plasma exchange may remove or dilute the antibodies implicated in GBS. In adults, plasma exchange reduced time to recover walking, reduced need for artificial ventilation, decreased duration of ventilation, and lowered the rate of severe sequelae at 1 year. Relapses are seen in ~10% of patients within 3 weeks of plasma exchange. It is contraindicated in patients with severe hemodynamic instability, bleeding diathesis, and septicemia.

Intravenous Immunoglobulin. IVIG has been shown to be of equivalent benefit (reduced mechanical ventilation and reduced length of stay) to plasma exchange in GBS in children. IVIG is easier to manage and more likely to be completed. The mechanism of action of IVIG is likely multifactorial (modulation of complement activation, binding and neutralization of idiotypic antibodies, saturation of Fc receptors on macrophages, and suppression of various inflammatory mediators). Minor side effects of IVIG include headache, myalgia, arthralgia, fever, and vasomotor reactions. IgA-deficient patients may develop anaphylaxis after the first course. Aseptic meningitis, congestive heart failure, vascular complications, and renal failure have also been reported. Plasma exchange is preferred in patients with IgA deficiency, hyperviscosity syndromes, and congestive heart failure.

Outcome

Children have a more favorable outcome than adults. The mortality in childhood GBS is <5%. Recovery begins 2–4 weeks after the plateau of symptoms and takes 3–12 months. Recurrence of symptoms can occur following IVIG therapy. Full recovery is seen in 75%–80% of children. Younger age (<9 years), rapid progression of weakness, and mechanical ventilation predict long-term deficits. Anti-GM1 antibodies and *Campylobacter jejuni* infection also predict poor outcome.

MYASTHENIA GRAVIS

Myasthenia gravis is a disorder of the neuromuscular junction characterized by fluctuating weakness and fatigability of skeletal muscles due to autoimmune destruction of acetylcholine receptors (AChRs) at the postsynaptic end plate. In childhood, MG is categorized by age or immunologic involvement as (a) autoimmune or juvenile MG (JMG), (b) congenital MG or genetic MG, or (c) transient neonatal MG (TMG). Autoantibodies against nicotinic AChR are detectable in 85%–90% of cases. The remaining cases involve antibodies against other targets (muscle-specific kinase or MuSK) or a genetic basis for abnormal neuromuscular transmission. Severity of weakness is proportional to the reduction in functional AChRs. Patients with antibodies against MuSK have atypical illness characterized by involvement of facial, bulbar, neck, shoulder, and respiratory muscles, with less involvement of ocular muscles. Microbial infections may trigger destruction of AChRs, and thymic hyperplasia is found in ~70% of cases.

Clinical Features

Juvenile Myasthenia Gravis

JMG is separated into subtypes: AChR antibody-positive JMG, MuSK antibody-positive JMG, and seronegative JMG. JMG has an onset between 3 months and 16 years (most <3 years). Onset is clinically similar to MG in adults, and symptoms are more evident late in the day. Ocular involvement is often asymmetric and presents as intermittent drooping of eyelids with a persistent upward gaze or as double vision. Weakness progresses to bulbar and generalized weakness within four years in 75% of those who present with isolated eye symptoms. Almost 75% of patients have bulbar weakness at presentation that results in slurred speech, difficulty chewing, or choking. Facial muscle weakness results in a flat, expressionless face and drooling. Weakness of neck muscles may cause the head to fall forward or backward. Leg involvement results in fatigability and weakness while climbing stairs or running. This weakness tends to be symmetrical and proximal. Weakness that involves diaphragm and muscles of respiration may be so severe as to cause respiratory failure. Physical findings are confined to the motor system, with no loss of sensation or coordination. Pupillary responses are not affected. Various maneuvers can unmask fatigability, including repetitive trips up and down stairs, repetitive exercises, or having the patient count to 100 or chew for 30 seconds.

MuSK Antibody-Positive JMG. JMG with MuSK antibodies is rare in young children, more common in the second decade of life, and females predominate. The thymus is usually normal or only mild altered. There are three phenotypes: (1) a phenotype indistinguishable from AChR antibody–positive patients, (2) a phenotype with prominent faciopharyngeal weakness, usually with marked muscle atrophy, and (3) a phenotype with relatively isolated neck extensor and respiratory weakness. Weakness is severe with more respiratory crises than non-MuSK MG.

Seronegative JMG. The frequency of seronegative MG is higher in childhood. The main differential diagnosis in seronegative children is congenital myasthenic syndrome (CMS), which usually presents in the first year of life.

Transient Neonatal Myasthenia Gravis

Transient neonatal MG presents shortly after birth in 10%–20% of babies born to mothers with autoimmune MG. Passive transplacental transfer of circulating AChR antibodies is the cause. Symptoms develop within hours of birth and range from mild hypotonia to generalized weakness, feeble cry, difficult feeding, ptosis, facial weakness, or life-threatening respiratory distress. The syndrome usually resolves in 3 weeks but can persist for months. Newborns of myasthenic mothers should be observed for signs of weakness. Treatment includes anticholinesterase, ventilatory support as needed, and plasmapheresis in severe cases.

Lambert–Eaton Myasthenic Syndrome

Lambert–Eaton myasthenic syndrome is rare in children and presents with proximal weakness, autonomic dysfunction, and areflexia. Diagnosis is based on repetitive nerve stimulation. The presence of serum antibodies to the P/Q-type voltage-gated calcium channel supports the diagnosis. Both immune-mediated and tumor-associated (neuroblastoma, Wilms tumor) cases have been described in children.

Congenital Myasthenic Syndromes

Congenital myasthenic syndromes (CMS) are genetic disorders of neuromuscular transmission produced by mutations that alter the expression and function of ion channels, receptors, enzymes, or other molecules necessary for neuromuscular transmission. Most present at birth, but some present later in childhood. Patients present with ptosis, ophthalmoparesis, dysphagia, dysarthria, weak cry, hypotonia, respiratory distress, or arthrogryposis multiplex. Anticholinesterase agents, such as pyridostigmine, are the first-line therapy. There is no role for immunotherapy.

Emergencies in Myasthenia Gravis

Myasthenic crisis is characterized by respiratory failure due to weakness of upper airway muscles, the diaphragm, or other respiratory muscles. It can be precipitated by respiratory infection, sepsis, aspiration, surgical procedures, rapid tapering of corticosteroid or immunotherapeutic drugs, initiation of corticosteroid therapy, and exposure to drugs. *Cholinergic crisis* is a severe weakness usually caused by overtreatment with cholinesterase inhibitors (CEIs). The weakness due to cholinergic crisis may be indistinguishable from myasthenic crisis. The muscarinic effects of CEIs increase bronchopulmonary secretions, which can obstruct the airway and cause aspiration. Patients show features of cholinergic excess, including excessive salivation, lacrimation, diarrhea, sweating, pupillary constriction, and muscle fasciculation. Patients with compromised renal function are more susceptible. CEI treatment should be withheld initially with either entity. Atropine is used to treat cholinergic crisis. Removal of triggers and institution of plasmapheresis or administration of IVIG may be necessary to treat myasthenic crisis. Steroids, immunotherapy, and thymectomy are not used for myasthenic crisis as they can take weeks to be effective.

Diagnosis

Edrophonium chloride (Tensilon) is an intravenous CEI with rapid onset (30 seconds) and short duration (15 minutes) of action. A Tensilon test involves administration of edrophonium in incremental doses and observing for improvement in function. Bradycardia can be a significant side effect. Relative contraindications are bronchial asthma or cardiac dysrhythmias. The test is most sensitive when using improvement in ptosis and double vision as end points. False-positive results can occur in other neuromuscular conditions (e.g., botulism, GBS, motor neuron disease, and lesions of brainstem). Edrophonium is not recommended in infants, for whom neostigmine is an alternative testing agent. Some patients may not show a response to edrophonium, but they may show improvement to neostigmine or pyridostigmine.

AChR antibody measurement is used to test for MG. Normal levels do not exclude MG and levels may be raised in autoimmune liver disease, systemic lupus erythematosus, inflammatory myopathies, and first-degree relatives of patients with acquired MG.

Antibodies to MuSK are present in 40%–60% of seronegative patients with JMG. Other antibodies may include low-affinity anti-AChR, anti-titin, and anti-ryanodine receptor antibodies.

Management

Respiratory compromise due to oropharyngeal and laryngeal muscle weakness may occur despite normal tidal volume and vital capacity. With diaphragm and accessory muscle weakness, vital capacity will be reduced, as will maximum inspiratory pressure measurements. An inability to produce >20 cm H_2O of NIF suggests the need for intubation. Neuromuscular-blocking agents (NMBAs) may have a prolonged and unpredictable action. Short-acting, nondepolarizing agents may be preferred, but prolongation of any paralytic should be anticipated. Medications that exacerbate muscle weakness should be avoided or stopped (**Table 30.3**).

Cholinesterase Inhibitors. In patients with moderately severe muscle weakness but without respiratory failure, it is reasonable to increase the dose of pyridostigmine every few days until a response is apparent. Side effects of CEIs include bronchospasm, excessive salivation, bradycardia, nausea, diarrhea, and miosis.

ACh Release Promoters. Guanidine and 4-aminopyridine enhance the release of ACh from nerve terminals. They improve ocular and limb muscle strength but without benefit for respiratory paralysis.

Immunosuppressive Therapy

If no improvement in weakness is seen with adequate CEI therapy, immunosuppressive drugs can be added. These include corticosteroids, azathioprine, cyclophosphamide, cyclosporine, and methotrexate. Corticosteroid treatment may offer short-term benefit. Other agents are used in individuals who relapse on corticosteroids or have disabling steroid side effects. In adults, oral prednisolone combined with azathioprine results in fewer relapses and less steroid usage. Mycophenolate mofetil, tacrolimus and cyclosporine have also been used. Rituximab has emerged as a promising treatment for seronegative JMG.

Plasmapheresis

Plasmapheresis removes AChR antibodies and leads to improvement within a few days that lasts for several weeks. It can also be used to prevent crises prior to thymectomy or surgery.

Intravenous Immunoglobulin

IVIG and plasmapheresis are equally effective. In patients in myasthenic crisis, IVIG is used if plasmapheresis is not available.

TABLE 30.3

Pharmaceutical Agents with the Potential to Aggravate Myasthenia Gravis

Antibiotics
Ampicillin, aminoglycosides (gentamicin, kanamycin, streptomycin, tobramycin), clindamycin, colistin, erythromycin, fluoroquinolones (e.g., ciprofloxacin, norfloxacin), lincomycin, neomycin, penicillin, polymyxin B, sulfonamides, tetracycline, trimethoprim-sulfamethoxazole, vancomycin
Anticonvulsants
Barbiturates, carbamazepine, gabapentin, phenytoin, trimethadione (no longer available in the US)
Antirheumatic Drugs
Chloroquine, penicillamine (could cause myasthenia gravis or elevation of antibodies)
Cardiovascular Drugs
Bretylium, calcium-channel blockers (nifedipine, verapamil), lidocaine, oxprenolol, procainamide, propranolol, and other β-blockers, quinidine
Psychotropic Agents
Chlorpromazine, diazepam, lithium, promazine
Replacement Hormones
Adrenocorticotropic hormone, corticosteroids, estrogens, oral contraceptives, thyroid hormones
Other Drugs
Diuretics (lower serum potassium), interferon-α, iodinated radiographic contrast agents, muscle relaxants, magnesium, opioids, neuromuscular-blocking agents, quinine

Thymectomy

Thymectomy is recommended in moderate and severe MG that is inadequately controlled on CEIs. The greatest benefit is in patients with early-onset, AChR antibody-positive MG.

Natural Course and Outcome of MG

Spontaneous remission can occur, especially in younger children. Thymectomy produces complete remission in 75% and improvement in 95% of cases. The course of congenital MG is static or slowly progressive.

ACUTE INTERMITTENT PORPHYRIA

The porphyrias are a group of disorders caused by defects in the enzymes of heme biosynthesis. Acute porphyria is characterized by acute, life-threatening attack of neurovisceral symptoms. Acute intermittent porphyria (AIP) is the most common form. Other acute porphyrias are hereditary coproporphyria, variegate porphyria, and 5-aminolevulinic acid (ALA) dehydratase-deficient porphyria. The porphyrias are classified as hepatic or erythroid types, based on site of the enzyme defect and as either acute or cutaneous, based on the clinical

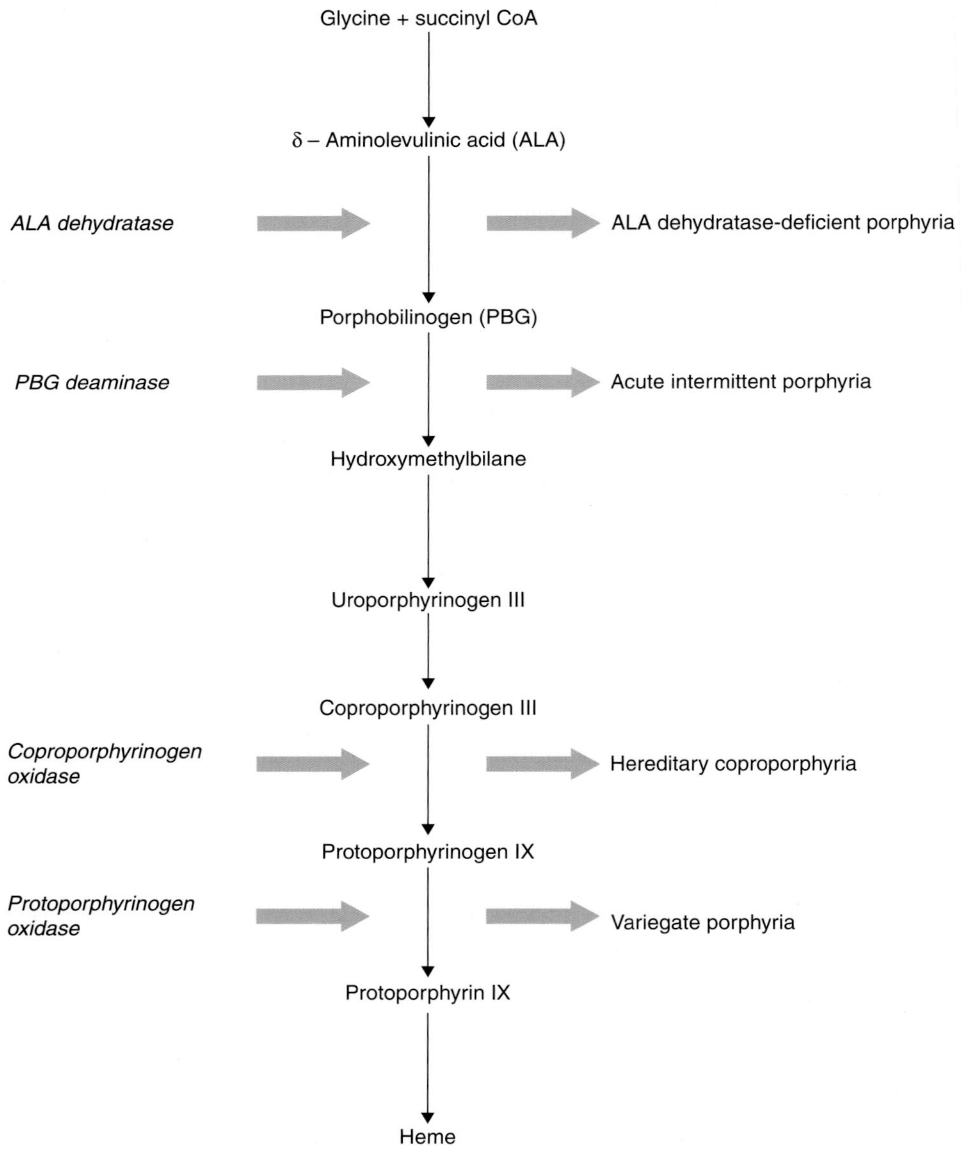

FIGURE 30.1. Heme biosynthetic pathway showing the enzyme defect causing acute hepatic porphyrias.

presentation. The enzyme defect associated with each porphyria and the metabolic by-products that accumulate are shown in **Figure 30.1**. Common to all acute porphyrias is overproduction and accumulation of ALA and porphobilinogen (PBG). Neurovisceral symptoms are due to the neurotoxic effect of PBG and ALA and interaction of ALA with γ-aminobutyric acid receptors.

Clinical Features

Classic features are abdominal pain, altered mental state, and peripheral neuropathy. Pain in the limbs, back, neck, and chest occur in 70% of cases. Nausea, vomiting, constipation, and occasionally diarrhea occur. Neurologic symptoms include paresthesias, myalgias, paresis, neuropathy, seizures, and coma. Deep-tendon reflexes may be lost. Respiratory failure occurs in 20% patients. Autonomic nervous system involvement (e.g., tachycardia, hypertension, sweating) is common. Hyponatremia and electrolyte disturbances may occur.

Precipitating Factors

Medications, starvation, hormonal factors, and infection can induce or worsen attacks. Bacterial and viral infections induce attacks by catabolizing heme, which induces ALA synthetase and the accumulation of porphyrin precursors.

Diagnosis

Misdiagnosis or delayed diagnosis is common. The presence of hypertension, dark urine, muscle weakness, and pain should heighten suspicion. When suspected, a rapid test for urine PBG levels should be undertaken. Measurement of enzyme activity and genetic testing can determine the type of acute porphyria and identify asymptomatic relatives.

Treatment of Acute Attack

β-Blockers are used to treat hypertension and tachycardia, unless the patient is hypovolemic. Benzodiazepines are used for seizures. Hyponatremia and hypomagnesemia should be carefully corrected. Enzyme activity is reversed by administering 10% glucose or carbohydrate-rich foods and hemin infusion. Hemin infusion may cause coagulopathy, bleeding diathesis, and transient renal insufficiency. Since the introduction of hemin therapy, case fatality has fallen from 10%–52% to <10% currently.

INTENSIVE CARE UNIT–ACQUIRED WEAKNESS

Intensive Care Unit–acquired weakness (ICUAW) refers to weakness with no plausible etiology other than critical illness. *Critical illness polyneuropathy* (CIP) refers to patients who have electrophysiologic evidence of an axonal polyneuropathy, and *critical illness myopathy* (CIM) indicates patients who have electrophysiologic or histologic defined myopathy. The term *critical illness neuromyopathy* (CINM) is for coexisting CIP and CIM. ICUAW is more common in adults than children. Risk factors include sepsis, systemic inflammatory response, multiorgan failure, mechanical ventilation, corticosteroids, neuromuscular-blocking drugs, aminoglycosides, hyperosmolality, parenteral nutrition, and hyperglycemia.

Prolonged Neuromuscular Transmission Blockade

Prolonged neuromuscular transmission blockade occurs in patients who receive muscle relaxants for days or weeks. Renal dysfunction, hypermagnesemia, and metabolic acidosis are other risk factors in prolonging neuromuscular blockade.

Critical Illness Polyneuropathy

CIP is an acute, generalized neuropathy often occurring after sepsis and multiorgan dysfunction. Clinical signs develop in 2–3 weeks. CIP is recognized when weaning from ventilation is difficult. Patients may complain of paresthesia or loss of sensation in a glove-and-stocking distribution. Bladder and bowel function are preserved. Limb edema may obscure atrophy.

Critical Illness Myopathy

CIM is a more common cause of ICUAW than CIP. Exposure to corticosteroids or NMBAs is the major risk factor. Other risk factors include sepsis and multiorgan failure. Patients have flaccid tetraparesis or tetraplegia. Deep-tendon reflexes may be normal or diminished. Cranial nerves and sensation are intact. Weaning from mechanical ventilation is difficult.

Diagnosis

Elevated creatine phosphokinase suggests a toxic or inflammatory cause of myopathy. In severely affected patients, electrophysiologic testing should be obtained. Nerve or muscle biopsy may be useful. The differences between CIP and CIM are summarized in **Table 30.4**.

Treatment and Prevention

Glutamine, glutathione, and branched-chain amino acid supplementation are associated with improved survival and shorter ICU stay. Strict glycemic control reduces the incidence of CIP/CIM in critically ill adults but is associated with hypoglycemia. Prolonged or high-dose corticosteroids and NMBAs should be avoided. It is thought that patients with CIM recover faster than those with CIP.

TABLE 30.4

Differences between Critical Illness Polyneuropathy and Critical Illness Myopathy

	CRITICAL ILLNESS POLYNEUROPATHY	CRITICAL ILLNESS MYOPATHY
Predisposing factor	Preceding systemic inflammatory response syndrome, sepsis, or multiorgan failure	Often received nondepolarizing muscle blocking agent, high-dose corticosteroid, or both
Clinical features	Sensory deficits present Weakness distal > proximal Tendon reflexes normal or ↓	No sensory deficit Weakness proximal > distal Tendon reflexes ↓ or absent Weakness of muscles supplied by the cranial nerves may occur
Electrophysiology	Low amplitude/absent sensory action potentials Normal motor unit potentials Reduced motor unit recruitment Normal muscle excitability Features of axonopathy without demyelination	Retained sensory nerve action potentials Small motor unit potentials Early motor unit recruitment Absent/reduced muscle excitability
Pathology	Axonal loss (sensory and motor nerve) Acute and chronic denervation of muscle	Loss of thick myosin filament Type II fiber atrophy (type I less common) or severe muscle fiber necrosis

Adapted from Khan J, Burnham EL, Moss M. Acquired weakness in the ICU: Critical illness myopathy and polyneuropathy. *Minerva Anesthesiol* 2006;72:401–6.

CHAPTER 31 ■ CHRONIC NEUROMUSCULAR DISEASE

ELENA CAVAZZONI, JONATHAN GILLIS, AND MONIQUE M. RYAN

Children with chronic neuromuscular diseases (NMDs) can have recurrent admissions to the pediatric intensive care unit (PICU) and a disproportionate use of healthcare resources. Their admissions often engender discussion about the appropriate use of intensive care support and the patient's quality of life. It is important for the intensivist to work with a neuromuscular neurologist to provide up-to-date information on diagnosis, disease trajectory, and prognosis and to develop a long-term care plan with the child and family.

OVERVIEW OF CHRONIC NEUROMUSCULAR DISEASES

Clinical Presentation and Differential Diagnosis

The presentation of chronic NMDs relates largely to their pathophysiology (**Table 31.1**). The chronic NMDs are discussed by categories of disorders

TABLE 31.1

Chronic Neuromuscular Disorders of Childhood

	■ ETIOLOGY	■ AGE OF ONSET	■ COURSE
Anterior Horn Cell			
Spinal muscular atrophy	Genetic (AR)	Variable (infancy–adulthood)	Progressive
Poliomyelitis	Infectious	Variable	Static
Acid maltase deficiency	Genetic (AR)	Variable (infancy–adulthood)	Progressive
Peripheral Nerve			
Congenital hypomyelinating neuropathy	Sporadic/genetic (AD/AR)	Neonatal	Static
Dejerine–Sottas disease	Sporadic/genetic (AD/AR)	Infancy	Static
Charcot–Marie–Tooth disease	Genetic (AD, AR, XL)	Childhood	Slowly progressive
Chronic inflammatory demyelinating polyneuropathy	Autoimmune	Variable (childhood)	Relapsing–remitting or progressive
Neuromuscular Disorders			
Congenital myasthenic syndromes	Genetic (AR, AD)	Neonatal or infancy	Static
Myasthenia gravis	Autoimmune	Variable (childhood)	Relapsing–remitting
Myopathies			
Congenital myopathies	Genetic (AR, AD, XL)	Variable (infancy–adulthood)	Static or slowly progressive
Congenital muscular dystrophies	Genetic (AR)	Infancy–childhood	Static or slowly progressive
Myotonic dystrophy	Genetic (AD)	Variable (neonatal–adulthood)	Static or slowly progressive
Duchenne and Becker muscular dystrophies	Genetic (XL)	Childhood	Progressive
Other muscular dystrophies	Genetic (AD, AR)	Variable (infancy–adulthood)	Progressive

AR, autosomal recessive; AD, autosomal dominant; XL, X-linked recessive.

primarily affecting nerves, the neuromuscular junction, or muscles.

Nerve Disorders

Spinal Muscular Atrophy

Spinal muscular atrophy type 1 (SMA 1) is the most common motor neuronopathy of childhood, with an incidence of 1 in 5000 live births. SMA is caused by recessive mutations in the survival motor neuron gene on chromosome 5. Four clinical subtypes with varying expression of modifying genes are defined on the basis of disease severity and progression. Infants with SMA 1 never sit unsupported, children with SMA type 2 sit but never stand, those with SMA type 3 are able to walk without assistance, and SMA type 4 is of adult onset.

Children with SMA type 1 present in the first months of life with hypotonia. Progressive weakness causes loss of antigravity strength and increasing difficulty breathing and feeding. Without ventilatory support, death from chronic respiratory insufficiency occurs before the age of 2 years. Noninvasive ventilatory support by nasal prongs or face mask may be successful in prolonging survival into the second decade of life. Invasive mechanical ventilation via tracheostomy can lead to longer survival.

Congenital Neuropathies

The congenital hypomyelinating or demyelinating neuropathies generally present in the first few years of life with hypotonia, weakness, and absent deep-tendon reflexes, often in association with congenital or acquired joint contractures. Complications include respiratory insufficiency, gastroesophageal reflux, and vocal cord paresis. Classification into congenital hypomyelinating neuropathy, Dejerine–Sottas syndrome, or forms of Charcot–Marie–Tooth disease is contingent on age at presentation and findings on nerve biopsy.

Neuromuscular Junction Disorders

Myasthenic Syndromes

The myasthenic syndromes are discussed in Chapter 30.

Muscle Disorders

Congenital Myopathies

The congenital myopathies are a heterogeneous group of rare disorders defined by distinctive histochemical or ultrastructural changes. The number of morphologically and genetically distinct congenital myopathies continues to grow (**Table 31.2**). Clinical severity varies widely. All may be associated with early-onset weakness, hypotonia, hyporeflexia, poor muscle bulk, dysmorphic features secondary to muscle weakness (e.g., pectus carinatum, scoliosis, foot deformities, high-arched palate, and elongated facies), and a distinguishing morphology on muscle biopsy. Late presentations include delayed motor milestones, frequent falls, or disease complications (e.g., contractures, scoliosis, and respiratory insufficiency).

Muscle weakness in the congenital myopathies is generally static. Facial weakness is common. Distal as well as proximal weakness may be present. The respiratory muscles are usually involved, but cardiac involvement is rare. Respiratory muscle involvement generally parallels the extent of limb weakness. Some disorders (e.g., myotubular myopathy and nemaline myopathy) may present at birth with severe hypotonia, little spontaneous movement, and respiratory insufficiency. Death from respiratory insufficiency, aspiration, or pneumonia occurs, but some infants survive with little residual disability. Increasing weakness of the axial musculature causes spinal deformity that rapidly progresses during adolescent skeletal growth. Paraspinal muscle rigidity and kyphoscoliosis can result in significant restriction of lung capacity and respiratory insufficiency.

Congenital Muscular Dystrophies

Some congenital muscular dystrophies affect only muscle, while others are associated with structural abnormalities of the brain and eyes (**Table 31.3**). The muscular dystrophies are caused by genetic abnormalities of the muscle membrane leading to progressive weakness, elevated creatine kinase, and dystrophic changes in muscle. Respiratory insufficiency is common. Some have a characteristic pattern of axial weakness, spinal rigidity, and early respiratory insufficiency with relative sparing of the limb muscles.

Myotonic Dystrophy

Myotonic dystrophy is caused by an abnormal expansion of a CTG trinucleotide repeat sequence in the myotonic protein kinase gene (*DMPK*). The size of the repeat sequence corresponds with severity of weakness (normal individuals, 5–37 repeats; childhood and adult onset, 50–350; infants with severe congenital myotonic dystrophy, >2000 repeats). The mother is the affected parent in cases of congenital myotonic dystrophy.

Infants with congenital myotonic dystrophy have congenital contractures, generalized hypotonia, and weakness. Facial weakness causes the characteristic tented upper lip and scaphoid temporal fossae. Swallowing difficulties are common; most children require gavage feeding. Respiratory insufficiency is common in children who present in the first few weeks of life and relates to lung hypoplasia caused by reduced intrauterine breathing movements, poor intercostal muscle action, and diaphragmatic hypoplasia. Bulbar weakness predisposes to aspiration. Approximately 50% of patients with congenital myotonic dystrophy require ventilation at birth. Children who require ventilation beyond the first month of life have a 25% mortality in their first year. Most survivors eventually become ambulant, with improved respiratory function with increasing age, but remain at risk of

TABLE 31.2

Congenital Myopathies

	■ INHERITANCE	■ MUSCLE BIOPSY FINDINGS	■ NATURAL HISTORY	■ ADDITIONAL FINDINGS
Central core disease	AD	Type 1 fiber predominance Cores in type 1 muscle fibers	Weakness static or slowly progressive Most patients remain ambulant	Scoliosis Congenital hip dislocation Predisposition to malignant hyperthermia
Nemaline myopathy	Variable: AD, AR, sporadic	Type 1 fiber predominance Nemaline bodies on trichrome stain	Weakness static or slowly progressive Variable severity Respiratory insufficiency common Bulbar involvement common	Scoliosis Acquired joint contractures
Myotubular myopathy	X-linked	Central nuclei in all muscle fibers	Severe congenital weakness Most patients are ventilator-dependent Significant early mortality	Ptosis Ophthalmoplegia Macrocephaly Pyloric stenosis
Centronuclear myopathy	AD, AR	Central nuclei in all muscle fibers	Variable weakness in childhood or later Most patients remain ambulant	Ophthalmoplegia in some Respiratory insufficiency may present late
Minicore myopathy	AR	Type 1 fiber predominance Multiple small cores in type 1 muscle fibers	Moderate weakness Most patients are ambulant Respiratory insufficiency in those with spinal rigidity	Ophthalmoplegia in some Spinal rigidity Hand involvement Cardiomyopathy in minority Predisposition to malignant hyperthermia
Congenital fiber-type disproportion	AD, AR, XL	Type 1 fiber predominance Type 1 fibers small	Variable weakness Respiratory insufficiency in some	Ophthalmoplegia in some Scoliosis common

AD, autosomal dominant; AR, autosomal recessive; XL, X-linked recessive.

later respiratory deterioration, cardiac arrhythmia, complications of poor gastrointestinal motility, diabetes, and mental retardation.

Duchenne Muscular Dystrophy

Duchenne and Becker muscular dystrophies are caused by mutations in the gene for dystrophin at Xp21. Duchenne muscular dystrophy (DMD) affects 1 in 5000 boys, is the most common muscular dystrophy of childhood, and usually presents at 3–5 years with an abnormal ("waddling") gait and frequent falls. Progressive weakness causes loss of independent ambulation at ages 8–13. Becker muscular dystrophy is less common and more slowly progressive. Long-term corticosteroid treatment slows the progression of DMD. Loss of ambulation is followed by the development of scoliosis and muscle contractures. Most young men with DMD die before the age of 30, because of respiratory insufficiency (90%) or cardiomyopathy (10%).

Other Muscular Dystrophies

The limb-girdle muscular dystrophies (LGMDs) usually present in adulthood. These uncommon neuromuscular conditions cause characteristic patterns of muscle weakness that affect the pectoral and pelvic girdle muscles and spare the face. Respiratory muscle involvement usually occurs late in the disease course (some LGMDs have preferential involvement of the axial musculature and early respiratory insufficiency).

TABLE 31.3

Congenital Muscular Dystrophies

SITE OF DEFECT	PROTEIN DEFECT	DISORDER/ INHERITANCE	NATURAL HISTORY	ADDITIONAL FINDINGS
Extracellular matrix protein	Laminin α_2 (merosin)	Merosin-deficient CMD (CMD type 1A) (AR)	Severe muscle weakness Respiratory insufficiency common	Leukodystrophy Demyelinating neuropathy
	Collagen VI	Ullrich (AD, AR) and Bethlem (AR) CMDs	Mild-to-moderate muscle weakness Respiratory insufficiency by late childhood—adolescence	Proximal joint contractures Distal hyperlaxity Follicular keratosis
Sarcolemmal proteins	Integrin α_7 (AR)		Congenital muscular dystrophy	
Glycosyltransferase enzymes	Fukutin (AR)	Fukuyama CMD (AR) Walker–Warburg disease (AR)	Severe muscle weakness Early respiratory insufficiency	Cerebellar dysgenesis Cobblestone lissencephaly Severe mental retardation
	POMGnT1	Muscle–eye–brain disease (AR)	Severe muscle weakness Early respiratory insufficiency	Cerebellar dysgenesis Cobblestone lissencephaly Severe mental retardation
	POMT1	Walker–Warburg disease (AR) LGMD with mental retardation (AR)	Severe muscle weakness Early respiratory insufficiency	Cerebellar dysgenesis Cobblestone lissencephaly Severe mental retardation
	Fukutin-related protein	CMD type 1C (AR) LGMD type 2I (AR)	Variable muscle weakness	Macroglossia Calf hypertrophy Cardiomyopathy
	LARGE	CMD type 1D (AR)	Moderately severe muscle weakness	Severe mental retardation Leukodystrophy
Endoplasmic reticulum protein	Selenoprotein 1 (*SEPN1*)	CMD with spinal rigidity (AR) Multiminicore disease (AR) Congenital fiber-type disproportion (AR)	Axial rigidity Axial weakness Respiratory insufficiency	Characteristic facies

CMD, congenital muscular dystrophy; AR, autosomal recessive; AD, autosomal dominant; LGMD, limb-girdle muscular dystrophy.

CLINICAL MANAGEMENT IN INTENSIVE CARE

Presentation to the PICU

Most presentations to the PICU will be for the management of respiratory compromise because of intercurrent illness, surgery, or disease progression. The severity of pulmonary compromise depends on the pattern and severity of involvement of respiratory muscles, the development of secondary thoracic wall abnormalities, and resultant changes in lung compliance.

Inspiratory muscle weakness limits the ability to take deep breaths and leads to peripheral airway collapse. An ineffective cough results in an inability to clear secretions and atelectasis. Superimposed upper respiratory tract infections also increase the volume of secretions, leading to frequent and rapid development of pneumonia.

In children with DMD and congenital myopathies, weakness of the diaphragm develops at the same rate as weakness of the intercostal and abdominal muscles. Significant respiratory compromise may occur, although paradoxical breathing is absent. Diaphragmatic weakness may be accentuated by supine positioning, exacerbating respiratory compromise in sleep.

In children with SMA, the intercostal muscles are more affected than the diaphragm. As the descent of the diaphragm during inspiration generates negative intrathoracic pressure, the thoracic cage will collapse (because of weaker intercostal muscles) at a time when the abdomen is expanding. This abnormal pattern—"paradoxical" breathing—can lead to chest-wall deformity and abnormal lung development.

Young children with chronic NMDs have abnormally high chest-wall compliance because of hypotonia and loss of muscle bulk. Intercostal muscle weakness makes the rib cage less able to withstand the elastic recoil of the lungs, leading to low end-expiratory volume and atelectasis. With increasing age, cartilaginous ossification causes a reduction in chest-wall compliance and increased chest-wall rigidity. Thoracic kyphoscoliosis may develop because of weak paraspinal musculature. Scoliosis further reduces chest-wall compliance and may lead to asymmetrical chest expansion. Together, these factors contribute to the development of ventilation/perfusion mismatch, increased work of breathing, and respiratory muscle fatigue.

Disease-Specific Aspects of Respiratory Care

Spinal Muscular Atrophy

Patients with SMA types 1 and 2 are at risk of respiratory complications. Ventilatory support during acute infectious exacerbations may be complicated by disease progression and thus difficult to withdraw.

Congenital Myopathies and Muscular Dystrophies

Most patients, even those who are asymptomatic, have restricted respiratory capacity and are at risk of insidious nocturnal hypoxemia. Sleep-related symptoms include sleep disturbance, nightmares, morning headache, daytime tiredness, and weight loss. Sudden respiratory failure may be precipitated by intercurrent infection or anesthesia and occur at any age. All patients with congenital myopathy should have baseline evaluation of their respiratory function as part of clinical and preoperative care. Regular chest physiotherapy, postural drainage, and assisted coughing techniques may improve respiratory toilet in patients with bulbar weakness, reduced vital capacity (VC), and recurrent aspiration. Respiratory infections should be treated early and aggressively.

Duchenne Muscular Dystrophy

The natural history of respiratory muscle involvement in DMD follows a characteristic pattern. First, an increase in VC that parallels somatic growth until the age of 10–12 years. During the next 2–4 years, most patients lose the ability to walk unaided and their respiratory function declines (VC decreases 8.5% per year). Sleep-disordered breathing is associated with a VC $< 60\%$ predicted for age. Sleep-disordered breathing and hypoventilation are associated with a VC $< 40\%$ predicted for age. In adults, a VC of <1.5 L or cough peak flow of <160 L/min predicts risk of respiratory failure, and a VC of <1 L is terminal without respiratory support.

Practical Issues during PICU Admission

Children with chronic NMD are particularly vulnerable to influenza, other viral respiratory infections, and aspiration. They require routine administration of pneumococcal and influenza vaccinations. Most children with chronic NMD admitted to PICU recover without needing invasive mechanical ventilation, but 25% require noninvasive respiratory support. The episode that necessitates admission may signify the inevitable decline in the underlying illness and prompt a decision about providing ongoing respiratory support.

ONGOING VENTILATORY SUPPORT

The indications for ongoing ventilatory support include CO_2 retention ($Paco_2 > 50$ mm Hg), chronic hypoxia ($Pao_2 < 90$ mm Hg), VC < 1 L, and recurrent pneumonia. The preferred method of home mechanical ventilation will depend on the clinical state of the patient, rate of progression of the underlying disorder, and quality of life considerations. Modes of support include bilevel positive-airway pressure by nasal mask or mechanical ventilation via tracheostomy. Home ventilation requires a large and ongoing support network for the patients and their families and may not be appropriate for all patients.

Long-term, Noninvasive Ventilation for Chronic NMD

Home noninvasive ventilation (NIV) is used increasingly in children with chronic NMD because it decreases hospitalization rates and improves respiratory function. NIV is not curative and does not prevent progression of the underlying neuromuscular disorder, but it may improve quality of life. The optimal time for introduction of NIV is controversial.

Delivery of Respiratory Support

NIV can be delivered by a nasal mask, face mask, or mouthpiece connected to bilevel, pressure-targeted ventilators. NIV is contraindicated in patients with upper airway obstruction and uncontrollable secretions. Severe swallowing impairment secondary to bulbar involvement is a relative contraindication. Complications of NIV include pneumothorax, facial irritation, gastric distension, and, in the long-term, midface hypoplasia.

Bulbar Dysfunction

Chronic NMDs may result in feeding difficulties, recurrent aspiration, dysarthria, poor articulation, and poor control of secretions. Feeding problems in the newborn period often necessitate gavage feeds and if persistent, insertion of a gastrostomy tube should be considered. Malnutrition can slow recovery after surgery or illness. Accelerated weight gain and improved respiratory function may follow gastrostomy placement.

Treatments for sialorrhea, such as anticholinergic agents and salivary gland botulinum toxin injections, may be effective but may cause increased viscosity of secretions and other side effects (**Table 31.4**).

Orthopedic Complications

Scoliosis and kyphosis are common complications of chronic NMDs and can affect mobility and respiratory function. Thoracic bracing does not prevent or reverse spinal curvature but can improve stability during sitting. Spinal fusion can halt progressive spinal deformity and preserves lung function. Postoperative complications are more common in children with VC of <30% predicted for age and those with a spinal curve of >100 degrees.

Orthopedic surgery may also be needed for congenital and acquired contractures and pathologic fractures secondary to disuse osteopenia. Passive stretching exercises, orthotics, splinting, and serial

TABLE 31.4

Management of Children with Chronic Neuromuscular Disorders

ASSOCIATED PROBLEMS	REFERRAL	POSSIBLE INTERVENTIONS
Skeletal Muscle Involvement		
Hypotonia Weakness Contractures	Physiotherapy Occupational therapy	Objective testing of muscle strength Regular exercise program Active and passive stretching Standing frame Orthotics/splinting—upper and lower limb Serial plaster casting Enhance mobility—walking frames or wheelchair Liaison with local services prior to discharge
Respiratory Muscle Involvement		
Reduced respiratory capacity Recurrent chest infections Aspiration Nocturnal hypoxia Respiratory failure	Physiotherapy Lung-function tests Sleep study Respiratory physician Occupational therapy	Breathing exercises Chest physiotherapy to clear secretions Seating assessment Influenza and pneumococcal vaccination Aggressive management of acute infections Nocturnal/daytime ventilation Liaise with local services
Bulbar Involvement		
Feeding and swallowing difficulties Failure to thrive Dysarthria Excessive drooling	Speech pathologist Dietitian Gastroenterologist Surgeon	Speech therapy Modified barium swallow Caloric supplementation/thickened feed Gavage feeding or gastrostomy feeding Anticholinergic medications Pharyngoplasty Salivary duct surgery/botulinum toxin injections
Cardiac Involvement		
Conduction defects Cardiomyopathy Cor pulmonale	Cardiologist	Electrocardiogram, Holter monitor, echocardiogram Medication if indicated
Other Areas of Associated Problems		
Developmental or psychosocial delay	Occupational therapy Physiotherapy Speech pathology Psychologist Developmental physician	Developmental stimulation Home programs Reassessment if deterioration

TABLE 31.4

Management of Children with Chronic Neuromuscular Disorders (*continued*)

ASSOCIATED PROBLEMS	REFERRAL	POSSIBLE INTERVENTIONS
Scoliosis	Physiotherapy Orthopedic surgeon	Spinal X-ray Monitoring of degree of curve Bracing Corrective surgery
Foot deformities	Physiotherapy Orthopedic surgeon	Splinting/serial casting Corrective surgery
Inability to perform activities of daily living Inability to achieve independence with bathing, toileting, dressing, feeding Difficulties with access Handwriting difficulties	Occupational therapy Community nurse	Aides for individual activities of daily living Wheelchair assessment Home nursing assistance Home and school modifications Typing and computer programs Car modifications Liaise with local services
Excessive weight gain Further limits mobility and exacerbates weakness	Dietitian Physiotherapy	Calorie-controlled diet Exercise program
Inability to participate in sport/leisure activities	Physiotherapy Occupational therapy	Liaison with/visit schools Sporting organizations for people with disabilities Hydrotherapy
Constipation	Dietitian Physician Gastroenterologist	High-fiber diet Laxatives/enemas
Depression or behavioral problems	Psychologist	Individual or family therapy Medication
Family financial and social difficulties	Social work Muscular Dystrophy Association Government assistance bodies	Disability allowance/pension Support groups Financial assistance with equipment and home modifications Transport and travel assistance
Planning future pregnancies	Geneticist Genetic counselor	Genetic counseling Planning prenatal diagnosis
Planning surgery	Consult with anesthesiologist Respiratory physician	Malignant hyperthermia precautions Lung-function tests and presurgical physiotherapy
Planning future employment	Vocational counseling service Occupational therapy	Planning school studies Vocational planning Training, work placement and support
Coordination of care	Pediatrician, pediatric neurologist, or rehabilitation specialist	Contact with general practitioner via telephone and letter Liaise with local services Arrange case conferences when necessary Determine timing of respiratory, orthopedic, and palliative interventions

Most ventilator-dependent adults consider that their quality of life is reasonable. Relatively few studies have been undertaken in children ventilated long term, but the information that is available suggests that their quality of life is considered good.

casting may be necessary in children who are immobilized for long periods by illness or surgery.

Cardiac Function

Symptomatic cardiac involvement is uncommon in the congenital myopathies and myasthenic syndromes, but cor pulmonale may be seen in those with advanced respiratory disease. Several of the congenital and LGMDs are associated with cardiomyopathy and conduction defects.

Advanced DMD is commonly associated with cardiac conduction defects, resting tachycardia, and cardiomyopathy. Mitral valve prolapse and pulmonary hypertension may also occur. Subclinical or clinical cardiac involvement is present in ~90% of Duchenne or Becker muscular dystrophy patients but is the cause of death in only 10% of men with DMD and 50% of patients with Becker muscular dystrophy. Progression of cardiomyopathy is prevented or slowed by early treatment with angiotensin-converting enzyme inhibitors.

Children with myotonic dystrophy rarely develop cardiomyopathy but commonly develop symptomatic or subclinical conduction disturbances that cause left ventricular dysfunction and may require a pacemaker.

Anesthesia

Subclinical respiratory insufficiency may be unmasked by anesthesia and exacerbated by postoperative atelectasis and spinal instrumentation. Preoperative assessment of respiratory state is important in helping to decide the timing of surgery. Patients should receive intensive preoperative physiotherapy, and must be mobilized as soon as possible after surgery (immobility exacerbates muscle weakness).

Children with myotonic dystrophy may be unusually sensitive to anesthetics and analgesics. Barbiturates, opiates, and nondepolarizing muscle relaxants risk prolonged postoperative sedation and apnea.

Malignant hyperthermia is an autosomal-dominant, pharmacogenetic disorder characterized by an increase in skeletal muscle metabolism in response to inhalation anesthetics and depolarizing muscle relaxants. The uncontrolled muscle contractions and hyperthermia may be fatal if untreated. Central core disease and minicore myopathy are associated with an increased risk of malignant hyperthermia. DMD is associated with a risk of life-threatening hyperkalemia after exposure to succinylcholine.

QUALITY OF LIFE IN CHILDREN VENTILATED FOR CHRONIC NMD

In a 15-year review of children with chronic NMD who were admitted to the PICU, most were discharged without the need for prolonged invasive ventilation, and only 9% of unplanned admissions ended in death. Nocturnal respiratory support was started in the PICU and continued after discharge in 23% of admissions. The authors concluded that "all children with underlying NMD should be provided with acute respiratory support in the anticipation that they are likely to recover. However, repeat admissions and chronic respiratory failure are likely and should be anticipated."

CHAPTER 32 ■ DEVELOPMENTAL NEUROBIOLOGY AND NEUROPHYSIOLOGY

LARRY W. JENKINS AND PATRICK M. KOCHANEK

Structural, biochemical, physiologic, and behavioral components of the brain differ from infancy to adolescence. Also, there are stages of development that are resistant or vulnerable to insults that affect neurologic outcome.

CENTRAL NERVOUS SYSTEM DEVELOPMENT

Brain Development Timeline

Central nervous system (CNS) development occurs through the process of neurulation during embryogenesis. The neural plate is formed by ectodermal tissue at ~2 weeks of gestation. By the 18th day of gestation, the neural plate forms the neural groove, which fuses, forming the neural tube in the 3rd gestational week, and is complete by the end of week 4. Throughout the first month of human gestation, specific CNS regions (e.g., forebrain, midbrain, and hindbrain) form. The hemispheres form in weeks 8–10. Neuronal proliferation is ongoing in weeks 8–18. Neuronal migration proceeds through weeks 12–24. Concomitant with regional CNS development, neurogenesis, proliferation, migration, differentiation, synaptogenesis, apoptosis, and myelination occur and continue up to 10 years of age (**Fig. 32.1**). Aberrations in any of these brain developmental processes may produce congenital CNS defects.

Development of Specific Brain Regions

Human brain growth starts in early gestation, peaks at 4 postnatal months, and continues for 2–3 postnatal years. The forebrain develops more slowly than the hindbrain (the medial hindbrain develops earlier than the lateral). The thalamus, hypothalamus, and mesencephalon develop during the early fetal and late embryonic periods. The pons and medulla of the hindbrain develop during gestational weeks 3–7.5. Neocortical and hippocampal structures grow mostly during the fetal period but do have some continuing neuronal and glial postnatal development.

Neurogenesis and Proliferation

The neural tube is formed by the neuroectoderm, with neuroepithelial cells differentiating into various types of neurons and glia. The mature human brain contains an estimated 10^{10} neurons. Neural precursor cells from the epithelium form the developing CNS and undergo mitotic arrest at various times during development. Prenatal brain development is characterized by rapid cell division under the control of numerous cell signaling pathways, including at least nine different growth factor cascades. It has been estimated that ~200,000 new neurons are produced each minute at between 8 and 18 weeks of gestation. After birth, neurogenesis occurs only in selected brain regions. Environmental or genetic stress during neurogenesis is a particularly vulnerable time for regional brain development. The CNS is more resistant to these stressors following neurogenesis. Fetal alcohol syndrome is a classic example of environmental stress that interferes with the developmental process of neurogenesis.

Programmed Cell Death

Neuronal cell type and number are regulated by apoptotic cell death during CNS development. Programmed cell death (PCD) begins in zones of proliferation and recurs as CNS remodeling proceeds. PCD persists postnatally owing to continued CNS development. Apoptotic regulation of neurons that undergo PCD prior to developing synaptic contacts (proliferative apoptosis) has been proposed to differ from target-dependent neuronal death pathways (neurotrophic-related apoptosis). Proliferative neuronal apoptosis prevents premature and dysfunctional neurogenesis from occurring.

Survival and death signals appear to play a key role in the evolution of neuronal death after CNS injuries such as asphyxia, TBI, seizures, infections, and other PICU-relevant insults. The Bcl-2 protein family, the adaptor protein Apaf1, and the cysteine protease caspase family are the principal regulators of PCD. As many as 70% of developing neurons die via PCD during embryogenesis to eliminate excess cell numbers and to assist in neural tube closure. Because of the upregulation of PCD during development, the developing CNS may be more prone to injury-related PCD than the adult brain.

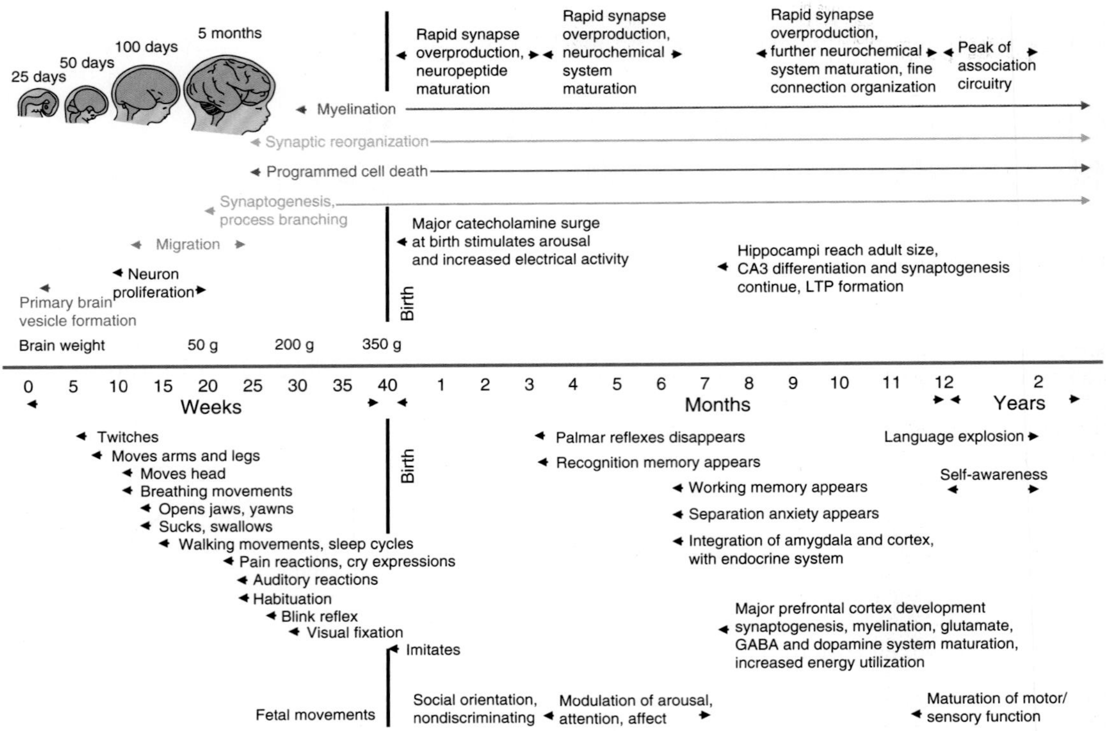

FIGURE 32.1. The key events of the human developmental timeline. The appearance of specific structural and functional developmental events is shown for the human fetus, infant, and young child up to 2 years of age. LTP, long-term potentiation; GABA, γ-aminobutyric acid. (Modified from Lagercrantz H, Ringstedt T. Organization of the neuronal circuits in the central nervous system during development. *Acta Paediatr* 2001;90:707–15; additional data from Levitt P. Structural and functional maturation of the developing primate brain. *J Pediatr* 2003;143:S35–S45; and from Herschkowitz N. Neurological bases of behavioral development in infancy. *Brain Dev* 2000;22:411–16.)

Migration, Differentiation, and Axonal Guidance

Neuronal migration occurs at between 12 and 24 gestational weeks and is modulated by neurotransmitters. Glutamate and *N*-methyl-D-aspartate (NMDA) receptor antagonists can inhibit neuronal migration and affect developmental neuronal apoptosis, CNS recovery, and plasticity. Stem cell commitment to neuronal lineage and neuronal progenitor specification are distinct steps of neurogenesis regulated by the same genes. Differentiated neurons possess unique and characteristic sizes, shapes, polarities, and expressions of neurotransmitters, neurotrophins, and receptors. Four primary types of signals guide axonal growth and target contact: chemoattractant, chemorepellent, contact attractive, and contact repellent. The first two classes are diffusible molecules that act over longer distances, while the latter two are within the extracellular matrix or membrane. Axonal pathfinding is most dependent on repulsive cues and pioneer axons that reach targets early in development. Some of these guidance molecules also affect cell migration, as both developmental processes tend to share common mechanisms.

Synaptogenesis, Gliogenesis, and Myelination

Synaptogenesis is one of the most important developmental processes and mechanism of recovery from CNS injury. Synaptogenesis is most rapid from ~20 to 24 weeks of gestation up to 8 months postnatally and continues at a high rate through puberty. Synaptogenesis persists throughout life (experience dependent rather than programmed) as does synapse loss. As a developing neuron reaches its destined position in the CNS, it extends dendrites and axons to distant targets via growth cones, which are guided by numerous extracellular molecules. On making target contact, presynaptic neurotransmitters or other secreted molecules diffuse and bind to the postsynaptic membrane. Synaptic vesicle accumulation in the presynaptic terminal of a brain region is a hallmark of the level of synapse maturation.

Glia are not passive during CNS development. Glia include astrocytes, oligodendrocytes, radial glia, and microglia. Astrocytic development occurs well after neuronal migration and differentiation, and oligodendrocytic development occurs after axonogenesis. Astrocyte functions in the CNS include structural support of neurons, ion homeostasis, ammonia detoxification, free radical scavenging, metal sequestration, growth factor production, immune response, and neuronal metabolic support. Astrocytes participate in synaptogenesis and neurogenesis as well as in cognitive function.

Microglia are CNS immune cells of myeloid origin that are similar to macrophages and represent 10% of the CNS cell populations in adults. They are normally in a resting state, but in response to infection or CNS injury, they enlarge and upregulate cytokines and chemokines, as well as surface antigens. They have been implicated in the response to encephalitis, ischemia, TBI, and demyelinating diseases.

Oligodendrocytes produce myelin, modulate axonal function in the CNS, and are vulnerable to excitotoxic injury, decreased trophin levels, and oxidative stress conditions. Neurons and oligodendrocytes signal each other during myelination to modulate neurofilament spacing, phosphorylation, and axonal diameter. Myelination continues at a high rate until 10 years of age, and to some degree throughout adulthood. New evidence suggests that myelination may even be an important mechanism of activity-dependent plasticity, influenced by environmental factors. Neural activity also affects myelination. White matter development in children correlates with motor skill and increased cognitive function. Magnetic resonance imaging (MRI) has shown correlation between white matter development and cognitive function. It has been postulated that increased white matter conduction speed may have as strong an influence on synaptic amplitude as do changes in pre- and postsynaptic elements and neurotransmitter function.

NEUROTRANSMITTER AND NEUROTROPHIN DEVELOPMENT

The synapse is the point of information flow between neurons where the release of and response to neurotransmitters occur. Synaptic activity mediated by neurotransmitters is a requirement for the survival of developing synaptic contacts in the immature brain. Neurotransmitters both mediate synaptic transmission and have trophic functions. An important role is played by glutamate, γ-aminobutyric acid (GABA), acetylcholine, catecholamines, serotonin, and opioids. The developmental neurotransmitter timeline displays considerable regional and temporal variation, which affects age- and regional-dependent injury, manipulations of the transmitter systems, and the possible effects of the transmitter systems on recovery. Insults to the brain at vulnerable developmental periods can produce long-term structural and functional CNS changes. The importance of neurotransmitters during CNS development is demonstrated by age-dependent adverse effects with the manipulation of neurotransmitter systems, especially glutamatergic and GABAergic systems, using sedatives, or anesthetics, after ischemia, status epilepticus, or TBI. Fetuses and newborn infants are particularly vulnerable. Before birth, the majority of neuromodulators and neurotransmitters increase during synaptogenesis. At birth, increased brain activity and a surge of catecholaminergic activity are associated with arousal. A decrease in adenosine occurs, along with a desensitization of adenosine receptors during the first postnatal days. In addition, periods of developmental "switches" in neurotransmitter function occur at birth, and sensitivity to glutamate toxicity may be especially high at this time.

Glutamate and GABA

Amino acids are the most abundant neurotransmitters in the CNS and have important functions in brain development. Many of the CNS behavioral and functional milestones during development can be correlated with the maturation of glutamatergic and GABAergic systems and their receptors.

Glutamate Receptor Development

Almost half of the synapses of the forebrain are glutamatergic, and excessive glutamate synapse creation occurs during the most active period of synaptogenesis in the first two postnatal years. The NMDA receptors (NMDARs) are a glutamate receptor subtype that regulates neuronal survival during development, axon and dendrite arborization, and synaptogenesis. Immature NMDARs are more excitable during early phases of development to promote use-dependent plastic changes necessary for normal development, learning, and memory. The brain is therefore more sensitive to excitotoxic insults, such as ischemia, TBI, and status epilepticus. Either too much or too little NMDAR activation can result in abnormal developmental processes and even neuronal death. Research is necessary in this area regarding the effects of long-term use of sedative and anesthetic agents in infants.

GABA and the GABA Switch

GABA also has trophic actions on synaptic and neuritic outgrowth and on neuronal viability during development. An estimated 25%–40% of all CNS synapses contain GABA, and its deficiency is fatal to infants. GABAergic inhibition of excitatory synaptic CNS activity occurs by neuronal hyperpolarization via postsynaptic $GABA_A$ (outward chloride channel) and $GABA_B$ (G-protein–coupled inward potassium channel) receptors in the adult brain. The inhibitory actions of GABA are also mediated by a reduction of excitatory neurotransmitter release via presynaptic $GABA_B$ receptors. In contrast, GABA is an excitatory neurotransmitter during prenatal development in humans. The $GABA_A$ receptor binds barbiturates, benzodiazepines, and ethanol, which alter chloride (Cl^-) flux through the channel. Thus, GABA is mainly excitatory during the fetal period but becomes inhibitory around birth in humans. The so-called "GABA switch" marks the point at which GABA becomes an inhibitory rather than excitatory neurotransmitter.

Glutamate synaptic transmission is initially based on NMDAR function at developmental stages when the CNS lacks functional α-amino-3-hydroxy-5-methyl-4-isoxazolepropionic acid (AMPA) receptors, and the $GABA_A$ receptor stimulates NMDAR calcium influx, a role usually performed in the mature brain by the AMPA receptor. $GABA_A$ receptor stimulation induces depolarization of immature neurons and increases NMDA-mediated intracellular Ca^{2+} during late human prenatal development. The switch from GABA excitation to inhibition that occurs at birth in humans is likely the result of a GABA-mediated induction of the expression and upregulation of the potassium–chloride cotransporter (KCC2), which serves to decrease the high Cl^- content of immature neurons. Several types of brain injury downregulate KCC2 and thus could affect the development of the GABA switch of the developing brain.

Adenosine

Adenosine is a neuronal, glial, and cerebrovascular transmitter that affects the excitability of neurons and the functional processes of oligodendrocyte progenitor proliferation and myelination during infancy and childhood. A_1 receptors are inhibitory and provide a line of defense against developmental excitotoxic cascades. A_{2a} receptors modulate dopaminergic D_2 receptor function, are concentrated in the basal ganglia, and may be an important therapeutic target in brain injury.

Acetylcholine

Acetylcholine is a major excitatory transmitter that is important in cognition and attention, motor function, and pain. Five muscarinic receptor subtypes have been identified, with $M_{1,2,5}$ coupled primarily to phosphoinositide turnover and $M_{2,4}$ coupled to cyclic AMP production. Abnormal cholinergic projections alter cortical development, plasticity, and function and are critical to cognitive function in the child. Cholinergic systems also participate in toxic excitatory neurotransmitter cascades in epilepsy, TBI, and cerebral ischemia.

Norepinephrine and Dopamine

Monoaminergic neurons form during telencephalic vesicle formation, and catecholamines are thought to play a significant role in early development. Norepinephrine is important in cognitive function, anxiety, arousal, and attention, and is necessary for normal brain development. Noradrenergic neurons appear at 5–6 weeks in humans, and adrenergic α_2 and β_1 receptors predominate in the CNS. In addition, a surge of catecholamine levels is associated with increased brain activity and arousal at birth (**Fig. 32.1**). Dopamine is also important in cognition, motor function, and addiction behavior. Dopaminergic neurons begin to develop at 6–8 weeks in humans. D_1 receptors, in particular, are critical for working memory function during the first year of life (**Fig. 32.1**). The use of catecholamines for blood pressure support in infants with immature or injury-altered blood–brain barrier (BBB) function warrants consideration owing to the potent catecholaminergic excitatory actions at birth, which in theory could be potentially excitotoxic at this critical developmental time.

Serotonin

Serotonin (5-HT) neurons have extensive contacts and synchronize complex motor and sensory information. Serotonin modulates developmental proliferation, differentiation, migration, and synaptogenesis. Aberrations in serotonin levels during development and early childhood result in CNS connectivity malformations and may contribute to later psychiatric disorders.

Neurotrophins

Growth factors, both intrinsic and extrinsic to the CNS, play a major role in normal brain function, development, injury, and repair. Nerve growth factor (NGF), brain-derived neurotrophic factor (BDNF), and neurotrophins 3–5 (NT3, NT4/5) are diffusible peptides that compose the neurotrophin family of trophic factors in mammalian brain. NTs are critical for neuronal survival, and the loss of NT activity after CNS injury can contribute to neuronal death and loss of function. NT receptors couple to a number of protein and lipid kinase intracellular pathways, such as the mitogen-activated protein kinase (MAPK), the phosphoinositide 3-kinase (PI3K), and the PKB pathways. This coupling is extremely important to the regulation of neural survival or death after ischemia, TBI, or other CNS insults.

SYNAPTIC AND BEHAVIORAL DEVELOPMENT

CNS electrical activity develops and matures with gestational and postnatal age. Even when preterm, infants show quantitative changes in electrical encephalogram (EEG) before and after birth. There can be a 30% increase in EEG amplitude and a 60% increase in continuity over the first postnatal weeks due to the arousal effects of neurotransmitters, neuromodulators, and neurotrophins. Behavioral and functional milestones correlate with the development of glutamatergic and GABAergic neurotransmission and synaptic maturity. As NMDA, AMPA, GABA, and neurotrophin systems mature, long-term potentiation (LTP) (an increase in synaptic strength that may correlate with memory storage) and long-term depression (LTD) (a decrease in synaptic strength that may also correlate with memory storage) are established. LTP and LTD are likely associated with cognitive function and occur at 7–10 postnatal months.

Primary behavioral and functional developments in the first 2 years (**Fig. 32.1**) include the cortical inhibition of brainstem reflexes and the development of recognition and working memory. The cortical inhibition of brainstem reflexes due to maturation of GABA inhibition and myelination occurs postnatally at ~3 months. Excessive cortical inhibition of brainstem nuclei, such as respiratory centers, may increase the risk for the sudden infant death syndrome. The development of recognition memory also takes place near the postnatal age of 3 months and requires adequate hippocampal and cortical visual development. Working memory (recent past memory that enables one to solve a current cognitive task) develops over the latter half of the first year of life, is dependent on prefrontal cortical function, and is modulated by glutamate, GABA, and dopamine. Between 7 and 10 months, infant prefrontal cortices undergo dramatic maturation in synaptic density and neurotransmitter systems and have increased glucose utilization required for both growth and activity-dependent processes. Similarly, the hippocampus reaches adult size, and synaptogenesis, coupled with the maturation of neurotransmitter systems, makes LTP development possible. During this time of rapid growth and activity-dependent synaptogenesis and maturation, the infant brain is especially vulnerable to injury, resulting in either short- or long-term changes in behavioral function. For example, at 2 years of age, rapid language development and acquisition occur, which has been further linked to increased connections between prefrontal cortex and associational cortical regions with the limbic and motor systems. Significant synaptogenesis also occurs in many of these same brain regions.

ANTIOXIDANT DEVELOPMENT

Major antioxidant enzyme systems include peroxyredoxins, thioredoxins, superoxide dismutase, catalase, and peroxidases. Glutathione, vitamin E, ascorbate, and coenzyme Q are water- or lipid-soluble low-molecular-weight antioxidants. The levels of these antioxidant enzymes and molecules in the brain are low during fetal development and increase at birth during the transition to a high-oxygen environment. Catalase appears to be more of a contributor to antioxidant defenses in the immature brain. Based on the antioxidant enzyme profile during brain development, the immature CNS may be at greater risk than the adult brain for oxidative injury.

CEREBROVASCULAR AND METABOLISM DEVELOPMENT AND FUNCTION

Vascular Development

The CNS vascular system develops in three phases: vasculogenesis, angiogenesis, and barrier genesis. The first functional organ to develop is the cardiovascular system, with blood vessels generated by mesodermal differentiated endothelial cells. These cells give rise to new blood vessels by a process called *vasculogenesis*, as compared to the generation of new blood vessels from existing vessels, called *angiogenesis*. The CNS developmental rate of angiogenesis is maximal around birth and early infancy. Vascular endothelial growth factor, its endothelial receptors, and the TGF-β family have major roles in CNS angiogenesis. Platelet-derived growth factor, numerous adhesion molecules, and factors/receptors that provide axonal cues also modulate CNS vascularization. Immature blood vessels are stabilized by *pericytes* (vascular mural cells) that are recruited to endothelial cells by these factors. Tissue oxygen levels are very important, low levels stimulate angiogenesis, and high oxygen levels inhibit this process.

Cerebral Blood Flow and Vascular Reactivity

Impaired cerebral blood flow (CBF) autoregulation may contribute to secondary injury across the age spectrum. Loss of pressure autoregulation could underlie the marked vulnerability of the acutely injured brain to otherwise tolerable hypotension that contributes to periventricular hemorrhagic venous infarction in preterm infants.

Perfusion Pressure Autoregulation of Cerebral Blood Flow

Pressure autoregulation is the major cerebrovascular response to acute changes in perfusion pressure, changes that result, at the extreme range, either in hypotension with hypoperfusion or in hypertension with hyperemia and BBB disruption. Vascular tone in the cerebral circulation compensates for changes in cerebral perfusion pressure (CPP) over a range of pressures to maintain CBF constant (between a CPP of ~40–160 mm Hg in adults) (**Fig. 32.2**). CPP is equal to the difference between mean arterial pressure and intracranial pressure. Autoregulation occurs instantaneously and is believed to be mediated by changes in vascular smooth muscle tension by a direct myogenic mechanism. Developmental studies of pressure autoregulation in newborns suggest a narrower perfusion pressure range, with a similar lower limit to adults—but an upper limit that is only ~90–100 mm Hg (**Fig. 32.3**). Resting mean arterial

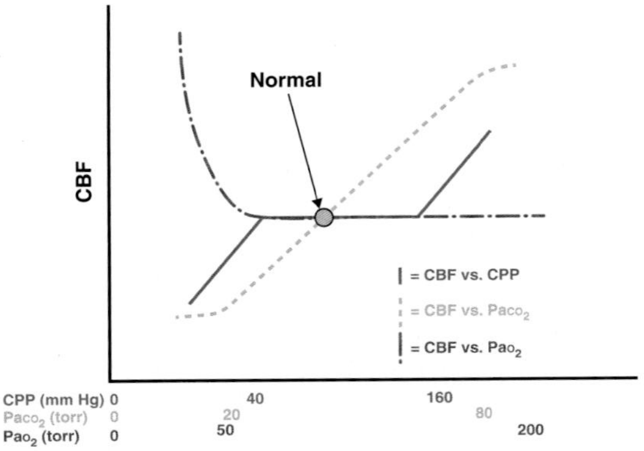

FIGURE 32.2. Relationships between CBF and CPP, Pa_{CO_2}, and Pa_{O_2} across therapeutic ranges generally encountered in the PICU. These values are provided based on normative data from adults. Pressure autoregulation maintains CBF constant between a CPP of between ~40 and 160 mm Hg. CBF is linearly related to Pa_{CO_2}, with an approximate 4% change in CBF per torr change in Pa_{CO_2} between ~20 and 80 torr. Below 20 torr, this curve dramatically flattens. Above ~80–100 torr, this relationship also more gradually flattens. The relationship between CBF and Pa_{O_2} is relatively flat until a Pa_{O_2} of ~50 mm Hg is reached, below which a dramatic increase in CBF is observed.

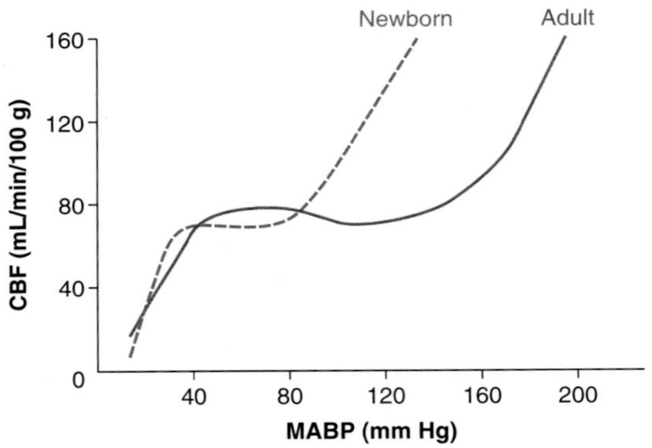

FIGURE 32.3. Comparison of the relative pressure: CBF autoregulatory curves from studies of subhuman primate newborns and adults. In the adult, CBF is maintained relatively constant when arterial blood pressure is between 50 and 160 mm Hg, while in newborns, CBF is maintained over a narrower range owing to a reduced upper limit of CBF autoregulation. CBF autoregulation of newborns makes them more vulnerable to both hypotensive and hypertensive episodes. MABP, mean arterial blood pressure. (From Hardy P, Varma DR, Chemtob S. Control of cerebral and ocular blood flow autoregulation in neonates. *Pediatr Clin North Am* 1997;44:137–52.)

blood pressure is substantially lower in the preterm than in the term newborn, demonstrating that the autoregulatory vascular reserve is much less. Evidence suggests that, in critically ill infants, the autoregulatory responses may be absent or significantly impaired and that early postnatal hypercapnia may further impair pressure autoregulation.

Cerebrovascular Response to Pa_{O_2}

The cerebrovascular response to changes in Pa_{O_2} is mediated locally and results in vasodilation under hypoxic conditions and in vasoconstriction with hyperoxia to maintain CBF constant over a range of Pa_{O_2} values (**Fig. 32.2**). This curve is relatively flat, except at reduced Pa_{O_2} levels (less than ~50 torr, 90% Sa_{O_2}), at which a steep rise in CBF curve occurs to maintain cerebral oxygen delivery. The cerebrovascular response occurs in parallel with carotid body sensors that adjust systemic blood pressure and respiration to compensate for changes in blood oxygen levels. The dramatic increase in CBF (and cerebral blood volume) when Pa_{O_2} is <60 torr is the basis for meticulously avoiding even mild hypoxemia in patients with reduced intracranial compliance.

Cerebrovascular Response to Pa_{CO_2}

The cerebrovascular response to changes in Pa_{CO_2} is mediated locally by changes in perivascular pH. In contrast to changes in perfusion pressure and Pa_{O_2}, a nearly linear relationship between Pa_{CO_2} and CBF exists between the range of Pa_{CO_2} values of 20 and 80 torr, with an approximate 4%/mm Hg change in Pa_{CO_2} (**Fig. 32.2**). Vasodilation increases with hypercapnia, and vasoconstriction with hypocapnia. At extremes of hypocapnia or hypercapnia, the response is blunted. This vasoreactivity is the basis of hyperventilation-mediated reduction in CBF and cerebral blood volume used therapeutically to reduce intracranial hypertension. The CBF response to changes in Pa_{CO_2} is related to the level of CBF at rest in a given brain region; thus, hyperventilation tends to equalize CBF throughout the brain. In addition, the CBF response to changes in Pa_{CO_2} is transient, lasting less than 24 hours for a given change and is believed to be mediated by compensatory changes in brain interstitial bicarbonate concentration, which take time to manifest. When a hyperventilation-mediated reduction in Pa_{CO_2} is used to reduce intracranial pressure, relative ischemia has been suggested to occur, in part because of a reduction in CBF. Relative ischemia may also result from limited off-loading of oxygen from hemoglobin as the dissociation curve shifts to the left. CO_2 reactivity appears to be less vulnerable to injury than is pressure autoregulation. Altered CO_2 reactivity may suggest substantial damage, and global loss of CO_2 reactivity is a concerning finding. Pressure autoregulation is maintained despite a new baseline CBF value when Pa_{CO_2} is altered.

Cerebrovascular Regulation—Developmental Issues

Birth involves a transition from a hypoxic to an oxygen-rich environment and it appears that, even in term neonates, it takes several days for vascular responses to mature. Studies in preterm human infants have confirmed that CBF increases over the first three postnatal days. Similarly, CO_2 reactivity increases from birth to early postnatal age, as do EEG amplitude and arterial blood pressure. CBF increases in children until 5–6 years of age, when it may be as much as 50%–85% higher than in adults, and then decreases to adult levels by 15–19 years of age. CBF parallels glucose metabolism; peak CBF and glucose metabolism occur at 3–9 years of age, corresponding to a very active growth period. It is estimated that human infants utilize up to 20% of their energy needs from ketones during the postnatal period.

Cerebral Blood Flow–Metabolism Coupling

CBF is tightly coupled to brain metabolism normally. It has been shown that CBF–metabolism coupling appears intact in normal newborn infants. The peak in cerebral glucose utilization during development correlates with the density of glucose transport proteins. Postnatal changes in regional CBF and cerebral metabolism occur in parallel in the human infant, with the highest rates of local cerebral metabolic rate for glucose (LCMRg) and CBF occurring at between 3 and 9 years of age during the well-recognized period of rapid cognitive development. Glucose is normally the lone cerebral substrate fueling active growth during this same period.

Cerebral Metabolism

Glucose serves as the major energy source for the developing brain. Glucose utilization through glycolytic and oxidative decarboxylation pathways parallels energy demands. Consequently, LCMRg increases during critical periods of growth and functional activity. Glucose entry into brain occurs via glucose transporter proteins (GLUTs). GLUT expression in the developing brain is proportional to energy demand, increases during maturation. Peak GLUT protein expression occurs during synaptogenesis, correlating with glutamate receptor maturity and learning and memory development.

The child's brain has a considerable metabolic demand compared to adults. Glucose utilization in 5-week-old infants in most brain regions is 71%–93% of that in the adult brain. LCMRg increases over the next 3 months, especially in the basal ganglia and the parietal, temporal, and occipital cortices. Frontal cortex LCMRg further increases by 8 months—at which time, cognitive function is rapidly developing. Adult levels of LCMRg are found by the time children are 2 years of age. LCMRg increases further until it reaches its highest levels, which are maintained until age 9. From this point forward, LCMRg declines until about age 20.

The immature brain can also utilize lactic acid, ketone bodies, and other metabolites (e.g., amino acids and free fatty acids). Brain monocarboxylate transporters for lactate and pyruvate develop over the midgestation period, providing another significant energy source, using both extracellular lactate and pyruvate as substrates. Lactate and pyruvate have also been shown to modulate the LTP and LTD that may be involved in synaptic plasticity critical to cognitive development at later stages of brain maturation. Due to the high fat ingestion of infants, more ketones are available in infant blood than in adult blood and can represent up to 20% of the carbon skeletons used in energy production. The BBB is quite permeable to ketones, and ketones play a more important role in bioenergetics of the immature CNS. CNS use of ketones may also be linked to amino acid and lipid biosynthetic pathway precursors, which are subsequently used in developmental membrane and myelin formation. Once the child is no longer dependent on maternal milk, the use of ketones as a metabolic fuel decreases as well.

BLOOD–BRAIN BARRIER AND CHOROID PLEXUS DEVELOPMENT

The BBB isolates brain blood compartments, provides selective transport of metabolites, ions, and molecules, and either metabolizes or modifies many blood- or brain-borne substances (**Fig. 32.4**). The BBB is impermeable to hydrophilic molecules, ions, and proteins, while key metabolic substrates (e.g., glucose) enter via transport proteins and water passes through the BBB via aquaporin-4 channels. Numerous metabolic barriers block the passage of molecules, including P-glycoprotein (involved in energy-dependent movement of hydrophobic drugs out of the CNS) and enzymes (e.g., monoamine oxidase), which protect synaptic function.

It is not clear if the BBB is "leaky" during fetal development and in the newborn infant. Tight junctions develop early during CNS maturation, and most proteins do not gain access to the extracellular compartment via the BBB during development. Cerebrospinal fluid (CSF) protein concentration is higher during early brain development and is thought to result from an immature choroid plexus; however, high CSF protein concentrations during development are not reflected in the extracellular space because of junctional complexes forming barriers at the CSF–brain interfaces that are not found in the adult brain. The BBB's permeability to ions and amino acids develops as transport systems mature in the brain; however, lipid-insoluble molecules are more permeable in the immature brain than in the adult brain. The fetal BBB permeability to macromolecules is similar to adults, but small molecules enter the fetal brain more readily.

Small lipophilic molecules, such as CO_2, O_2, and ethanol, can readily pass through the BBB. The mature BBB is impermeable to many molecules and substances due to cerebrovascular endothelial cell tight junctions,

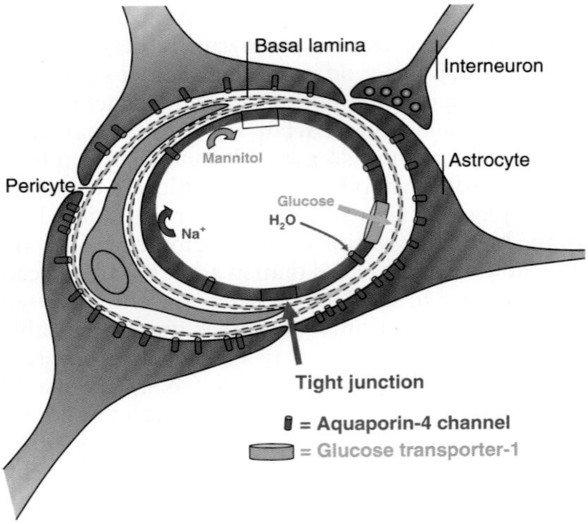

FIGURE 32.4. The structure of the mature BBB consists of endothelial cells connected by tight junctions, specialized supportive cells called pericytes, a basal lamina, and perivascular astrocytic end feet. (Modified from Abbott NJ, Ronnback L, Hansson E. Astrocyte-endothelial interactions at the blood–brain barrier. *Nat Rev Neurosci* 2006;7:41–53.)

which form the complete zona occludens (**Fig. 32.4**). Small polar molecules needed for brain function, such as glucose and amino acids, are transported across the barrier by carrier proteins, other small molecules and lipids are transported across by receptor-mediated endocytosis. The cerebrovascular endothelial cells contain monoamine oxidase and can defend brain synaptic function against circulating catecholamines. In addition, the barrier is surrounded by astrocyte foot processes that further modulate the movement of substances across the BBB via channels, transporters, and intracellular metabolism. Cerebrovascular tight junctions effectively prevent the movement of hydrophilic substances, such as cations (Na^+, K^+) and osmolar agents (e.g., mannitol), along with proteins, making osmolar gradients rather than oncotic gradients critical to water movement (**Fig. 32.4**). Water movement across the BBB is mediated via special water channels, termed *aquaporins*.

CEREBROSPINAL FLUID DYNAMICS

The major and minor pathways of CSF circulation differ in the developing brain compared to the adult. The major pathway of CSF absorption is via the arachnoid villi (arachnoid granulation) into the venous sinuses. The minor pathway includes drainage via ventricular ependyma, the interstitial and perivascular space, and perineural lymphatics. In adult humans, CSF production is around 500 mL/24 hours, and turns over 3–4 times a day. The two drainage pathways maintain normal homeostasis and neurochemical milieu. The CSF circulation begins in development, with choroid plexus formation at around 40–60 days of gestation. The arachnoid villi appear just before birth, and CSF reabsorption occurs at later ages. The minor CSF pathway is the primary route for CSF dynamics in the developing immature human brain because arachnoid villi function does not occur until the late infancy.

CHAPTER 33 ■ MOLECULAR BIOLOGY OF BRAIN INJURY

PATRICK M. KOCHANEK, HÜLYA BAYIR, LARRY W. JENKINS, AND ROBERT S. B. CLARK

INJURY RESPONSE IN THE IMMATURE BRAIN

The immature brain is more resistant to injury and more capable of recovery due to enhanced plasticity (ability to rewire or repair). Unfortunately, critical windows in development also represent periods of enhanced vulnerability. For example, the small size of the infant skull may predispose to a more diffuse pattern of injury from a traumatic impact. Despite increased plasticity, outcomes from brain injury in young children are often poorer than in adults. Mechanisms of injury differ in children, cardiac arrest is more likely due to asphyxia, and traumatic brain injury (TBI) is more likely due to abuse. Thus, although the developing brain exhibits resistance and resilience to injury, the mechanisms of injury are often more severe.

PATHWAYS AND APPLICATIONS TO PEDIATRIC INTENSIVE CARE

Secondary Injury

The essence of neurointensive care is the prevention of secondary injury. Two distinct types of secondary injury occur. Endogenous secondary injury cascades involve processes such as excitotoxicity, oxidative stress, and delayed neuronal death cascades that kill neurons and injure other components of the central nervous system (CNS). Exogenous secondary injury involves critically ill patients who suffer secondary insults in the field, emergency room, or ICU (e.g., hypotension and hypoxia). Normally tolerated secondary insults can exacerbate CNS consequences due to an enhanced vulnerability after cardiac arrest, stroke, TBI, status epilepticus (SE), or CNS infection.

Evolution of Secondary Injury

The five categories of secondary injury (**Fig. 33.1**) include those associated with (a) ischemia and energy failure, (b) excitotoxicity, (c) inflammation, (d) cerebral swelling, and (e) axonal injury. Within each category, a constellation of mediators of secondary damage is involved. Additional constituents are the roles of endogenous neuroprotectants, repair, and regeneration.

Ischemia

Global Cerebral Ischemia. The brain is exquisitely vulnerable to ischemia. Interruption in global cerebral blood flow (CBF), such as in cardiac arrest, initiates a stereotypic time course of events due to acute cellular energy failure. Phosphocreatine is depleted in 1 minute, and the adenylate energy charge is depleted in ~5 minutes. Membrane failure follows, with loss of ionic gradients, increases in intracellular calcium (Ca^{2+}) and sodium (Na^{+}), and a decrease in intracellular potassium (K^{+}). Free fatty acid release from the neuronal membrane occurs, and electroencephalogram (EEG) and evoked potentials fail. Sustained energy failure beyond a critical duration causes irreversible damage to neurons. During complete global brain ischemia, light microscopy of brain tissue reveals no pathologic derangements, and electron microscopy reveals only chromatin clumping. Damage to neurons, glia, and white matter does not manifest until reperfusion. The duration of irreversibility for global cerebral ischemia due to ventricular fibrillation (VF) cardiac arrest is 5–10 minutes, although it may be modified by factors such as temperature, blood glucose concentration, and pH.

Focal Cerebral Ischemia. Unlike global brain ischemia, focal ischemic insults (strokes) produce brain regions with differing blood flow reduction related to the vascular anatomy surrounding the area of occlusion. The typical result is an ischemic core, in which flow reductions are profound, surrounded by penumbral region that has less severe reductions. Protein synthesis and glucose utilization are impacted. Peri-infarct depolarization waves contribute to damage in the penumbra by transiently increasing metabolic demands. EEG fails at a CBF < 30 mL/100 g/min, hemiparesis is seen at CBF thresholds of ~23 mL/100 g/min, and anoxic depolarization occurs at CBF values 15–20 mL/100 g/min, resulting in ionic failure. If neuronal metabolic demands are increased (i.e., hyperthermia, seizures), neuronal death could be triggered at a higher CBF threshold. Neuronal death in focal cerebral ischemia involves necrosis in regions of permanent energy failure and mixed or apoptotic phenotypes in penumbral regions. However, biochemical footprints of apoptosis are seen even in core regions.

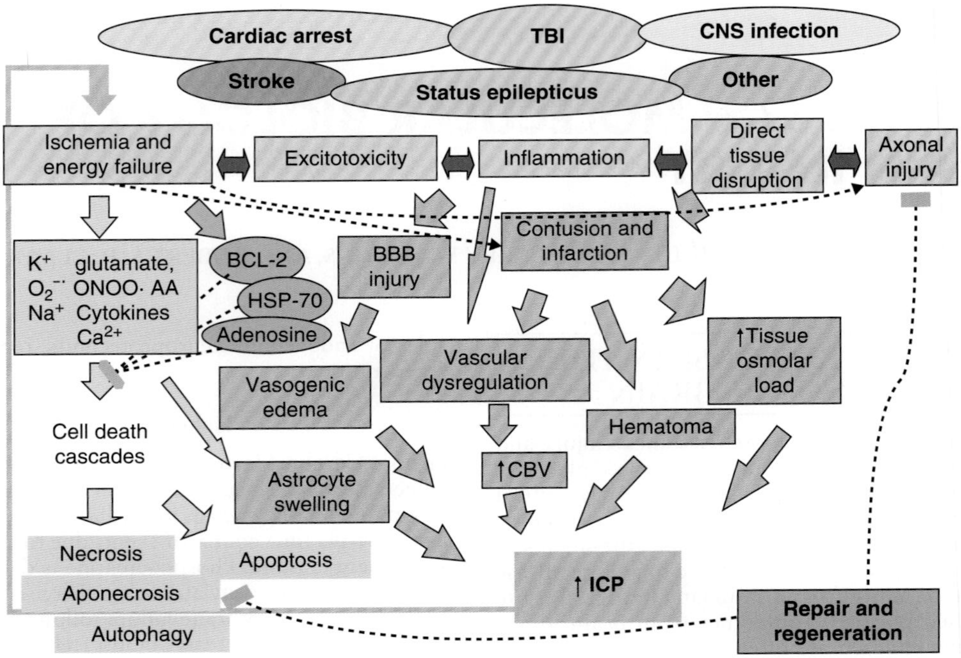

FIGURE 33.1. Secondary cascades triggered by the five initiators of secondary damage are shown for cell death cascades (*gray*), and for brain swelling–related process (*stippled gray*). In addition, a sixth category of endogenous neuroprotectants and repair and regeneration is initiated; the components of this cascade are shown in *black*. TBI, traumatic brain injury; O_2^-, superoxide anion; ONOO, peroxynitrite; AA, arachidonic acid; HSP-70, heat shock protein 70; ICP, intracranial pressure.

Posttraumatic Ischemia. Early hypoperfusion or ischemia after severe TBI in infants and children is associated with poor outcome. Regional hypoperfusion is common in contused brain regions and may be mediated by a reduced vasodilatory response to nitric oxide (NO), cyclic guanosine monophosphate (cGMP), cyclic AMP (cAMP), and prostanoids, reduced NO production by endothelial NO synthase (NOS), or the release of vasoconstrictors, such as superoxide anion or endothelin-1.

Ischemia in Other PICU-Relevant Central Nervous System Insults. Ischemia in other disorders, such as meningitis and SE, is less well defined. In meningitis, vascular dysregulation may be mediated by superoxide anion, endothelin, and disturbed regulation of NO production. In SE, metabolic coupling causes CBF to increase early, as much as fourfold, to meet increased metabolic demands.

Cell Death Pathways

Selective Vulnerability. Neurons in specific brain regions that are exceptionally vulnerable during global brain ischemia include the CA1 region of the hippocampus; cerebral cortex layers 3, 5, and 6; cerebellar Purkinje cells; and some brainstem nuclei in infants. That these neurons lack a unique vascular distribution suggests intrinsic vulnerability. A process known as *delayed neuronal death* causes these highly vulnerable neurons to die after threshold insults. During ischemia, cellular membrane failure occurs, with Ca^+ and Na^+ accumulation and K^+ efflux. In delayed neuronal death, electrophysiologic studies have revealed neuronal hyperexcitability in these regions after reperfusion, followed by a second wave of irreversible Ca^{2+} accumulation at ~48 hours.

Different neurons are selectively vulnerable after experimental TBI and models of epilepsy, predominantly the hippocampal neurons in the dentate hilus and the CA3 region. In experimental SE, limbic structures, including hippocampus, the piriform cortex, temporal cortex, and amygdala, are vulnerable. In meningitis models, the granular layer of the dentate gyrus of the hippocampus is highly vulnerable, which may underlie learning deficits seen in this condition.

Necrosis and Apoptosis. Neuronal death can occur through multiple pathways including necrosis, programmed cell death (PCD) or apoptosis, and mixed phenotypes. Necrosis involves progressive derangements in energy and substrate metabolism, followed by morphologic changes that include swelling of cells and organelles, subsurface cellular blebbing, amorphous deposits in mitochondria, condensation of nuclear chromatin, and, finally, breaks in plasma and organellar membranes. Neuronal death after hypoxic–ischemic insults can also occur through PCD or two additional forms of delayed neuronal death (necroptosis and pyroptosis). Local factors and the severity of ischemia determine whether injured neurons recover or undergo PCD or necrosis.

Autophagy. Autophagy mediates normal turnover of cellular constituents, such as organelles and membranes, using lysosomal degradation. It is associated with cell death during starvation. After ischemia and TBI, disruption of this process may lead to "autophagic stress," a disequilibrium between autophagic vacuole formation and degradation.

Key Initiators

Energy Failure. Energy failure sustained beyond a critical period produces neuronal membrane failure, Na^+ and Ca^{2+} accumulation, K^+ efflux, cellular swelling, and acute failure of organelles such as mitochondria and the endoplasmic reticulum (ER). Three pathways are involved. First, Ca^{2+} activates several degradative enzymes (including calpain proteases and phospholipases) that modify mitochondrial proteins and lipids. Second, oxidative stress further modifies mitochondrial constituents. Finally, unchecked Ca^{2+} sequestration in mitochondria leads to mitochondrial permeability. Links between mitochondrial failure, excitotoxicity, and oxidative stress play a key role. Cyclosporine-A blocks formation of the mitochondrial permeability transition pore and is neuroprotective in experimental models. The ER normally sequesters Ca^{2+}, and the resultant high concentration is important to activating enzymes that control protein folding. Ischemia induces Ca^{2+} release from the ER when stimulated by inositol 1,4,5-triphosphate (IP3) or activation of ryanodine receptors. IP3 is produced in the activation of metabotropic glutamate receptors in the excitotoxic process. Reduced ER Ca^{2+} concentration can trigger apoptosis.

Excitotoxicity. Excitotoxicity is the process by which glutamate and other excitatory amino acids (EAAs) cause neuronal damage. Glutamate levels increase in the brain early after ischemia or TBI as a result of release and/or failure of reuptake. The three main ionotropic glutamate receptors are the *N*-methyl-D-aspartate (NMDA), kainate, and α-amino-3-hydroxy-5-methyl-4-isoxazoleproprionic acid (AMPA) receptors. NMDA receptors allow Ca^{2+} influx, both directly and through voltage-gated channels, whereas the non-NMDA receptors mediate Na^+ influx with secondary action on voltage-gated Ca^{2+} channels and reverse action of the Na^+/Ca^{2+} transporter. Glutamate also acts at metabotropic receptors, which trigger second messenger systems and increase intracellular Ca^{2+} levels by causing a release of intracellular stores. Increased intracellular Ca^{2+} triggers processes that lead to cell injury or death, including oxidative and nitrative stress, mitochondrial or ER failure, and activation of Ca^{2+}-dependent proteases. Physiologic levels of glutamate are essential to neuronal survival, whereas excessive levels are neurotoxic. NMDA receptor subunits (NR2A and NR2B) may have different roles. Developmental differences in these two receptor subtypes may underlie age-related differences in neuronal vulnerability to anesthetics.

Therapies that have antiexcitotoxic properties include hypothermia, barbiturates, inhaled anesthetics, calcium channel blockers, and anticonvulsants. Other drugs that affect glutamate physiology include NMDA and AMPA receptor antagonists, glutamate release inhibitors, NMDA channel blockers, NMDA glycine-site antagonists (glycine is a co-agonist at the NMDA receptor), magnesium (which regulates NMDA receptor activation), γ-amino butyric acid (GABA) agonists (which reduce glutamate release), and selective NR2B receptor antagonists.

Apoptotic pathways play a greater role in secondary neuronal death in the developing brain. Whether strategies such as selective NR2B receptor blockade could allow antiexcitotoxic benefit to be facilitated without exacerbating apoptotic neuronal death is undetermined.

Oxidative Stress. After cardiac arrest, stroke, TBI, and in CNS infection, a number of biochemical pathways contribute to a marked increase in free radical production. Excitotoxicity-mediated increases in intracellular Ca^{2+} are believed to contribute to mitochondrial sequestration of Ca^{2+}, disruption of electron transport, and the production of reactive oxygen species (ROS) either linked to, or independent of, opening of the mitochondrial permeability transition pore. Other sources of free radicals include the cyclooxygenase-2, peroxidases (myeloperoxidase and cytochrome-c), and invading and resident inflammatory cells. Free radicals cause lipid peroxidation, protein and DNA oxidation, protein dimerization, and activation of transcription factors with dysregulation of neuronal homeostasis. Free radicals can be grouped into ROS and reactive nitrogen species (RNS). ROS include superoxide anion, hydrogen peroxide, and hydroxyl radicals. Among the RNS is NO, which is lipid soluble and readily crosses cell membranes. NO can act as an endogenous antioxidant. However, the reaction of NO with superoxide anion leads to peroxynitrite formation, a highly reactive radical species that can produce lipid, protein, and DNA nitration. Oxidation of the mitochondrial lipid cardiolipin releases cytochrome-c from the mitochondrial membrane, a seminal event that links oxidative stress and the intrinsic pathway of apoptosis. DNA damage from peroxynitrite in both the nucleus and mitochondria can activate the enzyme poly(ADP-ribose) polymerase (PARP), which results in energy failure via the PARP-mediated cellular suicide pathway. In experimental cardiac arrest, hyperoxic resuscitation plays a role in the level of oxidative stress.

Trophic Factor Withdrawal. Trophic factor withdrawal has relevance in the evolution of secondary damage after CNS insults. Neurotrophins, such as nerve growth factor, brain-derived neurotrophic

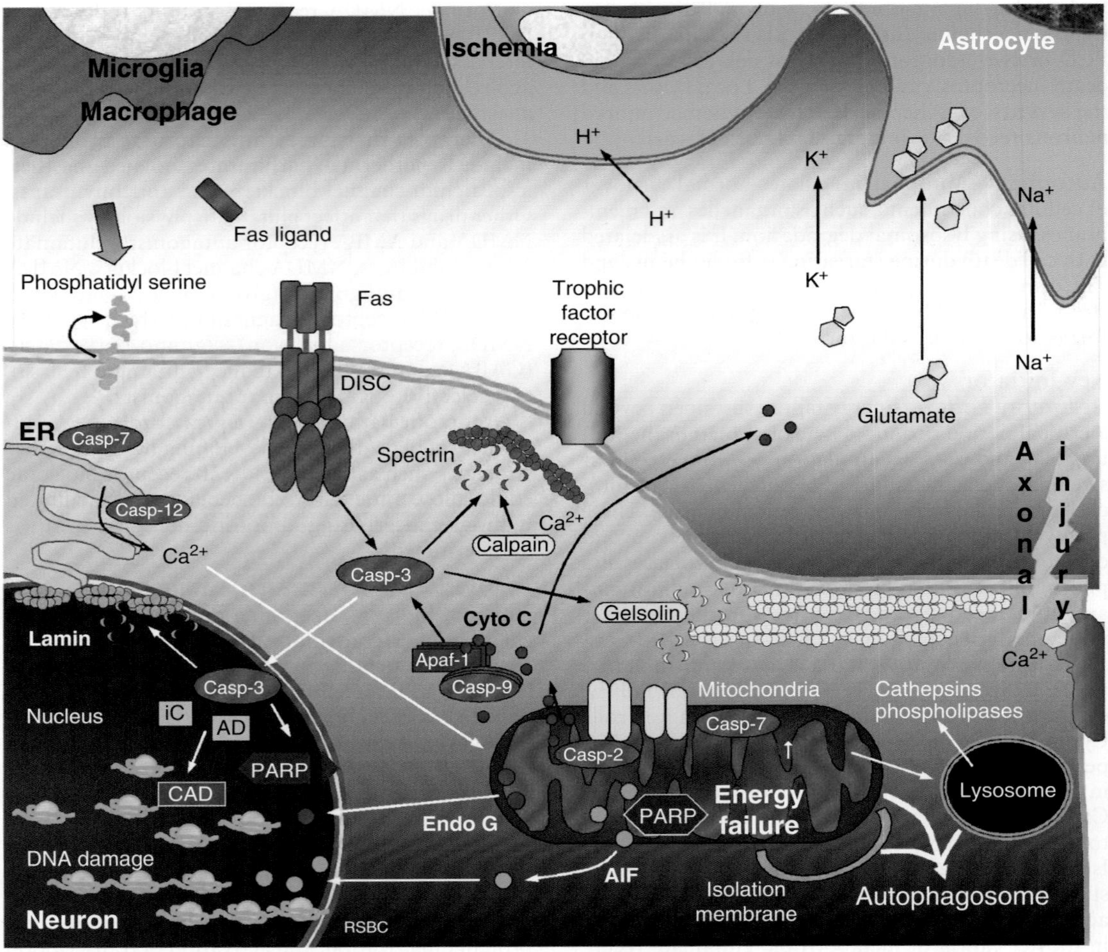

FIGURE 33.2. Neuronal death cascades resulting from necrosis, apoptosis (intrinsic, extrinsic, and apoptosis-inducing factor [AIF] pathways), and autophagy in CNS injury. ER, endoplasmic reticulum; Casp, caspase; CAD, caspase-activated deoxyribonuclease; Endo G, endonuclease G; ROS, reactive oxygen species; PARP, poly(ADP-ribose) polymerase; DISC, death-inducing signaling complex; iC/AC, inhibitor of caspase-activated deoxyribonuclease.

factor, basic fibroblast growth factor, and others, are constitutively produced by neurons and glia, bind to receptors on target neurons, and are essential to survival and plasticity. Loss of trophic input to a target neuron can trigger target neuron death several days after injury.

Neuronal Death Effector Pathways. In mature tissues, PCD requires initiation by either intracellular or extracellular signals. These signals have been characterized in vitro and are becoming better characterized in vivo (**Fig. 33.2**).

Intrinsic (Mitochondrial) Pathway of Apoptosis. Mitochondrial dysfunction, triggered by ATP depletion, oxidative stress, or calcium flux, leads to egress of cytochrome-c from the inner mitochondrial membrane into the cytosol. Oxidation of cardiolipin plays a role in cytochrome-c release. Cytochrome-c release can be blocked by antiapoptotic members of the bcl-2 family (bcl-2, bcl-XL, Mcl-1) and promoted by proapoptotic bcl-2 family members (bax, bad, bid). Cytochrome-c in the presence of dATP and a specific apoptotic protease–activating factor (Apaf-1) in cytosol activates the initiator cysteine protease caspase-9. Caspase-9 then activates the effector cysteine protease caspase-3, which cleaves cytoskeletal proteins, DNA repair proteins, and activators of endonucleases. Caspase inhibitors and mild hypothermia attenuate neuronal death in experimental models.

Apoptosis-inducing Factor Pathway. Another intracellular cascade of PCD linked to mitochondrial injury is the apoptosis-inducing factor (AIF) pathway. AIF release leads to large-scale DNA fragmentation (50–700 Kbp in size). Pharmacologic inhibitors of this pathway are lacking.

Endoplasmic Reticulum Stress-triggered Apoptosis. Synthesis of unique proapoptotic factors associated with ER stress can trigger apoptosis independent of mitochondrial failure. The reduction in ER Ca^{2+} concentration that results from IP3-mediated Ca^{2+} release from the ER leads to induction of proteins which mediate apoptosis.

Extrinsic Pathway Apoptosis. Extracellular signaling of apoptosis occurs through the tumor necrosis factor (TNF) superfamily of cell surface death receptors that includes TNFR1 and Fas/Apo1/CD95. Receptor–ligand binding of TNFR1-TNF-α or Fas-Fas-L facilitates caspase recruitment. The proximity of multiple caspases allows activation of the effector cysteine protease, followed by activation of caspase-3, where the mitochondrial and cell death receptor pathways converge.

Cellular Signaling Pathways. Neurotrophic factors, neurotransmitters, cytokines, and ROS activate multiple upstream signaling pathways linked to either pro-survival or pro-death activities. Important participants in the cell death cascades include the mitogen-activated protein kinases (MAPKs). MAPK cascades are complex and mediated by successive protein kinases that sequentially activate each other by phosphorylation. They are linked to two key components of the cell death cascade: c-Jun kinase (JNK) and p38 MAPK. JNK and p38 MAPK pathways activate caspase-3. Activation of JNK leads to induction of pro-death genes, including Fas-L. JNK increases p53 and Bax levels, which increase cell death. JNK and p38 function in different stress-signaling pathways, and both target similar nuclear transcription factors that can be activated by pro-death stimuli (e.g., ROS). MAPKs are also linked to survival signals through the ERK pathway, highlighting the complex cross talk between these cascades. PI3-K, PKB, and protein kinase A (PKA) pathways also have a major survival role. PKB may help mediate hypothermic neuroprotection.

Poly(ADP-Ribose) Polymerase Activation. The enzyme PARP plays a role in neuronal death after ischemia and TBI. It is located in mitochondria and the nucleus where it repairs DNA. A deleterious consequence of PARP activation in CNS injury is the consumption of nicotine adenine dinucleotide (NAD) that depletes mitochondrial energy stores. PARP knockout mice are highly protected from neuronal damage in experimental models of stroke and TBI.

Protease Activation. Increase in intracellular Ca^{2+} in neurons activates calpain proteases that initiate the "calpain–cathepsin cascade." Calpains are located in dendrites and in axons. Activated calpains cleave spectrin, kinases, phosphatases, membrane receptors, and lysosomes. Lysosomal rupture leads to release of >80 hydrolytic enzymes, of which cathepsins B, D, H, and L play a role in executing neuronal death by necrosis or autophagy.

Necroptosis. A novel form of programmed neuronal necrosis is necroptosis. In this pathway, TNF-α or Fas activates necrosis (evidenced by loss of neuronal membrane integrity) via a receptor-mediated process. Necroptosis is inhibited by necrostatin in experimental TBI.

Endogenous Neuroprotectant Pathways. The endogenous response to ischemic and excitotoxic insults is being defined in children (**Fig. 33.1**). Adenosine is an endogenous neuroprotectant produced in response to ischemia and excitotoxicity that decreases neuronal metabolism and increases CBF. Its release minimizes excitotoxicity via A_1 receptors by increasing K^+ and Cl^- and decreasing Ca^{2+} conductances in the neuronal membrane. Binding of adenosine to A_2 receptors (on cerebrovascular smooth muscle) causes vasodilation (binding to A_{2a} receptors on neurons may be detrimental). Adenosine A_1 receptor knockout mice develop lethal SE after experimental TBI, supporting an endogenous neuroprotectant effect. Another endogenous neuroprotectant is heat shock protein 70 (HSP70). HSP70 is induced in classic preconditioning in brain and is increased in CSF and brain tissue after severe TBI in children. HSP70 plays an important role in optimizing protein folding as a molecular chaperone. It also inhibits proinflammatory signaling. Bcl-2 is an important endogenous inhibitor of PCD. Its induction in experimental TBI reduces cortical tissue loss. CSF levels in clinical studies correlate with survival. Nitrite may be another powerful cytoprotective molecule.

Brain Injury without Neuronal Death

Several processes that result from injury lead to functional impairments (e.g., synaptic damage, disturbances in cell signaling and glial–neuronal cross talk, and alterations in neurotransmitter balance) without cell death. These injuries may be highly responsive to therapeutic interventions.

Brain Swelling. Cerebral edema or increased cerebral blood volume (CBV) following injury can cause secondary ischemia from raised intracranial pressure (ICP), local compression, or herniation. Brain edema develops via cellular swelling, blood–brain barrier (BBB) injury (vasogenic edema), or osmolar swelling (**Fig. 33.3**).

Cellular Swelling

Astrocyte Swelling. Cellular swelling (supplanted the term cytotoxic edema) occurs in astrocyte foot processes. Astrocyte-mediated reuptake of glutamate from the extracellular space is coupled to Na^+ and water accumulation. Similarly, acidosis, K^+, cytokines, and arachidonic acid mediate astrocyte swelling. Cellular swelling may predominate after secondary insults.

Aquaporins. Aquaporins are endogenous water channels that have a role in the molecular aspect of brain edema. Aquaporins 1–9 are a ubiquitous family of integral membrane proteins serving as water transport pathways. Aquaporin-1 is involved in membrane transport of water across osmotic

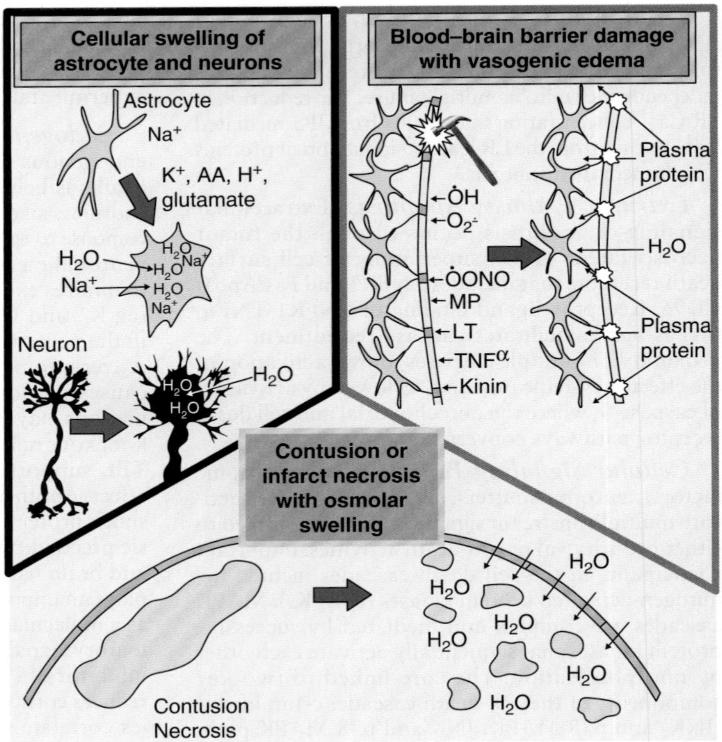

FIGURE 33.3. Three major mechanisms underlying the development of cerebral edema, including cellular swelling, BBB injury with vasogenic edema, and osmolar swelling that develops in both contusions and infarcts. AA, arachidonic acid; O_2^-, superoxide anion; ONOO, peroxynitrite; OH, hydroxyl radical; MP, metalloproteinase; LT, leukotriene; TNF-α, tumor necrosis factor α.

gradients, while aquaporins 4 and 9 are localized in astrocyte end-feet. Astrocyte swelling may be mediated by aquaporins and these water channels may represent a key new therapeutic target for control of raised ICP after TBI, ischemia, and CNS infections.

Vasogenic Edema

BBB permeability that results in vasogenic edema contributes to secondary brain swelling. This mechanism is less important after cardiac arrest. In bacterial meningitis, the acute inflammatory cascade (cytokine-mediated induction of leukocyte adhesion molecules, neutrophil accumulation, and related oxidative injury to vascular endothelium) contributes to BBB damage. In addition, matrix metalloproteinases (MMPs) have an important role in degrading the extracellular matrix.

Osmolar Swelling. Osmolar swelling in areas of contusion necrosis greatly contributes to the development of edema, particularly in TBI. Ironically, reconstitution of the injured BBB or development of an osmolar barrier around a necrotic focus may increase focal edema as the local tissue osmolar load increases when macromolecules are degraded to constituents. This mechanism may explain the benefit of osmolar therapy in cerebral contusion (**Fig. 33.4**). Osmolar swelling also underlies mass effect in the evolution of hemispheric stroke.

Cerebral Blood Volume. Increased CBV may have a role in pediatric brain swelling; however, adult data suggest that posttraumatic brain swelling is most likely edema rather than vascular engorgement. A role for hyperemia in cerebral swelling in meningitis is controversial. Increased CBV after CNS injury may contribute to raised ICP and result from *hyperglycolysis* (local increases in cerebral glycolysis). In regions with increases in glutamate levels (e.g., contusions), increase in the astrocyte uptake of glutamate is coupled to glucose utilization. Hyperglycolysis may mediate a coupled increase in CBF, CBV, and local brain swelling.

Inflammation and Regeneration

The major components of the CNS inflammatory response are leukocytes, microglia, and regeneration. Contributions to secondary damage can be mediated by circulating leukocytes in the inflammatory response. An endogenous inflammatory response mediated by microglia along with neurons and astrocytes has been recognized. The inflammatory response appears to have a delayed beneficial role, in the signaling of regenerative processes and neurogenesis.

Role of Inflammation in Secondary Injury. CNS infections are associated with robust acute inflammation. The inflammatory process also makes important contributions in stroke and TBI. Nuclear factor (NF)-κB activation, TNF-α, IL-1β, eicosanoids,

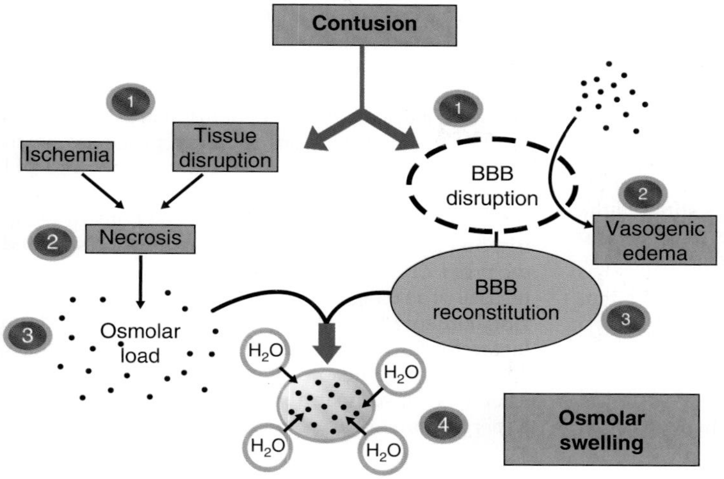

FIGURE 33.4. Temporal pathway involved in osmolar swelling in brain contusions or infarcts. Temporal profile shown by numbers 1–4. Necrotic brain regions generate a large osmolar load as they are degraded to constituent molecules. Early after the insult, BBB damage allows influx of additional proteins. With time, usually within 24–72 hours, an osmolar barrier re-forms, and water is then osmotically drawn from the surrounding brain regions into the contused or infarcted area, resulting in expansion of the mass lesion. BBB, blood–brain barrier.

neutrophils, and macrophages contribute to both secondary damage and repair. Damage-associated molecular patterns (DAMPS) initiate the innate immune response and interact with receptors to form a multiprotein complex called the inflammasome, which leads to IL-1β production. IL-6, IL-8, and IL-10 increase in CSF after severe TBI. Contusion and local tissue necrosis trigger upregulation of leukocyte adhesion molecules and neutrophil influx that add to secondary tissue damage.

Role of Inflammation in Repair and Regeneration. Possible beneficial aspects of inflammation occur during the subacute or chronic injury phases. The biphasic role of inflammation in CNS injury is seen in mice deficient in TNF-α that exhibit reduced brain edema and improved early functional outcome (vs. wild type) after TBI, but their long-term functional and histologic outcome is worse. Similarly, despite a detrimental role for iNOS early after cerebral ischemia, iNOS-deficient mice show impaired long-term outcome versus controls. It is unclear if anti-inflammatory therapies can improve outcome in CNS injury. Inhibition of the inflammatory response may exacerbate infection risk and any deleterious consequences on the link between inflammation and regeneration must be addressed.

Other Aspects of Repair and Plasticity. Neurotransmitter replacement may be a therapeutic avenue in the subacute period. Functional recovery in adults after moderate or severe TBI was seen with treatment with the dopaminergic agonist amantadine. Augmenting other transmitter systems (e.g., cholinergic or glutamatergic pathways) may also have merit.

Axonal Injury

Axonal injury plays an important role in TBI, perinatal brain injury, and stroke. Traumatic axonal injury (TAI) is the most established type of white matter damage. Injury due to physical shearing is present in severe injury in which frank axonal tears occur. TAI may also occur by a delayed process termed "secondary axotomy." Two hypothetical mechanisms include axolemmal permeability with calcium influx as the initiating event or a direct cytoskeletal abnormality that impairs axoplasmic flow. Hypothermia and cyclosporin A reduce TAI in experimental models.

Mechanisms of Enhanced Vulnerability of Injured Brain

Hypotension and Hypoxemia

The injured brain is extremely vulnerable to secondary physiologic derangements such as hypotension and hypoxemia. Hemorrhagic shock exacerbates intracranial hypertension after experimental TBI and worsens long-term functional outcome. Similarly, hypoxemia to $Pa{O_2}$ levels between 40 and 50 mm Hg for periods as short as 30 minutes exacerbates neuronal death in experimental TBI. In the initial minutes to hours after cardiac arrest, TBI, or stroke, CBF is compromised and metabolic demands are increased. Mechanical factors (e.g., thrombosis, vascular disruption, or vascular compromise from glial swelling), biochemical/molecular mechanisms (e.g., loss of endothelial NOS), or increases in levels of vasoconstrictors (e.g., endothelin-1) may hinder the ability of the vasculature to respond to challenges. Similar mechanisms may also underlie the loss of CBF autoregulation seen in some insults. Increased metabolic demands early after these insults are substantial. Metabolic demands several days after the insult are generally reduced, and the enhanced vulnerability during this phase may be secondary to brain swelling, which peaks between 24 and 72 hours. Hypotension or hypoxemia results in compensatory vasodilation, increased CBV, and further increased ICP, leading to a vicious cycle. Compromised CBF can also impair protein synthesis as regeneration is beginning.

Hyperthermia

Hyperthermia consistently exacerbates damage in experimental ischemia or TBI. The biochemical and molecular mechanisms have not been fully elucidated; however, exacerbation of the inflammatory response may be involved. An inability to compensate for increases in CBF to meet heightened metabolic demands could also be occurring. These findings support the need to prevent fever after cardiac arrest, stroke, and TBI (this is less clear in CNS infections).

Hypoglycemia and Hyperglycemia

The vulnerability of the brain to hypoglycemia is well described in experimental brain injury. Recent clinical data suggest enhanced vulnerability to hypoglycemia in injured brain; this is anticipated, as endogenous protective mechanisms, such as vasodilation, are often compromised after cardiac arrest, stroke, and TBI. Brain glucose levels can reach critically low values after TBI, particularly in pericontusional brain regions. Astrocyte-dependent homeostatic processes, such as uptake of excitatory neurotransmitters and pH regulation, are dependent on glycolytic rather than oxidative metabolism. Tight glucose control using insulin (serum glucose 90–120 g/dL) was associated with more critically low brain glucose levels than looser control (<150 mg/dL). Tight glucose control was also associated with increases in brain glutamate and the lactate/pyruvate ratio, suggesting metabolic failure. Although care must be taken to avoid hypoglycemia after CNS insults, it also must be recognized that hyperglycemia exacerbates CNS injury.

CHAPTER 34 ■ EVALUATION OF THE COMATOSE CHILD

NICHOLAS S. ABEND AND DANIEL J. LICHT

Coma is an altered state of consciousness which may result from a variety of insults to the brain. Morbidity and mortality are dependent on the coma etiology. Coma involves loss of both wakefulness (arousal, vigilance) and awareness of self and environment. Sleep–wake cycles are absent. Coma is characterized by sustained, pathologic, eyes-closed, unarousable unresponsiveness.

Between normal consciousness and coma is the spectrum of diminished consciousness. *Lethargy* is a state of reduced wakefulness with attentional deficits. *Obtundation* is characterized by blunted alertness and diminished interaction with the environment. *Stupor* is a state of unresponsiveness with little or no spontaneous movement, resembling deep sleep, but differs from coma because vigorous stimulation induces temporary arousal.

A patient in the *persistent vegetative state* (PVS) has sleep–wake cycles but is unaware of self and environment. Although such patients may make sounds, facial expressions, or body movements, detailed testing does not demonstrate reproducible purposeful responses to stimulation. The diagnosis of a PVS may be made 3 months following nontraumatic brain injury but should not be made until 12 months following traumatic injury. Children in the vegetative state 1 month after traumatic brain injury (TBI) had outcomes at 1 year of death (9%), PVS (29%), and recovery of consciousness (62%). Outcome for a nontraumatic etiology was worse with death (22%), PVS (65%), and recovery of consciousness (usually with severe cognitive disabilities) in only 13%. Functional neuroimaging and electrophysiologic studies have indicated that some patients considered to be in the vegetative state demonstrate reproducible physiologic changes in response to tasks, indicating some awareness despite the absence of behavioral signs of responsiveness. A patient in a *minimally conscious state* has severely altered consciousness but has behavioral evidence of self or environmental awareness, such as following simple commands or making simple nonreflexive gestures.

Akinetic mutism is a condition of extreme slowing or absence of bodily movement with loss of speech. Wakefulness and awareness are preserved, but cognition is slowed. Causes include extensive bihemispheric disease and lesions involving the bilateral inferior frontal lobes, paramedian mesencephalic reticular formation, or the posterior diencephalon. The *locked-in syndrome* is a state of preserved cognition with complete paralysis of the voluntary motor system. Eye movements may be preserved, allowing for some communication. It may result from lesions of the corticospinal and corticobulbar pathways at or below the pons or severe peripheral nervous system disease such as Guillain–Barré syndrome, botulism, or critical illness polyneuropathy. *Psychogenic unresponsiveness* may also mimic coma. Coma must also be distinguished from *brain death*, which is the permanent absence of all brain activities, including brainstem function. *Delirium* is an acute confusional state characterized by changes in level of consciousness, impaired attention, and a fluctuating course.

ANATOMY

Maintaining consciousness depends on interactions between the reticular activating system (RAS), thalamus, posterior hypothalamus, and cerebral hemispheres. The RAS constitutes the central core of the brainstem and extends from the caudal medulla to the thalamus and the basal forebrain. The RAS receives input stimulation from all sensory pathways and projects to vast areas of the cerebral cortex. Ascending portions of the *medial RAS* emanating from the Raphe nuclei regulate sleep cycles and use *serotonin* as the major neurotransmitter. The descending pathways regulate automatic motor functions, including rhythms of breathing. The *lateral RAS* projects to the reticular nucleus of the thalamus, which relays signals to the cortex, maintaining wakefulness. These projections are both *cholinergic* and *noradrenergic*. A second cholinergic pathway ascends through the hypothalamus to influence basal forebrain structures, including the *limbic* system, which influences conscious behavior. Noradrenergic pathways originating in the *locus ceruleus* have an excitatory effect on most of the brain, mediating arousal. Wakefulness is maintained by the RAS and thalamus, whereas awareness is dependent on the cortex.

ETIOLOGIES OF COMA

The main causes of coma are listed in **Table 34.1.** The prevalence of nontraumatic coma etiologies in children includes infection (~40%), intoxication (~10%), epilepsy (~10%), complications of congenital

TABLE 34.1

Etiologies of Coma

Traumatic Etiologies (Accidental or Abusive)
Cerebral contusion
Intracranial hemorrhage
Epidural hematoma
Subdural hematoma
Subarachnoid hemorrhage
Intraparenchymal hematoma
Diffuse axonal injury
Nontraumatic Etiologies
Hypoxic–ischemic encephalopathy
Shock
Cardiopulmonary arrest
Cardiac or pulmonary failure
Near drowning
Carbon monoxide poisoning
Cyanide poisoning
Vascular
Intracranial hemorrhage (subdural, epidural, subarachnoid, parenchymal)
Arterial ischemic infarct
Venous sinus thromboses
Vasculitis
Carotid or vertebral artery dissection (cervical or intracranial)
Mass lesions
Primary neoplasms
Brain metastases
Abscess
Granuloma
Hydrocephalus
Infections
Meningitis and encephalitis: bacterial, viral, rickettsial, fungal, protozoal
Abscess
Inflammatory/autoimmune/postinfectious
Acute disseminated encephalomyelitis
Multiple sclerosis
Sarcoidosis
Sjogren disease
Cerebritis (e.g., systemic lupus erythematosus)
Sepsis-associated encephalopathy
Autoimmune-mediated encephalitis
Paroxysmal neurologic disorders
Seizures, status epilepticus, nonconvulsive seizures, postictal state
Acute confusional migraine
Hypertensive encephalopathy
Posterior reversible encephalopathy syndrome
Systemic metabolic disorders
Substrate deficiencies
Hypoglycemia
Cofactors: thiamine, niacin, pyridoxine, folate, B_{12}
Electrolyte and acid–base imbalance: sodium, magnesium, calcium
Hypoglycemia
Diabetic ketoacidosis
Endocrine
Acute hypothyroidism
Addison disease
Acute panhypopituitarism
Uremic encephalopathy
Hepatic encephalopathy
Reye syndrome
Sepsis-associated encephalopathy
Porphyria
Inborn errors of metabolism
Urea cycle disorders
Aminoacidopathies
Organic acidopathies
Mitochondrial disorders
Toxins
Medications: narcotics, sedatives, antiepileptics, antidepressants, analgesics, aspirin, valproic acid encephalopathy
Environmental toxins: organophosphates, heavy metals, cyanide, mushroom poisoning
Illicit substances: alcohol, heroine, amphetamines, cocaine, and many others
Drug induced
Neuroleptic malignant syndrome
Serotonin syndrome
Malignant hyperthermia
Psychiatric
Conversion disorder
Catatonia
Other
Hypothermia

abnormalities (~10%), nontraumatic accidents (e.g., smoke inhalation and drowning) (~6%), and metabolic causes (~6%). Multiple interrelated factors crossing these subdivisions may be present in one patient.

EVALUATION OF THE COMATOSE CHILD

The evaluation of coma begins with stabilization of vital functions and identification of immediately reversible etiologies. An algorithm for initial evaluation of coma is outlined in **Table 34.2**, and practice guidelines are available at www.nottingham.ac.uk/paediatric-guideline.

Patient History

The history must include a detailed description of events, with particular attention to timing, exposures, and accompanying symptoms. Preceding somnolence

TABLE 34.2

Initial Evaluation of Coma

- Resuscitation and medical stabilization
  - Airway, breathing, and circulation assessment and stabilization
  - Ensure adequate ventilation and oxygenation
  - Determine whether hypertension is reactive (maintaining cerebral perfusion pressure) or problematic
- Bedside glucose assessment
  - Draw blood for glucose, electrolytes, ammonia, arterial blood gas, liver and renal function tests, complete blood count, lactate, pyruvate, and toxicology screen
- Neurologic assessment
  - GCS (modified for children) or FOUR score or coma description
  - Assess for evidence of raised intracranial pressure and herniation
  - Assess for abnormalities suggesting focal neurologic disease
  - Head CT scan (and possibly MRI when stable)
- Identify and treat critical elevations in intracranial pressure
  - Neutral head position, elevated head by 20 degrees, sedation
  - Consider hyperosmolar therapy (mannitol or hypertonic saline)
  - Hyperventilation as temporary measure
  - Consider need for intracranial monitoring and/or neurosurgical intervention
- Lumbar puncture if concern for infection or coma etiology unknown
  - Generally head CT scan first and defer lumbar puncture if concern for elevated intracranial pressure
  - If there is concern for infection and lumbar puncture must be delayed, then provide broad-spectrum infection coverage (including bacterial, viral, and possibly fungal)
  - If infection suspected, also draw blood and urine cultures
- Consider clinical and electrographic seizures
  - Treat seizures with anticonvulsants
  - Consider EEG monitoring to identify persisting nonconvulsive seizures
- Give specific antidotes if toxic exposures are known
  - Opiates = naloxone
  - Benzodiazepine = flumazenil
  - Anticholinergic = physostigmine
- Investigate source of fever and use antipyretics and/or cooling devices to reduce cerebral metabolic demands
- Detailed history and examination
- Consider additional metabolic, autoimmune, and endocrine testing

or headache suggests metabolic abnormality, toxin, infection, hydrocephalus, or expanding mass lesions. Sudden onset without trauma suggests seizure, intracranial hemorrhage, or hypoxic–ischemic encephalopathy caused by a cardiac event. A slowly progressive loss of consciousness suggests hydrocephalus, an expanding mass lesion, or indolent infection. Fluctuations in mental status may occur with metabolic etiologies, seizure, or subdural hemorrhage. Preceding headache aggravated with positional changes or Valsalva maneuver implies increased intracranial pressure (ICP) from hydrocephalus or a mass lesion. Headache with neck pain or stiffness suggests meningeal irritation from inflammation, infection, or hemorrhage. Fever suggests infection, but its absence does not rule it out, particularly in infants <3 months of age or immunocompromised children. Recent fevers or illnesses suggest autoimmune processes such as acute disseminated encephalomyelitis (ADEM) or possibly Reye-like illness (rare). A survey is included of medications and poisons kept in the places in which the child has been.

A history or multiple episodes of coma, developmental delay, or prior neurologic abnormalities suggest inborn errors of metabolism or epilepsy. Recent weight or constitutional changes suggest endocrine dysfunction. Prior cardiac disease raises the possibility of dysrhythmia or cardiac failure leading to hypoxic–ischemic encephalopathy. Travel history may explain exposure to infections. Exposure to kittens and lymphadenopathy may be clues to infection with *Bartonella henselae* (cat-scratch encephalopathy).

Physical Examination

Numerical scales of conscious level provide efficient standardized communication of a child's state, but a detailed description of the clinical findings is often more useful. The most widely used instrument is the Glasgow Coma Scale (GCS) score, which was initially developed to evaluate adults with head injury. Pediatric adaptations include the Pediatric Coma Scale, the Children's Coma Scale, and the GCS-Modified for Children (**Table 34.3**). The Full Outline of UnResponsiveness (FOUR) score was developed for use in adults with coma, and may have better interrater reliability than the GCS-Modified for Children.

Hyperthermia suggests an infectious etiology, a lesion impacting temperature control mechanisms, heat stroke, or anticholinergic ingestion. Hypothermia may be due to intoxication, sepsis, hypothyroidism, adrenal insufficiency, chronic malnutrition, or environmental exposure. Hypotension may be due to sepsis, cardiac dysfunction (which may be secondary to neurogenic stunned myocardium), toxic ingestion, or adrenal insufficiency. Hypotension may lead to poor cerebral perfusion, resulting in diffuse or watershed hypoxic–ischemic injury. Hypertension can be a physiologic response (to increased ICP) that functions to maintain cerebral perfusion pressure, and acutely lowering blood pressure may worsen the neurologic injury. Hypertension with bradycardia and a change in breathing pattern (Cushing triad) is a sign of elevated ICP and may signal impending herniation. Management may require temporary emergent measures to lower ICP (e.g., hyperventilation to reduce carbon

TABLE 34.3

Glasgow Coma Scale and Modification for Children

SIGN	GLASGOW COMA SCALE	MODIFICATION FOR CHILDREN	SCORE
Eye opening	Spontaneous	Spontaneous	4
	To command	To sound	3
	To pain	To pain	2
	None	None	1
Verbal response	Oriented	Age-appropriate verbalization, orients to sound, fixes and follows, social smile	5
	Confused	Cries, but consolable	4
	Disoriented—inappropriate words	Irritable, uncooperative, aware of environment—irritable, persistent cries, inconsistently consolable	3
	Incomprehensible sounds	Inconsolable crying, unaware of environment or parents, restless, agitated	2
	None	None	1
Motor response	Obeys commands	Obeys commands, spontaneous movement	6
	Localizes pain	Localizes pain	5
	Withdraws	Withdraws	4
	Abnormal flexion to pain	Abnormal flexion to pain	3
	Abnormal extension	Abnormal extension	2
	None	None	1
Best total score			15

dioxide and induce cerebral vasoconstriction and hyperosmolar therapy) followed by more definitive neurosurgical therapy. Hypertension in the setting of coma may also be the product of nonspecific sympathetic response or of stimulant intoxication. Primary or secondary hypertension may cause hypertensive encephalopathy that can manifest as coma. Primary hypertensive encephalopathy is suggested by a history of hypertension or renal disease, or by preceding headache, visual complaints, or seizures. Differentiating reactive/compensatory hypertension from a primary hypertensive encephalopathy may be difficult but is crucial in determining how to manage blood pressure. Bradycardia may occur with intracranial hypertension, cardiac disease, hypothermia, toxin exposure (sedating drugs), uremic coma, or myxedema coma. Tachycardia may occur with hypovolemic or cardiogenic shock, sepsis, pain, toxin exposure (amphetamines, cocaine, nicotine, and caffeine), malignant hyperthermia, anemia, heart failure, hyperthyroidism, pheochromocytoma, or pulmonary embolism. Abnormalities in respiratory rate and pattern of breathing may indicate pathology originating in the lungs, acid–base derangement, or nervous system dysfunction. *Cheyne–Stokes respiration* describes a rhythmic pattern of accelerating hyperpnea followed by fall in amplitude of breathing culminating in decelerating rate of breathing and apnea. It can be seen with extensive bihemispheric cerebral dysfunction, diencephalic (thalamic and hypothalamic) dysfunction, or cardiac failure. Pontine or midbrain tegmental lesions may result in central neurogenic hyperventilation. *Apneustic breathing* is characterized by a pause at the end of inspiration and reflects damage to respiratory centers at the mid- or lower pontine levels, at or below the level of the trigeminal motor nucleus. Apneusis occurs with basilar artery occlusion (leading to pontine infarction), hypoglycemia, anoxia, or meningitis. *Ataxic breathing* is completely irregular in rate and tidal volume, and occurs with damage to the reticular formation of the dorsomedial medulla.

A complete general examination is important in elucidating coma etiology and identifying medical issues requiring management. Involuntary hip flexion with passive flexion of the neck (*Brudzinski sign*) and resistance to knee extension with hips flexed (*Kernig sign*) indicate meningeal inflammation/irritation. Skin examination provides information about accidental or abusive trauma (bruises, lacerations), systemic medical disease (jaundice in liver failure, uremic frost, hyperpigmentation in adrenal insufficiency), and infection (superficial lacerations in cat-scratch fever, erythema migrans in Lyme disease, petechiae and purpura in meningococcemia). Clear fluid emanating from the nose or ears may indicate a cerebrospinal fluid (CSF) leak due to skull fracture. Organomegaly raises suspicion of metabolic, hematologic, and hepatic diseases. Abusive head trauma is suggested by retinal hemorrhages, metaphyseal fractures, rib fractures, and subdural hemorrhages.

In a comatose child, much of the examination that requires patient cooperation (such as mental status and sensory testing) cannot be performed. Thus, the neurologic examination is aimed at assessing response to stimuli and function of the brainstem and motor systems. Evaluation of responsiveness must include vigorous auditory and sensory stimulation. Nail-bed pressure, pinching, and sternal rubbing may be required.

Fundoscopic examination may show papilledema with increased ICP. However, papilledema may take

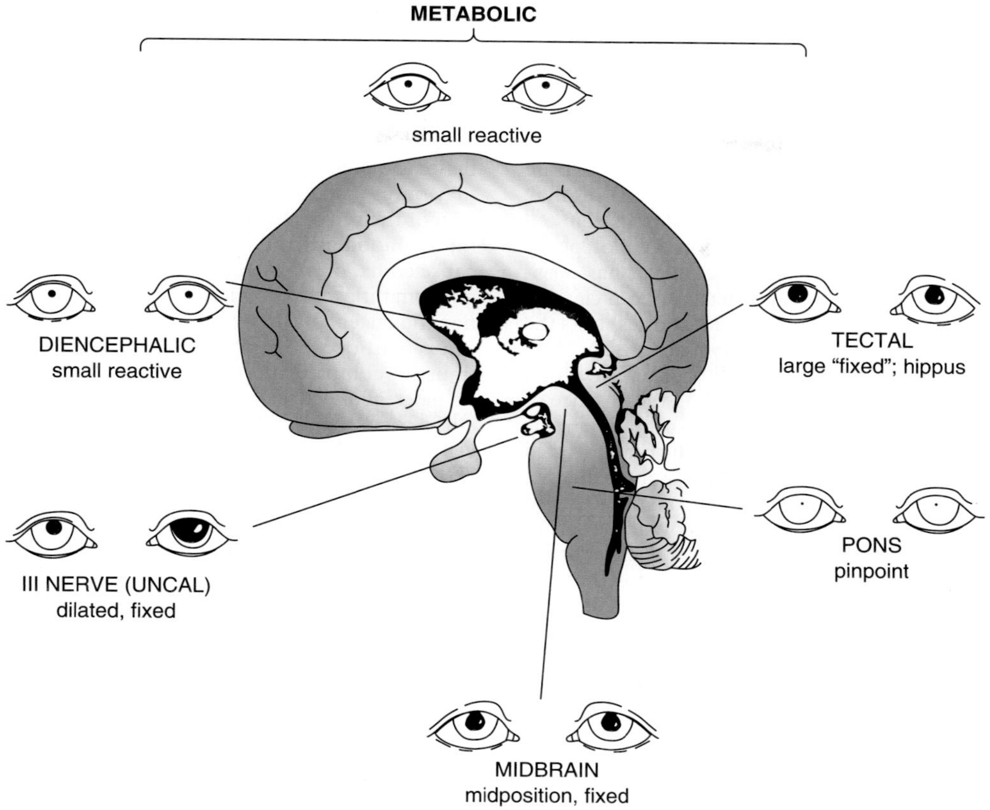

FIGURE 34.1. Pupil abnormalities characteristic of specific lesion locations.

hours or days to develop, and so its absence does not indicate normal ICP. Retinal hemorrhages may be seen in inflicted childhood neurotrauma. Flame-shaped hemorrhages and cotton-wool spots are seen in hypertensive encephalopathy.

Pupils (**Fig. 34.1**) are examined first by observing the size of both pupils in dim light and then by assessing reactivity to a bright light shined in each eye. Anisocoria (asymmetric pupils) is caused by either oculomotor nerve (cranial nerve III) disruption or impairment of sympathetic fibers (Horner syndrome). Oculomotor nerve palsy also results in ptosis and ophthalmoparesis and may be a sign of uncal herniation. Horner syndrome describes disruption of the sympathetic innervation to the face, characterized by mild ptosis over an abnormally small pupil (meiosis). In traumatic coma, Horner syndrome may be a clue to dissection of the carotid artery (sympathetic fibers are adjacent), or an injury to the lower brachial plexus (C8–T1).

Conjugate lateral eye deviation may be caused by destructive lesions of the ipsilateral cortex or pons, or by focal seizures in the contralateral hemisphere. Rarely, thalamic lesions may cause "wrong-way eyes," in which the eyes deviate away from the side of the destructive lesion. Tonic down gaze suggests dorsal midbrain compression. The complete dorsal midbrain syndrome of Parinaud (usually associated with pineal gland or midbrain tumors in children) includes pupillary light-near dissociation, lid-retraction, and convergence-retraction nystagmus.

Dysconjugate gaze suggests extraocular muscle weakness or, more commonly, abnormalities of the third, fourth, or sixth cranial nerves or nuclei. Unilateral or bilateral abducens nerve (cranial nerve VI) palsies are commonly seen in increased ICP (causing diplopia). An eye with oculomotor nerve (cranial nerve III) palsy is ptotic, depressed, and abducted, and has a dilated pupil. Oculomotor nerve palsy in a comatose patient suggests uncal herniation with midbrain compression, requiring urgent intervention. Trochlear nerve (cranial nerve IV) palsy causes hypertropia (one eye has higher visual axis) in the affected eye.

Roving eye movements are seen in comatose patients with intact brainstem function. Their disappearance may signal the onset of brainstem dysfunction. Periodic alternating gaze (ping-pong gaze) describes conjugate horizontal eye movements back and forth with a pause at each end. It may be seen with extensive bilateral hemispheric, basal ganglia, or thalamic–midbrain damage with an intact pons, and is thought to result from disconnection of cortical influences on oculovestibular reflex generators. It has also been reported in reversible coma from monoamine oxidase and tricyclic antidepressant toxicity.

Oculocephalic and oculovestibular reflexes are useful for assessing the integrity of the midbrain and pons in a comatose patient without spontaneous eye movements. To test oculocephalic reflexes, the examiner holds the patient's eyelids open and quickly moves the head to one side. In a comatose patient with an intact brainstem, the eyes will move in the direction opposite the head motion. After several seconds, the eyes may return to a neutral position. The head should be tested in both horizontal and vertical directions. Oculocephalic reflexes should not be tested if the patient has cervical spine trauma or if the spine has not been cleared.

The oculovestibular reflex (cold calorics) tests the function above the pontomedullary junction. The child must have an open external auditory canal with an intact tympanic membrane (including the absence of pressure equalization tubes), so visual inspection of the canal is an important first step. With the head elevated at 30 degrees, up to 120 cc of ice water is introduced in the ear canal with a small catheter. A conscious patient would experience nystagmus with slow deviation of the eyes toward the irrigated ear and a fast corrective movement away from the ear. In a comatose patient, the eyes will deviate slowly toward the irrigated ear and remain fixed there. If the brainstem vestibular nuclei (located at the pontomedullary junction) are impaired, no movement will be seen. In brain death, there is no brainstem function, and so no eye movement is seen with both ears tested. Five minutes should be allowed before the second ear is tested to allow return of temperature equilibrium between the two ears.

The corneal reflex is tested by tactile stimulation of the cornea, which should elicit bilateral eyelid closure. The afferent (sensory) signal is carried by the trigeminal nerve (cranial nerve V), and the efferent (motor) pathway is carried by the facial nerve (cranial nerve VII). Completion of the reflex loop requires intact trigeminal and facial nerve nuclei in the mid- and lower pons. The cough reflex (may be elicited with stimulation of the carina when a patient is intubated or undergoes suctioning) is mediated by medullary cough centers; sensory and motor signals are carried by glossopharyngeal (cranial nerve IX) and vagus (cranial nerve X) nerves. When the soft palate is stimulated, the gag reflex is elicited, manifested as elevation of the soft palate. As in the cough reflex, afferent and efferent signals are carried by the glossopharyngeal and vagus nerves, with processing in the medulla.

A comatose child may be flaccid, or may display an abnormal flexor or extensor posture. *Decorticate* posturing describes flexion of the arms and extension of the legs. *Decerebrate* posturing describes extension and internal rotation of the arms and legs. Decorticate posturing is related to dysfunction primarily in the supratentorial compartment, whereas decerebrate posturing is related to brainstem dysfunction.

Testing

Investigation should continue with laboratory, neuroimaging, and electrophysiologic testing (**Table 34.4**). Hypoxia, hypotension, hypoglycemia or hyperglycemia, hyperthermia, hypothermia, and anemia worsen the prognosis of coma and must be treated aggressively. Hypotonic fluids can worsen cerebral edema and should not be administered.

Testing of glucose should occur, since hypoglycemia may cause coma and worsen outcome. Hyperglycemia may occur in diabetic ketoacidosis or as a manifestation of the sympathetic response to systemic illness/injury. Blood gas and electrolyte abnormalities may cause coma, or may occur secondary to intracranial abnormalities. Liver function should be tested since hepatic encephalopathy may cause coma, and liver injury can occur from systemic hypoxic–ischemic injury. A complete blood count with differential can help detect infection, anemia, disseminated intravascular coagulopathy, lead encephalopathy, or sickle cell disease. Blood, urine, and stool cultures may help. Toxin screens should be performed if the etiology is unknown. Specific testing for medications found in the home may be indicated. Ammonia, lactate, and pyruvate testing can screen for metabolic disorders. Measurement of organic acids, amino acids, very long chain fatty acids, and acylcarnitine profile may be indicated. Some patients may require endocrine testing, including cortisol levels and thyroid function studies.

A normal head computed tomography (CT) scan does not rule out all structural intracranial processes. Magnetic resonance imaging (MRI) is superior to CT in assessing the subcortical structures, brainstem, and spinal cord and in detecting ischemic stroke and venous disease, early hypoxic–ischemic injury, hypertensive encephalopathy, demyelinating disease, toxic leukoencephalopathies, encephalitis, and diffuse axonal injury.

If infection is suspected, or no other etiology can be determined, a lumbar puncture should be performed. If there is suspicion of intracranial hypertension, then lumbar puncture should be deferred and treatment should be initiated for possible infections (bacterial and viral). CSF should be tested for cell count (both the first and the last tubes need to be tested to help differentiate true findings from a traumatic tap), glucose, protein, Gram stain, bacterial culture, viral polymerase chain reaction (PCR), and additional cultures when suspected clinically (fungal or tuberculosis). If the cause of coma remains unknown, additional studies may be directed at uncommon causes of coma in pediatrics such as Hashimoto encephalitis (thyroid function tests and thyroid autoantibodies), cerebral vasculitis (erythrocyte sedimentation rate, antinuclear antibody panel, and possibly angiography), or paraneoplastic disorders.

Most EEG findings are nonspecific, but they may help distinguish between focal and diffuse etiologies. An unexpectedly normal or only mildly abnormal EEG may raise concern for psychogenic, neuromuscular, or locked-in conditions. EEG may also identify nonconvulsive seizures or nonconvulsive status epilepticus. Continuous EEG monitoring has a better yield than standard EEG for identifying nonconvulsive seizures.

TABLE 34.4

Investigation of Nontraumatic Coma

INVESTIGATIONS	INDICATION/ CLINICAL CLUES	POSSIBLE ABNORMALITY	FURTHER INVESTIGATION IF ABNORMAL	POSSIBLE DIAGNOSES	ACTION
Dextrostix	All	Low	Blood glucose, liver function tests, blood ammonia, blood lactate, blood and urine amino acids, urine organic acids	Hypoglycemia secondary to: Fasting Severe illness Reye syndrome organic aciduria Fatty acid oxidation defect Hemorrhagic shock and encephalopathy	IV dextrose
Blood glucose	Previous polydipsia/ polyuria	High		Diabetic ketoacidosis	Fluids, insulin
Blood sodium	All	Low/high	Urinary sodium	Hypo/hypernatremia ± dehydration	Appropriate fluids
Blood urea	All	High	Blood creatinine, blood film	Dehydration Hemolytic uremic syndrome	Rehydrate, dialysis, plasmapheresis
Aspartate transaminase	All	High	Blood ammonia	Reye syndrome Hypoxia–ischemia	
Blood ammonia	All (unless cause known)	High	Blood orotic acid, urine organic acids	Urea cycle defect Organic acidemia	Sodium benzoate Hemodialysis
Full blood count and film	All	Low Hb			Transfusion
		High WBC		Infection	Third-generation cephalosporin
		Low platelets		DIC infection	
		Sickle cells on film	Hb electrophoresis	Sickle cell disease	
		Burr cells on film		Hemolytic uremic syndrome	Dialysis, plasmapheresis
	Residence in endemic area	Parasites on thick/thin films		Malaria	Quinine
	Pica	Basophilic stippling	Wrist X-ray—lead line	Lead encephalopathy	Chelation
	Pica	Basophilic stippling	Wrist X-ray—lead line	Lead encephalopathy	Chelation
Blood culture	All				Appropriate antibiotics
Stool culture	All	Shigella, enteroviruses			
Mycoplasma IgG, IgM	All (unless cause known)		Chest X-ray	Mycoplasma encephalitis	Azithromycin, prednisolone
Viral titers	Analyze if unexplained		Repeat at discharge		
Urine for toxin screen	Analyze if unexplained			Poisoning	Antidote

(continued)

TABLE 34.4

Investigation of Nontraumatic Coma (*continued*)

INVESTIGATIONS	INDICATION/ CLINICAL CLUES	POSSIBLE ABNORMALITY	FURTHER INVESTIGATION IF ABNORMAL	POSSIBLE DIAGNOSES	ACTION
Blood lead	Analyze if unexplained		Blood film—basophilic stippling, wrist X-ray—lead line		Chelation
Head CT scan without contrast	All (after resuscitation, afebrile patients should ideally be transferred for CT scan to a unit with neurosurgical facilities)	Blood: Subdural/Extradural/ Intracerebral	Skull X-ray/skeletal survey/clotting screen	Nonaccidental injury, tumor	Neurosurgical referral, child protection
		Space-occupying lesion		Space-occupying lesion	Neurosurgical referral
		Hydrocephalus: Obstructive/ Communicating	CSF examination	Meningitis, especially tuberculous	Antituberculosis coverage, neurosurgical referral
		Abscess	Contrast CT/MRI, culture aspirate		Neurosurgical referral, anaerobic coverage
		Swelling			Mannitol, hypertonic saline
		Focal low density		Cerebral abscess, herpes simplex, stroke, ADEM	
		Abnormal basal ganglia	Plasma/CSF lactate, blood gas	Leigh syndrome, hypoxic–ischemic, striatal necrosis	
Lumbar puncture	In febrile patient if no clinical or radiologic evidence of raised ICP (delay and treat if in doubt)	Gram stain, CSF cultures, PCR for viruses, TB			
		Pressure measurement: High	CT scan		Hypertonic therapy, hyperventilate
		Microscopy: High WBC		Meningitis/encephalitis	Third-generation cephalosporin, acyclovir
		Microscopy: High RBC	CT (traumatic tap should clear by third bottle)	Hemorrhage/encephalitis/nonaccidental injury	Neurosurgical referral, acyclovir, child protection
		Glucose: Low		Tuberculous meningitis	Immediate and prolonged antituberculosis therapy
		Protein: High		Tuberculous meningitis	Immediate and prolonged antituberculosis therapy

Prolonged search for acid-fast bacilli, culture for TB on Lowenstein–Jensen agar	Prodrome > 7 days, optic atrophy, focal signs, abnormal movements, CSF polymorphs < 50%, hydrocephalus and/or basal enhancement on contrast CT			Tuberculous meningitis	Immediate and prolonged antituberculosis therapy
Antibodies; e.g., herpes simplex, mycoplasma				Encephalitis	Acyclovir, Azithromycin
Lactate	Abnormal breathing/eye movements, basal ganglia lucencies		Muscle biopsy	Leigh syndrome	
EEG	All, especially if ventilated or evidence of subtle seizures (nystagmus, tonic deviation of eyes, clonic jerking limbs)	Epileptiform discharges		Status epilepticus	IV benzodiazepines, fosphenytoin, barbiturates
		Asymmetrical foci of spikes or periodic lateralizing epileptiform discharges on slow background		Herpes simplex encephalitis (many patients do not have characteristic EEG)	High-dose IV acyclovir for 2 wk
MRI	Unexplained encephalopathy	Frontotemporal abnormality	CSF for herpes simplex, PCR	Herpes simplex encephalitis	High-dose IV acyclovir for 2 wk
		Thalamic abnormality	CSF for EBV (arboviruses in endemic area)		

Hb, hemoglobin; WBC, white blood cell; RBC, red blood cell; DIC, disseminated intravascular coagulation; CSF, cerebrospinal fluid; TB, tuberculosis; EBV, Epstein–Barr virus.
From Kirkham FJ. Non-traumatic coma in children. *Arch Dis Child* 2001;85:303–12, with permission.

CHAPTER 35 ■ NEUROLOGIC MONITORING

ROBERT C. TASKER, MATEO ABOY, ALAN S. GRAHAM, AND BRAHM GOLDSTEIN

GENERAL ENGINEERING ASPECTS OF NEUROMONITORING

Medical instrumentation systems are often composed of sensors, signal conditioning hardware and software, output displays, and auxiliary signals. Sensors are used to convert physical measurements into electrical signal outputs. Many sensors are designed to be minimally invasive and to respond to the source of energy present while excluding other sources. Signal conditioning and processing (e.g., amplification and analog filtering) are typically required. Sensor outputs are analog (A) signals that must be converted to digital (D) form before they can be processed using more advanced techniques.

Most signals are filtered with analog integrated circuits before A/D conversion. During A/D conversion, analog signals are sampled at a rate determined by the manufacturer (i.e., the sampling rate or sampling frequency). To accurately represent the signal on the patient's monitor display, the sampling rate must be high enough so that a linear interpolation between the sample points results in a visually smooth and representative signal. In addition to the sampling rate requirements, quantization requirements must be met to avoid error that results from using the quantized signal rather than the true signal amplitude.

Once physiologic signals have been converted to digital form, digital signal processing algorithms are used to extract clinically significant parameters. Heart rate is estimated from the electrocardiogram (ECG) signal using automatic QRS detection algorithms, and diastolic and systolic pressures are obtained from pressure signals. Digital signal processing algorithms generally use a moving window of the physiologic signal to generate estimates. These moving-window segments (signal frames) range from 3 to 10 seconds in duration. Consequently, clinical parameters obtained represent an average over past values of the signal. Thus, patient monitors typically generate alarms *after* the alarm condition has persisted for several seconds. The obverse is also true. For example, after a successful resuscitation from cardiopulmonary arrest, the arterial oxygen saturation value will typically lag a few seconds after the patient's cyanosis has resolved.

CLINICALLY IMPORTANT PHYSIOLOGIC SYSTEMS AND SIGNALS

A limited number of physiologic systems may be monitored within the central nervous system (CNS). **Table 35.1** provides a list of commonly used monitoring modalities, according to frequency of usage in the pediatric intensive care unit (PICU). The electroencephalogram (EEG) and intracranial pressure (ICP) monitors have been available for decades. Newer techniques that assess cerebral oxygen delivery include ultrasound, transcranial Doppler (TCD), near-infrared spectroscopy (NIRS), and jugular venous oxyhemoglobin saturation ($Sjvo_2$). Monitoring of cellular and extracellular processes includes local brain tissue oxygen tension ($Pbto_2$) and extracellular fluid concentrations of glutamate, glucose, lactate, and pyruvate using microdialysis. *Multimodality neuromonitoring* refers to the simultaneous use of different combinations of these methods to provide a more complete physiologic picture of CNS activity.

DIAGNOSTIC EEG AND EVOKED POTENTIALS

The EEG monitors the electrical activity of the brain observed via scalp electrical potentials. The sources of this electrical activity are the neurons located in the outermost layers of the cerebral cortex. The information provided can be diagnostic of certain forms of encephalopathy (e.g., hepatic) or indicative of the severity of encephalopathy.

Vision, hearing, sensory, and motor functions may be discretely monitored to assess peripheral and CNS damage in patients with suspected injury. The integrity of the complete neural pathways may be assessed using evoked potentials, with abnormalities assigned to specific levels or sites of injury. Information from evoked potentials may help prognostication after severe brain injury, but the risk of false positives and negatives needs to be considered. Caution is needed when predicting unfavorable outcomes in patients with an absence of somatosensory evoked potentials (SEPs).

TABLE 35.1

Monitoring Systems

SYSTEM	TYPE	FEATURES	MEASURE	APPLICATIONS	USAGE
Clinical	Coma scale scores	Noninvasive Regional or global Intermittent	Change in clinical parameters	Very sensitive in awake, nonintubated patients	*Common* in all cases
ICP	Invasive pressure transducer	Invasive Regional Continuous	Change in pressure with known norms	Guides treatment in intracranial hypertension algorithm	*Common* in severe TBI
EEG	Brain activity (focal and global)	Noninvasive Focal or global Intermittent or continuous	Seizure detection, depth of anesthesia, and severity of injury	Guides treatment and prognostic	*Common* in seizure cases and encephalopathy
NIRS	Light absorption in near-infrared range	Noninvasive Regional Continuous	Estimate of frontal region cerebral venous oxygen saturation	Identification of unappreciated cerebral hypoxia; desaturation associated with outcome	*Less common* with most data in cardiac cases
TCD	Ultrasound of cerebral arteries	Noninvasive Regional Intermittent or continuous	Assessment of CBF-velocity; assessment of vasospasm	Noninvasive assessment of CBF-velocity, ICP, and autoregulation	*Rarely used* in pediatrics since lack of norms
$Pbto_2$	Intraparenchymal electrode measurement	Invasive Focal Continuous	Focal assessment of oxygen tension	Level III recommendation in adult severe TBI, with certain thresholds	*Rarely used* in pediatrics
$Sjvo_2$	Assessment of cerebral venous oxygen saturation	Invasive Global Intermittent or continuous	Global assessment of cerebral oxygen extraction	Level II recommendation in adult severe TBI, with certain thresholds	*Rarely used* in pediatrics
Pupillometry	Pupil assessment with standardized light source	Noninvasive Regional Intermittent	Quantified pupillary diameter and reactivity	Detects pupillary constriction even in small pupils	*Rarely used* in pediatrics
Cerebral microdialysis	Measurement of cerebral analytes	Invasive Focal Intermittent	Focal assessment of bioenergetics and tissue glutamate	Some recommendation for use in adults with severe TBI or poor-grade SAH	*Rarely used* in pediatrics

CBF, cerebral blood flow; EEG, electroencephalography; ICP, intracranial pressure; $Pbto_2$, partial pressure of oxygen in brain tissue; NIRS, near-infrared spectroscopy; SAH, subarachnoid hemorrhage; $Sjvo_2$, oxyhemoglobin saturation in jugular vein (bulb); TBI, traumatic brain injury; TCD, transcranial Doppler.

Continuous EEG Monitoring

Although 1-hour EEG is used in most circumstances, continuous 24-hour EEG or video-EEG monitoring is increasingly used in the ICU. Indications include surveillance for subclinical seizures, the effectiveness of therapy in refractory SE, the achievement of electrical silence in the treatment of severe TBI, metabolic encephalopathies, and neurologic conditions that limit a patient's ability to respond. The depth of impaired consciousness or coma can be assessed, as can the degree to which ongoing electrographic seizures contribute to that state.

The most common configuration is a 20-lead EEG with continuous recording and simultaneous digital video recording. Clinical annotations are made by bedside observers, usually a PICU nurse or parent. A variety of channel configurations can be used. A *channel* is simply a representation of the potential difference between two recording electrodes.

Additional electrodes may include eye leads to discern ocular movements, electromyography, ECG, and a measurement of respiratory frequency.

A variety of software packages are available to interpret EEG data. Specialized software can identify numerous epileptiform abnormalities and detect electrographic seizure activity. Some software systems include the ability to trigger alarms when a seizure or abnormality of interest is detected. Most digital EEG monitoring systems also acquire simultaneous digital video and audio signals.

The amount of useful clinical information gained through prolonged recordings (including simultaneous video monitoring) has proven superior to routine EEGs. Prognostic information can be gained in patients with hypoxic–ischemic encephalopathies. EEG monitoring can also be used as an ancillary study in the determination of death by neurologic criteria.

Limitations of continuous EEG monitoring primarily involve the level of expertise required for data interpretation. PICU staff can be taught to identify seizures and patterns of interest, but full review and analysis usually require a neurophysiologist or neurologist. The time required for interpretation remains significant but has been reduced by technologic advances in digital acquisition, the use of spike- and seizure-detection algorithms, and networked systems. Automatic detection software remains error prone, delays in analysis reduce the benefits of anticipatory care, the application and maintenance of electrodes requires trained technologists, and prolonged electrode placement using collodion can cause scalp breakdown.

Clinical Reports of Continuous EEG Monitoring in the PICU

Seizures may be difficult to detect in comatose children, especially if the episodes are subtle or if neuromuscular blocking agents are used. In these situations, emphasis is on detecting brief electroencephalographic seizures (ES) or prolonged episodes of electroencephalographic status epilepticus (ESE). Typically, ES activity is described as an abnormal paroxysmal event that differed from background activity "lasting longer than 10 seconds with a temporal–spatial evolution in morphology, frequency, and amplitude, and with a plausible electrographic field." ESE is defined as "either a single 30-minute ES or a series of recurrent independent ES totaling more than 30 minutes in any one hour."

In recent PICU series, ES has been identified in 7%–46% and ESE in 18%–35% of the cases. The wide range reflects the case mix in different series. Groups at high risk for ES are patients with epilepsy, CNS infection, structural brain lesions, encephalopathy after cardiac arrest, and TBI. When therapeutic hypothermia is used after cardiac arrest, it is common for seizures to occur during the period of rewarming because treatments that suppressed or treated the EEG activity (sedation, hypothermia) are discontinued.

The presence of ESE (rather than ES alone) is associated with increased mortality and worsened neurologic outcome. Debate about the significance of ES and ESE in comatose, sedated, paralyzed, and possibly postictal patients has led to substantial variation in treatment. ESE may merely be a biomarker of disease severity, with the underlying pathology having the major effect on outcome. Others suggest that early antiepileptic drug management is warranted, and that this seizure burden could be used as a potential therapeutic target in future studies. Instituting continuous EEG monitoring in the PICU requires significant resources including availability during nights and weekends. Additional evidence is needed to determine whether the interventions guided by the use of continuous EEG monitoring improve outcomes.

ICP MONITORING

A full discussion of ICP and cerebral perfusion pressure management is found in Chapter 38. Raised ICP is the most common cause of death in neurosurgical patients, and is extremely common in patients who suffer severe TBI. Elevated ICP following TBI often results in decreased cerebral perfusion pressure (CPP) and secondary injury due to ischemia. The major aim of monitoring and managing elevated ICP is the prevention of cerebral ischemia.

ICP monitoring devices are categorized by site of placement and the method of pressure signal transduction. Catheters can be placed in the lateral ventricles or within brain parenchyma. An intraventricular drain connected to a pressure transducer can be adjusted to zero externally and is the gold standard for measuring ICP. Catheter-tipped ventricular, subdural, or intraparenchymal microtransducers have less infection rate and risk of hemorrhage, but cannot be recalibrated after insertion and zero drift can occur in long-term monitoring.

ICP Trend and Waveform Data

When monitored continuously, changes in the time-averaged mean ICP may be classified into relatively few patterns (**Fig. 35.1**). The first pattern, low and stable ICP (below 20 mm Hg), is seen after uncomplicated TBI (**Fig. 35.1A**) or early after brain trauma before swelling evolves. The second pattern, high and stable ICP (above 20 mm Hg), is the most common pattern after TBI (**Fig. 35.1B**). The third pattern is vasogenic waves and includes B waves (**Fig. 35.1C**) and plateau waves (**Fig. 35.1D**). The fourth pattern is ICP waves related to changes in arterial blood pressure (ABP) and hyperemic events (**Fig. 35.1E–G**). The final pattern, refractory intracranial hypertension (**Fig. 35.1H**), leads to death unless surgical decompression is undertaken. In addition to these patterns, more information can be gained from analyzing the ICP waveform.

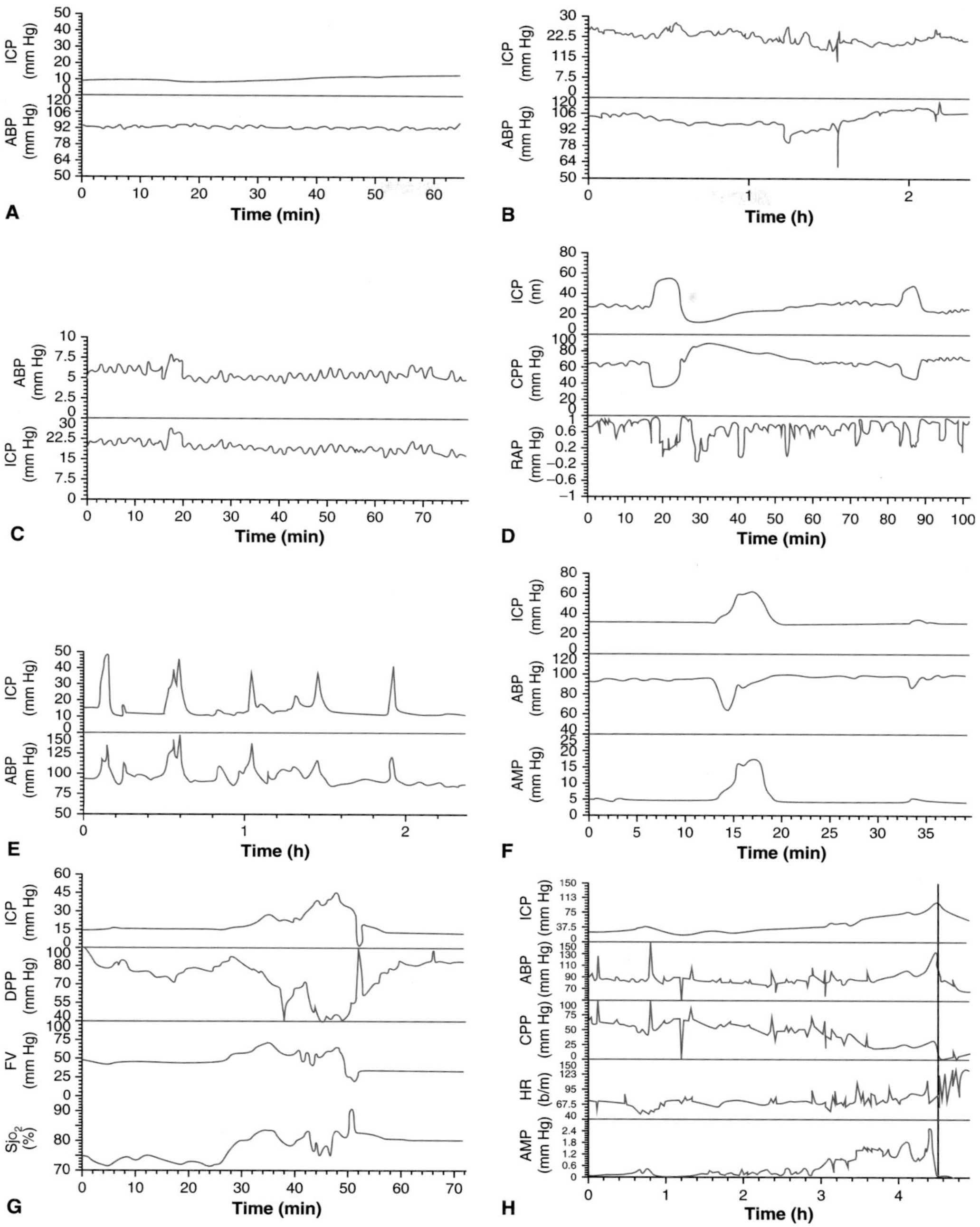

FIGURE 35.1. Examples of intracranial pressure (ICP) recording in various clinical scenarios after head trauma; note the different scales. **A:** Low and stable ICP: mean arterial blood pressure (ABP) is plotted in the *bottom panel*. **B:** Stable and elevated ICP: such a picture can be seen most of the time in patients with head injuries. **C:** B waves of ICP: these are seen both in mean ICP and spectrally resolved pulse amplitude of ICP (AMP). They are also usually seen in a plot of time-averaged ABP, but not always. **D:** Plateau waves of ICP: cerebrospinal compensatory reserve is usually low when waves are recorded (the correlation coefficient between AMP and mean ABP, RAP, is close to +1). At the top of the waves, during maximal vasodilatation, integration between pulse amplitude and mean ICP fails, as indicated by a fall in RAP. After the plateau wave, ICP usually falls below the baseline level and cerebrospinal compensatory reserve becomes better. **E:** High, spiky waves of ICP caused by sudden increases in ABP. **F:** Increase in ICP caused by temporary decrease in ABP. **G:** Increase in ICP of hyperemic nature: both blood flow velocity (FV) and jugular bulb oxygen saturation (SjO_2) increase in parallel with ICP. **H:** Refractory intracranial hypertension: ICP increases within a few hours to 100 mm Hg. The *vertical line* denotes the likely moment when the vasomotor centers in the brainstem became ischemic. At this point, the heart rate (HR) increased and CPP decreased abruptly. Note that pulse amplitude of ICP (AMP) disappeared around 10 minutes before this terminal event. CPP, Cerebral perfusion pressure. (From Kirkham FJ, Wade AM, McElduff F, et al. Seizures in 204 comatose children: Incidence and outcome. *Intensive Care Med* 2012;38:853–62.)

Assessment of Pressure–Volume Compensatory Reserve and Cerebrovascular Pressure Reactivity

The compensatory reserve in intracranial hydrodynamics can be studied through the relation between ICP and changes in volume of the intracerebral space, known as the pressure–volume curve. For example, an index of reserve based on the correlation coefficient (*R*) between amplitude (*A*) and mean pressure (*P*) can be derived (the RAP index). A RAP index close to zero indicates lack of synchronization between changes in amplitude (AMP) and mean ICP. This index denotes good pressure–volume compensatory reserve at low ICP (i.e., a change in volume produces little or no change in pressure) (**Fig. 35.2**). When the RAP index

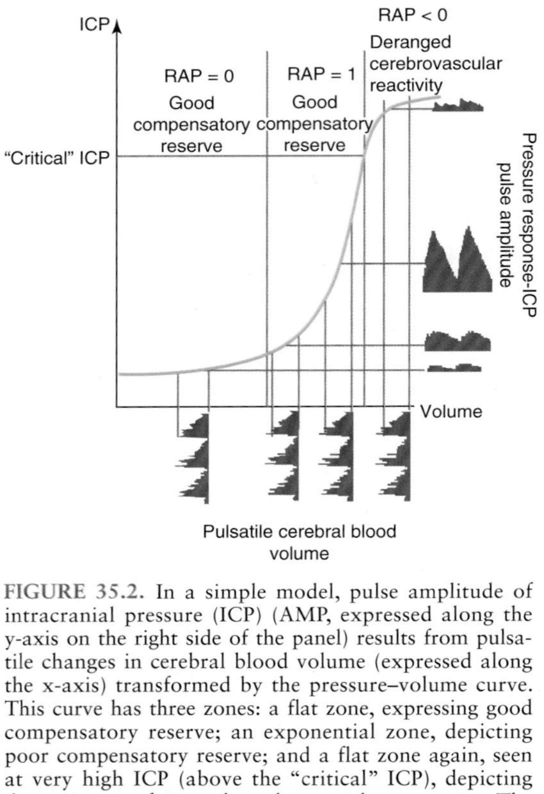

FIGURE 35.2. In a simple model, pulse amplitude of intracranial pressure (ICP) (AMP, expressed along the y-axis on the right side of the panel) results from pulsatile changes in cerebral blood volume (expressed along the x-axis) transformed by the pressure–volume curve. This curve has three zones: a flat zone, expressing good compensatory reserve; an exponential zone, depicting poor compensatory reserve; and a flat zone again, seen at very high ICP (above the "critical" ICP), depicting derangement of normal cerebrovascular responses. The pulse amplitude of ICP is low and does not depend on mean ICP in the first zone. The pulse amplitude increases linearly with mean ICP in the zone of poor compensatory reserve. In the third zone, the pulse amplitude starts to decrease with rising ICP. RAP, index of compensatory reserve. (From Abend NS, Dlugos DJ, Hahn CD, et al. Use of EEG monitoring and management of nonconvulsive seizures in critically ill patients: A survey of neurologists. *Neurocrit Care* 2010;12:382–9; Kirkham FJ, Wade AM, McElduff F, et al. Seizures in 204 comatose children: Incidence and outcome. *Intensive Care Med* 2012;38:853–62.)

rises to +1, compensatory reserve is low; therefore, a further rise in volume produces a rapid increase in ICP. After TBI with brain swelling, the RAP index is usually close to +1. When cerebral autoregulatory capacity is exhausted, the pressure–volume curve bends to the right, the capacity of cerebral arterioles to dilate in response to a fall in CPP is exhausted, and the arterioles tend to collapse passively. This phenomenon indicates terminal cerebrovascular derangement with a decrease in pulse pressure transmission from the arterial bed to the intracranial compartment.

Another ICP-derived index is the pressure-reactivity index (PRx), which incorporates the idea of assessing cerebrovascular reaction by observing the response of ICP to slow spontaneous changes in ABP. For example, when the cerebrovascular bed is normally reactive, any change in ABP produces an inverse change in cerebral blood volume and thus ICP. When cerebrovascular reactivity is disturbed, changes in BP are transmitted passively to ICP. A positive PRx signifies a positive slope of the regression line between the slow components of BP and ICP and signifies a loss of cerebral pressure autoregulation. A negative value of PRx reflects a normally reactive vascular bed, because ABP waves provoke inversely correlated waves in ICP and signifies the presence of cerebral pressure autoregulation. Abnormal values of both PRx and RAP are indicative of poor autoregulation or deranged cerebrospinal compensatory reserve, and are predictive of poor outcome in adults with severe TBI.

TRANSCRANIAL DOPPLER

TCD allows for portable, noninvasive, and repeatable measures of regional CBF. A multidirectional probe has been constructed for simultaneous TCD of the middle cerebral artery (MCA), ophthalmic artery, and/or posterior cerebral artery. The MCA is most commonly studied in children, it is readily accessible to the ultrasonographer, it is the most convenient for probe fixation and long-term monitoring, and it delivers the largest percentage of supratentorial blood. Although the blood flow velocity cannot express a baseline volume of flow, dynamic changes of CBF are reflected in TCD readings. If the ratio of flow velocity in the MCA to the velocity in the ipsilateral internal carotid artery is greater than 3, vasospasm is likely. A ratio below 2 indicates hyperemia. TCD can also be used to assess autoregulation with changes in blood pressure.

Clinical Context of TCD in Pediatric TBI

The incidence of impaired cerebral pressure autoregulation is greatest following moderate-to-severe TBI and is associated with poor outcome. Hyperemia is associated with both impaired autoregulation and poor outcome. Cerebral autoregulation often changes over the course of severe critical illness, worsening autoregulation mirrors progression of injury. In children, bilateral assessment of cerebral autoregulation is required because hemisphere differences are common with an isolated focal injury. Considerable variability in the blood flow velocity (for age and gender) occurs despite a normal CPP (i.e., >40 mm Hg). Patients with high mean blood flow velocity have lower hematocrit than patients with normal mean blood flow velocity, reflecting the sensitivity of the technique to physiologic change and a target for optimization of hemoglobin level. Future studies are needed to establish the relationship between vasospasm and long-term functional outcomes and to evaluate preventative or therapeutic options.

MONITORING BY NIRS

NIRS uses a modification of the Beer–Lambert Law, which describes the relationship between absorption of light and the concentration of deoxyhemoglobin (Hb), oxyhemoglobin (Hbo_2), and cytochrome aa3. NIRS technology differs from pulse oximetry in that it does not require a pulse; therefore, cerebral NIRS monitoring can be used during cardiopulmonary bypass.

NIRS can be accomplished by three mechanisms. A continuous-wave spectrometer is most common in clinical devices. Investigational devices measure "time-of-flight," which have the added benefit of accurately measuring the path length of the light. Phase-resolved spectroscopy emits light that is modulated at a known frequency and assesses the phase shift of the transmitted light to derive the path length.

Commercially available NIRS monitors use two detector optodes at fixed distances (**Fig. 35.3**). The shorter inter-optode distance is designed to represent extracerebral (scalp and bone) tissue infrared absorption. In an effort to better represent intracranial tissue absorption, the extracerebral component is subtracted from the absorption data received by the longer inter-optode distance. From the light absorption data generated, regional cerebral oxyhemoglobin saturation (rSo_2) is calculated. A scaled absolute hemoglobin concentration (oxygenated hemoglobin to total hemoglobin ratio), the tissue oxygenation index, is also available.

The range of baseline rSo_2 values is wide, 68% ± 10% in healthy children. In children with cyanotic heart disease, baseline values range from 38% to 57%. Current usage of NIRS includes detection of superior vena cava occlusion during cardiopulmonary bypass and assessing the effect of carotid ligation during initiation of venoarterial extracorporeal life support.

Limitations of NIRS include its inability to account for patients' varying ratios of brain and extracerebral tissues and variations with age and pathologic state. Icteric patients have depressed cerebral rSo_2 values due to absorption of light by bilirubin. Ongoing blood loss is associated with a decrease in rSo_2, despite $Sjvo_2$, indicating that a changing Hb level confounds cerebral oximetry. The reproducibility of cerebral oxygenation measurements in infants is poor. The major limitation is that no "gold standard" exists to compare NIRS-derived rSo_2. Poor-to-moderate correlation is seen in comparing rSo_2 to global cerebral oxygenation measures, such as $Sjvo_2$, central venous saturation, and invasively monitored cortical brain tissue $Pbto_2$.

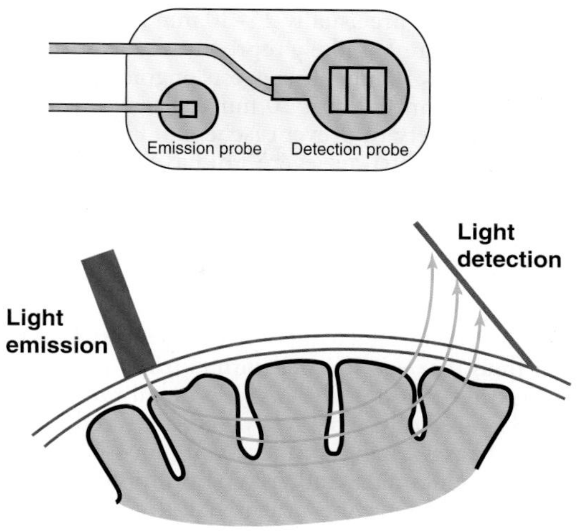

FIGURE 35.3. Near-infrared spectroscopy uses light between 700 and 1000 nm wavelengths, similar to other forms of oximetry. The tissue oxygenation index can detect differences between the left and right frontal hemispheres of the brain at a tissue depth of 2–3 cm. (Illustration courtesy L. Ibsen, MD, MediaLab@Doernbecher).

Clinical Context of NIRS in the PICU

The most robust data for NIRS and outcome in critically ill children come from the cardiac surgical population, typically involving complex repairs under deep hypothermic circulatory arrest. Recent studies showed that NIRS measurements correlated with neurocognitive outcome. Taken together, it is possible that targeting rSo_2 >50% may improve outcome.

REGIONAL BRAIN TISSUE OXYGEN MONITORING

A tissue-monitoring catheter (0.5 mm diameter) may be placed alongside the ICP catheter in the frontal cortex to a depth of 1.5–3 cm to measure regional *brain partial pressure tissue oxygen* ($Pbto_2$) changes. The technology uses a fluorescent dye that responds to O_2, or it can be used with a Clark electrode for measurements of partial pressure in O_2. A temperature probe may be added. Measurements reflect regional rather than global changes and may not correlate with other metabolic measures, such as $Sjvo_2$. Adult studies in TBI suggest that differences in $Pbto_2$ are associated with outcome. With normal CPP and ICP, threshold values in $Pbto_2$ are usually 25–30 mm Hg; measurements <15 mm Hg likely represent tissue at risk of hypoxia and <10 mm Hg suggests ongoing ischemia; therefore, a threshold of 20 mm Hg may provide a margin of safety to prevent ischemia. PICU reports on the use of $Pbto_2$ in severe TBI have been limited.

BRAIN TISSUE MICRODIALYSIS

A microdialysis catheter may be inserted into brain tissue and connected to a pump that delivers a perfusion fluid that equilibrates with extracellular brain tissue fluid through the dialysis membrane. Fluid samples are collected hourly and analyzed at the point of care. Changes in levels of glucose, lactate, pyruvate, glutamate, and various amino acids in the interstitial fluid may be measured. Extracellular concentrations of lactate and glutamate increase during episodes of jugular venous desaturation. Adult studies suggest that changes in these levels may precede the onset of symptomatic vasospasm in subarachnoid hemorrhage, may signal ischemia before detection by changes in either ICP or CPP, and may be predictive of outcome in TBI. Studies also show that increasing the fraction of inspired O_2 results in decreased levels of lactate and glucose, suggesting a potential role for hyperoxygenation as an early therapy. A pediatric catheter is available, but clinical experience is limited.

MULTIMODALITY NEUROMONITORING

Multimodal neuromonitoring refers to a practice described in adult neurocritical care that combines use of the multiple monitoring systems described in **Table 35.1**. High-quality pediatric studies or case series on the use of multimodal monitoring are lacking. Examination is needed of the critical thresholds for each neuromonitoring modality (singularly and in combination) and determination of the risk-to-benefit ratio and impact of such monitoring on patient outcome.

CHAPTER 36 ■ NEUROLOGIC IMAGING

DAVID J. MICHELSON AND STEPHEN ASHWAL

TECHNIQUES OF NEUROIMAGING

Computed Tomography

Computed tomography (CT) images are generated by the analysis of X-ray beams as they are sent through tissues from multiple angles. In comparison with magnetic resonance imaging (MRI), CT images can be quickly and easily obtained. Helical (spiral) scanners have shortened acquisition time of high-quality images, and sedation is rarely needed. Radiation exposure is a disadvantage for young patients and those who require repeated studies, given the risk of radiation-associated neoplasia and possible risk of developmental impairment. Alternative studies, such as ultrasound, MRI, or CT of lower resolution (and thus lower radiation dose), may be preferable. Acute allergic reactions to contrast agents can occur in older children and those with asthma. Portable CT machines make it possible to safely acquire images in patients too unstable for transport to a fixed scanner.

Conventional Anatomic Imaging

Axial images of the head are routinely obtained with a slice thickness of 5 mm; thinner slices can be obtained if greater detail is required, and images can be reformatted into other planes or into three dimensions. The brightness of each voxel (a pixel representing a three-dimensional [3D] volume) on a CT image reflects tissue density. Fatty tissue, water, and air appear dark; soft tissues appear as intermediate shades of gray; and mineralized bone, concentrated blood, iodinated contrast, and metallic objects appear bright. CT is limited by streaking artifacts in areas around metal prostheses, fragments (such as dental fillings or gunshot pellets), and dense bone (such as the temporal petrous bones in the posterior fossa). Areas of abnormal signal can be characterized as hypodense, isodense, or hyperdense relative to neural tissue. The differential for hypodense parenchymal lesions includes edema, infarction, neoplasia, demyelination, inflammation, and cyst formation. Hyperdensity is found in areas of contrast enhancement, hemorrhage, calcification, and hypercellularity. Abnormal calcification can be seen with congenital or chronic infections, tumors and hamartomas, abnormal blood vessels, areas of ischemia, metabolic disorders, and endocrine disorders.

CT Angiography

CT angiography images the vascular anatomy using an intravenous iodinated contrast agent. Thinly cut source images can be reformatted into 2D and 3D images that are nearly as detailed as MR angiograms. CT angiography is faster than MR angiography and can usually be done without sedation in older children.

Magnetic Resonance Imaging

MR images are generated by analysis of signals produced by hydrogen nuclei of molecules in varying tissues, as the spins of the nuclei are aligned in a strong external magnetic field and then perturbed by radiofrequency pulses. MRI is the modality of choice when resolution of fine anatomic detail is desired. Specialized sequences can highlight metabolic changes within the brain. MRI is the imaging test of choice for spinal cord injury. CT images are superior for visualizing fractures and dislocations but do not allow for adequate assessment of the cord. MRI also allows for far more precise imaging of posterior fossa structures, as it is not subject to the artifact produced by the dense temporal petrous bones on CT.

The principal disadvantage of MR imaging is the long acquisition time, necessitating sedation for young children. An audiovisual system within the scanner reduces the need for sedation in children >3 years old. Another disadvantage of MRI is the incompatibility of ferromagnetic materials with the electromagnetic field in the imaging suite. Plastic and aluminum MR-compatible monitors, ventilators, and anesthesia machines are available. Patients with metallic bullet fragments or implants, including cardiac pacemakers and neurostimulators, may not be able to undergo MRI safely. Information regarding the MRI compatibility of implanted medical devices is maintained at http://www.MRIsafety.com. Metallic objects that pose no safety risk (tracheostomy tubes with spiral metal reinforcement) may create artifacts. Gadolinium contrast for MRI studies is safe for most patients but does pose a risk of nephrogenic systemic fibrosis for patients with severely impaired renal function. Detailed guidelines regarding the safe use of contrast agents for CT and MRI are published by the American College of Radiology (http://www.acr.org/quality-safety/resources/contrast-manual).

Conventional Anatomic Imaging

As with CT, MR images are gray-scale maps, and the shade of each voxel reflects the composition of the tissue it represents. The shade of a voxel on an MR image is referred to as its *intensity*, rather than its *density*, because it is determined by factors beyond proton density, including proton mobility (T1 relaxation) and local magnetic effects (T2 relaxation). Various sequences, such as spin echo (SE), gradient-recalled echo (GRE), and fluid-attenuated inversion recovery (FLAIR), use programmed pulses of radiofrequencies and gradient magnetic fields to produce images that highlight T1 or T2 signal effects. On T1-weighted images, fat, methemoglobin, and gadolinium-containing contrast agents appear bright (hyperintense), while cerebrospinal fluid (CSF), muscle, deoxyhemoglobin, and hemosiderin appear dark. On T2-weighted images, CSF, edema, extracellular methemoglobin, areas of hypercellularity, infarction, and demyelination appear bright, while muscle, cortical bone, deoxyhemoglobin, and hemosiderin appear dark.

Routine brain imaging typically begins with a sagittal T1-weighted sequence that serves as a localizer for subsequent sequences and allows evaluation of the corpus callosum, pituitary gland, cerebellar vermis, and other midline structures. Axial T1- and T2-weighted images are also routinely acquired. Coronal images may be particularly helpful for investigation of the cerebellum, temporal lobes, and skull base. FLAIR sequences have improved sensitivity in older children for areas of abnormal intracranial T2 brightness in close proximity to CSF-filled spaces (e.g., ventricles and sulci). High-resolution volumetric 3D T1-weighted scans are useful for evaluation of developmental abnormalities and surgical planning.

Diffusion-weighted Imaging

The diffusion of water molecules can be measured along any 2D plane to which a strong magnetic field gradient has been applied. In standard diffusion-weighted imaging (DWI), bright areas reflect decreased or restricted movement of water. The apparent diffusion coefficient (ADC) map summarizes the diffusion in all three dimensions with the coloring reversed, such that areas of restricted water movement appear dark. DWI is useful in the early evaluation of ischemia, as diffusion restriction becomes apparent minutes after cytotoxic injury. DWI is also used to distinguish cystic tumors from epidermoid tumors and recurrent tumors from areas of peritumoral edema. Diffusion restriction is also seen within cerebral abscesses and empyemas.

Susceptibility-weighted Imaging

Gradient echo T2-weighted imaging can detect blood and blood breakdown products, but it is not as sensitive as susceptibility-weighted imaging (SWI) which makes these same paramagnetic artifacts far more apparent (**Fig. 36.1**). SWI shows areas of cerebral

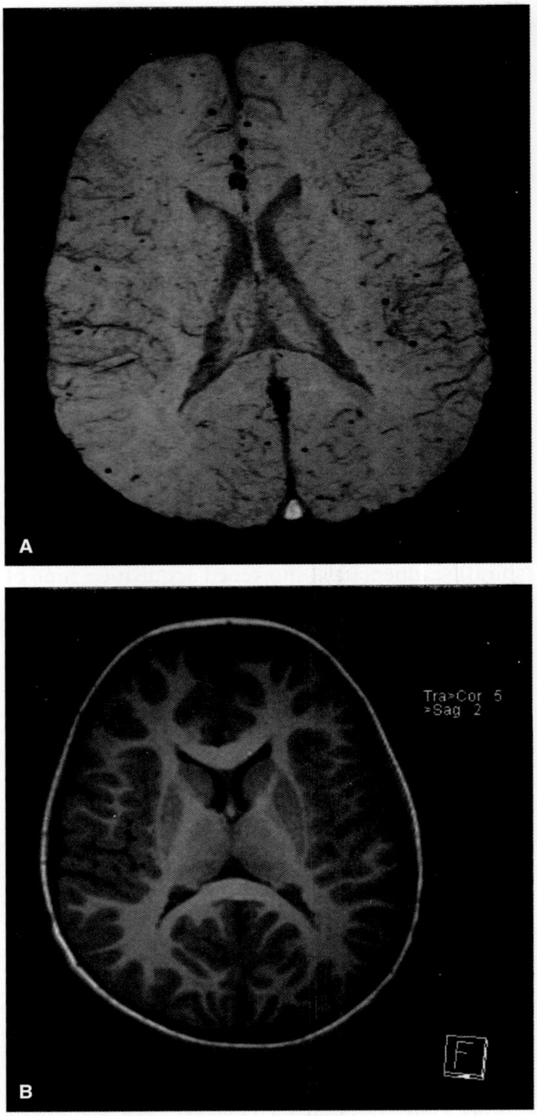

FIGURE 36.1. Four-year-old boy with a history of complex congenital heart disease (including a double-outlet right ventricle) who underwent cardiac bypass for an arterial switch procedure. Diffusely scattered punctate hemorrhages at the cortical–subcortical junction are visible on MRI using the SWI sequence (**A**) that would not have been identified using T1-weighted (**B**) or FLAIR sequences.

ischemia due to greater oxygen extraction in areas with slowed or diminished blood flow.

Diffusion Tensor Imaging

Because water diffuses more freely parallel to white matter fiber tracts, DWI using multiple planes can create color-coded maps that visualize tract disruption by mass lesions, traumatic shearing, and ischemic injury. These images are sometimes called fractional anisotropy (FA) maps. Clinical applications include presurgical planning for resection of brain tumors and epileptic regions of cortex. DWI may also help in the identification of subtle cortical and subcortical abnormalities in patients with medically intractable epilepsy.

MR Angiography/Venography

Reconstructions of the arterial supply and venous drainage of the brain can be obtained from maximum intensity projections (MIPs) from 2D or 3D time-of-flight images. The images created represent blood flow better than luminal diameter and can overstate the degree of stenosis in a vessel. As the process of generating MIP images may produce artifacts, suspected abnormalities should be confirmed in the source images.

MR Spectroscopy

Spectroscopic imaging most often analyzes the signals generated by protons of clinically important neuronal and glial metabolites, including *N*-acetyl aspartate (NAA), choline and phosphatidylcholine (Cho), creatine and phosphocreatine (Cre), myoinositol (mI), and lactate. Short echo images demonstrate a wider variety of metabolites and are useful for assessing inborn errors of metabolism. Longer echo times provide more accurate quantification of the principal brain metabolites, potentially useful in the assessment of prognosis.

MR Perfusion

A number of MR methods measure cerebral perfusion. Perfusion imaging is used to assess the risk of ischemia in tissues with decreased perfusion, identify decreased perfusion in primary and secondary vasculopathies, and grade the vascularity of tumors.

SELECTED CLINICAL APPLICATIONS

Trauma

The initial workup of children with head trauma usually begins with a CT of the head and neck, looking for acute hemorrhage, fracture, or displacement of vertebrae. Young children who suffer traumatic brain injury (TBI) are at particular risk of upper cervical spine injury because of the relative weight of the cranium, weakness of the paraspinous muscles, elasticity and redundancy of the interspinous ligaments, and horizontal orientation of the incompletely ossified facet joints.

Spinal MRI should be considered in children even without evidence of misalignment or fracture of the vertebrae on plain imaging in a neutral position, as soft tissue and cord edema, ischemia, and hemorrhage may only be visible on spinal MRI. The primarily pediatric entity, spinal cord injury without radiologic abnormality (SCIWORA), refers only to plain-film and CT imaging. As children reach adolescence, they are increasingly likely to sustain bony injuries with spinal trauma, but less severe injuries can still occur without plain-film evidence of fractures. Brain MRI provides greater sensitivity than CT for brainstem injury, edema and petechial hemorrhages from axonal shearing, small extra-axial fluid collections, and older blood products and is, therefore, the study of choice once a patient has been stabilized.

Imaging may show traumatic hemorrhage that is parenchymal, due to contusion or axonal shearing, or extraparenchymal, with the development of an epidural or subdural hematoma. When blood cells layer within a hematoma, the upper layer appears bright on T1- and T2-weighted images, while the bottom appears isointense to brain on T1-weighted images and dark on T2-weighted images. Finding signs of both old and new TBI adds to the suspicion for abusive head trauma in infants. Subarachnoid blood due to trauma is most commonly seen layering along the falx cerebri in the posterior interhemispheric fissure or the tentorium cerebelli and is best detected in the acute stage by CT. Subacute hemorrhage can be detected by FLAIR sequences on MRI, although high signal intensity on FLAIR can also be caused by rapid CSF flow, normally seen around the ventricular foramina, the aqueduct of Sylvius, and the prepontine cistern. CT and MRI may appear normal in the first 12 hours after severe TBI, with cerebral edema becoming evident later. DWI can show restricted diffusion due to cytotoxic edema within hours of injury.

Hypoxic–Ischemic Injury

The imaging of infarction depends more on the vascular distribution, degree, and duration of substrate deprivation than on the etiology and risk factors involved. Thrombosis of the superior sagittal sinus can result in parasagittal infarction, of the transverse sinus and vein of Labbé thrombosis in temporal lobe infarction, and of the deep cerebral veins, the straight sinus, or vein of Galen in thalamic infarction. Progressive venous obstruction causes vasogenic edema, infarction, and hemorrhage, all of which appear different on neuroimaging. CT may show areas of subcortical white matter hypodensity due to edema and areas of hyperdensity due to hemorrhage. Intravenous contrast is often necessary to detect venous thrombosis, with the flow of contrast around the thrombus described as the *empty delta sign*. MRI can often visualize venous thrombosis system without contrast.

Focal arterial infarction appears on CT as a wedge-shaped area of hypodensity that involves the cortex and white matter supplied by the occluded artery (**Fig. 36.2A**). Posterior circulation infarctions may be difficult to appreciate in infants whose temporal and occipital white matter normally appears hypodense from hypomyelination. MRI is more sensitive than

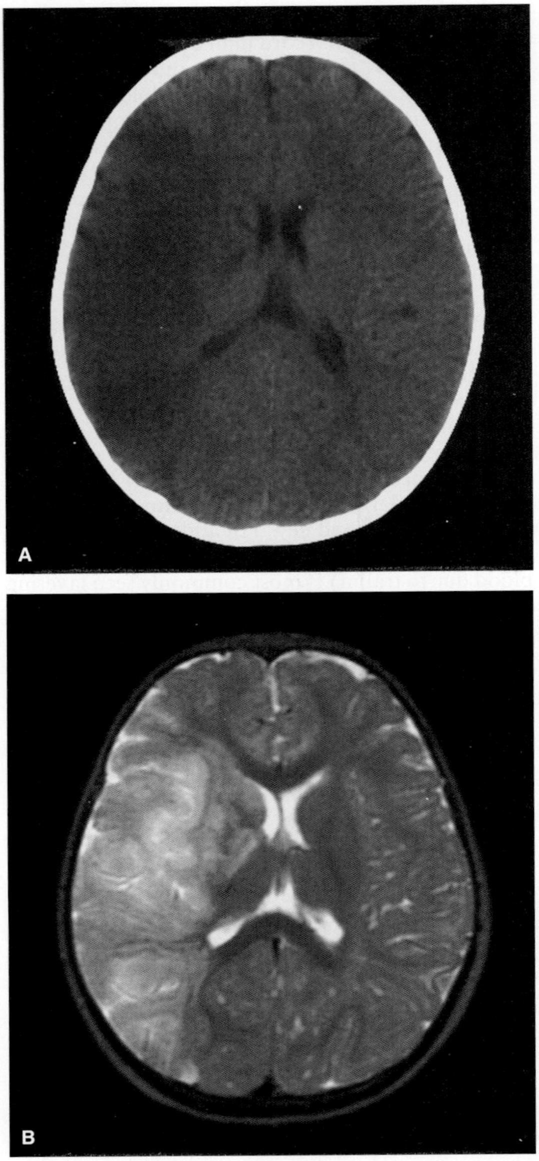

FIGURE 36.2. Two-year-old girl who awoke with left hemiparesis and right gaze preference. **A:** A wedge-shaped area of hypodensity is seen on axial CT. MRI shows (**B**) T2 hyperintensity, indicative of an ischemic stroke in the distribution of the right middle cerebral artery.

CT for the detection of early ischemia-related cerebral edema (**Fig. 36.2B**). DWI shows restricted water movement from cytotoxic edema as soon as 1 hour after injury. Angiography, using either CT or MR, can assess medium-to-large vessel abnormalities, such as occlusion, thrombosis, dysplasia, inflammatory vasculopathy, or dissection. Neither method is likely to detect the narrowing of arterioles and smaller vessels seen with inflammatory diseases.

Diffuse hypoxic–ischemic injury can result from cardiopulmonary arrest, severe hypotension, or hypoxemia. A decrease in cerebral perfusion initially causes shunting of blood flow to the posterior circulation to protect the brainstem. The cortex supplied by branches of the carotid artery, especially the intervascular boundary zones, is vulnerable to ischemic injury, often resulting in a "watershed" distribution pattern (**Fig. 36.3**). Profound decreases in cerebral blood flow do not allow preferential shunting and put regions with the high basal metabolic rates (including the thalami, basal ganglia, and sensorimotor cortex) at the greatest risk of injury.

CT within the first 24 hours may be read as normal even when severe ischemic injury has occurred. The earliest appreciable changes, such as basal ganglia hypodensity and effacement of the perimesencephalic cisterns, may be very subtle, with poor interobserver reliability. Later CT scans will show evidence of cerebral edema, with decreased differentiation between the cortex and white matter, effacement of the sulci and cisterns, and hypodensity of the deep and cortical gray matter. Particularly ominous for prognosis is the "reversal sign," with white matter appearing denser than cortex, possibly due to congestion from impaired venous drainage. Early changes of global ischemia can also be subtle with conventional MRI, although diffusion restriction can usually be seen in infarcted areas and proton MR spectroscopy can show a rise in glutamate and glutamine, with or without the presence of lactate. Very early DWI can significantly underestimate the extent of ischemic injury. Prognosis is best assessed by the presence of lactate

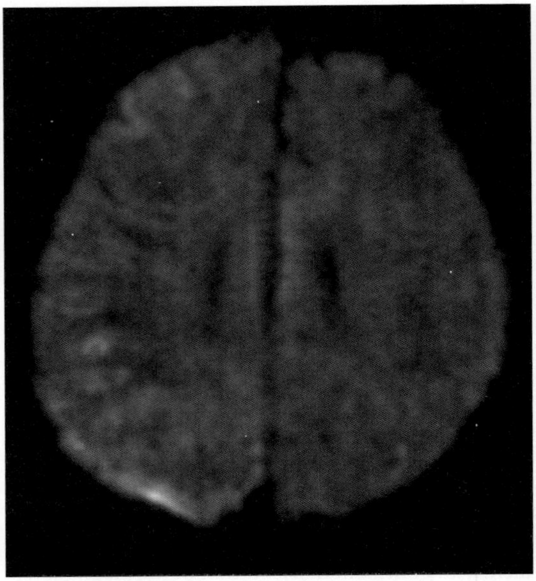

FIGURE 36.3. Thirteen-month-old boy presenting with pneumococcal meningitis and mild left-sided weakness. DWI shows restriction within the interarterial or watershed regions of the right frontal and parietal cortex.

or reduced NAA-to-Cre ratios on MR spectroscopy 3–5 days after injury.

Infection and Inflammation

When CNS infection is suspected and a lumbar puncture (LP) is contemplated, it is common to first obtain a head CT to determine if a mass lesion is present that might predispose to cerebral herniation. Studies in adults suggest that imaging prior to an LP is unlikely to be abnormal in patients with normal neurologic examinations. The presence of a mass lesion on CT is poorly predictive of the risk of imminent cerebral herniation, whether or not LP is performed.

Meningitis

CT in patients with meningitis can show meningeal contrast enhancement (especially in later stages) and show sources of infection such as mastoiditis, sinusitis, and skull-based fractures. Complications of meningitis (e.g., ischemic stroke from vasculitis, obstructive and communicating hydrocephalus, and hemorrhage from venous thrombosis) are also evaluated well by contrast-enhanced CT. MRI is more likely to show meningeal contrast enhancement in uncomplicated meningitis, and MRI with DWI is superior to CT in demonstrating some infectious and vasculitic complications of meningitis including encephalitis, cerebritis, abscess, empyema, ventriculitis, and ischemia (**Fig. 36.4**).

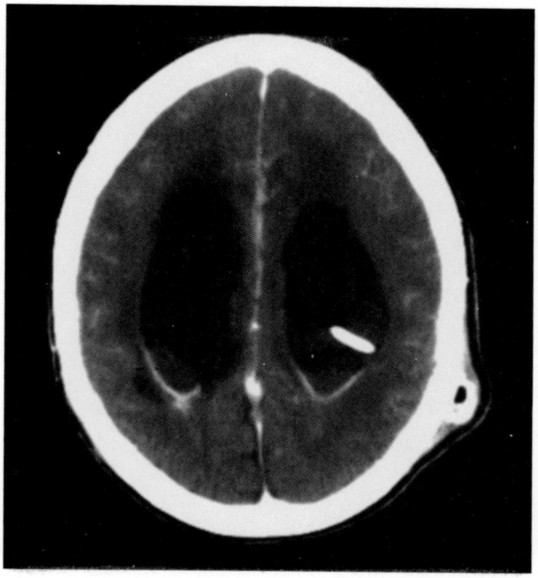

FIGURE 36.4. Thirteen-year-old boy with lumbar myelomeningocele and congenital hydrocephalus presenting with fever and obtundation. Brain MRI with contrast shows expanded lateral ventricles due to shunt failure and contrast enhancement of the lining of the posterior horns of the ventricles due to ventriculitis and pseudomonas meningitis. A portion of the ventriculoperitoneal shunt is visible in the left lateral ventricle.

Meningoencephalitis

MRI with DWI is highly sensitive for the cytotoxic edema and necrosis associated with infection and predictive of the long-term neurologic prognosis. Imaging findings in encephalitis due to herpesvirus are often focal, but with other viral agents, including enteroviruses and arboviruses, are often nonspecific and may be limited to subtle T2 hyperintensity within cortical and subcortical gray matter. Ring-enhancing lesions should raise the possibility of fungi (*Cryptococcus*, *Aspergillus*, *Candida*), parasites (toxoplasmosis, cysticercosis, amoebae), and *Mycobacterium tuberculosis*. The differential is expanded in patients who are immunocompromised.

Spinal Infections

Spinal CT with contrast enhancement has better detection of paraspinal infection than plain X-ray, but it is insufficiently sensitive to exclude early discitis or epidural abscess and does not assess spinal cord integrity. Urgent surgical intervention may prevent permanent injury, and MRI should be performed early in suspected spinal infection if no contraindication exists (**Fig. 36.5**).

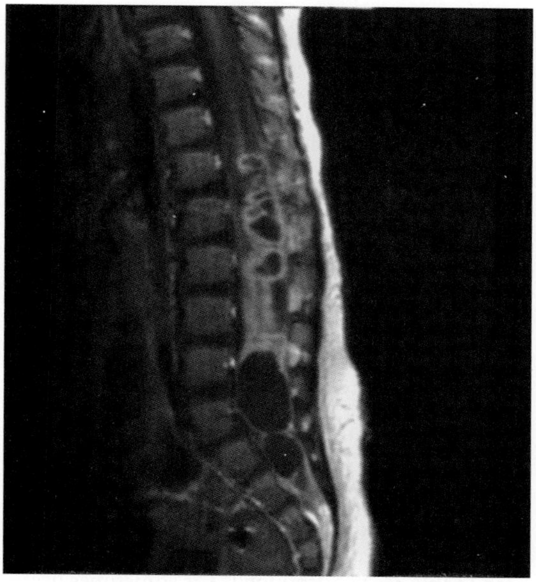

FIGURE 36.5. Fourteen-month-old boy presenting with fever, irritability, and sudden refusal to walk. MRI of the thoracolumbar spine shows multiple loculated ring-enhancing abscesses within the spinal epidural space. Imaging also revealed a dural sinus tract associated with a small conus medullaris lipoma and tethering of the spinal cord.

Postinfectious Encephalomyelitis

Autoimmune inflammatory neuropathies may follow infections, vaccinations, and traumatic

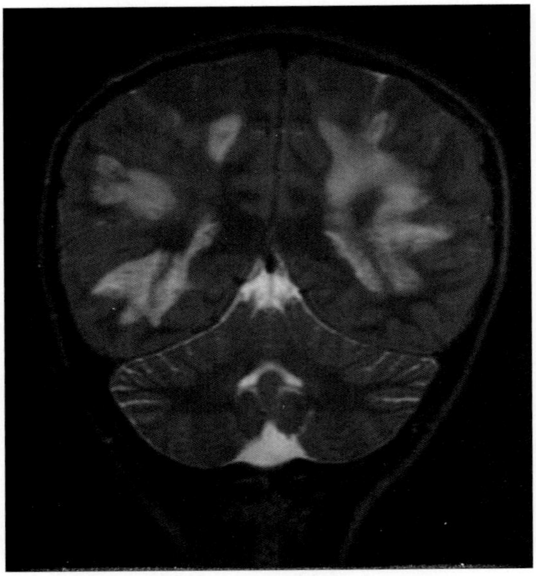

FIGURE 36.6. Seven-year-old girl who presented with hallucinations and obtundation due to ADEM. T2-weighted coronal MR images show diffuse T2 hyperintensity within the subcortical white matter, right thalamus, and pons.

injuries. Any portion of the central or peripheral nervous system can be involved in such isolated syndromes as optic neuritis, acute cerebellar ataxia, transverse myelitis, and Guillain–Barré syndrome. Alternatively, multiple areas of the nervous system can undergo autoimmune demyelination in cases of acute disseminated encephalomyelitis (ADEM). MRI is well suited for the detection of ADEM lesions in the brain and spinal cord. The differential of ADEM includes atypical infection (e.g., cryptococcal meningitis), neoplasia (e.g., lymphoma), ischemia (e.g., vasculitis), and demyelination from multiple sclerosis (MS) (**Fig. 36.6**).

Toxic and Metabolic Injury

A variety of metabolic disorders (from inborn errors of metabolism to acquired endogenous or exogenous toxins) can show nonspecific patterns characterized by whether they affect gray matter, white matter, or both (**Table 36.1**). Although CT is sometimes useful to detect calcifications that can occur in these disorders, MRI is superior for identifying the pattern of injury and may provide a specific diagnosis. While nonspecific, detection of otherwise unexplained deep gray matter lactate contributes to the diagnosis of mitochondrial disorders.

TABLE 36.1

Metabolic Disorders That Produce Gray and White Matter Imaging Abnormalities

Cortical Gray Matter Only
Cortical Dysgenesis
Congenital CMV infection
Congenital muscular dystrophy
Peroxisomal disorders
No Cortical Dysgenesis
Mucopolysaccharidoses
Lipid storage disorders
Deep Gray Matter
Early Thalamic Involvement
Krabbe disease
GM1 or GM2 gangliosidosis
Wilson disease
Profound neonatal hypotensive encephalopathy
Early Globus Pallidus Involvement
Canavan disease
Kearn–Sayre syndrome
Methylmalonic academia
Toxins (carbon monoxide and cyanide)
Maple syrup urine disease
L-2-hydroxyglutaric aciduria
Dentatorubropallidoluysian atrophy
Urea cycle disorders
Cree leukoencephalopathy
Early Striatal Involvement
Mitochondrial disorders (Leigh and MELAS syndrome)
Wilson disease
Organic acidurias
Molybdenum cofactor deficiency
β-Ketothiolase deficiency
Biotinidase deficiencies
Hypoxia–ischemia or hypoglycemia
Cockayne syndrome
Toxins

Adapted from Barkovich AJ. *Pediatric Neuroimaging*. Philadelphia, PA: Lippincott Williams & Wilkins, 2005.

Posterior Reversible Encephalopathy Syndrome

This syndrome of vasogenic edema in the parietal and occipital cortical and subcortical regions, also known as reversible posterior leukoencephalopathy syndrome (RPLS), is usually reversible. It has been associated with hypertensive crisis and other factors seen in critically ill children (e.g., sepsis, multiorgan dysfunction, anemia, and exposure to cytotoxic medications), all of which may cause endothelial injury

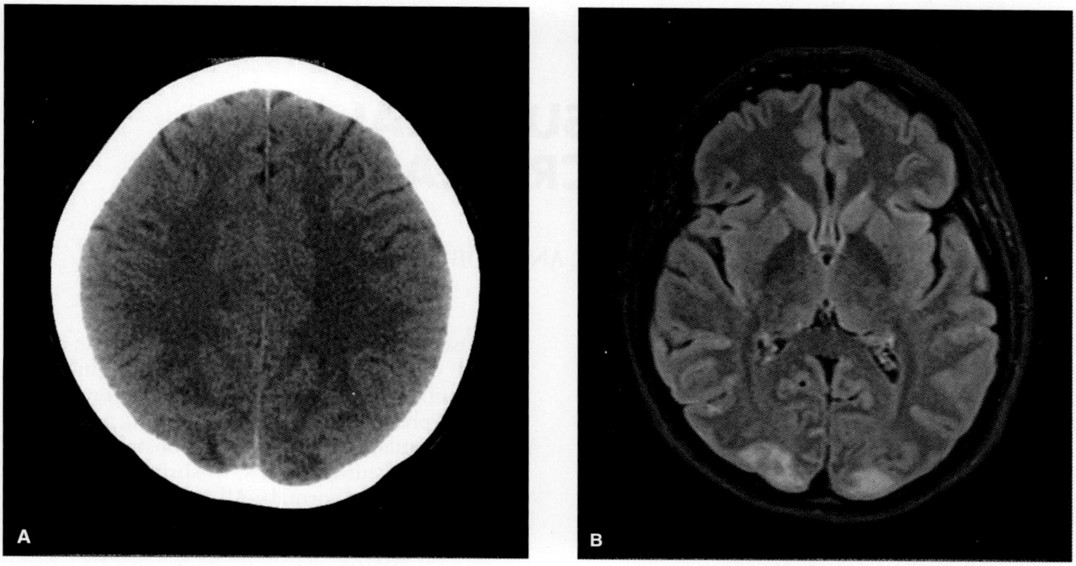

FIGURE 36.7. Twenty-two-year-old woman with hypertensive crisis in the postpartum period, presenting with a severe headache, transient loss of vision, and a generalized tonic–clonic seizure. Subcortical edema is visible as subtle hypodensity in the occipital cortex on head CT (**A**) and is more evident as hyperintensity on the FLAIR sequence of a head MRI (**B**).

or impair cerebral autoregulation. MRI using FLAIR sequences is particularly sensitive for this condition (**Fig. 36.7**). MRI with SWI and DWI sequences can also identify atypical or complex cases in which there is an unusual distribution of lesions or associated hemorrhage or ischemia.

CHAPTER 37 ■ NEUROSURGICAL AND NEURORADIOLOGIC CRITICAL CARE

MICHAEL L. MCMANUS, CRAIG D. MCCLAIN, AND ROBERT C. TASKER

CLINICAL SCIENTIFIC FOUNDATIONS

General Anesthetic Considerations

In neuroanesthesia, the goals include appropriate levels of oxygen and carbon dioxide, adequate cerebral blood flow (CBF), and avoidance of exacerbations of intracranial hypertension. Hyponatremia, hypo-osmolarity, and hyperglycemia are prevented as they contribute to cerebral swelling and neurologic injury. Anesthetic premedication is cautiously used to avoid respiratory depression and is avoided when significant intracranial hypertension is present. Induction agents are carefully titrated to avoid hypotension and decreased CBF. Thiopental, propofol, etomidate, and ketamine are common induction agents, and their effects on blood pressure (BP), intracranial pressure (ICP), CBF, and cerebral metabolic rate for oxygen ($CMRO_2$) are considered prior to use. Previous concerns about the deleterious effects of ketamine have been questioned, and its use is increasing. To minimize vasodilation from volatile agents, *anesthesia maintenance* usually involves a "balanced" technique of nitrous oxide, narcotic, and low-dose volatile agent. The effect of volatile agents on CBF can vary with the dose of agent (increased vasodilation at higher dose), the region of brain studied (more pronounced on surface vessels), and the use of hyperventilation to cause vasoconstriction (often requested by neurosurgeons, to shrink brain tissue, even when ICP is normal). All volatile agents cause dose-dependent increases in CBF that can be attenuated with controlled ventilation. There is long-standing debate around the use of nitrous oxide since it can cause some degree of cerebral vasodilation, may contribute to postoperative vomiting, and is contraindicated when air collections that it may expand are present (i.e., recent craniotomy). Ultra-short-acting agents (e.g., remifentanil or dexmedetomidine) are increasingly used. Anesthetic agents are managed to permit immediate neurologic assessment upon emergence. The effects of common anesthetics on $CMRO_2$, CBF, pressure autoregulation, and ICP are listed in **Table 37.1**.

Pre- and Intraoperative Fluid Management

Euvolemia is preferred before induction of anesthesia to avoid hypotension. Intraoperative fluids are predominantly isotonic as vasodilation and acute blood

TABLE 37.1

Effects of Anesthetics, Benzodiazepines, and Opioids on Cerebral Metabolism, Circulation, and Intracranial Pressure

■ AGENT	■ $CMRO_2$	■ CBF	■ PRESSURE AUTOREGULATION	■ ICP
Inhaled anesthetic	↓↓	↑	Absent	↑
Sevoflurane				
Isoflurane				
Desflurane				
Inhaled nitrous oxide	↑ or no change	↑	Present	↑
Intravenous anesthetic	↓↓	↓↓	Present	↓↓
Propofol				
Thiopental				
Dissociative anesthesia	No change	↑↑	?	↑↑
Ketamine				
Sedative benzodiazepines	↓↓	↓	Present	↓
Analgesic opioids	No change	No change	Present	No change

The direction of arrows indicates increased or decreased, and the number of arrows indicates the strength of the derangement above "no change" qualitatively.

loss can necessitate sudden infusion of large volumes. Fluid replacement is best guided by heart rate, BP, and perfusion since urine output can be profoundly influenced by stress-related changes in antidiuretic hormone (ADH) secretion, and oliguria can arise from many sources. Maintenance of euvolemia supports CBF and helps avoid venous air embolism (VAE) via skull dural sinuses. The stress response should maintain normal serum glucose levels without exogenous glucose administration. Glucose-containing fluids should be used to meet baseline needs for neonates and susceptible infants. Older children usually tolerate 18–24 hours of fasting before requiring glucose-containing fluid. Hyperglycemia may worsen injury due to ischemia, but it remains unclear if tight glycemic control offers significant benefits.

Hemodynamic Management

Intravenous anesthetic agents generally preserve CBF and autoregulation, while volatile agents cause some degree of vasodilation and autoregulatory impairment (**Table 37.1**). As depth of anesthesia increases, so too does the impact on the circulation and CBF. In cerebrovascular surgery, vasoactive medications are always kept available to manipulate the circulation.

Surgical Considerations

Cranial surgeries may require skull fixation using pin placement. Complications of pins include increases in heart rate, BP, and ICP, as well as skull fractures and intracranial hemorrhages. The sitting position is associated with an increased risk of VAE. Blood loss can be particularly challenging in hemispherectomies and craniofacial reconstruction. Anticonvulsant use may predispose to platelet dysfunction, thrombocytopenia, and factor deficiencies that can increase blood loss.

Emergence

Regardless of the neuroanesthesia technique, rapid *anesthesia emergence* is important. When extubation is not possible, it is still prudent to confirm responsiveness upon arrival in the PICU. Interlocking cycles in pathophysiology may lead to hemodynamic instability, cerebral edema, and intracranial hemorrhage in the immediate postoperative period (**Fig. 37.1**). Emergence

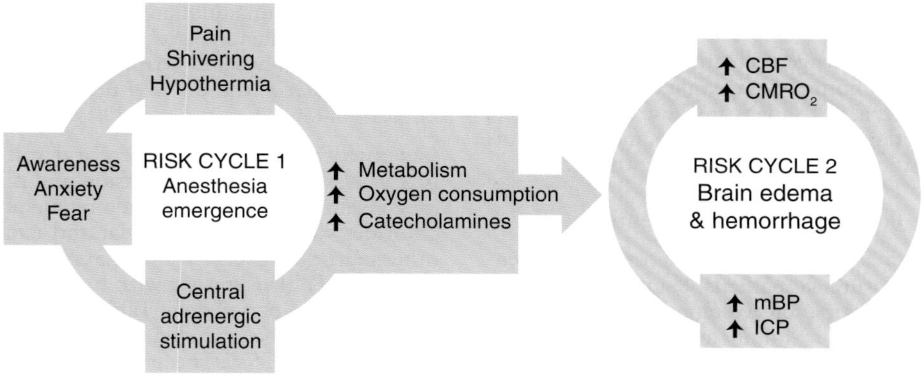

FIGURE 37.1. Potential stress-induced pathophysiology during emergency from anesthesia. mBP, mean blood pressure.

TABLE 37.2

Factors to Consider in the Patient Failing to Wake up at the End of Neurosurgery

FACTOR	INTERVENTION
Neuromuscular blockade	Impaired hepatic and/or renal metabolism may prolong the effect
Altered drug metabolism	Consider drug dosing and drug clearance of continuous infusions (also see hypothyroid)
Seizure	Assess and treat accordingly
Intracranial bleeding	Imaging required and surgery
Intracranial pressure/ischemia	Imaging required
Hypothermia	Warm patient
Hypoglycemia	Check blood glucose and treat accordingly
Hypercapnia	Check blood gas and support ventilation as needed
Hypo-osmolality	Check serum electrolytes and treat accordingly
Hypothyroidism	Thyroid hormone required for benzodiazepine metabolism; support patient until full emergence and thyroid function tests available

agitation may be due to pain, a full bladder, dysnatremia, drug reaction, or emergence delirium. When a patient unexpectedly fails to awaken at the end of surgery, a number of factors need to be considered and corrected (**Table 37.2**) and emergency imaging obtained.

POSTOPERATIVE NEUROSURGICAL CARE IN THE PICU

Initial PICU Care

Mechanical Ventilation

If postoperative mechanical ventilation is necessary, the goals are to support gas exchange and permit neurologic assessment. When inflation pressures are high, decreased BP and cerebral perfusion pressure (CPP, mean BP – ICP) should be avoided. ICP monitoring may be necessary if sedation interferes with neurologic examination or administration of PEEP increases ICP.

Hemodynamic and Fluid Management

Hemodynamic management targets BP within 20% of preoperative or normal-for-age values. When increased ICP is a concern, CPP targets are those used in trauma. Because of the risk of hyponatremia, many clinicians choose isotonic fluids (particularly normal saline).

Postoperative Dysnatremia

Disorders of salt and water homeostasis are common in neurosurgical patients. Pain, stress, nausea, vomiting, narcotics, and volume depletion may all have the potential to stimulate vasopressin production and induce a state of euvolemic hyponatremia not dissimilar to the syndrome of inappropriate antidiuretic hormone (SIADH). Hypotonic fluid administration or fluid restriction may contribute. Urine tonicity is often fixed in the postoperative period, and urine output is maintained constant at ~1 mL/kg/h. Hypotonic fluids decrease serum sodium concentration, and CSF drainage can cause sodium loss and hyponatremia.

Syndrome of Inappropriate ADH Secretion. Postoperative hyponatremia, euvolemia, and ADH excess define the SIADH. Screening approach includes serum sodium concentration < 135 mmol/L, urine output < 2 mL/kg/h, variable urinary sodium concentration (spot urine sodium > 20 mmol/L), and variable urine osmolarity. Other causes of hyponatremia that need to be excluded are volume depletion, edematous states (congestive heart failure, cirrhosis, and nephrosis), renal dysfunction, adrenal insufficiency, and hypothyroidism. SIADH occurs due to free water retention at the same time as natriuresis, with fluid balance maintained at the expense of serum osmolality. ADH excess leads to increased water permeability in the collecting duct, water retention, and subclinical volume expansion, with an increase in total body water of 7%–10%. The treatment of SIADH is to reduce free water excess by fluid restriction and diuretics. If a hyponatremic seizure occurs, then hypertonic saline is used to correct serum sodium to ≥130 mmol/L. A 3–5 mmol/L increase in serum sodium is anticipated with an IV bolus of 4–6 mL/kg (2–3 mmol/kg) of 3% saline.

Cerebral Salt Wasting. Cerebral salt wasting (CSW) is a diagnosis of exclusion and often overdiagnosed. The features include renal sodium and chloride wasting, hypovolemia, and exclusion of other causes of excess sodium excretion. Patients with SIADH also present with hyponatremia, but exhibit mild hypervolemia. **Table 37.3** lists diagnoses that should be excluded before concluding that the patient has CSW. The atrial natriuretic peptide level is high in cerebrovascular patients who have

TABLE 37.3

Differential Diagnosis of Salt Wasting

Physiologic extracellular fluid volume expansion (e.g., hyperhydration with 1.5 times maintenance followed by abrupt decreases in intake)
Diuretics
Hypoaldosteronism (Note: Aldosterone stimulates sodium reabsorption.)
Adrenocortical insufficiency
Renal tubular disorders (including congenital salt-losing disorders—Bartter or Gitelman syndrome)
Presence of an inhibitor of renal reabsorption of sodium such as osmotic agents, high concentration of ligands for the calcium receptor in the loop of Henle (e.g., hypercalcemia, gentamicin)
Obligatory excretion of sodium by the excretion of anions other than chloride
High-output renal failure (renal tubular damage such as obstructive uropathy, interstitial nephritis, and acute tubular necrosis)
Sodium wasting from cerebrospinal fluid drainage
Pressure natriuresis from adrenergic agents
Downregulation of renal sodium transport by chronic hypervolemia

received perioperative hypervolemic fluid management, and natriuresis is a response to homeostatic volume control, and not CSW. CSW has been reported in association with calvarial remodeling, tumor resection, and hydrocephalus. Hyponatremia (<135 mmol/L) with brisk diuresis (>3 mL/kg/h), elevated urine sodium (>120 mmol/L), or elevated urinary osmolarity (>300 mOsm/L water) is seen. The physiology involves inappropriate and excessive release of natriuretic peptides that leads to a primary natriuresis and volume depletion. A secondary hormonal response occurs with an increase in the renin–angiotensin system and arginine vasopressin production. Patients with CSW are more likely to have suffered postoperative stroke, have chiasmatic or hypothalamic tumors, or are younger than patients with normal postoperative sodium concentration. Almost half of the patients with CSW have postoperative hyponatremic seizures. The treatment of CSW involves sodium administration to match urinary losses and correction of intravascular volume contraction. More rapid resolution of hyponatremia after volume expansion may be achieved with fludrocortisone.

Diabetes Insipidus. Diabetes insipidus (DI) results from a deficiency of vasopressin and is expected after surgical procedures near the pituitary or hypothalamus. It is frequently associated with craniopharyngiomas and is a presenting symptom in 40% of cases. The diagnosis should be suspected when serum sodium is >145 mmol/L in association with urine output >2.5 mL/kg/h for three consecutive hours, or >4 mL/kg/h in any 1 hour. The urine osmolality is hypotonic (<300 mOsm/L) with increased plasma osmolality (>300 mOsm/L), in the absence of glycosuria, mannitol use, and renal failure. Severe dehydration and hypovolemia can occur. There are a variety of approaches to treating DI. Deficiencies of thyroid and/or adrenocortical hormones can coexist. Patients respond to an infusion of aqueous vasopressin, which has a rapid onset of action and brief duration of effect. Doses are titrated up rapidly until a response is seen. The potential for hypervolemia, hyponatremia, and hypertension requires close observation in a monitored setting. The infusion produces a "functional SIADH" state. Because urine output is then minimal (0.5 mL/kg/h), other clinical markers of volume status must be followed closely. Excessive fluids (oral or intravenous) can lead to intravascular volume overload, and the administration of hypotonic fluids can result in dangerous hyponatremia. Restricting fluids to replacement of insensible losses may prevent these complications. In children at risk for permanent DI and tolerating oral intake, IV fluids and the vasopressin infusion can be discontinued and free oral intake permitted. DDAVP is started when polyuria develops. DDAVP is a synthetic vasopressin that lasts 12–24 hours. It is administered orally or intranasally. Antidiuresis begins within 1 hour. DDAVP treatment is effective once an intact thirst mechanism has returned without vomiting.

Analgesia and Sedation

The ideal sedation regimen in neurosurgical patients would include short-acting or reversible agents that can be withdrawn intermittently to permit neurologic assessment. A single agent suitable for children is not available. Propofol is a potent, short-acting, sedative–hypnotic that is extremely useful in adult neurocritical care but has only limited utility in pediatrics because of an association with a fatal syndrome of bradycardia, rhabdomyolysis, metabolic acidosis, and multiple organ failure when infused over extended periods. This complication is related to the duration of therapy and the cumulative dose, and it is much less common in adults.

Dexmedetomidine, an α-2 agonist, has many of the advantages of propofol as an ultra-short-acting, single-agent, postoperative sedative. Unlike with propofol, spontaneous breathing is usually maintained. Because dexmedetomidine is both an α-2a and α-2b agonist, its central effects cause sympatholysis while its peripheral effects cause vasoconstriction. Transient increases in BP can be seen with boluses followed by hypotension and bradycardia as sedation deepens. Both hypo- and hypertension can be observed with long-term infusions, and a withdrawal syndrome results when extended infusions are discontinued. The mainstay of sedation in the PICU remains a combination of opioid and benzodiazepine. Titration to a validated sedation score is advised and regular "drug holidays" help insure that excessive sedation is avoided. Infants and children receiving sedative infusion for more than 3–5 days develop tolerance and experience symptoms of withdrawal when infusions are discontinued.

SURGERY-SPECIFIC PICU MANAGEMENT

Brain Tumors

Brain tumors are the most common solid tumors in children (the leukemias are the most common pediatric malignancy). The majority are in the posterior fossa, and obstruction of CSF flow occurs frequently. Symptoms include early morning vomiting and irritability or lethargy. Cranial nerve palsies and ataxia are common, and respiratory and cardiac irregularities usually occur late. Perioperative seizures may occur, with a 7.4% incidence following tumor resection. Factors associated with perioperative seizures include supratentorial tumor, age < 2 years, and hyponatremia due to SIADH or CSW. The role for seizure prophylaxis, especially in patients younger than 2 years of age, deserves further study. Posterior fossa surgery can be complicated by loss of airway protective reflexes and delayed awakening. Other complications include mutism, oculomotor palsies, hearing loss, ataxia, and hemiparesis. Vomiting is very common and hydrocephalus or CSF leak may occur.

The *posterior fossa syndrome* consists of a range of symptoms including aphasia, mutism, dysphagia, weaknesses, oculomotor palsies, and neurobehavioral abnormalities. Symptoms may appear hours or days (typically 24 hours to 4 days) after surgery and be of unpredictable duration. Long-term cognitive sequelae can occur.

Hydrocephalus

Eighty percent of CSF is produced in the choroid plexus of the lateral and fourth ventricles. The remainder is produced in the interstitial space and ependymal lining. Normal CSF volume is 150 mL (50% intracranial, the rest intraspinal) in adults and 50 mL in neonates. The rate of CSF production across ages is 0.15–0.30 mL/min (up to ~450 mL/day). CSF circulation occurs by two pathways. In the major, *adult*, pathway CSF is absorbed through arachnoid villi (arachnoid granulation) into the venous sinuses; in the minor, *infantile*, pathway CSF drains through the ventricular ependyma, the interstitial and perivascular space, and perineural lymphatics.

Hydrocephalus reflects a mismatch of CSF production and absorption that results in an increased intracranial CSF volume. Except for rare instances of excess CSF production (e.g., choroid plexus papillomas), the majority of cases of hydrocephalus are secondary to some type of obstruction to CSF flow or absorption. This commonly results from hemorrhage (neonatal intraventricular or subarachnoid), congenital problems (aqueductal stenosis), trauma, infection, or tumors (especially in the posterior fossa). Hydrocephalus can be classified as nonobstructive (communicating) or obstructive (noncommunicating) based on the ability of CSF to flow around the spinal cord. The rapidity of hydrocephalus expansion and the intracranial compliance determine the severity of symptoms. In the young infant, if hydrocephalus develops slowly, the skull will expand until massive craniomegaly (often with irreversible neurologic damage) occurs. However, if the cranial bones are fused or the cranium cannot expand fast enough, neurologic signs and symptoms appear quickly. The child may become progressively lethargic and develop vomiting, cranial nerve dysfunction ("setting sun" sign), bradycardia, brain herniation, and death.

Perioperative care is directed at controlling ICP and relieving the obstruction as soon as possible. When intubating, a rapid-sequence technique is used due to the risk of emesis and pulmonary aspiration. Maintaining normoventilation is important to avoid exacerbating ICP. The use of ketamine as an induction agent has been thought to exacerbate intracranial hypertension, but growing evidence indicates that it may actually offer some relief of elevated ICP. Children who develop a shunt infection usually have their entire system removed and external ventricular drainage established. The height of the drainage bag should not be significantly changed in relation to the child's head to avoid sudden alterations in ICP. When transporting children with CSF drainage, it is often best to close off the ventriculostomy tubing during these brief periods.

Slit Ventricle Syndrome

Slit ventricle syndrome (SVS) includes headache, small ventricles, and slow refill of pumping chambers in shunted children. It is an important long-term complication of ventriculoperitoneal shunts. SVS results from chronic CSF overdrainage, low CSF volume, and diminished compensation for acute alterations in brain or cerebrovascular volumes. It is important to avoid excess or hypotonic fluid administration and minimize any potential for brain swelling. Postoperative cerebral herniation has been reported after uneventful surgical procedures.

Cerebrovascular Surgery

Arteriovenous Malformations

Arteriovenous malformations (AVMs) are the most common cause of spontaneous intracerebral hemorrhage in children. These lesions are primarily congenital, arising during vasculogenesis in the third week of gestation. Familial cases can exist as in hereditary hemorrhagic telangiectasia (HHT or Osler–Weber–Rendu disease). AVMs consist of arterial feeding vessels, dilated communicating vessels, and draining veins carrying arterialized blood. Large malformations, especially those involving the posterior cerebral artery and vein of Galen, may present with congestive heart failure in the neonatal period. As vascular shunting grows, blood follows the path of least resistance and cerebrovascular territories served by feeder vessels become ischemic. Areas surrounding high-flow lesions may become pressure-passive and subject to severe postoperative hyperemia, edema, and hemorrhage. At the same time, obstruction of venous outflow may occur during surgery and small feeder vessels may be disrupted. Taken together, these mechanisms may precipitate a phenomenon termed "normal perfusion pressure breakthrough" that carries severe consequences (e.g., brain swelling, herniation, and death). Treatment involves therapy for increased ICP (diuretics, moderate hyperventilation, 30 degrees head-of-bed elevation) in addition to judicious use of moderate hypotension (while maintaining CPP) and moderate hypothermia. It remains to be determined whether staged reduction offers any advantage.

Malformations too small to produce congestive heart failure usually remain clinically silent unless they cause seizures or stroke. Intracranial hemorrhage is the most common presentation in children, with a mortality up to 25%. Subarachnoid or intracerebral hemorrhage usually results from acute rupture of a communicating vessel. Seizure is the second most common presentation of AVMs. Other presentations include macrocephaly, headaches, and altered mental status. Increasingly, AVMs are discovered as incidental findings or on prenatal ultrasound. Emergency evaluation begins with a noncontrast CT to localize hemorrhage, followed by MR imaging and angiography. Treatment may consist of embolization or stereotactic radiation for deep malformations, surgical excision of superficial ones, or a combination of modalities. Embolization may offer either definitive treatment or substantial flow reduction before surgery or radiotherapy. Platinum coils and/or ethylene–vinyl alcohol copolymer can serve as embolic agents once the malformation is accessed. Intraoperative complications include perforation, hemorrhage, vessel dissection, unintentional occlusion, and cerebrovascular end-artery "territorial" infarction. Tight BP control and heparinization is continued for 24 hours postoperative and low-molecular-weight heparin is maintained thereafter. Anticonvulsant therapy is often used. Bleeding, including that from the femoral arterial puncture site, is an even greater concern. In some centers, stereotactic radiosurgery is favored because of its low morbidity and mortality. However, this must be weighed against an obliteration delay of 2–3 years, an annual re-hemorrhage rate of 6%, and success rates that are highly variable due to differing treatment protocols.

Aneurysms

Intracranial aneurysms among children can be traumatic, infectious, or most often of unknown etiology (likely due to congenital malformations of an arterial wall). Children with coarctation of the aorta, polycystic kidney disease, fibromuscular dysplasia, Ehlers–Danlos syndrome, or systemic vasculopathy have an increased incidence. Aneurysms usually remain asymptomatic during childhood, but ruptures that occur in childhood are frequently lethal. Symptoms of subarachnoid or intracerebral hemorrhage appear suddenly, usually with intense headache, neurologic deficit, or unconsciousness. Occasionally aneurysms may present with symptoms related to ischemia or mass effect. Seizure and hydrocephalus are also reported. Surgical ligation or clipping is the treatment of choice, but the recent trend is toward endovascular therapy. Intraoperatively, a brief period of controlled hypotension is used to reduce vessel wall tension and the risk of surgical manipulation. Controlled hypotension should not be used in the presence of increased ICP when support of CPP is critical.

In patients with severe subarachnoid hemorrhage and vasospasm, treatment is controversial. Historically, adult centers have used hemodynamic augmentation therapy (hemodilution, hypervolemia, and induced hypertension). Evidence-based consensus recommendations, however, now call for nimodipine, euvolemia, induced hypertension, transcranial Doppler monitoring for vasospasm, advanced imaging to detect delayed cerebral ischemia, and cerebral angioplasty or intra-arterial vasodilators for symptomatic vasospasm.

Moyamoya Disease

Moyamoya disease is a steno-occlusive disease that results in progressive and life-threatening obstruction of intracranial vessels, primarily the internal carotid arteries near the circle of Willis. A dense vascular network of tiny collaterals subsequently develops, giving rise to the Japanese name (translated as "puff of smoke"). The dysplastic process may also involve systemic (especially renal) arteries. The acquired variety may be associated with meningitis, neurofibromatosis, chronic inflammation, connective tissue diseases, certain hematologic disorders, Down syndrome, sickle cell disease, or prior intracranial radiation. In children, moyamoya disease usually manifests as transient ischemic attacks progressing to strokes and fixed neurologic deficits. There is a high morbidity and mortality rate if left untreated.

Medical management includes antiplatelet therapy (aspirin) or calcium channel blockers. Surgical interventions restore blood flow by bypassing obstructions or stimulating angiogenesis. In children, the most common surgical intervention is pial synangiosis, wherein a scalp artery (usually the superficial temporal artery) is sutured directly onto the pial surface of the brain to enhance growth of new vessels in the brain. Because neovascularization requires months, postoperative stroke remains a high concern. EEG monitoring may help detect ischemia resulting from cerebral vasoconstriction. PICU care minimizes extremes of BP and maintains hydration while providing sufficient analgesia and sedation to prevent crying with hyperventilation. Treatment of nausea and prevention of vomiting are important. Some centers quickly restart antiplatelet therapy and begin or continue calcium channel blockers.

Epilepsy Surgery

Children requiring surgical management of seizures usually do so after chronically receiving multiple anticonvulsants. Postoperative care for hemispherectomy (partial or functional) or seizure focus excision or isolation emphasizes limiting intracranial fluid shifts and seizures.

Craniosynostosis and Craniofacial Surgery

Craniosynostosis, the premature fusion of one or more cranial sutures, results in cranial deformities with cosmetic and physiologic consequences. Premature closure of the sagittal sutures results in anterior–posterior elongation of the skull, referred to as scaphocephaly or dolichocephaly. Closure of the metopic suture fixes forehead growth, resulting in a triangular pattern or trigonocephaly. Fusion of a single coronal suture skews skull growth anteriorly or posteriorly to produce plagiocephaly, while fusion of both results in foreshortening of the skull or brachycephaly.

Repair of craniosynostosis is best undertaken as early in life as possible. Up to 6 months of age, endoscopic strip craniectomy with subsequent helmet modeling offers a minimally invasive solution for children with uncomplicated anomalies. Beyond infancy or when larger, more complex craniofacial reconstruction is required, there are numerous challenges. Half of children with syndromic craniosynostosis present with OSA, and for many of these, progressive airway obstruction is the primary indication for surgery. Patients with Apert, Pfeiffer, Crouzon, and related syndromes can present challenges for intubation; some require tracheostomy for safety through surgery. In many cases, even mask ventilation can be difficult. Return to the operating room for extubation under controlled conditions is common among patients with difficult airways. Blood loss during craniofacial reconstruction procedures can be significant. Depending upon the procedure, scalp incision, bone flap elevation, and continuous oozing may combine to produce losses totaling 50%–100% (or more) of the circulating blood volume. Massive blood loss and cardiac arrest occur suddenly, even without inadvertent sagittal sinus entry. VAE can occur during cranial remodeling. When blood loss reaches 50%–75% of the preoperative blood volume (or 40–60 mL/kg), some derangement in coagulation is likely. Some hospital protocols include the use of tranexamic acid, fresh frozen plasma, platelets, cryoprecipitate, and calcium gluconate. Crystalloid resuscitation may be so vigorous that saline-induced metabolic acidosis may occur. Buffered solutions such as lactated Ringers may offer advantages over normal saline. In the postoperative period, blood loss via drains should be followed closely, and signs of significant blood loss (tachycardia, hypotension, hypocapnia, and respiratory variation in systolic BP) recognized and acted upon.

CHAPTER 38 ■ HEAD AND SPINAL CORD TRAUMA

ROBERT C. TASKER AND P. DAVID ADELSON

EPIDEMIOLOGY

Worldwide, traumatic brain injury (TBI) is the leading cause of death and disability for children (>1 year old) and young adults. While most TBIs are mild concussions, >5 million people in the United States are living with TBI-related disabilities. The annual cost of TBIs is estimated at $76.5 billion. The prevalence of pediatric acute traumatic spinal cord injury (TSCI) averages 17.5 per million. The median age at presentation is 15 years, and 72% are male. Children ≤5 years are more likely than older children and adolescents to be injured from a road traffic accident (50%), present with cervical spine C1–C4 injuries (47%), and have concurrent TBI (24%).

HEAD INJURY PATTERNS

A *blunt head injury* occurs from forcible contact with a smooth surface. The curvature of the skull flattens at the point of impact tends, and the injury is spread over an area proportional to the deformation of the skull. When the deformity of the skull exceeds the limit of tolerance, fractures occur. Unfused cranial sutures may be involved and produce a "bursting fracture." Acceleration and deceleration are also important factors in injury production. An immediate, steep increase in pressure occurs at the point of impact, and a decrease in pressure at the opposite pole produces small areas of cavitation and hemorrhage in the superficial cortex.

In *sharp head injury*, the area of impact and extent of skull distortion are small. Laceration of the scalp, local depression or fragmentation of the skull, tearing of the dura, and bruising and laceration of the underlying brain may be seen. Intracerebral hemorrhage in these injuries usually arises from torn superficial vessels of the cortex.

A *compression or crush head injury* is unusual. Fractures tend to involve the foramina at the base of the skull and produce cranial nerve (CN) palsies. The internal carotid artery may be torn, leading to hemorrhage, dissection, or stroke. Side-to-side compression causes fractures across the sella turcica, which puts the pituitary at risk.

Development and Head Injury Patterns

The infant's large head and weak neck muscles increase the risk of rotational and acceleration–deceleration injuries. The soft cranial vault, anatomy of the dura, and rich vascular supply of the subarachnoid space place young children at risk for intracranial injury and bleeding, even in the absence of a skull fracture. The high water content and viscosity of the young brain increases the risk for axonal injury. With skull and brain maturation, adult patterns of intracranial injury are seen. Pediatric patients with thin skulls are more prone to skull fracture and *epidural hematoma* (EDH), whereas adult patients are prone to subdural and intraparenchymal hemorrhages.

TYPES OF INTRACRANIAL INJURY

Hemorrhage and Other Focal Brain Tissue Effects

Focal injury occurs when the brain impacts against the rigid inner table of the skull. Focal injury can produce mass effects from hemorrhage, contusion, or hematoma that induces herniation and brainstem compression. EDHs complicate 2%–3% of all pediatric TBI admissions. EDH of venous or bony origin may occur in the posterior fossa adjacent to the venous sinuses. They may have a delayed presentation in the setting of unfused sutures and open fontanelles. In older children, EDHs usually arise from arterial bleeding. Patients may have a short, lucid interval but then deteriorate rapidly from an expanding intracranial hematoma under arterial pressure. *Subdural hemorrhage* (SDH) is common in children, especially those with abusive TBI. The presentation depends on the size and location of the hemorrhage and associated brain injuries. The associated brain injuries account for unconsciousness at the time of accident or focal neurologic deficits. Traumatic *intraparenchymal hematomas* (contusions) increase in frequency with age. These lesions commonly involve the cortex and white matter of the frontal and temporal lobes, the body and splenium of the corpus callosum, and the corona radiata. It is likely that occult, diffuse white-matter changes are present (even in regions that appear normal on conventional brain imaging).

Diffuse Injury Involving Axons

Diffuse injury that involves axons (*diffuse axonal injury*, DAI) results from shearing forces that act at interfaces of the brain with differing structural integrity. This loss of connectivity, particularly in the fronto-parietal control network, can result in abnormal brain network function and impairments of self-awareness. Cranial CT imaging of DAI is variable in children. MRI is more sensitive to the white-matter changes usually seen.

Diffuse Swelling of the Cerebrum at Presentation

Cerebral swelling after pediatric TBI peaks between 24 and 72 hours. Focal or global swelling can cause shifts in brain tissue across intracranial compartments (**Fig. 38.1**). These *herniation syndromes* (**Table 38.1**) can exist despite normal intracranial pressure (ICP).

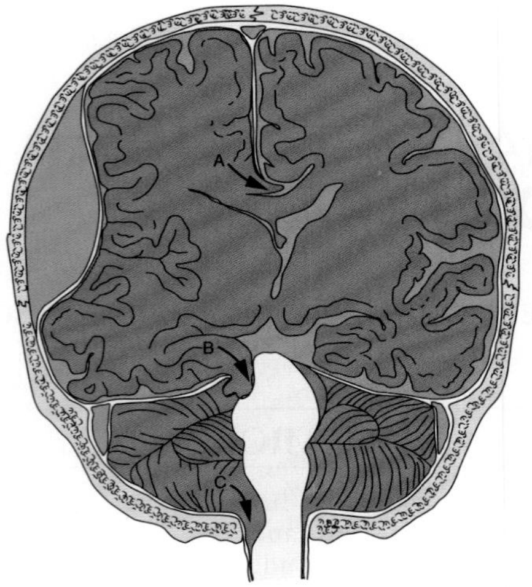

FIGURE 38.1. Herniation syndromes. **A:** Subfalcine and cingulate, occurs when one cerebral hemisphere is displaced under the falx cerebri across the midline; **B:** Uncal, supratentorial structures are displaced inferiorly under the tentorium cerebelli causing distortion and compression of the blood supply to infratentorial structures; **C:** Foramen magnum, downward herniation of the cerebellum causes compression of the brainstem (see **Table 38.1**).

TABLE 38.1

Types of Brain Tissue Herniation Syndromes

SYNDROME	MECHANISM	CLINICAL FEATURES
Foramen magnum	*Herniating tissue:* Downward mesial displacement of cerebellar hemispheres *Compression:* Unilateral or bilateral medulla by ventral parafollicular or tonsillae through foramen magnum	Episodic tonic extension with opisthotonic posturing, leads to quadriparesis Changes in blood pressure, heart rate, and arrhythmias Ataxic breathing Small pupils and disturbance of conjugate gaze
Central tentorial	*Herniating tissue:* Downward displacement of one or both cerebral hemispheres *Compression:* Diencephalon and midbrain through tentorial notch	ICP is usually raised Bilateral decorticate or decerebrate posturing An "upward" form of this syndrome may occur if supratentorial ventricles are decompressed in the presence of cerebellar mass
Uncal (lateral transtentorial)	*Herniating tissue:* Medial temporal lobe (uncus and parahippocampal gyrus) forced into the incisura *Compression:* Midbrain and posterior cerebral artery	ICP is usually raised Contralateral hemiparesis Ipsilateral dilated pupil and ptosis Unilateral or bilateral occipital lobe infarction Obstructive hydrocephalus from compression of aqueduct or perimesencephalic cistern Regions of necrosis and hemorrhage in tegmentum, subthalamus, midbrain, and upper pons
Cingulate	*Herniating tissue:* Cingulate gyrus herniates under the anterior falx *Compression:* Anterior cerebral artery	Infarction of regional tissue seen on imaging Contralateral lower extremity paresis

ICP, intracranial pressure.

Posttraumatic Ischemia, Tissue Oxygenation, and Metabolism

Brain swelling and intracranial hypertension can contribute to early secondary ischemia. Hypotension or hypoxemia can be devastating. The use of monitoring techniques that reflect the coupling between CBF and metabolism (e.g., brain microdialysis and oxygen probes) is increasing. Studies of brain metabolism suggest mitochondrial dysfunction after TBI.

Hypothalamic–Pituitary Injury

In moderate and severe TBI, the frequency of hypopituitarism is high. There is a subnormal response in at least one hypothalamic–pituitary axis in 23%–69% of cases. TBI-induced hypothalamic–pituitary dysfunction is associated with loss of consciousness, SDH, and skull fracture.

TRAUMATIC SPINAL CORD INJURY

Neurologic injury is associated with vertebral column injury in <50%, and complete SCI occurs in <25% of cases. Damage evolves over hours or days. Post-SCI ischemia or hypoxemia contributes to worsening injury. The clinician should be aware of the features and variety of spinal cord syndromes that occur in trauma (**Table 38.2**). In children <9 years, spinal injuries are more frequent in the atlas, axis, and upper cervical vertebrae. Ligamentous injuries that lead to atlanto-occipital dislocation (AOD) are more common than are bone injuries.

Spinal Cord Injury without Radiographic Abnormality

The anatomic characteristics of the young child (i.e., lack of neck musculature and large head size) lead to spinal cord injury without radiographic abnormality (SCIWORA). The clinical features range from tingling dysesthesias or numbness to frank weakness or paralysis. MRI demonstrates five categories of post-SCIWORA findings: complete transection, major hemorrhage, minor hemorrhage, edema only, and normal. Findings are predictive of outcome.

Traumatic Atlanto-Occipital Dislocation

AOD is disruption of the supporting ligaments that results in AO displacement. AOD is often missed on spine plain radiographs. Neurologic abnormalities that should prompt additional imaging with CT or MRI include CN paresis and motor or respiratory dysfunction. AOD is rare in children and adolescents, and most reported cases are fatal.

INITIAL CLINICAL MANAGEMENT

During the first hour after injury, management includes ensuring an adequate airway, maintaining normal blood pressure, protecting the cervical spine, undertaking cranial CT scan, and treating potential herniation syndromes. The most up-to-date *Brain Trauma Foundation Guidelines* are available at https://www.braintrauma.org/coma-guidelines/.

TABLE 38.2

Spinal Cord Syndromes in Trauma

SYNDROME	MECHANISM	FINDINGS
Complete cord transection	Trauma Secondary vascular	Loss of all motor function Loss of sensory function Above C3—apnea and death
Brown–Sequard (cord hemisection)	Penetrating trauma	Ipsilateral loss of proprioception Ipsilateral loss of motor function Contralateral loss of pain and temperature sensation Suspended ipsilateral loss of all sensory modalities
Central cord	Neck hyperextension	Motor impairment greater in upper limbs than in lower limbs Suspended sensory loss in cervicothoracic dermatomes
Anterior cord	Hyperflexion Anterior spinal artery occlusion	Variable motor impairment Pain and temperature loss with sparing of proprioception
Conus medullaris	Direct trauma	Extension to lumbosacral roots may produce both upper and lower motor neuron signs Spastic paraparesis Sphincter dysfunction Lower sacral "saddle" sensory loss

History, Diagnosis, and Classification of TBI

The most important part of the Glasgow coma scale (GCS) score is the motor component. The *best motor response* in either the upper or lower limbs is rated on a scale of 1–6. A score of 6 is given when the patient obeys commands. When there is no reaction to verbal stimuli and SCI is excluded, a noxious stimulus is applied. The preferred application of painful stimuli is the medial side of the arms or legs; this will help to differentiate a localization of pain response from abnormal flexor or extensor posturing. Movement toward the noxious stimulus is not localization.

Phase 1: Prehospital Care

Basic life support involves a rapid primary survey to identify and quickly treat life-threatening injuries. The protection of the cervical spine, correction of airway obstruction, and general cardiopulmonary resuscitation take precedence. Intubation and ventilation may be needed if a patient is obtunded. Intracranial hypertension with impending herniation is inferred from the presence of dilated, unresponsive pupils or a triad of systemic hypertension, bradycardia, and an abnormal breathing pattern. If physical findings suggest herniation, hyperventilation to lower ICP is provided. A complete SCI above C3 causes respiratory arrest and death unless ventilatory assistance is given. SCI at C3–C5 leads to respiratory failure (might be delayed onset).

Controlled Endotracheal Intubation

Rapid sequence intubation is used to secure the airway in children with suspected raised ICP, while protecting against the responses to laryngoscopy that raise ICP. Avoiding hypoventilation, hypotension, and hypoxemia is critical. Lidocaine pretreatment can attenuate the laryngeal reflex and sympathetic response.

Intubation for SCI

Every child with TBI is presumed to have TSCI. Intubation should be accompanied by in-line stabilization of the neck by an assistant or use of a cervical collar. Trauma patients may have delayed gastric emptying, and large-bore suction devices should be available. Injury above the upper thoracic spine levels may lead to loss of sympathetic tone and hypotension without a compensatory increase in heart rate. Atropine should be available.

Postintubation Procedures and Mechanical Ventilation

Immediately after intubation, the bed should be returned to the 30-degree-head-up position and the patient's head kept midline. Ventilation should achieve a pH of 7.35–7.45, with partial pressure CO_2 ($Paco_2$) 35–45 mm Hg. When life-threatening raised ICP or brain herniation is suspected, hyperventilation will be required until evaluated and definitively treated (e.g., hematoma evacuation, decompressive craniectomy). Maximal cerebral vasoconstriction occurs at a $Paco_2$ of 20 mm Hg, so hyperventilation below this is ineffective and may be harmful.

Secondary Survey of Other Injuries

Head

Evidence of skull-base fracture includes Battle sign (retro-auricular ecchymosis), raccoon eyes (periorbital ecchymosis), cerebrospinal fluid (CSF) otorrhea or rhinorrhea, and hemotympanum. Evidence of facial fracture includes instability of facial bones and zygoma (i.e., LeFort fracture) and step-off abnormality (i.e., orbital rim fracture). In infants, the tone of the fontanelle (bulging, soft, or sunken) may indicate ICP level. Abnormal carotid neck pulses, bruits, and Horner syndrome indicate traumatic carotid dissection.

Neck

TCSI must be assumed to have occurred until soft tissue or bony injury has been ruled out. The neck should be immobilized in an appropriate-size collar, and manipulation should be kept to a minimum. If the collar is removed, the neck should be held in midline position.

Thorax

Specific patterns of breathing after TBI may have localizing value (**Fig. 38.2**). SCI above C4 results in paralysis of all ventilatory muscles. Lower cervical injury may spare the diaphragm but abolishes accessory muscle strength, decreases vital capacity, and causes retention of secretions. With injuries at T11, respiratory function, vital capacity, and cough can be normal.

Pupillary Response

Pupillary size at rest and reaction to light should be noted. The light reflex is an afferent pathway through the optic nerve (CN II) and efferent pathway involving sympathetic and parasympathetic fibers along CN III. Bilateral dilated, unresponsive pupils indicate (in the absence of medication or poisoning) bilateral compression of CN III or severe cerebral hypoxia–ischemia. Unilateral or bilateral dilation that is unresponsive is an indication for emergent hyperventilation, brain imaging, and potential surgical intervention. Pinpoint pupils are associated with pontine lesions. Unilateral pupil dilation unreactive to direct stimulation but consensually reactive is caused by absent light perception in that eye or a deafferentated pupil. Ipsilateral pupillary constriction associated with ptosis and anhidrosis (i.e., Horner syndrome) may be a sign of transtentorial herniation,

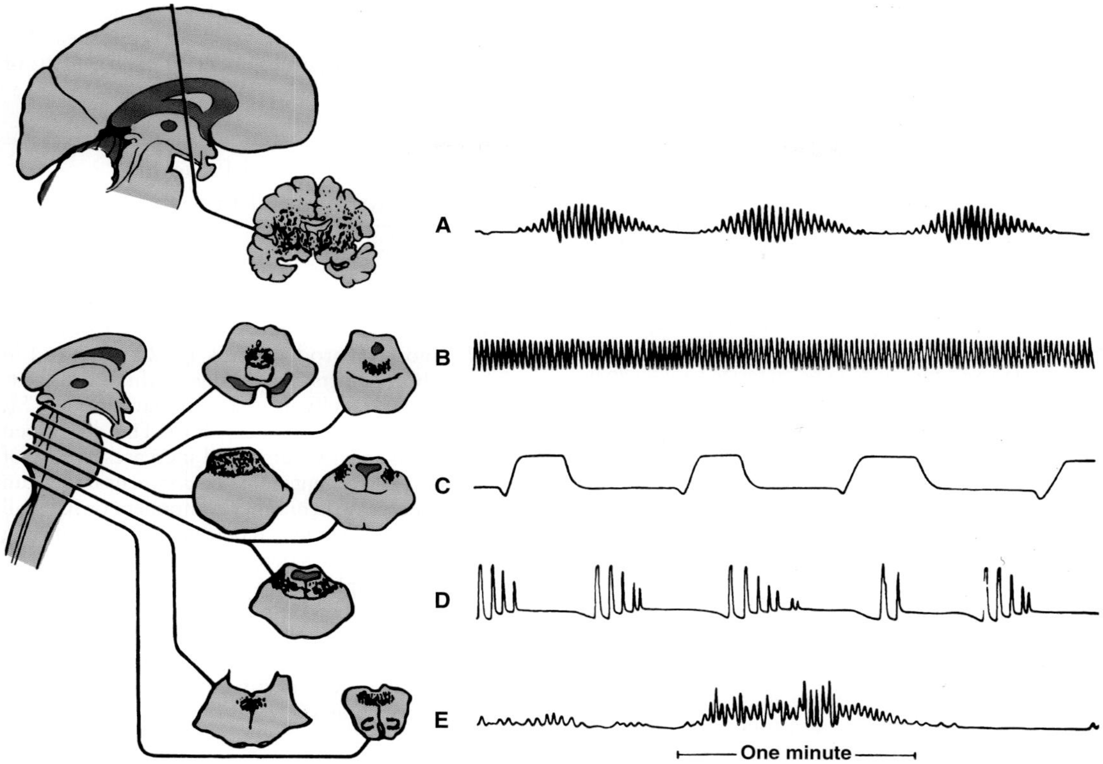

FIGURE 38.2. Injury to different portions of the brain leads to distinctive abnormal breathing patterns that may help localize the area of injury. **A:** Cheyne–Stokes respiration or alternating phases of hyperpnea indicate dysfunction deep within the cerebral hemispheres or diencephalon. **B:** Hyperventilation, or tachypnea, indicates damage in the rostral brainstem or tegmentum. **C:** Apneustic breathing or prolonged sustained end-inspiratory pauses indicate damage at the midpontine or caudal pontine level. **D:** Cluster breathing (periodic respirations that are irregular in amplitude) indicates lower pontine or high medullary injury. **E:** Ataxic respiration (completely random and irregular breathing) indicates medullary damage. (From Mettler FA. *Neuroanatomy*. St. Louis, MO: CV Mosby, 1948:816, with permission.)

damage to the hypothalamus with interruption of sympathetic pathways, or disruption of the cervical sympathetics. Injury to the midbrain tectum may result in pupils that are at midposition and fixed to light but retain hippus, the ciliospinal reflex, and response to accommodation.

Motor System

Focal weakness implies a structural lesion. Tone should be assessed in all four limbs. Patterns of decerebration should be looked for, and not mistaken as, seizures. Patterns must be assessed as unilateral, bilateral, spontaneous, or occurring only after stimulation. Appropriate localizing and flexor responses in a comatose patient imply that sensory pathways are functioning and that the pyramidal tract from the cerebral cortex to effector is functioning, at least partially. Unilateral absence of responses is consistent with an interruption of the corticospinal tract. *Decorticate rigidity* is flexion of the arms, wrist, and fingers, with adduction in the upper extremity and extension, internal rotation, and plantar flexion in the lower extremity. This motor pattern occurs if the impairment of brainstem activity is located *above the level of the red nucleus*, as seen with lesions involving the corticospinal pathways at the internal capsule, cerebral hemisphere, or rostral cerebral peduncle. *Decerebrate rigidity* consists of opisthotonus with the teeth clenched, the arms extended, adducted and hyperpronated, and the legs extended with the feet plantar flexed. This motor pattern occurs if the impairment of brainstem activity is located *between the levels of the rostral poles of the red nucleus and vestibular nuclei* (rostral midbrain to mid-pons), as seen during rostral–caudal deterioration with transtentorial herniation, expanding posterior fossa lesions, or neurotoxicity of the upper brainstem.

Functional Integrity of the Spine and Spinal Cord

The patient should be log-rolled (with the head kept in-line) to examine the entire spine. Ecchymoses should be noted. The spinal column should be palpated for widening of spaces or malalignment. The functional integrity of the spinal cord is evaluated by a thorough motor and sensory examination. The American Spine Injury Association (ASIA, at http://www.asia-spinalinjury.org) has tools for determining sensory and motor levels. *Complete injury* is signified by loss of motor function, segmental reflexes, and sensation below a given level. The *zone of partial preservation* is an area adjacent to the neurologic level in which abnormal sensory and motor findings are noted. An area of abnormal findings that is not contiguous with the postulated level qualifies as *incomplete injury*. As this lesion has the potential for improvement, a reassessment is vital. Flaccid areflexic paralysis and anesthesia to all modalities characterize *spinal shock*. This problem is found in half of TSCI patients and resolves within 24 hours in >90%. SCI above the seventh thoracic vertebra may mask the tenderness normally associated with an intra-abdominal injury.

INITIAL INVESTIGATIONS

A head CT scan should be performed after respiratory and hemodynamic stabilization. The CT scan serves to detect life-threatening abnormalities requiring urgent neurosurgery. The initial CT should visualize the craniocervical junction so that AOD, rotatory subluxation of C1 on C2, and other craniocervical disruptions can be evaluated. Patients with negative CT scans and mild neurologic disturbances, such as posttraumatic seizures (PTS), vomiting, headache, irritability, or GCS score of 12–15, can be observed. Imaging of the spine should be obtained in all patients with pain or tenderness of the neck or back, sensory or motor deficits, an impaired level of consciousness, or with painful, distracting injuries outside of the spinal region. The standard practice for cervical radiographs includes anteroposterior, lateral, and odontoid views. Lateral views should be screened for changes in vertebral alignment, bony structure, intervertebral space, and soft tissue. In neurologically intact patients, flexion–extension views may detect occult instability from ligamentous injury. Spinal CT scan is very sensitive in detecting bony injury. Spinal MRI is highly sensitive to changes in the soft tissues and is indicated in the presence of neurologic findings. In children with significant TBI or neck pain, a reasonable practice is to maintain cervical spine immobilization until an MRI can be performed to exclude ligament injury. In the conscious child, immobilization can be discontinued when the pain has resolved and flexion and extension radiographs reveal no apparent injury.

NEUROCRITICAL CARE MONITORING OF INTRACRANIAL PRESSURE

Children with severe TBI (GCS < 9) and a mass lesion should have the mass removed and, often, an ICP monitor inserted at the time of surgery. Children with moderate head injury (GCS 9–12) merit careful observation. Deterioration warrants repeat head CT to rule out interval development or enlargement of a mass lesion.

Cerebrospinal Fluid and Intracranial Pressure

The choroid plexus of the lateral and fourth ventricles produces 80% of CSF, and the remainder is produced in the interstitial space and ependymal lining. Adult CSF volume is 150 mL (neonatal is 50 mL) and CSF production is 10–20 mL/h (~450 mL/day). ICP reflects the volume of three compartments: brain parenchyma, extracellular fluid or CSF, and cerebral blood volume (CBV). The developed cranium is fixed in volume and increases in one of the intracranial contents must be compensated by an equivalent decrease in another component or ICP will increase. The point at which perfusion-compromising ICP elevation occurs is dependent on brain elastance and potential displacement of intracranial contents. Alterations may be compounded by brain edema, increased CBV, focal cerebral perfusion deficits around brain contusions, and variations in CBF and cerebrovascular CO_2 reactivity.

Invasive Intracranial Pressure Monitoring

ICP monitoring can be performed via a ventriculostomy or a fiberoptic monitor in the brain parenchyma. A ventriculostomy allows CSF drainage as a treatment. There is variation in practice, with observation rates of 14%–83%. Some centers follow clinical exam and serial CTs rather than monitoring ICP with similar outcomes.

Intracranial Pressure and Cerebral Perfusion Pressure Target Levels

Intracranial Pressure

In adults, the threshold for treatment of intracranial hypertension is 20–25 mm Hg. It is likely that the ICP threshold for poor outcome is similar across ages. Brief increases in ICP that return to normal in <5 minutes may be insignificant; but, sustained increases of ≥20 mm Hg for ≥5 minutes likely warrant treatment. The optimal ICP target for pediatric TBI is yet to be defined.

Cerebral Perfusion Pressure

Cerebral perfusion pressure (CPP) is calculated as the difference between mean arterial blood pressure and mean ICP. Normal values for mean arterial blood pressure and hence CPP are lower in children. Guidelines recommend a minimum CPP goal of 40 mm Hg or 40–50 mm Hg in slightly older children with weak evidence. In adult patients, 60 mm Hg is often targeted but goals may be individualized based on cerebral oxygenation and autoregulation.

NEUROCRITICAL CARE TREATMENTS

Phase 4: Initial ICP-Directed Therapies

Tier 1A: Sedation, Analgesia, and CSF Diversion Strategy

The first step to reduce ICP is to ensure adequate sedation, analgesia, and neuromuscular blockade. Other "first-tier" therapies include elevation of the head 30 degrees and keeping the head midline (reducing obstruction to cerebral venous return). If ICP remains elevated and a ventriculostomy is in place, CSF is drained.

Tier 1B: Hyperosmolar Therapies

If ICP is still elevated, hyperosmolar therapy using mannitol or hypertonic saline is instituted. A 3% hypertonic saline dose of 6.5–10 mL/kg IV, or a continuous infusion of 0.1–1.0 mL/kg/h, is given on a sliding scale. Serum osmolarity should be maintained <360 mOsm/L. Although mannitol is also commonly used, there are no studies to offer guidance. Intermittent mannitol doses are 0.25–0.5 g/kg. Hypertonic saline (typically 3%) may be better tolerated than mannitol can precipitate renal failure. Mannitol causes an immediate viscosity-reduction or pressure-mediated reflex vasoconstriction and a late osmotic effect to shift water out of brain tissue, but osmotic diuresis can lead to hypotension and hyponatremia. About 3% hypertonic saline may be better tolerated than mannitol, since sodium loading increases intravascular volume as opposed to diuresis and dehydration. Starting treatment with 3% hypertonic saline to gain acute control may avoid hypoperfusion when volume status is low. If the ICP becomes unresponsive to hypertonic saline, therapies for refractory intracranial hypertension must be considered.

Phase 5: Therapies for Refractory Intracranial Hypertension

Second Tier: Surgical Options

Surgical therapy may be required acutely to evacuate a mass lesion or as treatment for intracranial hypertension refractory to medical therapy. Early bifrontotemporoparietal decompressive craniectomy in adults with severe TBI decreased ICP and length of stay but worsened long-term outcome. Pediatric outcomes appear more favorable with decompression.

Third Tier: Other Medical Therapies

Third-tier medical measures include the use of barbiturate-induced coma, hypothermia, and hyperventilation. Barbiturates can induce electrophysiologic "burst suppression" and control ICP by reducing cerebral metabolic activity. The most common complication of barbiturate treatment is hemodynamic compromise and hypotension. Recent analysis raises concern for increased mortality with hypothermia but still suggested that hyperthermia be avoided. Controlled hyperventilation ($Paco_2$ 30–35 mm Hg) has been used in patients with cerebral hyperemia. Generally, earlier in the course of therapy, such management is avoided unless there is a temporizing treatment before emergency surgery.

SEIZURES AND ANTICONVULSANTS

Symptomatic seizures may occur following severe TBI. *Early seizures* occur within 7 days and *late seizures* occur after 7 days following injury. Recurrent seizures after 7 days following injury are labeled as *posttraumatic epilepsy* (PTE). In patients with severe TBI, the rate of clinical PTS may be as high as 12% and for subclinical PTS detected by EEG as high as 20%–25%. Seizure incidence increases with injury severity. The significance of subclinical seizures and the importance of early treatment are not understood. Prophylactic anticonvulsants are recommended in adults with severe TBI, but their role in children is controversial due to concerns that prophylaxis may impair functional recovery.

POSTTRAUMATIC MENINGITIS AND FEVER

Posttraumatic meningitis is a risk for mid-frontal, lateral–frontal, temporal–frontal, and posterolateral fractures. *Streptococcus* and *Staphylococcus* species predominate. Fever may be the earliest sign of meningitis, but hyperthermia occurs in ~30% of children with severe TBI within 24 hours of admission. Extracranial causes of fever are also possible (e.g., chest infection, fat embolism, wound infection). Irrespective of cause, hyperthermia must be controlled, as it may worsen neurologic outcome.

HYPOTHALAMIC–PITUITARY DYSFUNCTION

A low basal cortisol level, subnormal cortisol response, diabetes insipidus, or the syndrome of inappropriate antidiuretic hormone is common in the acute period and is usually transient. Cerebral salt wasting may cause hyponatremia. Adrenal insufficiency can be life-threatening. Growth-hormone, gonadal, and thyroid assessment is not necessary in the acute phase.

SCI-DIRECTED THERAPIES

In adults, high-dose methylprednisolone was the standard of care in the management of nonpenetrating acute SCI. Since 1998, concerns have been raised about the studies supporting steroid use and the increased incidence of infection and avascular necrosis with steroid treatment. Recent guidelines conclude that the administration of methylprednisolone is not recommended for the treatment of acute SCI and that high-dose steroids are associated with harmful side effects including sepsis and death.

CHAPTER 39 ABUSIVE HEAD TRAUMA

RACHEL P. BERGER, DENNIS W. SIMON, JENNIFER E. WOLFORD, AND MICHAEL J. BELL

Children with abusive head trauma (AHT) may present with an unclear or false history of present illness, making the rapid diagnosis of the brain injury one of many challenges in their management. Prior terms used to describe the constellation of abusive injuries include "shaken baby syndrome," "inflicted traumatic brain injury," "inflicted childhood neurotrauma," "nonaccidental traumatic brain injury," and "intentional traumatic brain injury." The term *abusive head trauma* represents an understanding that the mechanism of brain injury can include a combination of shaking, blunt impact, spinal cord injury, and hypoxic–ischemic injury.

EPIDEMIOLOGY

AHT is the leading cause of death from child abuse and the most common cause of severe traumatic brain injury (TBI) in infants. The incidence is 29.7 per 100,000 in the United States and 14.1 per 100,000 in Canada in <1-year-olds. The true incidence is likely underestimated.

Risk Factors

Peak incidence occurs in the first year of life (mean age 2–8 months). Approximately 25% of children with AHT are >1 year old. AHT is thought to be associated with the peak period of crying as this is the most common trigger. Circumstances related to caregivers also contribute to the risk of AHT. Stress, both for communities and for individuals, may be the most pervasive of these risks. Military deployment, natural disaster, and economic stress affect the rate of AHT. Individual stresses include young parental age, poor impulse control, lower levels of maternal education, substance or alcohol abuse, and mental illness (including postpartum depression). The absence of these risk factors should not remove AHT from the differential diagnosis.

Mechanisms of Injury

The mechanisms of injury in AHT include a combination of shaking, blunt force trauma, hypoxic–ischemic injury, and spinal cord injury. The effect of shear forces from shaking is most observable within the orbit. Retinal hemorrhages rarely occur in noninflicted TBI and, when present, do not have the same depth or affected area as seen in AHT. Shaking injury may explain subdural hematomas from tearing of bridging veins as the brain rapidly moves within the cranial vault. Blunt force trauma, alone or in combination with shaking, is another potential mechanism. Whether blunt force trauma is required to produce the forces necessary to cause severe (or fatal) brain injury is much debated. Contemporary experimental models suggest that previous models underestimate the complexity of the biomechanical forces in play as well as age-dependent differences in injury potential. Hypoxic–ischemic damage to the brain in AHT is common. Biomarkers of neuronal injury in AHT are more similar to those with hypoxic–ischemic injury than to TBI. It has been theorized that hypoxia–ischemia may result from a delay in seeking medical attention after an incident of abuse or due to injury to the brain stem and upper spinal cord injury with the development of apnea and hypoxic injury.

DIAGNOSIS

The history provided by the caregiver in cases of AHT is often unreliable, either because the informant is the perpetrator or because the informant is unaware that another person's actions caused the injuries. There may be no history of trauma. It is critical to obtain a detailed, time-focused history that includes the last time the child was healthy, the time when the child became symptomatic, what prompted the seeking of medical attention, and who was with the child when symptoms began. This information must be carefully documented so that changes in the caregiver's account can be determined in subsequent investigations.

Physical examination, including assessment of the airway, breathing, and circulation, is essential. Over half of the children with AHT have an initial Glasgow Coma Scale (GCS) score of 13–15; so it is important to consider AHT even if an infant or young child appears well. MRI, including diffusion-weighted imaging, may detect early edema and ischemia changes in the subacute stage of illness. MRI may also determine the timing of injuries and provide more complete information about diffuse axonal injuries and other forms of encephalomalacia. Imaging of the cervical spine may also be informative. Spinal canal subdural hemorrhage is present in >60% of children with AHT compared to 1% of children with noninflicted TBI.

An example of common head computed tomography (CT) findings is provided in **Figure 39.1**.

Nonneurologic traumatic injuries can help differentiate AHT from alternative diagnoses. Meticulous documentation (including photodocumentation) of bruises, petechiae, and abrasions aids future investigation. An acute or healing noncranial fracture is found in 25%–85% of children with AHT. Detection of fractures requires comprehensive imaging after the child has been stabilized. A postmortem skeletal survey is needed when any young child dies and AHT is in the differential diagnosis. An ophthalmologic examination should be performed as soon as it is feasible to use mydriatics (pupil diameter may be a key sign of intracranial hypertension). Multilayered hemorrhages or hemorrhages extending to the periphery of the retina are pathognomonic of AHT. Abdominal injuries must be considered in children with AHT and elevated transaminases should trigger diagnostic abdominal imaging. One-third of subjects with abdominal injury had no bruising, abdominal tenderness, or rebound on physical examination.

Differential Diagnosis

AHT must be considered in the differential diagnosis of any young child: (a) with abnormal head CT imaging, where the mechanism provided by the caretaker does not explain all of the injuries; or (b) with neurologic symptoms that cannot be explained by another disease process. The workup includes an evaluation for diseases that can be confused with AHT (**Table 39.1**). The most common mimic of AHT is noninflicted TBI. Much less common are glutaric aciduria type I, hemophagocytic lymphohistiocytosis, hemorrhagic disease of the newborn, arteriovenous malformations, and bleeding disorders. While these diseases resemble AHT, they rarely share all of its characteristics. Every patient being evaluated for AHT should have a baseline set of hematologic labs. Slight increases in PT/PTT are common after AHT as well as noninflicted TBI and do not represent an underlying bleeding disorder. In cases in which the only manifestation of abuse is bleeding (e.g., no fractures, no abdominal injury), when abnormalities of PT/PTT and/or platelets are persistent (or more severe than expected from TBI alone), or when patient history or family history raises concern, it is important to consider a bleeding diathesis. If there are other children in the home, reporting of suspicious cases should not be delayed while an evaluation is in process. The extent of the intensivist's involvement often depends on the availability of trained consultants in child maltreatment at the institution.

MANAGEMENT/TREATMENT

The overall management is similar to that of childhood TBI (reviewed in Chapter 38). Children with mild and moderate AHT (GCS > 8) receive supportive measures to avoid secondary insults (e.g., hypoxia, hypotension, hyperthermia, hyponatremia, and seizures). Children with "moderate" injuries have higher mortality than those with noninflicted TBI with a similar GCS. Cervical spine immobilization should be considered since the mechanism of injury may be unclear. Although many children with AHT will have membranous fontanels, AHT can lead to intracranial hypertension and cerebral herniation if compensatory mechanisms are overcome. Minimizing ICP and maintaining cerebral perfusion pressure (CPP) (mean arterial pressure − mean ICP) are as critical for AHT as for other TBI. An ICP target < 15–20 mm Hg is associated with best outcome.

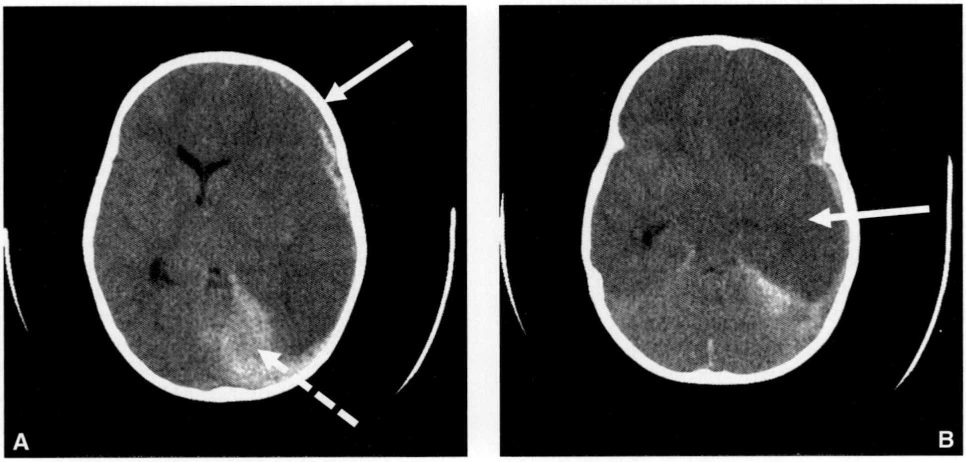

FIGURE 39.1. Head CT scan of a 3-month-old with AHT demonstrating acute subdural hematoma (**A**, *solid arrow*) with blood layering on tentorium (**A**, *dashed arrow*) and pronounced midline shift of cerebral contents. In (**B**), early evidence of cerebral hypoperfusion and infarction is noted (*solid arrow*).

TABLE 39.1

Recommended Evaluation for a Child with an Intracranial Injury Concerning for AHT

TEST	REASON	SPECIALIST RECOMMENDED TO EVALUATE RESULTS	OTHER
Dilated ophthalmologic exam[a]	To evaluate for retinal hemorrhages	Pediatric ophthalmologist	Strongly recommend photodocumentation
Skeletal survey including oblique views of ribs[b]	To evaluate for fractures	Pediatric radiologist	This should not be done as portable films
Follow-up skeletal survey	To evaluate for fractures (especially metaphyseal and rib fractures) that were acute at the time of the initial skeletal survey and could not yet be visualized	Pediatric radiologist	To be done 10–14 d after the initial skeletal survey (pelvis and skull can be omitted)[c]
Screening for possible hematologic etiology of intracranial hemorrhage[d]	PT/PTT/platelets/INR, Factor VIII, Factor IX, d-dimer, fibrinogen	Pediatric hematology consultation recommended if any abnormalities on screening evaluation	
Urine organic acids and serum amino acids	To rule out glutaric aciduria type I as an etiology in children with isolated intracranial hemorrhage		Glutaric aciduria type I is very rare and its presentation does not overlap entirely with AHT, but should be ruled out as a mimic. A report to CPS should not be delayed until the results of the tests are known
Brain MRI with imaging of the spine	Brain MRI can provide improved information about injury to the brain parenchyma, hypoxia. Spine MRI can provide important information about mechanism of injury	Pediatric neuroradiologist	
Screen for occult abdominal injury	Liver function tests, pancreatic enzymes		If AST or ALT > 80 IU/L, recommend definitive testing (e.g., abdominal CT)

[a]In children who are too unstable to have their eye dilated, recommend initial evaluation without dilation and/or sequential dilation of eyes.
[b]In children who die prior to being able to complete a skeletal survey, the skeletal survey should be done postmortem. Any abnormalities need to be relayed to the coroner performing the autopsy.
[c]In children who are too unstable to undergo a skeletal survey until 1 wk or more after admission, it is possible to perform a single skeletal survey 10–14 d after admission instead of both an initial and a follow-up.
[d]Measurement of Factors VIII and IX, fibrinogen, and D-dimer are not necessary in children who have other, nonhematologic manifestations of abuse as well (e.g., fractures).
AHT, abusive head trauma; PT, prothrombin time; PTT, Pediatric Triage Tape; INR, international normalized ratio; CPS, Child Protective Service; AST, aspartate aminotransferase; ALT, alanine aminotransferase.

Partial pressure of brain tissue oxygen ($Pbto_2$) monitoring is unavailable to many AHT victims due to their age and risk of skull fractures with monitor placement. Subclinical seizures may be more common, and continuous electroencephalography (EEG) monitoring can be helpful. Prophylactic anticonvulsants can be considered, but evidence that they improve outcome is lacking.

OUTCOMES

Mortality and morbidity after AHT is higher than after noninflicted TBI of similar severity. Possible reasons include the characteristics of the injury, delays by caretakers in seeking medical care, delays by medical providers in identifying trauma, effects of prior maltreatment or AHT, and developmental factors. Long-term neurocognitive outcome studies show severe morbidity from AHT.

REPORTING AND LEGAL ISSUES

In the United States, physicians are mandated to report suspected child abuse and are protected from ramifications of reporting as long as the report is made in good faith. Each state has unique laws and processes for filing a report of suspected abuse. Many institutions have dedicated social services staff or other personnel who can assist physicians in making a report to Child Protective Services (CPSs), or the relevant investigative body for the state. Ultimately, it is the physician's responsibility to ensure that a report is made. Information about reporting is available online for each state at www.childwelfare.gov/systemwide/laws_policies/statutes/. The goal of reporting is to provide authorities with the medical facts in language that is as simple and nonmedical, to inform them about the severity of injuries (e.g., whether or not they are life-threatening), and to provide information about the strength of the diagnosis (e.g., there is concern for abuse vs. the injuries are diagnostic of abuse). A report is not a static document and more information including a change in the assessment of the likelihood of abuse can be added as available (e.g., after a dilated eye exam or skeletal survey is performed). It is not the physician's responsibility to identify the perpetrator.

When discussing the CPS report with the family, the discussion can be brief, respectful, and forthright. Throughout the conversation, the physician's focus should remain on the child's well-being. Inclusion of a hospital social worker or support staff with expertise in the CPS system as part of the discussion can be very helpful. While notification of parents is important, if no parent is available, physicians should not delay reporting. Reporting of child abuse protects the child, and alerts CPS to the presence of a potentially violent environment. This is important for the safety of other children or adults in the home who may be victims of domestic violence.

PREVENTION

Unlike many conditions, measures to prevent AHT are generally societal in nature. The main way that an intensivist can prevent AHT is to have a high index of suspicion for possible cases, report them to the proper authorities, and work within this system to avert future cases by caregivers who are prone to this behavior.

CHAPTER 40 ■ STATUS EPILEPTICUS

KIMBERLY S. BENNETT AND COLIN B. VAN ORMAN

DEFINITION

The *classical definition* of status epilepticus (SE) is seizure activity, either continuous or episodic, without complete recovery of consciousness, which lasts for at least 30 minutes. SE can be conceptualized in stages: (a) *premonitory* or *prodromal SE*, characterized by an increasing frequency of serial seizures with recovery of consciousness between episodes; (b) *incipient SE*, defined as continuous or intermittent seizures that last up to 5 minutes without full recovery of consciousness; (c) *impending* or *early SE*, marked by seizure activity that persists 5–30 minutes; and (d) *established SE*, defined as seizures that last >30 minutes. When SE lasts longer than 30–60 minutes, *subtle SE* usually develops (clinical signs diminish, yet electroencephalographic [EEG] seizure activity persists). Finally, *nonconvulsive SE* (NCSE) refers to ongoing EEG seizure activity without associated clinical signs. An *operational definition* of SE is seizure activity lasting >5 minutes. In children, unprovoked, afebrile seizures typically last <4 minutes, and seizures that last >5 minutes are unlikely to remit spontaneously. SE that lasts >30 minutes is less likely to respond to anticonvulsants.

CLASSIFICATION

Generalized Convulsive Status Epilepticus

Generalized convulsive SE (GCSE) is tonic, clonic, or tonic–clonic seizure activity involving all extremities; it constitutes 73%–98% of pediatric SE. Seizures often begin focally but spread to involve the entire brain. *Focal motor SE* involves a single limb or side of the face, is less common than GCSE, and is frequently associated with focal brain pathology (**Table 40.1**). *Myoclonic SE* is characterized by irregular, asynchronous, small-amplitude, repetitive myoclonic jerking of the face or limbs. Myoclonic SE is more common in comatose patients and is often associated with anoxia or cardiac arrest (**Table 40.2**).

Nonconvulsive Status Epilepticus

NCSE is continuous, nonmotor seizures diagnosed by EEG. *Absence SE* is altered consciousness and a generalized 3-Hz symmetric spike-and-wave pattern on EEG. *Complex partial SE* is altered consciousness and focal EEG activity (usually in the temporal lobe). In comatose patients, NCSE should be considered in patients with prolonged obtundation after seizure cessation or coma of unclear etiology. Nonconvulsive seizures occur in 16%–46% and NCSE in 18%–33% of critically ill children with unexplained alterations of consciousness or suspected SE. NCSE and nonconvulsive seizures often occur in children with preexisting cerebral insults and epilepsy, but more than 40% of children with nonconvulsive seizures are previously healthy.

Refractory Status Epilepticus

SE of any classification that fails to remit despite treatment with adequate doses of two anticonvulsants is refractory status epilepticus (RSE). In children, 10%–40% of SE is refractory. Mortality for pediatric RSE is 13%–30%, and 33%–50% of survivors have neurologic sequelae. Almost half (46%) of neonates with SE develop RSE, and only

TABLE 40.1

Common Etiologies of Focal Motor Status Epilepticus

Brain Tumor
Astrocytoma
Oligodendroglioma
Glioblastoma
Infection
Brain abscess
Viral encephalitis
Cysticercosis
Tuberculosis
Vascular
Cortical vein thrombosis
Arteriovenous malformation
Cerebrovascular accident
Trauma
Posttraumatic cyst
Chronic subdural hematoma
Focal gliosis

TABLE 40.2

Common Etiologies of Myoclonic Status Epilepticus

Anoxic Injury
Cardiac arrest
Cardiopulmonary bypass
Carbon monoxide poisoning
CO_2 narcosis
Infection
Viral encephalitis
Acute demyelinating encephalomyelitis
Subacute sclerosing panencephalitis
Opportunistic infection
Injury
Heat stroke
Lightning
Intracranial hemorrhage
Metabolic
Hepatic failure
Renal failure
Hypoglycemia
Hyponatremia
Nonketotic hyperglycemia
Thiamine deficiency
Toxins
Tricyclic antidepressants
Anticonvulsants
Antibiotics (β-lactam, carbapenem, quinolone)
Opiates
Lithium
Heavy-metal poisoning
Genetic/Epilepsy Syndromes
Juvenile myoclonic epilepsy
Lennox–Gastaut syndrome
Absence epilepsy
Degenerative myoclonus epilepsy
Angelman syndrome

10% have good neurodevelopmental outcomes at 1 year of age. Super-refractory SE is defined as the persistence or recurrence of seizures despite 24 hours of pharmacologic coma.

Neonatal Status Epilepticus

Neonates are unlikely to demonstrate GCSE or continuous seizures. Frequent, serial seizures without recovery of consciousness can occur. Neonatal seizures are frequently polymorphic and may involve rapid extensor or flexor posturing, tremor of extended extremities, apnea, eye deviation, or automatisms. Conditions associated with neonatal SE are listed in **Table 40.3**.

TABLE 40.3

Common Etiologies of Neonatal Status Epilepticus

Perinatal or Acute Insults
Hypoxia-ischemia
Intracranial hemorrhage
Cerebral vascular accident
Infection
Meningitis
Encephalitis
Abscess
Metabolic
Hypoglycemia
Hypocalcemia
Hyponatremia
Hypomagnesemia
Bilirubin encephalopathy
Inborn Errors of Metabolism
Phenylketonuria
Nonketotic hyperglycemia
Pyridoxine deficiency
Histidinemia
Hyperammonemia
Homocitrullinemia
Maple syrup urine disease
Leucine-sensitive hypoglycemia
Toxins
Antibiotics (β-lactam, carbapenem, quinolone)
Anesthetics
Drug withdrawal
Heavy-metal poisoning
Cerebral Malformations
Neuronal migration defect
Neurocutaneous syndrome
Degenerative Diseases
Leigh encephalopathy
Leukodystrophies
Alpers disease
Sandhoff disease
Tay–Sachs disease
Benign Familial Syndromes
Benign familial neonatal seizures
Benign neonatal sleep myoclonus

EPIDEMIOLOGY

More than 40% of pediatric SE occur in children <2 years old, and 25%–40% occur in children with known epilepsy. Risk factors for SE in epileptic children include epilepsy induced by a neurologic insult (symptomatic epilepsy), previous episodes of SE, use of multiple anticonvulsant medications, psychomotor retardation, generalized background abnormalities on EEG, and tapering of anticonvulsant medications. However, 60% of SE in epileptic children occur despite therapeutic anticonvulsant levels and without any identifiable inciting event, such as fever or concurrent illness. SE is the presenting problem in 12% of children with new-onset, unprovoked seizures. New-onset SE, in 17% of children, has associated, treatable inciting events, such as electrolyte abnormalities or central nervous system (CNS) infections. Children with a preexisting neurologic abnormality are 3–24 times more likely to experience recurrence.

ETIOLOGIES

Febrile or acute symptomatic etiologies account for >80% of SE among children <2 years old. Cryptogenic and remote symptomatic etiologies (e.g., prior brain injury) account for more than 60% of SE in children >4 years of age. Tapering or withdrawal of anticonvulsant medications is a common inciting event among older children. CNS infection, metabolic abnormalities, traumatic brain injury, and anoxic brain injury are the common specific etiologies of acute symptomatic pediatric SE. Other inciting events are electrolyte abnormalities, toxic exposures, and congenital malformations. Identification and understanding of SE associated with fever and CNS inflammation in the absence of identified infection is increasing. Termed acute encephalopathy with inflammation-mediated status epilepticus (AEIMSE), the three most recognized disorders are idiopathic hemiconvulsive-hemiplegia syndrome in infancy (IHHS, age 0–4 years), fever-induced refractory epileptic encephalopathy in school-aged children (FIRES, age 4 years to adolescence and also known as acute encephalopathy with refractory, repetitive partial seizures [AERRPS]), and new-onset RSE (NORSE, age 20–50 years). These disorders typically involve fever that may abate days before seizure onset, often present as limbic encephalopathy (e.g., confusion or behavioral changes, movement disorders, and limbic seizures), and can be difficult to distinguish from other etiologies of RSE. Mortality is 12%, and refractory epilepsy and significant cognitive disability are typical.

MECHANISM OF DISEASE

Seizure Initiation and Progression

Seizure initiation and propagation involves a failure of γ-aminobutyric-acid (GABA)-mediated inhibition and/or an increase in glutamate-mediated excitation. Aberrant neuronal excitation commonly originates near regions of cerebral injury or scarring but may arise from uninjured neurons. As adjacent neurons begin firing, excitatory mediators, including glutamate, are released. Glutamate activates *N*-methyl-D-aspartate (NMDA) receptors, facilitating local neuronal synchronization, as well as seizure spread. The mechanisms that enable the self-sustained seizures necessary for SE remain poorly understood. Possible contributors include injury-induced axonal sprouting, a reduction of inhibitory interneuron activity, and receptor trafficking changes that favor excitability. Mechanisms implicated in seizure termination include a predominance of GABA activity, membrane stabilization by acidic extracellular pH, magnesium blockade of NMDA channels, activation of the sodium–potassium adenosine triphosphatase (Na/K-ATPase) pump system, and activation of potassium (K^+) conductance to allow membrane repolarization. Adenosine, an endogenous neuroprotectant, is thought to regulate basal neural inhibition and seizure termination.

Maturational Sequences in the Immature Brain

The immature brain is more susceptible to seizures, likely due to maturational differences of excitatory and inhibitory systems. Paradoxically, the immature brain is relatively resistant to seizure-induced cell death and synaptic reorganization. Despite a relative resistance to histologic injury, seizures during development can cause permanent, adverse effects, including cognitive impairment and lower seizure thresholds.

Cerebral Injury Induced by Status Epilepticus

Seizures that last 30–60 minutes are sufficient to cause neuronal injury. Both CSE and NCSE may be injurious. Neuronal injury induced by SE is likely mediated by excitotoxicity and is due to prolonged seizure activity, not to systemic complications, such as hypoxia, hypoglycemia, or hyperthermia. Cellular calcium influx plays an important role. An accompanying acute neurologic insult may shorten the seizure duration necessary to cause neuronal injury.

CLINICAL PRESENTATION AND DIFFERENTIAL DIAGNOSIS

Convulsive Status Epilepticus

Generalized Convulsive Status Epilepticus

GCSE may be tonic–clonic, clonic, or tonic in nature. Forty to eighty percent of GCSE in children present as continuous seizures, most commonly with generalized tonic–clonic activity. In children with epilepsy, GCSE often starts as increasing frequency of serial seizures, and prompt treatment may prevent progression. Neurologic examination may reveal abnormal cranial nerve function and unilateral or bilateral Babinski responses. Cerebrospinal fluid pleocytosis as a consequence of GCSE has been documented.

Clonic Status Epilepticus

Clonic SE may persist for hours or days, waxing and waning in intensity. Persistent postictal hemiplegia is common. Clonic seizures in young children are predominantly unilateral but may shift from side to side. Consciousness may be preserved, and autonomic involvement is generally less pronounced than with tonic–clonic seizures.

Tonic Status Epilepticus

Tonic SE is less common and occurs almost exclusively in children and adolescents with known epilepsy. Serial tonic seizures are typical, and autonomic manifestations, particularly increased bronchial secretions, may be pronounced. Over time, behavioral manifestations become limited to eye deviation, respiratory irregularities, and hypersecretion. A postictal confusional state may persist for days.

Focal Motor Status Epilepticus

Focal motor SE may affect children with acute inciting insults (**Table 40.1**) or those with epilepsy. Focal motor SE due to an acute illness (e.g., encephalitis) usually develops into secondary GCSE. In children with epilepsy, focal motor SE may manifest as jerking of the corner of the mouth or cheek, salivation, swallowing difficulties, and absent speech. Autonomic disturbance and impairment of consciousness may occur.

Myoclonic Status Epilepticus

Myoclonic SE is characterized by the incessant repetition of massive myoclonic jerks and can be difficult to control. Acute hypoxic–ischemic encephalopathy is the most common cause. Myoclonic SE also occurs with metabolic insults (e.g., hypoglycemia, hepatic or renal failure, or heavy-metal intoxication) (**Table 40.2**).

Nonconvulsive Status Epilepticus

NCSE can present with a variety of clinical features, including delirium, decreased speech, echolalia, blank staring with or without blinking, chewing and picking, tremulousness, subtle facial or limb myoclonus, rigidity or waxy flexibility, or vegetative features. Critically ill patients with unexplained coma or prolonged obtundation after CSE may have NCSE.

Absence NCSE

Generalized NCSE, widely known as absence SE, has also been called *petit mal status* and *spike-wave stupor* and 75% of cases occur before age 20. Absence SE is characterized by impairment of consciousness. Complex automatisms may occur and motor manifestations (e.g., myoclonic eyelid and facial twitching, bilateral or unilateral limb myoclonus, and/or atonic phenomena that produce falls, head nods, knee buckling, or other alterations of posture) are seen in about half of the cases. Patients are totally or partially amnestic of these episodes.

Complex Partial SE

Complex partial SE is also known as psychomotor status, focal NCSE, temporolimbic SE, or localized NCSE. Complex partial SE can present as frequently recurring partial seizures without full recovery of consciousness between seizures or continuous longstanding episodes of mental confusion and behavioral disturbance with or without automatisms. Complex partial SE is often marked by cyclic alterations between unresponsive staring and partial responsiveness with quasipurposeful automatisms.

Systemic Manifestations

During early SE, compensatory mechanisms to attenuate seizure-associated injury are prominent (i.e., increased catecholamines, tachycardia, hypertension, increased cerebral blood flow (CBF), increased central venous pressures, and hyperglycemia). Lactic acidosis is common, mild hypoxemia and modest hypercarbia may be seen. Other autonomic signs, including diaphoresis, hypersecretion, and mydriasis, are frequent. Late SE is marked by failure of compensatory mechanisms and seizure-associated injury (i.e., hyperthermia, hypotension, hypoglycemia, lost cerebral autoregulation). CBF becomes pressure dependent, making prompt correction of hypotension crucial. Cerebral edema may accompany late SE and is more common in pediatric than adult patients. Sustained motor convulsions may result in rhabdomyolysis and hyperkalemia. Hypoxia and hypercarbia frequently worsen. Apnea or poor handling of secretions is common. Pupillary and corneal reflexes may be absent in the ictal or postictal phases.

CLINICAL MANAGEMENT

Initial Stabilization

SE is a medical emergency that requires prompt intervention, as seizure duration is inversely associated with treatment responsiveness and favorable outcome. The first priority of initial stabilization is to ensure airway patency and control. The patient should be positioned so that ongoing seizure activity will not cause physical harm. Nothing should be placed into the patient's mouth due to the risk of aspiration. Supplemental oxygen should be provided and respiration assisted as needed. If neuromuscular blockade is necessary to facilitate intubation, a short-acting agent allows more rapid evaluation of continued seizure activity. If ongoing neuromuscular blockade is required, continuous EEG (cEEG) monitoring is indicated to assess for seizure activity. Hypotension or dehydration should be treated with isotonic fluid resuscitation or vasopressors. Hypertension is common with ongoing seizure activity, and should not be treated unless it persists after seizure activity has stopped. Thiamine may be considered prior to dextrose administration in older children at risk of nutritional deficiencies. Pyridoxine should be given to neonates with persistent seizures and suspected pyridoxine-dependent seizure activity. Empiric antibiotics and acyclovir should be administered to patients at risk of infection or with new-onset SE and fever. Hyperthermia (>38.5°C) should be treated with antipyretic medications or systemic cooling. Metabolic acidosis usually corrects spontaneously after seizure cessation and appropriate hydration.

Diagnostic Tests

Patients with SE should have serum glucose and electrolytes measured. Serum anticonvulsant levels should be measured in children on chronic therapy. Toxicology screening tests should be sent for patients with possible ingestions. A head computed tomography (CT) scan is appropriate in patients with new-onset seizures or those at risk for anatomic abnormalities, mass lesions, or cerebral edema. Lumbar puncture is indicated in patients at risk for meningitis or with a new-onset seizure disorder. Serum ammonia, lactate, and serum amino and urine organic acid levels should be checked in infants and children at risk for inborn errors of metabolism. More specific metabolic testing may be indicated. Evaluation for inflammation-induced or antibody-mediated SE should be considered in cases of super-refractory SE not attributable to other causes. Cerebral angiography or brain biopsy may be necessary to diagnose underlying microvascular cerebral vasculitis. The need for and extent of genetic testing should be evaluated with each case (>70 genes associated with epilepsy are identified and knowledge in this area is rapidly expanding).

Medications for Seizure Termination

Initial management should attempt to control SE within 30 minutes. Anticonvulsant choice is guided by clinician experience, clinical reports, and expert opinion. Benzodiazepines are the usual first-line agent, and levetiracetam, phenytoin, or valproate (for myoclonic or absence seizures) are often second line. Phenobarbital may be first line for neonates.

Benzodiazepines

Benzodiazepines facilitate GABA action by increasing the frequency of channel opening, which increases chloride permeability and leads to hyperpolarization. Commonly used benzodiazepines for SE include lorazepam, diazepam, and midazolam. Benzodiazepines lose potency during prolonged SE, possibly related to seizure-induced $GABA_A$ receptor downregulation. Additionally, benzodiazepines may precipitate myoclonus in a small percentage of neonates or tonic seizures in patients with Lennox–Gastaut syndrome. The peak effect of IV lorazepam occurs 15 minutes after dosing, and the duration is 3–6 hours. If a single dose is not effective, a second dose is recommended before (or concurrent with) administration of a second-line agent. For patients who do not have IV access, consider intramuscular, buccal, or intranasal routes of administration for midazolam. If rectal diazepam is used, the peak effect occurs 1.5 hours after administration.

Phenobarbital

Phenobarbital is the first-line agent for neonatal SE and a second-line agent for GCSE or complex partial SE. Phenobarbital is a barbiturate and acts by enhancing $GABA_A$ activity. The binding site for barbiturates differs from benzodiazepines, and reduced efficacy during prolonged SE has not been described. IV administration results in an onset after 5 minutes and peak levels after 15 minutes. Dose adjustment may be indicated in renal or hepatic failure. Phenobarbital can cause respiratory and hemodynamic depression.

Fosphenytoin

Fosphenytoin is a second-line agent for GCSE, complex partial SE, and neonatal SE. Fosphenytoin is a pro-drug that is dephosphorylated to phenytoin. Phenytoin acts as an antagonist of voltage-dependent sodium (Na^+) channels. Fosphenytoin has similar efficacy and fewer side effects (e.g., local injection site irritation and arrhythmias) than phenytoin. Peak levels of phenytoin are achieved roughly 20 minutes after IV dosing. Therapeutic levels of roughly 20 mg/L are targeted, although with hypoalbuminemia or concurrent valproate use, levels may underestimate free plasma concentrations.

Valproate

Valproate is the second-line agent for absence SE and is advocated by some as a second-line agent for GCSE. The precise mechanism of action of valproate remains unclear, but it increases endogenous GABA levels, enhances GABA response, and may stabilize neuronal membranes. Larger loading doses may be required in patients on liver enzyme-inducing drugs (e.g., phenobarbital, phenytoin, or carbamazepine). Therapeutic valproate levels are 50–150 mcg/mL. Hepatotoxicity and hyperammonemia are associated with valproate use, and transaminase levels and liver function should be monitored during treatment. It is also associated with thrombocytopenia, coagulation disorders, and pancreatitis.

Levetiracetam

Levetiracetam's mechanism of action remains poorly understood, but it is independent of GABA or NMDA activity and likely involves modulation of synaptic vesicle protein 2A and N-type calcium channel activity. It has a rapid onset of action, few drug interactions, minimal protein binding, lack of cardiorespiratory depression, and similar bioavailability with enteral and IV dosing. Reported seizure termination is 44%–75%. Adverse effects include sedation, aggression, and thrombocytopenia. Dose adjustment is recommended with renal insufficiency.

Nonconvulsive Status Epilepticus

Treatment of NCSE in comatose children is identical to that used for RSE, with rapid progression to pharmacologic coma. Consensus regarding the optimal EEG end point is lacking.

Refractory Status Epilepticus

Due to the ongoing risk for seizure-induced cerebral injury and systemic complications, RSE, whether convulsive or nonconvulsive, should be treated urgently. Consultation with a neurologist close monitoring, and interventions to maintain respiratory and hemodynamic stability are essential. Typically, pharmacologic coma is continued for 24–48 hours after seizure control. Pharmacologic coma is typically achieved using benzodiazepine or barbiturate infusions, guided by cEEG monitoring. The most efficacious EEG end point remains controversial. Midazolam infusion is the most common therapy and is associated with the longest duration of therapy, the highest incidence of breakthrough seizures, the greatest number of therapy changes due to lack of efficacy, but the least hemodynamic compromise. Pentobarbital is associated with the shortest duration of therapy, the lowest incidence of breakthrough seizures, the least changes in therapy, and the most hypotension. Dosing is usually titrated to burst suppression. Targeting the cessation of EEG seizure activity may provide similar efficacy with fewer side effects. The adverse effects of high-dose barbiturates include cardiovascular depression, hypothermia, ileus, and increased susceptibility to infections. In an effort to minimize adverse effects, recent guidelines advocate initial use of midazolam with transition to barbiturates should seizures persist.

Propofol, valproate, ketamine, topiramate, levetiracetam, lacosamide, and volatile anesthetics have been used as adjunctive therapies for RSE. Propofol controlled 64% of SE in one pediatric case series, but prolonged use is associated with propofol infusion syndrome (characterized by metabolic acidosis, lipidemia, arrhythmias, and cardiovascular collapse). Valproate has been added as adjunctive therapy in RSE. It may be particularly helpful in patients with myoclonic SE, absence SE, or Lennox–Gastaut syndrome. Ketamine is a noncompetitive NMDA receptor antagonist that is neuroprotective in experimental SE models and has been used in clinical RSE. Typically, ketamine has been added only after prolonged SE and failure of several other medications; some advocate earlier use may be advantageous. Ketamine may increase ICP so mass intracranial lesions should be excluded. Topiramate is a newer anticonvulsant medication that potentiates GABA activity, reduces glutamate release, and provides activity-dependent blockade of voltage-gated sodium channels. Topiramate is typically used for chronic seizure control but has been given to adult and pediatric patients with RSE via nasogastric tube. Levetiracetam use for RSE is described in one pediatric series of 11 patients, and was considered to be beneficial in 45% of cases. Lacosamide acts by enhancing slow inactivation of sodium channels. Lacosamide use in RSE shows promise with seizure termination in 38%–70% with rare adverse effects. Lacosamide may be particularly helpful for focal RSE, but it has also been given for NCRSE and GCSE. Finally, volatile anesthetics, such as isoflurane, may be used to treat RSE but these agents have not been subject to clinical trials. There are concerns for potential toxicity with long-term use, and technical expertise is required.

Additional Treatment Options

RSE that fails to respond to high-dose suppressive therapy is associated with high morbidity and mortality in children. Cerebral lobar resection or hemispherectomy can be considered in patients with discrete, localized seizure foci. Epilepsy syndromes commonly amenable to resection include hemimegalencephaly, Rasmussen encephalitis, prenatal cerebral artery infarction, tuberous sclerosis, malformations of cortical development, and Sturge–Weber syndrome. Other surgical options for patients without an identifiable discrete seizure focus may include multiple subpial transections, corpus callosotomy, and implantation of a vagal nerve stimulator. Additional nonsurgical therapies for RSE include electroconvulsive therapy (ECT), immunomodulation, and ketogenic diet. Immunomodulation may be helpful in cases of RSE due to inflammatory or autoimmune etiology (e.g., FIRES or antibody-mediated encephalitis). Available immunomodulation therapies include steroids, IV immunoglobulins, and plasma exchange. Therapeutic responses are best when treatment is initiated early after symptom onset.

OUTCOMES

In general, children with acute symptomatic or progressive encephalopathic etiologies have greater risk for mortality and morbidity. Conversely, children with febrile or cryptogenic etiologies tend to fare better. The risk of adverse outcome is particularly high among infants with perinatal difficulties or neurologic abnormalities prior to the development of SE. Reported mortality with cryptogenic or febrile SE is 0%–2%. Conversely, among children with acute symptomatic etiologies, mortality increases to 12%–16%. Anoxia and acute bacterial meningitis carry particularly high risks of mortality. Similarly, the risk of mortality is higher for younger children, ranging from 3% to 22.5% for those <2 years of age. A greater risk of developing epilepsy may occur in children in whom new-onset seizures present as SE. Cognitive or motor disabilities are reported after SE in 10%–35% of children. Risk factors for poor outcomes after SE include age <12 months, neuroimaging abnormalities, acute or remote symptomatic causes, progressive encephalopathy etiology or AEIMSE. Additional longitudinal prospective studies are necessary to further clarify the effects of SE on cognitive and motor outcomes in children.

CHAPTER 41 ■ CEREBROVASCULAR DISEASE AND STROKE

JOHN PAPPACHAN, ROBERT C. TASKER, AND FENELLA KIRKHAM

Approximately 3200 cases of stroke occur per year in children between 30 days and 18 years old in the United States. Although outcomes are better than in adults, 20% of children who suffer a stroke die and 50%–80% are left with significant disability.

PRESENTATION, EPIDEMIOLOGY, OUTCOME, AND COSTS

Overview of Childhood Presentation with Stroke and Cerebrovascular Disease

Acute focal neurologic signs in childhood can be symptomatic of a variety of pathologies (**Table 41.1**). The World Health Organization definition of stroke is *rapidly developing clinical signs of focal (or global) disturbance of cerebral function, with symptoms lasting 24 hours or longer, or leading to death, with no apparent cause other than of vascular origin.* Patients whose signs resolve within 24 hours have transient ischemic attacks (TIAs). Coma is a well-recognized presentation in children with subarachnoid hemorrhage (SAH) or intracerebral hemorrhage (ICH), large middle cerebral artery (MCA) territory infarction, vertebrobasilar circulation stroke, sinovenous thrombosis, bilateral border-zone ischemia, and reversible posterior leukoencephalopathy syndrome (RPLS). Seizures or headache may herald stroke and cerebrovascular disease (CVD), particularly sinovenous thrombosis. Silent infarction may be demonstrated in 25% of children with sickle cell disease (SCD) on magnetic resonance imaging (MRI) and may affect other "at-risk" populations (e.g., congenital heart disease (CHD).

Epidemiology

The prevalence of stroke and CVD in children appears to be increasing as a consequence of increased recognition and improved sensitivity of diagnostic neuroimaging using MRI or cranial computed tomography (CT) angiography and as more children survive with chronic conditions that predispose to cerebrovascular disease. Neonatal stroke affects 25–30 per 100,000 live births, and epidemiologic data suggest ongoing incidence rates of between 2 and 13 per 100,000 children/year. One-half to

TABLE 41.1

Differential Diagnosis in Children Who Present with Acute Focal Neurologic Deficit

Primary hemorrhagic stroke +/− mass effect
Acute ischemic arterial stroke +/− hemorrhage +/− **mass effect**
Acute venous stroke +/− hemorrhage +/− venous infarction +/− **mass effect**
Postictal (as Todd paresis is of short duration, if persistent, neuroimaging is essential; children with prolonged seizures may develop permanent hemiparesis)
Hemiplegic migraine (a diagnosis of exclusion, as migrainous symptoms are commonly seen in cerebrovascular disease)
Acute disseminated encephalomyelitis
Brain tumor
Abusive injury (subdural hematoma or strangulation with compression of internal carotid artery)
Encephalitis (e.g., secondary to herpes simplex—usually have seizures)
Rasmussen encephalitis
Posterior leukoencephalopathy (hypertension/hypotension or immunosuppression)
Unilateral hemispheric/focal cerebral edema (e.g., secondary to metabolic process)
Alternating hemiplegia
All stroke syndromes are potential neurosurgical emergencies and should always be discussed with a pediatric neurologist on presentation. Further management and any transfer must involve liaison with the nearest available PICU.

two-thirds are arterial ischemic stroke (AIS), and the remainder arise from hemorrhage or other diagnoses (e.g., sinovenous thrombosis without parenchymal involvement). The prevalence of AIS peaks in the first year of life, while SAH is more common in teenagers. Although childhood stroke is much more common in SCD, this condition does not entirely account for the greater incidence in children of African descent.

Definitions and Outcomes

Ischemic stroke occurs commonly in an arterial distribution, but superficial infarcts in the thalami or parietal, occipital, or frontal lobes thalami may be venous in origin (**Fig. 41.1**). Mortality is 6%–20%, and 50%–80% of events result in permanent cognitive or motor disability. Prognosis in pediatric stroke is significantly better than in the adult population. Seizure disorders complicate 15%–20% of ischemic strokes. Predictors of poor outcome include the presence of multiple etiologic risk factors, seizures at onset, an arterial stroke rather than a sinovenous thrombosis, cortical and subcortical infarction, and, for sinovenous thrombosis, the presence of venous infarcts. Hemorrhagic stroke includes ICH, most commonly due to arteriovenous malformation (AVM), and SAH (often secondary to aneurysm), but sinovenous thrombosis may cause either. Mortality of ICH and SAH is approximately twice that of ischemic stroke.

MECHANISM OF DISEASE

Risk Factors

About 50% of children presenting with an AIS have a known predisposing condition. Previously well children may have a recent history of trauma or infection (e.g., varicella), or may be found to have a vasculopathy or hereditary coagulopathy. Hemorrhagic stroke and sinovenous thrombosis may also occur in the context of acquired illnesses.

Stroke in Children with Recognized Diagnoses

Congenital Heart Disease

Embolization of air, thrombus, or infected vegetation may occur in children with CHD, particularly during cardiac catheterization, surgery, or secondary to infective endocarditis. Previously undiagnosed cardiac disease (e.g., a patent foramen ovale) may be discovered. Asymptomatic abnormalities of the aortic valve are associated with primary CVD such as cervicocephalic dissection and moyamoya.

Sickle Cell Disease

Most children with SCD and overt ischemic stroke have intracranial, large-vessel disease with intimal hyperplasia. Without prophylactic blood transfusion, 25% of patients suffer a stroke by age 45. Ischemic stroke predominates in children. The majority of adults have spontaneous ICH or SAH secondary to aneurysms. Sinovenous thrombosis, posterior leukoencephalopathy, watershed ischemia, and acute "silent" infarction have been underrecognized.

Intermediate-Risk Factors for Childhood Stroke

At least one-third of cases of childhood stroke occur in the context of infection (bacterial or tuberculous meningitis and varicella are well-recognized associations). Immunodeficiencies, both inherited and acquired, are associated with stroke. Stroke syndromes are well described in the hemolytic anemias, including intermediate forms of thalassemia, hereditary spherocytosis, paroxysmal nocturnal hemoglobinuria, and SCD. Iron deficiency appears to be a risk factor for stroke in children. Classical homocystinuria (deficiency of cystathionine β-synthase) is recognized as an important cause of arterial vascular disease. Homozygosity for the thermolabile variant of the methylene tetrahydrofolate reductase gene appears to be a risk factor for neonatal and childhood AIS, sinovenous thrombosis, and recurrence in childhood AIS. Supplementation of folate, vitamin B_{12}, and vitamin B_6 may reduce plasma homocysteine levels, although few data support efficacy in stroke prevention.

Hypertension is an important risk factor for stroke in adults but has been ignored in children. Systolic blood pressure above the 90th percentile is present in 54% of children with cryptogenic stroke and 46% with symptomatic stroke and is associated with cerebral arterial abnormalities. In childhood stroke, 9% have high random cholesterol levels, 31% have high triglyceride levels, and 22% have high lipoprotein, a risk factor for atherosclerosis and stroke in adults. The prevalence of inherited coagulopathies is ~10% in previously well patients. Polymorphisms such as factor V Leiden and Prothrombin 20210 may be associated with primary and recurrent neonatal and childhood sinovenous thrombosis and AIS. Adhesion of red blood cells, white blood cells, or platelets appears to be an important mechanism of endothelial damage in SCD and may play a role in stroke of other etiologies, such as moyamoya.

Between 30% and 80% of children with AIS have abnormal findings on cranial CT or MR angiographic studies. A less abrupt onset of stroke is characteristic of those with arteriopathy. A diagnosis of vascular disease predicts recurrent AIS. Spontaneous hemorrhage is most commonly secondary to an AVM, but aneurysms and pseudoaneurysms are not unusual and may occur in association with underlying conditions, including trauma.

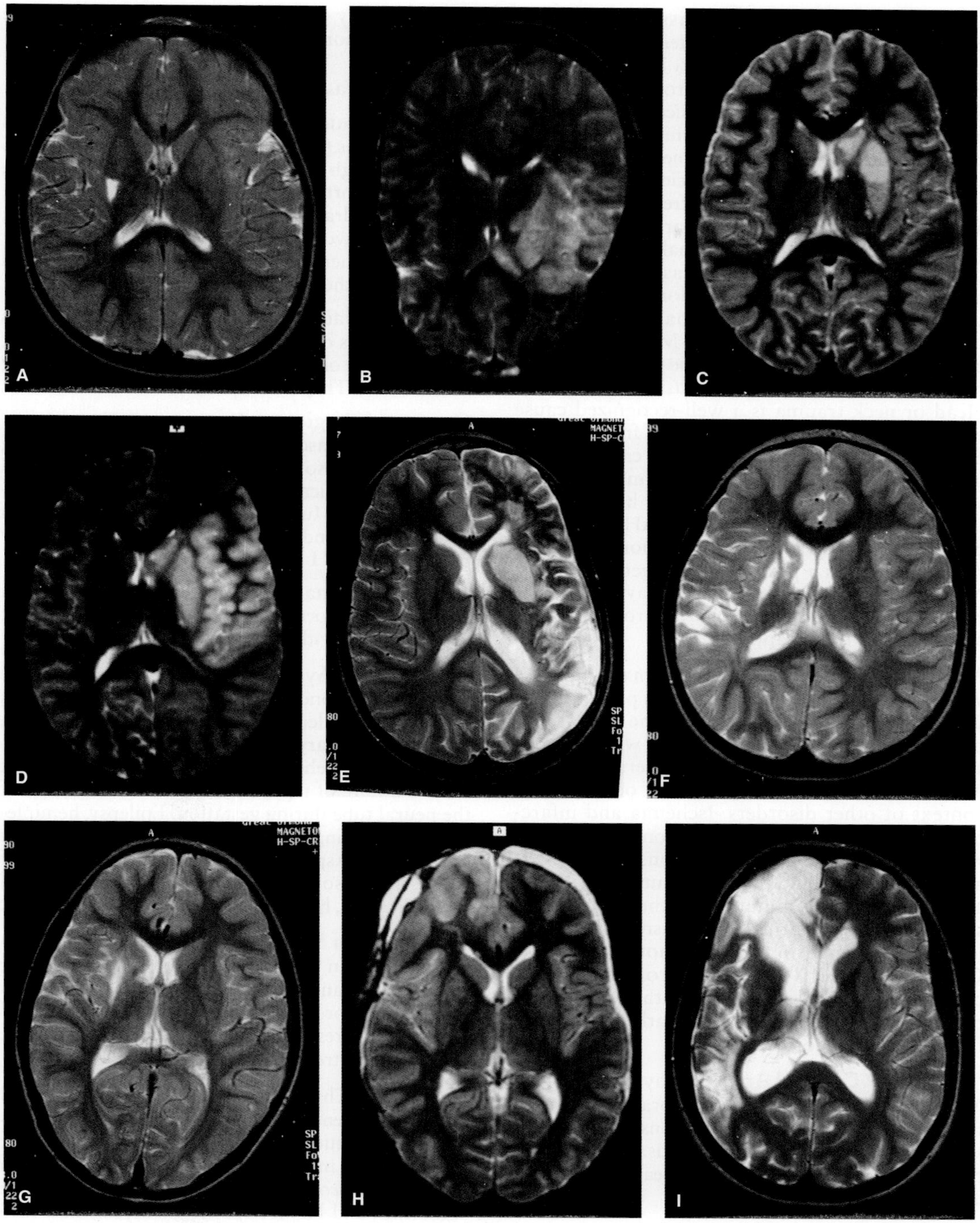

FIGURE 41.1. MRI scans from children with first and recurrent ischemic (arterial and venous) stroke. **A:** Basal ganglia infarct associated with transient cerebral arteriopathy after varicella. **B:** Temporal infarction associated with dissection. **C:** Small infarct associated with middle cerebral artery stenosis. **D:** Larger infarct after recurrence of stroke in **C.** **E:** Recurrent infarction after dissection. **F:** "Silent" posterior watershed recurrent infarction after embolic occlusion. **G:** Deep white matter infarct in *Haemophilus influenzae* meningitis. **H:** Right frontal cortical edema after craniopharyngioma surgery. **I:** "Silent" recurrent infarction in the posterior watershed territory in the same patient as in **H.**

Extracranial/Intracranial Dissection. Cervicocephalic dissections are reported in 6.5%–20% of childhood AIS and up to 50% of children with posterior circulation ischemic stroke. Risk factors include trauma, infection, anatomical variants of the neck, migraine, hyperhomocysteinemia, fibromuscular dysplasia, Marfan syndrome, Ehlers–Danlos syndrome, and α_1-antitrypsin deficiency. The internal carotid artery (ICA) is the most frequently affected artery followed by the vertebral artery. Dissections typically begin with a small intimal tear or primary intramural hemorrhage of the vasa vasorum. The intramural hematoma extends along the course of the artery. Intramural hematoma can be imaged using fat-saturated T1-weighted MRI of the neck, conventional arteriography may be required to demonstrate the tapering partial occlusion of the artery. Head or neck trauma is a well-recognized cause of dissection. Intraoral injuries (e.g., from a pencil carried in the mouth) can injure the carotid artery in the peritonsillar area. A dissection may compress surrounding nerves and disrupt their blood supply. Intracranial dissections can lead to SAH. Subintimal dissection results in stenosis or occlusion of the arterial lumen and is a potent thrombogenic stimulus. No randomized controlled trials have looked at reduction of microemboli or clinical stroke rate from antithrombolytic therapy.

Moyamoya. Moyamoya derives from the Japanese word meaning "something hazy, like a puff of smoke drifting in the air" and describes the appearance of the collaterals seen in association with bilateral severe stenosis or occlusion of the terminal ICAs. Moyamoya may be idiopathic or occur in the context of other disorders. Ischemia and infarction occur in the border-zone regions between the major cerebral arteries. Associations include SCD and Down syndrome. It also occurs in Williams syndrome (involves mutations in the elastin gene) suggesting that abnormal vessel distensibility may lead to hypoperfusion and promote collaterals. Other associations include neurofibromatosis, cranial irradiation, and arteriopathies. A genetic predisposition accounts for idiopathic, as well as familial, cases reported in Japan.

"Transient" Cerebral Arteriopathy in Previously Well Children. "Transient" cerebral arteriopathy may involve an inflammatory response to infections such as varicella, *Borrelia*, or tonsillitis. In many cases, the vasculopathy stabilizes or disappears; progression is associated with recurrent stroke.

Intracranial Arteriopathy in SCD. Narrowing of the distal ICA, proximal MCA, and anterior cerebral artery is characteristic of SCD. Gradual progression to occlusion commonly occurs with or without moyamoya collaterals. Pathologic examination shows endothelial proliferation, fibroblastic reaction, hyalinization, and fragmentation of the internal elastic lamina. The majority of clinical and silent infarcts occur in the MCA territory or in the border zones between the middle, anterior, and posterior cerebral territories.

Vascular Malformations

Arteriovenous Malformation. Arteriovenous malformations (AVMs) are high-flow arteriovenous shunts through a nidus of abnormal, thin-walled, coiled, and tortuous connections between feeding arteries and draining veins without an intervening capillary network. In children, AVMs commonly present with hemorrhage in deep areas of the brain (particularly the basal ganglia and thalamus).

Capillary Telangiectasias. Capillary telangiectasias are collections of dilated ectatic capillaries without smooth muscle or elastic fibers with normal intervening neural tissue. They rarely present with ICH or SAH.

Cavernous Angioma. Cavernous angiomas (cavernomas) are vascular malformations comprising thin-walled sinusoidal spaces, lined with endothelial tissue and calcifications without intervening parenchymal tissue. Multiple lesions are seen in 13% of sporadic cases and 50% of familial cases. They may present with ICH or epilepsy.

Venous Angioma. Venous angiomas are thin-walled channels with normal intervening neural tissue that are associated with a very low risk of bleeding.

Sturge–Weber Syndrome. Sturge–Weber syndrome is a sporadic condition characterized by a venous angioma of the leptomeninges, choroidal angioma, and facial capillary hemangioma involving the periorbital area, forehead, or scalp that probably result from a failure of regression of a vascular plexus of the neural tube during gestation. Epilepsy, hemiplegia, and learning disability are probably the result of ischemia. Aspirin may reduce the frequency of stroke-like episodes. If epilepsy cannot be controlled by medication, hemispherectomy may be beneficial.

Vein of Galen Malformation. Vein of Galen malformation is an embryonic choroidal AVM. It may be diagnosed antenatally, present in the neonate as heart failure, or present in older children as hydrocephalus, seizures, proptosis, or prominent scalp veins. Endovascular treatment is often possible.

Aneurysms. Three-quarters of patients with arterial aneurysms present with ICH. Approximately 10%–15% of arterial aneurysms are posttraumatic; a similar proportion are mycotic, and associated with infection (e.g., *Staphylococcus*, *Streptococcus*, gram-negative organisms, and HIV). Mycotic aneurysms may also arise secondary to embolization of infective thrombi into the intracranial circulation in patients with subacute bacterial endocarditis. Other associations with arterial aneurysms in children are polycystic kidney disease, SCD, tuberous sclerosis, Marfan syndrome, Ehlers–Danlos syndrome type IV, pseudoxanthoma elasticum, and hypertension. No underlying systemic disorder is found in a substantial proportion.

Cerebral Sinovenous Thrombosis

The venous drainage of the brain occurs through the "superficial" or "deep" cerebral sinovenous systems. In neonates, sinovenous thrombosis may be related to distortion of cranial bones during birth. In older children, trauma, sepsis, and underlying illnesses (e.g., malignancy or systemic inflammation) play a larger role. Septic foci include the inner ear, mastoid, or air sinuses. Dehydration, anemia, and inherited prothrombotic disorders (congenital or acquired) are recognized risk factors. Sinovenous thrombosis disrupts cerebrospinal fluid absorption within the superior sagittal sinus, resulting in diffuse cerebral swelling, communicating hydrocephalus, or pseudotumor cerebri (benign intracranial hypertension). "Outflow" obstruction causes regional venous hypertension and leads to focal cerebral edema. Risk factors for venous infarction include rapid onset of sinovenous thrombosis, complete luminal occlusion, and thrombosis located at the entry points of cerebral veins into the sagittal sinus.

Stroke Syndromes and Mimics

Posterior Circulation Arterial Stroke. Arterial disease associated with posterior circulation infarction in the cerebellum, brainstem, and parieto-occipital lobes is more common in boys than girls. A positive diagnosis of dissection may require conventional angiography in the acute phase, as MRI and angiography commonly miss the diagnosis in the posterior circulation (**Fig. 41.2**). Etiologic factors include minor trauma, subluxation of the cervical spine at the extremes of flexion and extension, chiropractic manipulation, frequent neck movements (e.g., secondary to athetoid cerebral palsy), hypertension, cardiac anomalies, and Fabry disease.

Reversible Posterior Leukoencephalopathy Syndrome and Border-zone Ischemia. RPLS is a cliniconeuroradiologic syndrome characterized by seizures, altered mental state, visual abnormalities, and headaches associated with predominantly posterior white matter abnormalities on CT and

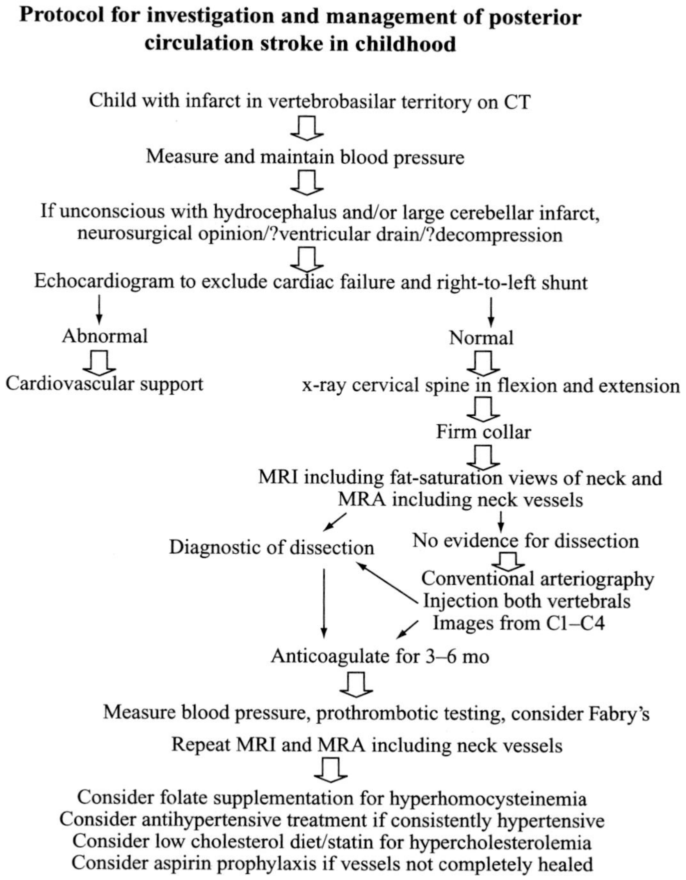
Protocol for investigation and management of posterior circulation stroke in childhood
Child with infarct in vertebrobasilar territory on CT
Measure and maintain blood pressure
If unconscious with hydrocephalus and/or large cerebellar infarct, neurosurgical opinion/?ventricular drain/?decompression
Echocardiogram to exclude cardiac failure and right-to-left shunt
Abnormal
Cardiovascular support
Normal
x-ray cervical spine in flexion and extension
Firm collar
MRI including fat-saturation views of neck and MRA including neck vessels
Diagnostic of dissection
No evidence for dissection
Conventional arteriography
Injection both vertebrals
Images from C1–C4
Anticoagulate for 3–6 mo
Measure blood pressure, prothrombotic testing, consider Fabry's
Repeat MRI and MRA including neck vessels
Consider folate supplementation for hyperhomocysteinemia
Consider antihypertensive treatment if consistently hypertensive
Consider low cholesterol diet/statin for hypercholesterolemia
Consider aspirin prophylaxis if vessels not completely healed

FIGURE 41.2. Algorithm for the management of posterior circulation stroke.

MRI examinations but without arterial or venous disease. RPLS is a common stroke mimic and has been recognized in an increasing number of medical settings, including hypertensive encephalopathy, eclampsia, acute chest crisis in SCD, and during use of immunosuppression. It is essential to distinguish RPLS from posterior circulation embolic stroke secondary to vertebrobasilar dissection. It is also important to exclude sinovenous thrombosis with venous infarction, particularly of the sagittal and straight sinuses. Many patients make a full clinical and radiologic recovery after conservative measures, including slow reduction of blood pressure and maintenance of normal oxygenation.

Acute Disseminated Encephalomyelitis. Acute disseminated encephalomyelitis (ADEM) is an immune-mediated process resulting in inflammation and myelin damage in the brain and spinal cord usually associated with infection or immunization. MRI may reveal demyelination.

Metabolic Stroke. Diabetes and inborn errors of metabolism can cause acute focal neurologic symptoms and signs (metabolic stroke) due to either vascular injury or direct tissue injury, which may be permanent or transitory. Metabolic diseases associated with stroke include homocystinuria, Fabry disease, Menkes disease, organic acidemias, and urea cycle disorders. Mitochondrial disorders can cause stroke-like episodes (i.e., mitochondrial encephalopathy with lactic acidosis and stroke-like episodes, MELAS) because of deficient energy supply and by the generation of oxygen free radicals. Targeted therapies may be available.

CLINICAL PRESENTATION AND DIFFERENTIAL DIAGNOSIS

In adults, controlled trials of thrombolysis have increased the need for rapid assessment. The concepts of "brain attack" and the management of acute stroke in stroke centers have received widespread publicity. Thrombolysis for anterior circulation stroke must begin within 4.5 hours. In contrast, in many children, the correct diagnosis is not made for days or weeks. Children may present with status epilepticus resistant to first-line therapy, with a reduced level of consciousness, with signs of intracranial hypertension or imminent central or uncal herniation.

Initial management goals include maintaining oxygen-hemoglobin saturation, cardiac output, systemic and cerebral perfusion pressure (CPP), temperature, and avoidance of hypo- and hyperglycemia. Endotracheal intubation may be needed. The head of the bed should be flat; this maneuver optimizes perfusion to the brain but risks aspiration in those with nausea and vomiting and compromised airway protection. At the same time as the above interventions and evaluations, the initial investigations should include a noncontrast cranial CT scan in order to rule out ICH. In AIS, CT scan changes may not become apparent until 3–24 hours after symptom onset. MRI should be deferred until after a decision has been made about the use of IV recombinant tissue plasminogen activator (rTPA). Additional tests include an electrocardiogram, arterial blood gas, serum electrolytes, renal function tests, liver function tests, a complete blood count including platelets, toxicology studies, and clotting studies (prothrombin time, international normalized ratio, and activated partial thromboplastin time).

The Four Targets of Early "Ischemic Stroke" Care

The four targets for ischemic stroke care include acute therapy to optimize neurologic status, etiologic workup for secondary prevention, prevention of neurologic deterioration or medical complications, and recovery and rehabilitation.

Optimizing the Neurologic Status

In instances where there is no hemorrhage, emergency therapy focuses on reestablishing blood flow. Treatment with rTPA is rarely an option in children due to timing of presentation and little evidence to support a benefit. Blood pressure management depends on the presenting blood pressure. A hypertensive patient may be "autoregulating" at a new set-point for blood pressure and regional cerebral blood flow. However, emergency control of hypertension is required when there is evidence of hypertensive end-organ damage (e.g., encephalopathy, dissection of the aorta, heart failure, or myocardial injury). When antihypertensive treatment is used, a short-acting IV agent is preferred and a gradual, 10%–15%, reduction is the target.

Prevention of Propagation of Thrombus and Early Recurrence. Approximately half of the children who present with AIS and a similar proportion of those with sinovenous thrombosis have a known predisposing condition, particularly SCD, cardiac disease, bacterial meningitis, and malignancy. Some are candidates for emergency management, such as exchange transfusion for patients with SCD or anticoagulation for venous sinus thrombosis.

Anticoagulation. Anticoagulation is required for cardiac embolic disease, documented large artery occlusive clot (e.g., ICA, MCA, or basilar artery), arterial dissection, and venous thrombosis. The major concern and risk is hemorrhagic transformation in the evolution of a large infarct. Several observational studies suggest that anticoagulation therapy is safe in children with AIS and sinovenous thrombosis. It is usually used with extracranial dissection. Aspirin is often preferred for AIS. The use of anticoagulation in patients with cardiac disease is more controversial and influenced by the cardiac pathology and by neurologic and imaging findings.

Workup for Secondary Prevention

MR angiography is very useful to exclude alternative pathology or confirm arterial disease. It is important that the vascular pathology is defined so that conditions requiring urgent management (e.g., arterial dissection) are not missed. Despite the need for general anesthesia, in most cases MRI has advantages over CT, as in addition to the essential exclusion of hemorrhage, ischemia may be documented within minutes (using diffusion-weighted imaging) or hours (using T2-weighted imaging) rather than days. The addition of magnetic resonance arteriography (MRA) and venography (MRV) often guides management. Most conditions that mimic ischemic stroke, such as ADEM, metabolic disease, and posterior leukoencephalopathy are recognized on MRI. Thrombosis in the large venous sinuses (sagittal, lateral, or straight) may be diagnosed on MR or CTV. Conventional angiography is required to diagnose small-vessel vasculitis, cortical venous thrombosis, and, sometimes, dissection, particularly in the posterior circulation.

Neurologic Deterioration in AIS

Deterioration in AIS can result from a number of mechanisms that include recurrent stroke, enlargement of the stroke, hemorrhagic transformation of the ischemic region, development of cerebral edema, midline shift with mass effect, a drop in perfusion pressure, anemia, hypoxemia, hypoglycemia, hyperglycemia, hyponatremia, seizures, infection, inflammation, and fever.

Surgical Decompression in Acute Stroke

Surgical decompression is considered with large MCA or cerebellar/posterior fossa infarcts. Clinical trials of decompressive craniectomy for adults with malignant ischemic stroke have shown increased survival and improved functional outcome when surgery is performed within 48 hours of stroke onset. Reports in children suggest that good outcome is possible even in the presence of signs of herniation. Intracranial pressure (ICP) monitoring should not delay surgery.

Intracranial Hemorrhage and Hemorrhagic Stroke

Patients with ICH or hemorrhagic stroke may require immediate neurosurgery. The main priorities are to prevent cerebral herniation if the blood collection is space-occupying, reverse coagulopathy, exclude sinovenous thrombosis, and to treat vasospasm with volume expansion. If an underlying AVM is present, the recurrence risk for hemorrhage is 2%–3% per year for life if untreated, and a careful decision regarding management (neurosurgery, neuroradiology with coils, or stereotactic radiotherapy) must be made once the patient has recovered from the acute phase. Although less common, aneurysms are associated with a significant rebleeding risk, particularly soon after presentation. A vascular team should evaluate these children so that an individualized management strategy, targeted at preventing recurrence, can be implemented.

Neurologic Deterioration and Surgical Clot Removal in Acute Hemorrhage

The principles of medical care for patients with ICH or hemorrhagic stroke are similar to those described for AIS. Additional risks include hydrocephalus (with resultant impaired cerebral perfusion) and hematoma enlargement with deterioration or herniation. Some of these patients will require ventricular drain insertion. Consideration should be given to the effects of bed position on hemodynamics, oxygenation, and neurologic status. If neurologic findings worsen with elevation of the head, the patient should remain flat. In cases of cerebellar or posterior fossa hemorrhage, the indications for surgery include a displaced fourth ventricle, early obstructive hydrocephalus, compression of the brain stem, and decreased level of consciousness. In cases of supratentorial hemorrhage, the indications for surgery include location close to the brain surface, hematoma volume >20 mL, and decreased level of consciousness.

DISEASE-SPECIFIC THERAPIES

Stroke Due to SCD

Children with SCD and high transcranial Doppler velocities (>200 cm/s) have a 40% stroke risk over the next 3 years. Primary prevention of stroke is possible if these children are screened appropriately and transfused indefinitely. With any neurologic deterioration, the goal is to begin transfusion within 2–4 hours of presentation, particularly if the deficit persists or progresses. If available, exchange transfusion (using a manual regime or erythrocytapheresis) is recommended over simple transfusion. In the first 48 hours, the goal is to reduce the hemoglobin S percentage to <20% and raise the hemoglobin to 10–11 g/dL (hematocrit of >30%).

CHAPTER 42 ■ HYPOXIC–ISCHEMIC ENCEPHALOPATHY

ERICKA L. FINK, MIOARA D. MANOLE, AND ROBERT S. B. CLARK

Hypoxic–ischemic encephalopathy (HIE) is a complex spectrum of brain injury from hypoxemia and/or ischemia with or without reperfusion injury. HIE is a major cause of pediatric morbidity and mortality that often results in disability, high costs, and lifelong healthcare needs.

CORE PATHOPHYSIOLOGY AND PATHOBIOLOGY

Global HIE can result from respiratory arrest, cardiac arrest, strangulation, poisoning, sagittal sinus thrombosis, or profound shock states. Cardiac arrest due to asphyxia is the most common cause in infants and children. Cardiac arrest due to arrhythmias is the most common cause in adults. Focal HIE can result from embolic or thrombotic stroke, or intracerebral hemorrhage.

Parenchymal cells (neurons, astrocytes, oligodendrocytes, or microglia) do not tolerate prolonged durations of ischemia. Neuronal and glial cell death can result from necrotic, apoptotic, and autophagic pathways. Necrosis is characterized by mitochondrial energy failure leading to cellular swelling, loss of membrane integrity, and an inflammatory response in surrounding tissues. Apoptosis is an energy-requiring process that requires new protein synthesis. Autophagy is an adaptive response to starvation, and results in autodigestion of cellular proteins and organelles to feed the cell. The degree of brain injury and outcome correlate with the duration of the no-flow state. The clinical goal is to restore cerebral blood flow (CBF) as rapidly as possible.

Cardiac Arrest

Mortality after cardiac arrest is very high, and despite the plasticity of the developing brain, neurologic outcomes can be dismal. Poor outcomes may be related to the hypoxemia and hypoperfusion prior to no-flow ischemia seen during asphyxial cardiac arrest. Death after successful return of spontaneous circulation (ROSC) is usually due to brain death, multiorgan system failure, or withdrawal of support (usually based on projected neurologic outcome). Survivors of cardiac arrest often develop some degree of HIE. Common manifestations of HIE include cerebral palsy, mental retardation, dysphagia, cortical vision impairment, hearing impairment, microcephaly, temperature instability, chronic ventilator dependence, and seizures.

Of the children who attain ROSC, prediction of survival and neurologic outcome after cardiac arrest is difficult. The need for three or more doses of epinephrine or >30 minutes of resuscitation is associated with poor neurologic outcome. Patients with witnessed cardiac arrest have better outcomes than those with unwitnessed cardiac arrest. Survival rate to hospital discharge is higher for in-hospital versus out-of-hospital cardiac arrest patients, with 65% of survivors having good neurologic outcome.

Absent pupillary and motor response predict poor outcome when measured several days after ROSC. Children with an EEG that exhibited discontinuous activity and/or was nonreactive have worse outcome in the first 72 hours after ROSC. In children who drown, any hypoxic–ischemic abnormality on brain computed tomography (CT) is associated with death or persistent vegetative state. Serum biomarkers of brain injury such as neuron-specific enolase (NSE) from neurons and S-100B from astrocytes show utility in preliminary studies. Children with basal ganglia lesions on conventional brain magnetic resonance imaging (MRI) or in the brain lobes on diffusion-weighted MRI had poor outcome. The use of hypothermia has confounded much of the outcome prediction data gleaned from adults with cardiac arrest; however, somatosensory-evoked potentials (SSEPs) have demonstrated good reliability.

CBF after Cardiac Arrest in Experimental Models

Asphyxial arrest produces a physiologically different milieu compared with arrest due to arrhythmia, because of the hypoxemia, acidosis, hypercarbia, and hypotension that precede cardiac arrest. During cardiac arrest, there is global ischemia, with no flow (or low flow when CPR is being provided). Immediately following reperfusion, there can be heterogeneous return of CBF in spite of normal or increased cerebral perfusion pressure (CPP). Areas of failed brain reperfusion after ROSC increase with increasing duration of cardiac arrest. At a microscopic level, there are areas of "no-reflow" interspersed with areas of restored blood flow and microinfarcts. Brain regions that are selectively vulnerable include the thalamus, amygdala, hippocampus, and striatum. It is hypothesized that vasospasm, perivascular edema, and increased blood viscosity play a role in the development of this "no-reflow" phenomenon. The second phase of CBF after cardiac arrest is characterized by increased global CBF immediately after ROSC, referred to as the "hyperemia" phase. This hyperemic phase may be essential for neuronal functional recovery, and postarrest hypotension worsens neurologic outcome. The third phase of CBF after cardiac arrest, the "delayed hypoperfusion" phase, begins ~15–30 minutes after ROSC and can persist for several hours. During this phase, there is regional heterogeneity of the CBF, with areas of high, normal, and low flow. The duration and degree of delayed hypoperfusion is associated with impairment of functional recovery, especially if not matched by a lower metabolic rate. Therefore, interventions that increase CBF and minimize delayed hypoperfusion after ischemia may improve neurologic recovery.

CBF after Cardiac Arrest in Humans

Normal CBF in infants is less than in children or adults and peaks at age 7 years. Most available data on CBF patterns after cardiac arrest in humans are recorded >6 hours after ROSC, since these patients require intensive stabilization. Furthermore, serial measurements of CBF have been rarely reported. In neonatal asphyxia, the development of high CBF velocities after 24 hours is predictive of poor prognosis. In adult patients, the CBF at 24 hours after ROSC can be low, normal, or high, and persistently high CBF values may be reflective of completely disrupted autoregulation and indicate the onset of irreversible brain damage.

Cerebral Metabolism after Cardiac Arrest

Whether cerebral metabolism is coupled to CBF after cardiac arrest is controversial. Nonoxidative or anaerobic cerebral metabolism adds an additional level of complexity. Cerebral metabolic rate for glucose (CMRGlu) is also reduced, in a magnitude similar to cerebral metabolic rate for oxygen ($CMRO_2$), after cardiac arrest.

Systemic Variables Affecting CBF after Cardiac Arrest

CBF is influenced by systemic physiologic variables, in particular $Paco_2$, Pao_2, blood pressure, and temperature (**Fig. 42.1**). Low $Paco_2$ produces vasoconstriction and decreased CBF, while high $Paco_2$ produces vasodilatation and increased CBF. Extreme hyperventilation and hypocarbia could exacerbate hypoperfusion, and should be avoided in the early postresuscitation period. Defining the optimal $Paco_2$ early after resuscitation is complex, and issues such as profound acidosis and response to catecholamines must be considered. Pao_2 has little effect on CBF until it is less than ~55 mm Hg, in which case CBF dramatically increases. Controversy surrounds the target Pao_2 during resuscitation and the postresuscitation period; supplementary oxygen may increase oxidative stress on reperfusion. It is logical to target normocarbia and normoxia in patients during and after cardiac arrest.

In general, CBF is maintained constant by autoregulation over a range of CPP, ~50–150 mm Hg in adults. Adults resuscitated from cardiac arrest may have compromised autoregulation. Pressure autoregulation may be absent or the lower limit of autoregulation increased (range 80–120 mm Hg). Higher mean arterial pressure (MAP) in the first 2 hours after cardiac arrest is associated with better outcome. The relationship between pressure autoregulation and outcome is not clear in infants and children.

Hypothermia decreases CBF via a coupled reduction in cerebral metabolism. It also suppresses excitatory neurotransmission and oxygen radicals. Animal models support hypothermia and induced hypertension to improve survival. Two randomized clinical trials in adult patients after VT/VF cardiac arrest support the use of postarrest hypothermia.

Prolonged central hypoxia and depressed ventilation stimulate chemoreceptors and a vagal response that leads to bradycardia, PEA, or asystole. Oxygen stores are depleted ~20 seconds after cardiac arrest, and there is loss of consciousness. Glucose and adenosine triphosphate (ATP) stores are depleted within

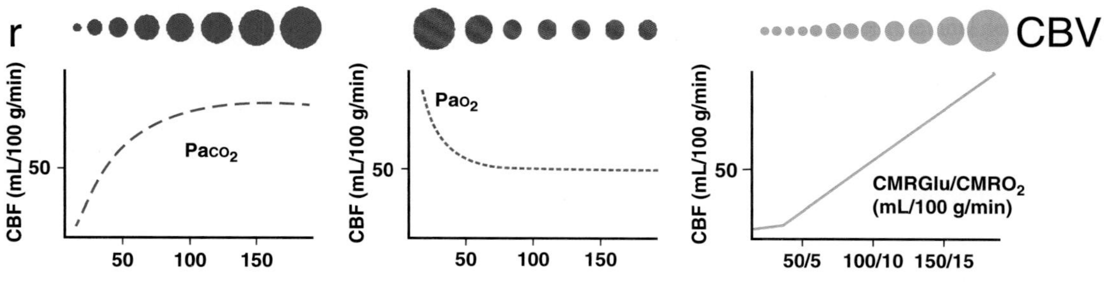

FIGURE 42.1. Physiologic factors affecting normal cerebral blood flow (CBF). Under a constant cerebral perfusion pressure, CBF changes occur via changes in the diameter of the cerebral blood vessels (r = radius), resulting in changes in cerebrovascular resistance and cerebral blood volume (CBV). $Paco_2$, partial pressure of carbon dioxide; Pao_2, partial pressure of oxygen; CMRGlu, cerebral metabolic rate for glucose; $CMRO_2$, cerebral metabolic rate for oxygen, X-axis units are mmHg for each of the three graphs. (From Robert S. B. Clark.)

5 minutes, whereupon the patient's brain crosses the threshold for cerebral ischemia. Following ROSC and reperfusion, transient hyperemia is followed by global hypoperfusion. This is a period when the brain is at risk of secondary injury, and may represent a therapeutic target.

Pathobiology after Reperfusion

Reperfusion and restoration of oxygen delivery to injured brain leads to increases in free radicals, and initiation of redox-sensitive cell-signaling pathways. The metabolic and electrical failure can result in coma despite restoration of CBF or oxygen and substrate delivery during reperfusion. Neuronal populations vulnerable to hypoxia–ischemia include the CA1 region of the hippocampus, cerebral cortical layers 3 and 5, amygdaloid nucleus, basal ganglia, and cerebellar Purkinje cells. Unique aspects in cellular energy metabolism and connectivity play a role in this susceptibility, since these regions do not have especially vulnerable microcirculatory patterns.

CLINICAL ASPECTS OF HYPOXIC–ISCHEMIC ENCEPHALOPATHY

Acute Management of Cardiac Arrest

The goals for pediatric cardiac arrest are provision of effective high-quality CPR, rapid ROSC, and prevention of secondary injury. Time to initiation of resuscitative efforts can strongly impact survival and neurologic outcome. Community education in bystander CPR may influence outcome after out-of-hospital arrests. Establishment of an airway for ventilation and oxygenation is imperative to the pediatric population, since most pediatric arrests have an asphyxial etiology. Hyperventilation should be avoided unless there are signs and symptoms of brain herniation. Circulatory failure should be treated aggressively following published pediatric shock guidelines. After stabilization, a quick neurologic assessment should be performed. This should include pupillary responses and Glasgow Coma Scale (GCS) score. The GCS, validated in traumatic brain injury, may also be useful in the assignment of severity of injury after cardiac arrest. The motor score is the most sensitive predictor for brain injury severity after trauma.

Pediatric Intensive Care Unit Management

PICU management after cardiac arrest consists of supportive care and prevention of secondary insults. Maintenance of normoxia, normocapnia, and normotension are bedrocks of supportive care. Titration of oxygen administration should maintain Spo_2 around 94% to avoid hyperoxia. Adults in whom Pao_2 was >300 mm Hg or <60 mm Hg had an associated increased risk of mortality. Hypoxia after ROSC was also associated with increased risk of death in children.

Cerebral edema after cardiac arrest and reperfusion is variable but is more common after asphyxia than arrhythmia arrest. Intracranial pressure is often increased after global ischemia, and can be severe enough to cause intracranial hypertension and herniation syndrome. Intracranial hypertension may be a consequence, rather than the cause, of cerebral ischemia and intracranial pressure monitoring is not routinely used. Revisiting the use of such monitoring (particularly in combination with monitoring of CBF, cerebral metabolism and brain tissue oxygenation) during evolving neurologic injury may be warranted. Recurrence of edema during rewarming from protective hypothermia is another reason to reconsider the use of monitors.

A CT may be helpful in situations where the etiology of arrest is unclear or where there may be concomitant trauma. Serial head CT scans after cardiac arrest are indicated only if new or evolving pathology is suspected, such as hemorrhage, evolving mass lesion, or herniation.

Contemporary Neurointensive Care Monitoring

Cerebral Blood Flow and Estimation of Cerebral Perfusion

CBF can be measured directly, but intermittently, using techniques such as stable Xenon CT, positron emission tomography (PET), or perfusion MRI. The few available reports focus on the relationship of CBF to outcome rather than the use of CBF measurements to guide clinical management. Transcranial Doppler (TCD) ultrasonography is a noninvasive, bedside method to measures middle cerebral artery (MCA) blood flow velocity as a surrogate for CBF. It provides no information about regional heterogeneity of CBF after cardiac arrest.

Cerebral Metabolic and Brain Activity Monitoring

Brain oxygenation can be measured using near-infrared spectroscopy (NIRS), a noninvasive and continuous estimate of cerebral oxygen extraction. Current disadvantages of NIRS include limited depth of penetration, focal rather than global information, and lack of definitions of target and critical values. Invasive brain tissue oxygenation can be determined using a fiberoptic catheter placed into brain parenchyma to measure the partial pressure of brain tissue oxygen ($Pbto_2$). The utility of $Pbto_2$ is being studied in traumatic brain injury and its use in cardiac arrest remains investigational. Global cerebral metabolism can also be measured if a jugular bulb catheter is placed and CBF is measured simultaneously. Cross-brain extraction of oxygen and glucose can be used to calculate $CMRO_2$ and CMRGlu. Like $Pbto_2$ monitoring, $Sjvo_2$

monitoring in patients after cardiac arrest remains investigational. Electroencephalography (EEG) is a noninvasive bedside method increasingly used after HIE to diagnose and guide management of nonclinical seizures. Seizures occur in as many as 30% of adults after cardiac arrest. Continuous monitoring during periods of muscle relaxation is also indicated. Presence of discontinuous EEG activity, epileptiform spikes, or discharges correlate with poor outcome. SSEPs may be more sensitive and specific in predicting unfavorable outcome after cardiac arrest. Cerebral microdialysis uses a catheter equipped with a dialysis membrane inserted into the brain parenchyma to do intermittent or continuous sampling of extracellular fluid to measure changes in brain chemistry. Currently, cerebral microdialysis is used as a research tool.

Magnetic Resonance Imaging/Spectroscopy

MRI provides detailed information about ischemic brain injury, is noninvasive, and does not use ionizing radiation. Diffusion-weighted imaging (DWI) uses differences in water diffusivity to acutely diagnose ischemia which may not be discernible on T2-weighted images. MRI requires longer scan times than CT, an increased need for sedation to prevent motion artifact, and the restriction of metal objects. Detection of injury in the cortical lobes and the basal ganglia has been associated with poor outcome after pediatric cardiac arrest. Magnetic resonance spectroscopy (MRS) has been used to demonstrate the relationship of metabolites (e.g., lactate, pyruvate, glutamate, *N*-acetylaspartate, and phosphocreatine) to outcome in patients with HIE.

Biomarkers

Serum and urine biomarkers are surrogates of brain injury that present a promising approach to detecting injury and predicting outcome. Most work has focused on NSE, a glycolytic protein from neurons and neuroectodermal cells, S-100B (a calcium-regulated protein released by injured astrocytes to modulate differentiation of neurons and glia), and myelin basic protein (MBP). A combination of GCS score, NSE, and S-100B predicts vegetative state or death in adults after cardiac arrest.

Therapies Targeting the Prevention and Treatment of Hypoxic–Ischemic Encephalopathy

Temperature Management

Fever (>38°C) after acute brain insult from trauma or hypoxia–ischemia exacerbates injury and may lead to worse outcomes. Mild, induced hypothermia has become a promising strategy for improving survival and neurologic outcome after cardiac arrest in adult patients. Benefits may occur through reductions in brain metabolic needs, excitotoxicity, oxidative stress, and inflammation. Hypothermia is used for comatose adult patients with VF/VT cardiac arrest. Whole-body hypothermia (or selective head cooling) is endorsed in the neonates for reduction of morbidity and mortality after birth asphyxia. Selective head cooling may not be effective outside the neonatal period. Extrapolating these studies, therapeutic hypothermia (32°C–34°C) is considered for children remaining comatose after cardiac arrest and ROSC.

During induction of hypothermia, particular attention should be given to electrolyte abnormalities, volume state, shivering, coagulopathy, dysrhythmias, and any effects on drug metabolism. Hypothermia decreases the systemic clearance of cytochrome P450 and CYP2E1-metabolized drugs. Additionally, the use of hypothermia requires a delay in the timing of clinical testing for prognostication of neurologic outcome and brain death. Previous concerns about adverse effects of hypothermia on successful defibrillation/cardioversion appear unfounded. A range of duration of hypothermia (12–72 hours), time to rewarming (12–24 hours), and target temperatures (32°C–34°C) have been used. Further study is needed to determine the optimal timing for initiation, duration, degree of cooling, rewarming interval, and whether patients benefit.

Cutting-Edge Strategies

Centers with extracorporeal membrane oxygenation capabilities are applying it as rescue therapy for imminent of ongoing in-hospital cardiac arrest (called ECPR) and for impending heart failure post–cardiac surgery. ECPR reestablishes cardiac output, allows for heart–lung rest, and can be combined with hypothermia (bypass enables temperature control and alleviates concern for arrythmogenicity or myocardial depression due to hypothermia). ECPR can be implemented during active CPR but requires significant resources and highly skilled personnel. Good neurologic outcome is sometimes possible even with prolonged resuscitation, and the survival rate is higher in patients with isolated cardiac disease.

Cognitive Rehabilitation

Environmental enrichment and exercise improve cognitive outcome in animal models of brain ischemia. Since synaptogenesis occurs until late childhood (peaking at 4 years of age), rehabilitation could make a significant impact, particularly in younger children with mild-to-moderate disability. Treatment in the form of therapies can help with muscle tone and control, oral muscle development, and vision.

FUTURE DIRECTIONS AND EMERGING THERAPIES

Reestablishment and Maintenance of Cerebral Blood Flow

The mechanism of postischemic hypoperfusion is not well understood, but it is thought to result from vasospasm, tissue edema, and cell aggregation. Postresuscitation hemodilution (hematocrit to 25%) and hypertension improves CBF and survival in animals. Pharmacologic agents beneficial for CBF promotion in animal studies include endothelin A antagonists, remifentanil, nitrous oxide, and nitric oxide (NO) donors. Studies in humans are lacking.

Antiexcitotoxic Strategies

Many antiexcitotoxic therapies have been tried after cerebral ischemia. Hypothermia is thought to exert its effects by reducing excitotoxicity and cerebral metabolism. Pharmacologic antiexcitotoxic strategies such as barbiturates or agents targeting *N*-methyl-D-aspartate and α-amino-3-hydroxy-5-methylisoxazole-4-propionic acid receptors have not shown benefit in preventing or reducing HIE.

Optimization of Bioenergetics and Preventing Energy Failure

Repletion of energy substrates and oxidative metabolism after ROSC may restore function to vulnerable cells. After reperfusion, selectively vulnerable neurons have a second wave of ATP depletion that coincides with cell death by apoptosis. The administration of ketones has shown promise in preventing energy failure and lactic acidosis after global ischemia in juvenile mice.

Antiapoptotic Strategies

Developing neurons may be at higher risk of apoptotic cell death after brain injury, as demonstrated by their increased sensitivity to irradiation. Thus, antiapoptotic strategies may be more effective in infants and children compared with adults. Treatment with caspase inhibitors decreases infarct size in animal models of global and focal ischemia. Gender may play a prominent role in apoptosis and response to antiapoptotic treatments in the developing brain.

Regeneration and Repair

Children have superior adaptive plasticity, as seen in their ability to recover from resection of portions of the brain (e.g. for seizure management), ability to learn multiple languages, and the increased potential for gains in function with targeted rehabilitation. The young brain may be at a greater risk of injury, and yet also have a greater potential for regeneration and repair. Neural stem cells reproduce throughout life, but their ability to replicate, migrate, and survive in areas of injury declines with age. In addition, gradual change in the cellular environment with aging does not favor regeneration. Cellular transplants and growth factor replacement remain potential adjuvant therapies after hypoxic–ischemic injury and require investigation. Agents such as erythropoietin are currently in clinical trials in traumatic brain injury and in birth asphyxia studies, but concerns include a possibility that abnormal axonal migration may cause seizures and promote the growth of tumors.

CHAPTER 43 ■ METABOLIC ENCEPHALOPATHIES IN CHILDREN

LAURENCE DUCHARME-CREVIER, GENEVIEVE DUPONT-THIBODEAU, ANNE LORTIE, BRUNO MARANDA, ROBERT C. TASKER, AND PHILIPPE JOUVET

EPIDEMIOLOGY AND MECHANISM OF DISEASES

The mechanisms responsible for neurologic impairment in metabolic encephalopathy divide broadly into (a) endogenous intoxication due to accumulation of neurotoxic metabolites; (b) energy failure secondary to the lack of metabolites essential for brain function; and (c) acute water, electrolyte, and/or endocrine disturbances.

Encephalopathies with Endogenous Intoxication

Liver failure and several inborn errors of metabolism (IEM) can induce metabolic encephalopathy by endogenous intoxication. In these diseases, intermediate products of amino acid catabolism are not detoxified by the liver (and/or the kidney) and contribute to neurologic symptoms. Cerebral edema due to cytotoxic mechanisms is frequent in these disorders. Specific therapeutic strategies can decrease toxic metabolite accumulation and restore brain function.

Hyperammonemia and Liver Diseases

Blood ammonia concentration ≥300–500 μmol/L is associated with severe central nervous system (CNS) dysfunction, including cerebral edema and coma. When the hepatic urea cycle is nonfunctional, ammonia is not transformed into urea and ammonia-free base (NH_3) crosses the blood–brain barrier (BBB). Once in the brain, ammonia is buffered by the formation of glutamine in the astrocytes. Glutamine and glutamate are eventually transformed into γ-aminobutyric acid (GABA). One hypothesis (extrapolated from animal studies) for the induction of brain edema during hyperammonemia is the trapping of glutamine inside the astrocyte, resulting in cell swelling and brain edema. Glutamine is also thought to disrupt mitochondrial permeability by interference with the mitochondria-permeability-transition process and liberation of free radicals through hydrolysis of ammonia, both leading to mitochondrial swelling and dysfunction. Another hypothesis for hyperammonemia-induced encephalopathy is injury through the increased production of glutamine that leads to excess extracellular glutamate, which induces neuronal hyperexcitability through activation of the *N*-methyl-D-aspartate (NMDA) receptors. Finally, a high level of ammonia has the potential for causing brain injury and cerebral edema by inducing hyperemia in cerebral blood flow (CBF) and impairing cerebral autoregulation. Human IEMs associated with hyperammonemia include primary urea cycle enzyme defects and secondary inhibition of urea cycle metabolism by organic acidurias (i.e., propionic, methylmalonic aciduria). The urea cycle is the final pathway for the excretion of waste nitrogen.

Reye-Like Illness

Reye-like illness is characterized by the combination of liver disease and metabolic encephalopathy. It can be defined by four criteria: (a) an acute noninflammatory encephalopathy with microvesicular fatty metamorphosis of the liver, confirmed by biopsy or autopsy; (b) a threefold increase of transaminases and/or ammonia; (c) absence of cerebrospinal fluid (CSF) pleocytosis; and (d) no other reasonable explanation for neurologic presentation with hepatic abnormality. The clinical features and electron microscopy of liver biopsy in patients with Reye syndrome are compatible with hepatotoxicity caused by acute, reversible mitochondrial failure. Reye syndrome has a number of potential causes, and it is likely that these involve a mechanism in which mitochondrial failure results in impaired glucose homeostasis, ammonia metabolism, and hepatocyte function.

Hepatic Encephalopathy

Hyperammonemia is not the only mechanism of hepatic encephalopathy since some patients with severe hepatic encephalopathy have normal ammonia levels. The other potential mechanisms are multiple and complex, involving (a) the combined toxic effects of accumulated ammonia and glutamine, mercaptans, fatty acids, and phenol; (b) increased "GABAergic tone"; (c) changes in BBB; and (d) disturbances in neurotransmission. The "increased GABAergic tone" hypothesis is supported by the presence of increased benzodiazepine receptor ligand levels in patients with hepatic encephalopathy. It is possible that a GABA receptor agonist (or precursor) is contained within the food cycle or is synthesized by gastrointestinal flora or that there is occult ingestion of benzodiazepine. Also, endogenous levels of the neurosteroid hormone dehydroepiandrosterone sulfate (decreased in humans with cirrhosis) may contribute to increased GABAergic tone.

Amino and Organic Acids Disorders

The amino and organic acid disorders that frequently cause acute metabolic encephalopathy are maple syrup urine disease (MSUD), propionic aciduria (PA), and methylmalonic aciduria (MMA). Hyperammonemia and/or the accumulation of intermediate metabolites (due to downstream enzyme defects) are involved in the pathophysiology of acute encephalopathy and may be reversible with specific treatment. In MSUD, deficiency of *branched-chain ketoacid dehydrogenase* disrupts the normal breakdown of branched-chain amino acids (i.e., leucine, isoleucine, and valine). In acute encephalopathic crises, there is a high risk of cerebral edema and brain stem herniation. Energy failure is likely responsible for cerebral edema because the Na^+/K^+-ATPase fails to maintain membrane gradients leading to cell swelling. Depletion of neurotransmitters such as dopamine and serotonin may be responsible for early neurobehavioral changes. In patients with PA and MMA, selective and symmetrical necrosis of the globi pallidi is observed during acute decompensation. Many toxic products accumulate, and their neurotoxic mechanisms may involve mitochondrial injury. Hyperammonemia is frequently observed.

Wilson Disease

Wilson disease is associated with an initial neurologic presentation between the ages of 10 and 20 years in one-third of cases. In this disorder, oxidative damage may be caused by accumulation of copper in the basal ganglia.

Encephalopathy Associated with Energy Failure

Any mechanism that reduces brain energy supply may lead to encephalopathy. Cerebral energy is supplied by mitochondria, and the principal metabolic fuel in the brain is glucose (**Fig. 43.1**). Specific therapeutic strategies that decrease cerebral energy demands and increase energy production are required to restore brain function.

Hypoglycemia

Under normal conditions, the brain relies on a constant supply of glucose from the blood for oxidative metabolism and function. It stores only a little glycogen in astrocytes and does not perform gluconeogenesis. Glucose has to be transported across the BBB via glucose transporter proteins expressed in the brain, mainly as the GLUT-1 glucose transporter. Disorders of carbohydrate metabolism, glycogen storage disease, hyperinsulinism, fatty acid oxidation disorders (FAODs), and disorders of amino acid metabolisms may present with severe hypoglycemia. During prolonged

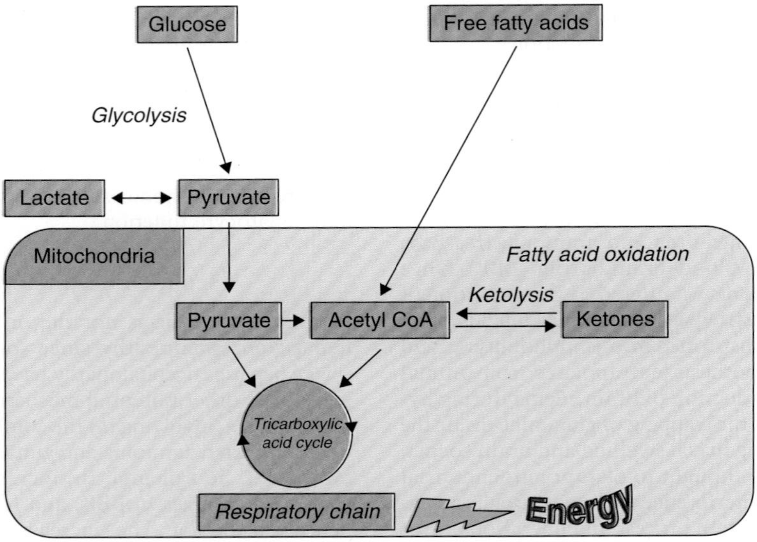

FIGURE 43.1. Energy failure model of metabolic encephalopathy. Hypoglycemia and any enzyme defect in mitochondrial energy production may result in metabolic encephalopathy. The pathophysiology of metabolic encephalopathy by fatty acid oxidation defect is multifactorial.

fasting, the brain can switch to lactate oxidation and increase ketone body uptake to restore energy balance. Specific neurons of the superficial cerebral cortex, basal ganglia, and hippocampus are most vulnerable to injury from hypoglycemia. Reactive oxygen species are generated in neurons at the time of glucose reperfusion.

Primary Mitochondrial Energy Metabolism Defects

Cellular respiration's first stage takes place in the inner mitochondrial membrane and consists of glycolysis of carbohydrates into pyruvate. The pyruvate is transported to the inner mitochondrial matrix, where it is converted to acetyl coenzyme A (acetyl CoA). The Krebs cycle achieves complete oxidation of acetyl CoA to produce two molecules of carbon dioxide and conserve free energy in the form of NADH (reduced form of nicotinamide adenine dinucleotide) and $FADH_2$ (reduced form of flavin adenine dinucleotide). Amino acids, fatty acids, and carbohydrates can enter mitochondria as intermediates of the Krebs cycle. Oxidative phosphorylation takes place in the mitochondrial matrix, for which NADH and $FADH_2$ are the "substrates." The electron transport chain results in phosphorylation of the majority of cellular ADP to ATP.

Mitochondrial disorders result in impaired respiratory chain activity or impaired oxidative phosphorylation. Tissues with high-energy demand are most commonly involved in mitochondrial diseases: neurons, myocardium, skeletal muscle, liver, and kidneys. The brain is particularly vulnerable, given the neuronal requirement for ATP to maintain ionic gradients. The basal ganglia and their high metabolic needs are particularly at risk. Primary defects in mitochondrial energy metabolism include pyruvate dehydrogenase (PDH) complex deficiency, tricarboxylic acid cycle deficiencies, and respiratory chain defects. The clinical presentation of a mitochondrial disease is often nonspecific with myopathy associated with CNS involvement, such as cognitive impairment, ataxia, seizures, and impaired consciousness. Altered consciousness is particularly frequent in Leigh syndrome. Necrosis of the basal ganglia and brain stem nuclei and stroke-like cortical lesions are often features. Most of these diseases are currently untreatable. FAODs comprise another group of diseases with impaired mitochondrial energy metabolism. The encephalopathy observed in these diseases may result from multifactorial insults, including limited fuel for the brain due to hypoglycemia along with abnormally low ketones, hyperammonemia, and a decrease in CBF due to circulatory failure.

Thiamine Deficiency

Thiamine (vitamin B_1) is an essential coenzyme in the pentose phosphate pathway and the tricarboxylic acid (Krebs) cycle. Thiamine deficiency decreases the amount of energy available to the brain and increases concentration of several metabolites. Patients nourished with total parenteral nutrition are at risk for thiamine deficiency if they have renal loss of thiamine or increased thiamine requirements because of systemic illness. Other causes of thiamine depletion include organ transplant, gastrointestinal surgery, malignancy, and acquired immunodeficiency syndrome. In adults, thiamine deficiency is in chronic alcoholism. Administration of glucose to severely thiamine-deficient patients can deplete stores further and exacerbate encephalopathy and heart failure. It is prudent to administer thiamine in the at-risk population before glucose administration and refeeding after starvation. The features are variable, and it may manifest by sudden collapse, seizures, or by the rare triad of gait ataxia, confusion, and ocular abnormalities. If missed, it can lead to death.

Encephalopathies with Acute Water, Electrolyte, and/or Endocrine Disturbances

Disorders of Osmolality

Sodium, glucose, and urea are the primary osmoles of the extracellular space and potassium the primary osmole of the intracellular space. Because cell membranes are permeable to water, an osmotic equilibrium is maintained, and the volume of intracellular fluid is determined by the osmolality of the extracellular space. Hypernatremia and hyperglycemia are the major causes of serum hyperosmolality. Hyponatremia is the major cause of serum hypo-osmolality. Any modification of brain water volume may result in acute encephalopathy.

Diabetic Ketoacidosis and Nonketotic Hyperosmolar Coma

Cerebral edema in *diabetic ketoacidosis* (DKA) typically occurs in the first 12 hours after the onset of treatment, but can present before treatment. The mechanism of cerebral edema is not well understood, but may be via a vasogenic process and perturbed BBB function, rather than osmotic cell swelling. Mechanisms leading to cerebral vasodilation and consequent vasogenic edema include an inflammatory process caused by vasoactive cytokines produced by ketones; reperfusion injury of ischemic cerebral tissues during rehydration; and loss of cerebral autoregulation. Endogenous intracellular osmoles are also generated in response to serum hyperosmolarity. They take 12–24 hours to dissipate and may induce cytotoxic edema as rehydration and insulin therapy decrease serum osmolarity. Initial rehydration in DKA should be limited to that needed to restore hemodynamic stability. *Hyperosmolar hyperglycemic nonketotic coma* is increasing in frequency because of increasing obesity in childhood. This condition shares a similar pathogenesis to the coma of DKA, but without ketone body accumulation.

Hyponatremia

Osmotic disequilibrium between a low-osmolality plasma and higher osmotic pressure within glial cells results in astrocytic water accumulation and brain edema. Rapid decrease in sodium concentration or a sodium level <120 mEq/L may cause severe edema. Too rapid correction of hyponatremia can induce central pontine myelinolysis (osmolar demyelination), a syndrome characterized by confusion, cranial nerve dysfunction, "locked-in" syndrome, and quadriparesis.

Hypernatremia

Hypernatremia is associated with cellular dehydration that affects brain function. Because the brain compensates for slow or chronic increases in osmolality by producing intracellular idiogenic osmoles to retain water, acute changes (e.g., salt poisoning) should be treated quickly and chronic changes treated slowly to avoid rebound cerebral edema. Patients with serum sodium greater than 160 mmol/L or serum osmolality greater than 350 mOsm/L may experience symptoms of lethargy, coma, and seizures. The most serious complication is dural sinus thrombosis, which happens with dehydration and hypovolemia but not saline toxicity.

Acute Uremic Encephalopathy—Dialysis Encephalopathy

Uremic encephalopathy typically occurs when renal glomerular function is less than 10%. It is worse in patients with acute rather than chronic renal failure and in patients with hepatorenal syndrome, given the kidney's inability to excrete ammonia. Osmotically active toxins and compounds with GABA and NMDA receptor effects participate in the pathogenesis. Disturbances in monoamine metabolism, decreased transport function, and increased permeability also participate, and hypertension and altered drug metabolism can contribute to neurotoxicity. The treatment is dialysis. *Dialysis encephalopathy* is caused by the rapid shift of fluids and electrolytes between intracellular and extracellular spaces during, or within 24 hours of, dialysis and is associated with acute, transitory neurologic disturbances. Clinical symptoms consist of confusion, headache, nausea, vomiting, tremor, and myoclonus. Cerebral edema may be seen secondary to a urea gradient between brain cells and blood.

Calcium, Magnesium, and Phosphate Disorders

Calcium is an important regulator of cellular function and is essential for many cellular processes, especially neurotransmission. Severe hypo- or hypercalcemia may induce encephalopathy. Magnesium is a cofactor of numerous enzymes vital for energy metabolism. Hypomagnesemia (usually in association with other electrolyte abnormalities, such as hypocalcemia) or hypermagnesemia may induce encephalopathy. Hypophosphatemia may also cause neurologic dysfunction.

Other Causes of Encephalopathy

Autoimmune thyroid disorders, both hyperthyroidism (Grave disease) and hypothyroidism (Hashimoto thyroiditis), affect the CNS and may lead to encephalopathy and coma. Intestinal intussusception and abdominal surgery in children may be associated with altered levels of consciousness from endogenous opioid poisoning caused by release of endorphins during paroxysms of pain or the release of neurotoxic vasoactive peptides and neuroactive gut hormones in reaction to gastrointestinal ischemia, dehydration, and electrolyte imbalance. In burn encephalopathy, awareness and responsiveness decline a few days after injury. The mechanism may be related to an outpouring of stress hormones and cytokines after the massive inflammatory response, or to high doses of narcotics and/or sleep deprivation. Sepsis-related encephalopathy is a common form of brain dysfunction. Its pathophysiology may involve the inflammatory cascade, mediator-induced cellular damage to the brain, mitochondrial and endothelial dysfunction, disturbed neurotransmission, derangement in calcium homeostasis or altered CBF.

DIAGNOSIS

The possibility of metabolic encephalopathy must be considered in parallel with other common conditions, such as sepsis, hypoxic–ischemic encephalopathy, encephalitis, exogenous intoxication, and brain tumors.

General Clinical Presentation

Metabolic encephalopathy may present with progressive confusion, diverse motor and sensory abnormalities, and rarely hallucinations. As the metabolic illness progresses, there may be increasing stupor or coma associated with progressive neurologic abnormalities of tone, posture, and movements. At a more advanced state, problems with respiratory control and abnormalities such as hiccups, apnea, and bradypnea may occur. In addition, other autonomic and homeostatic functions may be lost and result in bradycardia and hypothermia.

Patients with undiagnosed IEM may present during prolonged fasting, anesthesia, surgery, infections, prolonged exercise, medication exposure, and high protein intake. Valproic acid may worsen the state of patients with urea cycle disorders and respiratory chain disorders because of drug-induced enzyme inhibition. Steroids and adrenocorticotropic hormone increase protein catabolism. In patients with urea cycle disorders, noncompliance with a protein-restricted diet leads to acute deterioration. An IEM should be suspected with (a) recurrent or episodic lethargy and coma; (b) unexplained death in the family or any neonatal death; and (c) consanguinity. Infants may present with poor feeding, lethargy, hypotonia, vomiting, or failure to thrive.

Intracranial hypertension, secondary to cerebral edema and seizures, is a frequent presenting symptom in metabolic encephalopathies. Focal signs can mimic a stroke in mitochondrial encephalopathies. Patients with organic acidemias and urea cycle defects can present with focal neurologic signs and cerebral edema that are mistakenly diagnosed as cerebrovascular accident or cerebral tumor. *Hepatomegaly* may be observed in organic acidemia, FAOD, Wilson disease, hyperinsulinism, and glycogen storage diseases. An *abnormal urine or body odor* is present in some diseases in which volatile metabolites accumulate. Important examples are the fruity smell of ketoacids in DKA, the maple syrup odor of MSUD, and the sweaty feet odor of isovaleric acidemia.

Laboratory Investigations

Most disorders produce only intermittent abnormalities, so if rapid metabolic and genetic analysis is impossible, critical samples of blood and urine can be obtained and analyzed later. Venous blood should be collected in an ammonia-free, heparinized blood tube, quickly placed on ice, and transferred to the laboratory. IEM are difficult to diagnose and biologic signs should prompt consideration (**Table 43.1**). The determination of plasma ammonia level is crucial because hyperammonemia is life-threatening and requires urgent management. *Moderate hyperammonemia* (80–150 μmol/L) is common in IEM owing to a

TABLE 43.1

Algorithm for the Diagnosis of IEM Revealed by Encephalopathy

CLINICAL PRESENTATION	PREDOMINANT METABOLIC DISTURBANCE	ASSOCIATED METABOLIC/ NEUROLOGIC DISTURBANCE	MOST FREQUENT DIAGNOSES (DISORDER/ ENZYME DEFICIENCY)	DIFFERENTIAL DIAGNOSIS
Metabolic coma without focal neurologic signs	Metabolic acidosis	With ketosis	Organic aciduria (MMA, PA, IVA, GA I, MSUD) PC **MCD** **Ketolysis, gluconeogenesis**	Diabetes Exogenous intoxication Encephalitis
		Without ketosis	**PDH** **Ketogenesis defect** **FAO** **FDP**	
	Hyperammonemia	Normal glucose	**Urea cycle defects**	Reye syndrome Encephalitis Exogenous intoxication
		Hypoglycemia	**FAO** **HMG CoA lyase**	
	Hypoglycemia	With acidosis	**Gluconeogenesis, MSUD, HMG CoA lyase** **FAO**	
		Without acidosis	**FAO** **Hyperinsulinism**	
	Hyperlactatemia	Normal glucose	PC **MCD** Krebs cycle **PDH** Respiratory chain disorder	
		Hypoglycemia	**Gluconeogenesis** **FAO** **GSD**	

(continued)

TABLE 43.1

Algorithm for the Diagnosis of IEM Revealed by Encephalopathy (*continued*)

CLINICAL PRESENTATION	PREDOMINANT METABOLIC DISTURBANCE	ASSOCIATED METABOLIC/ NEUROLOGIC DISTURBANCE	MOST FREQUENT DIAGNOSES (DISORDER/ ENZYME DEFICIENCY)	DIFFERENTIAL DIAGNOSIS
Neurologic coma with focal signs, seizures, severe intracranial hypertension, strokes or stroke-like episodes	Biologic signs are variable, can be absent or moderate	Cerebral edema wo other lesions	**MSUD** **OTC**	Cerebral tumor Migraine Encephalitis
		Hemiplegia or hemianopsia	**MSUD** **OTC** **MMA** **PA**	
		Extrapyramidal signs	**MMA** **GA I** **Wilson** **Homocystinuria**	
		Caudate nucleus and putamen necrosis	**BBGD** **Urea cycle defect** **MMA** **PA** **IVA**	
		Stroke-like	Respiratory chain disorder CDG syndrome **Thiamine responsive megaloblastic anemia**	Moya moya syndrome, Vascular hemiplegia Cerebral sinus thrombosis Cerebral tumor

Treatable disorders appear in bold type.
MMA, methylmalonic academia; PA, propionic aciduria; IVA, isovaleric aciduria; GA I, glutaric aciduria type I; MSUD, maple syrup urine disease; PC, pyruvate carboxylase; MCD, multiple carboxylase deficiency; PDH, pyruvate dehydrogenase; FAO, fatty acid oxidation; FDP, fructose-1,6-diphosphatase; HMG CoA lyase, 3-hydroxy-3-methylglutaryl coenzyme A lyase; GSD, glycogen storage disorder; OTC, ornithine transcarbamylase; BBGD, biotin-responsive basal ganglia disease; CDG, carbohydrate-deficient glycoprotein.

secondary blockade of the urea cycle. *Severe hyperammonemia* (>300 μmol/L) is observed in primary urea cycle defects, organic acid disorders, and FAOD. Falsely high levels may be due to problems in sampling or transfer to the laboratory. Hyperammonemia with abnormalities in liver function tests is seen in acute liver failure and Reye syndrome. *Metabolic acidosis with increased anion gap* is observed in intermediate acid accumulation, such as organic acid disorders (PA and MMA). Metabolic acidosis also may be present in amino acid disorders, mitochondrial disorders, and disorders of carbohydrate metabolism. Elevated lactic acid, in the absence of sepsis or tissue hypoxia, is often observed in organic acid disorders and glycogen storage disorders (GSDs). Extreme elevation can be seen in primary mitochondrial energy metabolism defects. Ketones (acetoacetate and 3-hydroxybutyrate) are a product of fatty acid oxidation. *Hypoglycemia without ketonuria* is observed in FAOD and hyperinsulinism. *Neutropenia* can be seen in organic acidemias. *Myoglobinuria* is an indicator of FAOD.

Neurophysiology and Neuroimaging

Neurophysiology

Electroencephalography (EEG) during acute encephalopathy usually shows slow activity. Triphasic waves are characteristic of but not specific for hepatic coma. When clinical seizures occur, the EEG can provide information as to the severity of the epileptic condition. Rarely, an EEG reveals subclinical epileptiform activity. A burst-suppression pattern (not due to medication) is associated with poor prognosis.

Neuroimaging

Cerebral computed tomography (CT) is essential when evaluating a comatose patient. The absence of CSF spaces above the tentorium and obliteration of the basal cisterns are associated with cerebral edema and raised intracranial pressure. Characteristic lesions may be observed in white matter in organic acid disorders or basal ganglia in mitochondrial disorders. Magnetic resonance imaging (MRI) of the brain may suggest diagnosis of certain pathologies, such as mitochondrial encephalopathies. Magnetic resonance spectroscopy (MRS) can evaluate various brain metabolites, such as brain tissue lactate. Proton MRS can monitor response to therapy.

MANAGEMENT

Neurologic support includes attention to adequate oxygenation, perfusion, fluid and electrolyte balance, temperature control, seizure control, management of intracranial hypertension, and prevention of infection.

Management of Intracranial Hypertension

In severe hyperammonemia (>300 μmol/L), we recommend avoiding respiratory alkalosis from excessive hyperventilation. The target pH level is ~7.35 since the BBB has a lower permeability to NH_4^+ than to NH_3. Intracranial pressure monitoring is not routine in metabolic encephalopathy because of the potential for rapid improvement with treatment. No consensus exits on the indications of intracranial pressure monitoring for patients with acute liver failure. The use of near-infrared spectroscopy for cerebral oxygenation monitoring and the use of transcranial Doppler may help to detect changes in cerebral hemodynamics and guide management.

Seizure Control

In the case of hyperammonemia or suspicion of mitochondrial disorder, seizures should be treated to prevent secondary neurologic insult; however, valproic acid is contraindicated.

Temperature Control

The use of therapeutic hypothermia in metabolic encephalopathy has not been studied extensively, although the concept of reducing brain metabolism and secondary toxin production is appealing. Fever should be prevented and treated.

TABLE 43.2

Specific Treatments of Inborn Errors of Metabolism

DRUG	EFFECT	INDICATION(S)	DOSE	ADMINISTRATION ROUTE
Sodium benzoate	Ammonia removal	NH_3 > 200 μmol/L	500 mg/kg/d	IV
Phenylbutyrate	Ammonia removal	NH_3 > 200 μmol/L	600 mg/kg/d	IV or PO
Arginine	Ammonia removal	NH_3 > 200 μmol/L	500 mg/kg/d	IVC
Carglumic acid	Ammonia removal	NAGS defect, MMA, PA, FAOD, and NH_3 > 200 μmol/L	50 mg/kg/6 h	PO
Carnitine	Primary or secondary deficiency compensation	Organic aciduria, hyperlactatemia, FAOD	100 mg/kg/d	IVC or PO
Glycine	Increased urine excretion	IVA	500 mg/kg/4 h	IVC or PO
Vitamin B12	Enzyme cofactor	MMA	1–2 mg/d	IM
Metronidazole	Decreased toxin production by intestine bacteria	MMA, PA	20 mg/kg/d	PO
Biotin	PC cofactor	Hyperlactatemia, PA	10–20 mg/d	IV or PO
Riboflavin	Cofactor of acyl CoA dehydrogenase	FAOD	20–40 mg/d	IV or PO
Dichloroacetate or dichloropropionate	PDHk inhibitor	Hyperlactatemia >10 mmol/L	25 mg/kg/12 h	IV or PO

IV, intravenous; PO, orally; IVC, continuous intravenous infusion; NAGS, *N*-acetylglutamate synthase; MMA, methylmalonic aciduria; PA, propionic aciduria; IVA, isovaleric aciduria; PC, pyruvate carboxylase; FAOD, fatty acid oxidation disorder; PDHk, pyruvate dehydrogenase kinase.

Initial Treatment of Suspected Inborn Error of Metabolism

If an IEM is suspected, the aim is to reduce formation of toxic metabolites by decreasing substrate availability, and to prevent catabolism by providing adequate calories. Adequate hydration is important. Oral intake should be stopped to eliminate protein, galactose, and fructose ingestion. Calories should be provided as high-dose IV glucose to limit protein catabolism. Insulin may be necessary. This therapy also applies to FAODs and ketoacidosis. Once a diagnosis is made, special amino acid formulations may be indicated. Steroids should be avoided because they promote protein catabolism (**Table 43.2**). Sodium benzoate and sodium phenylacetate may enhance nitrogen/ammonia excretion. A metabolic specialist can guide specific therapies. Toxin removal by dialysis may be necessary to prevent brain injury, particularly for hyperammonemia or intractable metabolic acidosis. The more severe the cerebral edema, the higher the risk of cerebral herniation during therapy, especially with hyperammonemia. If neurologic deterioration occurs during renal replacement therapy, then the rate of toxin clearance should be reduced.

CHAPTER 44 ■ THE DETERMINATION OF BRAIN DEATH

THOMAS A. NAKAGAWA AND MUDIT MATHUR

Advancements in medical treatment improved care of the critically ill but obscured neurologic, respiratory, and circulatory parameters used to determine death. These medical advancements led to the development of additional criteria to determine death based on irreversible coma (brain death). The 1967 Harvard committee definition of irreversible coma included patients who were unresponsive, exhibited no movement, breathing, or reflexes, and had an isoelectric electroencephalogram (EEG). Criteria were further defined in a report from the President's Commission that stated: "[A]n individual who has sustained either (a) irreversible cessation of circulatory and respiratory functions or (b) irreversible cessation of all function of the entire brain, including the brainstem, is dead." These brain death criteria differed from those used in other countries because they required the loss of function of the entire brain, not just the brain stem. In 1987, pediatric-specific guidelines emphasized the history and clinical examination to determine the etiology of coma so that remediable or reversible conditions were excluded. Age-related observation periods and specific neurodiagnostic testing were recommended for children <1 year old. Little guidance was provided for the infant <7 days of age because of the lack of sufficient clinical experience in this age group. A 2011 update to the pediatric guidelines clarified issues such as observation intervals, determination of brain death for term newborns (37 weeks' gestational age to 30 days of age), and use of ancillary studies for all age groups (**Table 44.1**). Determination of death by neurologic criteria and consensus-based brain death guidelines has gained legal and medical acceptance, but no national brain death law exists. Physicians and healthcare providers are encouraged to become familiar with relevant laws and institutional policies intended to provide consistency for the determination of brain death in infants and children.

PREREQUISITE CONDITIONS THAT MUST BE SATISFIED PRIOR TO BRAIN DEATH TESTING

Determination of brain death for any infant or child requires establishing and maintaining normal age-appropriate physiologic parameters. The clinical examination can be affected by hypotension, shock, hypothermia, severe metabolic disturbances, sedation, or neuromuscular blockade. Hypothermia depresses central nervous system (CNS) function, metabolism, and clearance of medications. A minimum core body temperature of at least 35°C (95°F) should be maintained during the examination and testing period to determine brain death. Reversible conditions (e.g., severe hepatic or renal dysfunction, or inborn errors of metabolism) may play a role in the clinical presentation of comatose children. Organ dysfunction can reduce metabolism of sedative and neuromuscular blocking agents affecting the neurologic examination. Severe metabolic disturbances capable of causing coma such as glucose, pH, and electrolyte disturbances should be treated and corrected prior to initiating brain death testing. Hypernatremia has been implicated as a potential cause for coma, resulting in recommendations to correct sodium to "relatively normal" levels prior to determining brain death. Drug intoxication from barbiturates, opioids, sedative-hypnotics, anesthetic agents, antiepileptic agents, and alcohols can mimic brain death. Sedative agents should be discontinued for >24 hours in children and 48 hours in neonates prior to examination. Observation periods may need to be extended following termination of continuous infusions of sedative agents for several elimination half-lives to allow adequate drug clearance prior to brain death testing. Serum levels of sedative agents or antiepileptic medications in the low-to-mid-therapeutic range prior to testing should not interfere with the determination of death. Adequate clearance of neuromuscular blocking agents can be confirmed using a nerve stimulator. Unusual causes of coma such as neurotoxins and chemical exposure (e.g., organophosphates and carbamates) should be considered in cases when an etiology has not been established. Neuroimaging studies should demonstrate evidence of an acute CNS insult consistent with loss of brain function, but CT and MRI are not considered ancillary studies and should not be relied on to make a determination of death.

CLINICAL EXAMINATION CRITERIA TO DETERMINE BRAIN DEATH

Brain death determination is a clinical diagnosis that relies on the coexistence of coma and apnea

TABLE 44.1

Recommendations for the Determination of Brain Death in Infants and Children

1. Determination of brain death in term newborns, infants, and children is a clinical diagnosis based on the absence of neurologic function with a known irreversible cause of coma. Because of insufficient data in the literature, recommendations for preterm infants <37 wk gestational age are not included in this guideline.
2. Hypotension, hypothermia, and metabolic disturbances should be treated and corrected, and medications that can interfere with the neurologic examination and apnea testing should be discontinued, allowing for adequate clearance before proceeding with these evaluations.
3. Two examinations, including apnea testing with each examination, separated by an observation period are required. Examinations should be performed by different attending physicians. Apnea testing may be performed by the same physician. An observation period of 24 h for term newborns (37 wk gestational age) to 30 d of age, and 12 h for infants and children (31 d to 18 y) is recommended. The first examination determines whether the child has met the accepted neurologic examination criteria for brain death. The second examination confirms brain death based on an unchanged and irreversible condition. Assessment of neurologic function following cardiopulmonary resuscitation or other severe acute brain injuries should be deferred for 24 h or longer if there are concerns or inconsistencies in the examination.
4. Apnea testing to support the diagnosis of brain death must be performed safely and requires documentation of an arterial $Paco_2$ 20 mm Hg above the baseline *and* 60 mm Hg with no respiratory effort during the testing period. If the apnea test cannot be safely completed, an ancillary study should be performed.
5. Ancillary studies (electroencephalogram [EEG] and radionuclide cerebral blood flow [CBF]) are not required to establish brain death and are not a substitute for the neurologic examination. Ancillary studies may be used to assist the clinician in making the diagnosis of brain death (a) when components of the examination or apnea testing cannot be completed safely because of the underlying medical condition of the patient, (b) if there is uncertainty about the results of the neurologic examination, (c) if a medication effect may be present, or (d) to reduce the interexamination observation period. When ancillary studies are used, a second clinical examination and apnea test should be performed and components that can be completed must remain consistent with brain death. In this instance, the observation interval may be shortened, and the second neurologic examination and apnea test (or all components that are able to be completed safely) can be performed at any time thereafter.
6. Death is declared when the above criteria are fulfilled.

From Nakagawa TA, Ashwal S, Mathur M, Mysore M; Committee for Determination of Brain Death in Infants and Children. Guidelines for the determination of brain death in infants and children: An update of the 1987 task force recommendations. *Crit Care Med* 2011;39:2139–55.

during a period of observation after exclusion of confounding diagnoses. The foundation of brain death determination is the neurologic examination, which is consistent across the pediatric age spectrum. Neurologic examination criteria, including motor, brain stem, and autonomic assessment that must be met to make a determination of brain death in infants and children, are listed in **Table 44.2.** The clinical examination to determine brain death should be pursued only after all prerequisite conditions have been satisfied. Clinical criteria to determine brain death are based on the absence of neurologic function that includes deep unresponsive coma, loss of all brain stem reflexes (including apnea), and a lack of motor function (excluding spinal reflexes).

Testing for bulbar muscular activity should produce no grimacing or facial muscle movement when applying deep pressure on the mandibular condyles at the level of the temporomandibular joints or when applying deep pressure on the supraorbital ridge. Pharyngeal or gag reflex is tested by stimulation of the posterior pharynx with a tongue blade or suction device. Care should be exercised not to dislodge the artificial airway. The cough reflex can be reliably tested by examining the response to tracheal suctioning. Testing for corneal reflexes is achieved by touching the edge of the cornea with a piece of tissue paper or a cotton swab, or using small squirts of water to stimulate a reflex response. The oculovestibular reflex is tested by irrigating each ear with ice water (caloric testing) after the patency of the external auditory canal is confirmed. The head is elevated to 30 degrees, and each external auditory canal is irrigated separately with approximately 10–50 mL of ice water. Lack of movement of the eyes during at least 1 minute of observation means the reflex is absent (consistent with brain death criteria). Both ears should be tested, with an interval of several minutes separating each test. Oculocephalic testing may be performed in the absence of cervical fracture or instability. Caution is advised in patients with potential cervical spine injury to reduce risk of exacerbating a preexisting injury. The oculocephalic reflex is assessed by holding the eyes open and turning the head rapidly to each side and observing for eye movements. Absence of eye movement relative to movement of the head means the reflex is absent (consistent with brain death criteria). Oculocephalic and oculovestibular testing evaluate the integrity of the medial longitudinal fasciculus.

TABLE 44.2

Checklist for Documentation of Brain Death

Brain Death Examination for Infants and Children
Two physicians must perform independent examinations separated by specified intervals

AGE OF PATIENT	TIMING OF FIRST EXAMINATION	INTEREXAMINATION INTERVAL
Term newborn 37 weeks gestational age and up to 30 days old	☐ First examination may be performed 24 hours after birth or following CPR or severe brain injury	☐ At least 24 hours, OR ☐ Interval shortened because ancillary study (Section 4) is consistent with brain death
31 days to 18 years old	☐ First examination may be performed 24 hours following CPR or severe brain injury	☐ At least 12 hours, OR ☐ Interval shortened because ancillary study (Section 4) is consistent with brain death

Section 1. PREREQUISITES for Brain Death Examination and Apnea Test

A. IRREVERSIBLE AND IDENTIFIABLE Cause of Coma (Please Check)

☐ Traumatic brain injury ☐ Anoxic brain injury ☐ Known metabolic disorder ☐ Other (Specify) ________

B. Correction of Contributing Factors That Can Interfere with the Neurologic Examination	**Examination One**		**Examination Two**	
a. Core body temperature is over 95°F (35°C)	☐ Yes	☐ No	☐ Yes	☐ No
b. Systolic blood pressure or MAP in acceptable range (systolic BP not less than two standard deviations below age-appropriate norm) based on age	☐ Yes	☐ No	☐ Yes	☐ No
c. Sedative/analgesic drug effect excluded as a contributing factor	☐ Yes	☐ No	☐ Yes	☐ No
d. Metabolic intoxication excluded as a contributing factor	☐ Yes	☐ No	☐ Yes	☐ No
e. Neuromuscular blockade excluded as a contributing factor	☐ Yes	☐ No	☐ Yes	☐ No

If ALL prerequisites are marked YES, then proceed to Section 2, OR
——— confounding variable was present. Ancillary study was therefore performed to document brain death (Section 4)

Section 2. Physical Examination (Please Check) **NOTE: SPINAL CORD REFLEXES ARE ACCEPTABLE**	Examination One Date/Time: ———		Examination Two Date/Time: ———	
a. Flaccid tone, patient unresponsive to deep painful stimuli	☐ Yes	☐ No	☐ Yes	☐ No
b. Pupils are mid-position or fully dilated, and light reflexes are absent	☐ Yes	☐ No	☐ Yes	☐ No
c. Corneal, cough, gag reflexes are absent	☐ Yes	☐ No	☐ Yes	☐ No
d. Sucking and rooting reflexes are absent (in neonates and infants)	☐ Yes	☐ No	☐ Yes	☐ No
e. Oculovestibular reflexes are absent	☐ Yes	☐ No	☐ Yes	☐ No
f. Spontaneous respiratory effort while on mechanical ventilation is absent	☐ Yes	☐ No	☐ Yes	☐ No

The ——— (specify) element of the examination could not be performed because ———.
Ancillary study (EEG or radionuclide CBF) was therefore performed to document brain death (Section 4)

Section 3. APNEA Test	Examination One Date/Time———	Examination Two Date/Time———
No spontaneous respiratory efforts were observed despite final $Paco_2 \geq 60$ mm Hg and a ≥ 20 mm Hg increase above baseline (Examination One) No spontaneous respiratory efforts were observed despite final $Paco_2 \geq 60$ mm Hg and a ≥ 20 mm Hg increase above baseline (Examination Two)	Pretest $Paco_2$: ——— Apnea duration: ———min Posttest $Paco_2$: ———	Pretest $Paco_2$: ——— Apnea duration: ———min Posttest $Paco_2$: ———

Apnea test is contraindicated or could not be performed to completion because ———. Ancillary study (EEG or radionuclide CBF) was therefore performed to document brain death (Section 4)

Section 4. ANCILLARY testing is required (a) when any components of the examination or apnea testing cannot be completed; (b) if there is uncertainty about the results of the neurologic examination; or (c) if a medication effect may be present. **Date/Time:** ———

Ancillary testing can be performed to reduce the interexamination period; however, a second neurologic examination is required. Components of the neurologic examination that can be performed safely should be completed in close proximity to the ancillary test.

☐ EEG report documents electrocerebral silence, OR	☐ Yes ☐ No
☐ CBF study report documents no cerebral perfusion	☐ Yes ☐No

Section 5. Signatures

Examiner One

I certify that my examination is consistent with cessation of function of the brain and brainstem. Confirmatory examination to follow

———	———	———	———	———	———
(Printed Name)	(Signature)	(Specialty)	(Pager #/License #)	(Date mm/dd/yyyy)	(Time)

Examiner Two

I certify that my examination and/or ancillary test report confirms unchanged and irreversible cessation of function of the brain and brainstem. The patient is declared brain dead at this time
Date/Time of Death: ———

———	———	———	———	———	———
(Printed Name)	(Signature)	(Specialty)	(Pager #/License #)	(Date mm/dd/yyyy)	(Time)

EEG, electroencephalogram; CBF, cerebral blood flow; CPR, cardiopulmonary resuscitation; MAP, mean arterial pressure.
From Nakagawa TA, Ashwal S, Mathur M; Committee for Determination of Brain Death in Infants and Children. Guidelines for the determination of brain death in infants and children: An update of the 1987 task force recommendations. *Crit Care Med* 2011;39:2139–55.

Either test is considered sufficient under the current pediatric brain death guidelines.

Based on clinical experience and published reports, the current brain death guidelines recommend the performance of two neurologic examinations separated by an observation period. The 2011 guidelines recommend shorter observation periods than previously described for children. The recommended intervals between examinations are 24 hours for neonates (37 weeks gestational age to 30 days of age) and 12 hours for children older than 30 days of age to 18 years of age. The first examination determines that the child meets neurologic criteria for brain death. The second examination confirms brain death based on an unchanged and irreversible condition. If uncertainty about the examination exists, the time interval between observations and examinations warrants extension based on the physician's judgment. The examination results should remain consistent with brain death throughout the observation and testing period. Adult guidelines recommend a single clinical examination, but the pediatric examination criteria remain more conservative.

It is now recommended that neurologic evaluation and testing for brain death be deferred for at least 24 hours or longer from admission following cardiopulmonary arrest or severe traumatic brain injury to allow hemodynamic and metabolic stabilization prior to evaluation. If there are concerns about the validity of the examination (e.g., flaccid tone or absent movements in a patient with high spinal cord injury or severe neuromuscular disease) or if specific examination components cannot be performed because of medical contraindications (e.g., apnea testing in patients with significant lung injury or hemodynamic instability) or if examination findings are inconsistent and changing, continued observation until these issues are resolved is warranted to avoid improperly diagnosing brain death. An ancillary study can be pursued to assist with the determination of brain death in situations where certain examination components cannot be completed. The 2011 pediatric guidelines recommend that two different attending physicians perform the neurologic examinations. This change was made to reduce the chance of diagnostic error and avoid potential conflicts of interest when determining death. Apnea testing can be performed by the same physician who conducts the clinical examination, or by the attending physician who is managing ventilator support of the child.

APNEA TESTING

The 2011 guidelines to determine brain death recommend two apnea tests be performed, one with each neurologic examination, unless a medical contraindication exists. Conditions that invalidate the apnea test or that may prevent the apnea test being completed safely include high cervical spine injury, severe hypoxemia, hemodynamic instability, elevated ventilator settings, or the use of advanced ventilation modalities such as high-frequency oscillatory or jet ventilation. The apnea test evaluates the ability of the respiratory center in the brain stem to respond to elevated levels of carbon dioxide (CO_2). The normal $Paco_2$ threshold for establishing apnea in children ($Paco_2 > 60$ mm Hg) has been assumed to be the same as adults.

Apnea testing for infants and children is conducted in a manner similar to that for adults. Clearance of sedative and paralytic agents must be allowed prior to testing. Apnea duration must be sufficient for $Paco_2$ to increase to levels that normally stimulate respiration. Normal oxygenation and hemodynamics should be maintained. Patients should be preoxygenated with 100% oxygen to prevent hypoxia. If safe, $Paco_2$ should be normalized and documented prior to initiating testing. The typical CO_2 rise during apnea of 3–5 mm Hg/min may be variable since injured or dead brain may not contribute to CO_2 production. Mechanical ventilation is discontinued when apnea testing is initiated. The patient may be placed on continuous positive airway pressure (CPAP), a T piece attached to the ETT, or a self-inflating bag valve system (e.g., a Mapleson circuit). Newer ventilators provide backup ventilation rate when apnea is detected and may not allow completion of the apnea test. Another concern is the false appearance of spontaneous ventilation during CPAP administration with mechanical ventilation due to trigger sensitivity. If a self-inflating bag valve system is utilized, positive end-expiratory pressure (PEEP) should be titrated to maintain oxygenation. Tracheal insufflation of oxygen using a catheter inserted through the ETT has also been used, but care must be taken that the diameter of the insufflating catheter allows adequate exhalation of gas to prevent barotrauma. CO_2 washout can delay the rise in CO_2 with this technique. The physician(s) must continually observe the patient for spontaneous respiratory movements over a 5- to 10-minute period after disconnecting the ventilator and watch for deterioration in hemodynamic parameters and oxygen saturation. The $Paco_2$ should be measured by arterial blood gas analysis prior to and during the apnea test. $Paco_2$ should be allowed to rise to ≥ 60 mm Hg *and* ≥ 20 mm Hg above the baseline $Paco_2$. Achieving the increase of 20 mm Hg is especially relevant in children who may have elevated $Paco_2$ levels at baseline. If no respiratory effort is noted during the apnea examination despite an adequate increment in $Paco_2$, the test is consistent with brain death. The patient should be placed back on mechanical support until death is established with a repeat clinical examination or ancillary testing. Regardless of the spontaneous tidal volume generated, any respiratory effort is inconsistent with the current clinical definition of apnea and precludes the determination of brain death. If there is any concern regarding the validity of the apnea test, an ancillary study should be pursued.

Hypercarbia, hypotension, and hypoxemia can have deleterious effects on an injured brain, affecting CBF and ICP. Apnea testing should be undertaken only after the patient has met clinical criteria for brain death testing with loss of all brain stem reflexes and only by a physician experienced in managing ventilator support and capable of responding to hemodynamic or respiratory deterioration. Preoxygenation and attention to pretest conditions such as hypovolemia can minimize potentially adverse circulatory effects. The apnea test should be aborted if oxygen saturations fall below 85% or if hemodynamic instability occurs. If apnea testing cannot be completed, the patient should be placed back on appropriate ventilator support and apnea testing may be repeated later or an ancillary study can be performed.

ANCILLARY STUDIES USED TO ASSIST WITH THE DETERMINATION OF BRAIN DEATH

The current guidelines for infants and children state that ancillary studies are not required unless a complete neurologic examination and apnea test cannot be completed. Ancillary tests are not a substitute for the neurologic examination. An ancillary study is indicated: (a) when components of the neurologic examination and apnea test cannot be completed, (b) when conditions or confounding variables (e.g., medications) interfere with the neurologic examination and apnea test, (c) when there are concerns about the validity of the neurologic examination, and (d) to reduce the observation period between examinations. An ancillary study can shorten the interval between examinations if it is performed after a first neurologic examination and apnea test that are consistent with brain death, and if it supports the determination of brain death. The second neurologic examination and apnea test (or components that can be completed safely) can be performed and documented at any time thereafter to determine brain death for children of all ages. Ancillary studies may also allow family members to better comprehend the diagnosis of brain death and may be important as additional supportive evidence in situations where death is the result of homicide.

The most common ancillary studies to help determine brain death in infants and children are the documentation of electrocerebral silence (ECS) by EEG and the absence of CBF by radionuclide study. Four-vessel angiography remains the gold standard ancillary test, but is rarely used as the technical expertise to perform this test in children is not available in every facility. EEG can be performed at the bedside of a critically ill child in most institutions. Radionuclide CBF studies have been used extensively with good experience but may require transport of the critically ill child to a nuclear medicine suite. Data suggest that EEG and CBF are of similar confirmatory value, although CBF may be more sensitive in infants. EEG testing evaluates cortical and cellular function while radionuclide CBF testing evaluates flow and uptake into brain tissue. Each of these tests requires appropriate experts who understand the limitations of these studies to avoid misinterpretation. The goal of radionuclide CBF study is to determine if CBF is present. Tc99m hexamethylpropylene–amineoxime (HMPAO) has become the radiotracer agent of choice in many institutions performing radionuclide CBF studies because of its brain-specific uptake and ability to adequately visualize the posterior fossa on static imaging.

Normal hemodynamic parameters based on age and a minimum core body temperature of 35°C (95°F) should be attained and maintained during the neurodiagnostic testing period. Pharmacologic agents and significant drug intoxication (e.g., alcohol, barbiturates, opiates, and sedative-hypnotic agents) can affect EEG testing. Sedatives should be discontinued for ≥24 hours prior to EEG testing and clinical examination in the older patient, and ≥48 hours in the neonate. Barbiturate levels in the low-to-mid-therapeutic range should not preclude the use of EEG testing. While barbiturates reduce CBF, evidence suggests that a radionuclide CBF study can demonstrate absence of CBF and establish brain death in patients with high-dose barbiturate therapy.

The use of transcranial Doppler (TCD), brain stem auditory evoked potentials, and CT angiography as ancillary studies has been described in adults, but has not been validated in children. Single-photon emission computed tomography (SPECT) has also been studied, but limited data exist for its use. CT perfusion study measuring CBF, nasopharyngeal somatosensory evoked potentials (SSEPs), magnetic resonance angiography (MRA)-MRI, bispectral index, and perfusion MRI for children lack sufficient studies or clinical experience to validate their use.

If the EEG shows electrical activity or the radionuclide CBF study shows cerebral flow or cellular uptake, the patient cannot be pronounced dead. Observation of the patient should continue until death can be declared by a second clinical examination and apnea testing, or a follow-up ancillary study is performed with results consistent with brain death. It is important to note that ancillary studies are an adjunct to the clinical examination and apnea testing. Continued coma and apnea during an extended observation period is ultimately the final determining factor to determine brain death. If a radionuclide CBF study needs to be repeated, waiting at least 24 hours is recommended to ensure clearance of the radiotracer.

DETERMINATION OF BRAIN DEATH FOR TERM NEWBORNS (37 WEEKS GESTATION) TO 30 DAYS OF AGE

There is limited clinical experience determining brain death in neonates. Anatomically, the newborn has patent sutures and an open fontanel, resulting in less dramatic increases in ICP after acute brain injury, compared with older patients. The cascade of events associated with increased ICP ultimately leading to herniation is less likely to occur in the neonate. The physician declaring brain death in term newborns (37 weeks gestation or above) must be aware of the limitations of the clinical examination and ancillary studies in this age group. Careful, repeated examinations are important, with particular attention to assessment of brain stem reflexes and apnea testing. The recommended observation period between neurologic examinations is 24 hours for term newborns (37 weeks gestation) to 30 days of age. The clinical assessment may be unreliable immediately following an acute catastrophic neurologic injury or cardiopulmonary arrest. The metabolism of sedative agents may also be prolonged in the newborn. As with older children, brain death testing should be deferred for a period of 24 hours or longer in these situations and especially following therapeutic hypothermia.

As with any patient, a thorough neurologic examination including apnea testing must be performed to make the determination of death. The limited neonatal data evaluating $Paco_2$ thresholds for apnea suggest that the threshold of 60 mm Hg is also valid in the newborn. Profound bradycardia affecting hemodynamics may occur quickly and limit testing. If the apnea test cannot be completed, the examination and apnea test can be attempted at a later time, or an ancillary study may be performed. Ancillary studies in newborns are less sensitive than in older children. Recommendations for preterm infants <37 weeks gestational age have not been described owing to lack of sufficient data and clinical experience in this age group.

DIAGNOSTIC ERRORS AND DETERMINATION OF BRAIN DEATH

Some case reports have suggested that brain death is reversible, but on critical review, it is apparent that these patients would not have fulfilled brain death criteria by currently accepted standards in the United States. Review of these cases reveals that apnea testing was not appropriately performed or completed, imaging studies did not reveal a significant intracranial injury, EEG testing did not reveal ECS, or radionuclide CBF study did not demonstrate absence of flow. Hypothermia is known to depress CNS function and alter drug metabolism that can lead to a false determination of brain death if the patient is examined soon after being rewarmed. It is also important to consider that clearance of pharmacologic agents can be affected by the presence of organ dysfunction, total amount of medication administered, elimination half-life of the drug and any active metabolites, and other contributing factors such as hypothermia. Based on emerging literature and experience, waiting at least 24 hours following rewarming to ensure adequate metabolism of pharmacologic agents is strongly suggested before initiating brain death testing for all ages.

DETERMINATION OF BRAIN DEATH IN SPECIAL CIRCUMSTANCES

Little information is available to guide the clinician in the determination of brain death when advanced therapies, such as ECMO, are utilized. A potential indicator of brain death on ECMO is an increase in mixed venous oxygen saturation that is suspicious for decreased brain oxygen consumption. Performing apnea testing to determine brain death in a patient supported by ECMO may present a challenge because oxygenators are highly efficient and may not allow the $Paco_2$ to rise to appropriate levels. Reducing sweep gas flow or blending CO_2 into the oxygenator to elevate $Paco_2$ to required levels to demonstrate apnea has been reported.

Determining brain death in a child with cyanotic heart disease poses another challenge. Current brain death guidelines recommend termination of the apnea test if hemodynamic instability occurs or oxygen saturations fall below 85%. These patients are already in a desaturated state at baseline, and the apnea test cannot be completed as currently recommended. Ancillary testing may be needed to determine brain death, but many of these patients will be neonates in whom ancillary testing lacks sensitivity when compared with older children.

DOCUMENTATION AND DETERMINATION OF DEATH

Determination of brain death should be carried out by experienced clinicians (attending physicians) familiar with the care of neonates, infants, and children. Current guidelines recommend two examinations and apnea tests separated by an observation period. Death is declared after the second neurologic examination and apnea test confirm an unchanged and irreversible condition. In some countries, the time of death may be based on the first examination. When ancillary studies are used, all components from the second clinical examination that can be completed must remain consistent with brain death and documented. The determination of brain death has profound medical and legal consequences. Care must be taken to ensure that all parts of the clinical examination, including the apnea test, are performed properly and appropriately documented. Current pediatric guidelines include a checklist in an attempt to standardize documentation of the clinical examination, apnea test, and ancillary studies to determine brain death (**Table 44.2**). Use of this checklist is highly recommended to improve standardization and reduce diagnostic error when making a determination of brain death. Determination of brain death should never be rushed or take a priority over the needs of the patient or the family. It should be the expectation of medical providers that patients will continue to be actively managed until a determination of death has been made or a decision to withdraw medical therapies is agreed on between the family and the healthcare team. Appropriate emotional support for the family should be provided during this process. State law in certain situations may require consultation or referral to the medical examiner or coroner when death occurs.

Physicians must be open and honest in discussions with parents and families, and never allow a family to leave the hospital thinking they were responsible for allowing their child to die. Clear, concise, and simple terminology should be used so that the parents and family members understand that their child has died. *Brain death* is a medical term and is poorly understood even by some healthcare professionals. The term *brain death* should be avoided, and discussions with parents and families should center on the death of the child, not the death of an organ. Allowing families to be present during the brain death examination and apnea test can assist families in understanding that their child has died. It should be made clear that once death has occurred, continuation of medical therapies, including mechanical ventilation, is no longer an option unless organ donation is planned. A reasonable grieving period should be allowed for family members to spend with their child before discontinuing mechanical ventilation and other supportive medical therapies.

CHAPTER 45 ■ CARDIAC ANATOMY

STEVEN M. SCHWARTZ, ZDENEK SLAVIK, AND SIEW YEN HO

SEGMENTAL APPROACH TO CONGENITAL HEART DISEASE

Two primary systems are used to describe complex cardiac defects. These systems are based on morphologic analysis of various segments, but with differences in nomenclature, analysis, and definition of connections or junctions between segments.

Atrial Situs

The terms *right* and *left* atria are based on morphologic characteristics and not on their location in the heart or their venous and ventricular connections. The right atrium features a blunt atrial appendage with a *wide* connection to the smooth-walled part of the atrium, while the left atrium is characterized by a hooked appendage with a *narrow* connection. *Atrial situs* refers to the arrangement of the morphologic right and left atria within the heart. *Situs solitus* is the normal arrangement (right atrium is to the right, and left atrium is to the left). *Situs inversus* is the opposite arrangement. The *Andersonian system* suggests that atrial situs can be identified in all cases as *solitus*, *inversus*, and *right isomerism* or *left isomerism*. The *Van Praagh system* contends that atrial situs can be described as *solitus*, *inversus*, or *ambiguus*, in which ambiguus refers to the situation where separate right and left atria cannot be differentiated. *Polysplenia syndrome* is often used to mean the same thing as left atrial isomerism, and *asplenia syndrome* the same atrial arrangement as right atrial isomerism although these syndromes refer to more than just cardiac defects. Right atrial isomerism (asplenia syndrome) usually includes anomalies of pulmonary venous return, atrioventricular canal–type defects, double-outlet right ventricle (DORV), and transposition. Left atrial isomerism is more commonly associated with abnormalities of systemic venous connections (interrupted inferior vena cava), DORV, and normally related great arteries.

The Atrial Septum

The atrial septum contains a foramen ovale on the right side and the flap valve of the foramen on the left. The foramen ovale is the remnant of the ostium secundum, and the foramen primum is the embryologic opening between the early atrial septum (septum primum) and the area where the endocardial cushions normally form.

Ventricular Morphology and Topology

The morphologic right ventricle is heavily trabeculated, contains the moderator band of the septum, and has septal attachments of the associated atrioventricular (AV) valve. The left ventricle is smooth walled, is more bullet shaped, and has no septal attachments of the AV valve. Ventricular topology refers to the spatial anatomy of the inflow and outflow of the ventricle. One can imagine placing the palm of the hand on the septal surface of the right ventricle with the thumb extended toward the inflow and the fingers pointed toward the outflow. If this is accomplished with the right hand, the ventricle is "right handed" (normal orientation); if it is accomplished with the left hand, the ventricle is "left handed" according to the Andersonian scheme of nomenclature.

Atrioventricular Connections, Junctions, and Alignments

In a discordant connection or alignment, the morphologic right atrium opens into the morphologic left ventricle and vice versa. When there are two atria, two AV valves, and two ventricles, the tricuspid valve (TV) is always associated with the morphologic right ventricle, and the mitral valve is always associated with the morphologic left ventricle.

Ventricular Arrangements

The Van Praagh nomenclature system uses an embryologic approach to segmental anatomy. Transition from the straight heart tube requires the tube to loop, usually with the apex of the loop rightward (*dextro* or *d-loop*). Abnormal looping, with the apex of the loop to the left (*levo* or *l*-loop), results in the left ventricle located rightward of the morphologic right ventricle.

The Ventricular Septum

The ventricular septum is normally composed of an *inlet portion* (formed by endocardial cushion tissue), a *trabecular* or *muscular portion,* and the *outflow* or *conal portion*. The junction between these parts is the *membranous septum*, the common site of ventricular septal defects (VSDs).

The Great Arteries

Normally related great arteries occur when there are concordant ventriculo-arterial connections with the aorta posterior and slightly rightward of the pulmonary artery (**Fig. 45.1A**). In the case of double-outlet ventriculo-arterial connection, one of the ventricles gives rise to both great arteries, or in the case of a single great artery arising from a discordant ventricle, the artery with improper orientation is said to be *malposed*. Using the Andersonian nomenclature system, each great artery is assigned to the ventricle to which it is more than 50% committed. DORV occurs when both the great arteries are more than 50% committed to the right ventricle. Using the embryologic approach of Van Praagh, one describes the great arteries as normally related, transposed, or malposed (**Fig. 45.1B**). When there is a double-outlet connection, the great artery (usually the aorta) that is committed to the improper ventricle is said to be malposed.

SYSTEMIC AND PULMONARY VENOUS CONNECTIONS

Abnormalities of systemic venous connections include bilateral superior vena cava, left superior vena cava, interrupted inferior vena cava, and major alterations of venous connection such that a right-to-left shunt occurs. Pulmonary venous return to sites other than the left atrium may be either partial or totally anomalous, with supracardiac, cardiac, or infracardiac connections.

CARDIAC POSITION

Levocardia is the normal positioning of the heart on the left side of the thorax, *dextrocardia* occurs when the heart located predominantly in the right chest, and *mesocardia* is an intermediate situation with a more midline position.

CLINICAL EXAMPLES

Using the Van Praagh segmental approach for the description of cardiac anatomy, a normal heart can be referred to as atrial situs solitus, *d*-loop ventricles, and arterial situs solitus (S, D, S). The most common form of transposition of the great arteries is designated as atrio-ventricular concordance, ventriculo-arterial discordance in the Anderson system and as atrial situs solitus, *d*-loop ventricles, and *d*-transposition of the great arteries (S, D, D) or *d*-TGA in the Van Praagh system (**Fig. 45.1C**). Congenitally corrected transposition (**Fig. 45.1D**), also called *isolated ventricular inversion*, can also be described as atrioventricular discordance and ventriculo-arterial discordance (Anderson) or as atrial situs solitus, *l*-looped ventricles, and *l*-transposition of the great arteries (S, L, L) (Van Praagh).

CONGENITAL CARDIAC DEFECTS

The prevalence of congenital heart defects is 6–8 per 1000 live births (1 in 130–145). Congenital heart defects result in 10% of all infant deaths and 50% of deaths due to congenital malformations. Up to 85% of neonates born with congenital heart disease survive to adulthood.

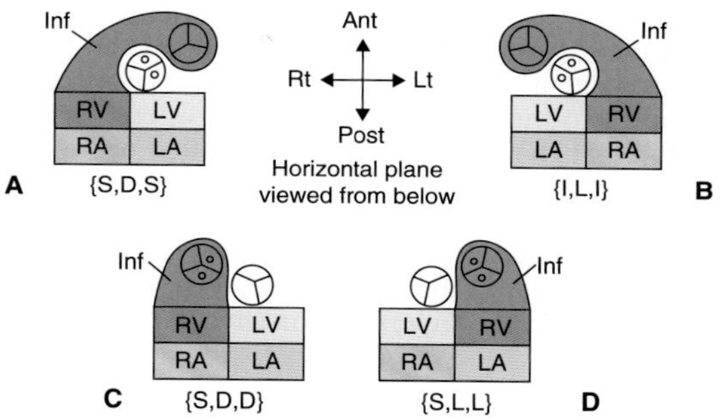

FIGURE 45.1. Schematic diagrams of normally related and transposed great arteries using segmental nomenclature scheme proposed by Van Praagh. **A:** Normal heart: atrial situs solitus, *d*-loop, situs solitus normally related great arteries (S, D, S). There is atrioventricular and ventriculo-arterial concordance. The aorta (designated by the coronary orifices on the diagram) is posterior and rightward. There is subpulmonary infundibulum (Inf) or conus. **B:** Mirror image normal: atrial situs inversus, *l*-loop, situs inversus normally related great arteries (I, L, I). There is atrioventricular and ventriculo-arterial concordance. The aorta is posterior and leftward of the pulmonary artery. There is a subpulmonary infundibulum or conus. The difference from normal is that the right atrium and ventricle are on the left, the left atrium and ventricle are on the right, and the aorta is leftward of the pulmonary artery. **C:** Usual form of transposition of the great arteries (*d*-TGA): atrial situs solitus, *d*-loop, *d*-transposition of the great arteries (S, D, D). There is atrioventricular concordance and ventriculo-arterial discordance. The aorta is anterior and rightward of the pulmonary artery, and there is subpulmonary conus. **D:** Congenitally corrected transposition of the great arteries (*l*-TGA): atrial situs solitus, *l*-loop, *l*-transposition of the great arteries (S, L, L). There is atrioventricular and ventriculo-arterial discordance. The aorta is anterior and leftward of the pulmonary artery, and there is subpulmonary infundibulum. (Modified from Foran RB, Belcourt C, Nanton MA, et al. Isolated infundibulo arterial inversion (S, D, I): A newly recognized form of congenital heart disease. *Am Heart J* 1988;116:1337–50.)

Congenital Heart Defects with Left-to-Right Shunts

Ventricular Septal Defects

VSDs are the most common congenital heart defect (30%). VSDs are divided into *inlet* (atrioventricular septal or endocardial cushion), *muscular*, *outlet* (doubly committed juxta arterial), and *perimembranous* defects. Eighty percent of VSDs are small (<3 mm diameter), with a high rate of spontaneous closure (particularly in the muscular and membranous septums). Large unrepaired defects with increased pulmonary-to-systemic blood flow ratio (>2:1) are at risk of developing pulmonary vascular obstructive disease in later childhood and adolescence.

Atrial Septal Defects

ASDs are classified into *ostium primum* ASD (part of atrioventricular septal defect [AVSD]), *ostium secundum* (within oval fossa and around the foramen ovale), and *sinus venosus* (superior or inferior adjacent to the orifice of superior or inferior caval vein, or at the coronary sinus [so-called unroofed coronary sinus into the left atrium]). The superior sinus venosus defect is commonly associated with partial anomalous pulmonary venous drainage involving the right upper pulmonary vein joining the lateral wall of the superior vena cava.

Patent Ductus Arteriosus

The ductus arteriosus is part of the normal fetal circulation joining the main pulmonary artery (MPA) with the descending aorta. Patency beyond 1 month of age (3 months in premature infants) is considered abnormal. The PDA can be the only source of pulmonary blood flow in some complex congenital heart defects (e.g., pulmonary valve atresia), but it can be absent in other defects (e.g., truncus arteriosus [TA]). Pulmonary vascular obstructive disease and subacute bacterial endocarditis are risks when the PDA is left unligated in childhood.

Atrioventricular Septal Defects

The complete form of atrioventricular septal defect (AVSD) (also called *endocardial cushion defect*) is characterized by a single AV valve spanning the inlet of both ventricles. Defects are present in the primum atrial septum and the inlet ventricular septum and result in interatrial and interventricular shunting. Three subtypes (*Rastelli A–C*) are recognized based on the chordal attachments of the AV valve to the septum. A partial AVSD is deficiency in either the interatrial or the interventricular septum in isolation. The complete form of AVSD is often associated with trisomy 21 and can lead to the early development of pulmonary vascular obstructive disease. If the left and right ventricles are approximately equal in size, the ASVD is "balanced" and a two-ventricle repair is possible. If one ventricle (usually the left ventricle) is hypoplastic, the ASVD is "unbalanced" and a single ventricle–staged palliation may be necessary.

Common Truncus Arteriosus

TA is a single arterial trunk with a single truncal valve (multiple leaflets) that arises from the heart and divides into the ascending aorta and pulmonary arteries. *Type I TA*, the MPA arises from the common truncus and then divides into the left and right pulmonary arteries. *Type II TA*, both left and right pulmonary arteries arise together from the common truncus without a discernible MPA. *Type III TA*, the right and left pulmonary arteries arise separately from the lateral walls of the TA. TA is the lesion most highly associated with *DiGeorge syndrome* (chromosome 22q11 deletion), and there is a high incidence of a right aortic arch in this lesion.

Aortopulmonary Window

An aortopulmonary window (APW) is a direct communication between the ascending aorta and the MPA usually in the form of a circular diaphragm and represents a high risk of early onset of pulmonary vascular obstructive disease.

Partial or Total Anomalous Pulmonary Venous Connection

One, or all, four pulmonary veins can connect anomalously with the systemic venous system, right atrium, or coronary sinus, resulting in partial or total anomalous pulmonary venous connection (PAPVC or TAPVC). PAPVC often involves the right upper pulmonary vein connecting to the superior vena cava and is often associated with a superior sinus venosus ASD. The various forms of TAPVC are classified into *supracardiac* (into the innominate vein; returns via superior vena cava), *intracardiac* (into the coronary sinus or directly to the right atrium), and *infracardiac* (into the umbilical, hepatic, or portal veins; returns via the orifice of the inferior vena cava). An obligate right-to-left shunt at the atrial level is necessary through an unobstructed secundum ASD for survival. Obstruction of the venous return pathway, most commonly at the vertical vein, leads to severe hypoxia and pulmonary hypertension postnatally. Unobstructed forms present with congestive heart failure and mild cyanosis.

Cyanotic Congenital Heart Defects

Tetralogy of Fallot

Tetralogy of Fallot (TOF) is the most common cyanotic congenital heart defect. It is a combination of four lesions that include an *outlet VSD, overriding aorta, right ventricular outflow tract obstruction* (*RVOTO*), and right ventricular *hypertrophy* although this is really all the result of a single defect, which is anterior deviation of the conal septum. There is a significant incidence of DiGeorge syndrome, especially if a right-sided aortic arch is present.

Pulmonary Atresia with Intact Ventricular Septum

Pulmonary atresia with intact ventricular septum (PA/IVS) includes a spectrum from mild to severe right ventricular hypoplasia due to outflow tract atresia with variable degrees of TV hypoplasia. The branch PAs are usually of reasonable size in contrast to patients with TOF with PA. The PDA is typically the only source of pulmonary blood flow. *Coronary arterial fistulae*, which are often stenotic, connect to the right ventricular cavity and can result in coronary steal.

Transposition of Great Arteries

Ventriculo-arterial discordance leads to aorta arising from the right ventricle and pulmonary artery from the left ventricle. Postnatal mixing of blood depends on the presence of a PDA and interatrial communication (**Fig. 45.1**).

Obstructive Congenital Heart Defects

Pulmonary Valve Stenosis

A variable degree of commissural fusion between the valvar cusps is the most common cause of pulmonary stenosis.

Aortic Valve Stenosis

Stenotic aortic valves can be described as unicuspid, bicuspid, or tricuspid depending on the number of functional commissures between valvar cusps. Unicuspid valves are usually the most severely stenosed. Aortic coarctation is the most common associated defect.

Aortic Coarctation or Interruption of the Aortic Arch (IAA)

In coarctation of the aorta (CA), the narrowing in the distal part of aortic arch around the aortic isthmus may be accompanied by a variable degree and extent of arch hypoplasia (**Fig. 45.2A** and **B**). The

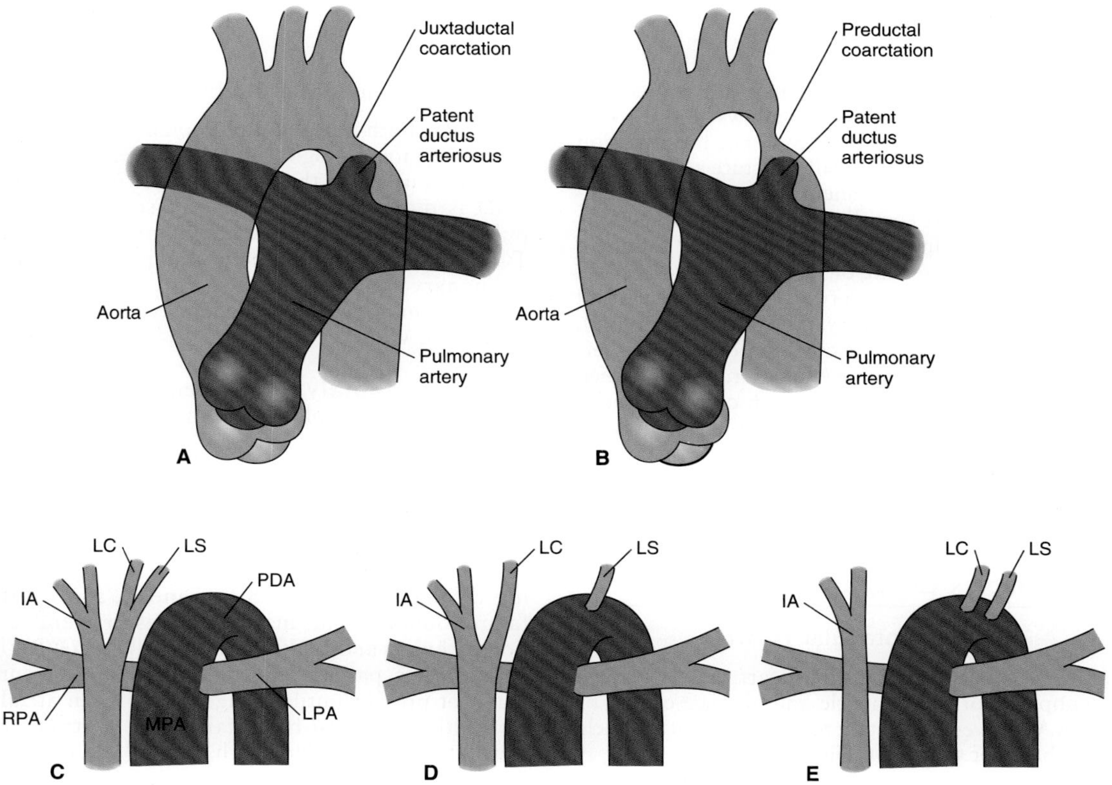

FIGURE 45.2. Coarctation and interruption of aortic arch. **A:** Juxtaductal coarctation of the aorta. **B:** Preductal coarctation of the aorta. **C:** Interrupted aortic arch type A. **D:** Interrupted aortic arch type B. **E:** Interrupted aortic arch type C. MPA, Main pulmonary artery. RPA, Right pulmonary artery. LPA, Left pulmonary artery. PDA, Patent ductus arteriosus. IA, Innominate artery. LC, Left carotid artery. LS, Left subclavian artery.

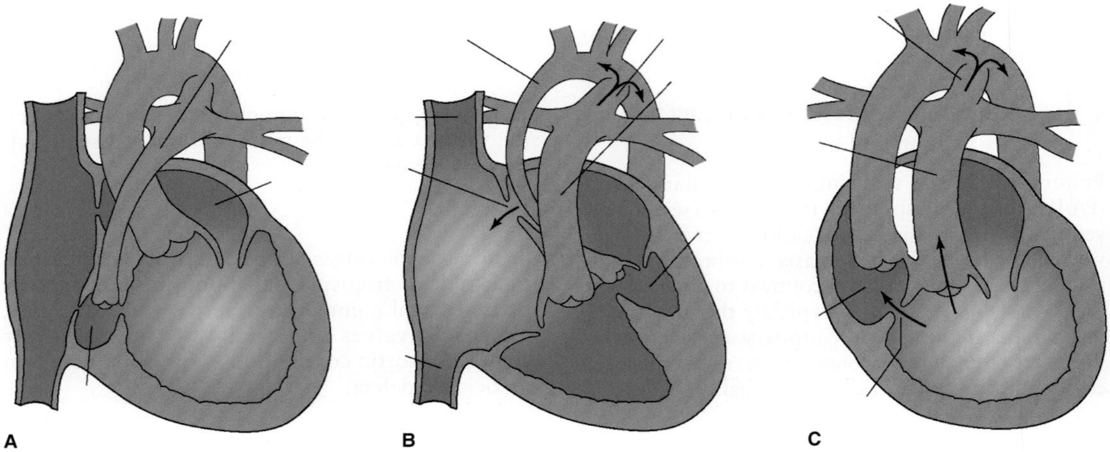

FIGURE 45.3. Variants of hearts with one functional ventricle. **A:** Hypoplastic right heart. There is severe tricuspid stenosis with a hypoplastic right ventricle, small ventricular septal defect, hypoplastic pulmonary artery, and a patent ductus arteriosus that provide pulmonary blood flow. The great arteries are normally related. **B:** Hypoplastic left heart syndrome. There is mitral and aortic stenosis with a hypoplastic left ventricle and ascending aorta. There is a ventricular septal defect and patent foramen ovale/secundum atrial septal defect. There is a patent ductus arteriosus that provides systemic blood flow. **C:** Double-inlet left ventricle with a ventricular septal defect or bulboventricular foramen providing flow to the right ventricle or outlet chamber. There is transposition of the great arteries. RVOT, right ventricular outflow tract.

PDA plays an important role in cases with severe neonatal aortic coarctation as it allows blood flow to reach lower part of the body. Systemic hypertension due to abnormal arterial wall structure and function and intracranial arterial aneurysms represent a long-term risk of severe complications even in successfully treated patients. In aortic arch interruption, a segment of aortic arch is missing or replaced by a solid cord. The defect is divided into: type A, interruption distal to the left subclavian artery; type B (most common), interruption between the common carotid and left subclavian arteries; and type C, interruption between the brachiocephalic and common carotid arteries (**Fig. 45.2C–E**). A PDA with right-to-left shunt is the only source of blood supply for lower body postnatally. Chromosome 22q11 deletion is strongly linked with type B interruption.

Complex Congenital Heart Defects

Univentricular Hearts

A wide variety of congenital heart defects involve hypoplasia of one ventricle and absence of one or both AV valves connecting to the dominant ventricle (double-inlet ventricle) (**Fig. 45.3**).

Double-Outlet Right Ventricle

In DORV, both aorta and pulmonary artery arise from the morphologic right ventricle. A VSD is the only outlet for the left ventricle. A subaortic VSD is more common and if associated with pulmonary stenosis has hemodynamics similar to TOF. With a subpulmonic position of the VSD, pulmonary stenosis is rare (aortic coarctation is more common) and hemodynamics are similar to TGA with VSD.

Ebstein Anomaly. In, Ebstein anomaly, the TV leaflets are displaced downward toward the RVOT, which separates the RV into a large upper "atrialized" segment and a lower (true) RV that is smaller—often consisting only of the RVOT. With severe downward displacement of the TV, patients can present with combined TV regurgitation and stenosis, increased RA pressures, right-to-left shunting through a PFO or ASD, cyanosis, and heart failure. Some patients may have accessory conduction pathways and *Wolff–Parkinson–White (WPW)* syndrome. A patient with mild TV displacement may not present until teenage years, when atrial fibrillation leads to heart failure or ventricular fibrillation and sudden death.

CHAPTER 46 ■ CARDIOVASCULAR PHYSIOLOGY

PETER E. OISHI, REBECCA J. KAMENY, JULIEN I. HOFFMAN, AND JEFFREY R. FINEMAN

HEMODYNAMIC PRINCIPLES

Flow, Velocity, and Cross-Sectional Area

Velocity is proportional to flow and inversely proportional to the cross-sectional area. Thus, peak velocity occurs in the aorta and reaches its nadir in the huge cross-sectional area of the capillary beds. Velocity increases again as blood moves from the capillaries toward the central veins.

Pressure, Flow, and Resistance

The primary determinants of flow (Q) through a vascular segment are the inflow pressure (P_i), the outflow pressure (P_o), and the vascular resistance (R). Flow through a vessel increases as the pressure difference across the vessel increases or the diameter of the vessel increases. Increased viscosity or vessel length decreases flow. Resistance is greatest at the level of the arterioles (not at the capillary bed) if blood flow is constant through the circulation. This is because capillary beds are vessels in parallel, while the arterial system feeding capillary beds is in series.

Compliance

The incremental change in volume (ΔV) per unit change in pressure (ΔP) defines the compliance (C) of a vessel, as indicated by the equation: $C = \Delta V/\Delta P$. Veins have thin walls that are less organized, contain less elastic tissue, and are ~20 times more compliant than arteries. Thus, most of the circulating blood volume resides in the venous system, and therapeutic volume expansion has a disproportionate effect on venous volume.

INTERACTION OF THE CARDIAC PUMP AND THE VASCULATURE

Cardiac output is determined by heart rate, contractility, preload, and afterload.

Vascular Function Curve

The vascular function curve describes how changes in cardiac output affect central venous pressure (CVP), or venous return. Maximal Q (flow) is achieved at a point when further reductions in the volume of the venous compartment are not possible. This point is termed the *critical closing pressure* (P_{cc}) and represents the lowest possible CVP and highest possible Q for any given blood volume. Maximum CVP is achieved when Q becomes zero and a steady state occurs in which pressures within the arterial and venous compartments are determined solely by compliance (combined vascular function and cardiac function curves are discussed below).

Cardiac Function Curve

The cardiac function curve is the reverse of the vascular function curve (**Fig. 46.1**). On the steep portion of the

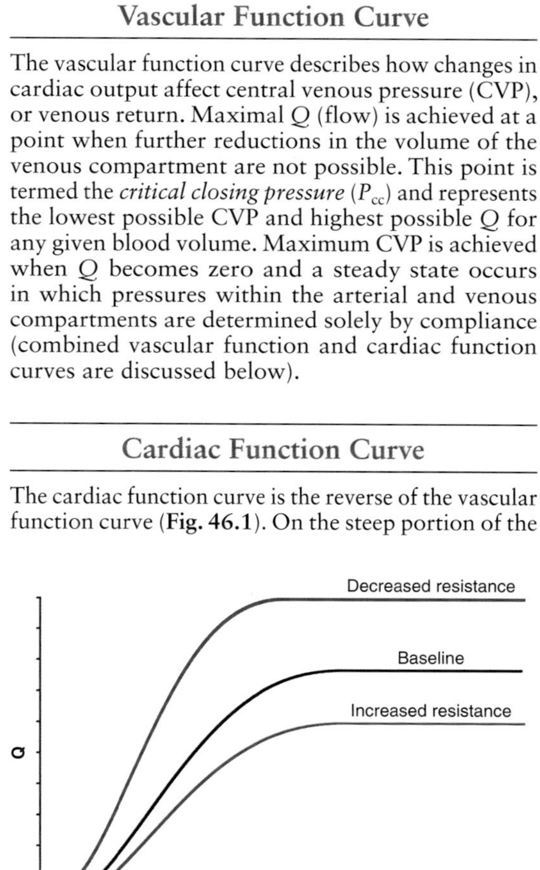

FIGURE 46.1. Cardiac function curves shown under conditions of varying degrees of systemic vascular resistance (afterload). The cardiac function curve describes how changes in CVP or venous return affect cardiac output (Q). On the steep portion of the curve, increases in CVP augment ventricular contractility. Increases in systemic vascular resistance (increased afterload) shift the curve downward, while decreases in systemic vascular resistance (decreased afterload) shift the curve upward.

curve, increases in CVP (preload), through increased venous return, distend the right ventricle (RV), which augments RV contractility and flow through the pulmonary circuit, ultimately increasing left ventricular preload and output. Changes in vascular resistance can also be reflected in the curve (**Fig. 46.1**).

Interaction of Vascular and Cardiac Function Curves

The superimposition of these curves in various physiologic states is useful, as it illustrates relationships between contractility, preload (including blood volume), and afterload. For example, **Figure 46.2** shows that alterations in vascular resistance affect both the vascular and cardiac function curves, whereas a single cardiac function curve can intersect with several vascular function curves with changes in blood volume (**Fig. 46.3**).

Pressure–Volume Loops

The hemodynamic and mechanical events of the cardiac cycle in the left ventricle (LV) can be graphically represented by the relationship between pressure and volume (**Fig. 46.4**). End-diastole is represented by point A (the point when the mitral valve closes). From points A to B, the ventricle undergoes isovolumic contraction. At point B, the aortic valve opens, and there is ejection with relatively little decrease in pressure until aortic valve closure (end-systole, point C). Then, diastole begins with isovolumic relaxation until point D (the mitral valve opens). From points D to A, there is filling of the ventricle. By imposing a change in preload or afterload without altering cardiac contractility (e.g., transient vena caval occlusion or phenylephrine administration), an informative series of pressure–volume loops can be generated (**Figs. 46.5** and **46.6**). The *end-diastolic pressure–volume relationship* (EDPVR) is defined by connecting the end-diastolic points of the family of loops (**Fig. 46.5**). EDPVR is altered in patients with diastolic dysfunction, but, unlike ESPVR, EDPVR is less adaptable to physiologic state and altered hormonal control. Unlike LV pressure–volume loops, RV pressure–volume loops do not normally contain an isovolumic relaxation or contraction phase, giving them a triangular shape. This property is load-dependent, and with elevated RV afterload (e.g., pulmonary hypertension or stenosis),

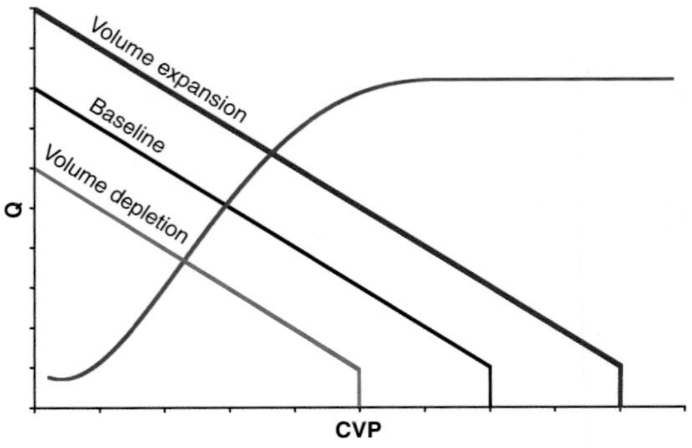

FIGURE 46.3. Effects of intravascular volume on the vascular and cardiac function curves. Intravascular volume expansion increases and intravascular volume depletion decreases the vascular function curve. The cardiac function curve is not altered by changes in intravascular volume. Because the cardiovascular system operates at the point of intersection between the two curves, the functional state of the system is affected by the volume status.

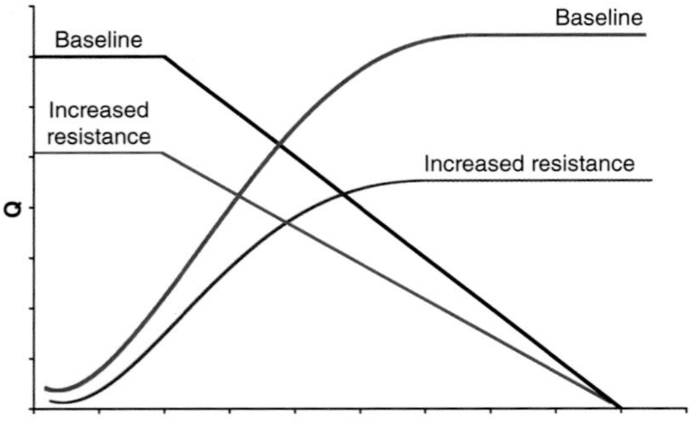

FIGURE 46.2. Effects of increased systemic vascular resistance on the vascular and cardiac function curves. Increased systemic vascular resistance (or afterload) shifts both curves downward, moving the operating state of the system that occurs at the point of intersection between the two curves downward. Increased systemic vascular resistance does not alter the vascular function curve at zero *Q*, as the CVP at this point is determined solely by the compliance of the venous compartment, at any given volume.

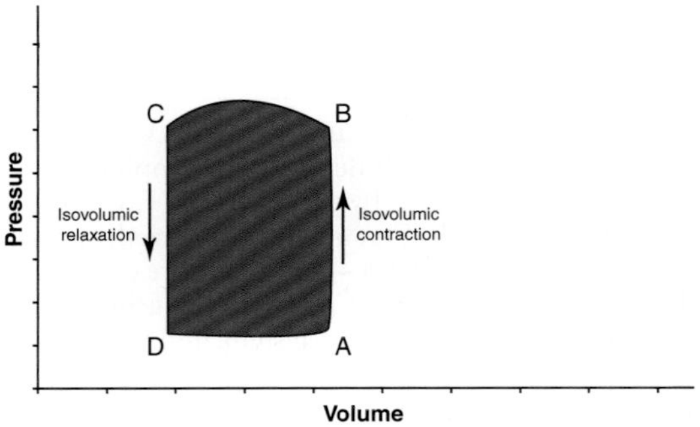

FIGURE 46.4. Left ventricle pressure–volume loop demonstrating the events of the cardiac cycle. Systole begins after point A with mitral valve closure. Then, the ventricle undergoes isovolumic contraction, followed by aortic valve opening (point B). Systole concludes after ejection and aortic valve closure (point C). Diastole begins with isovolumic relaxation, followed by mitral valve opening at point D. After filling of the ventricle, diastole ends at point A.

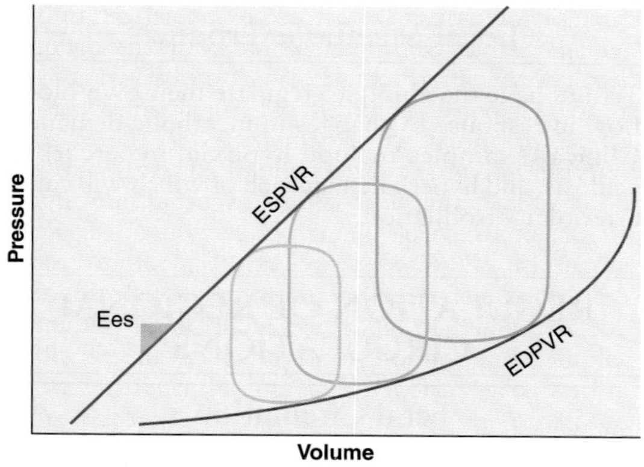

FIGURE 46.5. With acute alterations in preload (i.e., caval occlusion) or afterload (i.e., phenylephrine administration), a family of pressure–volume loops is generated. The linear ESPVR (end-systolic pressure–volume relationship) is defined by the connected end-systolic points of this group of curves; the slope of ESPVR is Ees (end-systolic elastance). The nonlinear EDPVR (end-diastolic pressure–volume relationship) describes the line generated by connecting the end-diastolic points of this group of loops.

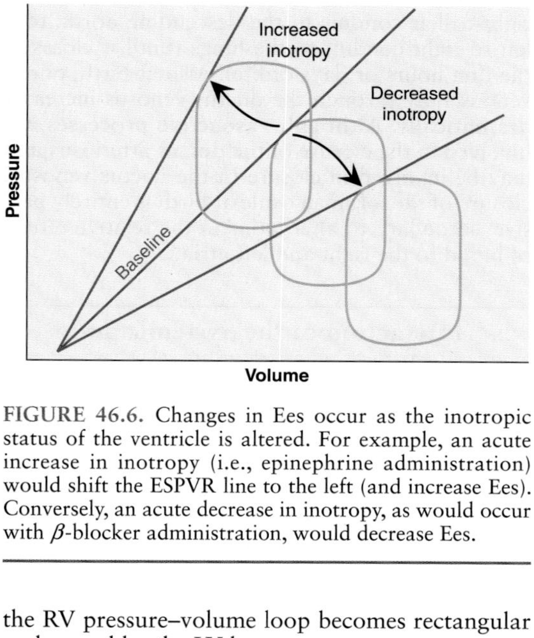

FIGURE 46.6. Changes in Ees occur as the inotropic status of the ventricle is altered. For example, an acute increase in inotropy (i.e., epinephrine administration) would shift the ESPVR line to the left (and increase Ees). Conversely, an acute decrease in inotropy, as would occur with β-blocker administration, would decrease Ees.

the RV pressure–volume loop becomes rectangular and resembles the LV loop.

Ventricular–Ventricular Interactions

Under normal conditions, the LV can contribute significantly to RV systolic function, while the RV minimally effects LV function. However, the elevated RV pressures and end-diastolic volumes in patients with pulmonary hypertension change septal position with flattening and eventual bowing into the LV, which affects LV diastolic function.

Ventricular–Arterial Coupling

Elevated vascular resistance increases afterload and decreases stroke volume if contractility and preload remain constant. Pressure–volume loops can be used to quantify this relationship. Ea is *effective arterial elastance* and is defined by the ratio of ESPVR to stroke volume (**Fig. 46.6**).

REGULATION OF VASCULAR RESISTANCE

Vascular resistance affects afterload and preload, two of the four determinants of cardiac output.

Autoregulation

Blood flow to tissues remains relatively constant over a wide range of arterial blood pressures owing to autoregulation. The mechanisms of this phenomenon are largely unknown. Autoregulation is essential for normal function of the brain, heart, and kidneys, and can become significant for other organs during times of increased metabolic demand.

Neural Control

Neural control for nearly all blood vessels in the body consists of feedback (afferent limb) and regulation (efferent limb) through the autonomic nervous system. The afferent limb of the neural control mechanisms consists of baroreceptors in arterial walls and stretch receptors within heart muscle. These receptors respond to stretch of the arterial wall and send nerve impulses to cardioinhibitory and vasomotor centers of the medulla. Atrial stretch receptors are located in the walls of both atria at the venoatrial junctions. These stretch receptors provide feedback to the hypothalamus and inhibit secretion of antidiuretic hormone (vasopressin) and play an important role in regulating intravascular volume. Two types of ventricular stretch receptors are found in ventricular myocardium, one type of which responds to mechanical stimulation, drugs, and chemicals through nonmyelinated afferent nerves (*C fibers*). Stimulation of C fibers located in the LV causes hypotension and bradycardia from parasympathetic stimulation and sympathetic inhibition. The efferent limb of neural control of the circulation, the autonomic nervous system, is divided into the sympathetic and parasympathetic systems. Two different types of sympathetic nerve fibers exist: vasoconstrictor and vasodilator. Sympathetic stimulation of the arterioles by vasoconstrictor fibers increases vascular resistance (the *resistance vessels*). Sympathetic vasoconstriction of larger arteries and of veins changes their volume and thus changes the circulating volume; these vessels are known as *capacitance vessels*.

Hormonal Control

The vasculature in the peripheral circulation is responsive to various circulating substances, including catecholamines, angiotensin II, vasopressin, eicosanoids, nitric oxide (NO), neurokinins, endothelin, bradykinin, and other peptide hormones. *Catecholamines* are the hormones of the adrenergic system. Stimulating α-receptors causes vascular smooth muscle contraction (vasoconstriction) and stimulating β-receptors causes vascular smooth muscle relaxation (vasodilation). Centrally controlled preganglionic sympathetic fibers innervate the adrenal medulla and stimulate norepinephrine secretion. Epinephrine is also secreted by the adrenal medulla, but it is a weaker vascular stimulant and tends to exert a β-agonistic effect at physiologic concentrations. *Angiotensin II*, a powerful vasoconstrictor, is produced by activation of the renin–angiotensin–aldosterone system. Angiotensin II has direct vasoconstrictor properties, acts centrally to stimulate the vasoconstrictor centers of the brain, and stimulates the secretion of antidiuretic hormone (vasopressin). *Prostaglandins* and other eicosanoids play a small role in regulating flow in the systemic circulation. Increased circulating levels of *atrial natriuretic factor* (ANF) are detected when left atrial pressure is elevated, even when the right atrial pressure is normal. In the circulatory system, ANF has vasodilator and cardioinhibitory effects. Circulating levels of ANF are increased in certain pathophysiologic conditions, such as congenital heart disease associated with elevated atrial pressures, congestive heart failure, valve disease, hypertension, coronary artery occlusion, and atrial arrhythmias. In addition, *β-type natriuretic peptide*, which is produced by the ventricular myocytes in response to stretch, has natriuretic, diuretic, and vasoactive properties.

Endothelial-Derived Factors

The vascular endothelial cells produce a variety of vasoactive substances that produce vascular relaxation and/or constriction, modulate the propensity of the blood to clot, and induce and/or inhibit smooth muscle migration and replication. *Nitric oxide* is a labile humoral factor produced by NO synthase from L-arginine in the vascular endothelial cell. NO diffuses into the smooth muscle cell, activates soluble guanylate cyclase, increases production of cGMP, and produces vascular relaxation. *Endothelin-1* (ET-1) is produced by vascular endothelial cells and is the most potent vasoconstrictor known (potency 10 times >angiotensin II). The breakdown of phospholipids within vascular endothelial cells results in the production of the important byproducts of arachidonic acid, including *Prostaglandin I_2* (PGI_2) and *thromboxane* (TXA_2). PGI_2 activates adenylate cyclase, resulting in increased cyclic AMP production and subsequent vasodilation, whereas TXA_2 results in vasoconstriction via phospholipase C signaling.

Local Metabolic Products

Tissues have the ability to regulate their own blood flow in response to changes in metabolic demands. Clinical examples include hypoxia, hypercarbia, acidosis, and hyperkalemia; each of which will cause arteriolar vasodilation.

REGULATION OF REGIONAL CIRCULATIONS

Fetal Circulation

The fetal RV supplies the majority of its blood via the ductus arteriosus and descending aorta to the placenta for oxygen uptake, and the LV supplies the majority of its blood via the ascending aorta to the heart and brain for oxygen delivery.

Transition from the Fetal to the Postnatal Circulation

At birth, the ductus arteriosus changes from a right-to-left conduit to the descending aorta, to a left-to-right conduit to the lungs (until it closes in the first hours or days of life). Also at birth, portal venous flow through the ductus venosus increases dramatically. Although vasoactive processes are involved in the closure of the ductus arteriosus and may be involved in closure of the ductus venosus, closure of the foramen ovale at birth is entirely passive, secondary to alterations in the relative return of blood to the right and left atria.

Interaction of the Systemic and Pulmonary Circulations

The pulmonary vascular resistance is normally 10%–20% of the systemic vascular resistance. Therefore, under normal conditions, only the total systemic resistance needs to be considered as a factor that affects cardiac output. However, if the RV fails, pulmonary vascular resistance is added in series to systemic vascular resistance.

Pulmonary Circulation

Morphologic Development

In the fetus and newborn, small pulmonary arteries have a thicker medial smooth muscle layer in relation to diameter than do similar adult arteries. This increased muscularity is partly responsible for the increased vascular reactivity and pulmonary vascular resistance in the neonate immediately after birth. In the first 4–6 weeks following birth, there is a reduction in medial muscular thickness of the walls of the small pulmonary arteries. A number of neonatal pulmonary vascular disorders (e.g., congenital heart disease with increased pulmonary blood flow) are associated with a failure of the normal involution of medial smooth muscle and/or a precocious progression to the adult morphologic state.

Pulmonary Blood Flow in the Fetus

In the fetus, gas exchange occurs in the placenta and the reduced pulmonary blood flow supplies nutritional requirements for lung growth (the lungs serve a metabolic or paraendocrine function). Fetal pulmonary arterial mean blood pressure increases progressively with gestation and, at term, is ~50 mm Hg (1–2 mm Hg > mean aortic pressure).

Regulation of Pulmonary Vascular Resistance in the Fetus and during the Perinatal Transition

The most prominent factor associated with high fetal pulmonary vascular resistance is the low blood O_2 tension (pulmonary arterial Po_2, 17–20 mmHg). At birth, with initiation of pulmonary ventilation, pulmonary vascular resistance decreases rapidly and pulmonary blood flow increases by 8- to 10-fold. By the first day of life, mean pulmonary arterial blood pressure is generally half systemic, with adult levels reached after 2–6 weeks.

Regulation of Postnatal Pulmonary Vascular Resistance and Blood Flow

The successful transition from the fetal to the postnatal pulmonary circulation is marked by the maintenance of the pulmonary vasculature in a dilated, low-resistance state. Decreasing oxygen tension and decreases in pH elicit pulmonary vasoconstriction. The response to alveolar hypoxia in which pulmonary arterioles constrict and divert blood flow away from hypoxic segments is unique to the pulmonary vasculature. In most vascular beds (e.g., cerebral vasculature), hypoxia is a potent vasodilator.

To characterize the unique relationship of pulmonary vascular pressure and position within the lung, West divided the lung into three theoretical zones based on the relationship between PAP (pulmonary artery pressure, inflow pressure), P_{alv} (alveolar pressure), and P_{ven} (pulmonary venous pressure, outflow pressure). In theory, no blood flows to zone I (upper zone) because P_{alv} > PAP > P_{ven}. Zone I conditions probably do not exist in a healthy lung. In zone II (middle zone), PAP > P_{alv} > P_{ven}. In this zone, blood flow increases down the lung, as PAP, but not P_{alv}, is influenced by gravity. In zone III (lower zone), blood flow does not change as it does in zone II because gravity affects PAP and P_{ven} equally, or PAP > P_{ven} > P_{alv}. Under normal conditions, pulmonary blood flow is largely determined by zone III conditions. Positive-pressure ventilation with high levels of peak end-expiratory pressure results in increased alveolar pressure, which may expand zone II and produce zone I conditions.

Coronary Circulation

Myocardial oxygen demand is almost exclusively met by increased myocardial blood flow.

Coronary Anatomy

The right coronary artery supplies the right atrium, RV, and part of the LV. The left coronary artery, which divides into the left anterior descending artery and the circumflex artery, supplies the left atrium and the rest of the LV, although some redundancy does exist. Venous return to the right atrium occurs principally through the coronary sinus.

Regulation of Coronary Blood Flow

Alterations in coronary blood flow are largely determined by alterations in vascular resistance.

Physical Factors That Regulate Coronary Blood Flow

Coronary perfusion pressure is directly related to aortic pressure. During early left ventricular systole, flow is transiently reversed by extravascular compression of the subendocardial arteries that supply the LV. Under normal conditions, subepicardial and subendocardial vessels are equally perfused during diastole. If diastole is excessively shortened, such as with severe tachycardia and/or if perfusion pressure is decreased, subendocardial ischemia can occur.

Myocardial Oxygen Demand–Supply Relationship. The LV extracts an almost maximal amount of oxygen from the blood that passes through the myocardium so that coronary blood flow must increase with myocardial oxygen demand. During maximal exertion, left ventricular oxygen consumption and left coronary blood flow increase fourfold. Increased flow is achieved by a decrease in coronary vascular resistance.

Coronary Reserve. Under normal conditions, coronary blood flow is autoregulated such that there is a range of perfusion pressure over which almost no change in flow occurs; a rise in pressure evokes vasoconstriction, and a fall in pressure evokes vasodilatation. Coronary flow reserve indicates the amount of extra flow that the myocardium can receive at a given pressure to meet increased demands for oxygen. Coronary reserve can be reduced by a number of conditions, such as when autoregulation is normal but the maximal possible flow is decreased, when maximal flows are normal but autoregulated flows increase, or when autoregulated flow and maximal flows are reduced at the same time.

Right Ventricular Myocardial Blood Flow. Right ventricular myocardial blood flow follows the general principles of coronary blood flow, but differences exist that are related to the low right ventricular systolic pressure and to the fact that alterations in aortic pressure change coronary perfusing pressure without altering right ventricular pressure work.

Neural Factors. Coronary blood flow increases with sympathetic stimulation; however, vasoconstriction is the predominant effect of sympathetic activation of the coronary arteries. Thus, even though α- and β-receptors are located on coronary vessels, coronary blood flow is most strongly influenced by local metabolic processes that match oxygen supply and demand.

CHAPTER 47 ■ CARDIORESPIRATORY INTERACTIONS IN CHILDREN WITH HEART DISEASE

RONALD A. BRONICKI AND LARA S. SHEKERDEMIAN

THE INVASIVE STUDY OF CARDIORESPIRATORY INTERACTIONS

Pressure–Volume and Pressure–Flow Relationships

The study of the interactions between cardiovascular and pulmonary systems requires an understanding of pressure–volume and pressure–flow relationships applied to elastic structures, such as blood vessels, cardiac chambers, and alveoli. The fundamental property of an elastic structure is its ability to offer resistance to a distending or collapsing force and to return to its resting volume after the force has been removed. The extent to which a structure undergoes a change in volume depends on the transmural pressure and its compliance. The transmural pressure (P_{tm}) is equal to the difference between intracavitary and surrounding pressures ($P_i - P_s$); a positive transmural pressure distends the cavity, and a negative transmural pressure reduces cavity size.

When a tube has a positive transmural pressure throughout, it is widely patent and blood flow (*Q*) is proportional to the perfusion pressure inflow–outflow gradient ($P_{in} - P_{out}$). These are known as *zone III conditions* for the flow of fluid. When P_{in}, P_{out}, and compliance are constant, as P_s increases, the transmural pressure decreases. As a result, the volume inside the tube decreases and resistance to flow increases, and flow is now proportional to the pressure gradient $P_{in} - P_s$. These are known as *zone II conditions*. As P_s increases further, the transmural pressure becomes negative, the tube collapses, resistance to flow increases further, **and flow ceases**, producing *zone I conditions*. The pressure at which $P_{in} = P_s$ is called the *critical closing pressure*. The different "zone" conditions may be created not only by changes in P_s but also from changes in P_{in}, P_{out}, and compliance. The physiologic significance of these concepts is that changes in P_s are analogous to changes in intrathoracic, intra-abdominal, or intravascular pressures with corresponding effects on systemic and pulmonary blood flow.

INTRATHORACIC PRESSURE AND RIGHT VENTRICULAR PRELOAD

Systemic venous return to the right heart is driven by a pressure gradient between the systemic venous circulation and the right heart, and is opposed by resistance to venous return (R_{VR}) or:

$$\text{Venous Return} = (P_{MS} - P_{RA})/R_{VR},$$

where P_{MS} is the mean systemic pressure and P_{RA} the right atrial pressure. *Mean systemic pressure* (P_{MS}) is defined as the circulatory pressure that results from arresting the heart and allowing for the equilibration of volume and pressure throughout the circulation and represents the P_{in} for venous return. The function of the venous capacitance vessels (not the arterial resistance vessels) is the principal determinant of P_{MS}. P_{RA} represents the P_{out} for venous return. An increase in P_{RA} causes systemic venous return and right ventricular output to decrease, unless there is a compensatory increase in P_{MS}. Venoconstrictors and intravascular volume expansion increase the P_{MS} while the converse occurs with venodilators and diuresis. Pharmacologic agents such as furosemide, nitric oxide donors, and angiotensin-converting enzyme inhibitors, and pathologic conditions such as sepsis vasodilate venous capacitance vessels, decrease the P_{MS}, and thus decrease venous return.

Spontaneous Inspiration and Right Ventricular Preload

During spontaneous inspiration, the pleural pressure (P_{pl}) becomes negative and the P_{tm} of the right atrium increases. As a result, the right atrium distends and the pressure within falls, increasing the pressure gradient for venous return. Spontaneous inspiration *in a euvolemic patient* displaces abdominal blood volume into the central circulation, contributing to venous return from the inferior vena cava. During inspiration *in a hypovolemic patient* with decreased abdominal compliance, venous return may decrease if zone II and III conditions are

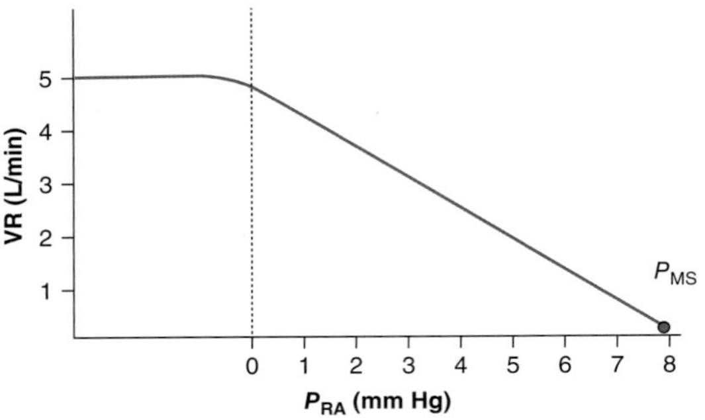

FIGURE 47.1. The relationship between right atrial pressure, mean systemic pressure, and venous return. Venous return (VR) increases as right atrial pressure (P_{RA}) decreases and then plateaus as P_{RA} falls below zero. The negative intrathoracic pressure is transmitted to the vena cava just outside the chest. As the transmural pressures in the vena cava become negative, they collapse at the thoracic inlet, creating zone I and II conditions, which limit or suspend venous return. Further decreases in P_{RA} have no effect on venous return because flow is now a function of the difference between the mean systemic pressure (P_{MS}) and atmospheric pressure or abdominal pressure.

created within the inferior vena cava. Similarly, Guyton showed that as right atrial pressure falls, venous return increases and then plateaus as zone II and III conditions are created as the vena cava enter the chest (**Fig. 47.1**).

Positive-Pressure Ventilation and Right Ventricular Preload

As ITP increases, right atrial pressure increases and the pressure gradient for venous return decreases. Systemic venous return may decrease if compensatory circulatory (acutely venoconstriction and over time fluid retention) reflexes do not generate an adequate P_{MS}. A noncompliant ventricle, or one surrounded by elevated ITP (due to the decrease in the P_{tm} during ventricular diastole), requires a higher-than-normal intracavitary pressure to maintain an adequate end-diastolic volume and right ventricular stroke volume.

INTRATHORACIC PRESSURE AND RIGHT VENTRICULAR AFTERLOAD

As lung volume is increased from residual volume to functional residual capacity (FRC), the radial traction provided by the pulmonary interstitium increases the diameter of the extra-alveolar vessels. In addition, with resolution of atelectasis, hypoxic pulmonary vasoconstriction is released, contributing to a decrease in the resistance of the extra-alveolar vessel. The net effect is reduction of right ventricular afterload as lung volume approaches FRC. As lung volumes increase above FRC, the caliber of alveolar vessels decreases as alveolar transmural pressure increases. As alveolar pressures increase further, zone II and III conditions are created, increasing the resistance to blood flow. As lung volumes approach total lung capacity, zone I conditions are created and alveolar vessels collapse and blood flow ceases.

Changes in the alveolar distending pressure (i.e., alveolar transmural or transpulmonary pressure), lung compliance, and the resulting changes in lung volume during ventilation affect pulmonary vascular resistance. Changes in the inflow and outflow pressures of the pulmonary circulation (i.e., pulmonary arterial and venous pressures, respectively) also determine the extent to which changes in lung volume alter pulmonary blood flow.

INTRATHORACIC PRESSURE AND LEFT VENTRICULAR PRELOAD

Spontaneous inspiration increases systemic venous return and right ventricular diastolic volume and pressure. As the right ventricle fills, the interventricular septum (normally bowed into the right ventricle because of higher left ventricular pressures) occupies a more neutral position between the two ventricles during diastole. This decreases left ventricular compliance and cavitary volume resulting in reduced stroke volume during inspiration. The mechanism by which the filling of one ventricle affects the filling of the other is diastolic ventricular interdependence, and contributes to *pulsus paradoxus*, the fall in systemic arterial pressure that occurs during spontaneous inspiration. Over the next few cardiac cycles, the increase in systemic venous return leads to an increase in left ventricular filling and output.

INTRATHORACIC PRESSURE AND THE LEFT VENTRICULAR AFTERLOAD

Spontaneous Ventilation and Left Ventricular Afterload

Left ventricular afterload is primarily determined by its systolic transmural pressure (aortic systolic pressure minus pleural pressure). Thus, an increase in afterload may result from an increase in aortic blood pressure or from a fall in pleural pressure (**Fig. 47.2**).

During spontaneous respiration, while thoracic arterial pressure decreases, pleural pressure falls to

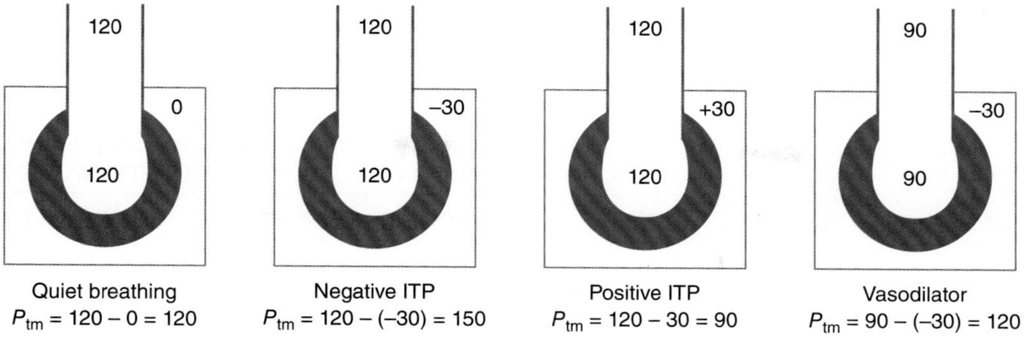

FIGURE 47.2. The relationships between changes in intrathoracic pressure and aortic pressure on left ventricular afterload. During periods of quiet breathing in which intrathoracic pressure (ITP) is 0, the left ventricular (LV) transmural pressure (P_{tm}) is equal to the LV systolic pressure (120) (left-hand panel). When ITP is negative, the transmural pressure is increased (P_{tm} is now 150) and wall stress within the ventricle is elevated. The opposite occurs when ITP is positive (P_{tm} then becomes 90). The increase in transmural pressure imparted by a negative ITP can be reversed by vasodilator treatment, which restores transmural pressure to baseline levels (right-hand panel).

a greater extent, resulting in a net increase in the left ventricular systolic transmural pressure and hence an increase in left ventricular afterload. In health, the impact of spontaneous breathing on the left heart is minimal. However, the impact of changes in pleural pressure on the LV becomes much more significant in the presence of excessively negative pleural pressures (e.g., in severe airway obstruction) and in patients with left ventricular systolic dysfunction.

Positive-Pressure Ventilation and Left Ventricular Afterload

During positive-pressure ventilation (PPV), an increase in ITP unloads the LV while increasing aortic pressure, so-called *reverse pulsus paradoxus*.

Variation in Systolic Pressure and Pulse Pressure during the Respiratory Cycle

During mechanical ventilation, the systolic arterial pressure and the pulse pressure increase during inspiration due to the effect of the increase in ITP on the P_{tm} of the thoracic arterial vessels. The greater the differences in systolic pressures (or pulse pressures) over a respiratory cycle the more likely the patient is to be responsive to volume administration.

CARDIORESPIRATORY INTERACTIONS IN CHILDREN WITH HEART DISEASE

A number of common pediatric critical care scenarios in which PPV can impact cardiovascular function are discussed below and summarized in **Table 47.1**.

CARDIORESPIRATORY INTERACTIONS IN CHILDREN WITH SYSTOLIC HEART FAILURE

Cardiopulmonary interactions play a major role in the symptomatology, hemodynamic manifestations, and management of systolic heart failure.

Cardiorespiratory Interactions during Spontaneous Respiration

Even at rest, the work of breathing of children with systolic heart failure is increased due to pulmonary venous hypertension and pulmonary edema. Their decreased lung compliance and exaggerated negative pressure breathing increase respiratory muscle oxygen consumption and circulatory demand. As ITP becomes increasingly negative, left ventricular afterload and ventricular wall stress increase, further increasing myocardial oxygen demand.

Positive-Pressure Ventilation in Systolic Heart Failure

PPV reduces right ventricular preload through effects on the right heart and reduces left ventricular afterload by eliminating exaggerated negative pressure breathing and decreasing the LV systolic transmural pressure. Unloading the respiratory musculature (pump) with mechanical ventilation is also beneficial in the treatment of heart failure. Under normal conditions, the respiratory pump receives <3% of global oxygen consumption and receives <5% of cardiac output. However, with an increase in respiratory load, the oxygen demand of the respiratory pump may increase

TABLE 47.1

Cardiorespiratory Interactions in Children with Heart Disease During Spontaneous and Positive-Pressure Ventilation

HEART DISEASE	KEY CONCERNS	SPONTANEOUS VENTILATION		POSITIVE-PRESSURE VENTILATION/CPAP	
		ISSUES	RESULT	ISSUES	RESULT
Heart failure (acute or chronic)	Elevated LV afterload Systolic LV dysfunction	Increased work of breathing Exaggerated negative intrapleural pressure swings	Increased LV afterload	Reduced work of breathing Removed negative swings in pleural pressure	Reduced venous return Reduced LV afterload Improved LV function
Postoperative—tetralogy of Fallot	Good systolic function Diastolic RV dysfunction Preload dependent	Increased RV preload Improved diastolic pulmonary artery flow	Improved cardiac output	Reduced RV preload Reduced diastolic pulmonary artery flow	Reduced cardiac output
Postoperative—Fontan/BCPS	Good systolic function Preload dependent Cardiac output depends on pulmonary blood flow	Increased preload Negative intrathoracic pressure improves pulmonary blood flow	Improved cardiac output	Reduced preload Reduced pulmonary blood flow	Reduced cardiac output
Duct-dependent systemic flow	Excessive pulmonary flow, leading to reduced systemic flow	Tachypnea and oversaturation are common Limited control of pulmonary flow	Possible excessive pulmonary flow and reduced systemic cardiac output	Better control of pulmonary flow, pH, and pulmonary resistance	Improved systemic cardiac output

CPAP, continuous positive airway pressure; BCPS, bidirectional cavopulmonary shunt; LV, left ventricle; RV, right ventricle.

to >50% of total oxygen consumption, necessitating an increase in respiratory muscle perfusion. Mechanical ventilation unloads the respiratory pump allowing for a redistribution of a limited cardiac output to other vital organs while decreasing myocardial work and oxygen consumption.

Positive-Pressure Ventilation in Children with Post–Cardiotomy Systolic Ventricular Dysfunction

Cardiac surgery inevitably results in myocardial injury due to intraoperative factors (e.g., cardiopulmonary bypass-induced inflammation, myocardial reperfusion injury, and cardiotomy) that lead to a degree of early postoperative systolic and diastolic ventricular dysfunction. Most infants and children require PPV after surgery, which provides respiratory support and hemodynamic support through its effects on ventricular loading conditions and work of breathing.

Positive-Pressure Ventilation in the Nonsurgical Patient with Systolic Ventricular Dysfunction

Noninvasive positive-pressure respiratory support (e.g., bi-level positive airway pressure [BiPAP] and continuous positive airway pressure [CPAP]) is now a mainstay of therapy in adults with acute cardiogenic pulmonary edema, as it has been shown to decrease the incidence of tracheal intubation and mortality.

CARDIORESPIRATORY INTERACTIONS IN CHILDREN WITH DIASTOLIC VENTRICULAR DYSFUNCTION

Diastolic ventricular dysfunction is relatively common in children with heart disease, in whom cardiac output may be compromised due to inadequate ventricular filling. When systemic ventricular systolic function is intact, the impact of changes in ITP on systemic venous return and ventricular filling predominate over the effects on ventricular afterload.

Diastolic Dysfunction in Children with Cardiomyopathy

Patients with restrictive cardiomyopathies have adequate if not normal systolic function, but as a result of diastolic disease are very sensitive to interventions that may decrease systemic venous return and right ventricular preload such as venodilators and PPV. The same is true of patients with hypertrophic cardiomyopathy. An emphasis should be placed on maintaining adequate ventricular preload and avoiding excessive PEEP in patients with diastolic dysfunction.

CARDIORESPIRATORY INTERACTIONS IN CHILDREN WITH CONGENITAL HEART DISEASE

Cardiorespiratory Interactions in a Functionally Univentricular Circulation

The unifying feature of the circulatory physiology of infants with these lesions is that the perfusion of the pulmonary and systemic circulations is from the output of a single or functionally single ventricle. PPV should be used to optimize ventricular loading conditions and improve myocardial and global oxygen transport balance, as already described. Ventilation should be manipulated to provide a normal arterial pH (avoiding both acidosis and alkalosis) remembering that alveolar hypoxia and acidemia increase pulmonary vascular resistance while alkalosis and supplemental oxygen reduce it.

Cardiorespiratory Interactions after the Fontan Operation

In the Fontan circulation, the mean systemic pressure is responsible for driving systemic venous return across the pulmonary circulation, rendering it much more susceptible to changes in pulmonary vascular resistance and to ventricular dysfunction. Diastolic dysfunction may complicate the early postoperative course following the Fontan procedure. In patients following the Fontan procedure, pulmonary blood flow increases by nearly two-thirds during inspiration, as the pleural pressure becomes negative. Flow can reverse, implying a brief complete cessation of pulmonary blood flow, when these patients perform a Valsalva maneuver.

Cardiorespiratory Interactions after the Bidirectional Cavopulmonary Shunt

In these patients, pulmonary flow is derived from the upper body venous drainage, and is driven by the upper body venous pressure. Pulmonary flow is exquisitely sensitive to changes in cerebral vascular resistance, ITP, and pulmonary artery pressure. Routine postoperative ventilation after the bidirectional cavopulmonary shunt should be directed at early initiation of spontaneous respiration, and extubation as soon as feasible. If pulmonary blood flow and oxygenation are inadequate, control of minute ventilation may be indicated to allow for a mild elevation of arterial carbon dioxide tension, which uncouples cerebral blood flow from cerebral metabolism. The resultant increase in superior caval return increases pulmonary blood flow.

Cardiorespiratory Interactions Following the Repair of Tetralogy of Fallot

Most infants have an uncomplicated postoperative course after repair of tetralogy of Fallot (TOF). However, right ventricular diastolic dysfunction is common, and a minority of patients may develop reduced cardiac output secondary to diastolic dysfunction with elevated right heart filling pressures, fluid retention, and pleural effusions. Minimizing ITP promotes venous return and right ventricular filling and increases right ventricular stroke volume. Left ventricular systolic function is typically intact in patients following repair of TOF; thus, changes in ITP impact primarily the right heart.

CHAPTER 48 ■ HEMODYNAMIC MONITORING

RONALD A. BRONICKI AND NEIL C. SPENCELEY

PHYSICAL EXAMINATION

The physical examination is essential in determining cardiovascular function. A *depressed or altered mental status* signifies that compensatory hemodynamic mechanisms are failing. *Capillary refill time* (CRT), when prolonged on presentation of a critically ill child, represents shock and increased mortality risk (≤2 seconds is normal). Examination of *central and peripheral pulses* provides volume, rate, and regularity of the pulse. The *core (rectal) to peripheral (great toe) temperature gradient* can be an indicator of adequacy of peripheral circulation, particularly in infants after cardiac surgery.

ELECTROCARDIOGRAM

Deciphering an underlying rhythm abnormality with bedside monitoring may be difficult (see Chapter 54). High heart rates and limited monitor fidelity may conceal p waves, blur QRS morphology, and conceal atrioventricular (A-V) dissociation. Incorrect lead placement is the most common technical problem of ECG monitoring.

CAPNOGRAPHY

Capnography is the graphic display of the concentration or partial pressure of CO_2 measured continuously in both inhaled and exhaled gases over time. It provides important information on changes in pulmonary blood flow (see Chapter 22). The CO_2 concentration is measured by infrared spectroscopy and sampled by either aspiration from the breathing circuit (sidestream analyzer) or inline measurement by a flow-through adapter and sensor (mainstream analysis). The normal baseline on the capnogram should have a CO_2 concentration of zero, reflecting inspiratory as well as early expiratory (anatomic dead space) gas; this is followed by a sharp upstroke, reflecting mid-exhalation and increasing alveolar gas; this is followed by the plateau phase, which represents a leveling off of alveolar gas. The capnogram then abruptly falls to zero, as the expiratory phase is terminated and inspiratory gas dilutes out the remaining CO_2. The point on the capnogram plateau just prior to the abrupt fall-off is called the end-tidal CO_2 ($ETCO_2$) concentration and approximates the arterial Pco_2 ($Paco_2$) under conditions of normal ventilation ($\dot{V}$) to perfusion ($\dot{Q}$) matching in the lung. The most common technical problem is a leak around the endotracheal tube, which lowers the $ETCO_2$ measurement and increases the arterial to $ETCO_2$ gradient.

Normally, the arterial to end-tidal CO_2 gradient ($Paco_2$-$ETCO_2$) is <2–3 mm Hg, and thus $ETCO_2$ levels approximate arterial CO_2 levels. $Paco_2$-$ETCO_2$ increases when $\dot{Q}$ is low compared with V (i.e., elevated $\dot{V}$:$\dot{Q}$ ratios). Diseases characterized by a decreased $\dot{V}$:$\dot{Q}$ ratios and intrapulmonary shunt (perfusion without ventilation) do not contribute significantly to $Paco_2$-$ETCO_2$. $ETCO_2$ monitoring can also be used to assess the effectiveness of chest compressions and the return of circulatory function during cardiac arrest.

ARTERIAL PRESSURE

Blood pressure is related to cardiac output (CO) and systemic vascular resistance (SVR). *Noninvasive oscillometric arterial pressure measurement* is the most common method used. The cuff should cover at least two-thirds of the upper arm. A cuff that is too small overestimates blood pressure and vice versa. The frequency of blood pressure measurement depends on the severity of disease. Technical difficulties occur with improper cuff placement, patient movement, and low arterial pressure.

Invasive arterial monitoring is the "gold standard" of blood pressure measurement. To ensure accuracy and counteract baseline drift, the pressure transducer must regularly be zeroed to atmospheric pressure at the level of the right atrium (RA) (mid-axillary line). If the transducer is placed below the RA, the arterial pressure reading will be falsely elevated and vice versa.

All monitoring systems produce natural energy at rest through oscillation, which can create artifact and possible distortion of the resultant waveform. Too much (*overdamping*) or too little (*underdamping*) may falsely lower or elevate systolic pressures. Overdamping is commonly encountered in the intensive care unit (ICU) due to obstruction or excessive compliance in the system and results in a narrow pulse pressure and flattened waveform. The mean arterial pressure is usually unaffected. Causes include bubbles, clots, tubing that is compliant, cracked, lengthy, or kinked, a soft transducer diaphragm, three-way taps, or a poorly secured transducer. Smaller-diameter cannula causes overdamping but cannot be avoided in younger children. Underdamping has the opposite effect. The mean pressure remains largely unchanged.

Placement of the tip of an invasive arterial line in or near the aorta may give a more consistent reading for a longer period. Placement of the catheter in a more peripheral position causes the pressure wave reflection from the extremity to augment the waveform, which results in a higher systolic pressure, lower diastolic pressure, and later appearance of the dicrotic notch. The mean arterial pressure remains fairly constant regardless of measurement site.

Complications of invasive arterial monitoring include bleeding, infection, nerve damage, arterial–venous fistulae, and vascular compromise. Most clinicians avoid the brachial and ulnar arteries because of decreased collateral circulation in the event of vascular injury. The temporal artery is contraindicated because of the risk of intracranial embolization. The axillary artery may be cannulated when access at other sites has failed, but the care team must consider the increased risks of retrograde embolization (resulting in stroke) compared to more distal sites.

Invasive blood pressure monitoring provides a continuous display of the arterial waveform (**Fig. 48.1**). A slow upstroke of the arterial waveform can be indicative of poor cardiac function but is also seen in aortic stenosis and elevations in SVR. A low pulse pressure may reflect a low stroke volume. A widened pulse pressure (elevated systolic and decreased diastolic pressures) is seen in lesions characterized by low SVR, such as an aorta-to-pulmonary artery runoff (e.g., patent ductus arteriosus or aortopulmonary artery window), and in aortic insufficiency.

CENTRAL VENOUS AND ATRIAL PRESSURES

The central venous catheter (CVC) may be inserted in the subclavian, femoral, basilic, jugular, or umbilical (newborn) veins using the Seldinger technique or by a cut-down procedure. There are risks associated with the insertion of CVCs, including infectious and thrombotic complications.

A normal central venous pressure (CVP) or RA pressure in the spontaneously breathing patient is −2–5 mm Hg. The atrial pressure waveform (**Fig. 48.2**) normally demonstrates three positive and two negative waves: the "*a*" wave follows the p wave on ECG and is produced by atrial contraction; the "*c*" wave is produced by ventricular contraction and bulge of the tricuspid valve upward into the RA; the "*x*" descent results from atrial relaxation; the "*v*" wave results from RA filling in late systole before opening of the tricuspid valve; and the "*y*" descent results from opening of the tricuspid valve and passive filling of the right ventricle (RV). The CVP is the mean RA pressure, which approximates the RV end-diastolic pressure when RV compliance and tricuspid valve function are normal. When ventricular function and compliance are diminished, atrial systole generates an end-diastolic pressure (reflected in the "*a*" wave) that is disproportionately higher than the mean pressure. Cannon "*a*" waves are produced when RA contraction occurs against a closed tricuspid valve (AV dissociation). Prominent "*v*" waves may be seen in tricuspid insufficiency, and rapid "*x*" and "*y*" descents are suggestive of pericardial disease and restraint.

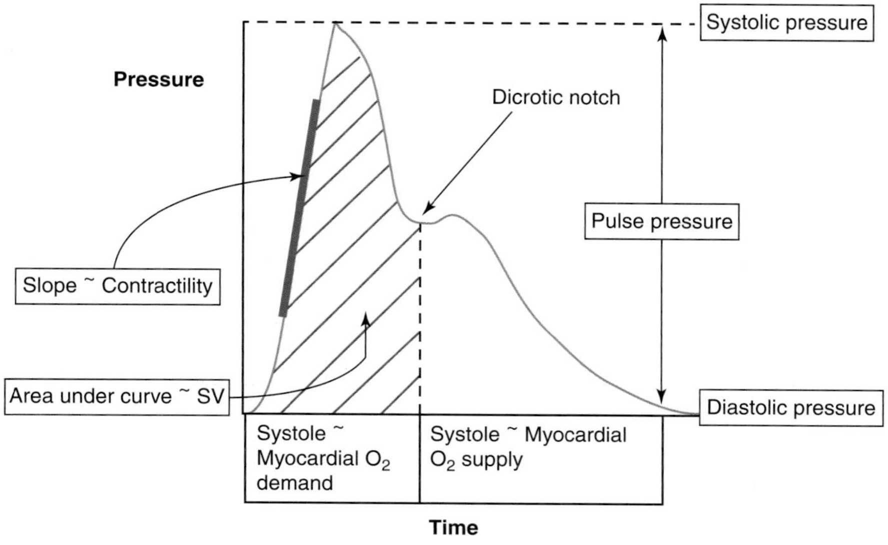

FIGURE 48.1. Arterial pulse waveform. Inspection of the arterial pulse waveform provides a *first approximation* of various aspects of hemodynamic function. The slope of the systolic upstroke may be proportional to myocardial contractility and inversely proportional to systemic vascular resistance. The area under the systolic curve approximates stroke volume. The duration of systole relative to the duration of the entire cardiac cycle reflects myocardial O_2 demand. The duration of diastole relative to the duration of the entire cardiac cycle reflects myocardial O_2 supply. Pulse pressure is the difference between systolic and diastolic pressures.

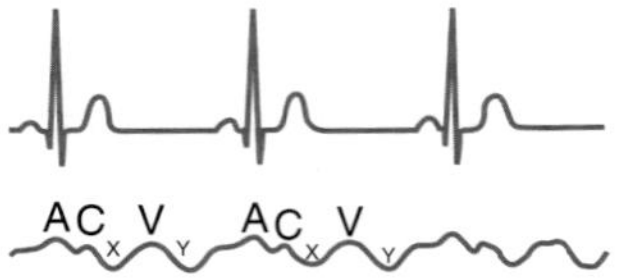

FIGURE 48.2. Central venous pressure tracing with corresponding ECG. See text for explanation. (From O'Rourke RA. The measurement of systemic blood pressure: Normal and abnormal pulsations of the arteries and veins. In: Hurst JW, ed. *The Heart*. New York: McGraw-Hill, 1990:159, with permission.)

Ventricular compliance is the ratio of the change of ventricular pressure (ΔP) to the change in ventricular volume (ΔV). Ventricular compliance may be diminished as result of myocardial disease (e.g., hypertrophic or ischemic myocardium), elevated operating volumes (e.g., systolic heart failure and elevated afterload), pericardial disease, increased intrathoracic pressure (positive pressure ventilation), lower airway disease that result in excessive lung volumes, large pleural effusions, and diastolic ventricular interdependence. When ventricular compliance is reduced, a higher than normal end-diastolic pressure is needed to maintain an adequate stroke volume.

In the presence of underlying cardiopulmonary disease, there may be no correlation between RA and left atrial (LA) pressures. In these situations, intraoperative placement of an *LA catheter* can help evaluate postoperative systemic ventricle filling. The exception is in patients with single-ventricle anatomy and a nonrestrictive interatrial communication, where the CVP is a measurement of the systemic ventricular filling pressure. It is safest to use the LA catheter strictly for pressure monitoring and avoid aspiration of blood or intermittent flushing of the line due to the risk of stroke.

PULMONARY ARTERIAL CATHETER

With a pulmonary artery catheter (PAC), ventricular filling pressures (RA and pulmonary artery occlusion pressures, PAOP), pulmonary artery pressures, mixed venous oxygen saturation, and temperature are directly measured (**Table 48.1**). With the addition of heart rate and systemic arterial blood pressure, a number of hemodynamic parameters may be derived including CO, stroke volume, SVR and pulmonary vascular resistance (PVR), oxygen delivery, and oxygen consumption.

TABLE 48.1

Common Hemodynamic Variables

PARAMETER	FORMULA	NORMAL RANGE	UNITS
Cardiac index	CI = CO/body surface area	3.5–5.5	L/min/m^2
Stroke index	SI = CI/heart rate	30–60	mL/m^2
Systemic vascular resistance index	SVRI = 79.9 × (MAP − CVP)/CI	800–1600	dyne-sec/cm^5/m^2
Pulmonary vascular resistance index	PVRI = 79.9 × (MPAP − PAOP)/CI	80–240	dyne-sec/cm^5/m^2
Left ventricular stroke work index	LVSWI = SI × MAP × 0.0136	50–62 (adult)	g-m/m^2
Right ventricular stroke work index	RVSWI = SI × MPAP × 0.0136	5.1–6.9 (adult)	g-m/m^2
Arterial oxygen content	$Cao_2 = (1.34 \times Hb \times Sao_2) + (Pao_2 \times 0.003)$		mL/L
Oxygen delivery index	$Do_2I = CI \times Cao_2$	570–670	mL/min/m^2
Fick principle	$CI = \dot{V}o_2I/(Cao_2 - C\bar{v}o_2)$	160–180 (infant $\dot{V}o_2I$) 100–130 (child $\dot{V}o_2I$)	mL/min/m^2 mL/min/m^2
Mixed venous oxygen saturation		65%–75%	
Oxygen extraction ratio[a]	$O_2ER = (Sao_2 - Svo_2)/Sao_2$	0.24–0.28	

CI, cardiac index; CO, cardiac output; SI, stroke index; SVRI, systemic vascular resistance index; MAP, mean systemic arterial pressure; CVP, central venous pressure; PVRI, pulmonary vascular resistance index; MPAP, mean pulmonary arterial pressure; PAOP, pulmonary artery occlusion pressure; LVSWI, left ventricular stroke work index; RVSWI, right ventricular stroke work index; Cao_2, arterial oxygen content; Hb, hemoglobin concentration (g/L); Sao_2, arterial oxygen saturation; Pao_2, partial pressure of dissolved oxygen; Do_2I, oxygen delivery index; $\dot{V}o_2I$, oxygen consumption index; $C\bar{v}o_2$, mixed venous oxygen content; O_2ER, oxygen extraction ratio; Svo_2, mixed venous oxygen saturation.

[a]The equation given for O_{2ER} is only valid if the contribution from dissolved oxygen is minimal. If this is not the case, oxygen content (Cao_2, $C\bar{v}o_2$) must be substituted for saturation (Sao_2, Svo_2).

The general consensus on the use of the PAC suggests that the PAC be used as infrequently as possible in children, but may be used to clarify cardiopulmonary physiology in selected patients with: (a) pulmonary hypertension; (b) shock refractory to fluid resuscitation and/or low-to-moderate doses of vasoactive agents; and (c) severe respiratory failure requiring high airway pressure.

The PAC comes in several sizes; the 5-French catheter is used for children weighing between 10 and 18 kg (with the proximal port located 15 cm from the catheter tip) and a 7-French catheter is used in patients weighing over 18 kg (with the proximal port located 30 cm from the catheter tip). The proximal port is used to measure the RA pressure and allows for the injection of an indicator solution (cold saline in the thermodilution method) to measure CO. The distal port allows for sampling blood to measure mixed venous oxygen saturations and for the measurement of pulmonary artery pressures and PAOP. The thermistor is located just proximal to the balloon and measures changes in the temperature of pulmonary arterial blood during thermodilution-derived CO measurements. The fourth lumen allows for the inflation of the balloon (located 1 cm proximal to the catheter tip).

The catheter is inserted through an introducer sheath and advanced by inflating the balloon with CO_2 or air and "floating" the tip while continuously monitoring the distal port pressures and waveforms (**Fig. 48.3**), as well as the ECG for dysrhythmias. When withdrawing the catheter, the balloon should be deflated to avoid valvular or vessel rupture. The catheter should be allowed to "float" (i.e., balloon inflated) into the wedged position *only* when actively obtaining a PAOP in order to minimize the risk of pulmonary infarction or rupture.

Interpretation of Thermodilution-Derived CO

Thermodilution to determine CO involves injecting a known volume of cold saline into the RA and measuring the resultant temperature change with the thermistor located in the pulmonary artery. CO is determined

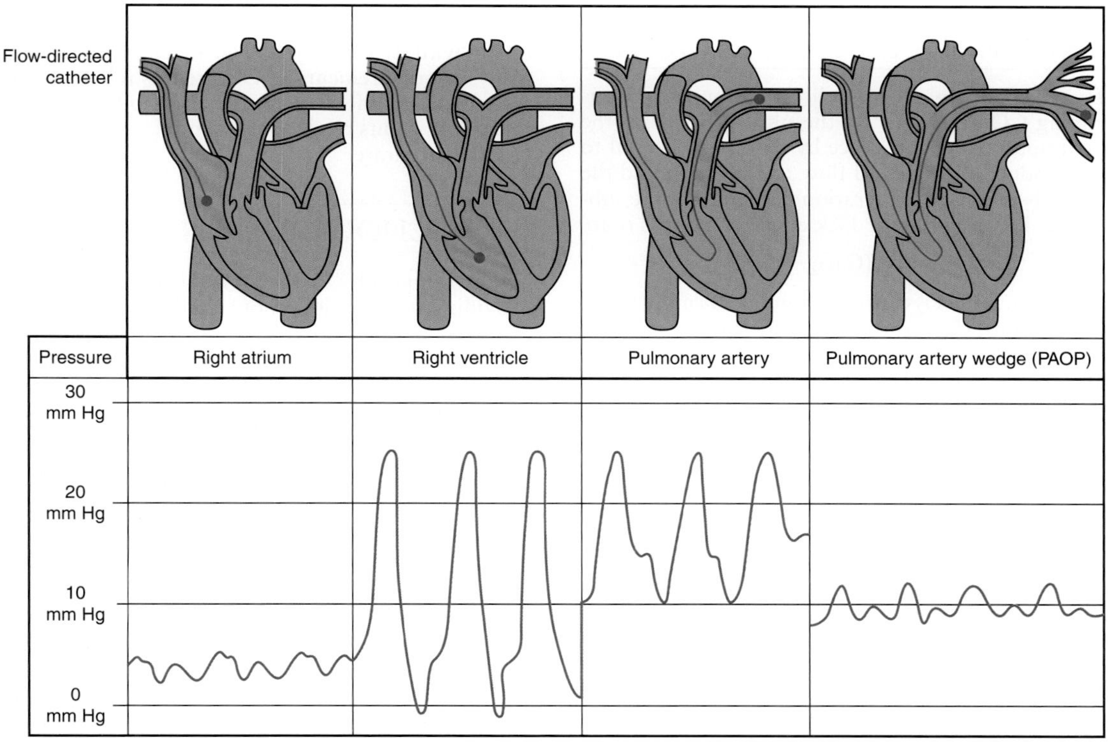

FIGURE 48.3. Pulmonary artery catheter waveforms. When the balloon is inflated and the catheter is advanced, a series of characteristic waveforms appear. As the catheter passes from the right atrium (RA) through the tricuspid valve into the right ventricle (RV), the low-amplitude RA waveform suddenly changes to a high-amplitude (high pulse pressure, high systolic pressure, low diastolic pressure) RV waveform. Further advancement through the pulmonary valve into the pulmonary artery (PA) yields a waveform with a higher diastolic pressure than in the RV while the systolic pressure is unchanged. Ultimately a position is reached where the systolic and mean pressures decrease, the tracing becomes damped, and the appearance of an "*a*" and "*v*" venous waves become more pronounced. This is the PA occlusion (or wedge) pressure (*PAOP*). When the balloon is deflated, the tracing should immediately return to a PA waveform.

by the amount of indicator divided by the change in concentration over time. Conditions in which the thermodilution method may prove unreliable have backward flow of blood on the right side, such as tricuspid and pulmonary valve regurgitation, and ventricular or atrial septal defects (with left-to-right and/or right-to-left shunting).

Interpretation of Other Hemodynamic Measurements from the PAC

The PAOP is used to indicate left ventricular (LV) end-diastolic volume; however, in patients with poor ventricular compliance, as discussed above, the correlation between the two parameters may be poor. Further, the PAOP will underestimate the LV end-diastolic pressure, which is reflected in the "*a*" wave, when LV compliance is low. The PAOP may also be used to distinguish cardiogenic (PAOP > 18 mm Hg) from permeability pulmonary edema (PAOP < 12 mm Hg).

THE FICK EQUATION AND INDIRECT CO MEASUREMENTS

The Fick principle is an indirect method for determining CO and relies on the observation that the total uptake of a substance by an organ is equal to the product of the blood flow to the organ and the arterial–venous concentration difference of the substance. Rearranging the Fick equation reveals that:

$$Q = \dot{V}O_2/(CaO_2 - C\bar{v}O_2)$$

where $\dot{V}O_2$ is the O_2 consumption (mL O_2/min), Q the CO (L/min), CaO_2 the arterial O_2 content (mL O_2/dL blood), $C\bar{v}O_2$ the *mixed* venous O_2 content (mL O_2/dL blood), and (Ca − Cv) O_2 = arteriovenous O_2 content difference. The CaO_2 is directly proportional to hemoglobin concentration and the arterial oxygen saturation. The dissolved O_2 in blood is a function of the partial pressure of O_2 (dissolved $O_2 = 0.003 \times PO_2$) and is negligible under most circumstances.

CaO_2 (mL O_2/dL) = [1.34 (mL/g) × hemoglobin concentration (g/dL) × [SaO_2 (%)/100]] + [0.003 (mL/dL/mm Hg) × PaO_2 (mm Hg)] and $C\bar{v}O_2$ (mL O_2/dL) = [1.34 (mL/g) × hemoglobin concentration (g/dL) × [SvO_2 (%)/100]] + [0.003 (mL/dL/mm Hg) × PvO_2 (mm Hg)], where the SaO_2 is the arterial O_2 saturation and $S\bar{v}O_2$ is the *mixed* venous O_2 saturation. In practice, $\dot{V}O_2$ is usually based on norms for age, gender, and size.

Calculation of the Q_p:Q_s Ratio

Another benefit of the Fick principle is that it allows separate calculations of systemic (Q_s) and pulmonary (Q_p) blood flow. Q_p and Q_s are nearly equal (Q_p:Q_s = 1) in the child with a structurally normal heart (except for the very small right-to-left shunt from the Thebesian and bronchial veins). Children with right-to-left shunts have a Q_p:Q_s < 1 (pulmonary undercirculation and hypoxemia), whereas those with left-to-right shunts have Q_p:Q_s > 1 (pulmonary overcirculation and heart failure). The magnitude of the shunt is described by the Q_p:Q_s ratio, such that Q_p:Q_s ≈ ($SaO_2 - SvO_2$)/($SpvO_2 - SpaO_2$), where $SpvO_2$ is the pulmonary vein O_2 saturation, and $SpaO_2$ the pulmonary artery O_2 saturation.

Pulmonary venous blood is difficult to sample, such that the $SpvO_2$ is presumed to be 100% in patients without significant lung disease. The use of an assumed value for $\dot{V}O_2$ from standardized tables is commonly used during cardiac catheterization, but is less useful in the critical care setting as oxygen demand and consumption vary considerably.

PULSE CONTOUR ANALYSIS

Another method for measuring CO is pulse contour analysis, which is based on the principle that the area under the curve of a central arterial waveform correlates with stroke volume (**Fig. 48.1**). Pulse contour analysis measurements of CO are less reliable than those from pulmonary arterial thermodilution. Intracardiac shunts render pulse contour measurement of CO inaccurate.

ECHOCARDIOGRAPHY

Echocardiography is an essential diagnostic tool, providing information about cardiovascular function that is not available from other monitoring modalities. LV systolic function can be assessed by determining the *fractional shortening* (FS), which is the change in LV short-axis diameter based on one-dimensional wall motion analysis or M-mode echocardiography (FS = End-Diastolic Dimension − End-Systolic Dimension/End-Diastolic Dimension; normal LVFS = 0.28–0.40). The primary limitation of this technique is that the contraction of the LV cannot be assumed to be entirely uniform or symmetric and M-mode interrogation may not capture regional differences in wall motion and wall thickening. Similarly, a flattened interventricular septum nullifies the measurement. Calculation of the *ejection fraction* (EF) is based on two-dimensional imaging of LV systolic function by quantifying changes in ventricular volume during the cardiac cycle. (EF = End-Diastolic Volume − End-Systolic Volume/End-Diastolic Volume; normal LVEF = 0.68 ± 0.09.) This technique relies on the modified Simpson rule method for measuring volumes.

Doppler techniques enable clinicians to estimate intracardiac and vascular pressures by measuring the velocity of blood in relation to the ultrasound beam. Based on a modified *Bernoulli's equation*, the pressure gradient that exists across an obstructive lesion is:

Pressure gradient = $4V^2$, where "V" is the velocity of blood as it accelerates across a narrowed orifice. Studies have shown that with systolic flattening of the interventricular septum, RV systolic pressure is at least half systemic. Other uses of echocardiography include a qualitative assessment of valvar regurgitation, pericardial effusion, and intracardiac shunting.

VENOUS OXIMETRY

Assuming minimal amounts of dissolved oxygen in blood and constant hemoglobin levels, the equations for the *ratio* of oxygen demand to oxygen delivery ($\dot{V}O_2/DO_2$) and the oxygen extraction ratio (O_2ER) can be simplified to:

$$\dot{V}O/DO_2 = O_2ER = SaO_2 - SvO_2/SaO_2$$

An increased O_2ER results from a reduction in DO_2 and/or increase in $\dot{V}O_2$. Oxygen consumption ($\dot{V}O_2$) can be maintained over a wide range of decreasing oxygen delivery (DO_2) with a compensatory increase in oxygen extraction, which is reflected in an increasing O_2ER. This phenomenon is shown in the *oxygen supply independent* portion of the $\dot{V}O_2/DO_2$ curve. However, there is a *critical* DO_2, which is defined by the onset of anaerobic metabolism and the accumulation of serum lactate; it occurs when the increase in oxygen extraction no longer suffices, oxygen demand exceeds oxygen supply (the beginning of the *oxygen supply dependent* portion of the $\dot{V}O_2/DO_2$ curve), and anaerobic metabolism ensues. It is not until the critical O_2ER is reached and the production of lactate exceeds its clearance that the serum lactate level begins to accumulate. Therefore, a rising O_2ER provides an indication of impending shock while a lactic acidosis usually signifies a shock state. The critical DO_2 is the same whether the decrease in DO_2 results from anemia, hypoxemia, or low CO. The corresponding percent oxygen extraction represents the critical O_2ER and remains constant at >60% or so, as it looks at the DO_2 in relation to $\dot{V}O_2$.

Systemic Compensatory Circulatory Responses to Maintain Tissue Oxygenation

There are several different scenarios involving alterations in $\dot{V}O_2$, DO_2, and oxygen extraction: (1) As oxygenation decreases, stimulation of chemoreceptors leads to neurohormonal activation and a compensatory increase in CO that maintains DO_2 and a normal O_2ER. (2) As oxygen-carrying capacity decreases (anemia), resistance to ventricular ejection and venous return decreases, allowing a compensatory increase in CO. Anemia also stimulates aortic chemoreceptors, leading to neurohormonal activation and increases in heart rate and contractility. DO_2 is maintained and the O_2ER remains normal. (3) With a decrease in oxygen content (from either arterial hypoxemia or anemia), there is a compensatory increase in CO, which preserves DO_2 and a normal O_2ER. If the decrease in oxygen content is so large as to result in reduced DO_2 despite increased CO, then the O_2ER will increase. (4) Increases in oxygen demand are met by a commensurate increase in CO and the O_2ER remains stable unless the increase in oxygen demand is severe and/or the compensatory circulatory response is limited.

Regional Compensatory Circulatory Responses to Maintain Tissue Oxygenation

A redistribution of CO is another mechanism by which the systemic circulation maintains oxygenation of vital organs. Vital organs (e.g., brain, myocardium, and diaphragm) have sparse sympathetic innervation and, therefore, are less responsive to sympathetic control, and their flow is maintained (if not augmented) by a redistribution of CO. When regional perfusion becomes limited, tissues compensate by recruiting previously closed capillaries, which enables tissue to extract a greater amount of oxygen. There are situations in which a normal or reduced O_2ER is associated with a pathologic state of impaired oxygen utilization, such as cyanide poisoning and some cases of septic shock.

The Oxygen–Hemoglobin Dissociation Curve

The affinity of hemoglobin for oxygen can change in situations associated with inadequate oxygen delivery (acidosis, hypercarbia, hypoxia, fever). A shift in the curve to the right represents a decreased affinity of oxygen for hemoglobin, whereas a shift to the left represents an increased affinity.

Central Venous Oximetry

The normal O_2ER in the superior vena cava is 25%–30%, 30%–35% in the jugular vein, and 15%–20% for the right atria–inferior vena cava junction. Oxygen extraction and O_2ER can be calculated using central venous oximetry.

NEAR-INFRARED SPECTROSCOPY

The oximeter uses differential absorption of at least two wavelengths of light and a dual-detector system that subtracts the effects of shallow signals, enabling estimation of deep tissue oxygenation. The algorithm evaluates a nonpulsatile signal of the microcirculation where 75%–85% of the blood volume is venous and thus near-infrared spectroscopy (NIRS) oximetry functions as a surrogate for tissue venous oxygen saturation.

Cerebral oximetry values correlate well with superior vena cava and jugular saturations. The normal cerebral O_2ER is 35% and the critical cerebral O_2ER, corresponding to the onset of neurologic deficits and a rise in brain lactate levels, is similar to the global critical O_2ER at 60% or so. As discussed above, as CO becomes limited, blood flow is redistributed to maintain perfusion of the most vital organs, rendering cerebral oximetry a relatively late indicator of a falling CO.

Renal oximetry and *mesenteric oximetry* provide an earlier indication of a falling CO than systemic or global parameters of tissue oxygenation (central or mixed venous oximetry and serum lactate levels) or cerebral oximetry. The normal mesenteric oxygen extraction is ~25%–35% and the critical O_2ER is similar to the global O_2ER at 60% or so. However, as CO falls and blood flow is redistributed, the mesenteric O_2ER increases first and becomes critical sooner than systemic or global parameters. The renal O_2ER increases appreciably only with significant decreases in renal Do_2. Multisite NIRS oximetry (combined cerebral, renal, and mesenteric) may provide a more sensitive indication of a falling CO than isolated cerebral oximetry.

LACTATE

The majority of lactate is produced in muscle, skin, brain, intestine, and red blood cells. In severe illness, the lungs and leukocytes can be a significant source, even in the absence of hypoxia. Hypoxia blocks oxidative phosphorylation by halting the donation of electrons. ATP production falls, NADH fails to regenerate, and proton numbers overwhelm the mitochondrial capacity for their consumption. Lactate dehydrogenase (LDH) is induced, converting significant quantities of pyruvate into lactate. Lactate clearance principally occurs in the liver and to a lesser extent the kidney. Once the renal threshold is exceeded (usually around 5 mmol/L), renal excretion occurs. Therefore, hepatic or renal dysfunction in any disease state can contribute to lactatemia.

CHAPTER 49 ■ HEART FAILURE: ETIOLOGY, PATHOPHYSIOLOGY, AND DIAGNOSIS

MARY E. MCBRIDE, JOHN M. COSTELLO, AND CONRAD L. EPTING

ETIOLOGY

The causes of pediatric heart failure are diverse but can be broadly divided into structural and myocardial heart diseases (**Table 49.1**).

Structural Heart Disease

Heart failure in patients with structural heart disease is often caused by chronic ventricular volume or pressure overload. Volume overload can be due to left-to-right shunting or valvar regurgitation. Pressure overload can be due to left or right ventricular outflow tract obstruction or high systemic or pulmonary vascular resistance. Infrequently, coronary ischemia or incessant arrhythmias are the fundamental problem.

Volume Overload

Significant left-to-right shunts at the ventricular or great vessel level lead to left ventricular volume overload and signs and symptoms of heart failure. The resultant left ventricular distension increases muscle fiber length, myocardial contractility, and stroke volume. Increased return to the left side eventually results in remodeling, leading to an elevation of diastolic pressure and contributing to left atrial hypertension. Increased pulmonary venous pressures, coupled with increased pulmonary blood flow, contribute to interstitial lung water, pulmonary edema, and tachypnea. Sinus tachycardia helps preserve cardiac output, and the constant workload (tachycardia, tachypnea) increases caloric consumption, contributing to failure to thrive. Ventricular systolic function is preserved, and thus a low cardiac output state does not occur. In addition to left-to-right shunts, patients at risk for developing left-sided heart failure include those with severe aortic or mitral insufficiency or atrioventricular septal defects with significant valvar regurgitation. Right-sided heart failure may be caused or exacerbated by regurgitation of the tricuspid or pulmonary valves.

Pressure Overload

Significant obstruction to systemic or pulmonary blood flow leads to ventricular myocyte hypertrophy, reduced end-diastolic volume (EDV), increased ventricular wall stress, decreased ventricular compliance, subendocardial ischemia from insufficient coronary

TABLE 49.1

Etiology of Pediatric Heart Failure

I. Structural heart disease
  a. Volume overload
    i. Left-to-right shunts
      1. Ventricular septal defect
      2. Atrioventricular septal defect
      3. Patent ductus arteriosus
      4. Aortopulmonary window
      5. Systemic arteriovenous malformation
    ii. Valvular regurgitation
      1. Aortic regurgitation
      2. Mitral regurgitation
      3. Tricuspid regurgitation
      4. Pulmonary regurgitation
  b. Pressure overload
    i. Right ventricular outflow tract obstruction
      1. Pulmonary stenosis
      2. Peripheral pulmonary stenosis
    ii. Left ventricular outflow tract obstruction
      1. Critical aortic stenosis
      2. Critical coarctation
  c. Complex congenital heart disease
    i. Congenitally corrected transposition of the great arteries
    ii. Common arterial trunk (truncus arteriosus)
    iii. VSD with IAA
    iv. Functionally single ventricle
      1. Fontan physiology
II. Myocardial heart disease
  a. Cardiomyopathy
    i. Dilated cardiomyopathy
    ii. Hypertrophic cardiomyopathy
    iii. Restrictive cardiomyopathy
    iv. Tachycardia-induced cardiomyopathy
    v. Arrhythmogenic right ventricular cardiomyopathy
    vi. Left ventricular noncompaction
    vii. Myocardial ischemia
  b. Systemic disease
    i. Sepsis/septic shock
    ii. Postarrest myocardial dysfunction
    iii. Systemic hypertension
    iv. Pulmonary hypertension
    v. Thyrotoxicosis
    vi. Transient dysfunction after cardiopulmonary bypass

VSD, ventricular septal defect; IAA, interruption of the Aortic Arch.

blood flow, and, ultimately, poor cardiac output. This physiology may be seen in neonates with critical aortic stenosis, in whom cardiac output is dependent on ductal flow and the work of the right ventricle. Right ventricular failure from pressure overload may develop in neonates with critical pulmonary valve stenosis (who may also have hypoxemia related to right-to-left shunting at the atrial level), pulmonary artery stenosis, conduit stenosis, and pulmonary hypertension. Right ventricular pressure load can ultimately affect left ventricular performance due to *interventricular dependence*. As the right ventricle ejects against significant outflow tract obstruction or increased PVR, the interventricular septum begins to flatten and then bow into the left ventricle. This in turn decreases left ventricular compliance, which ultimately leads to biventricular failure.

Complex Congenital Heart Disease

A combination of volume and pressure overload, reduced ventricular muscle mass, and primary myocardial dysfunction may be present in patients with congenital heart disease. Fifty percent of patients with a systemic right ventricle develop heart failure by age 20. Single-ventricle patients at greater risk include those with a systemic right ventricle, significant atrioventricular valve regurgitation, or a nonsinus rhythm. These patients typically exhibit exercise intolerance.

Myocardial Heart Disease

Cardiomyopathy

In patients with structurally normal hearts, primary cardiomyopathies are the most common etiology of heart failure. Cardiomyopathies are classified as dilated, hypertrophic, or restrictive subtypes, with 10% of patients having features of more than one subtype.

Dilated Cardiomyopathy

Of pediatric cardiomyopathies, the dilated phenotype is most common (approximately one-half of cases). Risk factors for the development of dilated cardiomyopathy include male gender, African-American heritage, and age less than 1 year. Dilated cardiomyopathy is characterized by a dilated, poorly functioning left ventricle without compensatory left ventricular wall hypertrophy. In two-thirds of cases, the cause is not identified, and are deemed idiopathic. Of cases with known etiologies, myocarditis and neuromuscular disorders are most common.

Hypertrophic Cardiomyopathy

Hypertrophic cardiomyopathy is characterized by a hypertrophied, nondilated ventricle in the absence of other disease processes. Approximately one-third of children with cardiomyopathy have a hypertrophic phenotype. Most cases are diagnosed in the first year of life. While the majority of cases of hypertrophic cardiomyopathy are idiopathic, others result from inborn errors of metabolism (e.g., Pompe disease), malformation syndromes (e.g., Noonan or Costello syndrome), and neuromuscular disorders (e.g., Friedrich ataxia). Children with hypertrophic cardiomyopathy may present with chest pain, arrhythmias, or exercise intolerance. Infants are likely to die from congestive symptoms, whereas older children do so suddenly. The risk of sudden death is 1%–8% per year, depending on age and other factors.

Restrictive Cardiomyopathy

Restrictive cardiomyopathy presents with significant diastolic dysfunction. Marked biatrial enlargement is present due to chronically elevated ventricular filling pressures. Restrictive cardiomyopathies may have genetic (e.g., sarcomeric mutations), acquired (e.g., sarcoidosis), and mixed (e.g., amyloidosis) etiologies. Restrictive cardiomyopathy is very rare (approximately 3% of pediatric cardiomyopathies). Children with restrictive cardiomyopathy may present with congestive failure, failure to thrive, or syncope. These patients are at risk for sudden death due to ischemia and ischemia-related complications. Pulmonary hypertension may be a significant issue.

Tachycardia-Induced Cardiomyopathy

The presence of a prolonged rapid heart rate can result in a phenotypic presentation that mimics dilated cardiomyopathy. Supraventricular tachycardias (e.g., atrial flutter or orthodromic reciprocating tachycardia) are most common. Sustained ventricular arrhythmias occasionally precipitate heart failure. Catecholaminergic polymorphic ventricular tachycardia and Brugada syndrome are examples of genetic disorders resulting in mutations in myocardial ion channels (ion channelopathies). These patients can present with sudden death or malignant ventricular arrhythmias resulting in acute myocardial dysfunction. If an arrhythmia is the primary disease process, conversion to sinus rhythm or rate control almost always improves cardiac function.

Arrhythmogenic Right Ventricular Cardiomyopathy/Dysplasia

Arrhythmogenic right ventricular cardiomyopathy/dysplasia (ARVC/D) is characterized by fatty infiltration of the right ventricular free wall. Roughly one-third of cases are familial, and several gene mutations have been identified. The electrocardiogram shows T-wave inversions, an epsilon wave, and QRS duration greater than 110 milliseconds in V_1–V_3. A cardiac MRI may show fibrous and fatty changes in the right ventricle. Afflicted patients present with decreased right ventricular function, arrhythmias, and sudden death.

Ventricular Noncompaction

Left ventricular noncompaction is categorized as a unique cardiomyopathy. Noncompaction refers to the pathologic finding of a developmental failure to form compact ventricular myocardium, leading to excessive and unusual trabeculations, most evident in the apical aspect of the left ventricle. Noncompaction cardiomyopathy may exist in isolation or in association with congenital heart disease, specifically AV septal defects, pulmonary stenosis, and hypoplastic left heart syndrome. The diagnosis is established by echocardiogram or cardiac MRI. Noncompacted left ventricles may have decreased systolic function, chamber dilation, and hypertrophy with characteristic heavy trabeculations.

Myocardial Ischemia

Ischemic cardiomyopathy is common among adults but rare in children. In patients with an anomalous left coronary artery from the pulmonary artery, myocardial ischemia develops as PVR falls, decreasing the perfusion pressure driving coronary blood flow. Although uncommon, coronary ischemia may develop after any operation involving the aortic root or coronary arteries. In patients with Kawasaki disease who develop coronary aneurysms, luminal stenosis or thrombosis may occur, either of which may cause myocardial ischemia.

Rejection of the Transplanted Heart

Transplant rejection is an immune response against the myocytes and endothelial cells, resulting in myocardial inflammation, cytokine release, and cell death from necrosis. The incidence of rejection is higher in the first 3 months after transplantation. When compared with adults, rejection in children is twice as likely to cause hemodynamic compromise.

Systemic Diseases

A number of systemic diseases result in heart failure. Children with severe sepsis or septic shock may develop reversible myocardial dysfunction, likely due to mitochondrial dysfunction and myocardial inflammation. Postresuscitation myocardial dysfunction is characterized by myocardial edema that causes decreased contractility, reduced left ventricular EDV, and impaired relaxation. It improves over several days. Patients with significant systemic or pulmonary hypertension may develop heart failure. High-output cardiac failure may be seen with arteriovenous malformations or large coronary-cameral or arteriovenous fistulae. Thyroid disorders and other endocrinopathies, such as Addison disease, various drugs, and several toxins, can result in heart failure.

PATHOPHYSIOLOGY

Cellular Adaptations in the Heart Failure Syndrome

Contractile Apparatus

Myocardial contractility involves excitation–contraction coupling, a calcium-dependent process. Myocyte calcium handling becomes dysregulated in the failing heart, leading to a depletion of sarcoplasmic reticulum calcium stores, altered sensitization of the contractile apparatus, and ultimately impacts the amplitude and duration of calcium release and contractile force generation. In patients with ventricular dilation, as the myocardial fibers become excessively stretched, force generation becomes less efficient (Frank–Starling relationship) (**Fig. 49.1**), also secondary to an altered calcium set-point in the contractile apparatus. One common physiologic feature of heart failure is a shift in the diastolic pressure–volume relationship to preserve stroke volume at a higher EDV and filling pressure. With progressive increases in the EDV, the wall tension in the ventricle increases, driving up myocardial energy consumption and increasing stroke work during systole (Laplace's law).

Neurohormonal Response

The neurohormonal adaptation to stress is initially adaptive, yet maladaptive in the chronic state. The sympathetic nervous system is activated, leading to elevated levels of circulating epinephrine and norepinephrine, which promote tachycardia, myocardial contractility (via β_1-adrenergic receptors), and arterial and venous vasoconstriction (via α-adrenergic receptors). This surge in catecholamines is lifesaving in a "flight-or-fight" response but, when sustained, contributes to tissue injury, including myocyte apoptosis. Renin–aldosterone–angiotensin system (RAAS) outflow increases sodium and water retention, increasing the circulating volume. Angiotensin augments afterload through vasoconstriction and promotes cardiac hypertrophy. Systemic cortisol, vasopressin, and endothelin-1 are also increased, further enhancing vasoconstriction. Globally, vascular and cardiac nitric oxide production is increased through eNOS and iNOS, which acutely decreases preload, reduces afterload, and augments end-organ perfusion through vasorelaxation. However, chronic elevations in NO promote apoptosis and inflammation, decrease inotropy, and contribute to adrenergic desensitization.

Various natriuretic peptides, some released in response to myocardial wall tension, such as *B-type natriuretic peptide*, counteract the RAAS and promote sodium natriuresis, contributing to chronic hyponatremia. Natriuretic peptides also cause transient vasodilatation, suppress inflammation, and may promote lusitropy. Tumor necrosis factor, IL-1, and IL-6 are endogenously produced by cardiomyocytes and are produced systemically in heart failure patients. These cytokines, among others, trigger further proinflammatory cascades, which have negative inotropic effects and contribute to cardiotoxicity, apoptosis, hypertrophy, extracellular matrix remodeling, and altered calcium homeostasis.

Cellular Adaptation and Energetics

Sustained tachycardia to increase cardiac output comes with a high energy cost and generally occurs as a late response. Extreme, invariant, and sustained

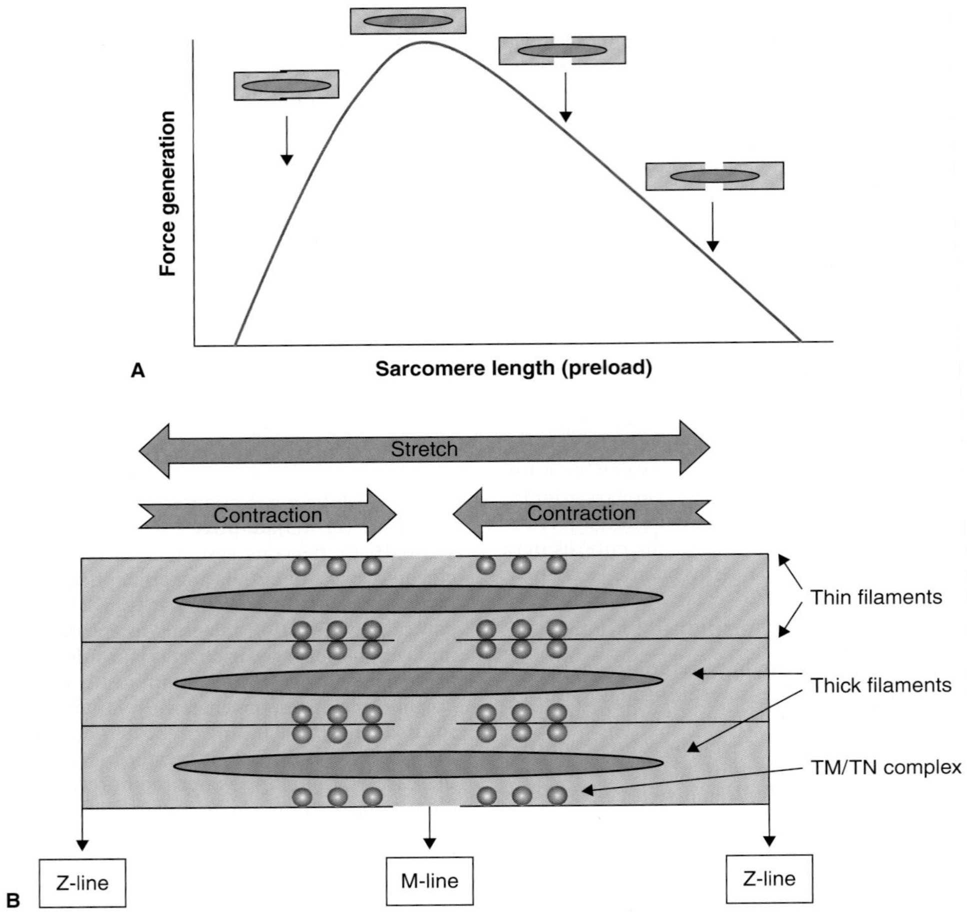

FIGURE 49.1. Frank–Starling relationship. **A:** As the sarcomere stretches, potential force generation increases, peaks, and diminishes with overstretch. Small stylized sarcomeric units demonstrate progressive stretch from left to right. **B:** A sarcomeric unit, demonstrating thick filaments (myosin heavy/light chains) and thin filaments (actin complexed with their associated tropomyosin/troponin [TM/TN] proteins). Lateral movement of the sarcomere during contraction brings the Z-lines closer together in systole. Excessive stretch in diastole, with progressive increases in EDV, decreases maximal force generation.

sinus tachycardia often portends cardiovascular collapse. After fetal life, individual cardiac myocytes respond to a wide variety of stressors (e.g., circulating catecholamines and increased afterload) with hypertrophy instead of proliferation. In response to stress, the myocytes are reprogrammed to express different isoforms of myosin heavy chain (MHC), switching to fetal α-MHC, which is poorly contractile and energetically inefficient. Thus, tachyphylaxis to hormonal mediators, inefficient and poorly contractile MHC, progressive hypertrophy, increased wall tension, and increased energy consumption set up a vicious cycle contributing to the heart failure syndrome.

Ventricular Remodeling

In response to decreased perfusion of critical tissues (e.g., brain, kidneys), the body signals the heart to increase stroke volume, contractility, and heart rate. The ventricles shift rightward along their end-diastolic pressure–volume relationship (EDPVR), increasing EDV and eventually elevating end-diastolic pressure (EDP) as limited by diastolic compliance (**Fig. 49.2**). In order for the ventricle to relieve wall tension under loaded conditions, the myocardium undergoes remodeling. Cardiac remodeling has been defined as "genomic expression resulting in molecular, cellular, and interstitial changes that are manifested clinically as changes in size, shape, and function of the heart after cardiac injury." Inflammation, matric metalloproteinase activity, and myofibroblast activation contribute to diastolic noncompliance. Decreased diastolic compliance and an elevated EDP further increase EDV to relieve pressure, contribute to further increases in wall tension, and set up a progressive process leading to detrimental myocardial remodeling.

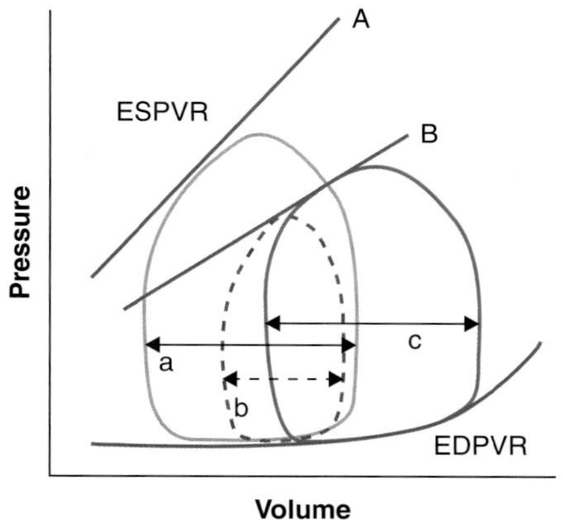

FIGURE 49.2. Compensation during systolic heart failure. Decreased inotropy (systolic failure) shifts the PV-loop along its end-systolic pressure–volume relationship (ESPVR) from *line A* to *line B*, resulting in a decreased stroke volume (SV, *arrow a* to *arrow b*). During compensation, the ventricle restores SV (*arrow c*) by increasing its end-diastolic volume (EDV), which necessitates operating at a higher filling pressure secondary to the shape of the end-diastolic pressure–volume relationship (EDPVR). Worsening diastolic compliance shifts the EDPVR upward or increases its slope, resulting in a similar decrease in SV (not shown), forcing the ventricle to increase inotropy to preserve SV, and drives tachycardia to preserve cardiac output.

CLASSIFICATION AND EVALUATION

Patient History

In a neonate or young infant, parents should be queried about the feeding history, including the volume of feeds, diaphoresis with feeding, and time to completion of feeds. Irritability with feeding may be a sign of underlying coronary ischemia or gut hypoperfusion. Failure to thrive is common in infants with heart failure. A careful maternal history is important. Maternal diabetes or exposure to lithium or alcohol is associated with congenital heart defects or cardiomyopathy. A maternal viral illness in late gestation may be associated with viral myocarditis in the neonate. Maternal nonsteroidal anti-inflammatory use may lead to premature closure of the ductus arteriosus that manifests as pulmonary hypertension and right heart failure soon after birth. Older children with acute heart failure may have signs or symptoms attributed to the respiratory or gastrointestinal systems that distract from considering a cardiac diagnosis. The history should include exposure to drugs or toxins, such as use of anthracyclines for treatment of malignancies.

A careful family history is also important in children with suspected heart failure. Inquiry should be made regarding relatives with congenital heart disease, cardiomyopathies, arrhythmias, sudden death, or muscular diseases (all of which are associated with hereditary transmission). Nearly one-fourth of pediatric cardiomyopathy patients have a family history of cardiomyopathy. Screening of first-degree relatives by echocardiogram, electrocardiogram, and/or genetic testing may be indicated following a diagnosis of a cardiomyopathy in an index case.

Physical Examination

A general assessment is made of the child's appearance (nutritional state, activity level, and color). Tachycardia is present in children with heart failure (compensatory response to limited stroke volume). The pulse pressure may be widened with low diastolic blood pressure in children with run-off lesions, such as a large ductus arteriosus, unrepaired common arterial trunk (truncus arteriosus), or an arterial-venous malformation. The systolic blood pressure is preserved except in patients with cardiogenic shock. Four extremity blood pressure measurements should be obtained in neonates with heart failure to assess for aortic arch obstruction. The systemic oxygen saturation should be measured via pulse oximetry to assess for hypoxemia and cyanotic congenital heart disease.

A detailed cardiac examination begins with an assessment of the precordium. Bulging just to the left of the sternum suggests long-standing cardiomegaly. A prominent right ventricular impulse or second heart sound may occur in children with right ventricular hypertrophy from pulmonary hypertension. A palpable thrill may suggest significant systemic ventricular outflow tract obstruction. In older children and adolescents, the neck should be assessed for signs of jugular venous distention.

The assessment of the respiratory system begins with a visual inspection for tachypnea, retractions, nasal flaring, or tracheal tugging. The abdomen should be inspected for hepatomegaly (common) or abdominal masses (rare, pheochromocytoma or medulloblastoma). In infants, the head and liver should be auscultated for bruits that suggest an arteriovenous malformation. A neurologic examination should assess muscle strength, bulk, and tone to screen for neuromuscular disorders.

Laboratory, Radiographic, and Cardiac Evaluation

The initial evaluation for all patients includes a chest X-ray, electrocardiogram, echocardiogram, and basic laboratory studies as discussed further below. Advanced testing may then be indicated in a subset of patients based on the clinical scenario and findings of these initial screening tests (**Table 49.2**). A cardiac-to-total-thoracic ratio on chest radiograph of greater than 0.55 in infants or greater than 0.5 in older children

TABLE 49.2

Diagnostic Testing for Children with Suspected Heart Failure

	ALL PATIENTS	SELECTED PATIENTS
Imaging	Chest radiograph Echocardiogram	Cardiac magnetic resonance imaging
Blood tests	Electrolytes Renal function Liver function tests Complete blood count Thyroid function tests Brain natriuretic peptide	Blood gases Troponin Viral serology ESR, CRP Lactate, pyruvate Ammonia Amino acids Carnitine/acylcarnitine Selenium Chromosomal analysis Genetic testing for cardiomyopathies
Other	Electrocardiogram	Cardiac catheterization Myocardial biopsy Urine (carnitine, ketones, amino and organic acids) Muscle biopsy

ESR, erythrocyte sedimentation rate; CRP, C-reactive protein.

is abnormal and suggests cardiomegaly. The cardiac silhouette size may be normal in fulminant viral myocarditis and severe cardiac dysfunction, if the chambers have not had time to dilate. In a minority of cases, a chest X-ray will give specific clues to the type of underlying cardiac disease.

EKG assessment may reveal left axis deviation, which can be seen in patients with complete atrioventricular septal defects. Those with acute viral myocarditis may have low voltage, ST segment changes, repolarization abnormalities, Q-waves, or arrhythmias. Patients with restrictive cardiomyopathy typically have prominent P-waves. Symptomatic patients with an anomalous left coronary artery from the pulmonary artery often have a deep, wide Q-wave in leads I, AVL, or V5–V7.

A complete echocardiogram is an important component of the evaluation. The normal left ventricular *shortening fraction* is 28%–40% and the *ejection fraction* 56%–78%. Gradients across the atrioventricular or semilunar valves and intracardiac shunting may be assessed using color Doppler interrogation. Intracardiac clots, which may develop due to stasis of blood flow in patients with poor myocardial function, may also be identified. In patients with dilated cardiomyopathy, the echocardiogram will demonstrate an enlarged and globally dysfunctional left ventricle, often associated with left atrial enlargement. Occasionally, the right ventricle and right atrium are dilated. In children with hypertrophic cardiomyopathy, echocardiographic findings include asymmetric hypertrophy of the interventricular septum, and less commonly hypertrophy of the free wall and apex. There may be systolic anterior motion of the mitral valve leaflets leading to dynamic left ventricular outflow tract obstruction. In restrictive cardiomyopathy, the striking finding on the echocardiogram is marked dilatation of both atrial chambers. Patients with noncompaction cardiomyopathy have a thin epicardial band of ventricular myocardium. Color flow by Doppler may be seen into the trabeculations of the noncompacted myocardium.

Initial laboratory studies include basic chemistries and a complete blood count. Hyponatremia and hypochloremia may be present due to free water retention. The blood urea nitrogen (BUN) and creatinine may be elevated in patients with inadequate renal perfusion. Anemia is present in approximately one-half of children with new onset acute heart failure. Polycythemia may suggest an unrecognized long-standing cyanotic heart defect. Thyroid function tests should be obtained as thyrotoxicosis may cause heart failure. Plasma brain natriuretic peptide (BNP) levels are typically elevated in patients with heart failure, and the trend of BNP may be a useful prognostic indicator of both disease progression and response to therapy.

Second-tier testing for many cardiomyopathy patients is warranted. Those with suspected inborn errors of metabolism should have blood tested for amino acids, a carnitine/acylcarnitine profile, lactate, pyruvate, and ammonia and urine tested for carnitine, ketones, and amino and organic acids. Genetic testing is available for a number of specific gene mutations or chromosomal abnormalities that cause dilated or hypertrophic cardiomyopathy.

Cardiac MRI has a growing role in the assessment of children with heart failure, although indications in critically ill children are less well established.

Right and left ventricular function and shunts can be precisely quantified and chamber volumes tracked serially. The presence of late gadolinium enhancement is suggestive of myocardial necrosis or fibrosis.

Cardiac catheterization for assessment of hemodynamic parameters may be useful in a subset of children with heart failure, but it is associated with a number of risks related to the procedure and sedation or anesthesia must be used judiciously. Patients with palliated or repaired congenital heart disease who present with acute heart failure warrant consideration for a diagnostic catheterization if noninvasive evaluation fails to establish a definitive diagnosis. In patients with suspected coronary artery abnormalities for whom the noninvasive imaging is inadequate, coronary angiography may be obtained. In heart transplant candidates with an elevated transpulmonary gradient (>15 mm Hg), assessment of the reactivity of the pulmonary vascular bed may be determined by vasodilator testing with oxygen, inhaled nitric oxide, and other drugs. Traditionally, those with a pretransplant baseline PVR greater than 6 Wood units per m^2 or greater than 4 Wood units per m^2 with vasodilator testing are at significant risk for posttransplant right ventricular failure. In patients with suspected myocarditis, a myocardial biopsy may be obtained for histology, viral polymerase chain reaction, and electron microscopy. In heart transplantation patients who present with acute heart failure, a myocardial biopsy should generally be obtained to evaluate for rejection. Samples should be assessed for cellular and antibody-mediated rejection.

CHAPTER 50 ■ CARDIOMYOPATHY, MYOCARDITIS, AND MECHANICAL CIRCULATORY SUPPORT

WILLIAM G. HARMON, APARNA HOSKOTE, AND ANN KARIMOVA

Cardiomyopathy is a disorder of cardiac myocyte structure or function. A cardiomyopathy can arise as a primary diagnosis, or result as a comorbidity from a systemic disease (e.g., systemic hypertension or infectious, rheumatologic, or metabolic disorders).

CARDIOMYOPATHIES

Dilated Cardiomyopathy

Incidence, Etiology, and Classification

After infancy, dilated cardiomyopathy (DCM) is the most common diagnosis leading to cardiac transplantation in both children and adults. Boys and African Americans are at a higher risk. DCM is most commonly diagnosed during the first year of life (41% of all patients), reflecting the genetic disease burden. The etiologic classifications include (a) idiopathic DCM (66%), (b) myocarditis (16%), (c) neuromuscular disorders (9%), (d) familial DCM (5%), (e) inborn errors of metabolism (4%), and (f) malformation syndromes (1%) (**Table 50.1**). With genetic testing, most children can now be placed into specific diagnostic categories.

Pathophysiology of Heart Failure in Dilated Cardiomyopathy

DCM arises as a result of an intrinsic or extrinsic cardiomyocyte abnormality or cell injury. Decreased ventricular function and progressive left-ventricular (LV) dilatation are the phenotypic hallmarks of DCM. Decreasing myocardial function and falling cardiac output (CO) initiate compensatory mechanisms to maintain blood pressure and organ perfusion. The baroreceptor response is a primary mechanism that opposes a fall in CO. Activation of the renin–angiotensin–aldosterone system augments preload (promotes fluid retention) and systemic vascular resistance (SVR) (renin-induced peripheral vasoconstriction). Over time (and with progressive myocardial dysfunction), these normal physiologic responses become maladaptive and harmful to a failing heart. A normal heart hypertrophies to compensate for chronic volume load as a means to decrease the luminal radius and lower wall stress and afterload. However, progressive LV dilation and wall thinning is the hallmark of DCM, representing a worsening cycle of increasing afterload, worsening energy balance, and progressive heart failure.

Diagnostic Testing

The intensivist is involved with DCM patients with uncompensated or fulminant heart failure. **Table 50.2** provides a summary of etiologic diagnostic testing for the presenting patient. A family history is paramount as inheritable conditions present at any age. Echocardiography, coronary CT imaging, cardiac magnetic resonance imaging (MRI), catheterization with myocardial biopsy, metabolic testing, and genetic analyses all play a role in diagnosis. MRI provides functional data and the presence and degree of acute myocardial inflammation, fibrosis, or ischemic injury. Serial monitoring of NT-proBNP levels correlates with patient status, and helps guide drug therapy for chronic DCM.

Therapeutic Strategies

The principles of treatment of DCM and myocarditis are similar, with the goal of stabilizing progression of decompensated heart failure (described in a subsequent section of this chapter).

Hypertrophic Cardiomyopathy

Incidence, Etiology, and Genetics

Hypertrophic cardiomyopathy (HCM) is a diverse set of disorders with a diagnostic phenotype of inappropriate cardiac hypertrophy with clinical effects that include asymptomatic hypertrophy, clinical heart failure, arrhythmia, or early *sudden cardiac death* (SCD) (see **Table 50.3**). HCM is the most common inherited cardiac disease and the most common specific cause of SCD in children (found in 36%). HCM represents ~42% of diagnosed pediatric cardiomyopathy cases. Hundreds of specific gene defects have been implicated in HCM, involving 30-plus genes encoding myofilaments (30%–50% of patients), Z-disc (~5% of patients), calcium-handling or mitochondrial proteins.

TABLE 50.1

Selected Causes of Dilated Cardiomyopathy (DCM) in Children

Gene Defects (Sarcomeric and Other, Often Classified as Familial DCM)
Myosin (MYH7)
Actin (ACTC)
Titin (TTN)
Troponin I (TNNI3)
Troponin T (TNNT2)
Tafazzin mutations
Many others. Can be tested for using research and commercial sources, as guided by a cardiac geneticist.
Infectious/Inflammatory
Previous viral myocarditis (acute and chronic)
Nonviral infections (Chagas disease, and others)
Inflammatory/toxic drug reactions (anthracycline, and others)
Neuromuscular
Duchenne muscular dystrophy
Becker muscular dystrophy
Emery–Dreifuss muscular dystrophy
Metabolic
Fatty acid oxidation defects (e.g., VLCAD, LCHAD, LCAD deficiency, others)
Propionic aciduria
Mitochondrial disorders
Carnitine deficiency
Nutritional deficiencies
(Many others, metabolic consultation is generally recommended)
Syndromes Associated with DCM
Barth syndrome
Friedrich ataxia
Noonan syndrome (HCM is more common)
Kearns–Sayre syndrome
Others—DCM is seen in many children with nonclassifiable syndromic features
Idiopathic
A primary genetic abnormality is presumed for many of these children. In previous decades, the majority of children were classified as having idiopathic disease. This is progressively decreasing and now an etiology is possible in the majority of children thoroughly studied.

VLCAD, Very long-chain acyl-CoA dehydrogenase; LCHAD, long-chain 3-hydroxyacyl-Co-A dehydrogenase; LCAD, long chain Acyl-CoA dehydrogenase deficiency.
Anatomical abnormalities (such as anomalous left coronary artery from pulmonary artery—ALCAPA or undiagnosed coarctation of the aorta) and arrhythmias (such as atrial ectopic tachycardia—AET) have to be excluded as underlying causes for left-ventricular dysfunction.

Diagnosis and Screening

HCM is often discovered in the PICU after an undiagnosed child is resuscitated from a sports-related cardiac arrest. HCM is also diagnosed during evaluation of an outflow murmur (from outflow tract obstruction), during evaluation for syncope, from a history that details risk factors such as sports-related syncope, or a family history of genetic heart disease or early sudden death.

Risk Stratification and Therapeutic Strategies

Treatment goals for HCM include alleviation of symptoms and prevention of SCD. If the risk of SCD is high, the child should receive an *automated implanted cardiodefibrillator* (AICD). Other interventions should include restricted physical activity, as exercise-induced catecholamine release exacerbates LV outflow tract (LVOT) obstruction, promotes LV ischemia, and induces lethal arrhythmia. Exertional symptoms are treated with β-adrenergic (e.g., propranolol) or calcium-channel blocking agents (e.g., verapamil). These agents improve diastolic filling by slowing heart rate, decrease dynamic LVOT obstruction by negative inotropic effects, improve angina symptoms by lowering myocardial oxygen demand, and in the case of calcium-channel blockers,

TABLE 50.2

Etiologic Agents in Myocarditis

VIRUSES	NONVIRAL INFECTIOUS PATHOGENS	NONINFECTIOUS ETIOLOGIES
Adenovirus	**Bacteria**	**Pharmaceuticals**
Arbovirus	*Borrelia burgdorferi*	Acetazolamide
Cytomegalovirus	*Brucella melitensis*	Amphotericin B
Enterovirus	*Chlamydia pneumoniae*	Anthracyclines
Coxsackie A and B	*Chlamydia psittaci*	Cephalosporins
Echovirus	*Clostridium*	Cocaine
Poliovirus	*Klebsiella*	Cyclophosphamide
Epstein–Barr virus	*Legionella pneumophila*	Digoxin
Hepatitis A, B, and C	*Leptospira*	Diuretics
Herpes simplex virus	*Meningococcus*	Dobutamine
Human immunodeficiency virus	*Mycobacteria*	Indomethacin
Influenza A	*Mycoplasma pneumonia*	Isoniazid
Measles	*Salmonella*	Methyldopa
Mumps	*Streptococcus species*	Neomercazole
Parvovirus B19	*Treponema pallidum*	Penicillin
Rabies	Tuberculosis	Phenylbutazone
Respiratory syncytial virus	Typhoid	Phenytoin
Rhinovirus	**Rickettsial**	Sulfonamides
Rubella	*Rickettsia rickettsii*	Tetracycline
Rubeola	*Rickettsia tsutsugamushi*	Tricyclic
Vaccinia virus	**Fungi and yeasts**	Antidepressants
Varicella	Actinomyces	**Hypersensitivity/autoimmune**
	Aspergillus	Celiac disease
	Candida	Diabetes mellitus
	Coccidioides	Hashimoto thyroiditis
	Cryptococcus	Mixed connective tissue disease
	Histoplasma	Myasthenia gravis
	Protozoa	Pernicious anemia
	Entamoeba histolytica	Rheumatoid arthritis
	Trypanosoma cruzi	Rheumatic fever
	Toxoplasma gondii	Scleroderma
	Parasites	Systemic lupus erythematosus
	Echinococcus granulosus	Takayasu arteritis
	Heterophyiasis	Thrombocytopenic purpura
	Plasmodium falciparum	Ulcerative colitis
	Schistosomiasis	Wegener granulomatosis
	Taenia solium (Cysticercosis)	Whipple disease
	Toxocara canis	**Toxins and others**
	Trichinella spiralis	Cornstarch
		Diphtheria
		Kawasaki disease
		Sarcoidosis
		Pertussis
		Scorpion venom
		Smallpox vaccine

improve microvascular perfusion. Vasodilators (e.g., angiotensin-converting enzyme inhibitors [ACEi]) should be avoided as afterload reduction can worsen dynamic LVOT narrowing. Digoxin is relatively contraindicated as increased contractility could worsen obstruction. Diuretics must be judiciously titrated to maintain sufficient preload and prevent dynamic outflow tract collapse; the stiff ventricle requires high filling pressures. In the PICU, phenylephrine or norepinephrine is used to treat acute hypotension in obstructive HCM (similar to use for tetralogy of Fallot "spells"). Inotropes (e.g., dopamine, dobutamine, and epinephrine) are relatively contraindicated. Septal reduction surgery should be considered for patients with symptomatic or severe resting outflow tract obstruction despite aggressive medication titration.

TABLE 50.3

Hypertrophic Cardiomyopathy—Selected Etiologies and Associations

Gene Defects Found to be Causative
Myosin heavy chain (MYH7)
Myosin light chain (MYL3)
Cardiac troponins (TNNTT2, TPMI, TNNI3)
Titin
Actin
Mitochondrial proteins
Calcium-handling proteins
Z-disc proteins
Others—specific gene defects are more commonly found in HCM, as opposed to DCM
Metabolic/Storage Disorders
Pompe disease
Danon disease
PRKAG2 familial glycogen storage disease
Hunter disease
Hurler syndrome
Fabry disease
Associated Syndromes
Noonan syndrome
Friedrich ataxia
Barth syndrome
LEOPARD (multiple lentigines) syndrome

HCM, hypertrophic cardiomyopathy; DCM, dilated cardiomyopathy; LEOPARD, lentigines, electrocardiographic abnormalities, ocular hypertelorism, pulmonary stenosis, abnormal genitalia, retarded growth, deafness.

Restrictive Cardiomyopathy

Incidence and Etiology

Restrictive cardiomyopathy (RCM) is a rare form of cardiomyopathy characterized by severe biventricular diastolic dysfunction and marked biatrial enlargement. Echocardiography demonstrates small-to-normal ventricular dimensions and profound atrial dilation, creating the "Mickey Mouse" appearance on apical four-chamber imaging. Gene defects in troponin (TTNI3) and the sarcomeric protein desmin have been implicated in familial cases.

Pathophysiology and Treatment Strategies

RCM leads to pulmonary venous congestion, and children often present with nonspecific respiratory symptoms. High filling pressures lead to rapid progression of pulmonary vascular disease. SCD can be the presenting sign. Echocardiography is the major diagnostic tool, and cardiac catheterization can define hemodynamics. MRI can rule out pericardial disease or further define and trend diastolic filling parameters. RCM is a high-risk disease, and many centers transplant early (40% undergo transplantation, 20% die without transplant within 2 years of diagnosis). Prior to transplantation, symptoms are treated with careful diuresis. No specific therapy is promoted to treat diastolic dysfunction.

Arrhythmogenic Right-Ventricular Cardiomyopathy

Arrhythmogenic right-ventricular cardiomyopathy (ARVC) is an increasing cause of SCD in children. It is a group of genetic heart diseases caused by several gene abnormalities of the desmosomal complex that lead to fibro-fatty infiltration of either ventricle, but classically affects the right side. Most cases are inherited in an autosomal dominant manner. Ventricular arrhythmias typically occur during adolescence or young adult years. *Epsilon waves*—low-amplitude signals between the end of the QRS complex to the onset of the T wave—are the most characteristic ECG findings. Many patients, particularly with near SCD, benefit from an ICD.

Left-Ventricular Noncompaction

LV noncompaction (LVNC) is a state of abnormal myocardial morphogenesis characterized by diffuse LV trabeculations and deep intertrabecular recesses, referred to as "spongy myocardium." LVNC as a cause of LV dysfunction is a phenotypic component in 9% of childhood cardiomyopathies. Approximately 20% of LVNC cases have an associated congenital heart defect (septal defects, Ebstein anomaly, or hypoplastic left heart syndrome). LVNC is diagnosed by echocardiography, showing deep intertrabecular recesses. Most patients demonstrate reduced LV function. Patients who develop heart failure should be treated similar to DCM, with attention to arrhythmia and thromboembolic prevention.

Acquired Cardiomyopathies

Primary pediatric cardiomyopathies result largely from inborn sarcomeric or metabolic abnormalities. In adults, cardiomyopathies occur secondary to atherosclerosis-induced coronary ischemia or chronic hypertension. Children at risk for secondary LV dysfunction include Kawasaki disease, renal disease, vitamin D deficiency, and cancer survivors.

Anthracycline-induced Cardiomyopathy

Anthracycline myocardial injury mechanisms include free radical generation leading to cardiocyte mitochondrial damage. Clinical cardiotoxicity can be acute or of late onset and requires echocardiographic monitoring throughout all stages of care. Current pediatric chemotherapy protocols limit anthracycline exposure to a cumulative dose (<300 mg/m^2).

Vitamin D Deficiency–induced Cardiomyopathy

DCM from hypocalcemia associated with vitamin D deficiency and rickets is described in dark-skinned infants, exclusively breastfed and not on calcium or vitamin D supplements. They present with a low serum calcium/ionized calcium, elevated parathormone, and low vitamin D.

MYOCARDITIS

Myocarditis is an inflammatory disease associated with lymphocytic infiltrate and cardiomyocyte degeneration not ischemic in origin. An endomyocardial biopsy diagnosis is not always available. A clinical definition is the presentation of new-onset heart failure with ventricular dysfunction with positive markers of inflammation, with or without positive virology in a previously well child, and with no structural heart disease.

Etiology

Myocarditis may be caused by a number of infective and noninfective agents (see **Table 50.4**).

Eosinophilic and Giant Cell Myocarditis

Eosinophilic myocarditis is a rare entity characterized by eosinophilia and myocardial inflammation with infiltrating eosinophils. It is attributed to eosinophilic syndromes, allergic reactions, autoimmune diseases, parasitic infections, and postvaccination. Patients present with congestive heart failure, ventricular arrhythmias, heart block, or myocardial infarction and have a characteristic endomyocardial biopsy. Steroid treatment may be helpful. *Idiopathic giant cell myocarditis* is a rare disease. Patients present with congestive cardiac failure, ventricular arrhythmias, or heart block and have an endomyocardial biopsy with giant cells and active inflammation. Despite institution of medical therapy, patients continue to have poorly

TABLE 50.4

Selected Etiologic Testing for a Child Presenting with Acute Myocardial Dysfunction

Immediate Evaluation

- Clinical and family history
- Basic chemistries (including total and ionized calcium, magnesium, glucose, renal profile, liver function tests including aminotransferases, lactic acid)
- Complete and differential blood count (neutropenia, lymphocytosis), coagulation profile
- Chest X-ray (cardiomegaly, pulmonary congestion/edema, persistent left lower lobe collapse from compression of left main bronchus by enlarged left atrium)
- 12-lead ECG (voltage changes, ST-T changes)
- Echocardiogram (to rule out anatomic abnormalities, assess degree of ventricular dysfunction)
- C-reactive protein, erythrocyte sedimentation rate
- Troponin, creatine kinase isoenzyme (CK-MB), B-type natriuretic peptide (BNP), *N*-terminal fragment (NT-proBNP)

Further Etiologic Testing

- **Microbiologic studies:** Viral IgM, PCR virology in serum, urine, stool, nasopharyngeal, tracheal aspirate (Enterovirus, Adenovirus, Parvovirus and then extended panel), Viral IgM, bacterial tests
- **Metabolic studies:** Urine organic acids, serum amino acids, ammonia, urine glycosaminoglycans, carnitine levels, acylcarnitine profile, cholesterol/triglycerides, RBC transketolase, red cell folate, transferrin, thiamine, selenium, vacuolated lymphocytes on peripheral smear
- Amino acid and organic metabolism, disorders of fatty acid metabolism, disorders of glycogen metabolism, glycoprotein metabolism, lysosomal storage disorders, mitochondrial disorders
- **Endocrine:** Thyroid studies, parathyroid hormone, vitamin D levels
- **Autoimmune:** Autoantibody screen, antinuclear antibodies, anti-DNA antibodies, anti-Ro
- **Genetic testing:** Barth syndrome

Testing for Further Management or Diagnosis in Selected Cases:

- Metabolic and genetic consultation
- Cardiac MRI
- Cardiac catheterization
- Endomyocardial biopsy (for both electron microscopy and viral PCR testing)
- Peripheral muscle biopsy
- Electrophysiologic studies and 24-hour Holter monitoring when primary arrhythmia suspected

controlled heart failure and arrhythmias that may respond to aggressive immunosuppressive therapy.

Epidemiology

The true incidence of myocarditis is underestimated. Acute viral myocarditis accounts for 7.5%–28% of SCD in children and young adults without previous heart disease (42% in infants with SCD). Myocarditis evolves into cardiomyopathy in ~10% of children and young adults. This may be an underestimation due to the lack of a biopsy or unknown subclinical cases.

Pathogenesis and Histology

The pathogenesis involves direct invasion by the cardiotropic virus, local inflammation, and activation of the humoral and cell-mediated innate immune responses. *Acute myocarditis* lasts up to 4 days with viremia, myocyte necrosis, macrophage activation, and release of cytokines. *Subacute myocarditis* is the next phase with proliferation of infiltrating mononuclear cells, cytotoxic T and B lymphocytes, and natural killer cells and lasts between 4 and 14 days with clearing of the virus. Finally, *chronic myocarditis* involves fibrosis and cardiac dilatation. The histologic findings used to define myocarditis (i.e., Dallas criteria) are described in **Table 50.5**.

Clinical Manifestations

Acute fulminant myocarditis (20%–30% of patients with myocarditis) involves a very acute onset of hemodynamic instability, congestive heart failure, and need for inotropic or mechanical circulatory support (MCS). The patients have a short viral prodrome with distinct onset of symptoms (<14 days), significant cardiac dysfunction requiring at least inotropic support to maintain CO and perfusion, normal cardiac size to less than moderate cardiomegaly on chest radiography, and normal LV end-diastolic volume by echocardiography (LV end-diastolic *Z*-score of <3). On histology, an intense inflammatory response is seen with significant lymphocytic infiltration and myocyte necrosis.

TABLE 50.5

Clinical Presentation, Histopathology, and Outcome of Myocarditis in Children

TYPE	CLINICAL PRESENTATION	HISTOPATHOLOGY	OUTCOME
Fulminant myocarditis	■ Viral prodrome ■ Distinct onset of illness within 2 wk of presentation ■ Severe cardiovascular compromise with ventricular dysfunction but not usually left-ventricular dilatation ■ Heart block or ventricular arrhythmias ■ Sudden death	■ Multiple foci of active inflammation and necrosis with lymphocytic infiltration, myocyte necrosis ± myocyte degeneration	■ Patients recover or die within 2 wk with complete histologic and functional recovery of the myocardium in survivors
Acute myocarditis	■ Less distinct onset of illness, with established ventricular dysfunction	■ Lymphocytic infiltration ± myocyte necrosis	■ May progress to dilated cardiomyopathy
Chronic active myocarditis	■ Less distinct onset of illness with clinical and histologic relapses; development of moderate ventricular dysfunction	■ Active or borderline associated with chronic inflammatory changes	■ Chronic heart failure
Chronic persistent myocarditis	■ Less distinct onset of illness (despite symptoms, e.g., chest pain, palpitations) but without ventricular dysfunction	■ Persistent histologic infiltrate with foci of myocyte necrosis	■ Chronic heart failure

Acute (nonfulminant) myocarditis has a longer prodrome and presents with a recent history of a nonspecific viral illness, associated with abdominal pain, nausea and vomiting, or coryzal symptoms. Because children are able to compensate for heart dysfunction, the diagnosis is frequently not suspected until acute collapse or sudden death occurs. Fulminant myocarditis usually recovers with supportive measures (93% survival after 5 years follow-up), while nonfulminant myocarditis, which has less intense inflammation but the virus persists in a more indolent form, has only 45% survival without transplant up to 11 years after biopsy.

Chronic myocarditis (from postinfectious immune or systemic autoimmune diseases) manifests as persistent or progressive ventricular dysfunction, arrhythmias, and chronic congestive heart failure. The disease often presents as an acute form of DCM.

Age-specific Differences in Presentation

Newborns and infants present with fever, poor feeding, vomiting, irritability or listlessness, periodic episodes of pallor, episodic cyanosis, tachypnea, or respiratory distress. The most common cause in neonates is enteroviral infection. Older children and adolescents commonly report a viral disease (10–14 days) prior to presentation. Initial symptoms are nonspecific and include lethargy, general malaise, diaphoresis, palpitations, rash, exercise intolerance, and low-grade fever. Physical examination is consistent with the findings of congestive heart failure. Dysrhythmias are common. Syncope or sudden death may occur.

Diagnostic Tests

Myocarditis should be suspected in any child (with a structurally normal heart) presenting with new-onset heart failure, unexplained shortness of breath or fatigue, or a new arrhythmia. Tachycardia without a clear cause is an important clue to myocarditis.

Electrocardiogram findings are variable but present in 93%–100% of patients. The most common ECG findings are (a) sinus tachycardia; (b) low-voltage (total voltage <5 mm) QRS complexes (standard and precordial leads) and Q-waves (lateral precordial leads); and (c) ST-T wave changes (flat or inverted T-waves in the standard or lateral precordial leads). Echocardiographic evaluation commonly reveals enlarged ventricular end-systolic and diastolic dimensions, reduced shortening and ejection fractions, and atrioventricular valve regurgitation (especially mitral).

Aspartate aminotransferase elevation is a sensitive marker (sensitivity of 85%). Creatine kinase isoenzyme (CK-MB) and cardiac troponin T (markers for myocardial damage) may be elevated. NT-proBNP is a good marker for persistent LV dysfunction. Viral studies including molecular (PCR) analyses of blood, nasopharyngeal aspirates, tracheal aspirates, and endomyocardial biopsy (when feasible considering hemodynamic conditions) should be performed. Tracheal aspirates have a high yield for viral identification, particularly adenovirus. Complications of biopsy include perforation, hemothorax, dysrhythmia, and death and increased in young patients with myocarditis (particularly those requiring inotropic support). Therefore, emphasis is placed on newer, less-invasive modalities myocarditis, such as MRI, although biopsy may be essential if eosinophilic or giant cell myocarditis is suspected.

THERAPEUTIC STRATEGIES IN CHILDREN WITH CARDIOMYOPATHY OR MYOCARDITIS

Treatment of Acute Decompensated Heart Failure

The initial management of children with acute heart failure is the same for both myocarditis and DCM. The use of diuretics (to reduce fluid overload) and vasodilators (to reduce SVR) may be used in stabilization. Dobutamine or milrinone infusions are administered via peripheral venous access and are first-line agents, if blood pressure allows. Patients in extremis have increased work of breathing due to pulmonary congestion and require positive-pressure ventilation, which also lowers LV afterload, improves energy balance, and increases LV stroke volumes. The process of stabilizing the airway and endotracheal intubation is a high-risk procedure for children with worsening hemodynamic status and has to be carefully managed, with access to emergency extracorporeal membrane oxygenation (ECMO) cannulation in the event of cardiac arrest. There is no ideal agent for induction of anesthesia for children in decompensating heart failure. The attending intensivist should use agents that they are familiar with, and in small doses in compromised patients with careful titration. Medications used for induction of anesthesia include (caveats in parentheses): fentanyl (minimal myocardial depression, short duration of action), etomidate (safe hemodynamic profile, risk of adrenocortical suppression, and limited familiarity), ketamine (increases heart rate and blood pressure, children with end-stage heart failure may not be able to mount a sympathetic response, in which case it can depress myocardial contractility), and midazolam (used with caution in a conservative and supplemental manner in the hands of experienced anesthetist).

In acute cardiogenic shock with acidosis, low-dose epinephrine (~0.05 mcg/kg/min), dopamine (~5 mcg/kg/min), or dobutamine, all increase CO by increasing the contractile state of the myocardium. $\beta 1$ stimulation is also chronotropic, and may be pro-arrhythmic. Milrinone is an inodilator that can increase the cardiac index (CI), lower the capillary wedge pressure, and prevent/lessen low CO syndrome after cardiac surgery. Milrinone is renally eliminated, with a variable elimination half-life of 30 minutes to 3 hours. Levosimendan is an inotropic agent that increases the sensitivity of myofilaments to calcium used outside of the United States as an alternative inotropic therapy in children with heart failure on prolonged catecholamine infusions that cannot be weaned. Diuretics help with reducing fluid overload and pulmonary congestion. Control of the heart rate by controlling temperature and reducing other causes of raised SVR improves filling and maintains preload. In most cases, the goal is to treat acute decompensation with intravenous vasoactive medications and transition to oral therapy using ACE inhibition, diuretics, β-blockade, and aldosterone antagonists. If a patient is not able to be transitioned to oral medications, this is considered to be end-stage, severe heart failure, and as such, mechanical support and cardiac transplantation should be considered as individually appropriate.

Specific Treatment for Myocarditis—Intravenous Immunoglobulin, Steroids, and Antiviral Agents

The use of intravenous immunoglobulin (IVIG) and steroids is favored but controversial. Improved ventricular function but without survival benefit is seen. Steroids have beneficial results in myocarditis associated with autoimmune disorders, vasculitis, dengue, eosinophilic syndromes, and giant cell myocarditis. Combination immunosuppression with monoclonal muromonab-CD3 (OKT3) has been used.

Management of Arrhythmias

Arrhythmias in myocarditis or DCM have to be vigorously treated.

Anticoagulation

Patients with myocarditis or DCM with an LV shortening fraction <20% are at risk of mural thrombi and embolization. Systemic heparin followed by aspirin or warfarin is often used.

Treatment of Chronic Heart Failure

Children are treated, based on adult protocols, using ACEi, β-blockers, aldosterone antagonists, and furosemide or similar diuretic for chronic heart failure. β-Blockers should be used with caution in children in the context of severe ventricular dysfunction. There is insufficient evidence to recommend the use of β-blockers in children with congestive heart failure.

Progressive Heart Failure Unresponsive to Conventional Management

Heart transplantation remains the final option for myocarditis and intractable severe heart failure (failure of conventional medical management). DCM is the most common diagnosis leading to heart transplantation beyond the first year of age. The indications for mechanical support are cardiogenic shock associated with dysrhythmias, severe hemodynamic compromise in fulminant myocarditis, and worsening end-organ function.

MECHANICAL CIRCULATORY SUPPORT

Devices

Extracorporeal Membrane Oxygenation

ECMO has two main advantages: a modification of cardiopulmonary bypass and the most robust form of MCS, ECMO is suitable for cardiopulmonary failure; second, ECMO can be initiated rapidly, even during active cardiopulmonary resuscitation, by insertion of arterial and venous cannulae either peripherally (cervical or femoral vessels) or centrally (via sternotomy). ECMO has a number of limitations. Its use is limited to a few weeks before complications increase and it often precludes ambulation and rehabilitation. The unloading of the failing left ventricle may be inadequate and an atrial septostomy may be necessary. ECMO is suited to patients with an anticipated recovery of native cardiac function within days to weeks.

Ventricular Assist Devices

Pediatric appropriate ventricular assist devices (VADs) include the Berlin Heart EXCOR VAD (most often used). It is a paracorporeal, pulsatile flow device, suitable for all ages with pump chamber volumes of 10–60 mL. Other devices include axial and centrifugal pumps (CentriMag or PediMag, HeartWare, and HeartMate II) that have good short- and long-term results. VADs are classified according to (a) mode of blood flow (pulsatile versus continuous), continuous flow may be driven by either centrifugal or axial pumps; (b) relative position of the pump and patient as extra- or paracorporeal versus intracorporeal (fully implantable), and (c) duration of intended use as temporary, short-term versus durable, long-term devices. Unlike venoarterial ECMO, patients supported with VAD are reliant on their own lung function (**Table 50.6**). Advantages of VADs include stable cannulae and excellent decompression of the left (systemic) atria, enabling extubation, discharge from ICU, and physical and nutritional rehabilitation.

TABLE 50.6

Comparison between Mechanical Support with ECMO versus VAD

	ECMO	VAD
Cardiac support	Yes (biventricular)	Yes (left or biventricular)
Respiratory support	Yes (oxygenator)	No
Decompression of left heart	Yes (via septostomy or vent), can be suboptimal	Yes, optimal
Initiation	Emergency or elective (peripheral or transthoracic access)	Elective (transthoracic access); few percutaneous devices
Anticoagulation	Yes (heparin)	Yes (heparin plus antiplatelet)
Transfusion requirements	Frequent	Less frequent
Duration of support	Days–weeks	Days–months–years

Choice of Device

ECMO is reserved for (a) the emergency institution of support for circulatory collapse when recovery is expected within days; (b) children with significant lung pathology requiring full cardiopulmonary support; or (c) stabilizing patients with unclear or severe end-organ dysfunction to determine reversibility with appropriate therapy. Most institutions consider transition from ECMO to VAD within 7–10 days; this decision depends on a patient's potential for recovery and duration of support.

Short-term centrifugal VADs (CentriMag, PediMag, Deltastream, and Tandem Heart) are suitable for acute processes such as myocarditis or acute cardiac allograft failure where recovery is expected within weeks. They are attractive initial selections for unstable patients in multiorgan system failure (particularly coagulopathy secondary to hepatic dysfunction) awaiting stabilization and transition to a long-term device ("bridge to bridge") or for patients requiring frequent flow titrations, such as those with single-ventricle physiology. Additionally, short-term VADs can be used for temporary support of severe right heart dysfunction following LVAD implantation. Short-term VADs are paracorporeal and patients are usually ICU bound.

Long-term VADs (Berlin Heart EXCOR, HeartWare HVAD and HeartMate II) have a role as a bridge to heart transplantation. In 2012, 25% of pediatric heart transplant recipients were bridged using VADs and ECMO use declined from 9.4% in 2005 to 2.6% in 2010. The survival rates (75%–92%) with long-term VADs are superior to ECMO (45%) for children reaching transplant. For infants and small children with BSA <0.7 m^2, Berlin Heart EXCOR is currently used worldwide, while in bigger children and teenagers there is a wider choice, including implantable pumps such as HeartWare or HeartMate II.

Timing

Optimal timing is critical and a delayed start of MCS in adults who are either in a progressive circulatory decline or in shock is associated with reduced survival. In children, renal and hepatic dysfunction at the time of initiation of MCS increased risk for death during bridge to transplant.

Patient Selection

MCS is considered in children requiring more than one inotrope or who have signs of heart failure with secondary organ dysfunction evidenced by need for a mechanical ventilation, feed intolerance, oliguria, or altered mental status and/or develop biochemical markers of low CO (elevated serum lactate, reduced mixed venous saturation, and renal or hepatic dysfunction). Resting tachycardia and arrhythmias are additional warning signs of a progressive heart failure. There are few absolute contraindications to MCS, and those include irreversible severe brain damage, chromosomal abnormality, prematurity, extremely small size, and conditions that preclude systemic anticoagulation (including implantation of VAD on cardiopulmonary bypass) such as recent hemorrhagic stroke.

Principles of Management

Peri-implantation Management

Preoperative ECHO. Pre-implantation ECHO is needed to exclude intracardiac thrombus, intracardiac shunts, and valvular regurgitation, which need to be addressed at implantation.

Cannulation. Long-term VAD implantation is performed on cardiopulmonary bypass. For LVAD, the cannulation is from the LV apex to the ascending aorta, while for RVAD the cannulae are from the right atrium into the pulmonary artery.

LVAD versus BiVAD. The majority of children can be supported with LVAD only and most centers restrict right heart MCS for severe RV failure with preoperative CVP >20 mm Hg, ascites, severe hepatic dysfunction, and poor RV function on preoperative ECHO.

Bleeding. Acute postimplantation bleeding is a common complication and can be exacerbated by preexisting hepatic dysfunction or the effects of cardiopulmonary bypass.

Adequacy of Mechanical Support. The primary goal of MCS is to restore oxygen delivery to peripheral tissues and the usual markers are followed.

Anticoagulation

Preoperative evaluation includes full clotting profile and thrombophilia screen. Once hemostasis has been achieved, an unfractionated heparin infusion is commenced and its effect monitored using anti-Xa levels and APTT. Long-term anticoagulation is maintained with warfarin or low–molecular weight heparin combined with antiplatelet agents. Most centers use thromboelastogram and platelet function tests to ensure efficacy of anticoagulation.

Weaning

Children with sufficient ventricular recovery should be considered for weaning from VAD. Interestingly, ventricular decompression with VAD combined with medical therapy might restore native heart function in children with end-stage heart failure due to cardiomyopathy. Thus, continuation of a heart failure medication on VAD with periodic checks of underlying ventricular function is common practice.

Complications

Neurologic

Stroke is the leading cause of mortality and morbidity of mechanical support in children. In children supported with pulsatile VAD, the stroke rate was 29%. Implantable continuous-flow devices have encouragingly lower stroke rates of less than 10% in adults.

Hematologic

Major bleeding occurs in 20%–40% of VAD recipients, and many require early surgical reexploration. Intravascular hemolysis caused by mechanical stress in continuous-flow devices can release free hemoglobin and lead to renal dysfunction.

Right-Ventricular Failure

Deterioration of right-ventricular (RV) function is an acute and unpredictable phenomena observed in some patients after LVAD implantation. Aggressive pharmacologic support of the RV with inotropes, pulmonary vasodilators, and diuretics, as well as rhythm control with pacing and/or antiarrhythmics, is often needed for days before the RV adapts.

Infection

Infection occurs in 30%–50% of pediatric VAD recipients and is a risk factor for reduced survival.

Other Adverse Events

Other adverse events in children supported with a pulsatile VAD include respiratory failure (continuous need for respiratory support) in 29%, hepatic dysfunction in 9%, and renal dysfunction in 12%. Arrhythmias are reported in 9% of patients and are usually well tolerated once the left ventricle is mechanically supported and the heart rhythm can be controlled pharmacologically. Device malfunction is relatively rare.

OUTCOMES FOR CHILDREN WITH MYOCARDITIS AND CARDIOMYOPATHIES (INCLUDING THOSE SUPPORTED WITH MECHANICAL CIRCULATORY SUPPORT)

Myocarditis

Ejection fraction <30%, shortening fraction <15%, and moderate-to-severe mitral regurgitation are associated with development of severe cardiac failure. Ventricular arrhythmias and heart block suggest significant myocardial damage and worse prognosis. Enterovirus and parvovirus etiologies are associated with worse prognosis. The outcome of acute lymphocytic myocarditis, in particular fulminant myocarditis, with appropriate intensive care is excellent with 80%–90% survival with almost full recovery of ventricular function.

Dilated Cardiomyopathy

One-third of affected children with DCM recover.

Hypertrophic Cardiomyopathy

Children who develop HCM as a result of an inborn metabolic defect have the worse outcomes (57% risk of death or transplant by age 2 years). Children diagnosed during infancy (less than 1 year of age) typically present with CHF, and appear to be at high risk, showing a 21% risk of death or transplant by the age of 2 years. In contrast to these high-risk groups, relatively good outcomes can be expected for patients with HCM who were diagnosed at an older age with idiopathic (likely sarcomeric) HCM. These children with "typical" hypertrophic disease have low rates of death or transplant (0.5% at 1 year, and 3% at 2 years following diagnoses).

Outcome Following Mechanical Circulatory Support

Preexisting hepatic and renal dysfunction (elevated bilirubin and reduced creatinine clearance) are associated with reduced survival, highlighting the impact of end-organ dysfunction on outcome. Patients of all age categories can be supported, and children <1 year have become the dominant age group in bridging. Neonates and infants <5 kg remain the biggest challenge, as their complication rates and subsequent mortality on bridge to transplant exceed 50%.

Timing of Transplant and Outcome

The 5-year outcomes for children with DCM, divided into etiologic subsets of (a) idiopathic disease, (b) neuromuscular disease, (c) familial isolated DCM, and (d) myocarditis, show myocarditis having the best outcomes. Available data predict that half of the children with DCM will stabilize over time on oral anti-heart failure medications, nearly one-third will go on to cardiac transplantation over the decade following their diagnosis, and ~20% will die without reaching or being eligible for transplantation.

CHAPTER 51 ■ TREATMENT OF HEART FAILURE: MEDICAL MANAGEMENT

JOSEPH W. ROSSANO, JACK F. PRICE, AND DAVID P. NELSON

Heart failure is a clinical syndrome characterized by a reduced ability of the heart to fill and/or eject blood to meet the body's metabolic demands. In children with structural heart disease, this can be the result of pressure or volume overload conditions and resultant ventricular dysfunction, especially in patients with a functionally univentricular heart or systemic morphologic right ventricle. Heart failure is also a common sequela of cardiomyopathies, where abnormal myocardial structure impairs the ability of the heart to contract and/or relax. Among the most common causes of heart failure in infants and children is low cardiac output syndrome (LCOS) after cardiac surgery, which is usually transient and reversible.

MANAGEMENT OF CHRONIC HEART FAILURE

Pharmacologic Agents Used for Treatment of Heart Failure

Heart failure is generally a chronic, progressive disorder, though certain types of cardiomyopathy such as left ventricular noncompaction can have an undulating phenotype. Another exception is acute myocarditis, especially the fulminant form, in which patients may have a complete recovery. The primary aim of therapy is to reduce symptoms, preserve long-term ventricular performance, and prolong survival primarily through antagonism of neurohormonal compensatory mechanisms. Since some medications may be detrimental during acute decompensation, the critical care physician should be knowledgeable of the medications and therapeutic goals of chronic heart failure treatment.

Diuretics

Diuretics are recommended for patients with symptoms of heart failure and evidence of volume overload. Although commonly used in the long-term management, there is a lack of studies that demonstrate long-term benefits of diuretic treatment. Animal models of cardiomyopathy indicate that furosemide activates the renin–angiotensin–aldosterone system (RAAS) and accelerates the decline of myocardial function. In adults, aldosterone antagonists (e.g., spironolactone) improve mortality when added to standard heart failure management, despite an increase in hyperkalemia.

Angiotensin-Converting Enzyme Inhibitors/ Angiotensin Receptor Blockers

Angiotensin-converting enzyme (ACE) inhibitors were the first agents to demonstrate improved survival in adults with symptomatic heart failure. These medications decrease the formation of angiotensin II, block the activation of the RAAS, and decrease adrenergic activity. Angiotensin receptor blockers (ARBs), primarily used in adults unable to tolerate ACE inhibitors, have also demonstrated reduction in mortality that is comparable, and possibly superior to the ACE inhibitors. The combination of ACE inhibitor and ARB treatment may provide additional benefits to improve left ventricular geometry, ejection fraction, and exercise capacity.

Although ACE inhibitors have been shown to reduce the Q_p:Q_s ratio in children with large left-to-right shunt lesions, long-term treatment has not been shown to be efficacious. There are multiple small studies to suggest efficacy of ACE inhibitors in the treatment of children with dilated cardiomyopathy (DCM). On the basis of the supportive pediatric evidence and abundant adult data, ACE inhibition is recommended for moderate or severe degrees of LV dysfunction in infants and children, and ARB therapy if ACE inhibition is not tolerated.

β-Blockers

As with ACE inhibitors, there is evidence that β-blockers in adults with chronic heart failure demonstrate improvement in symptoms, heart function, frequency of hospitalization, and survival despite negative inotropic properties. The presumed benefit of β-blockade is inhibition of the effects of the sympathetic nervous system. Although guidelines do not recommend β-blockers in children with heart failure, β-blockers are often empirically used with DCM on the basis of adult data and the supportive data in children.

Digoxin

Digoxin is a cardiac glycoside that improves contractility by inhibiting the Na–K-ATPase pump in the cardiac myocyte membrane. Although digoxin alleviates symptoms of heart failure, it has not improved mortality, and high doses are associated with increased mortality. Based on data from adult studies, the current recommendation is to use digoxin for symptomatic pediatric patients with the aim of reducing symptoms.

Electrophysiologic Management of Heart Failure

Arrhythmias can be a consequence of, or an unrecognized etiology of, heart failure in children. Tachycardia-induced cardiomyopathy is uncommon, but reversible. Over 90% of patients with tachycardia-induced cardiomyopathy had resolution of left ventricular dysfunction with medical therapy or radiofrequency ablation.

Antiarrhythmic Agents

There is limited evidence for the best choice of an antiarrhythmic agent in children with arrhythmias and heart failure. For arrhythmias where β-blockade is indicated (e.g., re-entrant tachycardia, ectopic focus tachycardia, and rate control for atrial fibrillation), metoprolol may be a good choice based on its dual efficacy for heart failure and antiarrhythmic agent. Although its antiarrhythmic efficacy is not well established, carvedilol decreases atrial and ventricular arrhythmias in adults after myocardial infarction. Amiodarone is an effective antiarrhythmic medication for a variety of arrhythmias. Although amiodarone decreases ventricular arrhythmias in adults with heart failure, effects on survival are contradictory. Patients with ventricular arrhythmias and depressed left ventricular function are at increased risk for sudden death, and an implantable cardioverter-defibrillator (ICD) should be considered (see below).

Cardiac Resynchronization Therapy

Disturbances in the normal electrical conduction of the heart are common in chronic heart failure, and often lead to dyssynchronous contraction. In adults, this is often due to left bundle branch block (uncommon in children). Restoration of ventricular synchrony with synchronized biventricular pacing is termed *cardiac resynchronization therapy* (CRT). In appropriately selected adults, CRT results in reverse remodeling and improved symptoms of heart failure. When combined with an ICD, CRT may improve mortality. There are limited data on CRT use in children, but short-term results demonstrate improved ventricular function with CRT. CRT may be useful in children or adults with congenital heart disease with an intraventricular conduction delay (e.g., tetralogy of Fallot or functionally univentricular hearts).

Implantable Cardioverter-Defibrillator

Ventricular arrhythmias and sudden cardiac death (SCD) are common in adults with heart failure. The limited data on SCD in children with heart failure indicate the incidence is lower than in adults. The use of an ICD as primary prevention of SCD is well established for adults with ischemic and nonischemic cardiomyopathy. The recommendations are for ICD placement in children with congenital heart disease with documented cardiac arrest or sustained ventricular tachycardia. An ICD should be considered for children with cardiomyopathy and recurrent syncope.

MANAGEMENT OF ACUTE DECOMPENSATED HEART FAILURE

Etiology and Pathophysiology

There is no universally accepted definition for acute decompensated heart failure. The incidence in children is not known, but as in adults, most admissions are for acute exacerbations of chronic heart failure. In contrast to adult patients, ischemic cardiomyopathy is rare and idiopathic DCM is more common. Other important causes of acute decompensated heart failure in children include tachycardia-mediated cardiomyopathy, acute myocarditis, DCM secondary to other etiologies (e.g., anthracycline toxicity, anomalous coronary artery, inborn errors of metabolism), and "high-output" cardiac failure (from arteriovenous malformation, thyrotoxicosis or anemia).

Irrespective of etiology, heart failure occurs after an index event produces an initial decline in heart function. This leads to compensatory mechanisms including activation of the sympathetic nervous system, salt and water preservation with activation of the RAAS system, and production of inflammatory cytokines (e.g., tissue necrosis factor, interleukin 1). The compensatory mechanisms delay the onset of symptoms for months or even years. The compensatory mechanisms are counterproductive over time and contribute to progressive myocardial damage, left ventricular remodeling, and eventual cardiac decompensation. Since symptoms of heart failure progress independently of hemodynamic status, treatment of heart failure should *not* be titrated on the basis of echocardiographic and/or catheterization results.

Diagnosis and Assessment of Acute Decompensated Heart Failure

The first signs of acute decompensated heart failure are typically respiratory symptoms such as dyspnea, tachypnea, and increased work of breathing. In children, gastrointestinal symptoms such as abdominal pain, vomiting, or diarrhea are also common. The cardiac examination may reveal jugular venous distention in older patients, a displaced point of maximal cardiac impulse, a gallop rhythm, or murmur of mitral regurgitation. The liver may be displaced inferiorly, and peripheral edema may be present in older children and adults. A chest radiograph is commonly used to evaluate cardiac size and the degree of pulmonary congestion.

The serum level of B-type natriuretic peptide (BNP) is a sensitive screening tool to differentiate cardiac dyspnea from other forms of dyspnea in adult patients. BNP is a cardiac neurohormone secreted in response to ventricular volume expansion and pressure overload. Serum BNP levels have also been shown to be elevated in pediatric patients with ventricular dysfunction in the acute and chronic setting. Although BNP may aid in making the diagnosis of acute decompensated heart failure, there are no data that the values at admission are predictive of outcome. Other useful laboratory data include assessment of renal function and serum electrolytes, as patients are frequently on chronic diuretics.

Although quantification of cardiac function is important, the severity of a patient's symptoms *cannot* be predicted by the degree of ventricular systolic dysfunction. Two-dimensional and M-mode echocardiography provides the standard assessment of function with an easily calculated ejection fraction and shortening fraction, but these measures are preload and afterload dependent.

Preload, an important determinant of cardiac output, is defined as the stretch of the myocardium at end diastole. The stretch on myocytes is determined by the end-diastolic volume (EDV), which correlates with atrial filling pressure. Because of ventricular diastolic stiffness, increases in stroke volume with increasing preload become limited at higher EDVs (**Fig. 51.1**). Filling pressures that are elevated above normal levels coincide with symptoms in patients with decompensated heart failure, and restoration of filling pressures to normal or near normal is an important endpoint of initial therapy. Elevated filling pressures can be estimated clinically with elevated jugular venous pulsations, hepatomegaly, and presence of pulmonary congestion.

Although most patients with acute decompensated heart failure have elevated filling pressures with adequate tissue perfusion, some patients present with cardiogenic shock. Svo_2 values from a central line in the superior vena cava can be a surrogate for mixed-venous saturation in patients with or without intracardiac shunting. Assessment of cardiac output with venous oximetry can improve outcome for postoperative patients with congenital heart disease. Additionally, near-infrared spectroscopy can provide a noninvasive surrogate for superior vena cava saturation.

Algorithm for Rapid Assessment and Management of Heart Failure

A simple and useful tool to help guide management of the patient with acute decompensated heart failure is the rapid assessment algorithm. As shown in **Figure 51.2**, patients are classified according to the signs of elevated filling pressures (wet or dry) and adequacy of perfusion (warm or cold). The goal of heart failure treatment is to transition a patient to the "warm and dry" category. Patients who present as "warm and wet" or "cold and wet" generally respond well to medical management. The "cold and dry" state is typically a dire condition, which may require aggressive treatment, such as mechanical support. This conceptual framework was designed for adults with heart failure, and its benefit for children with heart failure has not been validated. It is a useful conceptual framework to approach patient management.

Adequate Perfusion with Elevated Filling Pressures: "Warm and Wet"

The patient with congestion but adequate perfusion is the most common presentation of acute decompensated heart failure, and typically responds well to medical therapy. Diuresis is a critical component of the initial management of the patient with elevated filling pressures and may be the only therapy needed in the patient with adequate perfusion. Diuretics combined with vasodilators have also been shown to decrease mitral regurgitation and increase forward ejection fraction. Assessment of systemic perfusion is essential in determining whether to continue chronic therapy for heart failure during acute exacerbations. If perfusion is adequate, β-blockers and ACE inhibitors can generally be continued during hospitalization. If perfusion is marginal, the negative inotropic effects of β-blockers may necessitate discontinuation or dose reduction. Some patients may not tolerate acute withdrawal from β-blockade. In adults, continuance of chronic β-blocker therapy during hospitalization is associated with a decreased risk of death or rehospitalization. Initiation of a β-blocker is usually contraindicated while the patient is in decompensated heart failure. Delaying initiation of a β-blocker until the patient has been transitioned back to the "warm and dry" state is generally advised.

Poor Perfusion with Elevated Filling Pressures: "Cold and Wet"

Patients with congestion and poor perfusion typically require intensive care. The initial approach to these patients will depend on the degree of circulatory compromise. The cornerstone of therapy is afterload reduction. Vasodilators and diuretics may be adequate for many patients. Avoiding inotropic agents appears to be beneficial in adults; pediatric data are lacking, and milrinone tends to be first-line therapy for children with decompensated heart failure in the "cold and wet" state. In children with decompensated heart failure, the use of β-adrenergic agonists is avoided, especially at higher doses. There are no pediatric data to support the use of a specific vasodilator for acute decompensated heart failure. Nitroprusside is an effective agent for treatment of heart failure. It has a rapid half-life and can be quickly uptitrated to effect. Cyanide toxicity is a potential side effect, especially with chronic use or renal impairment.

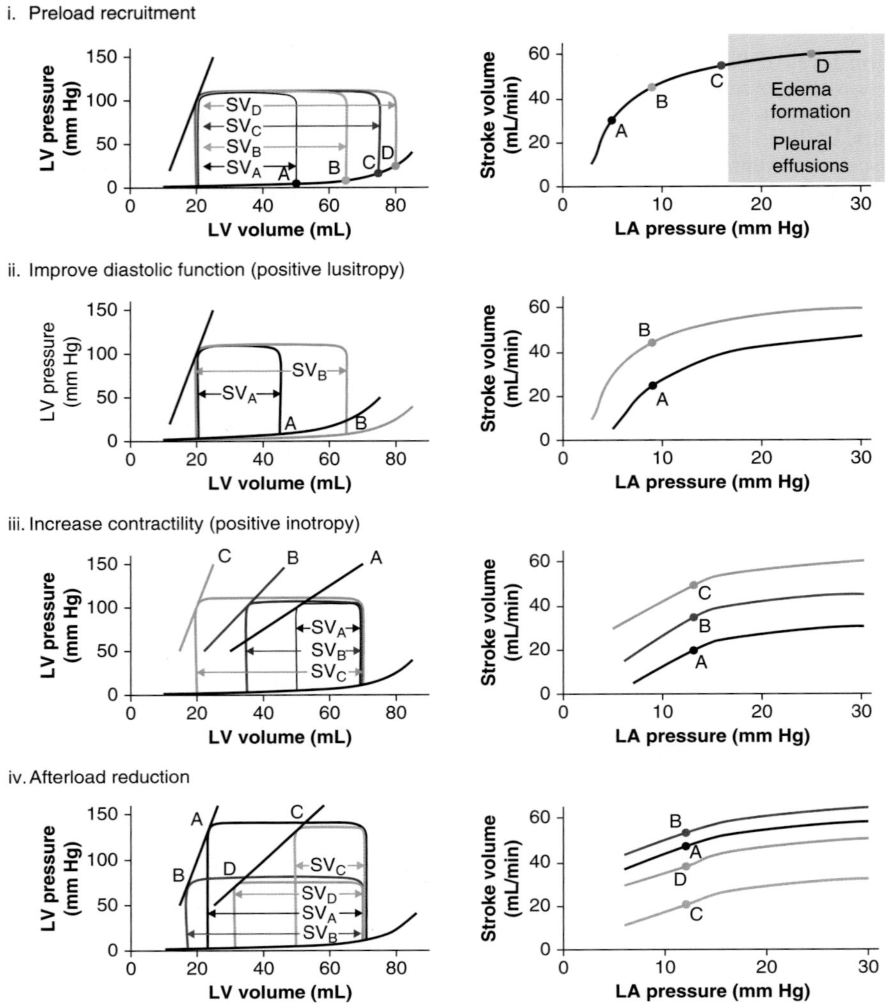

FIGURE 51.1. Paired changes in pressure–volume and Starling relationships with isolated manipulations in preload (i), lusitropy (ii), contractility (iii), and afterload (iv). End-diastolic point A and stroke volume A (SV_A) for each pair of graphs represent the initial baseline hemodynamic condition. **Panel i** demonstrates the effect of preload recruitment on the pressure–volume and Starling relationships. Fluid volume administration augments EDV from points A to B, with the increase in stroke volume shown as the difference between SV_A and SV_B. Since diastolic compliance is nonlinear, increases in stroke volume are progressively less with further fluid administration (SV_C and SV_D). EDVs A, B, C, and D define the diastolic compliance relationship. Preload augmentation is limited by elevations in left ventricular end-diastolic pressure (EDP), which can lead to impaired myocardial perfusion and elevations in atrial pressure, with resultant transcapillary leak and edema formation. **Panel ii** demonstrates beneficial effects of positive lusitropy on the pressure–volume and Starling relationships. Enhanced ventricular compliance corresponds to an increased EDV for the same EDP, thereby augmenting stroke volume without increasing atrial pressure. Enhanced lusitropy results in a greater stroke volume for a comparable atrial pressure. **Panel iii** demonstrates beneficial effects of positive inotropy on the pressure–volume and Starling relationships. Increases in contractility are shown as enhancement of the end-systolic pressure–volume relationship (ESPVR), demonstrated by increases in slopes of lines A to B to C on the left-hand graph. At constant preload, increased contractility enhances ejection during isovolumic contraction, decreasing the end-systolic volume and increasing stroke volume (from SV_A to SV_B to SV_C). Enhanced contractility results in a greater stroke volume for a comparable preload. **Panel iv** demonstrates beneficial effects of afterload reduction on the pressure–volume and Starling relationships. From baseline conditions A or C, afterload reduction allows the heart to eject to a lower systolic pressure and volume (points B and D), enhancing ejection and augmenting stroke volume (SV_A to SV_B and SV_C to SV_D). At normal contractility (slope AB), the ventricle responds to altered afterload with only a small change in stroke volume (SV_A to SV_B). On the other hand, neonatal and failing hearts are particularly sensitive to alterations in afterload. Benefits of afterload reduction are therefore more pronounced in neonatal hearts and in the setting of poor contractility. With reduced contractility (as shown by the reduced slope of ESPVR CD), the increase in stroke volume is greater for a comparable change in afterload. Afterload reduction results in a greater stroke volume for a comparable preload.

	No Congestion	Congestion
Adequate perfusion	"Warm and Dry" A Optimal profile: focus on prevention of disease progression and decompensation	"Wet and Warm" B Diuresis with continuation of standard therapy
Critical hypoperfusion	"Cold and Dry" L Limited further options for therapy	"Wet and Cold" C Diuresis and redesign of regimen with other standard therapies

FIGURE 51.2. Profile of resting hemodynamics. Patients frequently progress from profile A to profile B or profile C. Profile "L" refers to patients presenting with severely low cardiac output. The letter L was chosen rather than the letter D to avoid the implication that this profile necessarily follows profile C. (Reproduced with permission from Grady KL, Dracup K, Kennedy G, et al. Team management of patients with heart failure: A statement for healthcare professionals from The Cardiovascular Nursing Council of the American Heart Association. *Circulation* 2000;102:2443–56.)

Pediatric experience with other vasodilators such as nitroglycerin for heart failure treatment is limited.

Inotropes. Inotropic agents can be used to improve perfusion or treat hypotension in "wet and cold" patients. The decision to use inotropic agents should be based on clinical assessment of end-organ perfusion, and *not* on echocardiographic results (patients with significant ventricular dysfunction that remain compensated may be harmed by inotropes). Traditional inotropic agents used for decompensated heart failure include dobutamine, low-dose dopamine or epinephrine, milrinone, and calcium chloride (**Table 51.1**). *No trial of long-term therapy with a positive inotropic agent has demonstrated improved outcomes in patients with heart failure. Most trials have found increased mortality with positive inotropic agents.*

Dobutamine. Dobutamine is a β-adrenergic agonist, which stimulates both β_1- and β_2-receptors. β_1-Receptor stimulation increases intracellular cyclic adenosine monophosphate (cAMP), increasing contractility by release of calcium from the sarcoplasmic reticulum. β_2-Receptor activation results in peripheral vasodilation and decreased SVR. The decrease in SVR may cause a reflex tachycardia; an increase in heart rate and contractility may result in an undesired increase in myocardial oxygen consumption. Although short-term infusions of dobutamine improve symptoms, decrease filling pressures, increase ejection fraction, and improve exercise tolerance, tachycardia and arrhythmias are common side effects. Based on adult studies, routine use of dobutamine for heart failure has fallen out of favor.

Dopamine. Dopamine is an endogenous catecholamine. At low doses (2–5 μg/kg/min), there is stimulation of dopamine receptors in the renal, cerebral, coronary, mesenteric, and pulmonary vasculature. Higher doses of dopamine stimulate β-adrenergic receptors, increasing contractility, and heart rate. At higher doses ($\geq$10 μg/kg/min), there is α-adrenergic stimulation, resulting in vasoconstriction and increased systemic and pulmonary vascular resistance. There is no evidence to support the use of "renal dose" dopamine. The side-effect profile is similar to dobutamine (tachycardia, arrhythmias, and increased myocardial oxygen consumption).

Milrinone. The most commonly used agent for acute decompensated heart failure in children is milrinone, a phosphodiesterase (PDE) inhibitor with both vasodilatory and inotropic properties. Milrinone inhibits the breakdown of cAMP by the PDE III isozyme. By blocking breakdown of intracellular cAMP, calcium transport into the cell is enhanced and myocyte contractility improved. In addition, reuptake of calcium is a cAMP-dependent process, so these agents may enhance diastolic relaxation of the myocardium by

TABLE 51.1

Commonly Used Infusions for the Treatment of Heart Failure

AGENT	LOADING DOSE	INFUSION DOSE RANGE
Dopamine	None	3–10 μg/kg/min
Dobutamine	None	3–20 μg/kg/min
Milrinone	50–100 μg/kg over 60 min	0.25–1 μg/kg/min
Calcium chloride	None	5–20 mg/kg/h
Epinephrine	None	0.03–0.2 μg/kg/min
Arginine vasopressin	None	0.01–0.05 U/kg/h
Hydrocortisone	None	50 mg/m^2/d ÷ q6h
Triiodothyronine	None	0.05–0.1 μg/kg/h

increasing the rate of calcium reuptake after systole. PDE inhibitors increase cardiac muscle contractility, vascular smooth muscle relaxation, and cardiac output without increasing myocardial oxygen consumption or ventricular afterload.

Calcium. Calcium chloride can increase myocardial contractility in the postarrest setting. In the adult heart, calcium released from the sarcoplasmic reticulum accounts for the majority of the calcium that binds to troponin C. In the neonate, the sarcoplasmic reticulum is relatively sparse and undifferentiated, so the neonatal myocardium is more dependent upon extracellular calcium stores for contractile function. Contractility is proportional to the level of ionized calcium in the blood. In contrast to catecholamines, calcium chloride does not induce tachycardia or arrhythmias. The chronic use of calcium chloride for decompensated heart failure in children has not been studied, but it has been used extensively in perioperative patients with congenital heart disease. The use of calcium chloride can acutely improve myocardial contractility and cardiac output without excessive tachycardia, especially in younger patients.

Levosimendan. Levosimendan is a promising agent in a class of medications known as calcium sensitizers. It increases both inotropy and vasodilation without increasing calcium levels or myocardial oxygen demand. The enhancement of contractility occurs by binding to troponin C and increasing myofilament sensitivity to calcium. Levosimendan causes vasodilatation via opening of potassium-dependent adenosine triphosphate channels. The ability to improve cardiac function without increasing intracellular calcium or myocardial oxygen consumption may prove to be a breakthrough in the treatment of acute and chronic heart failure. Levosimendan has been used safely and effectively in adults with heart failure and shown improved mortality. There are isolated case reports of its use in children with severe heart failure postoperatively and in the setting of a DCM. The drug is not yet available in the United States.

Poor Perfusion with Normal Filling Pressures: "Cold and Dry"

Patients with inadequate perfusion and normal filling pressures represent a tenuous population. Vasodilators may worsen perfusion in patients with marginal blood pressure. In the setting of significantly compromised perfusion or cardiogenic shock, multiple inotropic agents may become necessary, including potent vasoconstrictor agents such as epinephrine or vasopressin. Addition of vasodilation therapy may become feasible if inotropic therapy improves perfusion. Inotropic agents rarely return these patients to an asymptomatic state and, although acutely life-saving, they may decrease long-term ventricular function and increase mortality. If there is an inadequate response to vasodilator therapy and increasing inotropic requirements are needed to maintain adequate perfusion, mechanical circulatory support should be considered.

Epinephrine. Epinephrine has dose-dependent actions on α- and β-adrenergic receptors. At low doses, the β-adrenergic receptor response predominates, resulting in vasodilation, increased heart rate, and contractility. At higher doses, α-receptor stimulation mediates vasoconstriction and increased SVR. Although, the increased SVR and contractility may acutely improve perfusion, this may occur at the expense of increased myocardial oxygen consumption and myocardial work. High-dose catecholamines often promote tachycardia and proarrhythmic effects, increase myocardial oxygen consumption, and depress the myocardial adrenergic response by downregulating β-adrenergic receptors. Prolonged use of high-dose catecholamines may further amplify cardiomyocyte and sarcomeric injury, thus aggravating diastolic and systolic ventricular dysfunctions.

Vasopressin. The use of arginine vasopressin during (and post) cardiac arrest has been shown to improve return of spontaneous circulation and survival. Endogenous vasopressin levels are elevated in children with heart failure, but reduced in patients after cardiopulmonary bypass. Vasopressin acts directly upon vascular smooth muscle to increase SVR, but does not have the associated tachycardia found with catecholamines. Vasopressin also acts directly on the myocardium by increasing cytosolic calcium via V_1 receptors. The use of vasopressin in children to improve low cardiac output in postoperative catecholamine resistant shock has been demonstrated. Even if vasopressin has direct myocardial effects, the increased afterload with vasopressin is unlikely to be well tolerated in the failing myocardium for long periods.

Mechanical Support. In the setting of increasing inotrope requirements for the failing myocardium, the situation is dire. Medical therapy is unlikely to return the patient to an asymptomatic state, and continuation of therapy will likely increase the stress on an already failing myocardium. At this point, mechanical support should be considered to "rest the myocardium." In children, mechanical support has generally been used as a bridge to cardiac transplantation. In the setting of a potentially reversible process, such as myocarditis, mechanical support has been used as a bridge for recovery. Mechanical support can reduce the stress on a failing heart to reverse some of the pathologic molecular changes characteristics of heart failure. When used in adults with severe heart failure as destination therapy or bridge to possible recovery of function, mechanical support is associated with increased survival and increased quality of life compared to medical therapy.

MANAGEMENT OF LOW CARDIAC OUTPUT SYNDROME AFTER CARDIAC SURGERY

Although LCOS is currently associated with lower mortality, it still results in increased hospital stay, resource utilization, and possible long-term cognitive dysfunction. Prompt recognition, diagnosis, and management of LCOS are fundamental to effective cardiac intensive care and essential for optimal patient outcome.

Causes of Low Cardiac Output after Surgery

Low cardiac output after congenital heart surgery is typically multifactorial. Defects in myocardial systolic or diastolic contractile function can be accompanied by altered ventricular loading and residual cardiac lesions. Ventricular preload is often inadequate, due to blood loss, perioperative fluid shifts, changes in diastolic compliance or physiologic changes resulting from the surgical procedure (e.g., Fontan or shunted single-ventricle physiology). Increases in intrathoracic pressure (e.g., tamponade or pneumothorax) will limit venous return and impede ventricular filling. Ventricular afterload is often increased after bypass procedures, resulting from bypass-mediated vascular injury and altered vascular reactivity. Cardiopulmonary bypass induces both systemic and pulmonary endothelial dysfunctions, presumably due to ischemia–reperfusion injury to the endothelium. Acute pulmonary hypertension episodes cause an acute rise in right ventricular (RV) afterload, shift the interventricular septum into the systemic ventricle, and decrease the preload of the systemic ventricle. Pulmonary hypertensive crises most often present with acute systemic hypotension and diminished perfusion. Arterial oxygen saturation decreases only if right-to-left intracardiac shunting can occur.

Residual anatomic or electrophysiologic abnormalities can diminish cardiac output after congenital heart surgery. Uncorrected anatomic defects (e.g., outflow obstruction or valvar insufficiency) reduce the effective stroke volume and increase myocardial demands. Similarly, persistence of a left-to-right intracardiac shunt will yield excessive pulmonary blood flow and diminish systemic blood flow. Low cardiac output could be exacerbated by arrhythmias, which limit ventricular filling and/or compromise atrioventricular synchrony.

Treatment of Low Cardiac Output after Surgery

Management of postoperative LCOS includes optimization of preload and afterload; prompt diagnosis of residual cardiac lesions; prevention of hypoxia as dictated by cardiac anatomy, anemia, or acidosis; and administration of pharmacologic agents to improve myocardial contractile function. In low cardiac output associated with right heart failure, some children benefit from pulmonary vasodilator therapy or the presence of an atrial level shunt to allow right-to-left shunting to augment LV preload.

Minimize Oxygen Requirements

Reduced cardiac output and increased systemic oxygen consumption can alter systemic oxygen balance adversely after cardiopulmonary bypass. Oxygen consumption correlates significantly with central temperature, so pyrexia should be treated aggressively. A cooling blanket may be useful, but shivering should be avoided. Induction of heavy sedation, paralysis, or mild hypothermia can reduce metabolism.

Ensure Adequate Preload

Inadequate preload is common in postoperative cardiac surgical patients. Potential causes of hypovolemia include bleeding, excessive ultrafiltration, diastolic dysfunction, vasodilation from rewarming, and afterload reduction. Cardiac tamponade or pneumothorax can impair preload and must be considered. Myocardial swelling that limits myocardial filling and prevents adequate output may necessitate sternal reopening.

Although true ventricular preload is the end-diastolic ventricular volume, preload assessment can be estimated from atrial pressure. **Figure 51.1**, panel i, shows how preload determination is predominantly a "trial and error" process. When atrial pressure is low, fluid administration augments EDV and increases stroke volume. With successive fluid administration, increases in stroke volume become limited due to the nonlinear nature of ventricular compliance. A stiff ventricle (e.g., RV dysfunction after tetralogy of Fallot repair) has higher end-diastolic and right atrial pressures and requires higher filling pressures to generate adequate output. These patients may also benefit from lusitropic therapy intended to improve diastolic ventricular filling.

Prompt Recognition of Arrhythmias

Early recognition of postoperative arrhythmias is imperative; a baseline postoperative surface electrocardiogram is needed for comparison with preoperative and subsequent postoperative tracings. Continuous electrocardiographic monitoring is essential. Since sinus bradycardia, bundle branch block, and atrioventricular block occur after many cardiac surgical procedures, temporary atrial and ventricular pacing wires are placed to facilitate pacing, if necessary. Nonsustained ventricular (22%) and supraventricular tachycardia (12%) are the most common arrhythmias in postoperative cardiac surgical patients. Next are sustained ventricular, junctional, and supraventricular arrhythmias (6%, 5%, and 4%, respectively).

Junctional ectopic tachycardia (JET) is a problematic tachyarrhythmia that usually occurs in the first 48 hours following surgery, especially after closure of a ventricular septal defect and in younger patients. It may be poorly tolerated, especially in patients with unstable hemodynamics. Early recognition of JET can be aided by surveillance of atrial pressure waveforms. The loss of distinct *a* and *v* waves is often the first indication of arrhythmia and/or atrioventricular dyssynchrony. Hypomagnesemia may contribute to the onset of JET, and administration of intravenous magnesium in the early postoperative period may reduce the incidence of JET. If the hemodynamics allow, adrenergic agents, which may exacerbate JET, should be reduced or discontinued. Restoration of atrial contribution with pacing, either atrial or dual chamber atrioventricular sequential, is the initial therapy of choice. If the junctional rate is too fast to allow pacing, the goal of pharmacologic therapy is to provide rate control to allow pacing. While intravenous amiodarone is considered the drug of choice, hypothermia or procainamide administration have also been effective. Since the risk of JET is increased in the presence of low output ("low cardiac output begets JET"), the diagnosis of JET should prompt the search for other causes of LCOS, including residual cardiac lesions.

Prompt Diagnosis of Residual Cardiac Lesions

Residual cardiac lesions in the postoperative patient can lead to LCOS and result in increased morbidity and mortality. In patients with LCOS following cardiopulmonary bypass, data from invasive lines and echocardiography should be used to rule out residual structural lesions. Catheterization should be considered if LCOS persists and the etiology remains elusive.

Treatment of Depressed Myocardial Contractility

Since low cardiac output after pediatric heart surgery is often associated with some level of contractile dysfunction, inotropic support in the early postoperative period is usually necessary. **Figure 51.1, panel iii** demonstrates the beneficial effects of positive inotropy on the pressure–volume and Starling relationships. At constant preload, increased contractility should enhance ejection during systole to increase stroke volume. **Figures 51.1** and **51.3** illustrate the use of Starling curves to assess efficacy of hemodynamic interventions.

Inotropic agents and vasodilators are used in pediatric cardiac surgical patients to help reestablish adequate myocardial function during and after surgery. Support is often initiated with milrinone and a low-dose infusion of epinephrine or dopamine. The infusion rate is titrated to produce the desired systemic blood pressure. Since high-dose epinephrine (>0.1 μg/kg/min) results in tachycardia and systemic vasoconstriction, it is often used in combination with vasodilators such as milrinone or sodium nitroprusside to treat ventricular dysfunction and decrease systemic afterload (or at least attenuate the α_1-effects of epinephrine).

PDE inhibitors improve cardiac index by enhancing both systolic and diastolic functions, and by reducing systemic and pulmonary vascular resistance. For patients at high risk for LCOS, some centers prefer to load with milrinone during bypass to avoid potential

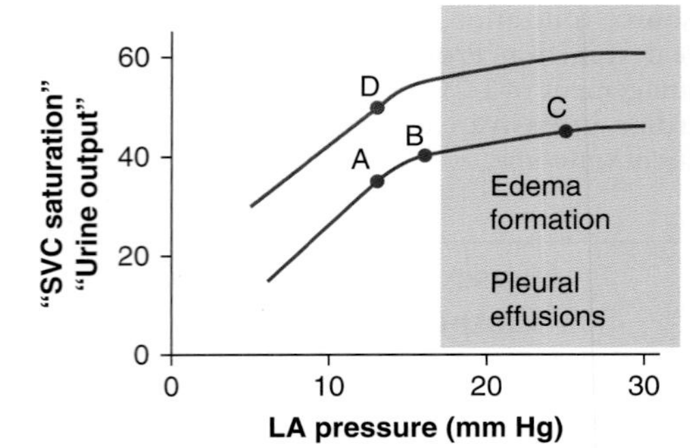

FIGURE 51.3. Modified Starling relationship. Since stroke volume is not easily monitored, indirect measures of cardiac output such as SVC saturation or end-organ perfusion such as urine output may be plotted against atrial pressure to create a "modified" Starling relationship. Fluid administration augments preload and leads to improvement in SVC saturation and end-organ perfusion (point A to point B). Preload augmentation is limited, however; progressive fluid administration ultimately leads to excessive atrial pressures, with resultant edema formation (point C). Alternate ways to improve SVC saturation or urine output include afterload reduction, lusitropic improvement, or inotropic augmentation, which all shift the Starling relationship upward and leftward (point D). The therapeutic goal of enhanced lusitropy, increased contractility, or afterload reduction is improvement in systemic blood flow for a comparable preload (reflected as improved SVC saturation and enhanced organ perfusion).

hypotension. The use of milrinone in children early after congenital heart surgery has been shown to reduce the incidence of LCOS. Since renal dysfunction results in delayed clearance of milrinone, patients with renal insufficiency are at risk for toxicity, so the dose should be adjusted based on creatinine clearance to avoid excessive vasodilation, especially in neonates.

Cardiac contraction and relaxation are mediated by cyclic fluctuations in cytoplasmic calcium concentration. Hypocalcemia may occur in the postoperative period, especially in patients with 22q11 deletion syndrome or neonates with transient hypoparathyroidism. Transfusion of citrate-treated blood products and administration of loop diuretics may exacerbate hypocalcemia. Ionized calcium, the physiologically active form of calcium, should be monitored frequently in the postoperative period and normal levels maintained with supplementation. Many centers use calcium infusions routinely in neonates after cardiopulmonary bypass to augment and stabilize extracellular ionized calcium (**Table 51.1**). Significant hypercalcemia, however, may be associated with increased cell death and decrease in myocardial relaxation.

Although the mechanism remains unclear, investigators have advocated thyroid hormone therapy as a potential treatment for LCOS. During cardiopulmonary bypass, circulating levels of the thyroid hormones triiodothyronine (T_3) and thyroxine (T_4) are reduced; these deficiencies can persist for several days and may play a role in postoperative myocardial depression. Administration of T_3 to children after congenital heart surgery results in hemodynamic improvement, although it is unclear if this improves clinical outcomes.

Arginine vasopressin has been advocated as a therapeutic option for pediatric patients with refractory hypotension after surgery, to improve systemic arterial blood pressure when conventional therapies fail. Cardiopulmonary bypass leads to decreased arginine vasopressin levels. Arginine vasopressin has also been shown to be effective for refractory hypotension in patients on mechanical circulatory support.

Both pre- and postoperative patients can develop prolonged low cardiac output that requires escalating inotropic support and is refractory to other therapy. Adrenal dysfunction may contribute to morbidity in critically ill patients, and stress-dose hydrocortisone (50 mg/m^2/d) can reduce inotropic requirements in pediatric patients with LCOS refractory to conventional therapy.

Afterload Reduction for Systemic Ventricular Failure

Elevated afterload is particularly detrimental to the neonatal heart, especially when compounded by postoperative myocardial dysfunction. Afterload reduction is often beneficial in postoperative patients showing signs of LCOS. Furthermore, if high-dose catecholamines cannot be avoided, afterload reduction/vasodilator therapy should be considered to counter catecholamine vasoconstrictor effects (**Figure 51.1, panel iv** demonstrates the beneficial effects of afterload reduction on pressure–volume and Starling relationships). The therapeutic goal of afterload reduction is improvement in systemic blood flow for a comparable preload (reflected as improved SVC saturation and enhanced organ perfusion).

Some centers use the potent vasodilator phenoxybenzamine, an α-adrenergic blocking agent, in selected pediatric patients after cardiac surgery. Phenoxybenzamine is a potent vasodilator with a very long half-life (>24 hours) and its use may be complicated by severe hypotension. Many centers prefer sodium nitroprusside for afterload reduction and vasodilator therapy in patients with congenital heart disease. Although it is a less potent vasodilator, the therapeutic effects of nitroprusside are easier to titrate due to its short half-life and rapid onset of action. PDE inhibitors are also commonly used for afterload reduction in pediatric patients with congenital heart disease. Their inotropic and lusitropic effects combined with systemic and pulmonary vasodilation make them particularly useful for LCOS. Sodium nitroprusside has also been advocated in patients with excessive pulmonary blood flow after Norwood palliation. In such patients, nitroprusside reduces afterload to improve myocardial performance and SVR to improve the balance of pulmonary and systemic blood flow.

Management of Right Ventricular Failure

Right heart failure is a common complication of congenital heart surgery and cause of LCOS. Factors contributing to postoperative RV dysfunction include difficulties with right heart myocardial protection and right ventriculotomy. Patients undergoing right heart procedures, including tetralogy of Fallot and Fontan procedures, often demonstrate restrictive physiology (diastolic RV dysfunction), characterized by antegrade diastolic pulmonary arterial flow coinciding with atrial systole.

Children with acute RV restrictive physiology have a decreased cardiac index because the stiff right ventricle has impaired diastolic filling. Alterations in LV filling may also occur, due to the hypertensive RV. Alterations in ventricular compliance make patients with RV failure particularly sensitive to alterations in venous return caused by intrathoracic pressure changes. As discussed below, these patients benefit from ventilation strategies that minimize intrathoracic pressure. Patients with RV failure may benefit from manipulation of pulmonary vascular resistance (PVR) to minimize RV afterload. PDE inhibitors are particularly beneficial in these patients, due to the combined lusitropic and pulmonary vasodilatory effects.

The ability to maintain a right-to-left shunt at the atrial level is beneficial in patients with RV dysfunction. In patients undergoing the modified Fontan procedure, fenestration between the Fontan pathway and atrium is associated with reduced pleural effusion and significantly shorter hospital stays. In patients who undergo tetralogy of Fallot repair, a right-to-left atrial shunt can be similarly facilitated by maintaining the patency of the foramen ovale or by creating a small fenestration in the atrial septum.

Ventilation Strategies after Pediatric Cardiac Surgery

Cardiopulmonary Interactions

Since the cardiorespiratory system functions as a unit, ventilation (both spontaneous and mechanical) has effects on hemodynamics. These effects may be pronounced in children following cardiac surgery and an understanding of the interaction between the cardiovascular and respiratory systems is crucial to their management. Alterations in intrathoracic pressure and lung volume affect dynamic and loading conditions of the right and left ventricle differently, often having opposing effects. A transient increase in intrathoracic pressure decreases RV preload and LV afterload, whereas spontaneous inspiration (a decrease in intrathoracic pressure) increases RV preload and LV afterload. The effect of ventilation on RV afterload depends primarily upon lung volume (PVR is lowest at functional residual capacity). Since intrathoracic pressure effects can be opposite for the right and left ventricles, the ventilation strategy depends upon whether right or left ventricular dysfunction predominates.

In patients with systemic ventricular contractile dysfunction, positive intrathoracic pressure may be beneficial because of the reduction in LV afterload. On the other hand, venous return effects of positive intrathoracic pressure are amplified in lesions with no right ventricle (Glenn and Fontan procedures) or in patients with RV failure (especially patients with restrictive physiology after tetralogy of Fallot repair).

Lung Recruitment in Patients with Congenital Heart Disease

Lung recruitment is an important principle for ventilation of patients with respiratory failure and is also important in management of patients with congenital heart disease. Ventilation strategies for patients with congenital heart disease should strive to maintain an "open lung" and a normal functional residual capacity.

Effects of Positive-Pressure Ventilation in LV Failure

Positive intrathoracic pressure is beneficial in patients with systemic ventricular dysfunction by reducing LV afterload. In addition to optimal lung recruitment, higher levels of positive end-expiratory pressure may thus be hemodynamically beneficial. Tidal volumes should be maintained in the range of 6–10 mL/kg to avoid overdistension and increased PVR and RV afterload. Furthermore, shorter inspiratory times may augment systemic ventricle filling in patients with systemic ventricular dysfunction.

Effects of Positive-Pressure Ventilation in RV Failure

Alterations in RV compliance make patients with RV failure sensitive to changes in systemic venous return caused by changes in intrathoracic pressure. Spontaneous inspiration enhances diastolic flow and overall cardiac output in these patients, so early extubation may be beneficial. Because of the detrimental effects of positive-pressure ventilation on RV dynamics, alternative modes of ventilation have been advocated (e.g., negative-pressure and high-frequency jet ventilation [HFJV]). These methods help reduce mean airway pressure but maintain a similar $Paco_2$ and may benefit patients with RV dysfunction and/or pulmonary hypertension (e.g., postoperative patients with restrictive RV physiology and Fontan physiology).

MEDICAL MANAGEMENT OF MYOCARDITIS

Care of a patient with possible myocarditis depends on the severity of myocardial involvement. Animal studies suggest that bed rest may prevent an increase in intramyocardial viral replication in the acute stage; thus, it appears prudent to limit activity at time of diagnosis. Supportive care should prevent hypoxemia, maintain cardiac output and prevent metabolic disturbances, use diuretics to remove excess extracellular fluid volume, and use anticoagulation (aspirin, warfarin, and/or heparin) to reduce thrombotic/embolic phenomena.

Afterload Reduction

Afterload reduction is the cornerstone of therapy for patients with myocarditis and clinically significant contractile dysfunction. Sodium nitroprusside can be used alone or in conjunction with inotropic agents (see below). PDE inhibitors (e.g., milrinone infusion) can provide both inotropy and afterload reduction. When chronic oral therapy is tolerated, ACE inhibition and diuretics are typically prescribed. Addition of a β-blocker such as carvedilol or metoprolol may also be beneficial (monitor hemodynamic effects closely).

Circulatory Support

Since catecholamines can aggravate myocardial injury, their use should be carefully assessed and doses minimized. Low-dose dopamine or dobutamine can help decreased ventricular function. Higher doses of catecholamines should prompt consideration for mechanical support, especially the more potent catecholamines epinephrine or norepinephrine. Low-dose epinephrine may be temporarily necessary to maintain blood pressure and/or systemic perfusion but mechanical circulatory support considered if prolonged high-dose epinephrine (>0.1 µg/kg/min) is necessary as these patients are at high risk for progressive shock or cardiac arrest. Since all inotropic agents have detrimental effects, goal-oriented therapy with SVC saturation monitoring to guide inotrope and vasodilator therapy is recommended. Mechanical circulatory support (MCS) is indicated for patients unresponsive to medical therapy (Chapter 52). Transplantation becomes necessary in patients who do not acutely recover despite medical and mechanical support.

Antiarrhythmic Agents

Arrhythmias in these patients should be vigorously treated. Antiarrhythmic therapy for supraventricular tachyarrhythmias include β-blockers, procainamide, and amiodarone (digoxin is usually avoided in patients with suspected myocarditis). Ventricular arrhythmias may respond to lidocaine. Intravenous amiodarone may be preferable for refractory arrhythmias. Despite aggressive treatment of arrhythmias, rapid deterioration to ventricular fibrillation may occur, especially in the very young. Complete atrioventricular block requires immediate temporary pacing with possible need for a permanent pacing system. Persistent or refractory arrhythmias may require MCS.

Immune Modulation

The use of immunosuppressive agents in suspected or proven viral myocarditis is controversial. No improvement was shown among patients treated with azathioprine versus cyclosporine along with prednisone and conventional medical therapy. A frequently used but unproven therapy for children with myocarditis is intravenous immunoglobulin (IVIG). Patients receiving IVIG are reported to have better left ventricular function at follow-up (1-year survival tended to be higher but was not statistically significant). At most centers, patients with myocarditis are typically treated with one to two doses of 1 g/kg of IVIG.

Although immunosuppressive therapy has not been shown to be beneficial in most patients with histologically confirmed myocarditis, combined treatment with (IVIG) and pulse-dose steroids is advocated for patients with the fulminant necrotic myocarditis phenotype because of anecdotal reports of benefit (IV methylprednisolone, 10 mg/kg every 8 hours for three doses).

MEDICAL MANAGEMENT OF CARDIOMYOPATHIES

Treatment Strategies for Dilated Cardiomyopathy

Acute management of a child newly diagnosed with DCM should include efforts to rule out myocarditis or surgically correctable causes (i.e., anomalous left coronary artery arising from the pulmonary artery, aortic arch obstruction). Supportive care (of heart failure symptoms) should be provided and risk of complications (thromboembolic events or arrhythmias) minimized. Intramural thrombus detected by echocardiography is an indication for systemic anticoagulation. Arrhythmias can cause sudden death in DCM patients, so patients should have telemetry or Holter monitoring. Supraventricular or ventricular arrhythmias should be treated to preserve cardiac output. Electrolyte imbalances should be identified and corrected. Short-term management of patients with heart failure consists of the same supportive care used in heart failure from other conditions (see above). This includes IV diuretics for symptomatic relief from venous congestion, and intravenous vasodilators or inotropes to augment cardiac output. Once the acute decompensation is controlled, treatment should transition to oral afterload reduction and neurohormonal inhibition (ACE inhibitors, β-blockers, and diuretics).

Treatment Strategies for Hypertrophic Cardiomyopathy

Therapy of hypertrophic cardiomyopathy (HCM) is directed at reduction of symptoms, prevention of untoward complications, and prevention of SCD. Patients with HCM should be assessed for risk of SCD. An ICD is recommended for patients who survive an SCD episode or who experience one or more episodes of sustained ventricular tachycardia. These high-risk patients represent a small percentage of patients with HCM.

Medical therapy with β-blockers or non–dihydropyridine calcium channel blockers is the first-line approach to patients with HCM. β-Blockers and verapamil may reduce severe LV outflow obstruction. Diuretics may alleviate symptoms in some patients but should be used with caution as a reduced preload may increase the outflow obstruction. Likewise, ACE inhibitors can alter loading conditions and worsen the outflow gradient. A subset of patients progresses to end-stage HCM characterized by decreased LV systolic function, thinning of the walls secondary to fibrosis and LV dilation. These patients should be managed for heart failure with standard accepted medical and/or surgical therapy. Not all arrhythmias are ventricular in nature; 20% of adult patients with HCM develop atrial fibrillation and require antiarrhythmic therapy and anticoagulation.

Nonmedical therapy includes surgical myomectomy, pacemaker therapy, and alcohol septal ablation (relieves outflow tract obstruction with varying degree of success). Regardless of the intervention, procedures to reduce outflow tract obstruction do not reduce the risk of SCD secondary to ventricular arrhythmias. Infective endocarditis is a rare complication that occurs in patients with severe outflow tract obstruction, in the region of the thickened anterior leaflet of the mitral valve.

Therapeutic Strategies for Restrictive Cardiomyopathy

There has been no consistent approach to therapy for restrictive cardiomyopathy (RCM) in children. A variety of medications have been administered in combinations, including digoxin, afterload reducing agents, calcium channel blockers, and β-blockers. Risks and benefits of ACE inhibition in pediatric RCM remain to be determined. Modulation of neurohormonal activation by ACE inhibitors may affect fibroblast activity, interstitial fibrosis, intracellular calcium handling, and myocardial stiffness. In adults with diastolic heart failure, the use of ACE inhibitors has been suggested, but data are limited. In adults with diastolic dysfunction, tachycardia is poorly tolerated; therefore, β-blockers or calcium channel blockers are part of the treatment regimen. Diuretics may be useful for symptoms of venous congestion, but over-diuresis should be avoided. Because of the high incidence of thromboembolic events, antiplatelet therapy or anticoagulants should be administered. Cardiac transplantation is the therapy of choice since medical therapy is ineffective and the development of pulmonary hypertension is common and mortality is high. Most patients should be evaluated and listed for transplantation at the time of presentation.

While listed for transplantation, Holter monitoring to evaluate for signs of ischemia, ventricular arrhythmias, or conduction disturbances should be done every 6 months. Implantable defibrillators should be considered for signs of ischemia or ventricular arrhythmias. Strenuous physical activity should be avoided.

Therapeutic Strategies for Arrhythmogenic Right Ventricular Dysplasia

Management of patients with arrhythmogenic right ventricular dysplasia (ARVD) consists of antiarrhythmic agents, but the only therapy with survival benefit is ICD placement. In addition, therapies for heart failure may be instituted as the disease progresses toward a pattern similar to DCM. Cardiac transplantation is required in some cases.

Therapeutic Strategies for Left Ventricular Noncompaction Cardiomyopathy

Treatment of left ventricular noncompaction cardiomyopathy (LVNC) is dependent on associated comorbidities. Patients with the hypertrophic or dilated phenotypes should be treated as outlined above. Aggressive anticoagulant therapy should be considered in cases of thrombus or systemic embolic events. In patients with associated mitochondrial myopathy, a combination of riboflavin, thiamine, coenzyme Q10, and carnitine may be considered. Serial Holter monitoring of patients with LVNC should be considered as there is an increased risk of arrhythmias. Ventricular arrhythmias may prompt ICD placement. Patients who are refractory to adequate medical therapy may require cardiac transplantation.

CHAPTER 52 ■ TREATMENT OF HEART FAILURE: MECHANICAL SUPPORT

IKI ADACHI, LARA S. SHEKERDEMIAN, PAUL A. CHECCHIA, AND CHARLES D. FRASER JR.

Mechanical circulatory support (MCS) for children has lagged behind the adult counterpart, with extracorporeal membrane oxygenation (ECMO) long being the mainstay or even the only modality for MCS in children. Pediatric-specific ventricular assist devices (VAD) have the potential to transform the outlook for children with end-stage heart failure awaiting transplantation. As children are so divergent in size and cardiac physiology, appropriate understanding and selection of devices are important for success.

HEART FAILURE IN CHILDREN

The number of children with heart failure has been increasing, resulting in growing demand for pediatric MCS. Possible explanations include better recognition of pediatric cardiomyopathy with earlier treatment and advancements in surgery and perioperative care for children with congenital heart disease (CHD), leading to increased survival. Improved survival of these patient groups could lead to an increased incidence of end-stage heart failure in children, adolescents, and young adults. Typical examples of end-stage heart failure in the setting of operated CHD involve children whose morphologic right ventricle is sustaining the systemic circulation and who progress to failure of that systemic ventricle. Cardiac transplantation remains the treatment of choice for end-stage heart failure, but this growing need cannot be addressed due to the static number of donor organs.

While pediatric MCS is in rapid evolution, there has been significant refinement of MCS therapy in adults over the last decade. The most significant change is the emergence of durable intracorporeal (implantable) devices. The impressive efficiency of these devices with relatively low morbidity makes early institution of the device a reasonable option in preference to escalating medical management. In adults, VADs are used as a bridge to transplant, as a bridge to recovery, or as destination therapy (for patients who opt against transplantation or for whom transplantation is not an option).

The scope of the use of intracorporeal devices in the pediatric population is limited by body size, and they can, therefore, only be used to provide MCS in larger children and adolescents. Although miniaturized intracorporeal devices for smaller children are on the horizon, the Berlin Heart EXCOR, a paracorporeal pulsatile device, is the only currently available option. It is likely that high success rates (~90%) can be achieved with very careful patient selection and management at high-volume centers. However, the Berlin Heart EXCOR is associated with significant morbidity profiles (stroke in ~30%, bleeding in 40%–50%, and infection in 50%–60%). The incidence of complications in children with pulsatile VADs is greater than in adults with intracorporeal devices. This significant complication rate in children suggests the need for careful assessments of the risks and benefits when considering device placement.

PATIENT SELECTION

MCS for any patient is indicated when the benefits outweigh the risks. Since each patient and device has a unique risk profile, the appropriateness and the timing are determined on a case-by-case basis by the multidisciplinary team, the family, and (when appropriate) the patient. Consideration should be given to medical and social aspects. MCS selection should also be influenced by the institutional experience.

Other confounding issues must be considered in providing MCS in children. Children with CHD may have anatomic variations that pose significant difficulty in cannulation (e.g., abnormal size and location of the aorta and unusual location or shape of the ventricle). Previous surgical procedures may jeopardize the application of MCS with derangement of anatomy and of circulatory physiology (e.g., systemic–pulmonary artery shunts and disconnected caval veins or pulmonary artery after Glenn or Fontan operations). In addition to the anatomy and circulatory physiology, a thorough understanding of the pathophysiologic features of pediatric heart failure is a prerequisite to a successful outcome.

At present, long-term VAD support in children requires candidacy for heart transplantation. Extreme prematurity, body weight <2.0 kg, significant neurologic injury, a constellation of congenital anomalies with unlikely survival beyond childhood, and major chromosomal aberrations are generally accepted contraindications for MCS. Multisystem organ failure may be a relative contraindication, but does not exclude patients if reversal of organ function is predicted after hemodynamic improvement. It has been well documented that liver and renal dysfunction improve after restoration of hemodynamic stability with MCS.

DEVICE SELECTION

Device selection for initial MCS in children with heart failure is ideally limited to cardiac support with VADs that support the left ventricle (LVAD), right ventricle (RVAD), or both (BiVAD). However, some children with acute decompensated heart failure also have significant pulmonary dysfunction, which is often reversible and may require cardiopulmonary support; in such cases, temporary support with ECMO may be indicated. Moreover, if the patient is in cardiopulmonary arrest with ongoing cardiopulmonary resuscitation, then ECMO is the support of choice as this can be rapidly initiated (peripherally) and will provide support to both ventricles and the lungs. The Texas Children's Hospital Pediatric MCS guideline is shown in **Figure 52.1**.

EXTRACORPOREAL MEMBRANE OXYGENATION

ECMO is separately covered in Chapter 17. ECMO is a temporary device and should be confined to short-term support for heart failure. Although it has been used for this purpose, ECMO has little or no real role in bridging children to heart transplantation. There is a significant survival benefit of long-term VAD support over ECMO support for patients waiting for heart transplantation. This is of increased importance because of longer waiting duration on the transplant list in the recent era. The negative effects of ECMO are evident even after patients are bridged to cardiac transplant. Mortality rate posttransplant is higher in patients supported with ECMO compared with those who had VAD support, irrespective of diagnosis.

Controversy exists, however, regarding the best mode of MCS if anticipated support duration is short (<2 weeks). Many pediatric heart centers utilize ECMO irrespective of the etiologies of heart failure. ECMO should not be a device for pure circulatory

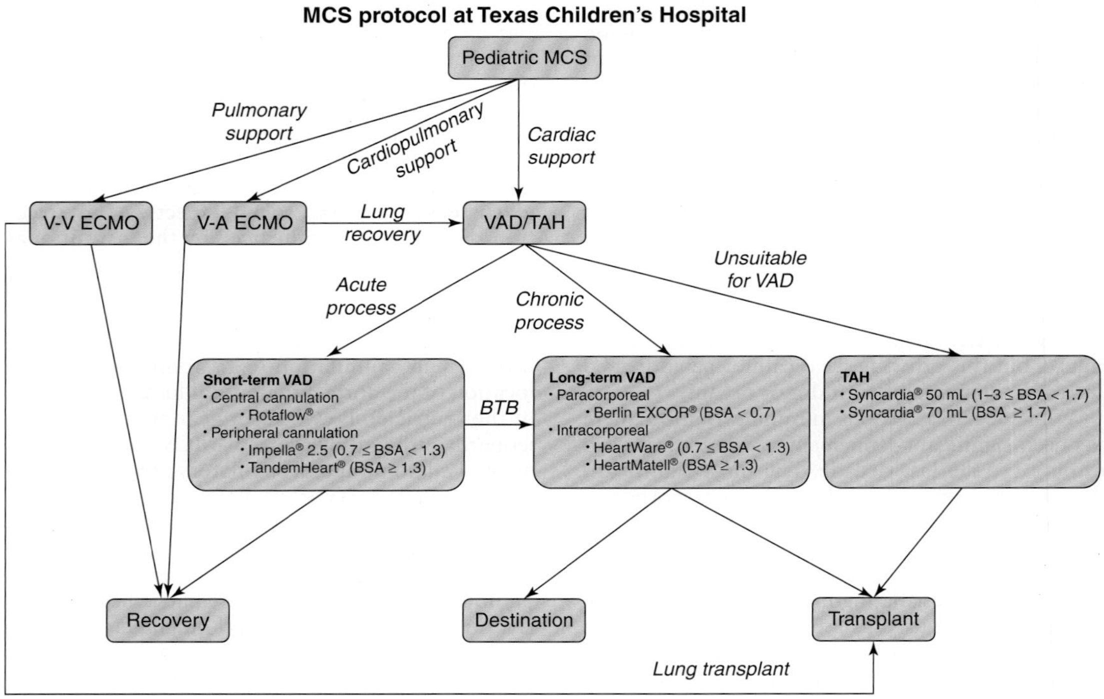

FIGURE 52.1. Mechanical circulatory support protocol from Texas Children's Hospital. Type of MCS support is determined by considering the following factors: (a) which organ(s) to support (e.g., heart only, lungs only, or both heart and lungs), (b) anticipated duration of MCS support based on the etiologies of heart failure, (c) patient's body size, (d) the goal of MCS support (e.g., recovery, destination, or transplant). MCS, mechanical circulatory support; V-V ECMO, veno-venous extracorporeal membrane oxygenation; V-A ECMO, veno-arterial extracorporeal membrane oxygenation; VAD, ventricular assist device; TAH, total artificial heart; BSA, body surface area.

support; it incorporates an oxygenator and should be considered for "cardiac *and* pulmonary" support. A fundamental question would be whether the patient needs pulmonary support. Because of disadvantages inherently associated with an oxygenator, it is preferable that ECMO be reserved for situations when there is a need to support the lungs. A clear example would be extracorporeal cardiopulmonary resuscitation (eCPR), as discussed earlier. Other applications of ECMO for circulatory support include the presence of significant pulmonary hypertension, hemodynamic instability due to septic shock, or severe pulmonary edema resulting from ventricular dysfunction. A very specific situation in which ECMO should be considered in the setting of isolated ventricular failure would be as temporary support for patients after stage 1 palliation of hypoplastic left heart syndrome. Even in this setting, however, a conversion to a short-term VAD might be an option provided that pulmonary function is preserved.

The advantages of short-term VADs compared with ECMO include the simplicity of the circuit and better decompression of the failing ventricle. The lack of an oxygenator and the simple circuit configuration invoke less inflammation and require less anticoagulation. Better ventricular decompression is critical in patients with acute heart failure with a reasonable chance of cardiac recovery (e.g., acute myocarditis). Short-term VAD support with a centrifugal pump provides excellent decompression of the left heart (or systemic ventricle), with immediate impact on left atrial pressure, pulmonary venous hypertension, pulmonary edema, and lung function. It is clear that a short-term VAD (directly drains the left heart) provides better decompression of a failing left ventricle than does ECMO (has only indirect effect on the left heart). **Figure 52.2** illustrates this principle; the inflow (venous) cannula of a VA ECMO circuit in the right atrium (RA) only drains the left heart if there is a patent foramen ovale. Conversely, inflow to the LVAD comes from a cannula placed directly on the left side of the heart. Hence, short-term VAD support provides a better chance of recovery based on anecdotal experience that suggests that better decompression is associated with a better chance of cardiac recovery.

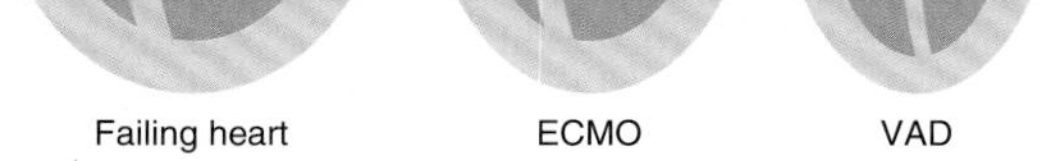

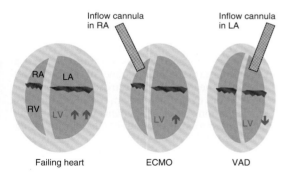

FIGURE 52.2. Improved decompression of failing heart by ventricular assist device. **Left:** Failing heart displaying left atria and ventricle volume distension. **Center:** Moderate improvement of left atria and ventricle volume distension by placing veno-arterial extracorporeal membrane oxygenator inflow (blood return to device) cannula in right atria (indirect decompression). **Right:** Marked improvement of left atria and ventricle volume distension by placing left ventricular assist device inflow (blood return to device) cannula in left atria (direct decompression). RA, right atria; RV, right ventricle; LA, left atria; LV, left ventricle; ECMO, extracorporeal membrane oxygenator; VAD, ventricular assist device.

There are, however, certain situations where ECMO support may be preferable to VAD in the setting of acute heart failure or shock with preserved oxygenation. ECMO is preferred when the right heart is unable to provide "adequate" flow in order to fill the left heart (and therefore the systemic circulation). Suboptimal right heart output can be due to inherent right ventricular dysfunction (e.g., severe cardiac allograft rejection), intractable ventricular arrhythmias, or pulmonary hypertension. Inadequacy of the right heart can also occur when the demand for total cardiac output is extraordinarily increased beyond what even a healthy ventricle can provide (e.g., septic shock). MCS for septic shock is very different in that the flow requirement can be exceedingly high (e.g., 150%–200% flow). Such a high cardiac output cannot be achieved with LVAD support alone since the right heart cannot cope with such high demands. Another example where ECMO would be preferred is when pulmonary blood flow is supplied by a ventricle to pulmonary artery conduit (e.g., stage 1 palliation for hypoplastic left heart syndrome with a right ventricle to pulmonary artery conduit). In this setting, VA ECMO support is necessary as pulmonary blood flow and oxygenation would not be adequate once the systemic ventricle were decompressed on VAD.

Management

Following initiation of VA ECMO, systemic vascular resistance (SVR) is elevated. This can be due to a combination of the low cardiac output with an elevated afterload or the need for high doses of vasoconstrictors prior to ECMO support. Once ECMO support is established, inotropic agents (particularly vasoconstrictors) should be discontinued and systemic vasodilators should be considered in order to optimize flows and perfusion to the organ beds. Ventilator settings are typically weaned to lung protective mode. Once "full-flow" (see **Table 52.1**) support is established, attention should be paid to the cardiac filling pressures (central venous or left atrial pressures, where available). Ideally, these should be low in keeping with the goal of unloading the heart when support is initiated. Furthermore, the waveform of the arterial line can provide insight into the adequacy of decompression of the systemic ventricle. If the heart is decompressed well, there should be minimal ejection from the patient's heart (a completely or nearly flat arterial waveform, loss of pulsatility). Continued pulsatility is associated with increased myocardial work, left atrial hypertension,

TABLE 52.1

Calculations Used to Determine "Full Flow" for Mechanical Circulatory Support

A. Patient's body weight < 10 kg
0.15 × (weight in kg) [L/min]
B. Patient's body weight ≥ 10 kg: based on patient's age
Age ≤2 years old: 3.0 × body surface area [L/min]
Age ≤4 years old: 2.8 × body surface area [L/min]
Age ≤6 years old: 2.6 × body surface area [L/min]
Age ≤10 years old: 2.5 × body surface area [L/min]
Age >10 years old: 2.4 × body surface area [L/min]

pulmonary edema, and a delay in cardiac recovery. Potential causes of inadequate decompression with "full-flow" support include volume overload during resuscitation, systemic vasoconstriction, inadequate size or suboptimal location of an inflow cannula, and aortic insufficiency. This can also be seen in the setting of significant systemic-to-pulmonary collaterals.

If the chest X-ray shows significant pulmonary venous congestion or if the patient displays pulmonary edema, a decision has to be made regarding how to decompress the systemic ventricle. There is controversy regarding how often left atrial decompression is necessary during VA ECMO support in children with severe heart failure. While some investigators estimated the frequency that pediatric patients would require left atrial decompression on ECMO to be ~22%, others reported that half the patients in their clinical series developed lung edema, thereby benefitting from left atrial decompression.

There are several options for left atrial decompression in patients placed on VA ECMO support for acute heart failure. Balloon atrial septostomy, or blade septectomy followed by balloon septostomy using the transcatheter technique, is widely used and minimally invasive. The procedure can be done using fluoroscopy or at the bedside with echocardiographic guidance. If ECMO has been established with central cannulation, addition of a left atrial cannula is an option. A potential complication with this approach is thrombosis within the cannula due to limited flow. Percutaneous left atrial vent placement is another option during ECMO support, but this technique can be challenging, especially in small children.

SHORT-TERM VENTRICULAR ASSIST DEVICE IN PATIENTS WITH HEART FAILURE

Indication

As mentioned, in many centers, ECMO remains the mainstay of MCS regardless of the etiology or the likely clinical course of heart failure. If expertise and experience allow, VAD should be the modality of choice and ECMO reserved for when there are clear clinical advantages such as in the presence of severe pulmonary dysfunction, following eCPR, or the presence of other factors already discussed. Aside from the advantage of a smaller circuit volume, smaller circuit area, and the need for less systemic anticoagulation, the most significant difference between the two modes of support is the degree of decompression of the left (systemic) ventricle.

Short-term VAD may be used in children with heart failure secondary to (a) acute processes (e.g., acute myocarditis or acute rejection of a cardiac allograft), (b) acute exaggeration of chronic heart failure (e.g., acute worsening of dilated cardiomyopathy due to superimposed infection), or (c) postoperative ventricular dysfunction (e.g., following reimplantation of anomalous left coronary artery arising from the pulmonary artery or late arterial switch operation with deconditioning of the left ventricle). If the etiologies are acute processes, it is highly likely that the cardiac function will recover with adequate decompression.

VAD Cannulation and Management

The most typical approach for the short-term LVAD support is left atria to ascending aorta cannulation via sternotomy. Obviously, the necessity of sternotomy is the big downside of this mode of MCS. Once the desired VAD flow has been established, inotropic support should be reduced appropriately but not discontinued. Similarly, inhaled nitric oxide should not be automatically discontinued. This is because, unlike ECMO support, the right ventricle typically requires ongoing pharmacologic support when the left heart is mechanically supported. Almost always, however, initiation of vasodilator drugs is necessary to achieve optimal mean arterial pressures since SVR is substantially elevated in most cases. Once full-flow perfusion is achieved with the target mean arterial pressure, adequacy of systemic perfusion is confirmed by physical examination, urine output, clearance of lactate, reversal of acidosis, near-infrared spectroscopy saturations, mixed venous oxygen saturation, end-organ function, etc. Ventilation settings in patients on LVAD should be optimized to maintain a low pulmonary vascular resistance (PVR), to maximize cardiac output from the right ventricle, and to provide better filling of the LVAD. Unlike an ECMO circuit, the short-term VAD circuit does not contain a heat exchanger. Therefore, desired temperature, usually normothermia, may not be always achievable, especially when the chest is left open in small children. Alternative strategies to maintain normothermia may be needed (e.g., overhead radiant heater or an external convective warmer).

The decision regarding when to discontinue or transition to other type of support requires clinical judgment. Most patients with acute etiologies of heart failure are expected to recover within a short period of time (typically <2 weeks), sufficiently short for the MCS to be discontinued. This recovery process should not be confused with reverse-remodeling that denotes favorable alterations in myocardial structure observed in patients with chronic heart failure (i.e., dilated cardiomyopathy) supported with long-term VADs. Some investigators have described functional recovery of the heart in the setting of acute heart failure as "rapid reverse-remodeling." However, short-term VAD use may be too short for the favorable structural changes to occur. Instead, the main purpose of short-term VAD use for acute heart failure is to support the circulation while protecting the lungs until the inflammatory storm subsides and other end-organs recover (i.e., bridge to recovery).

With the use of short-term VADs, the majority of patients with acute etiologies (85%) can be successfully bridged to recovery, while 100% recovery can be achieved in patients with acute myocarditis. Reports on ECMO support for acute myocarditis have survival rates of 63%–80%. Most patients with acute myocarditis can be supported reasonably well with either mode of MCS (ECMO or short-term VAD). The difference in left heart decompression, however, could make a difference in the severest end of the spectrum where there is virtually no cardiac contractility. The superior outcome with short-term VAD support is due to the capability of saving these sickest children who would not have survived without perfect decompression of the left heart.

In contrast, the goal of VAD support in the setting of chronic heart failure is different from that for acute heart failure. Chronic heart failure implies that cardiac recovery is unlikely. These patients will need a more chronic and durable form of heart failure treatment, such as long-term VADs or heart transplantation. Therefore, the major role of the short-term VAD support in the setting of chronic heart failure is initial salvage when the patient acutely deteriorates with an evidence of ongoing end-organ injury (i.e., INTERMACS 1 profile). (The Interagency Registry for Mechanically Assisted Circulatory Support scale is used to classify advanced heart failure patients according to hemodynamic status. Profile/level 1 is worst, 7 is best, see **Table 52.2.**) It has been shown that preoperative INTERMACS 1

TABLE 52.2

Interagency Registry for Mechanically Assisted Circulatory Support (Intermacs) Levels

Profile 1	Critical cardiogenic shock	Patient with life-threatening hypotension despite rapidly escalating inotropic support and critical organ hypoperfusion, often confirmed by worsening acidosis and/or lactate levels.
Profile 2	Progressive decline	Patient with declining function despite intravenous inotropic support, which may be manifest by worsening renal function, nutritional depletion, and inability to restore volume balance.
Profile 3	Stable but inotrope-dependent	Patient with stable blood pressure, organ function, nutrition, and symptoms on continuous intravenous inotropic support (or a temporary circulatory support device or both), but demonstrating repeated failure to wean from support due to recurrent symptomatic hypotension or renal dysfunction.
Profile 4	Resting symptoms	Patient can be stabilized close to normal volume status but experiences daily symptoms of congestion at rest or during activities of daily living (ADL). Doses of diuretics generally fluctuate at very high levels. More intensive management and surveillance strategies should be considered, which may in some cases reveal poor compliance that would compromise outcomes with any therapy. Some patients may shuttle between Profiles 4 and 5.
Profile 5	Exertion intolerant	Comfortable at rest and with ADL but unable to engage in any other activity, living predominantly within the house. Patients are comfortable at rest without congestive symptoms, but may have underlying refractory elevated volume status, often with renal dysfunction. If underlying nutritional status and organ function are marginal, patient may be more at risk than INTERMACS Profile 4 and require definitive intervention.
Profile 6	Exertion limited	Patient without evidence of fluid overload is comfortable at rest, and with ADL and minor activities outside the home but fatigues after the first few minutes of any meaningful activity. Attribution to cardiac limitation requires careful measurement of peak oxygen consumption, in some cases with hemodynamic monitoring to confirm severity of cardiac impairment.
Profile 7	Advanced NYHA III	A placeholder for more precise specification in the future, this level includes patients who are without current or recent episodes of unstable fluid balance, living comfortably with meaningful activity limited to mild physical exertion.

From Boyle AJ, Ascheim DD, Russo MJ, et al. Clinical outcomes for continuous-flow left ventricular assist device patients stratified by pre-operative INTERMACS classification. *J Heart Lung Transplant* 2011;30:402–7.

profile is a significant predictor of early mortality after long-term VAD implantation. By stabilizing the hemodynamics, it would be possible to minimize and ideally reverse pulmonary venous hypertension, to improve lung function, and to provide good systemic oxygen delivery to the tissues and organs, making the patient a better candidate for more invasive operation with a long-term VAD.

LONG-TERM VAD

Indication

When the etiology of heart failure is chronic in nature and the patient is relatively stable with respect to secondary organ function and functional status (INTERMACS profile 2 or 3), then long-term VADs are the devices of choice. The selection of device is mainly determined by the size of a patient. Currently, the only pediatric long-term VAD that has widespread acceptance worldwide is the Berlin Heart EXCOR (Berlin Heart, Inc. The Woodlands, TX). In older children, adult-sized intracorporeal devices such as HeartMate II (Thoratec Corp. Pleasanton, CA) or HVAD (HeartWare Inc. Framingham, MA) are additional options. The Berlin Heart EXCOR is used in patients with a body surface area (BSA) of 0.7 m^2 or smaller, whereas the HeartMate II (Thoratec Corp.; Pleasanton, CA) is used in patients with a BSA of 1.3 m^2 or larger. The HVAD can be used for intermediate range of patients ($0.7 < \text{BSA} < 1.3\ m^2$).

Prior to making the decision regarding VAD implantation, it is essential to assess carefully the function of the right ventricle as this will directly impact on the device strategy (i.e., LVAD vs. BiVAD). It is not always easy to accurately assess the RV function in the setting of severe LV dysfunction, and some degree of RV dysfunction is almost inevitable in patients with chronic heart failure. To this end, some centers advocate routine use of BiVAD for all patients. However, global experience would suggest that LVAD can provide adequate circulatory support for most children with severe heart failure as RV failure is typically secondary to LV failure. Studies show that clinical outcome with BiVAD is worse than that of LVAD and LVAD alone should be used if possible, except in scenarios when RV function is inherently compromised. Examples of compromised RV function include arrhythmogenic right ventricular dysplasia, posttransplant chronic graft dysfunction, and infarction of the right coronary artery territory. One specific population to consider BiVAD support rather than LVAD alone is in patients with restrictive cardiomyopathy, which is typically associated with biventricular dysfunction as well as elevated pulmonary vascular resistance.

Management of LVAD

If LVAD support is chosen, an important focus of postoperative care is directed at optimizing the right heart's cardiac output. Since most patients supported with an isolated LVAD have some degree of RV failure, right heart management is a key to success. The basic principles of preventing right heart failure on LVAD include optimizing cardiopulmonary interactions, minimizing pulmonary vascular resistance, and maintaining right heart cardiac output with the lowest possible central venous pressure. Inotropes are usually required during the early postoperative period, and many centers advocate the use of inhaled nitric oxide. A clinically important question is how to assess right heart cardiac output. Echocardiography is very useful in this regard. An advantage of a pneumatic paracorporeal device over an intracorporeal device is the fact that the filling status of a pump can be assessed under a direct vision. This is the most direct indicator of right heart cardiac output, provided that there is no significant aortic insufficiency or intracardiac shunting.

SPECIAL CONSIDERATIONS

Bridge to Recovery

As discussed earlier, most "recoverable" hearts have acute, temporary etiologies of heart failure, and are best supported by a short-term VAD. Cardiac function usually recovers within a short period of time (often after an acute insult such as acute inflammation secondary to infection, myocarditis, or cardiac surgery). However, there is a small subset of patients whose heart undergoes myocardial recovery in a gradual fashion and patients benefit from support with a long-term VAD without the ultimate need for transplantation. Recovery from chronic heart failure with a long-term VAD is not well described in children (largely anecdotal experience).

VAD as Destination Therapy

In adults, it is more common to employ long-term VAD support for patients who are deemed not to be transplant candidates and whose cardiac function is unlikely to recover. This strategy, termed "bridge-to-destination" or alternatively "chronic VAD therapy," is not a widely accepted option for children. In the near future, chronic VAD therapy will gain a more important role in the management of pediatric heart failure. Children who might benefit from this therapy include those with certain systemic diseases that preclude transplant candidacy (e.g., Duchenne or Becker muscular dystrophy; patients with malignancy) in whom improvement of quality of life may be offered with VAD support.

Functionally Univentricular Physiology

As discussed earlier, advancements in congenital heart surgery over the past few decades have resulted in a growing population of survivors, particularly those with a Fontan circulation, who develop circulatory failure late in adolescence or early adulthood. Although Fontan failure can be multifactorial, VAD support for a single systemic ventricle can improve the failing circulation when the primary etiology of circulatory failure is systolic ventricular dysfunction. This mode of usage is termed "systemic VAD (SVAD)." Since patients in this category have unique anatomic and physiologic features, SVAD treatment must be optimized individually. The location of the systemic ventricle and its apex is critical for device selection. In the presence of dextrocardia, it may be difficult to implant the HeartMate II as these devices are essentially designed to fit hearts with an apex on the left (levocardia). In patients with a functionally univentricular heart and Fontan circulation, the absence of a subpulmonary ventricle may result in suboptimal filling of an SVAD. Therefore, it is important to ensure almost complete systemic ventricular decompression with a higher VAD setting and optimal cardiopulmonary interactions to encourage passive flow into the pulmonary arteries.

If the primary reason for Fontan failure is pulmonary in origin (i.e., increased transpulmonary gradient), then the placement of a VAD at a subpulmonary position may be an option. When the problems are at multiple levels that would preclude the successful application of VAD use, an alternative option may be a total artificial heart (TAH).

Total Artificial Heart

There are certain situations where VAD support is not an ideal solution. An example would include chronic graft failure after heart transplantation (e.g., chronic rejection, transplant coronary artery disease, etc.). The necessity of immunosuppression for the cardiac graft poses a significant risk for infectious complications when VAD support is provided. In this scenario, the TAH (Syncardia Inc., Tucson, AZ) may make postoperative care much simpler since it eliminates the need of immunosuppressive therapy. The TAH may also be considered if VAD support requires multiple and complex concomitant procedures (e.g., repair or replacement of aortic and/or atrioventricular valves), in the presence of severe aortic regurgitation or if a VAD cannot be placed for anatomic reasons, most typically cardiac position. The TAH should be considered in a minority of patients with end-stage heart failure awaiting transplantation and who cannot be supported with more conventional VAD devices. The use of the TAH in children is technically challenging. The small thorax size in children poses a major limitation in patient selection, with the current system's 70-cc pump size. Soon a smaller system (with a 50-cc pump) will become commercially available and expand the pediatric application of the TAH.

CHAPTER 53 ■ THORACIC TRANSPLANTATION

STEVEN A. WEBBER, LAURA A. LOFTIS, AARTI BAVARE, RENEE M. POTERA, AND NIKOLETA S. KOLOVOS

CARDIAC TRANSPLANTATION

Transplantation offers survival and improved quality of life for selected children with end-stage heart disease due to acquired or congenital cardiac defects.

Indications for Cardiac Transplantation

Transplantation of the heart is considered to be indicated when expected survival is under 2 years and/or when the patient has an unacceptable quality of life. Diagnoses that lead to transplantation are age-dependent; congenital heart disease accounts for two-thirds of transplants in infants, and cardiomyopathy accounts for a similar proportion among adolescents. Norwood reconstruction and transplantation for hypoplastic left heart syndrome have survival rates >80% at 1 year. Because wait times for newborn heart transplant are ~2 months, costs of care are high prior to transplantation, there is significant pretransplant morbidity, and wait-list mortality is as high as 25%, most centers have moved away from transplantation. This strategy increases availability of organs for other infants with cardiac disease unsuitable for surgical palliation.

Contraindications to transplantation include chronic hepatitis B or C, or HIV infection; prior nonadherence with medical therapy; recent treatment of malignancy with inadequate follow-up to ensure likely cure; active acute viral, fungal, or bacterial infections; elevated and *fixed* pulmonary vascular resistance (PVR), inadequate intraparenchymal pulmonary vascular bed; diffuse pulmonary vein stenosis; and major extracardiac disease felt to be nonreversible with heart transplantation (e.g., severe systemic myopathy). Decision-making is based on consensus discussion among all team members, including intensive care staff.

Evaluation of the Cardiac Transplant Candidate

Many children who require an evaluation for cardiac transplantation are receiving care in the PICU. A typical evaluation protocol requires a thorough history and physical examination. Cardiac diagnostic studies usually include chest radiograph, electrocardiogram, echocardiogram, and cardiac catheterization (selected patients may need an exercise test, ventilation–perfusion scan, chest CT, MRI, or pulmonary function tests).

Anatomic and Hemodynamic Considerations

A significant anatomic and hemodynamic consideration is that the lung vasculature is adequately developed and PVR is acceptable. Important surgical anatomy includes abnormalities of cardiac and visceral situs (especially systemic and pulmonary venous return) and the size and anatomy of the main and branch pulmonary arteries (presence of stenoses, distortions, and nonconfluence). Cardiac catheterization is usually indicated pretransplant to assess PVR. Excessive fixed PVR will result in acute donor right ventricular failure and necessitate a right ventricular assist device in the immediate postoperative period. Children with an indexed PVR (PVRI) ≤ 6 indexed units (IU) are at low risk for acute donor right heart failure and a PVRI of 6–10 IU increases risks, but transplantation is not contraindicated. A PVRI > 10 IU is a contraindication to isolated heart transplantation, unless a major fall is achieved (well below 10 IU) with pulmonary vasodilator therapy (100% oxygen or nitric oxide). It should be noted that a rapid fall in PVR can acutely elevate left atrial pressure in patients with poor left ventricular function and may precipitate pulmonary edema. VADs can be used to lower PVR in selected wait-list candidates and allow successful bridge-to-transplant without posttransplant acute right ventricular failure.

Laboratory Investigations

The laboratory tests needed in a transplant candidate include blood type (ABO), HLA antibody screen, complete blood count with differential, coagulation screen, blood urea nitrogen, creatinine, glucose, electrolytes, calcium, magnesium, liver function tests, lipid profile, and brain natriuretic peptide. Blood typing ensures ABO compatibility with the transplanted organ. Isohemagglutinins against blood group antigens do not develop until later in infancy, and so infants with absent or low anti-A and anti-B isohemagglutinin titers can be transplanted across ABO barriers. This means that pre- and posttransplant transfusions must be planned to avoid blood products that contain inappropriate anti-A and anti-B antibodies. Preformed anti–human leukocyte antigen

(HLA) antibodies are checked to see if the patient is "sensitized."

Serologic screening should be done for antibodies to cytomegalovirus (CMV), Epstein–Barr virus (EBV), herpes simplex, varicella-zoster, HIV, hepatitis (A, B, C, and D), measles, and *Toxoplasma gondii.* The infectious diseases' serologic status guides prophylaxis and the evaluation of posttransplantation fever. Candidates in whom transplantation is not imminent should undergo appropriate immunizations (PPD/Mantoux placement, immunization with hepatitis B, pneumococcal, and influenza) during the pretransplant evaluation.

Consultations

A multidisciplinary team (transplant cardiologist and surgeon, cardiac anesthesiologist, social worker, transplant coordinator, and infectious disease expert) evaluates each candidate. A screening psychiatric/psychological examination of the patient and the family is also important to identify patients and families at high risk for poor psychosocial outcome while waiting for (and after) transplantation. Patients with Fontan circulation require evaluation for cirrhosis, and may require hepatology consultation. Additional consultations that may be needed include neonatology, genetics, neurology, dental, oncology, immunology, nephrology, nutrition, physical/occupational therapy, development, and hospital finance.

Evaluation of the Cardiac Donor

Evaluation of the donor heart requires a careful history including donor age, gender, IV drug use, cardiovascular disease, distance from transplant center, malignancy, body size, cause of death, presence of chest trauma, need for cardiopulmonary resuscitation, length of resuscitation, and evaluation of the hemodynamic status (including blood pressure, heart rate, central venous pressure, fluid balance, blood gas, types and doses of inotropes, electrocardiogram, chest radiograph, echocardiogram, cardiac enzymes). A history of cardiopulmonary resuscitation is not a contraindication to donation. Brain death results in physiologic disturbances, including temperature instability with hypothermia, circulatory volume changes (most commonly depletion), and neuroendocrine dysfunction (depletion of circulating thyroxine, cortisol, insulin, glucagon, and antidiuretic hormone).

Donor hearts with more than mildly impaired systolic function despite inotropic agent or thyroid hormone are usually avoided (e.g., shortening fraction < 26%, ejection fraction < 50%). Mild atrioventricular valve regurgitation (common after brain death) is not a contraindication to donation. Pericardial effusion may indicate myocardial contusion. Mild, nonspecific ST- and T-wave changes often reflect central nervous system effects, electrolyte disturbances, or hypothermia and do not contraindicate donation. Interpretation of cardiac enzymes is difficult following trauma. Elevation of troponin I may be a predictor of acute graft failure in infants. Use of donors >35 years of age risks posttransplant coronary disease and poor long-term survival.

Size matching is critical in the selection of donors. The cardiac output of an undersized donor (<75%–80% of recipient weight) may be insufficient for the needs of the recipient. Use of oversized donors is common. Recipient cardiomegaly leaves room in the chest for an oversized donor heart. Use of donor-to-recipient weight ratios of 2.5:1 is common in children, and ratios of 3:1–4:1 have been successfully used in newborns and infants. Marked oversizing results in delayed sternal closure. In infants, oversizing has been associated with a prolonged ventilator course and increased risk of primary graft failure. Oversized donor hearts may cause a high-output postoperative syndrome associated with systemic hypertension, raised intracranial pressure, and mental status changes. Oversizing donors may improve outcome when the recipient has significant preoperative pulmonary hypertension.

All donors should be screened for CMV, EBV, HIV-1, HIV-2, human T-lymphotropic viruses 1 and 2 (HTLV-1, HTLV-2), hepatitis A, B, and C, syphilis, *T. gondii*, and all culture results investigated since admission. The presence of antibodies to CMV, EBV, or *T. gondii* is not a contraindication to transplantation but guides posttransplantation therapy and surveillance. Evidence of retroviral infection (HIV or HTLV) is a contraindication to heart transplantation. The presence of hepatitis B surface antigen is usually considered a contraindication to heart donation; the use of hepatitis C-positive donors remains controversial.

Surgical Techniques of Graft Implantation

The *biatrial anastomosis* for cardiac transplantation has been applied to thousands of patients of all ages with excellent results. Despite great success, this technique yields nonanatomically correct results, with large atrial cavities that may contribute to dysfunction of the tricuspid valve and sinus node. Many centers now perform a *bicaval anastomosis* in children of all ages. Some forms of congenital heart disease lend themselves to the bicaval technique (e.g., patients who have had previous Mustard or Senning operations or Glenn anastomoses). The bicaval technique may be associated with superior caval vein stenosis, especially in infants. Transplantation for congenital heart disease (CHD) performed after multiple palliative procedures presents formidable surgical challenges.

Postoperative Management and Early Complications

Cardiovascular Considerations

Inotropic Agents. Cardiac dysfunction occurs due to hypoxic–ischemic insult to the donor heart. Recovery of systolic function is rapid, but diastolic dysfunction may persist for weeks. Most heart transplant recipients benefit from low-dose inotropic support in the postoperative period for 2–3 days. The choice of inotrope depends on physician preference, heart rate, PVR, and blood pressure. Low-dose vasodilator/inotropic agent therapy such as dobutamine or milrinone treats low cardiac output and high systemic vascular resistance.

Systemic Hypertension. Systemic hypertension is common and may result from vigorous function of an oversized donor organ or high-dose corticosteroids. It may be severe for 24 hours after a successful transplant. Treatment with IV vasodilators and β-blockers may be necessary. Epicardial pacing wires should be working if β-blockers are to be used, since the transplanted heart is at risk for transient sinoatrial disease.

Pulmonary Vascular Resistance. Nitric oxide is begun during surgery to wean from cardiopulmonary bypass. Acidosis must be avoided, and increased levels of inspired oxygen and generous sedation are provided in the early postoperative period. Prostaglandin E_1 (PGE_1) can also be used. The right heart may require inotropic support (epinephrine in addition to milrinone or dobutamine). If right ventricular dysfunction persists, mechanical support is provided.

Cardiac Rate and Rhythm. Sinus bradycardia, with or without an atrial or junctional escape rhythm, is common. The denervated sinus node responds to chronotropic agents (not atropine) or atrial pacing (all recipients should have temporary pacing wires). Ventricular ectopy and nonsustained ventricular tachycardia may occur in the first two weeks but rarely require treatment. The fresh cardiac allograft has limited ability to increase stroke volume; therefore, an adequate heart rate is important to maintain cardiac output. Target heart rates are 140–150 beats/min in infants and 100 beats/min in teenagers.

Primary Graft Failure. Failure to wean from cardiopulmonary bypass and early graft failure are associated with high mortality. *Primary graft failure* refers to acute left ventricular or biventricular failure not due to elevated PVR. Poor donor selection, prolonged ischemic time, poor preservation technique, and hyperacute rejection (rare after anti-HLA antibody screen) should all be considered. When primary graft failure occurs, recovery is possible with circulatory support, usually achieved with extracorporeal membrane oxygenation (ECMO). Early graft failure has a poor outcome, and may be a contraindication to retransplantation.

Respiratory Support. The principles of respiratory support do not differ from other open heart procedures. Early extubation should be the goal. The patient who required prolonged preoperative ventilation usually requires prolonged ventilatory support postoperatively to retrain respiratory muscles. Infants with long-standing cardiomegaly often have significant tracheobronchomalacia, and persistent or recurrent pulmonary atelectasis.

Renal Function. The combination of chronic heart failure, cardiopulmonary bypass, and low cardiac output and the use of cyclosporine or tacrolimus contribute to postoperative renal dysfunction. Oliguria is common but acute renal failure is rare in children, and dialysis is seldom required. Persistent oliguria is managed with loop diuretics and low-dose dopamine. Low cardiac output is managed with inotropic agents. Administration of a continuous furosemide infusion may be helpful. These maneuvers usually stimulate an adequate urine output (>1 mL/kg/h). In neonates and infants, IV PGE_1 may also provide a diuretic effect. The immunosuppressive agents, tacrolimus and cyclosporine, are highly nephrotoxic. When urine output remains low, it may be necessary to decrease dosage or hold calcineurin inhibitors. This is facilitated by the use of T lymphocyte–depleting agents (intravenous "induction therapy"), which provides effective immunosuppression in the first few days and allows more gradual introduction of calcineurin inhibitors.

Gastrointestinal Complications. All patients should receive intravenous or oral H_2 antagonists to decrease the risk of stress ulcers. These are usually continued until corticosteroids have been weaned or discontinued. Optimal calories are provided without excessive volumes to prevent fluid retention. Pancreatitis is common posttransplantation and should be suspected in the presence of abdominal pain or feeding intolerance. Immunosuppression that avoids azathioprine and corticosteroids may reduce this complication. Symptoms of gastrointestinal perforation may be subtle in small children on immunosuppression, especially corticosteroids. Gastroesophageal reflux disease is common and should be aggressively managed, but many drug interactions occur between immunosuppressants and drugs for gastroesophageal reflux.

Infectious Precautions. Infections are a leading cause of death and morbidity in the first year following heart transplantation. A short course of antibiotics (a first-generation cephalosporin) is given as prophylaxis against mediastinal and wound infection. Broader staphylococcal coverage (vancomycin) is considered for a prolonged intensive care unit (ICU) stay, long-standing vascular catheters, or colonization with methicillin-resistant *Staphylococcus aureus*. Oral nystatin is started to prevent Candida infections and ganciclovir to prevent early CMV infection if recipient or donor is seropositive for CMV. Patients at high risk for yeast infections (e.g., pretransplant ECMO) are prophylaxed with fluconazole ("azole" antifungals affect calcineurin-inhibitor metabolism via the cytochrome P450 system) requiring a reduction in tacrolimus or cyclosporine dosing (50%–90%). Initiation of prophylaxis against *Pneumocystis jiroveci* starts close to hospital discharge.

Immunosuppression and Early Acute Rejection. High-dose IV methylprednisolone (15–20 mg/kg) is given in the operating room, tapered over the next 1–2 weeks, and the patient discharged on maintenance corticosteroid therapy. Steroid-free immunosuppressive regimens are increasingly being used. Cyclosporine or tacrolimus is commenced within 24–48 hours of surgery once urine output is good. If anti–T-cell induction therapy is used (commonly antithymocyte globulin [ATG]; less often interleukin-2 receptor [IL-2R] antagonist), there is less urgency to introduce a calcineurin inhibitor in the first 1–5 days. Cyclosporine or tacrolimus can then be started orally rather than IV. Delaying these agents may be particularly useful when urine output is low or renal function is deteriorating.

Numerous strategies are available for maintaining immunosuppression. A calcineurin inhibitor is used as the primary immunosuppressive agent (~80% of children are on tacrolimus at discharge). Most centers use a second, adjunctive agent—most commonly mycophenolate mofetil (MMF)/mycophenolic acid. More centers are using steroid avoidance regimens or early steroid weaning in children. Agents of similar classes are not given together, as they enhance toxicities. Combination therapies use two or three agents of different classes with different mechanisms of action.

Daily assessment for rejection is required. Rejection is generally delayed with use of induction therapy and severe rejection before 7–10 days is rare (except in the sensitized patient). Infants and young children experience less acute rejection than do adolescents. Pallor, increasing tachycardia, abdominal pain, gallop rhythm, and oliguria all are suggestive of severe rejection. Ideally, rejection is identified by echocardiography and/or surveillance biopsy before such signs develop. The electrocardiogram may show reduced precordial voltages. The tempo of rejection can be quite abrupt in the early posttransplant period, and any deterioration after initial recovery from surgery is serious. If evidence of graft dysfunction is unequivocal, empiric bolus intravenous corticosteroids are given. Endocardial muscle biopsy generally shows lymphocytic infiltrates (predominantly T cells) with varying degrees of edema and myocyte damage or necrosis.

Medium-term and Late Complications

Immunologic complications fall into two groups: allograft rejection/graft dysfunction (acute and chronic), which reflects inadequate or ineffective immunosuppression, and nonspecific immunosuppression (infection and malignancy). Nonimmune side effects of immunosuppressive therapy (i.e., tissue and organ toxicities) are an important cause of morbidity, and occasionally mortality.

Acute Rejection

Patients remain at risk for acute rejection indefinitely. Acute rejection/acute graft failure is the most common cause of death between 30 days and 3 years after heart transplantation (a third of all deaths, peak between 1 and 3 months). By 3 years, half of recipients are free of acute rejection. Late acute rejection episodes (after the first year) carry a poor long-term prognosis, especially if associated with graft dysfunction. More than mild systolic failure requires IV milrinone, monitoring for dysrhythmias, treatment with IV methylprednisolone for 3–5 days, and an endomyocardial biopsy if the patient is stable. Plasmapheresis and anti–B-cell/plasma cell agents may be required. Treatment should not be delayed awaiting biopsy or results. Acute rejection with hemodynamic compromise can be rapidly fatal. Unless there are specific contraindications, full hemodynamic support, including mechanical support, should be used as the condition is often reversible.

Chronic Rejection and Posttransplant Coronary Arterial Disease

The terms *chronic rejection* and *posttransplant coronary arterial disease* are generally used synonymously. Coronary disease subsequent to transplantation is an accelerated vasculopathy and the leading cause of death among late survivors. Immune mechanisms are probably of central importance in young children. Use of older donors, donor cigarette usage, late acute rejection episodes, older recipient age, retransplantation, and black race are some of the risk factors reported for the development of posttransplant coronary arterial disease. CMV infection may also contribute to the development of graft vascular disease. Symptoms of ischemia are often absent, though some children experience episodes of abdominal pain and/or chest pain despite operative denervation of the heart. Syncope and sudden death are also common presentations of graft coronary disease in children. In the current era, the diagnosis is most often made during surveillance-selective coronary angiography.

Unfortunately, no curative treatment exists. Diastolic dysfunction develops early and once overt systolic failure ensues, survival is poor, and consideration should be given to retransplantation. Inotropic agents should be used with great caution. Patients with syncope should receive an automatic implantable cardioverter defibrillator. β-Blockers may be given for their anti-ischemic benefits if heart failure is not advanced. Percutaneous coronary interventions may have a role in select patients but are limited by the diffuse and small-vessel nature of the disease. Early outcomes for late retransplantation (more than 6 months after primary transplant) are similar to those for primary transplantation.

Infections

Infection is second to graft failure as a cause of death in the first 30 days and during the remainder of the first year. When there is evidence of pneumonia and deteriorating clinical status, bronchoalveolar lavage is performed to obtain deep cultures for viruses, fungi, and bacteria. In CMV infection in heart recipients, gastroenteritis, hepatitis, and bone marrow suppression are relatively common and pneumonitis is rare. CMV *disease* remains a tissue diagnosis, and when made early, treatment with IV ganciclovir and/or oral valganciclovir is usually effective. EBV can be asymptomatic or cause a nonspecific viral syndrome, mononucleosis, fulminant "viral sepsis," or post-transplant lymphoproliferative disorder (PTLD). The strongest risk factor for PTLD is development of primary EBV infection, although children who are seropositive for EBV at transplant are not completely protected. Therapy includes reduction of immunosuppression and the administration of antiviral agents (without proven benefit), monoclonal antibodies against B-cell antigens (rituximab), chemotherapy, and cellular (adoptive) immunotherapy.

Nonimmune Complications

Nonimmune toxicities of immunosuppressive therapies include systemic hypertension, hyperlipidemia, glucose intolerance, decreased bone density, and bone marrow suppression. Progressive renal dysfunction due to calcineurin inhibitor toxicity is increasingly problematic in long-term survivors (leading to renal transplantation).

Survival

Pretransplant comorbidities such as progressive end-organ dysfunction (especially renal), malnutrition associated with advanced heart failure, and progressive rise in PVR can have an important impact on outcomes. Children in all age groups have shorter waiting times for heart transplants than adults, but a greater risk of death while waiting (http://srtr.transplant.hrsa.gov/). The highest death rate is among infants <1 year of age. The improvement in survival over the last few years is due to reduction in early mortality. One-year survival is ~90%, with a relatively small drop over the following 3–4 years.

LUNG TRANSPLANTATION

Indications for Transplantation

In children, the most common diagnosis for lung transplantation is end-stage lung disease secondary to cystic fibrosis (>50% of lung transplant referrals) and the second is pulmonary hypertension. Disorders of surfactant protein synthesis may result in end-stage lung disease also prompting referral for lung transplantation.

Evaluation and Care of the Transplant Candidate

Careful selection and timing are essential to optimize outcomes. Patients are presented at a multidisciplinary conference such that laboratory testing, pulmonary function, and anatomic considerations can be taken into account. Nutritional status should be optimized, intercurrent infections prevented, and muscle mass maintained with regular exercise. Intubating a patient with impending respiratory failure secondary to end-stage lung disease, particularly those who have been maintained on noninvasive support, can be challenging. Prolonged desaturation and compromised cardiac output immediately following the procedure should be anticipated. Following intubation, patients with obstructive lung disease should be placed on ventilator settings that will allow for a prolonged expiratory phase. Deep sedation and, frequently, neuromuscular blockade are required to facilitate interaction with the ventilator.

Extracorporeal Support as Bridge to Lung Transplantation

Recent advances in devices and techniques have led to improvements in outcome. Studies in adults demonstrate 1-year survival posttransplant in patients bridged with ECMO of 60%–75%. Children requiring ECMO support in the period prior to transplant have poorer outcome (1-year survival 33%). Results of patients bridged to transplant using veno-venous ECMO (VV ECMO) have been encouraging. The ability to awaken and extubate these patients helps to minimize complications related to long-term ventilation and sedation (infection, muscle fatigue, and organ dysfunction). Novalung is not currently approved for pediatric use. Other devices have been used, such as a membrane oxygenator with cannulation of the pulmonary artery and left atrium.

Postoperative Management and Early Complications

Acute Complications

Reperfusion Injury/Graft Failure. Reperfusion injury occurs from restoring blood supply to the ischemic donor lungs during and after transplant. Reperfusion injury is characterized by infiltrates on CXR and poor gas exchange. It occurs in 20%–30% and can be self-limited or progress to early graft failure. Treatment includes inhaled nitric oxide (iNO), PGE_1, positive-pressure ventilation, and extracorporeal support. Acute graft failure is a major cause of death in the first 30 days.

Acute Rejection. Acute rejection can present with poor gas exchange, increasing chest tube drainage, frothy sputum, and worsening gas exchange. Pathologically, acute rejection is seen as infiltrates in the perivascular and interstitial regions with associated airway inflammation. Acute rejection is treated with intravenous methylprednisolone or ATG if refractory to methylprednisolone. Recurrent rejection warrants consideration of change in the immunosuppression regimen.

Systemic Inflammatory Response Syndrome. Varying degrees of systemic inflammatory response occur in the immediate posttransplant period. Treatment includes supportive care of hemodynamics and organ function.

Bleeding. Postoperative bleeding is common and arises from vascular anastomoses, surgical planes of dissection, or airways. Bleeding risk is related to preoperative infection, duration of surgery, and organ function.

Nerve Injury. Phrenic nerve injury is common especially after bilateral lung transplantation and can complicate postoperative respiratory recovery.

Posttransplant Surveillance: Bronchoscopy, Computerized Tomography, Radiographs, Pulmonary Function Testing

Daily chest radiographs are routine while chest tubes are in place and are used to follow lung parenchymal changes, assess lung volumes, check catheter and tube position, and to detect evolving effusions. Bronchoscopy is performed at 24 hours posttransplant to check mucosal and anastomotic integrity and graft perfusion, and to clear bronchial secretions/blood. Bronchoscopies with transbronchial biopsy, chest computerized tomography (CT), ventilation perfusion scans, and pulmonary function tests are performed on a scheduled basis posttransplant. CT scans can be used to assess growth of transplanted lungs in infants and young children.

Subacute Complications

Airway dehiscence was a common complication avoided by the use of donor and recipient peribronchial tissue approximated near the anastomotic site to restore some bronchial circulation. Bronchial stenosis can affect 10% of cases and can be treated with bronchoscopic dilation. Transplanted airways grow with somatic growth and bronchial stenosis is not affected by age or size of the recipient.

Cardiovascular Considerations

Inotropic Agents and Cardiopulmonary Interactions

The immediate posttransplant lung recipient is on pressors (e.g., epinephrine, vasopressin) as warranted by the hemodynamics. PGE_1 is administered for 48 hours to reduce reperfusion injury. Inhaled NO is used postoperatively until extubation to improve the PaO_2/FIO_2 ratio and to decrease pulmonary arterial pressure in patients with severe graft dysfunction ($PaO_2/FIO_2 < 150$).

Dysrhythmias

Atrial flutter or fibrillation is reported in nearly 10% of cases and thought to be generated by electrical aberrance from the suture lines for pulmonary venous anastomosis.

Systemic Hypertension

Hypertension is common due to high-dose steroids, calcineurin inhibitors, or acute kidney dysfunction (from cardiopulmonary bypass or nephrotoxic medications). Calcium channel blockers are often used to treat hypertension.

Respiratory Support

Control of Ventilation

Lung transplant recipients can have deep (hyperpnic) and infrequent (hypopneic) breaths due to the denervated donor organs. It may lead to patient–ventilator dyssynchrony, significant discomfort, and agitation. Allowing patient-dictated ventilator support may facilitate weaning.

Criteria for Extubation

Early extubation allows weaning of sedatives and facilitates pulmonary toilet. Adequate gas exchange, good mucosal perfusion and integrity, and hemodynamic stability are the criteria.

Gastrointestinal Complications

Gastrointestinal complications are common, especially gastroesophageal reflux disease and postoperative ileus. Aggressive prevention and treatment are indicated.

Endocrine Considerations

Hyperglycemia may result from pancreatic insufficiency in cystic fibrosis patients or from a high-dose steroid immunosuppressive regimen. Insulin infusion is the mainstay of therapy.

Renal Function

Acute kidney injury (AKI) is common due to exposure to cardiopulmonary bypass, fluid shifts, and nephrotoxic medications such as immunosuppressive agents (calcineurin inhibitors) and antibiotics (aminoglycosides).

Infectious Precautions

Lung transplant recipients are more susceptible than other solid-organ recipients to infections because of colonization of recipient and donor airways. Early posttransplant infections with bacteria, adenovirus, influenza, parainfluenza, or RSV are common. Pathogens responsible for late infections include CMV, EBV, and fungal organisms. Infections delay recovery, affect transplanted and other organ functions, hamper immunosuppression, and cause morbidity and mortality. Cystic fibrosis patients have increased risk of infections and are specifically prone to infections from colonization with resistant organisms prior to transplant.

Immunosuppression

Current immunosuppressive regimens target relatively specific steps in the stimulation or activation of T cells or eliminating alloreactive B cells. Attempts have been made to reduce high panel-reactive antibody titers with an induction schema using either intravenous immunoglobulin or plasmapheresis, although there is no currently accepted standard of practice. Another therapeutic strategy to limit antibody-mediated injury is to eliminate alloreactive B cells using therapeutic agents such as rituximab, an antibody specific for CD20 that is capable of depleting B cells.

Immunoprophylaxis

Infectious complications account for more than 40% of deaths in the first 12 post-op months. Children at high risk for CMV infection (positive recipient or donor serology) receive CMV prophylaxis for 3–6 months. Pulmonary fungal infection (10%) and *P. jiroveci* pneumonia are common infections. Vaccinations should be administered as scheduled, vaccine response may be decreased, and live virus vaccines avoided.

Outcomes

Survival after pediatric lung transplantation is worse than any other solid-organ transplant (similar to adults). In the first year, non-CMV infection and graft failure are the leading causes of death. Beyond 3 years, chronic rejection (bronchiolitis obliterans syndrome, BOS) accounts for ~42% of deaths. BOS is treated with azithromycin, altered immunosuppression, and photopheresis, and by prevention or treatment of gastroesophageal reflux disease.

CHAPTER 54 ■ CARDIAC CONDUCTION, DYSRHYTHMIAS, AND PACING

RICHARD J. CZOSEK, DAVID S. SPAR, JEFFREY B. ANDERSON, TIMOTHY K. KNILANS, AND BRADLEY S. MARINO

TACHYARRHYTHMIAS

Tachyarrhythmias (an abnormal mechanism of tachycardia) are classified as three electrophysiologic mechanisms: (a) reentry, (b) abnormal automaticity, and (c) triggered activity. In children, reentry is most often seen in supraventricular tachycardia (SVT), but can also be seen in ventricular tachycardia (VT) (e.g., postoperative congenital cardiac patients). The reentrant circuit requires two distinct conducting pathways with slow conduction in one and unidirectional block in the other pathway. Reentrant arrhythmias have a regular rate with a sudden onset and termination; they can also be provoked by an electrical stimulus (e.g., a premature atrial or ventricular contraction or pacing maneuvers) and can be terminated by pacing or direct current cardioversion. *Automaticity* refers to groups of cells that can spontaneously depolarize. Automatic arrhythmias are sensitive to the adrenergic and metabolic state and sympathomimetic agents, but pacing and direct current cardioversion do not convert these arrhythmias. Tachycardias that are derived from triggered activity share characteristics of reentrant and automatic arrhythmias; they may be induced or terminated with pacing maneuvers, have warm-up and cool-down phases, and are catecholamine sensitive.

Diagnostic Approach to Tachyarrhythmias

Narrow QRS complex tachycardia implies conduction through the His–Purkinje system and a supraventricular origin. A wide QRS complex tachycardia is assumed to be ventricular in origin (**Fig. 54.1**). It should be determined whether there is a one-to-one ratio of P waves to QRS complexes, and then the relationship between the QRS complex and the P wave should be examined.

Supraventricular Arrhythmias

The most common arrhythmia in the pediatric population is SVT. SVT may be either reentry (more common) or abnormal automaticity.

Atrioventricular Reciprocating Tachycardia. The most common type of reentrant SVT in children is atrioventricular reciprocating tachycardia (AVRT), which requires participation of both the atrium and ventricle in the reentrant circuit and involves an accessory pathway. Examples of AVRT include Wolff–Parkinson–White syndrome (WPW), orthodromic tachycardia from concealed bypass tracts, and atrioventricular nodal reentrant tachycardia (AVNRT). WPW is characterized by a short PR interval, a delta wave (represents ventricular preexcitation prior to normal activation of the AV node and His–Purkinje system), and episodes of tachycardia associated with an accessory pathway (**Fig. 54.2**). Patients with WPW are at increased risk of atrial fibrillation, hemodynamic instability, and sudden death. The best predictor for sudden death is a ventricular preexcited RR interval (SPRR) during atrial fibrillation of <250 milliseconds, which can lead to ventricular fibrillation. These patients are candidates for a catheter-ablation procedure.

The goal of acute therapy for AVRT is to terminate the reentrant circuit and restore sinus rhythm. If vascular access cannot readily be obtained or the patient is hemodynamically unstable, then direct current synchronized cardioversion is indicated (0.5–1.0 J/kg). In the hemodynamically stable patient with AVRT, vagal maneuvers should be attempted. First-line medical therapy is IV adenosine (0.1 mg/kg); in refractory cases, β-blockers (e.g., esmolol), procainamide, calcium-channel blockers (e.g., diltiazem), or amiodarone can be used. Calcium-channel blockers are contraindicated in young children (especially <1 year of age) due to reports of hemodynamic collapse and sudden death. Digoxin and β-blockers are first-line oral therapy for chronic prevention. Digoxin and calcium-channel blockers are contraindicated for WPW because they may enhance anterograde conduction down the accessory pathway and allow a more rapid ventricular response during atrial fibrillation. For SVT refractory to first-line oral therapy, flecainide, sotalol, amiodarone, and verapamil can also be considered. The success rate for catheter ablation of AVRT is 86%–97%, and >95% for AVNRT.

Atrial Flutter. Atrial flutter occurs in newborns and children with congenital heart disease (especially after

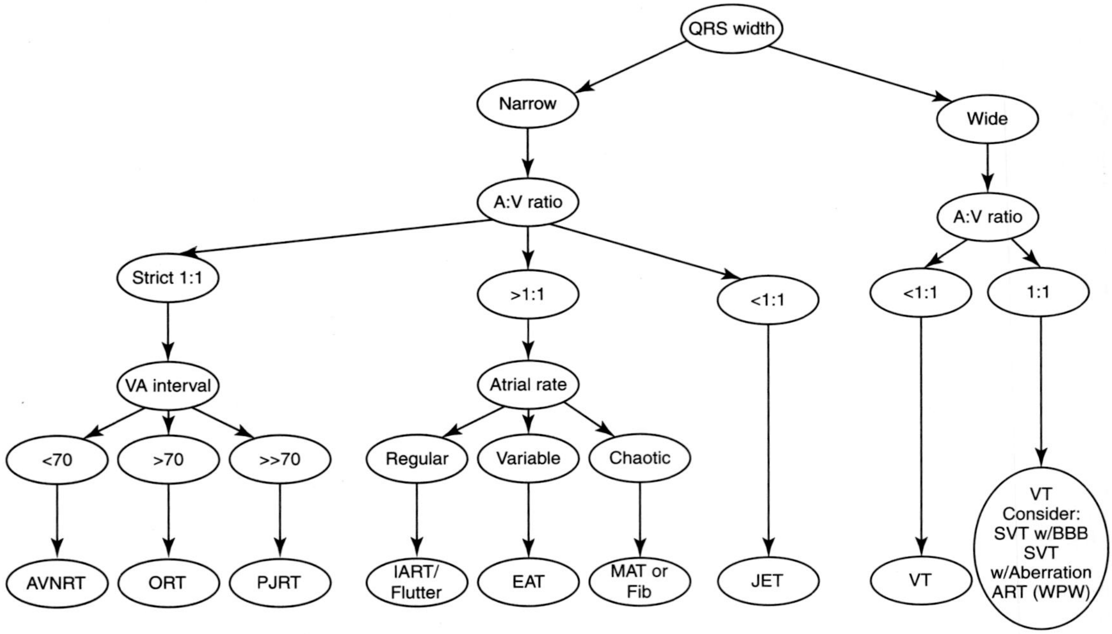

FIGURE 54.1. Diagnostic approach for determining tachycardia mechanism. VA interval (RP interval in text) is measured in milliseconds. ART, antidromic reciprocating tachycardia; AV, atrioventricular; AVNRT, atrioventricular nodal reentrant tachycardia; BBB, bundle-branch block; EAT, ectopic atrial tachycardia; IART, intra-atrial reentrant tachycardia; JET, junctional ectopic tachycardia; MAT, multifocal atrial tachycardia; ORT, orthodromic reciprocating tachycardia; PJRT, permanent junctional reciprocating tachycardia; SVT, supraventricular tachycardia; VA, ventriculoatrial; VT, ventricular tachycardia; WPW, Wolff–Parkinson–White. (From Walsh EP. Clinical approach to diagnosis and acute management of tachycardias in children. In: Walsh EP, Saul JP, Triedman JK, eds. *Cardiac Arrhythmias in Children and Young Adults with Congenital Heart Disease*. Philadelphia, PA: Lippincott Williams & Wilkins, 2001.)

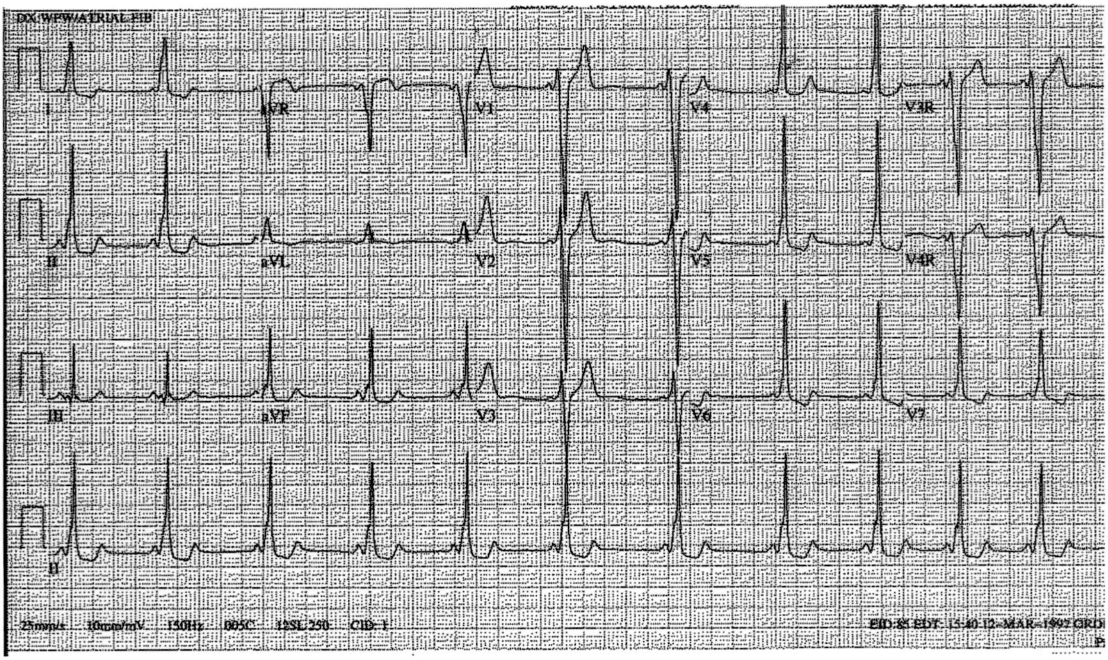

FIGURE 54.2. ECG from a child with Wolff–Parkinson–White syndrome. Note the short PR interval and delta wave.

atrial surgery for congenital heart defects). Characteristic saw-toothed flutter waves are usually present in leads II, III, and aVF. Atrial rates may reach 600 bpm. Direct current synchronized cardioversion (0.5–1.0 J/kg) is the primary treatment modality (high success, low recurrence) in the newborn. Second-line therapy includes digoxin, procainamide, amiodarone, and sotalol. Procainamide slows the flutter rate, results in more rapid AV conduction, and should be used with digoxin.

Intra-Atrial Reentrant Tachycardia. Reentrant atrial tachycardia in patients who have undergone surgery for congenital heart disease is referred to as intra-atrial reentrant tachycardia (IART). The procedures that predispose to IART involve the atria and include atrial septal defect repair, atrial baffling procedures (Senning or Mustard operation) for D-transposition of the great arteries, and the Fontan operation. Symptomatology is related to the ventricular response rate and myocardial function. A fast ventricular response rate results in palpitations, syncope, or sudden death. A slow ventricular response rate results in gradual fatigue or exercise intolerance, especially in the Fontan patient (AV synchrony may be crucial for adequate cardiac output). Long-standing IART results in sluggish flow in the atria or Fontan pathway and increases the risk for thromboembolic events. Prior to attempts to convert IART, the presence of an atrial thrombus should be ruled out unless the patient is in the rhythm <24 hours. Acute therapy includes synchronized cardioversion or transesophageal pacing. Antiarrhythmic medications such as propafenone, amiodarone, and sotalol are used in refractory cases. Postcardioversion, there remains a high risk for thrombus formation from "atrial stunning," and anticoagulation is recommended for 1 month. Medications for chronic IART include flecainide, propafenone, amiodarone, and sotalol.

Automatic Supraventricular Tachycardia. Atrial automatic tachycardias tend to present in children <6 years of age but can occur in older children. The heart rate is inappropriately high for the patient's activity and is sensitive to the adrenergic state. Persistence of the tachycardia may lead to a tachycardia-mediated cardiomyopathy.

Ectopic Atrial Tachycardia. Ectopic atrial tachycardia (EAT), or *automatic atrial tachycardia*, arises from a focus of increased automaticity within the atria. Heart rates range from 130 to 210 bpm in children and can reach 300 bpm in infants. While some cases spontaneously resolve, most patients require chronic therapy.

Multifocal Atrial Tachycardia. Multifocal atrial tachycardia (MAT), or chaotic atrial rhythm, is rare and arises from multiple foci of increased automaticity located within the atria. The tachycardia is defined by the presence of three or more P-wave morphologies. It commonly presents in neonates, with up to 50% of patients having an associated cardiac defect or other medical condition. It frequently spontaneously resolves during the first year of life.

Treatment of Ectopic Atrial Tachycardia/ Multifocal Atrial Tachycardia. Initial treatment of an automatic SVT involves decreasing the ventricular response rate by slowing AV conduction and decreasing automaticity of the abnormal focus or foci. Digoxin and calcium-channel blockers (if >1 year old) can slow conduction through the AV node. β-Blockers, which oppose adrenergic stimulation of the focus, may help suppress the tachycardia. Class IA (procainamide) and IC agents (flecainide) decrease automaticity and prolong refractoriness. Class III agents (amiodarone and sotalol) slow conduction. Spontaneous resolution of EAT is unlikely in older patients, and catheter ablation is first-line therapy. In young patients, resolution of EAT is common with low recurrence rates. Adenosine, overdrive pacing, and cardioversion are not successful in converting automatic tachycardias to sinus rhythm.

Junctional Ectopic Tachycardia. Junctional ectopic tachycardia (JET) is a result of enhanced automaticity in the region within or adjacent to the AV junction. JET is characterized by a narrow complex tachycardia with AV dissociation (usually a ventricular rate faster than the atrial rate). In children, JET may be familial and congenital, or may follow surgery for congenital heart disease. Postoperative JET is usually transient, lasting <72 hours, and commonly follows repairs near the AV node (ventricular septal defect, tetralogy of Fallot [TOF], and AV canal repairs). Treatment for congenital JET includes antiarrhythmic medications, with amiodarone being the most successful. Postoperative JET can be treated with amiodarone or procainamide. Nonpharmacologic measures include fever control, hypothermia to 35°C, sedation, and avoiding sympathomimetic medications. Atrial pacing faster than the junctional rate can allow for AV synchrony and improve hemodynamics.

Ventricular Arrhythmias

Ventricular Tachycardia. VT is defined as three or more ventricular ectopic beats in a row at a rapid rate. The possible mechanisms of a wide QRS complex tachycardia are listed in **Table 54.1**. The patient with a ventricular arrhythmia may be asymptomatic or present with cardiomyopathy or cardiac arrest. The mechanisms by which ventricular arrhythmias occur are the same as those for supraventricular arrhythmias: reentry, automaticity, and triggered automaticity. When a wide QRS complex tachycardia is irregular, occurs with a gradual onset and termination, and does not respond to cardioversion, an automatic mechanism should be suspected. Patients with an automatic VT may be treated with medical therapy to suppress the focus or curative catheter-ablation therapy. β-Blockers and verapamil (verapamil is

TABLE 54.1

Mechanisms of a Wide QRS Complex Tachycardia

Orthodromic atrioventricular reciprocating tachycardia with aberration or bundle-branch block
Antidromic atrioventricular reciprocating tachycardia
Atrial tachycardia with bystander accessory pathway, allowing antegrade conduction (WPW)
Atrioventricular reciprocating tachycardia involving a Mahaim fiber
Ventricular tachycardia

avoided in infants) may be effective and have a low side-effect profile. For those who require continued medical therapy, amiodarone and sotalol offer high success rates.

In patients with prior surgical repair of congenital heart disease, a reentrant mechanism of VT is most common, typically occurring after a ventriculotomy. The incidence of VT after repair of TOF ranges from 4% to 15% with late sudden death in 6%. Demographic (prior palliative shunt, older age at repair, right ventriculotomy), hemodynamic (higher NYHA class status, LV end-diastolic pressure > 12 mm Hg), and electrophysiologic (QRS duration > 180 milliseconds, QRS rate of change) variables are proposed risk factors. In patients with pulmonary regurgitation, pulmonary valve replacement reduces the incidence of sustained monomorphic VT. Aortic stenosis also increases risk for ventricular arrhythmia and mortality (associated with greater outflow tract gradient).

Hypertrophic Cardiomyopathy. Risk factors for sudden cardiac death (SCD) in adults with hypertrophic cardiomyopathy (HCM) include nonsustained VT, family history of sudden death, unexplained syncope, LV thickness > 30 mm, and abnormal blood pressure response during exercise. An implantable cardioverter defibrillator (ICD) is recommended for prevention of SCD in adults with one or more major risk factors, but data are limited in children.

Arrhythmogenic Right Ventricular Cardiomyopathy. Arrhythmogenic right ventricular cardiomyopathy (ARVC) is a less common cause of VT and SCD in apparently healthy victims. The pathologic findings are subtle, and the echocardiogram is frequently normal. The cardiomyopathy involves aneurysmal dilatation and dyskinesis of the right ventricular outflow tract. ICD therapy is recommended in patients with one or more risk factors for SCD (early and severe RV dysfunction, advanced disease with biventricular dysfunction, family history of SCD, and symptomatic VT).

Cardiac Tumors. Although cardiac tumors are rare, they are a source of ventricular arrhythmias with an automatic focus. Rhabdomyomas are the most common cardiac tumor in children, usually found in those with tuberous sclerosis.

Long-QT Syndrome. The congenital *long-QT syndrome* is due to cardiac ion channelopathies associated with abnormal cardiac repolarization resulting in QT prolongation, syncope, cardiac arrest, and SCD. These symptoms are due to polymorphic VT (torsades de pointes [TdP]). The presenting symptom can be a seizure and patients with a presumed seizure disorder should have a screening ECG. Patients at highest risk for SCD include a QTc > 500 milliseconds, history of TdP leading to syncope, prepubertal boys, postpubertal girls, and events occurring in infancy. Effective therapies include pacing (for bradycardia and pause-dependent episodes of ventricular arrhythmia), magnesium, and β-blockers (esmolol). Long-term therapy is usually β-blockers. Indications for an ICD include aborted cardiac arrest, breakthrough cardiac events despite adequate medical therapy, and prior LQT triggered events with a QTc > 550 milliseconds. It is important to avoid cardiac stimulants and medications that prolong the QT interval (some antiarrhythmics, psychotropic medications, erythromycin, and many antifungal agents).

Brugada Syndrome. Brugada syndrome is a familial, primary, electrical abnormality with ECG findings that consist of a right ventricular conduction delay and ST segment elevation ("coved" and "saddle" shape elevations) in the anterior precordial leads (V1–V3). Patients are typically young male adults with syncope, ventricular arrhythmias, and SCD. The only effective treatment for Brugada syndrome is an ICD.

Catecholaminergic Polymorphic VT. Catecholaminergic polymorphic VT (CPVT) has been associated with abnormalities in the cardiac ryanodine receptor (RYR2) (responsible for the release of calcium and calsequestin-2 from the sarcoplasmic reticulum). Patients develop polymorphic or bidirectional VT during exercise and increased adrenergic states. β-Blockers, flecainide, and ICD are the mainstay of therapy.

Systemic Causes of Ventricular Arrhythmia. Wide QRS complex rhythms and ventricular arrhythmias are caused by an assortment of systemic causes (**Table 54.2**). Management of acute ventricular arrhythmias is dependent on the etiology and hemodynamic stability of the patient. Medical management or synchronized direct current cardioversion (2 J/kg) may be used to treat a perfusing ventricular arrhythmia or a wide QRS complex arrhythmia with an organized electrical pattern. If the rhythm is pulseless or disorganized, CPR and asynchronous defibrillation are indicated.

Bradyarrhythmias

Bradyarrhythmias can be a primary electrical problem, but in the ICU they are often the manifestation of respiratory, medication, or metabolic issues.

TABLE 54.2

Systemic Causes of Ventricular Arrhythmia

Metabolic	Hyperkalemia Hypokalemia Hypomagnesemia Hypocalcemia Hypoxia Acidosis
Ischemia	Kawasaki disease
Infectious	Systemic viral infections causing myocarditis Systemic bacterial infections causing endocarditis
Toxic	Cocaine/catecholamine infusions/ stimulants Antiarrhythmic medications Digitalis toxicity Psychotropic medications
Traumatic	Commotio cordis Mechanical irritation/central catheters

TABLE 54.3

Treatment for Hemodynamically Significant Bradycardia

Trendelenburg position (supine with the head lower than the level of the pelvis and feet)
Volume expansion
Pharmacologic interventions
  Anticholinergic agents
    Atropine 0.02–0.04 mg/kg (maximum 1–2 mg) IV/IO
  β-adrenergic agonists and activators of adenylate cyclase
    Isoproterenol infusion: 0.01–2.0 μg/kg/min
    Epinephrine IV bolus: 0.05–0.01 mg/kg; infusion: 0.1–0.5 μg/kg/min
    Glucagon (for β-blocker overdose) 0.03–0.15 mg/kg IV
  Digoxin-specific antibody Fab fragments for digoxin toxicity
  Temporary transcutaneous or transvenous pacing
Treat reversible causes:
  6 Hs: hypoxia, hypovolemia, hydrogen ion (acidosis), hypoglycemia, hypo/hyperkalemia, and hypothermia.
  5 Ts: toxins, tamponade, tension pneumothorax, thrombosis (pulmonary), thrombosis (coronary)

Diagnostic Approach to Bradyarrhythmias

If the ratio between atrial and ventricular complexes is 1:1 and there is a normal PR interval, the rhythm is most likely sinus bradycardia or ectopic atrial bradycardia. If the PR interval is prolonged for age but each atrial beat is conducted to the ventricle, then first-degree AV block is present. If there is a relationship between atrial and ventricular activity, the relationship is not 1:1, and there are more atrial than ventricular complexes, then there is likely second-degree AV block. If there is no relationship between the atrial and ventricular activity and the atrial rate is faster than the ventricular rate, then there is complete or high-grade AV block. If the ventricular rhythm is faster than the atrial rhythm and the atrial rhythm is bradycardic for age, then the rhythm is likely an escape rhythm from either the junction or ventricle (most likely a junctional escape rhythm).

Bradyarrhythmia Etiologies

Sinus Node Dysfunction. Sinus node dysfunction (SND) in patients with congenital heart disease typically results from a surgical scar or suture line around sinoatrial (SA) nodal tissue. Following cardiac transplantation, SND is secondary to cardiac denervation or direct surgical SA nodal damage. Other cardiac operations that involve mechanical trauma to the SA node include atrial-switch operation, Fontan procedure, and atrial septal defect repairs (particularly sinus venosus defects). Although medications are used, the reliable long-term treatment for symptomatic SND is an atrial pacemaker. The treatment options for hemodynamically significant bradycardia are listed in **Table 54.3**.

Abnormalities of Atrioventricular Conduction. The multiple etiologies for first-degree AV block include: increased vagal tone, digoxin or β-blocker administration, viral myocarditis, Lyme disease, hypothermia, electrolyte abnormalities, congenital heart disease (before and after surgery), rheumatic fever, or associated cardiomyopathy. Mobitz type I second-degree AV block (Wenckebach) appears as progressive PR interval prolongation during the grouped beating, culminating in a nonconducted P wave followed by resetting of the grouped beating pattern. The sudden loss of AV conduction without preceding PR interval prolongation is indicative of Mobitz type II second-degree AV block. Mobitz type II heart block is a more concerning pattern. Third-degree AV block (complete heart block) may be congenital or acquired and results in complete AV dissociation with the atrial rate faster than the ventricular rate. Complete heart block can be associated with congenital heart diseases such as L-transposition of the great arteries (congenitally corrected transposition of the great arteries), heterotaxy syndrome (left atrial isomerism), or AV canal defect. It can also be associated with maternal autoimmune syndromes (systemic lupus erythematosus). Congenital complete heart block may cause hydrops fetalis dependent on the rate of the escape mechanism in utero.

Treatment for first-degree or Mobitz type I second-degree heart block is usually unnecessary except when patients are significantly hemodynamically compromised from concomitant illness or after cardiac surgery. In the patient with asymptomatic

Mobitz type II second-degree heart block, acute intervention is usually not required; the long-term risk of progression to complete heart block is treated with a permanent pacing system. The indications for permanent pacing prior to discharge in newborns include average heart rate below 55 bpm, wide complex escape mechanism, and hemodynamic instability secondary to bradycardia. In the presence of associated congenital heart disease, permanent pacing is indicated for infants secondary to an incidence of death as high as 29%.

PRINCIPLES OF TEMPORARY PACING

The three basic types of temporary pacemaker programming used are based on the goal and need of pacing (codes used on pacemakers are listed in **Table 54.4**).

- *Asynchronous or fixed-rate* is pacing of the atrium (AOO), ventricle (VOO), or both (DOO) at a set rate without the ability to sense intrinsic cardiac activity.
- *Single chamber synchronous (demand)* is pacing and sensing of either the atrium (AAI) or the ventricle (VVI). If there is native cardiac activity, the device will inhibit subsequent pacing until the rate drops below the lower rate limit.
- *Dual chamber AV sequential* is pacing that utilizes both atrial and ventricular (DDD) wires to sense and synchronously pace both the atrium and the ventricle.

ANTIARRHYTHMIC DRUGS

The *Vaughan Williams classification* organizes antiarrhythmic drugs by common electrophysiologic properties (**Table 54.5**).

Class I antiarrhythmic agents block the rapid sodium channel. *Class IA* agents include procainamide, disopyramide, and quinidine. Medications in this group delay repolarization and lengthen action potential and refractory periods. They are unique in their significant effects on the autonomic nervous system and carry a risk of proarrhythmia. They are used to treat atrial, ventricular, and AV reentrant tachycardia. *Class IB* medications include lidocaine, mexiletine, and phenytoin. They shorten the action potential and are primarily used for treatment of ventricular arrhythmias. *Class IC* agents include flecainide, propafenone, and encainide. They have a relatively high potential for proarrhythmia. When an atrial arrhythmia is treated with a class IC medication, it is important to also use an AV nodal slowing agent (β-blocker or digoxin).

Class II is designated for the β-blockers, which competitively inhibit the cardiac β-adrenergic receptor. They can be used to treat all automatic arrhythmias and some reentrant tachycardias as well. Atenolol has more cardiac β-receptor selectivity, less CNS penetration, and a longer half-life than other β-blockers. Nadolol has less penetration to the brain than other β-blockers and a low incidence of CNS side effects. Carvedilol and metoprolol are approved in the United States for the management of CHF in adults.

TABLE 54.4

Pacemaker Codes from the North American Society of Pacing and Electrophysiology and British Pacing and Electrophysiology Group

POSITION 1	POSITION 2	POSITION 3
Chamber paced	Chamber sensed	Response to sensed event
O = none	O = none	O = none
A = atrium	A = atrium	I = inhibited
V = ventricle	V = ventricle	T = triggered
D = dual (A + V)	D = dual (A + V)	D = dual (T + I)

The first two positions of this code are chamber paced and chamber sensed. The third position is described as follows:
D—(dual): In DDD pacemakers, atrial pacing is in the inhibited mode (the pacing device will emit an atrial pulse if the atrium does not contract).
In DDD and VDD pacemakers, once an atrial event has occurred (whether paced or native), the device will ensure that an atrial event follows.
I—(inhibited): The device will pulse to the appropriate chamber, unless it detects intrinsic electrical activity. In the DDI program, AV synchrony is provided only when the atrial chamber is paced. On the other hand, if intrinsic atrial activity is present, no AV synchrony is provided by the pacemaker.
T—(triggered): Triggered mode is used only when the device is being tested. The pacing device will emit a pulse only in response to a sensed event.
Adapted from Miller RD. *Miller's Anesthesia*. 6th ed. Philadelphia, PA: Elsevier, 2005.

TABLE 54.5

Vaughn Williams Classification of Antiarrhythmic Drugs

CLASS	EFFECT	DRUGS
I	Sodium-channel blockade	
Subclass IA		Procainamide, disopyramide, quinidine
Subclass IB		Lidocaine, mexiletine, phenytoin
Subclass IC		Flecainide, propafenone, encainide
II	β-adrenergic receptor blockade	Propranolol, esmolol, atenolol, nadolol, carvedilol
III	Potassium-channel blockade	Amiodarone, sotalol, bretylium
IV	Slow, inward, calcium-channel blockade	Verapamil, diltiazem, nifedipine
Other		Digoxin, adenosine

Class III agents include amiodarone, sotalol, and bretylium. These agents prolong the action-potential through action on potassium channels. Amiodarone and sotalol have additional effects on action-potential propagation and variable effects on the autonomic nervous system. Sotalol has a faster onset of action and shorter duration of activity.

Class IV antiarrhythmic drugs are calcium-channel blockers (specifically verapamil, diltiazem, and nifedipine). Their cellular activity decreases sinus node automaticity, slows AV node conduction, and prolongs refractoriness, resulting in sinus bradycardia and prolongation of the PR interval. Verapamil is most valuable for the treatment of reentrant SVT that involves the AV node in patients >1 year of age and those without WPW. Diltiazem is frequently used for control of the ventricular rate during atrial tachycardia or atrial fibrillation by slowing conduction through the AV node. Calcium-channel blockers are used for long-term therapy of pulmonary hypertension, preferably nifedipine, as it has little effect on the sinus node, AV node, and cardiac contractility.

Nonclassified Antiarrhythmic Medications

Digoxin may be used for atrial tachycardia, atrial fibrillation, premature atrial complexes, and blocked premature atrial complexes. The mechanism of action is mediated by an increase in vagus nerve tone and decrease in sympathetic efferent activity. Digoxin toxicity can result in almost any type of arrhythmia (a late indicator of toxicity). If toxic, serum electrolyte abnormalities should be corrected and atrial and ventricular arrhythmias treated with phenytoin or lidocaine. Atropine or a temporary pacemaker can be used to treat bradycardia or AV block. Digoxin-immune, antigen-binding Fab fragments are specific antibodies that may be used to bind digoxin and may be especially helpful in cases of potentially life-threatening toxicity.

Adenosine is an endogenous purine nucleoside that is useful for terminating AV reentrant tachycardia. The effects of adenosine are brief, with a half-life of <10 seconds. Patients with orthotopic heart transplant have a denervation-induced super-sensitivity to adenosine and it should be avoided in this population.

CHAPTER 55 ■ PREOPERATIVE CARE OF THE PEDIATRIC CARDIAC SURGICAL PATIENT

JENNIFER J. SCHUETTE, ALAIN FRAISSE, AND DAVID L. WESSEL

Congenital heart disease (CHD) occurs with a frequency of 1 in 100 live births, and accounts for 29% of deaths attributed to birth defects and 5.7% of overall infant mortality (57% of CHD infant mortality occurs during the neonatal period). Optimal preoperative care involves initial stabilization, airway management, establishment of vascular access, delineation of anatomy, and resuscitation of any secondary organ dysfunction. Surgical management begins when cardiac, pulmonary, renal, and central nervous systems are optimized.

PATIENT DEMOGRAPHICS

With emphasis on early primary repair for congenital cardiac defects, the demographic makeup of patients in the intensive care unit (ICU) has changed substantially. Interventions on even prematurely born neonates have become more commonplace with encouraging results with respect to morbidity and mortality. Many congenital defects are palliated or corrected but not cured, and more children with CHD are surviving into adulthood.

NEWBORN CONSIDERATIONS

Neonates respond more quickly and profoundly to physiologic stress (e.g., rapid changes in pH, lactic acid, glucose, and temperature). Neonates have diminished fat and carbohydrate reserves. Their high metabolic rate and oxygen consumption account for the rapid appearance of hypoxia when they become apneic. Immature liver and kidney functions are associated with reduced protein synthesis, glomerular filtration, drug metabolism, and hepatic synthetic function. The neonatal capillary system tends to leak fluid from the intravascular space. The neonatal myocardium is less compliant, less tolerant of increased afterload, and less responsive to increases in preload. The benefits of neonatal reparative operations in patients with two ventricles include the early elimination of cyanosis and congestive heart failure, optimal circulation for growth and development, reduced anatomic distortion from palliative procedures, reduced hospital admissions while awaiting repair, and reduced parental anxiety while awaiting repair.

Tolerance of hypoxia and plasticity of the neurologic system are well described in the neonate. Cognitive or psychomotor abnormalities associated with months of hypoxemia or abnormal hemodynamics may be eliminated by early repair. However, early reparative surgery that results in more exposure to CPB (e.g., repeated conduit changes) may be associated with cognitive or motor impairment and may require careful risk–benefit assessment. As a group, children with CHD are in the normal range for IQ despite being at increased risk for developmental delay and disabilities. In patients with complex CHD, neurobehavioral abnormalities such as hypo- and hypertonia, jitteriness, motor asymmetry, and absent suck are reported in more than 50% of newborns; up to 38% of infants have disabilities that include hypotonia, head preference, lethargy, restlessness, agitation, motor asymmetry, and feeding difficulties.

Neurologic pathology has been demonstrated preoperatively, including infants who have not suffered hemodynamic compromise or severe hypoxia postnatally. Preoperative electroencephalograms are frequently abnormal (1/5 have epileptiform activity and 1/3 have moderate-to-diffuse disturbances in background activity). Preoperative cranial ultrasound has found abnormalities in 30%–60%. Preoperative MRI has a lower false-positive rate and is considered the gold-standard for brain imaging in these infants. Abnormalities on MRI are noted in 30%–50% (infarction, hemorrhage, white matter injury, and periventricular leukomalacia).

PREOPERATIVE MANAGEMENT AND CARE

Physical Examination and Laboratory Data

A complete history and physical should examine the extent of cardiopulmonary impairment, airway abnormalities, and associated extracardiac congenital anomalies. Ten key features required to identify and treat low–cardiac output states in the perioperative period are described in **Table 55.1**.

Chest radiography shows heart size, pulmonary vascular congestion, airway compression, and areas of consolidation or atelectasis. The electrocardiogram may

TABLE 55.1

Ten Intensive Care Strategies to Diagnose and Support Low Cardiac Output States

1. Know the cardiac anatomy in detail and its physiologic consequences
2. Understand the specialized considerations of the newborn and implications of reparative rather than palliative surgery
3. Diversify personnel to include expertise in neonatal and adult congenital heart disease
4. Monitor, measure, and image the heart to rule out residual disease as a cause of postoperative hemodynamic instability or low cardiac output
5. Maintain aortic perfusion and improve the contractile state
6. Optimize preload (including atrial shunting)
7. Reduce afterload
8. Control heart rate, rhythm, and synchrony
9. Optimize heart–lung interactions
10. Provide mechanical support when needed

reveal rhythm disturbances and demonstrate ventricular strain patterns (ST- and T-wave changes) characteristic of pressure or volume overload on the ventricles.

Echocardiographic and Doppler Assessment

Echocardiography can provide accurate anatomic diagnosis without the need for cardiac catheterization in young children. The intensivist should be aware of the limitations of echocardiography and should consider alternative diagnoses when intra- or postoperative findings are inconsistent with the echocardiographic diagnosis.

Doppler measurements add greatly to the diagnostic capabilities. Measurements of pressure gradients across semilunar valves and obstructions are frequently accurate but may not always correlate with peak systolic ejection gradients measured at catheterization. The standard for assessment of physiology when other information is ambiguous or contradictory remains cardiac catheterization.

Quantification of left ventricular ejection and shortening fractions is made by geometric modeling using the Simpson rule. Assumptions inherent in this calculation can lead to inaccurate estimations of ventricular volumes and dynamics. Doppler techniques for assessing ventricular function are relatively independent of geometry and loading conditions.

Transesophageal echocardiography (TEE) can confirm preoperative diagnoses, assist in formulating surgical plans, identify residual defects, and guide surgical revisions. Smaller probe size allows the use of TEE in patients weighing ≤3.5 kg. Recent 3D technology optimizes the evaluation of the site of valve regurgitation.

Cardiac Catheterization

Cardiac catheterization may be necessary for physiologic assessment, interventional procedures such as balloon atrial septostomy or valvotomy, or anatomic definition not discernible by echocardiography. Catheterization is not typically performed before infant or neonatal operations for ventricular septal defects, complete atrioventricular canal defects, tetralogy of Fallot, interrupted aortic arch, hypoplastic left heart syndrome (HLHS), or coarctation of the aorta. However, in older patients with complex anatomy (e.g., a single ventricle), physiologic data from catheterization may be essential.

In the child with CHD, the superior vena cava gives the best indication of true mixed venous oxygen saturation; an increase ("step-up") in saturation of ≥5% downstream from the superior vena cava suggests the presence of a left-to-right shunt. The magnitude of the left-to-right shunt can be calculated from *the Fick equation*. The frequently used term Q_p/Q_s (pulmonary-to-systemic blood flow ratio) can be derived simply from the measured oxygen saturation values.

Fick equation for the calculation of Q_s and Q_p:

$$Q_s = \dot{V}o_2/(Cao_2 - Cmvo_2)$$

$$Q_p = \dot{V}o_2/(Cpvo_2 - Cpao_2)$$

where Q_s = systemic blood flow, Q_p = pulmonary blood flow, $\dot{V}o_2$ = oxygen consumption, Cao_2 = arterial oxygen content, $Cmvo_2$ = mixed venous oxygen content, $Cpvo_2$ = pulmonary vein oxygen content, $Cpao_2$ = pulmonary artery oxygen content, Sao_2 = arterial oxygen saturation, $Smvo_2$ = mixed venous oxygen saturation, $Spvo_2$ = pulmonary venous saturation, and $Spao_2$ = pulmonary artery saturation. By substituting the equations for oxygen content into the equations for Q_s and Q_p, one can derive a simplified Fick equation for Q_p/Q_s:

$$Q_p/Q_s = (Sao_2 - Smvo_2)/(Spvo_2 - Spao_2)$$

The patient whose aortic blood is fully saturated can be assumed to have no significant right-to-left shunting. Blood samples should also be obtained from the pulmonary veins, left atrium, and left ventricle for oxygen saturation determinations and ascertainment of the source of desaturated blood. Pulmonary venous desaturation implies a pulmonary source of venous admixture (e.g., pneumonia, atelectasis, or other pulmonary disease).

In the presence of a left-to-right shunt and elevated PVR, pressure and saturation measurements are repeated during ventilation with 100% oxygen or inhaled nitric oxide to assess reactivity of the pulmonary vascular bed and ventilation–perfusion abnormalities. If breathing 100% oxygen increases pulmonary blood flow and Q_p/Q_s (with a fall in PVR), reversible processes (e.g., hypoxic pulmonary vasoconstriction) are contributing to elevated PVR. Patients with a high, unresponsive PVR and small left-to-right shunt despite a large shunt orifice may have irreversible pulmonary vascular damage and surgical repair may be contraindicated.

In the newborn with single-ventricle physiology, mitral stenosis or atresia, and excess pulmonary blood flow, the large blood return to the undersized left atrium may be "restricted" across a patent (stretched open) foramen. The determinant for atrial septostomy is the systemic oxygen saturation level, not the Doppler-measured pressure gradient across the atrial septum.

Magnetic Resonance Imaging and Angiography

Cardiac magnetic resonance imaging (CMR) provides excellent segmental and anatomic analysis (particularly the pulmonary veins and thoracic aorta) through 3D angiography. Ventricular mass, volume, and function can be assessed using steady-state free-precession sequences. Phase-contrast flow-velocity mapping may provide adequate hemodynamic data obviating the need for cardiac catheterization. In younger children, temporal and spatial resolution is challenging; breath holding to avoid respiratory motion artifacts may require general anesthesia.

Contraindications to CMR include not MR-compatible pacemakers and recently implanted endovascular or intracardiac devices. Computed tomography (CT) is an alternative when shorter acquisition times are essential or the risks of anesthesia are too high. CT angiography provides better resolution than CMR and may be necessary to delineate small structures such as pulmonary veins, coronary arteries, and collateral vessels. CT is the modality of choice to assess the airway and surrounding vascular structures.

Assessment of Patient Status and Predominant Pathophysiology

Rather than trying to determine the management for each individual anatomic defect, a physiologic approach can be taken. The assessment should address (a) how the systemic venous return reaches the systemic arterial circulation to maintain cardiac output (the presence of intracardiac mixing, shunting, or outflow obstruction), (b) whether the circulation is in series or parallel and if the defects are amenable to a two-ventricle or single-ventricle repair, (c) whether pulmonary blood flow is increased or decreased, and (d) if there is a volume load or a pressure load on the ventricles.

Most pathophysiologic mechanisms pertinent to the perioperative plan and preparation involve severe hypoxemia, excessive pulmonary blood flow, congestive heart failure, obstruction of blood flow from the left heart, or poor ventricular function. Some patients present with multiple, interrelated problems.

Severe Hypoxemia

Many cyanotic forms of CHD present with severe perinatal hypoxemia ($Pa{O_2}$ < 50 mm Hg) without respiratory distress. Infusion of prostaglandin E_1 (PGE_1) maintains or reestablishes pulmonary flow through the ductus arteriosus. This may improve mixing of venous and arterial blood at the atrial level in patients with transposition of the great arteries. Neonates rarely require surgery while severely hypoxemic except those with obstructed total anomalous pulmonary venous connection. They present with severe hypoxemia, congested lungs, significant distress, and no benefit from PGE_1 and require emergency surgery.

PGE_1 can reopen a ductus arteriosus for several days after birth or maintain its patency for an extended period. Side effects of PGE_1 (apnea, hypotension, fever, and agitation) are easily managed. PGE_1 improves arterial oxygenation neonates with obstructed pulmonary flow (critical pulmonic stenosis or pulmonary atresia) by providing pulmonary blood flow from the aorta via the ductus arteriosus. The improved oxygenation reverses the lactic acidosis that developed during hypoxia and provides marked clinical improvement.

Neonates with transposition of the great arteries must have adequate mixing of blood at the atrial level to achieve oxygen delivery. A balloon atrial septostomy can create or enlarge an atrial septal defect using echocardiographic guidance and can be performed at the patient's bedside. It may also be used in any neonate with left atrial hypertension (e.g., HLHS with intact atrial septum). An intra-atrial stent may be necessary to maintain patency.

Cyanotic patients who present after infancy require hydration to prevent thrombotic problems caused by elevated hematocrits. The perioperative team should prepare for significant coagulopathy in cyanotic patients.

Excessive Pulmonary Blood Flow

Excessive pulmonary blood flow may be the primary physiologic problem in patients with CHD. Left-to-right shunts can cause chronic low-grade pulmonary infection and congestion that cannot be medically eliminated. Surgery should not be postponed; not correcting the defect risks recurrent infections, increased cardiovascular morbidity, and long-term pulmonary sequelae. Respiratory syncytial virus (RSV), human metapneumovirus, parainfluenza, and influenza infections are prevalent in this population. Palivizumab prophylaxis has decreased RSV hospitalization rates in CHD patients by 48%.

Increased pulmonary blood flow causes respiratory impairment and left heart dilation from pulmonary venous return that is several times normal. When the body requires more systemic blood flow, the heart responds inefficiently, much of the increased cardiac output is recirculated to the lungs, and symptoms of congestive heart failure appear. Children with failing hearts increase heart rate, redistribute cardiac output to favored organs, and decrease extremity perfusion. These symptoms suggest that profound pathophysiologic alterations have occurred. This information is used to assess the severity of the illness, formulate an anesthetic plan, a surgical or cath intervention, and predict postoperative course.

Obstruction of Left Heart Outflow

Patients with obstruction to left heart outflow are among the most critically ill. These lesions include interruption of the aortic arch, coarctation, aortic stenosis, and mitral stenosis or atresia as part of HLHS. They present with inadequate systemic perfusion and profound metabolic acidosis. Systemic blood flow is dependent on blood flow into the aorta from the ductus arteriosus and PGE_1 may be required for survival. Systemic circulation in these neonates is dependent on right ventricular contractile function and ductal patency. PGE_1 infusion restores perfusion and surgery can be deferred until the patient's condition improves. Other supportive measures include ventilatory and inotropic support and correction of metabolic and electrolyte abnormalities. Adequacy of resuscitation influences postoperative outcome.

Ventricular Dysfunction

Understanding the extent of ventricular dysfunction preoperatively provides insight into intraoperative and postoperative events. When the heart is dilated and volume overloaded, there is a propensity for ventricular fibrillation during sedation, anesthesia, and/or intubation of the airway. Assessment should include the patient's functional limitation (an indicator of myocardial performance and reserve), quantification of the degree of hypoxia, and amount of pulmonary blood flow (evaluation of PVR and Q_p/Q_s).

PREOPERATIVE MANAGEMENT OF PATIENTS WITH A SINGLE VENTRICLE

Single-Ventricle Anatomy and Physiology

For a variety of lesions, the systemic and pulmonary circulations are in parallel and a single ventricle supplies both systemic and pulmonary blood flow. The proportion of ventricular output to either vascular bed is determined by the relative resistances to flow. Pulmonary artery and aortic oxygen saturations are equal with mixing of the systemic and pulmonary venous return within a "common" atrium. Assuming adequate mixing, normal cardiac output, and normal pulmonary venous oxygen saturation, a $Sa{O_2}$ of 80%–85% with a $Sv{O_2}$ of 60%–65% indicates a Q_p/Q_s of ~1 and a balance between systemic and pulmonary flows. Although "balanced," the single ventricle receives and ejects twice the normal amount of blood: one part to the pulmonary circulation and one part to the systemic circulation. A Q_p/Q_s of >1 implies an intolerable volume burden on the heart.

Preoperative Management

Changes in PVR have a significant impact on systemic perfusion and circulatory stability, especially preoperatively, when the ductus arteriosus is widely patent. In preparation for surgery, systemic and pulmonary blood flow should be balanced to prevent volume overload and ventricular dysfunction. Resuscitation involves maintaining a patent ductus arteriosus with PGE_1. Intubation and mechanical ventilation are not necessary in all patients. Patients are usually tachypneic, but provided the work of breathing is not excessive and systemic perfusion maintained without a metabolic acidosis, spontaneous ventilation is preferable to achieve an adequate systemic perfusion and balance of Q_p and Q_s. Mild metabolic acidosis and low bicarbonate level may not indicate poor perfusion and lactic acidosis. If the presentation involves circulatory collapse and end-organ dysfunction, then surgery may be postponed to establish stability and return of vital organ function.

Intubation and mechanical ventilation may be required due to apnea secondary to PGE_1, to provide additional support in a low–cardiac output state, or for manipulation of gas exchange to assist in balancing the pulmonary and systemic flows. An $Sa{O_2}$ of >90% indicates pulmonary overcirculation, i.e., $Q_p/Q_s > 1.0$. PVR can be increased with controlled hypoventilation to induce a respiratory acidosis; it may necessitate sedation and neuromuscular blockade. Ventilation in room air is indicated. It is important to remember that these patients have limited oxygen reserve and may desaturate suddenly and precipitously. Controlled hypoventilation reduces the functional residual capacity and oxygen reserve, which would be further reduced by the use of a hypoxic inspired gas mixture. An alternate strategy to increase PVR is to add carbon dioxide to the inspiratory limb of the breathing circuit. While either a hypoxic inspired gas mixture or a hypercapnic strategy can decrease Q_p/Q_s to 1, the hypercapnic strategy is more likely to increase cerebral and systemic oxygen delivery. Patients who continue to have pulmonary overcirculation (high $Sa{O_2}$, reduced systemic perfusion) despite these maneuvers require early surgical intervention to control pulmonary blood flow.

Decreased pulmonary blood flow in a preoperative patient with a parallel circulation is reflected by hypoxemia with an SaO_2 of <75%. This may be due to restricted flow across a small ductus arteriosus, increased PVR secondary to parenchymal lung disease, or increased pulmonary venous pressure secondary to obstructed pulmonary venous drainage or a restrictive atrial septal defect. Sedation, paralysis, and manipulation of mechanical ventilation to maintain mild alkalosis may be effective if PVR is elevated. Nitric oxide may also be used as a specific pulmonary vasodilator. Systemic oxygen delivery is maintained by improving cardiac output with inotropes and a hematocrit >40%. Among some newborns, pulmonary blood flow may be insufficient because the mitral valve hypoplasia in combination with the occasional finding of a restrictive or nearly intact atrial septum severely restricts pulmonary venous return to the heart. The newborn is intensely cyanotic and has a pulmonary venous congestion pattern on chest X-ray. Urgent cardiac catheterization with balloon septostomy, dilation, or stent placement of a restrictive atrial septal defect may be necessary. Immediate surgical intervention and palliation may be preferred at some centers.

Systemic perfusion is maintained with volume and vasoactive agents. Inotropic support is necessary when ventricular dysfunction is secondary to shock associated with a closing ductus arteriosus. Systemic afterload reduction with phosphodiesterase inhibitors (e.g., milrinone) may improve systemic perfusion and reduce atrioventricular valve regurgitation in volume-loaded hearts. However, milrinone may also decrease PVR and not fully address the imbalance of pulmonary and systemic flows. Necrotizing enterocolitis is a risk secondary to splanchnic hypoperfusion, and many do not feed newborns with a wide pulse width and low diastolic pressure (<30 mm Hg) prior to surgery. Historically, enteral feeding has been avoided preoperatively in single-ventricle patients awaiting first-stage palliation, but that practice is now more varied among centers.

RISK STRATIFICATION IN PEDIATRIC CARDIAC SURGERY

Reliable tools and methods for preoperative risk stratification in pediatric cardiac surgery are essential to fully inform patients and their families, to compare institutions fairly, and to improve postoperative care. Several scoring systems have been developed for predicting outcome and guiding perioperative therapy. They include the Risk Adjustment in Cardiac Heart Surgery score (RACHS-1) and the Aristotle Comprehensive Complexity score. These scoring systems are limited in that they primarily focus on the specific surgical procedure with sparse additional clinical data. More recently, the Society of Thoracic Surgeons and the European Association of Cardiothoracic Surgery (STS-EACTS) established morbidity and mortality scores and categories, which include a broader array of pre-, intra-, and postoperative clinical data. Additionally, the Pediatric Cardiac Critical Care Consortium (PC^4) has created a multi-institution database, which provides real-time analysis on numerous quality and outcome metrics for medical and surgical pediatric CICU patients.

A valuable addition to the preoperative evaluation would be a blood marker capable of acutely predicting postoperative morbidity and mortality after congenital heart surgery. Though intra- and postoperative lactate trends detect low–cardiac output syndrome and predict outcome after CHD repair, preoperative values do not correlate with postoperative outcomes. Preoperative brain natriuretic peptide (BNP) and N-terminal pro-BNP (NTpro-BNP) plasma levels may provide an estimate of the risk of open-heart surgery in children with CHD.

CHAPTER 56 ■ POSTOPERATIVE CARE OF THE PEDIATRIC CARDIAC SURGICAL PATIENT

RONALD A. BRONICKI, JOHN M. COSTELLO, AND KATE L. BROWN

GENERAL POSTOPERATIVE CONSIDERATIONS

Respiratory Dysfunction

Infants have a high chest-wall-to-lung-compliance ratio that reduces the end-expiratory lung volume and predisposes to atelectasis and pulmonary venous admixture. The infant diaphragm contains fewer fatigue-resistant–type muscle fibers and immature sarcoplasmic reticulum, reducing the contractile reserve. The cross section of the subglottic region is also decreased compared with older children, predisposing infants to upper airway obstruction. Structural heart lesions that transmit systemic pressure to the pulmonary vasculature and allow for excessive pulmonary blood flow (e.g., large nonrestrictive ventricular septal defect [VSD]) increase extravascular lung water and contribute to a decrease in lung compliance. Left-sided heart defects, such as mitral stenosis and left ventricular dysfunction, produce pulmonary venous hypertension and contribute to interstitial pulmonary edema formation. Cardiopulmonary bypass (CPB) also contributes to respiratory dysfunction. CPB and the pulmonary ischemia–reperfusion injury can induce inflammatory-mediated changes in the pulmonary microvasculature that increase vascular permeability and interstitial edema formation. During cardiac surgery, *recurrent laryngeal nerve injury* may occur, resulting in *vocal cord dysfunction*, which may cause upper airway dysfunction. Injury to the thoracic duct may also occur during cardiac surgery, resulting in a *chylothorax, which may* present with respiratory distress, worsening oxygenation, or persistent chest tube drainage. If the infant has been fed, the pleural effusion appears creamy and the diagnosis is established with a triglyceride level > 1.2 mmol/L and total cell count > 1000 cells/μL (predominantly lymphocytes) in the pleural fluid. Neuromuscular competence may be compromised due to central nervous system depression, *diaphragm paresis* or *paralysis*, or disuse atrophy of the respiratory musculature (compounded by malnutrition, muscle relaxants, or steroid administration). Diaphragm paresis is usually secondary to *phrenic nerve injury* (left more commonly) and results from the application of ice to the area during surgery; from difficult dissection; from surgery in the area of the pulmonary arteries, aortic arch, or superior vena cava (SVC); or from attempts at central venous access.

Supportive care for parenchymal lung disease includes supplemental oxygen, strategies for reducing extravascular lung water, and the recruitment of atelectatic lung segments with end-expiratory pressure. Causes of hypoxemia unresponsive to these measures include intracardiac shunting and collaterals with right-to-left shunting.

Cardiovascular Dysfunction

Postoperative systolic dysfunction is in part due to CPB-induced inflammatory mediators such as tumor necrosis factor-α. The primary mechanism for myocardial dysfunction following surgery is an intraoperative period of ischemia (cardioplegic arrest) compounded by reperfusion injury (see section on Cardiopulmonary Bypass). Other factors that impact postoperative cardiac function include the surgical approach and preexisting ventricular dysfunction due to a volume or pressure load (see section on Specific-Lesion Management). The adverse effects of CPB have a disproportionately greater impact on the myocardium of infants, as they have less myocardial reserve. Infant myocardium contains poorly organized sarcoplasmic reticulum, leading to inefficiencies of calcium delivery to the myofilaments, and it possesses relatively few, poorly organized contractile proteins. As a result, the infant myocardium is less compliant, less responsive to fluid and inotropes, and more susceptible to increased ventricular afterload. *Pericardial tamponade* may lead to hypotension and cardiac arrest. Accumulation of blood in the pericardium or mediastinum usually accounts for tamponade in the first 24–48 hours after cardiac surgery. Echocardiography reveals right atrial and perhaps right ventricular collapse.

Pulmonary Hypertension

Pulmonary arterial hypertension following cardiac surgery occurs in cardiac defects associated with long-standing increased pulmonary pressure and blood flow (e.g., large, nonrestrictive VSDs). Patients with pulmonary venous hypertension resulting from left ventricular dysfunction or obstruction to pulmonary venous return are also at risk. CPB produces an inflammatory response, and pulmonary ischemia–reperfusion injury causes endothelial injury, reduced nitric oxide production, and an increase in pulmonary vascular resistance and reactivity.

Assessment of Hemodynamics and Oxygen Transport Balance

Measurement of central venous oximetry allows for assessment of the relationship between oxygen demand and delivery (oxygen transport balance). Serum lactate levels also assess global oxygen transport balance, but oxygen extraction increases and becomes critical well before lactate production exceeds clearance and begins to rise. Cerebral oximetry is used as a surrogate for cerebral venous oxygen saturations, allowing for an assessment of cerebral oxygen transport balance. Cerebral oximetry is also used to infer global or systemic oxygen transport balance.

Maintenance of Tissue Oxygenation

Low cardiac output may result from inadequate venous return, ventricular dysfunction, excessive afterload, or arrhythmias. A relatively inadequate preload may be due to diastolic dysfunction, where an elevated ventricular filling pressure is needed to maintain an adequate stroke volume, and volume administration results in a prompt improvement in cardiac output. A lack of improvement suggests that preload reserve is exhausted and either inotropic or afterload-reducing therapies are indicated to improve stroke volume. Another cause of inadequate preload is cardiac tamponade with collapse of the right atrium and cessation of right ventricular filling. Findings include hypotension that fails to respond to volume administration while right atrial pressure and heart rate rise. Low cardiac output following surgery may result from diastolic or systolic dysfunction. *Diastolic dysfunction* refers to an abnormality of diastolic distensibility, filling, or relaxation of the ventricle. The time course of ventricular filling is altered, and the filling pressure is elevated. In diastolic heart failure, an adequate stroke volume is not maintained, and in contrast to systolic failure, the ejection fraction is not depressed and the low-output state results from inadequate ventricular filling. The most common causes of diastolic dysfunction are ischemic myocardium and conditions that lead to ventricular hypertrophy such as hypertension or obstructive lesion. *Systolic dysfunction* is characterized by reduced ejection fraction and stroke volume despite an elevated ventricular end-diastolic pressure and volume. With either ventricle, systolic dysfunction renders the ventricle less responsive to volume and more sensitive to increases in afterload.

General strategies for supporting critically ill patients include therapies that decrease oxygen demand and improve oxygen transport balance such as mechanical ventilation and unloading of the respiratory pump, sedation and analgesia, and avoidance of hyperthermia. Therapy for diastolic dysfunction involves volume administration, optimization of heart rate and rhythm (ensuring atrial ventricular synchrony and adequate time for ventricular filling), and minimizing intrathoracic pressure. Inotropic and afterload-reducing agents are of little benefit, as systolic function is intact. Therapy for systolic dysfunction focuses on optimizing ventricular loading conditions. Reducing afterload enhances ventricular ejection and may be accomplished pharmacologically or mechanically (e.g., positive-pressure ventilation).

Vasoactive Therapy

Vasoactive agents that induce venodilation decrease systemic venous return and ventricular diastolic volume and pressure but have no effect on ventricular afterload. Thus, stroke volume and cardiac output do not increase. If, however, the ventricle is operating on the ascending portion of its pressure stroke volume curve, venodilation will cause stroke volume to decrease. Vasoactive agents that dilate arterial resistance vessels enhance ventricular ejection. Inotropic agents increase cardiac output as a result of an increase in ejection fraction and stroke volume and sometimes as a result of an increase in heart rate.

Catecholamines

The hemodynamic effects of catecholamines are dose-dependent and mediated by adrenergic receptors. Activation of β_2 receptors leads to vascular smooth muscle relaxation and vasodilation of arterial resistance and venous capacitance vessels. Activation of β_1 receptors enhances contractility and increases heart rate. Activation of α_1 receptors leads to vascular smooth muscle contraction and vasoconstriction. β-Adrenergic receptors experience agonist-mediated desensitization, and an attenuated response occurs with prolonged exposure to elevated levels of catecholamines. Catecholamines increase myocardial oxygen demand due to chronotropic and inotropic effects. The agents most associated with dysrhythmias are isoproterenol and epinephrine and, to a lesser extent, dopamine and dobutamine.

Dopamine is the immediate precursor of norepinephrine, and approximately half of the dopamine-induced response results from release of norepinephrine from sympathetic nerve terminals. Dopamine directly stimulates α, β, and dopaminergic receptors. Moderate doses (5–10 mcg/kg/min) have chronotropic and inotropic effects. At high doses (>10 mcg/kg/min), α-adrenergic effects predominate and systemic vascular resistance increases.

Dobutamine significantly increases cardiac output by increasing stroke volume and, to a lesser extent, by increasing heart rate and reducing systemic vascular resistance. In contrast to dopamine, dobutamine causes dilation of venous capacitance vessels and a reduction in ventricular filling pressures.

Epinephrine is an endogenous catecholamine produced by the adrenal medulla from norepinephrine in response to stress. Epinephrine provides inotropic support and, in low doses (<0.1 mcg/kg/min), decreases systemic and pulmonary vascular resistance and diastolic blood pressure through β_2 agonists activity. At much higher doses, activation of α_1 receptors leads to vasoconstriction of arterial resistance vessels.

Norepinephrine is the neurotransmitter of the sympathetic nervous system. It causes vasoconstriction of venous capacitance and arterial resistance vessels by activating α_1 receptors, while providing inotropic support. Norepinephrine is ideal for restoring an adequate perfusion pressure in the setting of vasodilatory shock.

Milrinone acts through inhibition of phosphodiesterase III and is unaffected by adrenergic receptor desensitization. It reduces cAMP degradation, causing vasodilation of venous capacitance and pulmonary and systemic arterial resistance vessels while providing modest inotropic support. The prophylactic use of high-dose milrinone has been shown to significantly reduce the risk of death or the development of a low–cardiac output syndrome relative to placebo in children after cardiac surgery. The half-life of milrinone is age-dependent and ranges from <1 hour in children to >3 hours in infants. Milrinone is predominantly cleared via renal excretion, and dosing may need to be adjusted in patients with renal insufficiency.

Nitroprusside spontaneously releases nitric oxide, which activates soluble guanylate cyclase producing increased levels of cGMP. Nitroprusside causes dose-dependent dilation of systemic and pulmonary arterial resistance and venous capacitance vessels. In congestive heart failure, nitroprusside increases stroke volume and cardiac output and reduces ventricular filling pressures. Nitroprusside decomposition releases cyanide, which undergoes transsulfuration to form thiocyanate. Cyanide toxicity can occur when using nitroprusside at high doses for long durations, especially with hepatic dysfunction, and should be anticipated and monitored.

Nitroglycerin undergoes biotransformation to yield nitric oxide. Nitroglycerin produces dose-dependent dilation of systemic and pulmonary arterial and venous capacitance vessels and is thus useful in the treatment of congestive heart failure. In low-to-modest doses (<3 mcg/kg/min), nitroglycerin increases venous capacitance, reducing ventricular filling pressures without significantly changing stroke volume. In high doses, systemic and pulmonary vascular resistances are reduced, increasing stroke volume and cardiac output.

Vasopressin has an antidiuretic effect, and physiologic levels are required for normal vascular tone. Vasopressin may have utility in cardiac arrest and vasodilatory shock.

Neurologic Issues

Children with cardiac disease may have congenital brain abnormalities linked to genetic or syndromic diagnoses. Nearly 20% of full-term neonates with congenital heart disease have periventricular leukomalacia on preoperative brain magnetic resonance imaging (MRI). Both CPB and deep hypothermic circulatory arrest (DHCA) contribute to impairments in cerebral pressure autoregulation. CPB techniques applying a pH-stat versus alpha-stat approach and a higher versus lower hematocrit goal appear advantageous, based on various indicators of neurologic well-being. Metabolic perturbations of hyperthermia and hyperglycemia may arise following CPB. Hyperthermia can exacerbate brain injury and should be treated. Aggressive treatment of hyperglycemia risks hypoglycemia, and there is no data that it benefits outcomes. Correlations have been identified between low cerebral NIRS values and postprocedural neurologic events, including seizures and cerebral MRI abnormalities. Prolonged periods of DHCA have been linked to seizures, and adverse scores on developmental tests. Low cerebral and mixed venous oxygen saturations have been linked to adverse events, such as cardiac arrest, which has a significant deleterious effect on neurodevelopmental scores of children with heart disease. The use of postoperative NIRS monitoring and treatment protocols aimed at averting or curtailing adverse events may improve neurologic outcomes. Cardiac arrest and low–cardiac output states may necessitate initiation of ECLS. Approximately 50% of children who survive ECLS and undergo formal neurodevelopmental evaluation have a range of disabilities.

Endocrine Disease

Transient postoperative hyperglycemia is a neuroendocrine response to stress and is very common in critically ill children with cardiac disease. It results from accelerated glucose production (exacerbated by glucocorticoids given during CPB) and the development of relative resistance to insulin. Current evidence does not support the use of insulin therapy to achieve *tight glycemic control* (glucose levels of less than 120–140 mg/dL) following pediatric cardiac surgery.

Adrenal insufficiency leads to hypotension resistant to fluid and inotropic therapy. Improvement with hydrocortisone supplementation following neonatal cardiac surgery has been reported. Some patients may have end-organ resistance to cortisol. It is unclear whether the administration of steroids improves cardiovascular function in this setting.

The *sick euthyroid syndrome* occurs to a variable degree in all children following cardiac surgery regardless of complexity. Transient reductions occur in thyroid-stimulating hormone, total triiodothyronine (T_3), free thyroxine (T_4), and reverse triiodothyronine (rT_3), with an elevation in T_3 uptake. Levels of rT_3 return toward normal before T_3 levels, which remain low beyond the critical postoperative period.

Gastrointestinal Issues

Poor nutritional states and failure to thrive are common in children with heart disease. Several factors contribute including poor intake (suck–swallow incoordination, gastroesophageal reflux disease [GERD]), high energy expenditure, impaired intestinal absorption, and reduced splanchnic blood flow. These factors render patients susceptible to postoperative infection, necrotizing enterocolitis (NEC), and prolonged recovery. Congenital gastrointestinal defects associated with congenital heart disease include malrotation in heterotaxy syndrome, hind gut atresia in VACTER(L) syndrome, esophageal atresia in VACTER(L) or CHARGE syndromes, and a range of malformations in children with chromosomal syndromes (trisomy 21, 8, 5). GERD is common in patients with heart disease and arises even more frequently in syndromic babies. The main treatment is inhibition of acid production from the gastric mucosa and promotion of gastric motility by pharmacologic agents. Patients with severe GERD symptoms may need surgical intervention with placement of a gastric tube and fundoplication in order to achieve adequate weight gain. The hypermetabolic state generated by CPB is associated with high resting energy expenditure. The use of fluid restriction immediately following surgery contributes to a caloric deficit. Feeding algorithms are beneficial in achieving shorter times to achieve full enteral nutrition and reach a better caloric balance during recovery.

Necrotizing enterocolitis is an inflammatory bowel condition associated with prostaglandin use, low–cardiac output syndrome, and prematurity. NEC is prevalent in the hypoplastic left heart syndrome (HLHS) and truncus arteriosus but has been reported in most forms of neonatal heart disease. Treatment consists of intravenous broad-spectrum antibiotics and bowel rest with parenteral nutrition, and surgical intervention if required for bowel necrosis or perforation.

Chylothorax arises in 1%–5% of children after cardiac surgery. Secondary immune deficiency may develop due to lymphocyte and plasma protein loss in the pleural drainage. The first line of therapy involves feeding with medium-chain triglycerides, which without caloric supplements will lead to a reduction in caloric intake. Refractory cases warrant cessation of enteral feeding and institution of parenteral nutrition.

Hematologic Issues

Immediately following CPB, hypofibrinogenemia, thrombocytopenia, residual heparinization, and poor clot formation predispose to mediastinal bleeding. The use of whole blood reduces bleeding compared to replacement with blood product components. Blood transfusion is common following cardiac surgery, with the potential adverse effects of transfusion including lung injury, immune modulation, and the potential transmission of infection. Antifibrinolytic agents reduce bleeding in high-risk patients (e.g., undergoing reoperation). Aminocaproic acid (Amicar) and tranexamic acid are derivatives of lysine and enzyme inhibitors against proteins such as plasmin.

Lower-flow venous pathways (Fontan) and synthetic material in the circulation (prosthetic heart valves, Gore-Tex shunts) necessitate anticoagulation to prevent thrombosis. Extracorporeal support devices (ventricular assist device and *extracorporeal membrane oxygenation* [ECMO]) require anticoagulation in order to maintain device and cannula patency and integrity, as do intravenous catheters in high-risk patients (for example, where the central veins have been injured by multiple previous interventions). Intravenous unfractionated heparin is the first-line anticoagulant in the ICU. Options for long-term anticoagulation include (a) coumadin, which inhibits the synthesis of vitamin K–dependent clotting factors. Coumadin has a gradual onset of effect; therefore, an overlap with heparin therapy is required, and is subject to drug interactions when administered in conjunction with hepatic enzyme inhibitors or enhancers; (b) low-molecular-weight heparin, which targets anti-factor Xa activity and is administered via subcutaneous injection; and (c) antiplatelet agents including aspirin and clopidogrel are orally administered and provide long-term inhibition of platelet aggregation in children at risk for thrombosis in synthetic intravascular material.

Infectious Issues

Healthcare-associated infections (HAIs) following cardiac surgery are linked to comorbid medical conditions (e.g., 22q11 deletion that impairs the immune system), preoperative ventilation, greater operative complexity, younger age, blood product exposure, and reoperations. Bundle approaches to decrease HAIs include removal of central venous catheters as soon as possible, head-up positioning to reduce the risk of ventilator-associated pneumonia, and optimal timing of antibiotics to prevent surgical site infections. Exposure to broad-spectrum antibiotics predisposes to fungal infections. Primary immune deficiency occurs with genetic syndromes such as trisomy 21 and 22q11 deletion; a secondary immune deficiency is induced after transplantation, and may also be seen in patients with a significant chylothorax and immunoglobulin leak. Prophylactic antifungal agents are recommended in patients on prolonged broad-spectrum antibiotics and immediately following heart transplantation.

Renal Issues

Renal injury and impairment of kidney function are common following cardiac surgery. The pediatric modification of Acute Kidney Injury Network (AKIN) graded classifications may be used to describe a patient's level of renal impairment. Kidney injury affects 40%–50% of patients following cardiac surgery and is more prevalent in younger children, single-ventricle physiology, those with preexisting renal disease, and following long CPB times. The etiology of postoperative renal failure is linked to low–cardiac output syndrome and affected patients tend to require higher doses of inotropes or even mechanical circulatory support. Postoperative renal impairment arises early after surgery and is reversible in the majority of cases (type 1 cardiorenal syndrome). Mortality rates are higher in patients with postprocedural renal impairment, reflecting their increased complexity and morbidity. The first line of therapy for mild renal impairment (AKIN grade 1) includes fluid restriction, judicious use of diuretics, optimization of preload and cardiac function, and avoidance of nephrotoxic agents. In a high proportion of patients, a diuresis evolves after 24–48 hours, with corresponding recovery of the renal injury.

Severe forms of renal failure (AKIN grade 3) effect 10%–15% of patients and frequently require supportive therapy with peritoneal dialysis, hemodialysis, or hemofiltration.

CARDIOPULMONARY BYPASS

Basic components of a CPB circuit include two venous cannulae that drain systemic venous blood from the superior and inferior vena cava (or one from the right atrium), a cardiotomy reservoir, a heat exchanger, a membrane oxygenator, a roller pump, and an arterial filter (**Fig. 56.1**). An arterial cannula returns oxygenated blood to the aorta (alternatively the innominate, axillary, or femoral artery is used). A second arterial cannula can be used during repair of an interrupted aortic arch, when one arterial cannula is placed in the ascending aorta and a second in the ductus arteriosus to perfuse the lower body. Before initiation of CPB, the circuit is "primed" with crystalloid solution, glucose, buffer, heparin, calcium, and either whole blood or packed red blood cells and albumin. The priming volume may exceed the blood volume of a neonate and lower the hematocrit, plasma proteins and clotting factors, decrease the oncotic pressure and cause interstitial edema and a propensity for bleeding. Heparin is administered for the duration of CPB to prevent thrombosis, consumption of clotting factors, and oxygenator dysfunction.

Prior to CPB, mediastinal dissection is performed and the thymus is subtotally resected. Infants have greater oxygen consumption, and initial flow rates are higher than in adults. Most children are cooled to minimize metabolic needs and oxygen consumption. Hypothermia provides protection to the brain and other organs, especially during low-flow states and periods of DHCA. Adverse effects of hypothermia include inflammation and changes in capillary permeability leading to interstitial edema. The degree of hypothermia varies depending on the age of the patient and complexity of the case. Mild hypothermia (30°C–34°C) is used for simple cases in older children, whereas deep hypothermia (15°C–22°C) is reserved for complex repairs such as aortic arch reconstruction in a neonate. Because hypothermia increases viscosity and red blood cell rigidity, hemodilution is

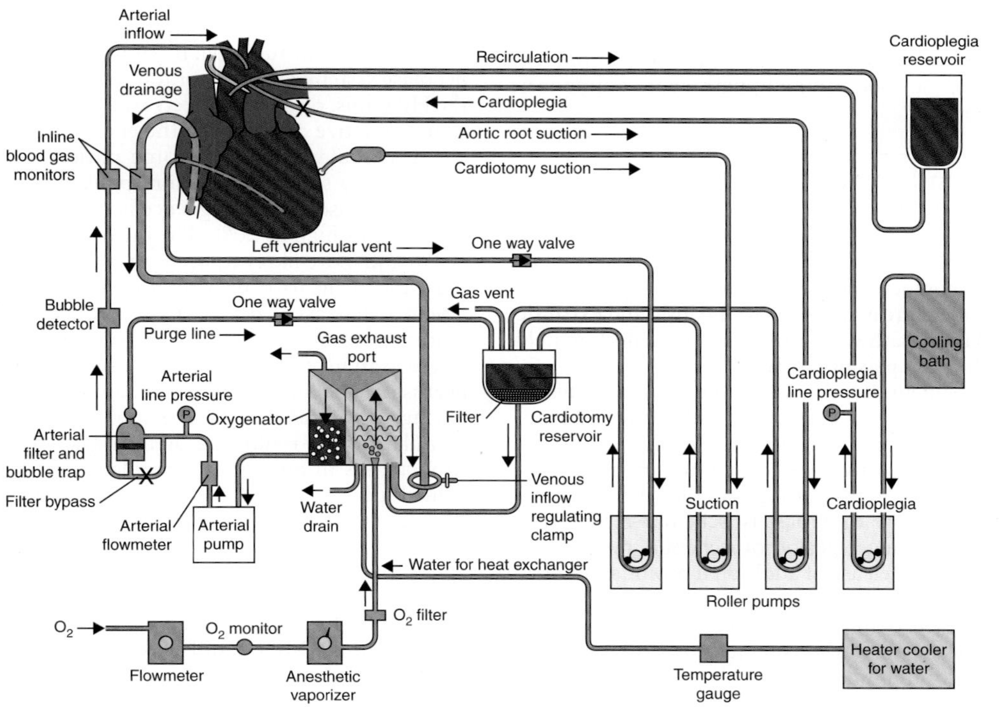

FIGURE 56.1. Extracorporeal cardiopulmonary bypass circuit.

used during moderate-to-deep hypothermic CPB. In infants, a nadir hematocrit of 25% is associated with favorable acute and neurodevelopmental outcomes. Temperature has an impact on blood pH. With increasing hypothermia, blood pH becomes progressively alkalotic. Using an alpha-stat strategy, pH is maintained at 7.40 without regard to temperature.

Selected right heart repairs, such as a pulmonary valve replacement or tricuspid valve surgery, may be performed on CPB with a beating heart provided that no intracardiac communication exists that would allow passage of an air embolus to the systemic circulation. Fibrillatory arrest may be used for right heart procedures in the event an atrial communication exists. To obtain a motionless heart for most intracardiac repairs, the aorta is cross-clamped proximal to the aortic cannula and a cold, potassium-rich cardioplegia solution is delivered via a smaller cannula into the aortic root. Alternatively, cardioplegia may be delivered retrograde through the coronary sinus. Asystole develops as the cardioplegia perfuses the coronary circulation. The combination of cardioplegia and hypothermia provides myocardial protection for several hours. Following placement of the aortic cross-clamp, blood from aortopulmonary collaterals will continue to return to the left atrium. DHCA may be used to eliminate left atrial blood return and facilitate repair of complex left heart disease. During circulatory arrest, pump flow ceases. Periods of circulatory arrest <40 minutes are usually well tolerated. Following rewarming and weaning from CPB, the surgeon ensures adequacy of the repair. Once separated from CPB, protamine is given to reverse the effect of heparin. Protamine administration is associated with vasodilation, hypotension, and occasionally with acute pulmonary hypertension.

The Inflammatory Response to CPB: Pathophysiology and Treatment

With exposure of plasma proteases to the CPB circuit, the contact system and the alternate pathway of complement are activated. The intrinsic and extrinsic coagulation pathways are activated, and ultimately thrombin and plasmin activate the classical pathway of complement. Byproducts of the plasma proteases activate endothelial cells, platelets, leukocytes, macrophages, and parenchymal cells, leading to the production of cellular-derived inflammatory mediators. Another factor in the pathophysiology of the inflammatory response to bypass is ischemia–reperfusion injury. Following a period of ischemia, reperfusion stimulates the release of additional proinflammatory mediators. At the conclusion of bypass, the formation of heparin–protamine complexes further stimulates the classical pathway of complement. With initiation of the proinflammatory cascade, a compensatory anti-inflammatory response limits the inflammatory response and extent of tissue injury.

End-Organ Injury and the Inflammatory Response to Cardiopulmonary Bypass

Inflammatory mediators bind to cerebral vascular and vascular-associated cells, increasing the permeability of the blood–brain barrier, resulting in cerebral edema. The primary mechanism of immune-mediated cerebral injury results from ischemia–reperfusion injury, which may also lead to impaired endothelial-dependent vasodilation and disturbed cerebral pressure autoregulation. The systemic inflammatory response and more importantly pulmonary reperfusion injury impair respiratory function. Damage to the pulmonary endothelium and alveolar epithelium leads to interstitial and alveolar edema and a decrease in lung compliance. Impaired surfactant production resulting from injury to type II alveolar pneumocytes and inactivation of surfactant by extravasated plasma proteins further decrease lung compliance. Preexisting lung disease, prolonged duration of CPB and ischemia, and pulmonary venous hypertension contribute to lung injury. The inflammatory response to CPB and pulmonary reperfusion injury also damage the pulmonary endothelium, leading to increases in pulmonary vascular resistance and heightened pulmonary vascular reactivity. The inflammatory response to bypass and much more importantly reperfusion injury following cardioplegic arrest lead to myocardial injury and impaired systolic and diastolic function. Inflammatory mediators, primarily cytokines produced by cardiomyocytes and interstitial cardiac leukocytes, exert a direct effect on the cardiomyocyte, contributing to impaired myocardial function.

The inflammatory response to CPB also affects systemic vascular function. Inflammatory mediators decrease systemic vasomotor tone and interfere with the HPA axis, resulting in decreased cortisol production, a relative adrenal insufficiency, and impaired cardiovascular function. Some patients develop vasodilatory shock that is unresponsive to volume and vasopressors. Vasoplegia occurs in adults with an incidence as high as 20%. The incidence in children is 3% and more likely to occur in children undergoing CPB for heart transplantation or placement of a ventricular assist device. Bypass-induced inflammatory response increases intestinal permeability. There is an inverse relationship between mesenteric perfusion and increases in intestinal permeability during CPB. This may be due to nonpulsatile flow stimulating the renin–angiotensin system, leading to increases in mesenteric vascular resistance and contributing to mesenteric ischemia. Inflammation and ischemia-related injury compromise the integrity of the mucosa, resulting in bacterial translocation and further stimulation of the inflammatory cascade.

The vast majority of pediatric centers have incorporated the use of glucocorticoids, modified ultrafiltration (MUF), and heparin-coated circuits to ameliorate the inflammatory response to CPB. Ultrafiltration removes water, reverses hemodilution, and eliminates low-molecular-weight substances, including inflammatory mediators. Heparinization of the contact surface of the circuit has been shown to modify the inflammatory response to bypass, decreasing cytokine release as well as inhibiting the contact system and complement activation.

LESION-SPECIFIC MANAGEMENT

Patent Ductus Arteriosus

Following ligation of a patent ductus arteriosus (PDA), chylothorax (related to thoracic duct injury) and injury to the recurrent laryngeal or phrenic nerves may occur. A subset of premature neonates develops a low–cardiac output state following PDA ligation, likely related to acute alterations in myocardial loading conditions.

Atrial and Ventricular Septal Defects

Most isolated secundum, primum, or sinus venosus atrial septal defects (ASDs) are electively repaired between 1 and 3 years of age. Patients with large VSDs typically have congestive heart failure and warrant referral for surgical repair in early infancy. Selected infants with large VSDs who are not thought to be candidates for primary repair because of the presence of multiple VSDs with anticipated difficult surgical exposure or noncardiac comorbidities may be palliated with a pulmonary artery band.

Residual defects following isolated ASD repair are uncommon. Obstruction to the SVC or pulmonary veins may occur following sinus venosus ASD repair. Following ASD or VSD closure, most patients are candidates for early extubation. Atrial arrhythmias may occur following ASD closure, including transient sinus node dysfunction following repair of sinus venosus defects. Junctional ectopic tachycardia (JET) and heart block may develop following VSD repair. Postpericardiotomy syndrome may develop in the days to weeks following septal defect repair.

Atrioventricular Septal Defects

Most complete atrioventricular septal defects (AVSDs) are referred for surgery between 3 and 6 months of life and use a one-patch, two-patch, or modified single-patch technique. Potential residual lesions include left-sided atrioventricular valve regurgitation, VSD, and pulmonary hypertension. Inotropic support and afterload reduction may be indicated to treat left-sided atrioventricular valve regurgitation and pulmonary hypertension. Arrhythmias such as JET and complete heart block may complicate the postoperative course. Partial AVSDs are repaired between 1 and 2 years of age with a patch closure of the ASD and suture closure of the cleft in the left-sided atrioventricular valve.

Truncus Arteriosus

Surgical repair of truncus arteriosus is typically undertaken in the newborn period and involves VSD closure, removal of the pulmonary arteries from the arterial trunk, and placement of a conduit from the right ventricle to the pulmonary arteries. Following repair of truncus arteriosus, potential residual lesions include right ventricular outflow tract obstruction, VSD, and pulmonary hypertension. Patients are at risk for developing a variant of right ventricular failure due to restrictive right ventricular physiology (**Table 56.1**). Treatment options are outlined in **Table 56.2**. Significant truncal valve regurgitation may compromise coronary blood flow and increase the

TABLE 56.1

Factors That May Contribute to Restrictive Right Ventricular Physiology Following Neonatal Right Ventricular Outflow Tract Reconstruction

RISK FACTOR	ETIOLOGIES
Diastolic dysfunction	Poorly elastic, hypertrophied right ventricle; right ventriculotomy; right ventricular muscle bundle resection; myocardial ischemia–reperfusion injury; noncontractile VSD patch
Deceased right ventricular preload	Tricuspid stenosis
Myocardial ischemia	Injury to conal branch of coronary artery crossing RVOT; inadequate coronary perfusion pressure
Volume load	Residual VSD; pulmonary regurgitation
Increased right ventricular afterload	Residual stenosis of the right ventricular infundibulum, pulmonary valve, or pulmonary arteries

VSD, ventricular septal defect; RVOT, right ventricular outflow tract.

TABLE 56.2

Treatment of Restrictive Right Ventricular Physiology

■ PHYSIOLOGIC GOALS	■ SPECIFIC TREATMENT STRATEGIES
Optimize ventricular preload	Patent foramen ovale, allowing for right-to-left shunting and left ventricular preload
	Ensure an adequate albeit elevated right atrial pressure
	Drain significant ascites
	Maintain atrioventricular synchrony
Inotropic support	Judicious use of dopamine, milrinone, and epinephrine
Lusitropy	Milrinone
Optimize myocardial oxygen supply and demand	Maintain coronary perfusion pressure
	Heart rate control
	Judicious use of inotropes
Maintain low right ventricular afterload	Use lowest possible mean airway pressure and maintain lung volume at functional residual capacity
	Avoid acidosis
	Drain pleural effusions, pneumothoraces, or hemothoraces
Minimize systemic oxygen consumption	Maintain normothermia
	Provide adequate sedation and analgesia
	Consider muscle relaxant

volume load on the left ventricle. Arrhythmias such as JET, ectopic atrial tachycardia, and complete heart block may occur. A state of low cardiac output may exist related to one or more of the above problems.

Coarctation of the Aorta

A prostaglandin E1 (PGE_1) infusion is indicated once a coarctation is suspected in a neonate. If the neonate presents in shock, supportive care is provided to recover end-organ function prior to surgery. In patients with a coexistent VSD or AVSD, management strategies may be needed to balance the systemic and pulmonary circulations. Several techniques are available for coarctation repair, including resection with end-to-end anastomoses, patch aortoplasty, and subclavian flap aortoplasty. Neonates with a critical coarctation are at risk for significant pulmonary hypertension in the early postoperative period. Beyond the neonatal period, postoperative systemic hypertension is common, due to a combination of pain, baroreceptor stimulation, and activation of the renin–angiotensin–aldosterone system. Hypertension may contribute to *postcoarctectomy syndrome* (mesenteric arteritis), which is characterized by abdominal pain, fever, ileus, melena, and leukocytosis. As pulsatile flow dramatically increases to vessels beyond the coarctation, thin-walled arterioles may overdistend and rupture, particularly those in the mesentery. Caution is warranted when advancing feeds during the first few postoperative days. Additional early complications include bleeding, chylothorax, phrenic nerve injury, and recurrent laryngeal nerve injury. Spinal cord ischemia leading to paralysis is a rare but important complication. Older patients with inadequate collateral formation may be at greater risk.

Interrupted Aortic Arch

Neonates with interrupted aortic arch have ductal-dependent systemic blood flow and require a PGE_1 infusion. Corrective surgery involving VSD closure and reconstruction of the aortic arch is performed within the first few days of life. Potential residual lesions include a VSD and subaortic or aortic arch obstruction. The extensive suture lines following reconstruction of the arch makes bleeding a postoperative concern and blood pressure should be controlled. Vigilance for pulmonary hypertension is warranted. The most common type of interrupted aortic arch (type B interruption between the left subclavian and left carotid arteries) is associated with a 30%–80% incidence of DiGeorge syndrome (at risk for hypocalcemia and immune deficiency).

Aortic Stenosis (Valvar, Subvalvar, Supravalvar)

Aortic valve stenosis is the most common type of left ventricular outflow tract obstruction. Subvalvar and supravalvar aortic stenosis are less frequent. Neonates with critical aortic valve stenosis may present with severe left ventricular dysfunction and shock and stabilization with PGE_1 may be indicated. Provided that other left-sided structures are adequate for a biventricular repair, treatment options include balloon valvuloplasty or surgical valvotomy. Balloon valvuloplasty is preferred, although evidence that outcomes are superior is lacking. Following the alleviation of critical aortic valve stenosis, most patients will have a marked improvement in clinical status with recovery of left ventricular function. However, low cardiac output may be present and inotropic support may be indicated. The PGE_1 infusion may be continued until the left ventricular function is adequate to support the systemic circulation, as evidenced by predominantly left-to-right ductal flow by lower-extremity pulse oximetry or echocardiography. Pulmonary hypertension may be problematic in the first few days following the intervention. If pulmonary hypertension persists, the adequacy of the intervention and other left-sided heart structures should be reassessed. For patients with a poorly functioning aortic valve but otherwise adequate left-sided structures, the aortic valve may be replaced with a homograft or autograft (Ross operation). Those with inadequate left-sided structures may require a Norwood operation. Following aortic root replacement (involving coronary artery reimplantation) or repair of supravalvar stenosis, vigilance should be maintained for coronary ischemia. In most patients, postoperative care is centered on controlling hypertension and monitoring for bleeding in those with extensive aortic suture lines.

Valvar Pulmonary Stenosis

Neonates with critical pulmonary valve stenosis have ductal-dependent pulmonary blood flow, necessitating a PGE_1 infusion. Balloon valvuloplasty is the intervention of choice, and surgical valvotomy is reserved for neonates who fail transcatheter intervention. The most common problem encountered following balloon dilation is ongoing cyanosis, which may worsen as the ductus arteriosus constricts after discontinuation of PGE_1. In such patients, right ventricular hypoplasia and poor compliance cause persistent right-to-left atrial shunting. Resumption of PGE_1 maintains ductal patency and pulmonary blood flow and provides time for right ventricular compliance to improve. Surgical intervention is required in 15%–25% of neonates with critical pulmonary stenosis, either for failure of the balloon valvuloplasty or persistent cyanosis. A systemic-to-pulmonary shunt can provide adequate pulmonary blood flow until right ventricle compliance and capacity improve. If infundibular hypertrophy or residual pulmonary valve stenosis is contributing to the cyanosis, an infundibular patch or pulmonary valvotomy may be required.

Tetralogy of Fallot

Neonates with tetralogy of Fallot and minimal obstruction to pulmonary blood flow are usually asymptomatic and well oxygenated. These lesions mimic the pathophysiology of a large VSD and develop congestive heart failure during the first weeks of life as pulmonary vascular resistance falls. More commonly, progressive right ventricular outflow tract obstruction and worsening cyanosis develop. Neonates with more severe right ventricular outflow tract obstruction or pulmonary atresia develop excessive cyanosis upon closure of the ductus arteriosus. Such patients may be stabilized with a PGE_1 infusion and referred for early surgical intervention. Indications for surgical intervention for older infants with tetralogy of Fallot include increasing cyanosis or the occurrence of a hypercyanotic episode (i.e., "TET spell"). Complete repair of tetralogy of Fallot includes VSD closure, resection of muscle bundles in the right ventricular outflow tract, a pulmonary valvotomy or leaflet resection, and, if necessary, patch augmentation of the pulmonary valve annulus (i.e., transannular patch) and proximal pulmonary arteries or placement of a right ventricular-to-pulmonary artery conduit. Some patients manifest restrictive right ventricular physiology following surgery (**Table 56.1**), which leads to systemic venous hypertension and may result in ascites and pleural effusions. Poor right ventricular compliance may lead to inadequate filling and output. Treatment options are discussed in **Table 56.2.** Minimizing intrathoracic pressure increases systemic venous return and right ventricular filling and output. JET is the most common arrhythmia seen early following tetralogy of Fallot repair.

Tetralogy of Fallot with Pulmonary Atresia

In tetralogy of Fallot with pulmonary atresia, the central pulmonary arteries may be diminutive or absent and one or more *major aortopulmonary collateral vessels* (MAPCAs) are present. The MAPCAs are variable in number and usually arise from the descending aorta, although their origin may be from the ascending aorta, aortic arch, brachiocephalic vessels, or coronary arteries. Pulmonary blood flow may be quite variable depending upon the size and number of MAPCAs and the severity of stenosis within these vessels. Generally such patients do not have ductal-dependent pulmonary blood flow. Although primary complete repair in early infancy is possible, in many cases, a staged series of surgical and transcatheter interventions are required. If the central pulmonary arteries are small but confluent, the initial operation may involve placement of a systemic-to-pulmonary shunt, an aortopulmonary window, or placement of a right ventricular-to-pulmonary artery conduit to promote growth of these vessels. Intervention for MAPCAs depends upon their size, the presence or absence of proximal stenosis within the vessel, and a determination as to whether the vessel represents redundant blood supply to individual lung segments. Redundant MAPCAs can be coil occluded in the catheterization laboratory or ligated at surgery to eliminate left-to-right shunting. If an MAPCA represents the sole source of pulmonary blood flow to a lung segment, the proximal end of the MAPCA is removed from its source and incorporated into the native or newly constructed central pulmonary arteries, such that blood flow to the lung is supplied from a single source (*unifocalization* procedure). Once the pulmonary vascular bed has been optimally recruited, intracardiac repair is completed including VSD closure and (if not previously completed) right ventricular outflow tract reconstruction. A patent foramen ovale or placement of a fenestrated VSD patch may be indicated in those patients with an inadequate pulmonary vascular bed to maintain left ventricular filling.

Tetralogy of Fallot Absent Pulmonary Valve Syndrome

In addition to the features of tetralogy of Fallot, patients with absent pulmonary valve syndrome have rudimentary pulmonary valve leaflets. The pulmonary arteries can be severely dilated from in utero to-and-fro flow (severe regurgitation) across the right ventricular outflow tract. Some neonates manifest severe respiratory compromise after delivery due to tracheobronchial compression by the aneurismal pulmonary arteries. Prone positioning may be beneficial as gravity may pull the pulmonary arteries off of the airways. Early surgery is indicated, which includes plication or replacement of the central pulmonary arteries and placement of a valved right ventricular-to-pulmonary artery conduit. The postoperative course may be complicated by respiratory failure and prolonged ventilation due to distal bronchomalacia and reduced number of alveoli.

Pulmonary Atresia with Intact Ventricular Septum

Pulmonary atresia with intact ventricular septum is characterized by a membranous or muscular obstruction of the pulmonary valve and varying degrees of right ventricular and tricuspid valve hypoplasia. The left and right pulmonary arteries are usually normal size. Right ventricle to coronary artery fistulae are present in half of cases, particularly in those with significant tricuspid valve and right ventricular hypoplasia. In one-third of patients with pulmonary atresia and intact ventricular septum, stenosis, interruptions, or ostial occlusions are present in coronary vessels. The myocardium supplied by these coronary arteries is dependent on flow from the right ventricle through the coronary fistulae, a condition known as *right ventricular dependent coronary circulation* (RVDCC). In patients with evidence of coronary-cameral fistula by echocardiogram, a cardiac catheterization is required to determine whether RVDCC is present. All neonates with pulmonary atresia have complete intracardiac mixing and ductal-dependent pulmonary blood flow, and PGE_1 is indicated. Provided that the tricuspid valve and right ventricle are reasonable size and there is no RVDCC, the right ventricular outflow tract is reconstructed to allow regression of right ventricular hypertrophy and promote right ventricular growth with the anticipation that more normal size right-sided heart structures will enable a biventricular repair. The ASD may be left open to allow for decompression of the right heart, ensuring adequate left ventricular filling. A systemic-to-pulmonary shunt may also be placed, ensuring adequate pulmonary blood flow. Alternatively, the right ventricle may be decompressed in neonates with membranous pulmonary atresia by transcatheter perforation of the pulmonary valve using a stiff wire or radiofrequency ablation catheter followed by balloon valvuloplasty. At best, transcatheter intervention avoids the need for early surgical intervention in one-third of patients due to persistent cyanosis. In this scenario, a systemic-to-pulmonary artery shunt with or without a right ventricular outflow tract patch is needed. If RVDCC exists, relief of right ventricular outflow obstruction is contraindicated, and the initial operation is a systemic-to-pulmonary artery shunt as the first stage of single-ventricle palliation. Cardiac transplantation may be considered for the unusual infant with severe RVDCC and myocardial dysfunction that precludes single-ventricle palliation. Residual lesions following intervention in neonates with pulmonary atresia and intact ventricular septum include residual right ventricular outflow tract obstruction and pulmonary regurgitation. Restrictive right ventricular physiology is common following a two-ventricular repair, and management is similar to that following repair of tetralogy of Fallot or truncus arteriosus (**Tables 56.1** and **56.2**).

D-Transposition of the Great Arteries

In D-transposition of the great arteries (D-TGA), the aorta arises from the anatomic right ventricle and the pulmonary artery arises from the anatomic left ventricle. In ~40% of cases, a VSD exists. Obligatory intercirculatory mixing takes place at the atrial, ventricular, or great artery level. A PGE_1 infusion may be needed to maintain ductal patency or a balloon septostomy to enlarge the atrial communication may be indicated if severe cyanosis is present. An additional benefit of PGE_1 is its pulmonary vasodilatory effect. Neonates with D-TGA and a moderate-to-large VSD are generally well oxygenated and do not require a PGE_1 infusion if the ventricular outflow tracts are unobstructed. Neonates with D-TGA and no significant outflow tract obstruction receive an arterial switch operation and septal defects are closed. Using the Lecompte maneuver, the pulmonary artery is translocated anterior to the aorta such that its branches drape over the aorta. The coronary arteries are mobilized with a button of periosteal tissue and reimplanted into the neoaorta. If a significant right ventricular outflow tract obstruction is present, a Damus–Kaye–Stansel procedure may be performed as an initial palliation, or as a part of the complete repair including closure of the VSD and placement of a right ventricle-to-pulmonary artery conduit. If significant left ventricular outflow tract obstruction exists, the Rastelli procedure (baffle to close the VSD to the aorta and placement of a right ventricle-to-pulmonary artery conduit) or Nikaidoh operation (aortic root translocation into a surgically enlarged left ventricular outflow tract, VSD closure, and right ventricular outflow tract reconstruction) may be performed. Potential residual lesions following the arterial switch operation include branch pulmonary artery stenosis. Coronary artery stenosis may manifest signs of coronary ischemia and left atrial hypertension. Until the morphologic left ventricle adapts to pumping against systemic vascular resistance, inotropic support and afterload reduction may be indicated. Volume should be administered cautiously, as ventricular compliance is impaired. Vigilance for bleeding is required given the extensive aortic suture lines. Infants with D-TGA and intact ventricular septum referred after 1–2 months of age often require a pulmonary artery band to "prepare" the left ventricle before the arterial switch operation. A systemic-to-pulmonary artery shunt is usually required at the time of the pulmonary artery band to ensure adequate pulmonary blood flow. These patients are often critically ill postoperatively with biventricular failure and low cardiac output. Right ventricular function is impaired due to the acute volume load created by the shunt and left ventricular function is impaired as a result of the acute increase in afterload. Inotropic support and measures to decrease pulmonary overcirculation may be indicated.

Total Anomalous Pulmonary Venous Return

Neonates with isolated obstructed total anomalous pulmonary venous return (TAPVR) present with pulmonary venous congestion, cyanosis, and pulmonary hypertension within hours of birth. They require stabilization including mechanical ventilation and inotropic support and emergent surgical intervention. Those with unobstructed TAPVR present with a murmur, mild cyanosis, and signs of right ventricular volume overload. Patients with obstructed TAPVR are predisposed to pulmonary hypertensive crises following surgery. The left atrium may be small and poorly compliant, and rapid volume infusions may exacerbate pulmonary edema and pulmonary hypertension. The reactive pulmonary hypertension following repair of TAPVR may be responsive to inhaled nitric oxide.

Single-Ventricle Physiology

Single-ventricle physiology is present when there is complete mixing of systemic and pulmonary venous return and the determinant of pulmonary and systemic blood flow (Q_p and Q_s, respectively) is the relative resistances. Single-ventricle–like physiology may be present in neonates with biventricular anatomy, such as interrupted aortic arch and truncus arteriosus, with the caveat that there may not be complete mixing of systemic and pulmonary venous return. The ratio of systemic and pulmonary blood flow may be calculated by using the modified Fick equation $Q_p/Q_s = Sao_2 - Scvo_2/Spvo_2 - Spao_2$ (Sao_2, arterial oxygen saturation; $Scvo_2$; central venous oxygen saturation; $Spvo_2$, pulmonary venous oxygen saturation; and $Spao_2$, pulmonary artery saturation). The Sao_2 and $Spao_2$ are the same value, as there is completing mixing of systemic and pulmonary venous return; cerebral NIRS oximetry or central venous oximetry may be used for $Scvo_2$; and an assumed value is used for the $Spvo_2$. The Q_p/Q_s ratio will be underestimated if one overestimates the $Scvo_2$ and/or $Spvo_2$ value. In any case, cerebral NIRS oximetry and the $Scvo_2$ assess the adequacy of Q_s.

Systemic-to-Pulmonary Artery Shunt

The most used systemic-to-pulmonary artery shunt is the *modified Blalock–Taussig shunt*. This entails placement of a Gore-Tex tube graft between the distal innominate artery or proximal subclavian artery and the pulmonary artery (usually without CPB). An alternative systemic-to-pulmonary artery shunt is a *central shunt*, the placement of a Gore-Tex tube between the ascending aorta and pulmonary artery. If the systemic-to-pulmonary artery shunt is relatively large, excessive pulmonary blood flow will subject the systemic ventricle to volume overload; conversely a relatively small shunt or pulmonary artery stenosis will result in cyanosis. The loss of a shunt murmur and an abrupt increase in the arterial to end-tidal carbon dioxide gradient (for intubated patients) suggests acute shunt thrombosis. Other causes of early postoperative cyanosis are listed in **Table 56.3**. Reported neurologic complications following shunt surgery include Horner syndrome, recurrent laryngeal nerve injury, and phrenic nerve injury.

Pulmonary Artery Band

In neonates with single ventricular physiology and unobstructed pulmonary and systemic blood flow, a band may be placed on the main pulmonary artery to decrease pulmonary blood flow and the extent of pulmonary overcirculation and congestive heart failure (from the volume load on the ventricle) and the development of pulmonary vascular obstructive disease.

Damus–Kaye–Stansel Procedure

In children with single ventricular physiology and subaortic or aortic stenosis, a Damus–Kaye–Stansel palliation provides unobstructed systemic blood flow. This procedure involves anastomosis of the

TABLE 56.3

Potential Causes of Excessive Cyanosis Following Single-Ventricle Palliation

	STAGE 1 (E.G., NORWOOD, PAB, SP SHUNT)	SUPERIOR CAVOPULMONARY ANASTOMOSIS	FONTAN
Inadequate pulmonary blood flow	Pulmonary hypertension Stenosis of systemic-to-pulmonary shunt Thrombosis of systemic-to-pulmonary shunt Excessive tightness of pulmonary artery band Obstruction to pulmonary venous or left atrial egress	Pulmonary hypertension Stenosis of Glenn/hemi-Fontan pathway Thrombosis in Glenn/hemi-Fontan pathway Pulmonary artery stenosis Veno-veno collaterals	Pulmonary hypertension Anatomic obstruction to Fontan pathway Thrombosis in Fontan pathway Pulmonary artery stenosis Veno-veno collaterals Pulmonary arteriovenous malformations Baffle leak Oversized fenestration
Pulmonary venous desaturation	Atelectasis Pulmonary edema Pleural effusions Pneumonia	Atelectasis Pulmonary edema Pleural effusions Pneumonia	Atelectasis Pulmonary edema Pleural effusions Pneumonia
Systemic venous desaturation	Anemia High $\dot{V}O_2$ Low cardiac output	Anemia High $\dot{V}O_2$ Low cardiac output	Anemia High $\dot{V}O_2$ Low cardiac output

PAB, pulmonary artery band; SP shunt, systemic pulmonary shunt; $\dot{V}O_2$, oxygen consumption.

proximal main pulmonary artery and ascending aorta. The distal main pulmonary artery is oversewn and a systemic-to-pulmonary shunt is placed to provide pulmonary blood flow. The postoperative physiology and complications are similar to the Norwood operation, discussed below.

Stage 1 Norwood Procedure

Neonates with HLHS and other single-ventricle heart defects with aortic arch obstruction typically undergo a Norwood operation within the first days of life. This operation entails anastomosis of the proximal pulmonary artery and the aorta, reconstruction of the aortic arch to allow unobstructed systemic blood flow, and an atrial septectomy to ensure unobstructed pulmonary venous return. Pulmonary blood flow is provided with either a modified Blalock–Taussig shunt or right ventricular-to-pulmonary artery conduit (*Sano shunt*). After the Norwood operation, the single right ventricle pumps blood to the systemic circulation and coronary arteries via the reconstructed aorta ("*neoaorta*"), and to the pulmonary circulation through the systemic-to-pulmonary artery *shunt*. Postoperatively, residual aortic arch obstruction may be associated with inadequate systemic perfusion and pulmonary overcirculation. Narrowing at the anastomosis of the aorta and pulmonary artery predisposes to coronary ischemia. Stenosis of the proximal or distal end of a systemic-to-pulmonary artery shunt contributes to cyanosis. Sano shunts may be obstructed by right ventricular muscle bundles, and are uncommonly associated with the development of aneurysms at their insertion site into the right ventricle. Myocardial dysfunction or atrioventricular valve regurgitation may cause inadequate systemic perfusion and a low–cardiac output state. Supportive care includes inotropic support, afterload reduction to improve ventricular ejection and to decrease the systemic-to-pulmonary vascular resistance ratio, and avoidance of excessive supplemental oxygen and hyperventilation. Potential causes of hypoxemia are outlined in **Table 56.4**.

Superior Cavopulmonary Anastomosis

A superior cavopulmonary anastomosis involves redirection of the SVC blood flow to both pulmonary arteries. The bidirectional *Glenn operation* (bidirectional cavopulmonary shunt operation) involves an end-to-side anastomosis between the SVC and the pulmonary artery. The *hemi-Fontan operation* involves the end-to-side anastomosis between the SVC and the pulmonary artery, the proximal SVC is anastomosed to the inferior surface of the pulmonary artery, and a patch is placed at the junction of the SVC and the right atrium. The functional result of this operation is the same as the bidirectional Glenn operation,

TABLE 56.4

Etiologies of Low Cardiac Output after the Fontan Operation

RA PRESSURE	LA PRESSURE	ETIOLOGIES
Low	Low	Hypovolemia (bleeding, inadequate preload)
High	Low	Fontan pathway or pulmonary artery obstruction Elevated pulmonary vascular resistance Clotted fenestration
High	High	Ventricular failure Atrioventricular valve stenosis or regurgitation Arrhythmia Ventricular outflow tract obstruction Tamponade

RA, right atrial; LA, left atrial.

but it facilitates later completion of the lateral tunnel Fontan operation. Because pulmonary blood flow is passive through a superior cavopulmonary anastomosis, it is not performed when pulmonary vascular resistance is elevated. Efforts to maintain a low transpulmonary gradient (i.e., mean pulmonary artery pressure − mean common atrial pressure) in the postoperative period are warranted. Cyanosis may be caused by pulmonary venous desaturation, systemic venous desaturation, inadequate pulmonary blood flow, and collaterals with physiologic right-to-left shunting (**Table 56.3**). Ventilator strategies that minimize airway pressure and maximize exhalation time will enhance pulmonary blood flow. Early extubation is desirable. Elevated $PaCO_2$ increases cerebral and thus pulmonary blood flow and arterial oxygenation with this anatomy. Following a superior cavopulmonary anastomosis, the *SVC syndrome* may develop, which is characterized by cerebral and upper extremity venous congestion, and is caused by a small cross-sectional area of the pulmonary vascular bed, stenosis of the Glenn pathway, or (uncommonly) increased pulmonary vascular resistance.

Modified Fontan Procedure

The Fontan procedure is performed at ~2 years of age. During this operation, the inferior vena cava is connected to the pulmonary arteries, which bypasses the heart, separates the systemic and pulmonary circulations, and eliminates cyanosis. The lateral tunnel and extracardiac modifications are the Fontan techniques. A 3–4-mm fenestration in the Fontan pathway may be placed, which allows for right-to-left shunting and maintenance of ventricular preload, and lowers systemic venous pressure. Residual obstruction to the Fontan pathway may contribute to a low–cardiac output state. General postoperative strategies are directed at optimizing cardiac output while minimizing the transpulmonary gradient (**Table 56.4**). Systolic function is generally preserved; however, there is often diastolic dysfunction that is compounded by a reliance on systemic venous pressure to drive blood across the pulmonary circulation. Other acute postoperative issues include arrhythmias (e.g., sinus node dysfunction, accelerated junctional rhythm, or JET), and prolonged chest tube drainage. Cyanosis may be caused by pulmonary venous desaturation and right-to-left shunting through collaterals (**Table 56.3**). Thrombosis may occur in the systemic venous pathway, causing an elevated transpulmonary gradient and low–cardiac output state.

Anomalous Origin of the Left Coronary Artery from the Pulmonary Artery

Patients with anomalous origin of the left coronary artery from the pulmonary artery (ALCAPA) often develop myocardial ischemia as pulmonary vascular resistance (and thus left coronary artery perfusion) declines during infancy. Preoperative mechanical ventilation, inotropic support, and diuresis may be required while urgent surgery is arranged. The common surgical approach is transfer of the left coronary artery from the pulmonary artery to the aorta. Postoperative management of myocardial dysfunction and mitral regurgitation may be required. ECMO is required in a minority of patients.

Ebstein Anomaly

In Ebstein anomaly of the tricuspid valve, the septal and posterior leaflets are displaced into the anatomic right ventricle and are variably adherent to the ventricular septum. The nondisplaced anterior leaflet may be fenestrated and redundant or "sail-like" and cause obstruction of the right ventricular outflow tract. The functional right atrium may be quite enlarged. ASDs (commonly) and pulmonary valve stenosis or atresia are associated with Ebstein anomaly. One or more accessory conduction pathways may exist at the tricuspid valve annulus, creating the necessary substrate for atrioventricular reentrant tachycardia. Right-to-left shunting at the atrial level occurs. In some neonates, functional pulmonary atresia develops when the pulmonary artery pressure exceeds the pressure generated by the Ebsteinoid right ventricle, and the pulmonary valve leaflets fail to open. Severe tricuspid regurgitation and extreme right atrial enlargement cause pooling of venous return in the compliant right atrium with limited shunting across the ASD to the left atrium. The enlarged and hypertensive right ventricle causes the interventricular septum to deviate into the left ventricle during diastole, decreasing the effective compliance and filling of the left ventricle. Neonates with Ebstein anomaly presenting with significant cyanosis (<75%–80% saturation) should receive PGE_1.

Decision-making for symptomatic neonates with severe Ebstein anomaly is complex. If pulmonary atresia is present, it must be determined whether it is anatomic or functional. If functional atresia is suspected, discontinuation of PGE_1 allows for ductal constriction and decreased pulmonary artery pressure and opening of the pulmonary valve leaflets. Anatomic pulmonary atresia may warrant attempted transcatheter perforation and balloon dilation or surgical placement of a systemic-to-pulmonary shunt.

For symptomatic neonates who fail medical management as outlined above, there is no single reparative or palliative procedure that is associated with widespread success. For neonates with both cyanosis and heart failure, one surgical option is to place a systemic-to-pulmonary artery shunt, oversew the tricuspid valve annulus, and perform an atrial septectomy as the first-stage procedure toward Fontan palliation. Plication of the right atrium is usually necessary to reduce its volume and promote right-to-left shunting across the atrial septum. Alternatively, a two-ventricle repair may be attempted consisting of a reduction atrioplasty, fenestrated closure of the atrial septum, and tricuspid valvuloplasty. Neonates with Ebstein anomaly who undergo early surgical intervention are at significant risk for developing a low–cardiac output state, and a number of factors may contribute. Neonates with a ductus arteriosus or systemic-to-pulmonary shunt and pulmonary and tricuspid regurgitation may develop a circular shunt, which is characterized by the shunting of blood from the aorta through the ductus arteriosus or shunt, retrograde through the pulmonary and tricuspid valves, across the atrial communication, and out of the left ventricle and aorta. In this situation, an emergent reoperation may be required to ligate the ductus arteriosus, limit the shunt size, ligate the main pulmonary artery, or reduce tricuspid regurgitation with a valvuloplasty. Neonates undergoing biventricular repair may have low cardiac output from a combination of residual tricuspid regurgitation and biventricular dysfunction. Interventions to maintain low pulmonary and systemic vascular resistance are warranted.

CHAPTER 57 ■ PULMONARY HYPERTENSION

JOHN K. MCGUIRE, SILVIA M. HARTMANN, AND APICHAI KHONGPHATTHANAYOTHIN

CLASSIFICATION

Pulmonary hypertension (PH) classification is based on clinical factors (**Table 57.1**), includes both adults and children, and uses the same *pulmonary arterial hypertension (PAH)* definition for both: mean pulmonary artery pressure ≥ 25 mm Hg, pulmonary capillary wedge pressure ≤ 15 mm Hg, and an increased pulmonary vascular resistance (PVR).

In this classification system, *idiopathic pulmonary arterial hypertension* (IPAH) is the most common category in group 1 and is diagnosed when a patient has no family history of PH, mutations associated with hereditable PAH (HPAH), or identified PAH

TABLE 57.1

WHO Classification of Pulmonary Hypertension

1.	Pulmonary arterial hypertension
1.1	Idiopathic PAH (IPAH)
1.2	Heritable PAH (HPAH)
1.2.1	Bone morphogenetic protein receptor type 2 (*BMPR2*) mutations
1.2.2	Activin receptor-like kinase (*ALK1*) and endoglin mutations
1.3	Drug- and toxin-induced
1.4	Associated with (APAH)
1.4.1	Connective tissue disease
1.4.2	HIV infection
1.4.3	Portal hypertension
1.4.4	Congenital heart disease
1.4.5	Schistosomiasis
1.4.6	Chronic hemolytic anemia
1.5	Persistent pulmonary hypertension of the newborn (PPHN)
1.6	Pulmonary veno-occlusive disease/pulmonary capillary hemangiomatosis
2.	Pulmonary hypertension due to left heart disease
2.1	Systolic dysfunction
2.2	Diastolic dysfunction
2.3	Valvular disease
3.	Pulmonary hypertension due to lung diseases and/or hypoxia
3.1	Chronic obstructive pulmonary disease
3.2	Interstitial lung disease
3.3	Other pulmonary disease with mixed restrictive and obstructive pattern
3.4	Sleep-disordered breathing
3.5	Alveolar hypoventilation disorders
3.6	Exposure to high altitude
3.7	Developmental abnormalities
4.	Chronic thromboembolic pulmonary hypertension
5.	Pulmonary hypertension with unclear multifactorial mechanisms
5.1	Hematologic disorders: myeloproliferative disorders
5.2	Systemic disorders: sarcoidosis, Langerhans cell histiocytosis, neurofibromatosis type 1, vasculitis
5.3	Metabolic disorders: glycogen storage disease, Gaucher disease, thyroid disorders
5.4	Other: obstruction by tumor mass, chronic renal failure on dialysis

Modified from Ivy D. Advances in pediatric pulmonary arterial hypertension. *Curr Opin Cardiol* 2012;27(2):70–81.

risk factors. PAH secondary to congenital heart disease and *persistent pulmonary hypertension of the newborn* (PPHN) are also included in group 1. Groups 2, 3, 4, and 5 comprise what was historically designated as secondary PH.

In 2011, a new classification system divided pediatric PH patients into 10 categories (**Table 57.2**, modification of Panama Classification).

Patients with PH are also classified by the limits the disease places on the individual. This *functional classification* (New York Heart Association system) is a strong predictor of mortality in adult patients and is an important factor in choice of PAH therapy in adults and children.

EPIDEMIOLOGY

The largest numbers of children with PH (82%) are those with transient disease processes, including PPHN

TABLE 57.2

Proposed Categorization of Pediatric Hypertensive Vascular Disease

GROUP	EXAMPLES
1. Prenatal or developmental pulmonary hypertensive disease	Associated with oligohydramnios/pulmonary hypoplasia Congenital diaphragmatic hernia Alveolar capillary dysplasia Lymphangiectasia Associated with oligohydramnios/pulmonary hypoplasia
2. Perinatal pulmonary vascular maladaptation	Idiopathic PPHN PPHN triggered by another disease process including sepsis or meconium aspiration syndrome Associated with trisomy 21
3. Pediatric cardiovascular disease	Associated with systemic-to-pulmonary shunt with increased PVRI Eisenmenger syndrome After repair of TGA, left heart obstruction
4. Bronchopulmonary dysplasia	
5. Isolated pediatric pulmonary hypertensive vascular disease	IPAH HPAH Secondary to drug or toxin PVOD/PCH
6. Multifactorial pulmonary hypertensive vascular disease in congenital malformation syndromes	Associated with VACTERL syndrome Associated with CHARGE disease Associated with DiGeorge disease Associated with Scimitar complex
7. Pediatric lung disease	Associated with cystic fibrosis Associated with sleep-disordered breathing Associated with chest wall and spinal deformities Associated with surfactant protein deficiency
8. Pediatric thromboembolic disease	Secondary to central venous catheters Associated with sickle cell disease Associated with methylmalonic acidemia and homocystinuria Due to malignancy After splenectomy
9. Pediatric hypobaric hypoxic exposure	
10. Pediatric pulmonary vascular disease associated with other system disorders	Associated with portal hypertension Associated with malignancy Due to metabolic disorders Due to autoimmune or autoinflammatory diseases Due to infectious diseases (HIV, schistosomiasis, pulmonary TB) Associated with chronic renal failure

PPHN, persistent pulmonary hypertension of the newborn; PVRI, pulmonary vascular resistance index; TGA, transposition of the great arteries; IPAH, idiopathic pulmonary arterial hypertension; HPAH, heritable pulmonary arterial hypertension; PVOD, pulmonary veno-occlusive disease; PCH, pulmonary capillary hemangiomatosis; VACTERL, vertebral, anus, cardiac, tracheoesophageal fistula, renal, and limb; CHARGE, coloboma, heart defect, atresia choanae (also known as choanal atresia), retarded growth and development, genital abnormality and ear abnormality.
Modified from Ivy D. Advances in pediatric pulmonary arterial hypertension. *Curr Opin Cardiol* 2012;27(2):70–81.

and systemic-to-pulmonary shunts. Most registries exclude patients with transient PH, and the majority of the remaining patients (57%–70%) have PAH, either IPAH or HPAH. The second most common cause of progressive PAH in children is associated with congenital heart disease (24%–36%) when excluding flow-related PH from systemic-to-pulmonary shunts. Patients with PH due to pulmonary diseases (11%–13%) include patients with bronchopulmonary dysplasia (5%) and obstructive sleep apnea (1.4%) as the cause of PH. Overall, chronic PAH is rare in children (3 cases/million children) especially compared with PPHN, which is about 30 cases/million children. The incidence of IPAH, the most common type of PAH, is 0.48–0.7 cases/million children, with a prevalence estimated at 2.2–4.4 cases/million.

PATHOPHYSIOLOGY OF PH

The Pulmonary Vasculature

In PH, both the function and structure of the pulmonary vasculature are abnormal (**Fig. 57.1**). Independent of etiology, PH in children is a combination of vasoconstriction, inflammation, structural remodeling of the pulmonary vessels, in situ thrombosis, and impaired vascular growth. Cell types that play key roles in acute and chronic PH include endothelial cells, smooth muscle cells, inflammatory cells, and platelets. Imbalances between the production of endogenous vasodilators and vasoconstrictors contribute to excess pulmonary vasoconstriction.

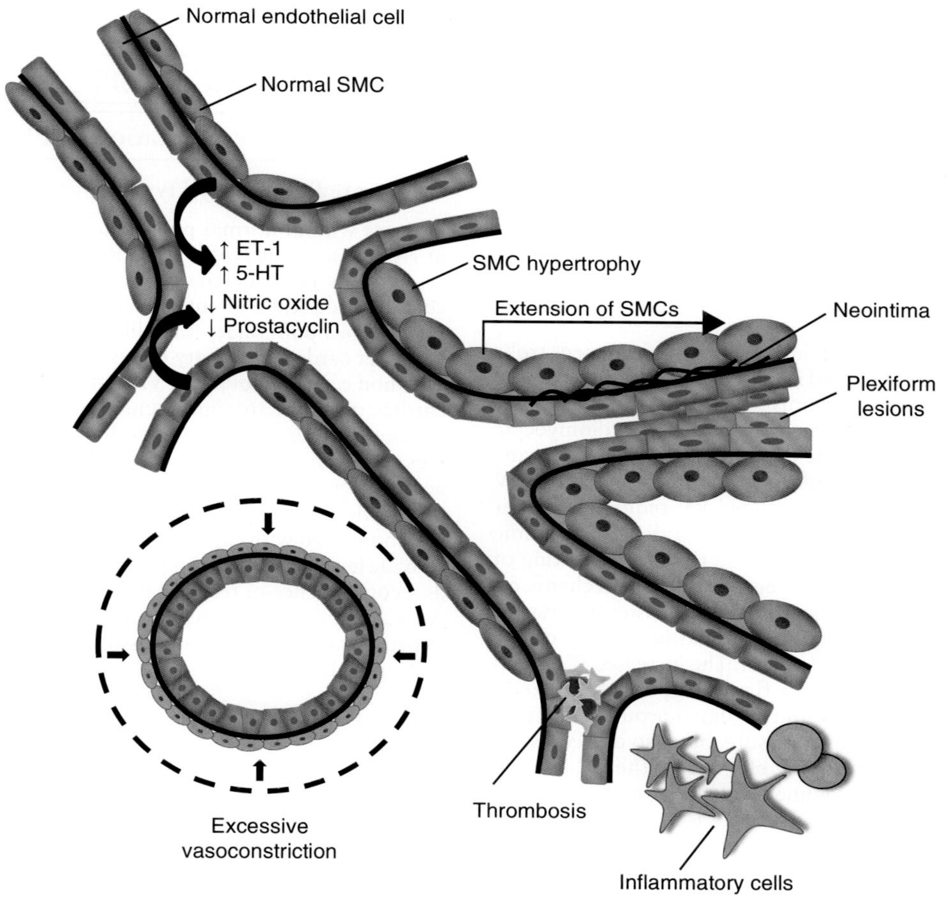

FIGURE 57.1. Pathophysiology of pulmonary hypertension: PH can be due to abnormal function of the pulmonary vasculature with excessive vasoconstriction, increased elaboration of vasoconstricting agents such as endothelin-1 and serotonin as well as decreased production of nitric oxide and prostacyclin from the endothelial cells. Smooth muscle hypertrophy and extension of smooth muscle cells onto arterioles that generally lack musculature also contribute to pulmonary hypertension. In some disease processes, plexiform lesions, monoclonal expansion of endothelial cells, can obstruct the lumen of pulmonary blood vessels. Chronic thrombosis of pulmonary vasculature and ongoing inflammation of the pulmonary parenchyma can also contribute to increased pulmonary vascular resistance in some instances. SMC, smooth muscle cell; ET-1, endothelin-1; 5-HT, serotonin.

The earliest change is often excessive vasoconstriction of the pulmonary arteriole in the setting of hypoxia. The mechanism is not fully elucidated but likely involves decreased vascular smooth muscle expression and activity of Kv1.5 potassium channels that close in response to hypoxia, leading to depolarization, calcium entry into the pulmonary vascular smooth muscle cell, and vasoconstriction. The vascular wall medial smooth muscle cell is the primary cell type implicated in pathologic vascular remodeling. Intimal thickening occurs due to abnormal proliferation of endothelial cells, likely in response to abnormal production of, and altered cellular responses to, growth factors. The endothelial cells in patients with PH produce increased amounts of vasoconstrictors, including endothelin-1 (ET-1) and serotonin (5-HT), while producing decreased amounts of vasodilators, such as nitric oxide and prostacyclin, leading to an imbalance that results in increased PVR. Additional structural changes include increases in fibroblasts and extracellular matrix between the endothelium and the internal elastic lamina, forming a "neointima." A reduced cross-sectional area of the vascular bed may be a result of reduced formation of blood vessels due to abnormal angiogenesis or from obstruction of blood vessels by in situ thromboses that form in the setting of an abnormal endothelium or in response to inflammatory mediators. Cytokines and chemokines may promote smooth muscle hypertrophy.

The Right Ventricle

PH increases RV afterload, leading to decreased stroke volume and increased RV end-diastolic volume. Initial compensatory mechanisms (e.g., Starling response) increase stroke volume in response to cardiomyocyte stretching. Over time this mechanism is inadequate, and to minimize loading of cardiomyocytes, the RV hypertrophies. The thickened RV requires a higher filling pressure for the same end-diastolic volume to maintain pulmonary blood flow in the setting of diastolic dysfunction. Neurohormonal mechanisms, including the renin–angiotensin–aldosterone system, are activated to increase circulating blood volume and maintain cardiac output. The increased RV blood volume leads to septal flattening, which not only decreases LV filling and cardiac output by increasing LV end-diastolic pressure, but also decreases the LV assistance in ejecting blood from the RV, thereby exacerbating the volume overload experienced by the RV. Eventual dilation of the RV is associated with the development of tricuspid regurgitation, which leads to further volume loading of the strained RV, and right atrial dilation that predisposes to atrial arrhythmias, which can impair RV filling and ultimately cardiac output. In general, the RV tolerates a volume load better than a pressure load without impairment of cardiac output as the RV is compliant and tolerates increased volume at relatively preserved end-diastolic pressures.

Genetics

Bone morphogenetic factor receptor type-II (BMPR-II) gene mutations are the most common identified genetic cause of PAH and have been found in 50%–90% of adults with HPAH. Presence of a BMPR-II mutation is associated with a 10%–20% lifetime risk of developing PAH. Other gene interactions or environmental triggers likely contribute to development of disease.

Pulmonary Hypertension in Acute Lung Disease

PH as a consequence of increased PVR is commonly present in severe lung disease associated with acute lung injury/ARDS, bronchiolitis, pertussis, and other acute pulmonary pathologies, and, if associated with RV dysfunction or failure, may be of significant clinical importance.

DIAGNOSIS

Clinical Presentation of PH

Acute Pulmonary Hypertensive Crisis

Patients with abnormal pulmonary vasculature are at risk of acute increases in PVR. These "acute PH crises" may be associated with pulmonary disease, central venous catheter infections in patients receiving intravenous pulmonary vasodilators, or postoperative after cardiopulmonary bypass. Hypotension is a common early sign of high PVR-induced reduction in cardiac output. Late signs include bradycardia with hypotension and signal impending cardiac arrest. Desaturation may not be evident in patients with acute increases in PVR in the absence of an atrial communication. In patients who are tracheally intubated and monitored with capnometry, the end-tidal carbon dioxide level decreases during acute increases in PVR as a consequence of reduced pulmonary blood flow. An acute increase in central venous pressure is also expected with acute increases in right ventricular end-diastolic pressure.

Chronic PH

Symptoms of chronic PAH are mainly due to the inability to increase cardiac output on exertion. The most common presenting symptom is dyspnea on exertion (65%–75%). Syncope (7%–20%) and near syncope (8%) reflect cerebral hypoperfusion due to inadequate cardiac output in the setting of exercise. Cyanosis with exercise (16%–18%) and pallor with exertion (5%) are also reported. Signs of RV dysfunction may manifest a loud pulmonic component of the second heart sound (P2) that is associated with high pulmonary artery pressure. Over time, the intensity of P2 may diminish if right ventricular function and right-sided cardiac output worsen. An early systolic or holosystolic murmur may be heard at the left lower sternal border consistent with tricuspid regurgitation as well as an early diastolic murmur indicative of pulmonary insufficiency. Abdominal exam can reveal hepatomegaly and ascites, and peripheral edema may be evident on inspection of the extremities.

PH Diagnostic Evaluation

Electrocardiogram

Almost 80% of patients with IPAH demonstrate right atrial enlargement, and 87% demonstrate right ventricular hypertrophy on ECG. Evidence of right ventricular strain may be present.

Echocardiogram

Echocardiography is necessary in patients who have suspected PH from history or physical examination. It is an excellent initial diagnostic tool to assess (a) presence and severity of PH, (b) RV function, and (c) presence of left heart disease and/or congenital heart disease. Peak right ventricular systolic pressure (RVSP) can be estimated by the maximal Doppler velocity of the tricuspid valve regurgitation (TR) jet. Using a simplified Bernoulli equation, the RVSP would be equal to $4V^2$ + RAP, where *V* is the peak velocity of the TR jet and RAP is the mean right atrial pressure. Diastolic pulmonary arterial pressure (dPAP) can be estimated by measuring the end-diastolic velocity of pulmonary regurgitation jet in the same manner. Estimation of the RVSP by TR is problematic when TR is trivial or absent. In a patient with ventricular septal defect (VSD) or patent ductus arteriosus (PDA), RV pressure can be estimated by measuring the peak flow velocity across the VSD or PDA. In absence of these defects, the position of the interventricular septum with the heart in short-axis view moves leftward with PH, giving the appearance of a D-shaped left ventricle. Presence of left heart disease must be evaluated in any patient with PH since the treatment and prognosis are very different from PAH.

Cardiac Catheterization

Patients suspected to have group 1 PH should undergo cardiac catheterization to define the presence and severity of PH and to rule out anatomic causes of PH not obvious from noninvasive evaluation. To rule out PH from left heart disease (group 2 PH), a left atrial pressure (LAP) or pulmonary arterial wedge pressure (PAWP) should be determined. Any patient with LAP or PAWP > 15 mm Hg qualifies for a diagnosis of PH secondary to left-sided heart disease.

Vasoreactivity Testing

Acute pulmonary vasoreactivity testing is done during cardiac catheterization using a short-acting pulmonary vasodilator such as nitric oxide, epoprostenol, or adenosine. A positive response in adult patients is a reduction in mean PAP at least 10 mm Hg below baseline with a final PAP ≤ 40 mm Hg. In pediatric practice, a positive response is a fall in mean PAP and PVRI by 20% with no change or an increase in cardiac output. Approximately 40% of children with IPAH demonstrated pulmonary vasoreactivity as opposed to 10%–26% in adults.

Imaging

Plain X-ray films of the chest may show an enlarged cardiac silhouette due to right ventricular hypertrophy and enlarged central pulmonary arteries in acute or chronic PH. The lung fields can also demonstrate reduced vascularity consistent with decreased pulmonary blood flow. High-resolution computed tomography (CT) scanning of the chest is helpful for excluding pulmonary causes of PH such as interstitial lung disease or emphysema. CT pulmonary angiography can be used to diagnose pulmonary thromboembolism. Ventilation-perfusion ($\dot{V}/\dot{Q}$) scanning is also useful for evaluating the possibility of pulmonary thromboembolic disease. Cardiac magnetic resonance imaging (MRI) may be superior to echocardiography for determining right ventricular volume and contraction and may be used for follow-up of patients with PAH on chronic therapy.

Lung Biopsy

Lung biopsy can be considered in patients who are suspected to have pulmonary veno-occlusive disease, undiagnosed parenchymal lung disease, or in patients with congenital heart disease in whom clinical and hemodynamic data are concerning for safety of cardiac surgical repair, as the presence of a severe arteriopathy on lung biopsy may influence the surgical repair strategy.

TREATMENT

Patients with PAH are admitted to the intensive care unit when there is acute decompensation with RV failure and/or syncope. Regardless of cause, cardiovascular decompensation due to an acute pulmonary hypertensive crisis is a medical emergency (**Fig. 57.2**).

Oxygen and General Supportive Measures

Oxygen has pulmonary vasodilatory effects and should be given to treat hypoxemia or as an adjunct to pulmonary vasodilators. Noninvasive positive pressure ventilation (NIPPV) may have a role in augmenting oxygenation, treating hypoventilation, providing LV afterload reduction, and reducing work of breathing. In the setting of acute right heart failure, inotropic

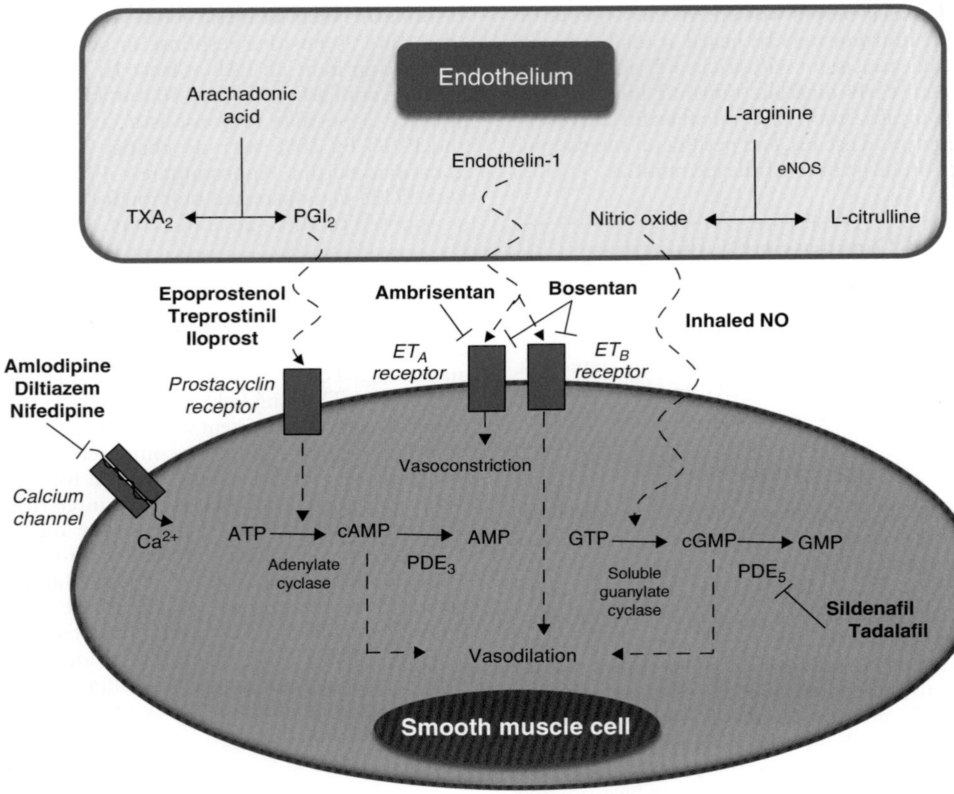

FIGURE 57.2. Pulmonary hypertension pharmacology. Activation of the prostacyclin receptor by endogenous prostacyclin or agonists (epoprostenol, treprostinil, or iloprost) increases the formation of cAMP from adenosine triphosphate (ATP) by enhancing activity of the enzyme adenylate cyclase, which ultimately leads to vasodilation. Endothelial cells also produce endothelin-1, which binds to two types of endothelin receptors on the smooth muscle cell—ETA receptors that lead to smooth muscle cell contraction and ETB receptors that promote smooth muscle cell relaxation. Bosentan is a nonselective endothelin receptor antagonist and ambrisentan is selective for the ETA receptor and both cause vasodilation by inhibiting the action of endothelin-1. Nitric oxide is elaborated in the endothelial cell and diffuses into the smooth muscle cell where it leads to vasodilation by increasing the production of cGMP through increased activity of soluble guanylate cyclase. Inhaled nitric oxide acts by the same mechanism. Extracellular calcium enters smooth muscle cells through calcium channels and participates in vasoconstriction, which is inhibited by various calcium-channel blockers. Sildenafil and tadalafil inhibit the enzyme PDE5 and thereby increase intracellular cGMP leading to vasodilation. TXA2, thromboxane; PGI2, prostacyclin; eNOS, endothelial nitric oxide synthase; ETA receptor, endothelin A receptor; ETB receptor, endothelin B receptor; ATP, adenosine triphosphate; cAMP, cyclic adenosine monophosphate; AMP, adenosine monophosphate; GTP, guanosine triphosphate; cGMP, cyclic guanosine monophosphate; GMP, guanosine monophosphate; PDE3, phosphodiesterase 3; PDE5, phosphodiesterase 5.

medications such as dobutamine and/or milrinone can be used to support RV function. Diuretics are used to treat congestive symptoms with careful titration to avoid excessive reduction in intravascular volume. Intubation and initiation of invasive mechanical ventilation is a high-risk procedure in the patient with acute pulmonary hypertensive decompensation. Anesthetic agents may depress respiration (exacerbating hypoventilation and respiratory acidosis) and vasodilate (reducing preload and further impairing RV output). Hyperventilation is useful for a severe, acute pulmonary hypertensive crisis in an intubated patient. Aggressive hyperventilation can cause decreased venous return, alveolar over distention, lung injury, and cerebral vasoconstriction; hence, it should be used sparingly. Hypoxic pulmonary vasoconstriction occurs in atelectatic lung regions and lung overdistention can compress alveolar pulmonary blood vessels, further contributing to elevated PVR.

Inhaled Nitric Oxide

Nitric oxide (NO) is produced endogenously by vascular endothelium and mediates vasodilatation by increasing 3′-5′-cyclic guanosine monophosphate (cGMP) within the vascular smooth muscle cells. Accumulation of nitrogen dioxide (NO_2) and methemoglobin are potential toxicities, though accumulation of these products is rarely dose limiting. The lowest effective dose should be used and the upper limit is usually not more than 20–30 ppm. Abrupt withdrawal or interruption of iNO may aggravate rebound PH; hence, it should be gradually decreased to a minimum before discontinuation. Nitric oxide has been shown to improve oxygenation and decrease the incidence of extracorporeal membranous oxygenation (ECMO) use in term newborns with hypoxic respiratory failure and PPHN, excluding patients with congenital diaphragmatic hernia.

Calcium-Channel Blockers

Despite the lack of randomized clinical trials, calcium-channel blockers (CCB) such as nifedipine, diltiazem, and amlodipine have been used successfully to treat adults and children with IPAH for many years. However, only a small number of patients with IPAH will respond to CCB, and careful selection of patients is required. Patients who do not respond to vasodilator testing may deteriorate with CCB due to negative inotropic effects.

Phosphodiesterase Type-5 Inhibitors

The cyclic nucleotide phosphodiesterases catalyze degradation of cyclic AMP and GMP. Phosphodiesterase type-5 (PDE5) specifically degrades cGMP in vascular smooth muscle cells. Inhibition of this enzyme by PDE5 inhibitors (sildenafil) results in increased intracellular cGMP and pulmonary vasodilatation. Sildenafil has been shown to reduce PAP and vascular resistance, and the effect is additive to that of nitric oxide. Although chronic use of sildenafil in children with PAH was generally well tolerated with mild to moderate side effects, long-term outcome data showed that high-dose sildenafil was associated with higher rates of death, prompting the FDA to issue a warning on prescribing sildenafil to children with PAH.

Prostacyclins

Prostacyclin (PGI_2) is produced by vascular endothelial cells and vasodilates by increasing 3′- and 5′-cyclic adenosine monophosphate (cAMP) within vascular smooth muscle cells. Synthetic prostacyclin analogs that have been used to treat PH include epoprostenol, treprostinil, and iloprost. Because of a short half-life (3–5 minutes), epoprostenol is administered by continuous intravenous infusion. Epoprostenol improves exercise capacity, quality of life, and survival in patients with IPAH. Abrupt withdrawal of the medication has been reported to cause rebound PH and acute deterioration and death. Treprostinil is a synthetic analog of epoprostenol with a longer half-life than epoprostenol, thus enabling it to be given either by subcutaneous or intravenous infusion. Iloprost is a synthetic prostacyclin analog used by inhalation.

Endothelin Receptor Antagonists

Endothelin (ET) mediates pulmonary vasoconstriction and possesses proinflammatory effects, which are thought to be the mechanisms by which elevated ET activity contributes to PAH. Bosentan is an oral, nonselective ET receptor antagonist that binds to both ET_A and ET_B receptors. The most significant side effect is dose-dependent elevation of liver transaminases in approximately 10% of patients. These changes were reversible after treatment discontinuation or dose reduction. Other side effects include anemia and peripheral edema.

Atrial Septostomy

In patients with severe, refractory PH, creation of a small hole in an atrial septum permits right-to-left atrial shunting at the time when the right ventricle is unable to pump against increased pulmonary pressure. Because of the palliative nature and the risks associated with the procedure, it is usually reserved for those with severe heart failure refractory to medical therapy with severe syncopal symptoms or while awaiting lung transplantation or when medical therapy such as prostacyclin analog infusion is not available.

Transplantation

Single lung, double lung, or heart–lung transplantation has been used for pediatric patients with PH refractory to other therapies. The 5-year survival is 49% for children receiving lung transplants. Among survivors, functional status is generally good, with 86% of children having no physician-reported activity limitations at 5 years after transplant.

PERSISTENT PH OF THE NEWBORN

PPHN occurs mainly in term or late preterm neonates due to a failure of PVR to fall at birth. It leads to right-to-left shunting through a patent foramen ovale or ductus arteriosus. Mechanisms proposed in idiopathic PPHN include impaired nitric oxide production, failure of arteriolar smooth muscle cell thinning, and the presence of increased extracellular matrix in the pulmonary vasculature that impairs blood vessel distensibility, leading to poor accommodation of the increase in pulmonary blood flow that occurs at birth. Treatment of infants with PPHN involves mechanical ventilation with sedation and neuromuscular blockade, inhaled nitric oxide, and high-frequency oscillatory ventilation. ECMO may be necessary for some patients. An 81% survival is seen in neonates with PPHN receiving ECMO. Patients with PH secondary to irreversible lung dysplasia is almost universally fatal. A need for initiation of ECLS on or after day 5 of life and a duration of ECLS therapy for greater than or equal to 10 days were predictors of an irreversible lung dysplasia.

CHAPTER 58 ■ THE IMMUNE SYSTEM

RACHEL S. AGBEKO, NIGEL J. KLEIN, AND MARK J. PETERS

THE IMMUNE SYSTEM

The convention is to describe the innate and the adaptive immune systems as separate entities. However, the two are intricately linked. The key features of the innate and adaptive immune system are outlined in **Table 58.1**. The initial step in host defense is determination of whether matter poses a threat to the host. The innate immune system serves as both a sensor and the initial removal apparatus of infection- or injury-associated matter. Targeting microorganisms in the innate system occurs through interactions between host-derived pattern recognition receptors (PRRs) and pathogen-associated molecular patterns (PAMPs) on microbes. Microbes, but not host tissues, express molecular sequences or PAMPs, such as lipopolysaccharide (LPS) or lipoteichoic acid. Endogenous danger-associated molecular patterns (DAMPs) are of host origin, and examples include the cytokine high-mobility group box 1 (HMGB-1), mitochondria, and heat shock proteins. PRRs are circulating free receptors (e.g., mannose-binding lectin [MBL]), membrane phagocytic receptors (complement receptor), cytoplasmic signaling receptors, and membrane-bound signaling receptors (e.g., toll-like receptor TLR4). In response to this PRR ligation, chemotactic substances or "alarmins" are released to draw polymorphonucleated neutrophils, phagocytes, and antigen-presenting cells (e.g., dendritic cells, DCs) to the site. Then, the innate immune system interacts with the adaptive immune system to induce an initially generic but rapidly more specific host response to microbial invasion. This includes the capacity to produce specific antibodies. In addition, the response includes elements to downgrade the response, including anti-inflammatory cytokines and monocyte deactivation.

IMMUNODEFICIENCY AND INTENSIVE CARE

Immunodeficiencies that may be seen in the critically ill are listed in **Tables 58.2** and **58.3**. Knowledge about specific immunologic defects in critically ill children can be vital to orchestrating the use of the increasing array of treatment modalities now available. These include modulators of cytokines, complement components, cellular and soluble receptors, and pathway signaling.

BALANCE OF SUSCEPTIBILITY VERSUS SEVERITY: CLUES FROM THE IMMUNE SYSTEM

Complement System

Working in concert with the adaptive immune system, activation of the three complement pathways (classical, lectin, and alternative) leads to the construction of membrane attack complexes that cause direct lysis and death of the microorganisms. During activation, opsonic and chemotactic factors are generated that facilitate the removal of live and dead organisms

TABLE 58.1

Characteristics of the Innate versus Adaptive Immune System

■ INNATE IMMUNE SYSTEM	■ ADAPTIVE IMMUNE SYSTEM
Older phylogenetically—present in all multicellular organisms	Evolved later—present only in vertebrates
Present from birth	Learned response
Does not require previous exposure	Slower but more definitive
No memory	Memory specific to antigen
Cellular components—phagocytic system (monocytes, macrophages, DCs) and natural killer cells	Cellular components—T and B lymphocytes
Soluble components—cytokines, complement, and acute-phase proteins	Soluble components—immunoglobulins

TABLE 58.2

Severe Combined Immunodeficiency Syndromes

DISORDER	PHENOTYPE	MUTATED GENE	MOLECULAR DEFECT
SCID-X1	T − B + NK−	Common g-chain	Absence of receptors for IL-2, IL-4, IL-7, IL-9, IL-15, and IL-21
JAK3 deficiency	T − B + NK−	JAK3	Defect of signaling via IL-2, IL-4, IL-7, IL-9, IL-15, and IL-21
IL-7 receptor deficiency	T − B + NK+	IL-7 receptor α	Absence of IL-7 receptor α
RAG-1, RAG-2 deficiency	T − B − NK+	*RAG-1* and *RAG-2*	Defective VDJ recombination
Artemis deficiency	T − B − NK+	Artemis	Defective VDJ recombination; radiation sensitivity
Ligase IV deficiency	T − B − NK+	Ligase IV	Defective VDJ recombination; radiation sensitivity
Cernunnos deficiency	T − B − NK+	Cernunnos	Defective VDJ recombination; radiation sensitivity
Adenosine deaminase deficiency	T − B − NK−	*ADA*	Block in purine salvage metabolism
Purine nucleoside phosphorylase deficiency	T − B + NK+	*PNP*	Block in purine salvage metabolism
T-cell receptor deficiencies	T − B + NK+	CD3€/$\delta/\gamma/\zeta$	Defective T-cell signaling
ZAP70 deficiency	T − B + NK+	*ZAP70*	Defective T-cell signaling
ORAI-1	T + B + NK+	*ORAI-1*	Defective T-cell signaling
CD45 deficiency	T − B + NK+	*CD45*	Defective T- and B-cell signaling
Coronin 1A	T − B + NK+		
P561ck	T − B + NK+		
WHN/Nude SCID	T − B + NK+		
DNA-PKcs	T − B − NK+		
Reticular dysgenesis (adenylate kinase-2 deficiency)	T − B − NK−		
MHC II	T + B + NK+		
CD3 deficiency	T − B + NK+		

VDJ, variable diverse joining.

from the circulation and from tissues. Patients with terminal complement component deficiencies are particularly susceptible to *Neisseria* sp., including *Neisseria meningitidis*; paradoxically, these infections are generally less severe than in normal populations. It appears that complement activation, while critical for host defense against meningococci, leads to more inflammation and clinical deterioration.

Mannose-Binding Lectin

MBL is a liver-derived plasma protein that recognizes repeating sugar arrays on the surface of many bacteria, fungi, viruses, and parasites. MBL binds to microbes, such as *Staphylococcus aureus* and *N. meningitidis*, and activates complement in an antibody- and C1-complex–independent fashion. Approximately one-third of the population is deficient in MBL, with 10% having profound deficiency. Children admitted to intensive care following infection, trauma, or surgery have a greatly increased risk of developing the systemic inflammatory response syndrome (SIRS) within the first 48 hours of PICU admission if they have MBL deficiency.

Endotoxin Recognition

The archetypal PAMP is the gram-negative bacterial cell wall component LPS, to which humans are exquisitely sensitive. On binding, the transmembrane receptor TLR4 signals to intracellular components, which, in turn, leads to NFκB-mediated downstream

TABLE 58.3

Other Congenital Immunodeficiency Syndromes

DISORDER	CHROMOSOME	GENE	FUNCTION/DEFECT	DIAGNOSTIC TESTS
X-linked chronic granulomatous disease	Xp21	*gp91phox*	Component of phagocyte NADPH	Nitroblue tetrazolium test *gp91phox* by oxidase-phagocytic respiratory burst immunoblotting; mutation analysis
X-linked agammaglobulinemia	Xq22	Bruton's tyrosine kinase (*Btk*)	Intracellular signaling pathways essential for pre-B-cell maturation	*Btk* by immunoblotting or FACS analysis and mutation analysis
X-linked hyper-IgM syndrome (CD40 ligand deficiency)	Xq26 (CD154)	CD40 ligand	Isotype switching, T-cell function	CD154 expression on activated T cells by FACS analysis mutation analysis
Wiskott–Aldrich syndrome	Xp11	*WASP*	Cytoskeletal architecture formation, immune-cell motility and trafficking	*WASP* expression by immunoblotting; mutation analysis
X-linked lymphoproliferative syndrome	Xq25	*SAP*	Regulation of T-cell responses to EBV and other viral infections	Mutation analysis *SAP* expression—under development
Properdin deficiency	Xp21	Properdin	Terminal complement component	Properdin levels
Type 1 leukocyte adhesion deficiency	21q22	CD11/CD18	Defective leukocyte adhesion and migration	CD11/CD18 expression by FACS analysis; mutation analysis
Chronic granulomatous disease (recessive)	7q11 1q25 16p24	*p47phox* *p67phox* *p22phox*	Defective respiratory burst and phagocytic intracellular killing	*p47phox*, *p67phox*, *p22phox*, expression by immunoblotting; mutation analysis
Chédiak–Higashi syndrome	1q42	*LYST*	Abnormalities in microtubule-mediated lysosomal protein trafficking	Giant inclusions in granulocytes; mutation analysis
MHC class II deficiency	16p13 19p12	*CIITA (MHC2TA) RFXANK*	Defective transcriptional regulation of MHC II molecule expression	HLA-DR expression; mutation analysis
RFX5			13q13	*RFXAP*
Autoimmune lymphoproliferative syndrome	10q24	*APT1* (Fas)	Defective apoptosis of lymphocytes	Fas expression; apoptosis assays; mutation analysis
Ataxia telangiectasia	11q22	*ATM*	Cell-cycle control and DNA damage responses	DNA radiation sensitivity; mutation analysis
Inherited mycobacterial susceptibility	6q23 5q31 19p13	IFN-γreceptor IL-12 p40 IL-12 receptor b1	Defective IFN-γproduction and signaling function	IFN-γreceptor expression; IL-12 expression; IL-12 receptor expression; mutation analysis

WASP, Wiskott–Aldrich syndrome protein; MHC, major histocompatibility complex; FACS, fluorescent activated cell sorting; EBV, Epstein–Barr virus.

gene expression and cytokine activation. Nonspecific protection against LPS can be provided by circulating humoral factors (e.g., LPS-binding protein and antibodies directed against the core of endotoxin [EndoCAb]). Higher preoperative levels of IgM EndoCAb are associated with better outcome following surgery, and higher IgG EndoCAb levels have been linked to survival in sepsis.

Cytokines

Many associations have been found between gene polymorphisms that control cytokine expression and susceptibility to, and severity of, critical illness. IL-10, an anti-inflammatory cytokine, is an important example, as these levels are critical in the modulation of the proinflammatory/anti-inflammatory balance.

The Inflammasome

The inflammasome is an intracellular macromolecular signaling complex that activates caspase-1, in turn activating pro-IL-1β and pro-IL-18 into the potent proinflammatory cytokines IL-1β and IL-18. Inflammasomes assemble in response to mitochondrial stress, reactive oxygen species, extracellular ATP, and potassium efflux.

THE BALANCE BETWEEN PROINFLAMMATION AND ANTI-INFLAMMATION

Systemic Inflammatory Response Syndrome and Sepsis

Systemic inflammation can be induced by any major insult that does not result in immediate death (**Tables 58.4** and **58.5**). Systemic inflammatory response syndrome was a term describing this response—that was called *sepsis* when it was the result of suspected or proven infection. Importantly noninfectious causes, such as burns, trauma, surgery, and pancreatitis, can also cause this clinical picture. SIRS was dropped from the Sepsis-3 definitions because of concern about it being too nonspecific. Sepsis is now reserved for a *life-threatening* organ dysfunction caused by a dysregulated host response to infection. Regardless of the terminology, it is clear that similar alterations in organ function (measured by standard platelet count, coagulation times, blood urea nitrogen, creatinine, hepatic enzymes, arterial blood gases, and lactate) may follow from the inflammatory response either to infection or to noninfectious insults (**Table 58.6**). Some degree of systemic inflammation (what we used to call mild-to-moderate SIRS) is most likely beneficial; for example, both a raised temperature and production of the cytokine TNF facilitate killing of microorganisms. However, a similar response may cause harm, either by being too severe or by spilling over into body compartments where they are not required. Examples include excessive body temperatures raising tissue oxygen demand beyond the available supply and causing rhabdomyolysis, while pathways that involve TNF or IL-6 may contribute to myocardial depression.

Excessive Proinflammation

It is widely held that sepsis-induced multiorgan failure results from an excessive, unchecked proinflammatory response typified by mediators such as TNF and IL-1. This response overlaps with the predominantly proinflammatory T-helper-1 (T_H1) pattern of immunity associated with cytotoxic T-cell and macrophage activation and suppression of humoral responses. A compensatory, anti-inflammatory response syndrome (CARS) is also initiated at the same time. This "arm" of the immune response is typified by such mediators as IL-10, and shares many characteristics with the T-helper-2 (T_H2) response, involving the suppression of macrophage activation and promotion of antibody production.

Excessive Anti-inflammation: "Acquired Immunoparalysis"

An excessive compensatory anti-inflammatory response to the primary insult leaves patients in a state of *acquired immunoparalysis*, in which they are unable to produce an adequate immune response to a new threat, such as a nosocomial infection. In part, this inadequacy is attributable to apoptosis of DCs and lymphocytes in response to the CARS/T_H2 mediators. Ongoing physiologic insults, such as nosocomial infection, endocrine abnormalities, and repeated tissue trauma during this time, propagate a state of immunoparalysis by attenuating recovery of HLA-DR expression, leaving the patient at risk of further infection, late morbidity, and mortality.

RESOLUTION VERSUS PERSISTENCE OF THE INFLAMMATORY RESPONSE

A key element in resolving the immune response is effective clearance of microorganisms. Inability of PMNs to get to the right place at the right time, or to achieve effective killing of bacteria, leads to persistence of the inflammatory response from unresolved infection.

Defects in the Removal of Microorganisms

Neutropenia

Restoration of neutrophil counts is required to clear many infections but (in a paradox similar to the balance of susceptibility versus severity discussed previously) is often associated with a clinical deterioration as the systemic inflammatory response worsens.

TABLE 58.4

Definitions of Systemic Inflammatory Response Syndrome, Infection, Sepsis, Severe Sepsis, and Septic Shock

SIRS	*Sepsis-3 Definition*
The presence of ≥2 of 4 criteria, one of which must be abnormal temperature or leukocyte count: Core temperature of ≥38.5°C or ≤36°C Tachycardia (a mean heart rate ≥SD above normal for age in the absence of external stimulus, chronic drugs, or painful stimuli) **OR** otherwise unexplained persistent elevation over a 0.5- to 4-h time period **OR** for children < 1 y old: bradycardia, defined as a mean heart rate < 10th percentile for age in the absence of external vagal stimulus, β-blocker drugs, or congenital heart disease, or otherwise unexplained persistent depression over a 0.5-h time period Mean respiratory rate ≥2 SD above normal for age or mechanical ventilation for an acute process not related to underlying neuromuscular disease or the receipt of general anesthesia Leukocyte count elevated or depressed for age (not secondary to chemotherapy-induced leukopenia) or ≥10% immature neutrophils	SIRS no longer used Criteria not specific to a dysregulated immune response
Infection	***Not defined***
A suspected or proven (by positive culture, tissue stain, or polymerase chain reaction test) infection caused by any pathogen **OR** a clinical syndrome associated with a high probability of infection. Evidence of infection includes positive findings on clinical exam, imaging, or laboratory tests (e.g., white blood cells in a normally sterile body fluid, perforated viscus, chest X-ray consistent with pneumonia, petechial or purpuric rash, or purpura fulminans)	
Sepsis	***Sepsis (not yet validated for children)***
SIRS in the presence of, or as a result of, suspected or proven infection	Life-threatening organ dysfunction caused by a dysregulated host response to infection characterized by acute change in organ failure score (≥2 SOFA score in adults)
Severe sepsis	
Sepsis plus one of the following: cardiovascular organ dysfunction **OR** acute respiratory distress syndrome **OR** two or more other organ dysfunctions. Organ dysfunctions are defined in **Table 58.5**	Severe sepsis term no longer used
Septic Shock	***Septic Shock***
Sepsis and cardiovascular organ dysfunction as defined in **Table 58.5**	Septic shock is a subset of sepsis in which underlying circulatory and cellular/metabolic abnormalities are profound enough to substantially increase mortality. E.g., In adults sepsis and vasopressor therapy needed to elevate MAP ≥65 mm Hg and lactate > 2 mmol/L (18 mg/dL) despite adequate fluid resuscitation

TABLE 58.5

Organ Dysfunction Criteria

Cardiovascular Dysfunction
Despite administration of isotonic IV fluid bolus ≥40 mL/kg in 1 h
Decrease in BP (hypotension) ≤5th percentile for age or systolic BP ≤2 SD below normal for age (**Table 58.6**)
OR Need for vasoactive drug to maintain BP in normal range (dopamine ≥5 mcg/kg/min, or dobutamine, epinephrine, or norepinephrine at any dose)
OR Two of the following:
Unexplained metabolic acidosis: base deficit > 5.0 mEq/L
Increased arterial lactate > 2 times upper limit of normal
Oliguria: urine output < 0.5 mL/kg/h
Prolonged capillary refill: >5 s
Core to peripheral temperature gap > 3°C
Respiratory
Pa_{O_2}/F_{IO_2} < 300 in the absence of cyanotic heart disease or preexisting lung disease
OR Pa_{CO_2} > 72 torr or 20 mm Hg over baseline Pa_{CO_2}
OR Proven need for >0.5 F_{IO_2} to maintain saturation >92%
OR Need for nonelective invasive or noninvasive mechanical ventilation
Neurologic
GCS ≤11
OR Acute change in mental status with a decrease in GCS ≥3 points from abnormal baseline
Hematologic
Platelet count < 80,000/mm^3 or a decline of 50% in platelet count from the highest value recorded over the previous 3 days (for chronic hematology/oncology patients)
OR International normalized ratio >2
Renal
Serum creatinine level > 2 times upper limit of normal for age or twofold increase in baseline creatinine
Hepatic
Total bilirubin > 4 mg/dL (not applicable for newborn)
OR ALT > 2 times upper limit of normal for age

BP, blood pressure; GCS, Glasgow Coma Scale; ALT, alanine aminotransferase.

Leukocyte Adhesion

Activated leukocytes are recruited into inflamed tissues by adhesion molecules present on neutrophils, platelets, and endothelial cells. Type 1 leukocyte adhesion deficiency results from a lack of surface protein CD18, necessary for the formation of the β_2 integrin heterodimers involved in firm adhesion. Failure of leukocytes to migrate into tissues results in delayed clearance of bacteria. Patients with <1% expression of CD18 present early with recurrent bacteremia, progressing to life-threatening infections and requiring bone marrow transplantation. Patients with a moderate phenotype (2.5%–6% of the normal concentrations of protein) have peritonitis, delayed wound healing, and skin infections. Leukocytes can form complexes with themselves or other cell types, including platelets and cell fragments, or "microparticles." In sepsis, these circulating platelet–neutrophil complexes are reduced due to binding to the endothelium or migration into the tissues. These primed platelet–neutrophil complexes cause tissue injury and initiate thrombus formation, explaining why the combination of low platelets and neutrophils is a predictor of poor outcome in meningococcal sepsis.

Bacterial Killing

Chronic granulomatous disease is a rare condition due to a deficiency in the enzyme NADPH oxidase, which is required for production of toxic conditions that effect bacterial killing. These patients suffer stubborn infections similar to those seen in patients with leukocyte adhesion deficiency or neutropenia.

TABLE 58.6

Age-Specific Vital Signs and Laboratory Variables

AGE GROUP	HEART RATE (Beats/min)		RESPIRATORY RATE (Breaths/min)	LEUKOCYTE COUNT ($\times10^3$/mm)	SYSTOLIC BLOOD PRESSURE (mm HG)
	Tachycardia	Bradycardia			
0 days–1 wk	>180	<100	>50	>34	<72
1 wk–1 mo	>180	<100	>40	>19.5 or <5	<75
1 mo–1 y	>180	<90	>34	>17.5 or <5	<100
2–5 y	>140	NA	>22	>15.5 or <5	<94
6–12 y	>130	NA	>18	>13.5 or <4.5	<105
13 to <18 y	>110	NA	>14	>11 or <4.5	<117

Lower values correspond to 5th percentile; upper values correspond to 95th percentile.
NA, not applicable.

Granuloma formation probably represents a failure to adequately remove microbial products. These lesions paradoxically may necessitate the use of steroids to reduce the ensuing inappropriate inflammatory response.

Effective Removal of Prokaryote and Eukaryote Material for Resolution of Infection and the Inflammatory Response

For the inflammatory response to resolve, effective removal of cellular (host and microbial) debris must occur without further release of proinflammatory elements (endotoxin). Importantly, "spent" PMNs undergo apoptosis after they have performed these useful functions—and therefore die "silently" without leaving inflammatory cellular debris. These apoptotic PMNs are then phagocytosed by tissue macrophages.

Hemophagocytic Lymphohistiocytosis

Hemophagocytic lymphohistiocytosis (HLH) describes a mix of congenital and acquired conditions in which high fever, lymphadenopathy, hepatosplenomegaly, pancytopenia, liver dysfunction, and central nervous system dysfunction are often prominent (**Table 58.7**). Abnormally large and activated cells of myeloid origin (hemophagocytes) are typically found on examination of bone marrow. Secondary HLH represents a sustained, systemic inflammatory response following a variety of primary insults (viral, bacterial, or fungal). Mutations in the genes for perforin are especially important, occurring in 20%–40% of HLH cases. Perforin is a protein found in granules of cytotoxic effector cells, including natural killer cells and activated lymphocytes. Lack of perforin prevents access of the cytotoxic enzymes, and the inflammatory stimulus of the infected target cell persists. *Macrophage activation syndrome* (MAS) may be seen as HLH in the

TABLE 58.7

Criteria for the Diagnosis of Hemophagocytic Lymphohistiocytosis

The diagnosis of HLH is established by fulfilling either or both of the following criteria:

1. A molecular diagnosis consistent with HLH (e.g., PRF1, RAB27A, STXBP2, STX11, SH2D1A, UNC13D, or XIAP)

and/or

2. Having ≥5 of the following 8 clinical criteria:
   a. Fever
   b. Splenomegaly
   c. Cytopenia affecting two cell lineages: hemoglobin < 9 g/dL (or 10 g/dL for infants <4 wk of age), platelets < 100,000/µL, and neutrophils < 1000 µL
   d. Hypertriglyceridemia (>272 mg/dL) and/or hypofibrinogenemia (<150 mg/dL)
   e. Hemophagocytosis in the bone marrow, spleen, or lymph nodes without evidence of malignancy
   f. Low or absent NK cell cytotoxicity (according to local laboratory reference values)
   g. Hyperferritinemia (>500 ng/mL)
   h. Elevated soluble CD25 (IL-2Ra chain > 2400 U/mL)

context of rheumatic disease. Although less common, MAS does occur in other rheumatologic disease, for example, systemic lupus erythematosus, Kawasaki disease, and inflammatory bowel disease.

THERAPIES FOR THE SYSTEMIC INFLAMMATORY RESPONSE IN THIS FRAMEWORK

Therapies That Can Modulate the Balance between Effective Microbial Killing and the Resultant Inflammatory Response

The use of intravenous immunoglobulin and clindamycin could be beneficial in *Staphylococcal* and *Streptococcal* toxic shock syndromes. Both agents neutralize the effect of exotoxins—intravenous immunoglobulin by binding to the exotoxins, and clindamycin by inhibiting the production of exotoxins.

Possible Therapies for Acute Severe Proinflammation

High-Dose Corticosteroids

Glucocorticoids inhibit production of the proinflammatory cytokines TNF-α, IL-1α, IL-1β, IL-6, IL-8, IL-12, IFN-γ, and granulocyte macrophage colony-stimulating factor (GM-CSF). In addition, glucocorticoids increase transcription of IL-1ra and IL-10, inhibit neutrophil activation, and suppress the synthesis of phospholipase A_2, cyclooxygenase, and inducible nitric oxide synthase. The option of high-dose steroids might be reconsidered in pediatric catecholamine-resistant septic shock, in which the risk of early cardiovascular collapse is greater than that of secondary infection. Observational studies suggest that relative adrenal insufficiency may be common and intensive cardiovascular support alone may be insufficient without replacing adequate doses of hydrocortisone.

Physiologic Doses of Corticosteroids

At physiologic levels, cortisol supports vascular adrenergic receptor function and inhibits cytokine-induced nitric oxide synthase, potentiating vasoconstriction and myocardial contractility. The use of corticosteroids in septic shock remains inconclusive. The Surviving Sepsis Campaign guideline recommends physiologic doses of hydrocortisone in patients with poor response to fluid resuscitation and vasopressor therapy.

Activated Protein C

Recombinant human activated protein C (rhAPC) possesses anticoagulant, profibrinolytic, and anti-inflammatory properties. Trials did not show benefit and the manufacturer removed APC from the market.

Anticytokine Therapies—Monoclonal Antibodies

Effective blockade of TNF is being assessed in clinical trials. A meta-analysis of trials in severe sepsis in adults showed that TNF blockade was safe and had a survival benefit (relative risk 0.93; 95% CI, 0.88–0.98; $p = 0.01$) though this has not translated into clinical practice. HLH poses a hyperinflammatory state in children that might be amenable to anticytokine therapy. A small case series on the use of recombinant IL-1-receptor antagonist (anakinra) in secondary HLH showed improvement. Given the nature of the study, it is too early to be able to attribute clinical benefit.

Possible Therapies for Immunoparalysis

Aggressive Deintensification of Patients

Priority should be given to removal of invasive monitoring lines, endotracheal tubes, and urinary catheters at the earliest possible time to reduce the risk of transient bacteremia in these vulnerable patients.

Stimulating Factors

GM-CSF and G-CSF are naturally occurring cytokines that stimulate the number and antimicrobial functions of both neutrophils and monocytes. Administration of GM-CSF appears to have minimal side effects, to restore monocyte HLA-DR expression and function, and to assist in reducing sepsis episodes, but to date, it has not been shown to affect mortality. *Immunonutrients*, such as glutamine, have been evaluated. Glutamine is critical for the integrity and function of metabolically active tissues. In models of sepsis and injury, glutamine supplementation increases survival, improves immune function, reduces bacteremia, increases gut barrier function, and decreases gastrointestinal mucosal atrophy. Studies have either shown benefit or no effect; it may be that glutamine supplementation is beneficial only when appropriately targeted. A mortality benefit has been suggested for enteral feeding with eicosapentaenoic acid, γ-linolenic acid, and antioxidants in adult septic shock cases. These lipids are reported to have both pro- and anti-inflammatory actions.

Removal of Inhibitory Plasma Mediators

Conventional plasma exchange has been used to remove plasma mediators; however, it does not consistently affect plasma levels of IL-6, IL-6R, TNF-α, TNF-αR, or C-reactive protein. By comparison, continuous hemofiltration has been shown to minimally reduce inflammatory mediators (complement activation, plasma thromboxane, and proinflammatory cytokines at high-volume filtration).

CHAPTER 59 ■ NEUROHORMONAL CONTROL IN THE IMMUNE SYSTEM

KATHRYN A. FELMET

THE NEUROHORMONAL RESPONSE TO ACUTE STRESS

Acute stress activates the release of epinephrine from the sympathetic nervous system (SNS), the release of cortisol from the hypothalamic–pituitary–adrenal (HPA) axis, and the release of endogenous opioids. The adrenal steroids and endogenous epinephrine and opioids have immunosuppressant properties. The acute stress response also triggers the release of proinflammatory peptides, such as vasopressin and prolactin.

There is a shared chemical language of the neuroendocrine and immune systems. Immune cells express receptors for neurotransmitters and hormones. Endocrine cells, peripheral nerves, and cells of the central nervous system (CNS) express receptors for immune-derived cytokines. Immune cells also produce hormones and signaling molecules resembling neurotransmitters. Brain cells produce a wide variety of cytokines.

The immune system can be thought of as a sensory organ that perceives microscopic threats. These peripheral stresses activate immune cells, send signals to the CNS via peripheral or autonomic afferent nerves, and initiate an immunoregulatory response.

RECENT NEUROENDOCRINE IMMUNE MEDIATORS APPLIED TO CRITICAL ILLNESS

Corticosteroids, growth hormone, and vasopressin are NEI (neuro-endo-immune) mediators with immunomodulatory effects that have been proposed as therapeutic agents for the critically ill.

Adrenal replacement therapy may have immunomodulatory affects. Recommendations for adrenal replacement therapy in children with sepsis are conservative. They are recommended for patients with fluid-refractory, catecholamine-resistant shock and suspected or proven absolute adrenal insufficiency (e.g., resulting from chronic steroid exposure or adrenal hemorrhage). Corticosteroids have immunosuppressive effects. It is unclear whether the doses used for adrenal replacement increase patients' susceptibility to nosocomial infection.

Growth hormone treatment increases mortality in sepsis. Trauma, sepsis, and surgery induce a state of growth hormone resistance. The hyperglycemic, catabolic state induced by growth hormone depletion and resistance is compounded by the normal stress response, the effects of immune-derived cytokines, and inadequate calorie delivery. Unfortunately, exogenous growth hormone treatment increases mortality. The reasons behind this unexpected outcome may relate to the immunomodulatory effect of growth hormone. At physiologic levels, growth hormone is immunostimulatory but has an immunosuppressive effect at supraphysiologic levels.

Vasopressin infusion use in vasodilatory shock also has immune effects. A large randomized controlled trial found that low-dose vasopressin did not offer a mortality advantage over norepinephrine in septic shock. In patients with less severe septic shock, vasopressin was associated with improved survival. As vasopressin has immunosuppressive effects in the CNS and immune-supportive effects in peripheral tissues, it is difficult to predict which effect would predominate during vasopressin infusion in the ICU.

PATHWAYS OF COMMUNICATION

Efferent Signals: How the Central Nervous System Communicates with the Immune System

Signals can travel between the brain and immune system on peripheral nerves or in the form of circulating chemical signals, such as hormones or cytokines.

Autonomic Control of Inflammation: The Cholinergic Anti-inflammatory Pathway

In the presence of endotoxin, macrophages release cytokines that promote inflammation and potentiate activation of the immune response. Macrophages express nicotinic acetylcholine receptors. Binding of an appropriate ligand to these receptors decreases the release of tumor necrosis factor (TNF)-α and other endotoxin-inducible proinflammatory cytokines (IL-1β, IL-6, and IL-18) without altering release of the anti-inflammatory cytokine IL-10 (**Table 59.1**).

TABLE 59.1

Proinflammatory and Anti-inflammatory Cytokines

	PRODUCED BY	ACTIONS ON IMMUNE CELLS	RELEVANCE IN CRITICAL ILLNESS
Proinflammatory Cytokines			
TNF-α	APCs, NK cells, T cells	Local inflammation, endothelial activation	An early mediator of inflammation and shock
IL-1β	APCs, epithelial cells	T-cell activation, macrophage activation	Causes fever and acute-phase protein production
IL-12	B cells, macrophages	Activates NK cells, induces CD4 T-cell differentiation into T_H1–like cells	Suppresses T_H2
IFN-γ	T_H1 cells, NK cells	Potent macrophage activation, suppresses T_H2 responses	Low levels associated with increased risk of infection
GM-CSF	Macrophages, T cells	Stimulates growth and differentiation of granulocytes and monocytes	Increases HLA-DR expression, may be clinically useful as an immune stimulant
Anti-inflammatory Cytokines			
IL-4	T_H2 cells, mast cells	B-cell activation, suppresses T_H1 cells, IGE switch	Suppresses T_H1 response
IL-10	T_H2 cells, APCs	Potent suppressor of macrophage functions	Suppresses T_H1 response
Other Important Cytokines			
IL-2	T cells	T-cell proliferation, supports T_H1 cells	Most important proliferative factor for T cells
IL-6	T cells, macrophages, endothelial cells	T- and B-cell growth and differentiation	Causes fever, and acute-phase protein production levels are related to severity of systemic inflammation
IL-8	Monocytes, endothelial cells	Chemotactic for neutrophils	Levels are related to severity of systemic inflammation
GCSF	Fibroblasts and monocytes	Stimulates neutrophil growth and differentiation	Exogenous GCSF safely increases neutrophil counts but does not alter mortality

APCs, antigen-presenting cells; HLA-DR, human leukocyte antigen-DR.

This acetylcholine-dependent downregulation of inflammation is reproduced by stimulation of the vagus nerve.

Autonomic Control of Inflammation: The Noradrenergic Pathway

The SNS also innervates the immune system. Postganglionic sympathetic neurons follow vasculature to innervate all primary and secondary lymphoid organs. Cells of the bone marrow, thymic epithelial and dendritic cells, monocytes, and macrophages express both α- and β-adrenergic receptors. B and T cells express the β_2-adrenergic receptors exclusively. In the bone marrow, β-adrenoceptor activation suppresses cell proliferation and differentiation, whereas a-adrenoceptor activation suppresses myelopoiesis but enhances lymphopoiesis. In dendritic cells, monocytes, and macrophages, β-adrenoceptor activation inhibits endotoxin-induced release of proinflammatory cytokines (IL-1β, TNF-α, IL-12, and interferon [IFN]-γ) and increases the release of anti-inflammatory cytokines (IL-10 and IL-6) in response to endotoxin. IgG transcription is enhanced by binding to β-adrenergic receptors on B cells. In general, catecholamines are believed to favor T helper cell (T_H)-2 cytokines and inhibit cellular immunity by suppressing T_H1 cytokine production.

Other Neurotransmitters

Opioids. Pain stimulates the immune response, and exogenous opioids and endogenous endorphins have immunosuppressive effects. Opioids induce immune suppression at analgesic doses by binding to naloxone-sensitive opioid receptors in the brain. Acutely, centrally acting morphine activates the SNS, and most of the immunosuppressive effects of morphine may occur via this pathway. Morphine also activates the HPA axis, which may lead to cortisol-mediated immune suppression, particularly during chronic administration.

Somatostatin and Somatostatin Receptor Ligands. Somatostatin analogs (e.g., octreotide) are used in the treatment of gastrointestinal hemorrhage. In addition to decreasing splanchnic blood flow, somatostatin inhibits the release of insulin and decreases secretion and absorption in the gastrointestinal tract. Somatostatin has direct immunosuppressive effects in vitro. In the bone marrow, somatostatin inhibits proliferation, particularly in response to granulocyte colony-stimulating factor (GCSF). Somatostatin strongly inhibits IFN-γ production by T cells, thereby decreasing macrophage activation and antigen presentation.

Other Neuropeptides. *Substance P*, a neuropeptide present in afferent nerves in the dorsal horn of the spinal cord, is a mediator of pain sensation. Substance P is powerfully proinflammatory via TNF-α and IL-12 and plays a role in chronic inflammation. Substance P counteracts glucocorticoid-mediated apoptosis and is one of a group of neuropeptides shown to have immunoregulatory function. Currently, no therapeutic agents are directed at these neuropeptides and their importance is poorly understood.

Humoral Efferent Pathways

The Hypothalamic–Pituitary–Adrenal Axis

Activation of the HPA axis begins with release of corticotrophin-releasing hormone (CRH) from the hypothalamus in response to cortical signals (generated by fear, pain, or hypotension) or immune-derived signal molecules (IL-1β, TNF-α, and IL-6). CRH leads to adrenocorticotropic hormone (ACTH) release by the pituitary, which causes cortisol release by the adrenal gland. Cortisol inhibits growth, increases catabolism, and enhances protein synthesis and acute-phase reactant generation in the liver. Cortisol potentiates catecholamine vasoconstrictive action and regulates body water distribution. Corticosteroids stabilize lysosomal membranes, decrease capillary permeability, impair demargination of white blood cells, impair phagocytosis, and decrease IL-1 release, preventing fever. Steroids support T_H2 (humoral immunity) over T_H1 (cellular immunity).

Peptide Hormones: Prolactin and Vasopressin

Prolactin and vasopressin are the immunostimulatory hormones associated with the CNS response to stress. These hormones are released simultaneously with HPA axis and SNS activation and represent an important counterbalance to the immunosuppressive effects of the stress response. *Prolactin* directly opposes many of the actions of corticosteroids. Prolactin release is stimulated by IL-1β, IL-2, IL-6, oxytocin, serotonin, and thyrotropin-releasing hormone. *Vasopressin* is released in response to hypotension and increased serum osmolarity. In children with septic shock, circulating vasopressin levels tend to be elevated. Vasopressin has different immunomodulatory effects in the periphery than in the CNS.

Afferent Signals: Alerting the Central Nervous System to a Microbial Threat

Immune Activation of Afferent Peripheral Nerves

Inflammation sensed by the vagus nerve increases inflammation-suppressing signals traveling back down the vagus and activating humoral responses via the HPA axis.

Circulating Cytokines

Humoral pathways of immune-to-brain communication involve circulating cytokines. Receptors, or receptor mRNA, in the brain are present for several cytokines. Proinflammatory cytokines are large, lipophobic, and their diffusion across the blood–brain barrier (BBB) is limited. When circulating concentrations are high, cytokines are carried across the BBB by saturable transport proteins. Cytokines also bind to surface receptors on the endothelium of brain capillaries, releasing soluble mediators (nitric oxide and prostaglandin).

Peripheral Responses: The Effects of Neuroimmunomodulation

The Sickness Response

In response to illness (TNF-α and IL-1 signals) the CNS initiates physiologic changes that include fever, increased white blood cell count, production of acute-phase proteins, increased slow-wave sleep, and behavioral changes (reduced feeding, drinking, activity, and social interaction). Alterations in pain sensation are also a part of the sickness response. The acute stress response rapidly induces analgesia, presumably by a neural route. Later, inflammatory cytokines induce hyperalgesia, signaling the individual to care for a wound.

Inflammation and Phagocytosis

Nonspecific immunity is rapidly initiated by microbial invasion or trauma and serves to limit tissue damage and infection to the wound or site of entry. Phagocytic cells recruited by inflammation produce proinflammatory cytokines (IL-1, IL-6, and TNF-α) amplifying the local immune response. The vasodilation, increased capillary permeability, coagulation, and phagocyte diapedesis that prevent local spread of disease can be disastrous globally, causing hypovolemic shock, disseminated intravascular coagulation, and acute respiratory distress syndrome. Recovery from sepsis depends on a balance between proinflammatory and anti-inflammatory signals. Antigen-presenting cells, such as macrophages and dendritic cells, engulf foreign matter and bacteria, break them down, and present their molecules as antigens to T lymphocytes. Antigen presentation is crucial in initiating adaptive immunity. Impaired antigen presentation is associated with mortality and secondary infection. Anti-inflammatory therapies downregulate proinflammatory cytokines, but can cause immune-cell apoptosis and modulate the specific immune response in ways that may not favor survival.

Humoral versus Cellular Immunity

The generation of a specific immune response takes several days, and during this time, the organism depends on the nonspecific immune response. T-cell proliferation is suppressed by catecholamines and supported by prolactin. Helper T (T_H) cells make cytokines that support other cells. T_H1 cells are stimulated by pathogens (e.g., *Mycobacterium tuberculosis*, *Helicobacter pylori*, and *Pneumocystis jirovecii*) that accumulate inside the vesicles of macrophages and dendritic cells. A T_H1 or cell-mediated immune response supports the production of immunoglobulin (Ig) G, an opsonizing antibody that facilitates uptake of these pathogens. Cytokines associated with T_H1 responses (IFN-γ, IL-12, and TNF-α) are proinflammatory. A T_H1 proinflammatory phenotype is associated with autoimmune disease.

Extracellular spaces are protected by the T_H2 or humoral immune response. In response to extracellular pathogens (e.g., *Staphylococcus* spp.), T_H2 cells activate naïve antigen-specific B cells to produce IgM antibodies that bind and neutralize viruses and intracellular pathogens that travel through these spaces. The cytokine profile associated with T_H2 humoral immune response is anti-inflammatory, with IL-4 and IL-10 predominating. The catecholamine and cortisol excess seen in the stress response favor T_H2 responses. Septic patients tend to have increased numbers of T_H2 cells relative to the normal T_H2–T_H2 balance.

Apoptosis and Lymphocyte Proliferation

A few days into sepsis, the catecholamine and cortisol excess of the acute phase suppresses the initial hyperinflammatory state, replacing it with a state of relative immune suppression. A syndrome of immune paralysis, which consists of lymphoid depletion, deactivation of antigen-presenting cells, and production of anti-inflammatory cytokines, has been dubbed the *compensatory anti-inflammatory response syndrome*.

IMMUNE COMPETENCE AND FAILURE IN THE PICU

The Acute and Prolonged Phases of Critical Illness

Critically ill patients need a balance between immunosuppressive and immune-supportive signals, between short-term improvement in blood pressure and long-term cell growth and repair (**Fig. 59.1**).

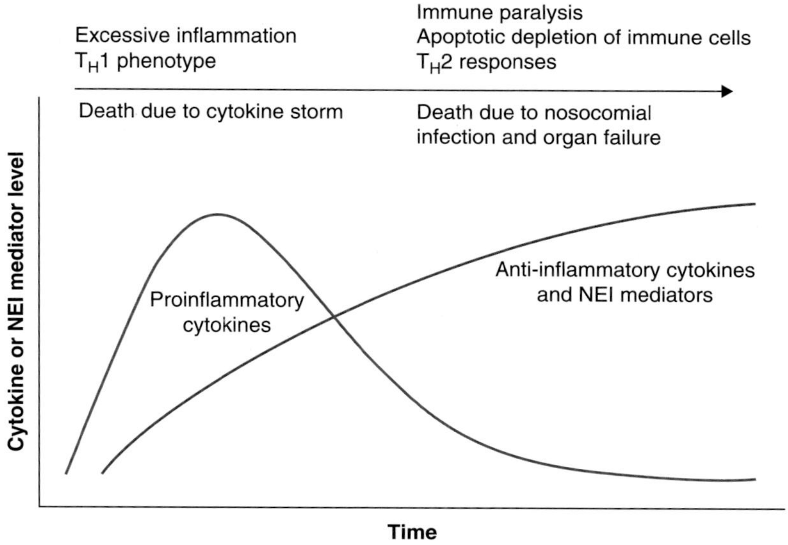

FIGURE 59.1. The acute and prolonged phases of critical illness and sepsis. Early death in sepsis can occur due to overwhelming inflammation with cytokine storm, which causes shock and tissue injury. Therapies directed at decreasing inflammation may be considered during this phase. Resuscitation medications used during this phase, including catecholamines and corticosteroids, are anti-inflammatory. During the prolonged phase of critical illness, patients developed immune paralysis with depletion of lymphoid elements due to apoptosis and decreased antigen-presenting capacity. During this stage, patients are at high risk for secondary infection. Therapies that enhance immune function by activating antigen-presenting cells or by blocking lymphocyte apoptosis may be considered in the future.

Neuroendocrine Immune Failure

Decreased anterior pituitary hormone levels and loss of their normal pattern of pulsatile release characterize the prolonged phase of critical illness. Cortisol levels remain elevated in chronic critical illness despite a fall in ACTH release. The metabolic consequence is an impaired ability to use fatty acids as fuel substrates and a tendency to store fat and to waste protein from muscle and organs. The immune consequences are impaired lymphocyte and monocyte function and increased lymphocyte apoptosis.

Immunomodulatory Effects of ICU Therapies

Circulating Catecholamines

Catecholamines exert an immunosuppressive effect. Dopamine at doses as low as 1 μg/kg/min has an inhibitory effect on prolactin release and decreases lymphocyte proliferation. Dopamine inhibits release of growth hormone and contributes to the catabolic state in critical illness.

Opioids

Opioids have inhibitory effects on lymphocyte function and survival and on NK cell and macrophage growth and activity.

Glucocorticoids and Adrenal Support

In the acute phase of critical illness, adequate cortisol is necessary to maintain vascular tone and catecholamine responsiveness. Adrenal replacement therapy has been advocated for catecholamine-resistant shock. Both endogenous and exogenous steroids suppress fever, promote an anti-inflammatory cytokine profile, cause immune-cell apoptosis, and promote a T_H2/humoral immunity phenotype.

The Vagus Nerve

Nonsteroidal anti-inflammatory drugs and the antiarrhythmic amiodarone increase vagal activity. Patients with vagal nerve stimulators and patients with transplanted organs have disruptions in their cholinergic anti-inflammatory pathways. Without the effect of the vagus nerve to inhibit TNF-α production in response to endotoxin, these patients may have intermittent elevations in inflammatory cytokines.

Assessment and Treatment of Immune Suppression due to Critical Illness

Withdrawal of Unnecessary Immune Suppressants

Drugs that mimic the acute stress response, such as catecholamines and steroids, should be tapered as soon as hemodynamics and underlying conditions allow. Morphine and other opioids should be used no more than necessary to control a patient's pain. Affinity at the μ-receptor correlates with degree of effect on immune function. Opioids specific for the χ- or ∂-receptors may induce less immune suppression; therefore, methadone and fentanyl may be slightly less immunosuppressive than morphine. Receptor affinity predicts that buprenorphine, hydromorphone, oxycodone, oxymorphone, and tramadol are the least immunosuppressive.

Immune Monitoring

Patients with impaired B-cell function, as evidenced by low immunoglobulin levels, may benefit from IVIG. Recombinant human prolactin may have therapeutic potential to reverse lymphopenia observed in the ICU and to speed hematopoietic reconstitution after bone marrow transplant. Metoclopramide and vasopressin increase pituitary prolactin release.

CHAPTER 60 ■ THE POLYMORPHONUCLEAR LEUKOCYTE IN CRITICAL ILLNESS

M. MICHELE MARISCALCO

Phagocytic leukocytes are critical in the acute inflammatory response. They mobilize to sites of infection or injury and release cytotoxic molecules to eliminate microbes. Phagocytes are also involved in repair of tissue injury. Deficits in phagocyte function or number cause impaired wound healing and recurring infections.

NEUTROPHIL PHYSIOLOGY

Granulopoiesis, Marrow Release, and Margination

The bone marrow is a large organ (70% larger than the liver), and 50% of its function is to produce neutrophils. The normal ratio of neutrophils to erythroid cells is 2:1–3:1. As cells differentiate from hematopoietic stem cells, they undergo five divisions and mature in the storage pool for ~5 days. The nucleus contracts from the ovoid shape of the promyelocyte to the "band," and finally the mature neutrophil with a three- to five-lobed nucleus. The elimination of foreign microorganisms through phagocytosis, generation of reactive oxygen metabolites, and release of microbicidal substances depend on the mobilization of neutrophilic granules and secretory vesicles. The mature neutrophil contains four granule populations. The primary (azurophil) granule forms early (myeloblast) and contains myeloperoxidase and neutrophil elastase. Secondary (specific) granules contain high concentrations of lactoferrin and low concentrations of gelatinase (matrix metalloproteinase 9, MMP-9). Tertiary granules (gelatinase) are low in lactoferrin and high in gelatinase. Secretory vesicle membranes contain cytochrome β_{558} (one of the components of the NADPH oxidase system), receptors for complement (CD35 [complement receptor 1, CR1], CD11b/CD18 [Mac-1, CR3]), receptor for complement component 1q, receptors for monovalent and polyvalent immunoglobulin (CD32, CD64, CD16), and receptor for bacterial lipopolysaccharide (CD14). Exocytosis of granules occurs in reverse order, with secretory granules being the easiest to mobilize and the primary granule the least easy, requiring strong phagocytic stimuli. The primary granule contains a number of antimicrobial peptides: the four α-defensins (human neutrophil peptide 1 through 4), bactericidal/permeability-increasing protein (BPI), and serprocidins (serine proteases with microbicidal activity: proteinase-3, cathepsin G, and elastase). The α-defensins have microbicidal activity against fungi, bacteria, enveloped viruses, and protozoa. BPI is highly cationic, kills gram-negative bacteria at nanomolar concentrations, and neutralizes lipopolysaccharide. The serprocidins are cationic polypeptides with proteolytic activity against extracellular matrix proteins (elastin, fibronectin, laminin, type IV collagen, and vitronectin). Specific granules are larger and rich in antibiotic substances. Gelatinase granules are smaller and more easily exocytosed. They are important as a reservoir of matrix-degrading enzymes and membrane receptors required during neutrophil extravasation. Neutrophils contain three metalloproteinases that degrade major structural components of the extracellular matrix and are important for the extravasation of neutrophils. The secretory vesicles are endocytic and constitute a reservoir of membrane-associated receptors required at the earliest phases of neutrophil localization.

Maturation of the neutrophil and granule protein synthesis are achieved by transcription factors. The most well known is granulocyte colony-stimulating factor (G-CSF), which promotes neutrophil proliferation and maturation and enhances neutrophil microbicidal activity in vivo. Granulocyte–macrophage colony-stimulating factor (GM-CSF) acts on progenitors that are committed to produce either neutrophils or monocytes but can also act on granulocyte precursors directly. As with G-CSF, GM-CSF can enhance neutrophil reactivity. Neutrophils continuously egress from the sinusoids of the bone marrow. Within the circulation, half of the neutrophils are in the flowing stream, and the other half are inaccessible to phlebotomy (the *marginating pool*). In response to stress, exercise, or IV epinephrine, the neutrophils in the marginating pool are released into the circulating pool. Neutrophilia occurs after the administration of glucocorticoids, with 60% of the response due to mobilization from the marginated pool, 10% due to increased bone marrow release, and 30% due to lengthened half-life in circulation. The administration of G-CSF shortens the transit time of neutrophils through the marrow, particularly in the postmitotic pool. In response to inflammatory stimuli or infection, neutrophil production and release significantly increase. "Mature" neutrophils released from the bone marrow have altered function after infection, compared with during the "noninfected" state. They have decreased chemotaxis, phagocytosis, and ability to upregulate CD10 (a neutral endopeptidase, present on only mature granulocytes).

Neutrophil Localization in Infection

The first defense against microbes is local immunity. The epithelial surface functions as a physical barrier and releases antimicrobial peptides. Secretory IgA is released from submucosal plasma cells. If the microbial burden exceeds these processes, then neutrophil recruitment is required to control the infection. Epithelial–bacterial interactions result in release of cytokines (IL-1 and tumor necrosis factor (TNF)-α and chemokines [IL-8, CXCL8, and G-CSF]). The cytokines activate macrophages that reside in the submucosa, which amplifies the proinflammatory signal with additional release of proinflammatory chemokines and cytokines. The endothelium of the nearby postcapillary venule, under the immunologic pressure of proinflammatory cytokines, transforms from a nonadhesive surface to a proadhesive surface through the expression of specific ligands on the endothelial surface. Selectins are responsible for the initial capture of the neutrophil from the free-flowing stream and their rolling on the endothelial surface. Members of the immunoglobulin superfamily (IgSF), intercellular adhesion molecule 1 (ICAM-1), and vascular cell adhesion molecule (VCAM) are critical for neutrophil slowing, arrest, and migration on the cell surface (**Fig. 60.1**). The endothelial surface secretes a number of chemokines and lipid-derived products, such as CXCL8 (IL-8) and platelet-activating factor (PAF), which activate neutrophils through specific receptors. This step is critical for the transition from rolling to arrest. Once the leukocyte has arrested, it polarizes and then "crawls" (also known as diapedesis) through the endothelial lining, either between endothelial cells (transendothelial migration [TEM]) or less commonly across the endothelial cell itself (transcellular migration). The neutrophil must breach the venular wall, including the pericyte sheath and the venular basement membrane. This requires the pericyte to express key adhesion molecules (e.g., ICAM-1 and VCAM-1) and chemokines. Perivascular mast cells and macrophages are also rich sources of neutrophil and monocyte chemoattractants. The egress across the venular wall is significantly slower than across the endothelium itself.

Neutrophils migrate toward chemotactic factors released by the bacteria itself (bacterial peptide, fMLF), anaphylatoxins (C5a, C3a) produced after complement activation, and chemokines and arachidonic acid metabolites produced by macrophages and fibroblasts present in the subendothelial matrix (**Fig. 60.1**). Locomotion through the subendothelial matrix requires additional integrins, which recognize matrix proteins, including fibronectin, collagen, vitronectin, and vimentin. Locomotion results in the release of both gelatinase granule and secretory vesicle contents. In many situations, neutrophil recruitment does not occur in the sequence just described. Neutrophils or platelets already recruited to an inflammatory focus can recruit other neutrophils. In vascular beds (such as the liver, kidney, and lung), geometric constraints affect neutrophil localization. As neutrophils are exposed to inflammatory mediators, as occurs in sepsis, they become more rigid. They are more easily trapped in lung capillaries and hepatic sinusoids. The physical trapping of an activated neutrophil alone may be sufficient to result in injury, as described in following sections.

Opsonophagocytosis and Microbial Killing

The ingestion and disposal of microbes is a major aspect of neutrophil function. To facilitate recognition of microbes by neutrophils, these targets are "decorated" with serum opsonins. Opsonins include proteolytic fragments derived from the complement cascade and specific immunoglobulins. Receptors that recognize opsonized bacteria are present on the neutrophil surface. Ligation of Fc portion of immunoglobulin (FCγ) or complement receptors initiate a cascade that results in the exocytosis of granules, the respiratory burst, and phagocytosis. As neutrophil receptors are activated, the plasma membrane "ruffles" and assumes a bipolar configuration, with the formation of a "head" (or pseudopod) and "tail" (or uropod). The pseudopod surrounds the microbe and fuses at the distal end to form a phagolysosome. The particle is internalized and generally completely surrounded by plasma membrane. Granules join this new vacuole and discharge their contents within seconds. Release of myeloperoxidase from the primary granule is important for oxygen-dependent killing. Release of other granule contents, such as BPI, lactoferrin, and defensins, is critical for oxygen-independent killing. The *respiratory burst* refers to the coordinated consumption of oxygen and production of metabolites when neutrophils are confronted with appropriate stimuli, actions that are the basis of all oxygen-dependent killing by neutrophils and other phagocytes. The NADPH oxidase system is a transmembrane electron system in which NADPH, the primary electron donor on the cytoplasmic side of the membrane, reduces oxygen in the extracellular fluid or within the phagolysosome to form superoxide (O_2^-). In turn, two molecules of O_2^- can spontaneously (or enzymatically through superoxide dismutase) form hydrogen peroxide (H_2O_2). While both H_2O_2 and O_2^- can directly kill bacteria, it is the hydroxyl radical ($OH^{\bullet}$) and hypohalous acids produced from O_2^- and H_2O_2, respectively, which are the most injurious to microbes (and to healthy tissue/cells, if directly exposed). Myeloperoxidase released from primary granules forms hypochlorous acid (HOCl), which is directly toxic to microbes. Hypochlorous acid can react with amines to form *N*-chloramines (RNHCl). RNHCl are lipophilic and readily penetrate cellular membranes. HOCl and RNHCl inactivate heme proteins, other proteins,

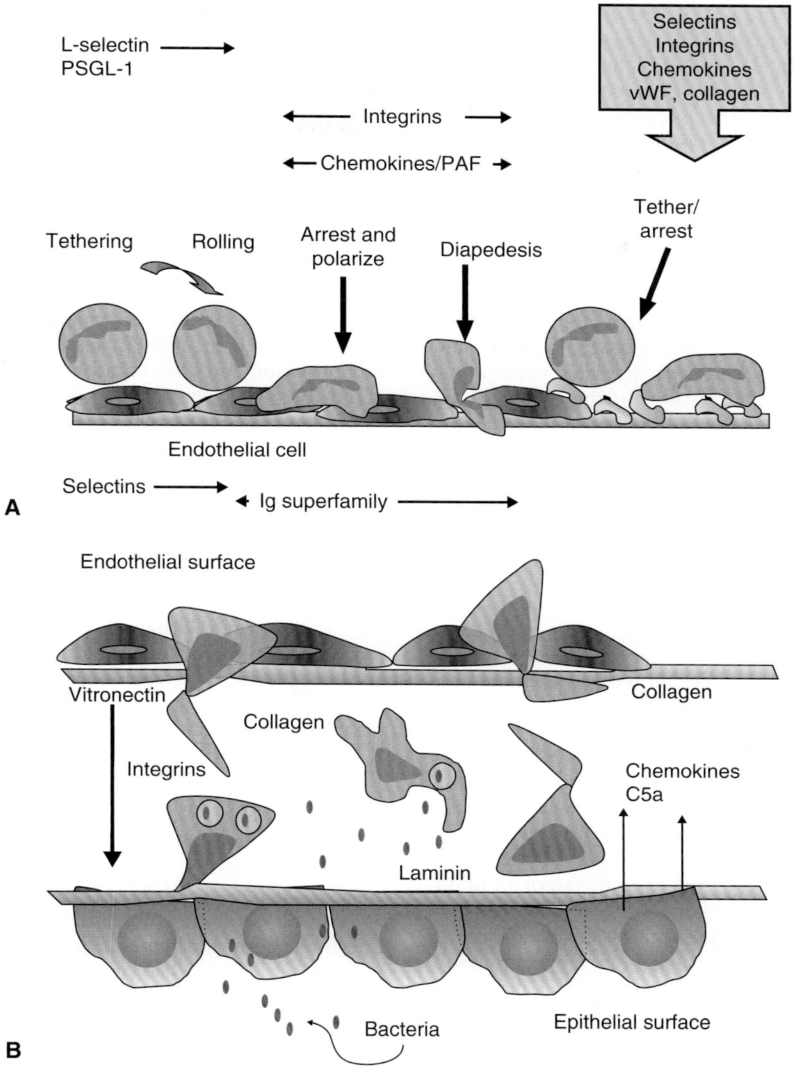

FIGURE 60.1. Neutrophil localization. **A:** In an inflammatory focus, the endothelium, which is normally nonadhesive, becomes proadhesive as a result of activation by cytokines, such as IL-1β and TNF. Neutrophils are tethered from the free-flowing stream and roll on the endothelial lining of the blood vessel, an interaction mediated by all three members of the selectin family. The neutrophils slow, arrest, and change shape (polarize). Integrins and their ligands, the immunoglobulin gene superfamily, mediate the transition from rolling to arrest. This transition is also dependent on the production of activating agents by the endothelial surface, such as PAF and IL-8. The neutrophils then crawl over the surface of the endothelium until they migrate through the endothelial monolayer. There is a hierarchy of molecules needed for transmigration, including PECAM, CD99, and JAM-1, and these specifically occur at the lateral border recycling compartment (LBRC). A neutrophil may be tethered by adherent platelets or another adherent leukocyte. Platelets themselves release chemokines, which activate neutrophils. Platelets may bind directly to von Willebrand factor (vWF) on the endothelial surface or on the basement membrane; alternatively, they may bind to collagen or fibronectin on the exposed basement membrane. In very select vascular beds (the blood–brain barrier for example), neutrophils may migrate directly through the cell body of an endothelial cell. **B:** Neutrophil localization in response to bacterial challenge. Bacteria present on the epithelial surface activate the epithelium to produce neutrophil chemokines NAP-2 (CXCL7) and ENA-78 (CXCL5); complement is activated, and the chemotactic factor C5a is produced. The epithelial surface also produces TNF-α and/or IL-1β, promoting the transition of the adjacent endothelial surface from an antiadhesive to a proadhesive surface. Neutrophils emigrate out of the blood vessel across the endothelial cell lining and crawl through the basement membrane and along the connective tissue. This is mediated by members of the β_1-integrin family and CD11b/CD18 (Mac-1, $\alpha_M\beta_2$). These integrins interact with their specific epitopes in the basement membrane structural proteins (e.g., laminin and vitronectin) and collagen. Neutrophils can continue to emigrate across the epithelial surface. Upon encountering bacteria, neutrophils surround them with plasma membrane, forming a phagolysosome. In the phagolysosome, both oxygen-dependent and oxygen-independent mechanisms are operative, resulting in bacterial killing.

and amino acids, and oxidize DNA. $OH^\bullet$ formed in the presence of iron ions (Fe^{3+}) from O_2^- is a strong oxidant. HOCl, H_2O_2, and $OH^\bullet$ participate in killing the microbe in the phagocytic vacuole.

A central feature of the inflammatory pathology of acute sepsis is accumulation of activated neutrophils within the microcirculation of highly vascular organs such as the liver, leading to immune-mediated tissue damage and organ dysfunction. However, accumulation of neutrophils in the liver enhances clearance of pathogens from the circulation (both viruses and bacteria). This occurs through a process called "NETosis." NETs (neutrophil extracellular traps) are large webs of decondensed chromatin coated with granule proteins that are expelled from activated neutrophils that capture and kill microbes in the extracellular space. This requires interactions with toll-like receptor 4–activated platelets, and is dependent on neutrophil LFA-1. These intravascular NETs ensnare bacteria and viruses decreasing the circulating pathogen load. However, the intravascular NETs can cause collateral liver damage in both bacterial and viral sepsis modes.

Modulation of the Immune Response

The neutrophil has key roles, in both the innate and acquired immune systems, beyond bacterial clearance. Mature neutrophils synthesize proinflammatory cytokines (IL-1α and IL-1$\alpha\beta$, IL-6, IL-17, IL-18); anti-inflammatory cytokines (IL-1ra, transforming growth factor β [TGF-β]); both CC and CXC chemokines; colony-stimulating factors (G-CSF and macrophage colony-stimulating factor [M-CSF]); angiogenic and fibrogenic factors (vascular endothelial growth factor [VEGF] and TGF-α) and TNF-superfamily (TNF-α, Fas Ligand, and BAFF or B lymphocyte–activating factor). Haptoglobin, an acute-phase protein, is present in the specific granules of neutrophils. Haptoglobin binds free hemoglobin, and haptoglobin–hemoglobin complexes are cleared by macrophages. Free hemoglobin serves as a source of iron, which enhances bacterial growth and virulence or participates in the generation of reactive oxygen species (ROS). In addition to being antimicrobial, defensins (from the primary granule) are chemotactic for lymphocytes and monocytes and contribute to the secondary wave of leukocytes required for resolution of infection. Neutrophils enter lymphoid organs and can modulate the adaptive immune response by inhibiting rather than augmenting the response of T and B cells to immunization. A specialized population of neutrophils reside in the spleen, secrete BAFF, and induce immunoglobulin switching of B cells. Neutrophils also regulate the maturing of the natural killer (NK) cells (patients with severe congenital neutropenia have abnormal NK cell development).

Clearance of Neutrophils

The half-life of neutrophils is very short, less than 12 hours in the circulation. Circulating neutrophils undergo apoptosis (programmed cell death) and are removed by the reticuloendothelial system of the spleen and bone marrow. Aging neutrophils return to the bone marrow, to be ingested by local macrophages. Neutrophils that migrate to an inflammatory source have a prolonged half-life and increased function. However, these neutrophils do undergo apoptosis and are cleared from the tissue by inflammatory monocytes that have transformed to macrophages. The rapid influx of neutrophils to an inflammatory site is followed by monocytes that mature into inflammatory macrophages. These macrophages either emigrate from the tissue into the lymphatics or proliferate and secrete reparative cytokines, such as TGF-β_1, resolving the neutrophil accumulation and inflammatory process. Circulating apoptotic neutrophils are almost exclusively cleared by Kupffer cells in the liver.

DEFECTS IN NEUTROPHIL NUMBER AND/OR FUNCTION

Neutrophils are important to host defense at epidermal/epithelial surfaces continuously exposed to bacteria. Children with neutrophil defects have recurrent bacterial infections of skin, lung, oropharynx, and rectal area.

Congenital and Developmental

Congenital Neutropenias

Congenital neutropenias are characterized by low neutrophil count (<500 neutrophils/µL). *Severe congenital neutropenia* appears after birth, with 90% of all children symptomatic within 6 months. The most common genetic defect is in neutrophil elastase, which may also result in cyclic neutropenia. Omphalitis is often the presenting sign. These children also have upper and lower respiratory infections and skin and liver abscesses. In *cyclic neutropenia/cyclic hematopoiesis*, a cyclic fluctuation occurs in all hematopoietic lines, though the neutrophil line is most marked. Neutrophil counts cycle at an average of 21 days, including periods of severe neutropenia that are 3–10 days in duration. Oral ulcerations, gingivitis, pharyngitis, and tonsillitis are common. In all of the diseases of severe congenital neutropenia, G-CSF greatly improves life span and the quality of life. Children and adults are at risk for developing myelodysplastic syndrome/acute myeloid leukemia. Other causes of intrinsic defects resulting in neutropenia are Shwachman–Diamond, albinism/neutropenia syndromes (including Chédiak–Higashi Syndrome), bone marrow failure syndromes (acquired and congenital), and neutropenia associated with metabolic abnormalities (organic acidemias).

Defects of Oxidative Metabolism

The most widely recognized and most prevalent defect of neutrophil function is *chronic granulomatous disease* (CGD), a heterogeneous disease characterized by recurrent life-threatening infections with bacteria, fungi, and the formation of abnormal granulomata. The defect is in the NADPH oxidase, the enzyme system responsible for the oxidative burst. The most common genotype of the CGD is the X-linked mutations of gp91^{phox} (70% of cases). Males are affected and females are carriers. With heavy lionization of the functional gene, an X-linked form of CGD has been reported in females. Clinically, CGD is variable and the age at presentation ranges from infancy to late adulthood. The most frequent sites of infection are lung, lymph nodes, and liver. The functional defect is the inability of the NADPH complex to generate superoxide (O_2^-) and the downstream ROS (H_2O_2 and $OH^\bullet$) resulting in defective microbial killing and recurrent infections with catalase-positive bacteria. Other granule functions in the CGD neutrophils are intact. However, ROS are required for the activation of the primary granule serine proteases cathepsin G and elastase. The overwhelming majority of infections result from *Aspergillus* (40%), *Staphylococcus aureus* (12%), *Burkholderia cepacia* (8%), *Nocardia* (7%), and *Serratia marcescens* (5%). As many as 32% of those with CGD have gastrointestinal involvement, and 38% have urogenital involvement. The cornerstone of treatment is trimethoprim/sulfamethoxazole prophylaxis. Itraconazole prophylaxis is routinely recommended in patients with CGD, regardless of age or previous fungal infections. A multicentered trial of IFN-γ demonstrated 70% fewer infections, compared with placebo. In severe infections, granulocyte infusions have been used. As the deletion for X-linked CGD is encoded next to the *Kell blood antigen*, deletion of the Kell locus may also occur, resulting in CGD with the McLeod phenotype. Hence, a potential transfusion hazard may exist in X-linked CGD patients. If Kell blood antigen-negative individuals are transfused with Kell-positive blood products (or granulocytes), antibodies to Kell antigen may develop. Therefore, all patients with CGD should be screened for Kell antigen. If they are found to be Kell negative, transfusion is best avoided, or Kell-negative erythrocytes or granulocytes should be used.

Defects of Leukocyte Adhesion and Trafficking

Children with recurrent, necrotic bacterial infections, impaired pus formation, and impaired wound healing may have leukocyte adhesion deficiency 1 (LAD-1) with defects in the β_2 integrins. LAD-1 is an autosomal-recessive disorder with mutations in the common chain of the β_2 integrin CD18, which results in a deficiency in number or function of adhesion molecules Mac-1 (CD11b/CD18), LFA-1 (CD11a/CD18), and p150,95 (CD11c/CD18) on the cell surface. Neutrophils cannot adhere and transmigrate to the inflammatory focus. Some patients have <1% of expression of these adhesion molecules. With this severe type, children present within the first months of life with omphalitis and delayed cord separation. They have severe infections, impaired pus formation, and impaired wound healing. They have neutrophilia at baseline, but with infections, the neutrophil count may rise >100,000/µL. Recurrent infections of the skin, upper and lower airways, bowel, and perirectal area are common and usually due to *S. aureus* or gram-negative bacilli. Pathognomonic for neutrophil-adhesion defects, the skin lesions are necrotic, and almost no pus is seen surrounding them. In patients with a moderate phenotype, β_2-integrin expression may be up to 30% of normal adult controls. Infections are less ominous, but periodontal disease, leukocytosis, and delayed wound healing are the rule. Treatment for these children is early and aggressive. Bone marrow transplantation is the only definitive treatment for children with LAD-1. In LAD-2, or congenital disorder of glycosylation IIc (CDGIIc), defects occur in glycosylation. Selectins must be appropriately glycosylated for full function. In these children, neutrophils cannot be captured from the free-flowing stream; therefore, transition to an arrested cell cannot occur. Although these children have severe recurrent infections, they also have neurodevelopmental defects due to glycosylation abnormalities. In LAD-3 (also known as LAD-1/variant), the defect occurs because of the inability of the integrins to be activated. Children with LAD-3 have defects in both neutrophil extravasation and also with platelet aggregation. Hematopoietic stem cell transplantation is curative for LAD-1 and LAD-3. Children with LAD-2 also have severe neurologic defects, and stem cell transplantation will not have an effect on the neurologic defects.

Developmental Defects in Neutrophil Function

Newborn infants, whether term or premature, have peripheral blood counts similar to older children and adults. However, they differ dramatically from adults in their response to sepsis. The profound, sustained neutrophilia with sepsis seen in adults is not found in neonates and premature infants. Instead, neonates and premature infants frequently become neutropenic during infection due to low neutrophil cell mass and an apparent inability to increase the proliferation of the early progenitor pool. Neutrophils from neonatal cord blood have diminished chemotaxis due, in part, to a decreased amount of Mac-1 from the secretory vesicles and gelatinase granules. Term infants rapidly establish normal chemotactic function within 1–2 weeks, whereas premature infants' chemotactic defect remains for weeks. In contrast, if bacteria are sufficiently opsonized, neonatal neutrophils demonstrate normal phagocytosis. However, term or preterm plasma is unable to fully opsonize bacteria. Even adult neutrophils have defective phagocytosis if infant plasma is used for opsonization.

NEUTROPHILS AND CRITICAL ILLNESS

Neutrophil Function in Critical Illness

Circulating neutrophils from infected or traumatized patients are not the "same" as neutrophils from those individuals in the noninflamed or noninjured state. In many ways, these neutrophils have already been stimulated. However, they may also be more prepared to fight infections. In infection and trauma, circulating neutrophils have decreased markers of apoptosis and decreased L-selectin. Thus, the proportion of aged cells that would normally undergo apoptosis under noninflamed conditions decreases in those individuals with infections. G-CSF and IL-6 increase transit time of neutrophils in the maturational pools and delay apoptosis, and the levels of both are dramatically elevated in sepsis. Neutrophils obtained from individuals with infection and trauma have diminished chemotactic function, compared with neutrophils from those individuals after the infection has resolved. In patients with sepsis and multiple organ failure, chemotactic response to the chemokine IL-8 is also reduced. Neutrophil rigidity is increased in patients with sepsis. Neutrophils from patients with sepsis have increased spontaneous oxidative burst activity. In traumatized patients, chemotaxis is delayed, spontaneous oxidative burst activity is increased, oxidative activity with stimulation is diminished, and opsonophagocytosis is decreased. Strong evidence exists that trauma or ischemia results in "activated" neutrophils, and these neutrophils can sequester in remote organs, leading to injury.

Transfusion-Related Acute Lung Injury

The neutrophil is the effector cell in transfusion-related acute lung injury (TRALI). TRALI is caused by activation of pulmonary neutrophils by activating substances in transfused blood products. Studies suggest that, for TRALI to develop, multiple "hits" must occur. The first hit results in activation of the endothelium, and a normal antiadhesive surface becomes proadhesive for neutrophils. Neutrophils become activated and sequestered in the lung. This first hit can occur from sepsis, trauma, or massive blood transfusion. The second hit is the infusion of specific antibodies directed against antigens on the neutrophil surface and/or biologic modifiers in the stored blood component, which activate the adherent or trapped neutrophils in the lung, causing neutrophil–endothelial injury, capillary leak, and ALI. Differentiating TRALI from transfusion-associated circulatory overload (hydrostatic pulmonary edema) may be difficult and require invasive studies (measurement of filling pressures). Blood component and donor management strategies appear to prevent some of TRALI, including the avoidance of blood products from individuals with known leukocyte antibodies, leukoreduction of blood components, shortening the storage time of cellular components to reduce accumulation of cytokines and other biologic response modifiers, and washing cellular components prior to transfusion.

Neutropenia and the ICU

Neutropenia clearly disposes patients to bacteremia, fungemia, and sepsis, but its effect on outcome in patients in the ICU is not completely clear. The use of colony-stimulating factors in patients with febrile neutropenia due to cancer chemotherapy reduced the amount of time spent in the hospital and time for neutrophil recovery, but did not benefit survival. In a large cohort of ICU pediatric oncology patients, neutropenia was not associated with increased mortality (fungal infections and higher Pediatric Risk of Mortality scores were associated with increased mortality). Recommendations regarding the use of G-CSF in neutropenic, critically ill patients must be individualized. In neutropenic children with proven or suspected fungal infections in whom mortality is high, G-CSF appears prudent. If neutropenic patients have sepsis (bacteremia and organ failure), G-CSF would be indicated. However, those who have pneumonia or another pulmonary process and neutropenia may be at risk for developing worsening respiratory status with the use of G-CSF.

Use of Colony-Stimulating Factors in Non-neutropenic ICU Patients

There is no conclusive evidence that either G-CSF or GM-CSF improves outcome in the non-neutropenic patient. G-CSF differs from GM-CSF in its specificity of action on developing and mature neutrophils, its effects on neutrophil kinetics, and its toxicity profile. GM-CSF results in priming of monocytes/macrophages and release of inflammatory cytokines. G-CSF also results in production of anti-inflammatory factors. G-CSF or GM-CSF in the non-neutropenic ICU patient should be used only in the context of therapeutic trials.

Use of Granulocyte Transfusion

Currently, there is no evidence to support the generalized use of granulocyte transfusions with neutropenia and infection.

Critical Care Therapies and Neutrophil Function

Mechanical Ventilation

Mechanical stretch of the alveolar epithelium can lead to the production of proinflammatory cytokines, in particular chemokines for neutrophils. In humans with ALI, the use of conventional ventilation strategy (compared with a protective ventilation strategy) for as little as 36 hours results in increased production of plasma IL-6 and bronchoalveolar fluid, which activates donor neutrophils.

Hypothermia

Mild hypothermia (32°C–34°C) is used in adult patients after cardiac arrest and neonates with hypoxic encephalopathy. Hypothermia decreases neutrophil motility, respiratory burst, and phagocytosis, thus potentially decreasing secondary inflammatory injury at the cost of increasing infection risk. Therapeutic hypothermia delays C-reactive protein response and suppresses white blood cell and platelet count in infants with neonatal encephalopathy compared with standard care. In a meta-analysis of therapeutic hypothermia for neonatal encephalopathy, cooling resulted in decreased risk for sepsis despite an increased risk of leukopenia. In a meta-analysis of trials of adult patients who suffered a cardiac arrest, mild hypothermia resulted in a better neurologic outcome and there was no difference in pneumonia or sepsis.

Cardiopulmonary Bypass

In cardiopulmonary bypass (CPB), the interaction of the blood elements with the oxygenator membrane and the mechanical stress of the circuit on the cells result in complement activation, production of PAF and other arachidonic intermediates, and activation of the kallikrein system. Neutrophils are activated with increased oxidative burst, and myeloperoxidase, elastase, and lactoferrin are found in the plasma. This inflammatory process is also seen in extracorporeal membrane oxygenation (ECMO). Blood neutrophils from neonates who are treated with ECMO are activated, and neutrophil elastase is increased in the plasma, compared with those same neonates before ECMO is initiated. In addition, lung injury worsened once they were placed on ECMO.

Drug Effects

Barbiturates and Anesthetics. Barbiturates, midazolam, and propofol all inhibit respiratory burst, and barbiturates inhibit chemotaxis, opsonophagocytosis, and intracellular killing.

Pentoxifylline and Cyclic AMP Modulators. Pentoxifylline, a xanthine derivative, is a phosphodiesterase inhibitor used for treatment of claudication. It also decreases *TNF* gene transcription in sepsis, prevents necrotizing enterocolitis in neonates by preserving small-vessel function, prevents endothelial dysfunction in sepsis, enhances prostacyclin release, and attenuates the release of thromboxane. Pentoxifylline increases erythrocyte and leukocyte deformability, presumably by increasing cyclic AMP levels. In a meta-analysis of pentoxifylline in neonatal sepsis as an adjunct to antibiotics, mortality was reduced with pentoxifylline, and no adverse events were found. Given the few patients studied, no recommendation for pentoxifylline use in neonates can be made, but larger trials should be developed. Activation of neutrophil β_2-adrenergic receptors results in decreased IL-8-induced chemotaxis. Catecholamines, including epinephrine, norepinephrine, dobutamine, and dopamine, depress neutrophil phagocytic ability and production of ROS.

Corticosteroids. The main anti-inflammatory effects of corticosteroids result from changes in the function of macrophages, monocytes, and granulocytes, including the decreased production of anti-inflammatory cytokines, inhibition of arachidonic acid metabolism, and decreased granulocyte adherence and migration. Lymphocyte number and function are also markedly affected by corticosteroids.

Modulating Neutrophil Function

Anti-integrin Therapy

Animal studies demonstrate that antiadhesive strategies are successful. However, human studies in traumatic shock, stroke, burns, myocardial infarction, and transplant have demonstrated no benefit of β_2-integrin, LFA-1, or ICAM-1 blockade. Use of anti-α_4 or anti-$\alpha_4\beta_7$ therapy in inflammatory bowel disease has been successful. Anti-integrin therapy has also been of great use in oncology.

Neutrophil Elastase Inhibition

When neutrophils have reduced deformability (in sepsis, severe trauma, and ALI) they are potentially trapped in capillaries. These neutrophils may then secrete neutrophil elastase, reactive oxygen products, and other soluble mediators of tissue injury. A selective inhibitor of neutrophil elastase, sivelestat, attenuates leukocyte adhesion in pulmonary capillaries and also attenuates the decreased neutrophil deformability in sepsis. In humans with ALI, sivelestat infusion attenuated diminished neutrophil deformability. A systematic review and meta-analysis found no effect of sivelestat on survival at 30 or 180 days in subjects with ALI or ARDS.

Leukocyte Depletion

Neutrophils from patients with sepsis are primed by inflammatory factors, they are more rigid, and are more easily trapped in the microcirculation; they readily mobilize secretory granules, ROS, and proteolytic enzymes. Leukopheresis has been promulgated for Crohn disease, ulcerative colitis, and systemic lupus erythematosus. Filters used for leukopheresis selectively adsorb neutrophils expressing CD64 and complement receptors, which are abnormally elevated in patients with inflammatory and autoimmune disorders. Studies are not of sufficient strength to make recommendations.

CHAPTER 61 THE IMMUNE SYSTEM AND VIRAL ILLNESS

LESLEY DOUGHTY

Viral replication and destruction of protective epithelial barriers "open the door" for bacterial infection, and the antiviral immune response alters our ability to mount an appropriate antibacterial immune response. Common viral infections can set the stage for bacterial coinfection that carries the risk of severe morbidity and significant mortality.One example is the immunomodulation by viral infection seen in bacterial coinfection with influenza. Significant immune compromise can occur during critical illness of many etiologies in patients not receiving immunosuppressive medications (septic shock, acute lung injury, and trauma). During this time, latent viruses (e.g., cytomegalovirus, CMV) can reactivate and contribute to the severity and mortality from critical illness.

SCIENTIFIC FOUNDATIONS

Immune Response to Viral Infection

Mucous membrane surfaces, respiratory epithelium, and skin are portals of entry for viruses. Examples of mechanisms shared by multiple viruses are fusion with cell membrane (enveloped viruses) or endocytosis after binding to cell-surface molecules. Many cell-surface molecules are exploited by viruses to gain entry into cells. Expression of such molecules is cell-type specific and can determine tissue tropism for certain viruses. After contact with cells, viral replication and the antiviral immune response begin. Replication of lytic viruses directly injures mucosal and epithelial protective barriers by cell lysis upon release of viral particles (**Table 61.1**). Via killing of virus-infected cells, expression of inflammatory mediators, and leukocyte infiltration, the antiviral immune response further injures tissue by releasing damage-associated molecules (DAMPs) that add to the immune system activation. The earliest and least specific is the innate immune response followed by a pathogen-specific adaptive immune response leading to immunologic memory. Recognition of viruses by the innate immune system begins with recognition of viral pathogen-associated molecular patterns (PAMPs) (expressed during viral replication) with pattern recognition receptors (PRRs) (e.g., toll-like

TABLE 61.1

Mechanisms of Bacterial Adherence to Host Cells during Viral Infection

Respiratory epithelial disruption	Loss of mucociliary function
	Basement membrane exposure
Bacterial features	Fimbriae
	Capsule
Expression of viral glycoproteins	Neuraminidase (influenza/parainfluenza)
	Hemagglutinin (influenza/parainfluenza)
	Glycoproteins F and G (RSV)
Upregulation of host cell receptors	CD14, CD15, and CD18
	PAFR
	Complement protein C3
	Fimbriae-associated receptors
	IgA translocating receptor
	PentamericIgM
Proteins from injured ECM	Fibrinogen
Other	Coupling bacteria to epithelium by RSV
	Altered bacterial adhesins

ECM, extracellular matrix; RSV, respiratory syncytial virus; PAFR, platelet-activating factor receptor.
Adapted from Mashayekhi A, Shields CL, Shields JA. Transient increased exudation after photodynamic therapy of intraocular tumors. *Middle East Afr J Ophthalmol* 2013;20(1):83–6.

receptors [TLRs]). The innate response is critical for recruitment of effector cells, containment of viral particles, and initiation of the adaptive (antigen-specific) immune response necessary for viral eradication and immunologic memory. Binding to TLRs initiates intracellular signal transduction leading to production of proinflammatory cytokines, including type I interferons α and β (IFN-α/β), type III interferons (IFN-λ subtypes), TNF-α, IL-1β, IL-6, and chemokines, such as CCL2, CCL20, and CCR7, which facilitate trafficking of alveolar macrophages, dendritic cells (DCs), and neutrophils to sites of viral invasion. Anti-inflammatory cytokines, such as IL-10, soluble TNF-α receptor, and IL-1 receptor antagonist, are also induced.

IFN-α/β activates NK cells and macrophages, induces maturation of DCs, and upregulates proteins important in antigen presentation to T cells. Activated CD8 cells differentiate into cytotoxic T cells (CTLs) that contribute to lysis of virus-infected cells and to viral clearance. Once activated by viruses, DCs mature as they migrate to draining lymph nodes where they present viral antigens to CD4 T cells (via MHC I) and CD8 cells (via MHC II). Antigen-activated CD4 cells differentiate to Th1 (proinflammatory), Th2 (anti-inflammatory), regulatory T cells (Tregs), or Th17 depending on the inflammatory milieu. Cytotoxic CD8 T cells eliminate virus by induction of the antiviral cytokine IFN-γ, by perforin-induced lysis of virus-infected cells, and by induction of apoptosis through Fas ligand with Fas (CD95) on the virus-infected cells. The ideal result of this immune cascade is eradication of the virus, production of antibodies specific for multiple viral peptides, and creation of memory T cells and B cells important in protection against subsequent infection with the same virus. IFN-α/β is a critical antiviral cytokine. In the absence of IFN-α/β signaling, viral replication is unchecked and overwhelming viral infection occurs. In chronic viral infection, a lower but sustained IFN-α/β response continues (despite this, the virus persists). Evidence of IFN-α/β pathway activation in hepatitis C, HIV, and latent tuberculosis is associated with disease progression and poor response to IFN therapy.

The respiratory tract is continually challenged by inhaled particulate matter, and immunosuppressive Tregs are critical in this process. In respiratory syncytial virus (RSV) and influenza, Tregs are activated and secrete excessive IL-10 that dampens Th1 proinflammatory responses. Other cell types that contribute to dampening the inflammatory response incited during viral infections include plasmacytoid DCs, neutrophils (by facilitating viral clearance), and airway epithelial cells (AECs) (via expression of CD200). When the virus is eradicated and the proinflammatory response is resolving, an anti-inflammatory environment evolves to promote healing. Th2 cytokines IL-4 and IL-13 are important mediators, and IL-13 is critical to changing macrophage phenotype to "alternatively activated macrophages" (M2) that are anti-inflammatory and important to tissue repair.

IMPACT OF VIRAL INFECTION ON ANTIBACTERIAL DEFENSE

The immune response to respiratory viral infection can compromise antibacterial function, creating a permissive state for bacterial superinfection. Many changes occur that are associated with decreased bacterial killing. In addition, altered differentiation of T cells, suppressed DC, CD4 proliferation, and CD8 T-cell cytotoxicity are seen. In contrast, there is enhancement of suppressive Tregs ($CD4^+ CD25^+$) (**Table 61.2**). Unfortunately, IFN-α/β produced during viral infection suppresses differentiation to Th17 cells, important for neutrophil activation, bactericidal protein production, and tissue remodeling that result in antibacterial protection.

Respiratory Viruses

When viral infection disrupts protective epithelial barriers, mucociliarydysfunction as well as exaggerated bacterial colonization by adherence to exposed basement membrane elements permit penetration into deeper tissues. Specifically, bacterial adherence is enhanced in areas where epithelium has been denuded. Mechanisms of bacterial adherence to infected/disrupted epithelium can be nonspecific as exemplified by bacteria binding to fibrinogen- and fibronectin-binding protein of the exposed extracellular matrix as seen with group Aβ-hemolytic streptococcus (GAβHS) in influenza A infection. Some mechanisms for increased bacterial adherence during viral infection can be specific for bacterial features. For example, in models of RSV and influenza, enhanced fimbriae- and capsule-mediated binding of nontypeable*Haemophilus influenzae*, GAβHS, and *Neisseria meningitidis* to alveolar epithelial cells can occur. Native host cell-surface protein/receptor expression can be upregulated during many viral infections and have been associated with increased adherence of *N. meningitidis* and *Streptococcus pneumoniae* to virus-infected epithelial cells. Viral infection can also result in the host cell expression of viral glycoproteins. The best-characterized glycoproteins are hemagglutinin (HA) and neuraminidase (NA) expressed on the host cell surface during influenza infections. HA binds to terminal sialic acid residues of host cell surface permitting internalization of virus and fusion of viral envelope with cell membrane leading to penetration into host cells. NA is critical for replication of influenza and parainfluenza because it cleaves sialic acid residues from host glycoproteins during viral budding from infected cells facilitating release of newly synthesized virus. These sialic acid residues on host proteins provide protection against bacterial adherence and once cleaved by NA, bacteria adhere and invade. NA activity is a key determinant of the virulence of a given strain and a determinant of the severity of an epidemic. Other viral glycoproteins implicated in susceptibility to bacterial superinfection

TABLE 61.2

Immunomodulatory Effects of Viral Infections

■ CELL TYPE	■ DECREASED	■ INCREASED
Macrophages	MHC expression Activation and recruitment Phagocytosis Bacterial killing Antigen presentation	Inflammatory cytokines
Neutrophils	Bacterial killing	TLR 2 expression Apoptosis
Dendritic cells	Altered IFN-α/β production Altered IFN-γ signaling MHC expression Antigen presentation	Apoptosis
NK cells	Activation	
T cells	CD4 proliferation CD8 cytotoxicity Th2 cytokines Treg activation DTH response	Th1 cytokines Apoptosis
Other	Bone marrow suppression Complement activation	

include glycoproteins F and G that are inserted into the host cell membrane during RSV infection. RSV virions bind pneumococci to form complexes that exhibit enhanced adherence to uninfected epithelial cell layers. In this way, RSV directly acts as a coupling agent between bacteria and host cells. **Table 61.1** lists many factors induced during viral infection that promote bacterial adherence and facilitate invasion.

Other Viruses

Measles virus (MV) infection suppresses many aspects of the immune response leading to vulnerability to secondary infections. The mechanisms reported include depressed delayed-type hypersensitivity (DTH) reactions, poor antigen presentation and poor lymphocyte proliferative response to mitogens, accelerated apoptosis of DCs and lymphocytes, bone marrow suppression, altered IFN-α/β production and signaling, and diminished DC IL-12p70 production with a long-lasting shift toward a Th2 response with sustained elevated levels of IL-4. The consequence of these factors is prolonged immunosuppression from a transient viral infection resulting in a high frequency of secondary infections. Human CMV is capable of modulating the immune response permitting its persistence in a latent state. Numerous alterations in host immune function occur, including loss of DTH response to recall antigens, reduced lymphoproliferative responses and NK cell activity, and suppressed bone marrow myelopoiesis. CMV can infect DCs directly and modulate the function of this critical aspect of host defense contributing to viral persistence and subsequent immunosuppression.

CLINICAL CONSEQUENCES OF VIRAL AND BACTERIAL COINFECTION

Influenza

The association between viral infection and bacterial infection has been repeatedly described for respiratory viruses (influenza, RSV, human metapneumovirus, and parainfluenza) and secondary bacterial pneumonia. Antecedent or concurrent viral and bacterial infection has been associated with severe morbidity and high mortality. Recently, *Streptococcus pneumoniae* is the most common secondary infection, but early methicillin-resistant *Staphylococcus aureus* infection was a risk factor for mortality.

Respiratory Syncytial Virus

Studies have shown a low incidence of bacterial coinfection in RSV-infected infants and children. In contrast, mechanically ventilated infants with severe RSV have a high incidence (38%–44%) of bacterial coinfection. Coinfection of RSV with another viral pathogen occurs with rhinovirus(RV) and metapneumovirus.

Cytomegalovirus

In an immunocompetent host, CMV causes asymptomatic or very mild illness; in some, a mononucleosis-like syndrome. In an immunosuppressed individual, it can cause severe/fatal disease, involving liver, lung, GI tract, and CNS. Overall, CMV occurs in childhood with 30%–40% incidence within the first year of life increasing thereafter to 60%–70% in adults. CMV infection results in a dormant infection after the acute phase and typically remains in this state. Immunosuppressed individuals are at significant risk for primary infection (if seronegative), and reactivation is commonly seen. With active CMV disease, there is increased risk for secondary infections, malignancies such as posttransplantlymphoproliferative disease, and cardiovascular disease, and overall in this setting active CMV disease is associated with increased mortality. There is a strong association between critical illness in previously immunocompetent patients and CMV reactivation, and 33% of critically ill patients developed detectable CMV by12 days in the ICU. There is also an increased incidence of nosocomial infection in the presence of reactivated CMV.

Other Viruses

Serious bacterial superinfection is a known complication of varicella, including necrotizing fasciitis, toxic shock syndrome, septic shock, bacteremia, epiglottitis, spinal epidural abscess, pyogenic arthritis, osteomyelitis, meningitis, orbital cellulitis, and subdural empyema. The primary bacterial culprits are GAβHS and *Staphylococcus aureus*. Measles causes profound immunosuppression during infection and is a significant cause of measles-related mortality.

VIRAL INFECTIONS AND ASTHMATIC EXACERBATIONS

Viral infections, especially RSV and RV early in life, are associated with the development of asthma over time. Respiratory viral infections precipitate 60%–85% of acute asthma exacerbations in children. In pediatrics, RSV and RV are the most common. RV, specifically, is a major destabilizer of asthma, and found in 50%–70% of asthma exacerbations. In the asthmatic, RV can extend beyond the upper respiratory tract and persist longer. Asthmatics are more susceptible to RV infections, and viral replication in bronchial epithelial cells (BECs) obtained from asthmatics is increased. Asthma exacerbations are more severe in the children with persistence of viral RNA suggesting that the severity of asthma exacerbations may be linked to prolonged RV infection. BECs but not peripheral blood mononuclear cells (PBMCs) from asthmatics have defective production of IFN-β and IFN-λ (type III interferons) during RV infection, indicating that an important antiviral and immunomodulating cytokine is defective in the respiratory compartment when it is needed most. IFN-β and -λ are important inducers of apoptosis of RV-infected cells. The induction of other proinflammatory cytokines was similar in asthmatic versus healthy BECs, suggesting that all antiviral pathways were not deficient. It has been suggested that in the presence of an impaired interferon response, a more vigorous inflammatory response (other mediators) may be necessary for virus eradication and in this way may contribute to asthma exacerbation. The asthmatic airway is characterized by the presence of eosinophils and T cells expressing Th2 cytokines, including IL-4, IL-5, and IL-13. This environment may also contribute to ineffective antiviral responses (**Fig. 61.1**). Recently, a therapeutic trial using IFN-β in asthma has been done, and results are pending.

VIRAL INFECTIONS AND AUTOIMMUNE DISEASE EXACERBATIONS

The viruses most closely associated with autoimmune phenomenon include CMV, herpes simplex virus (HSV), Epstein–Barr virus (EBV), human herpesvirus (HHV) 6 and 7, hepatitis C, parvovirus B19, and MV (**Table 61.3**). Many of these viruses remain in the host in a latent fashion and become activated during stress or systemic inflammation by proinflammatory cytokines or during immunosuppressed states. It is unclear whether reactivation of these viruses is a product of the inflammatory response during an autoimmune exacerbation or if viral reactivation is provocative for autoimmune exacerbations. Another association for which there is considerable data is between coxsackie B4 (CB4) and type 1 diabetes mellitus.

There are several proposed mechanisms for aggravation of autoimmune diseases by the above viruses. One frequently hypothesized mechanism is referred to as *molecular mimicry* where the immune response to viral infection cross-reacts with self-antigens. This results in activation of T and B cells leading to the production of self-reactive autoantibodies capable of mediating tissue injury. Alternatively, viruses such as CMV, during primary or reactivated disease, can activate antigen-presenting cells (APCs) and virus-specific T cells resulting in activation of preexisting autoreactive T cells in susceptible individuals. This phenomenon is called *bystander activation*. A key antiviral cytokine produced during the immune response to most viruses is IFN-α. There is a great deal of data implicating IFN-α in the development of autoimmune diseases, such as systemic lupus erythematosus (SLE), thyroid disease, and type 1 diabetes. In addition, there are many reports of patients receiving therapeutic IFN-α for diseases, such as hepatitis C, who develop autoimmune phenomenon, such as SLE, type 1 diabetes, psoriasis, inflammatory arthritis, or Sjögren syndrome and autoimmune thyroid diseases. IFN-α is known to potentiate immune responses through differentiation of monocytes to macrophages, augmented capacity for antigen presentation, and increased T cell stimulation and survival. These effects may promote survival of autoreactive T cells and B cells leading to autoantibody-mediated tissue

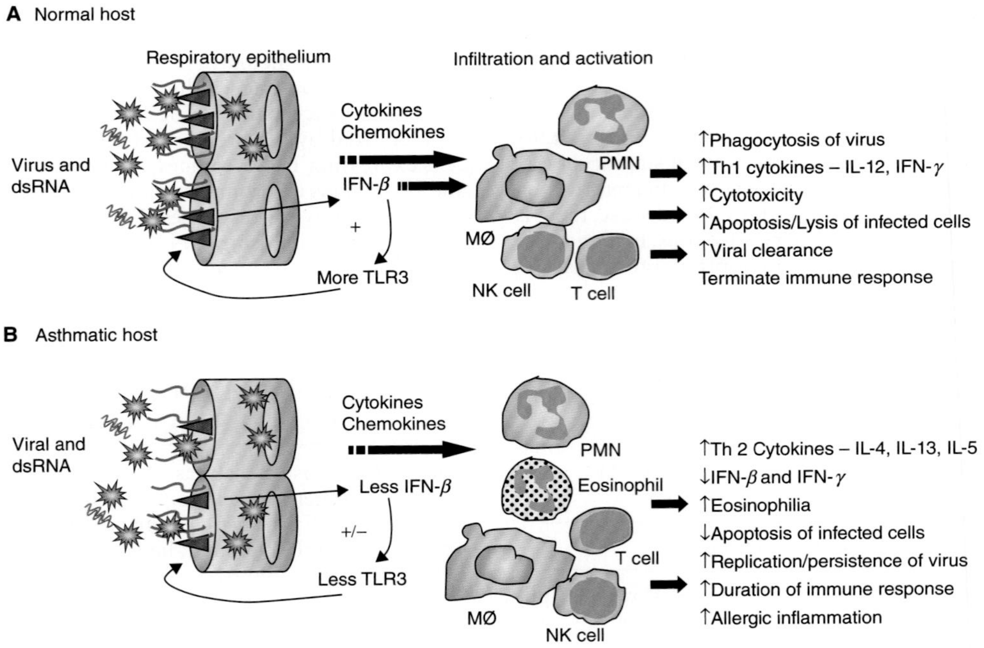

FIGURE 61.1 The antiviral immune response in asthma. Viruses infect respiratory epithelium and dsRNA (released during replication of most viruses) signals through TLR 3, which is constitutively expressed on epithelial cells. Both lead to production of a multitude of cytokines and chemokines, including IFN-β by epithelial cells. IFN-β upregulates TLR 3 leading to further induction of IFN-β. IFN-β induces IFN-α, both of which are pleiotropic cytokines activating a multitude of inflammatory cells, kinases, and regulatory proteins critical for viral containment. **A:** Under normal circumstances, activation and infiltration of inflammatory cells leads to a proinflammatory response including Th1 cytokines that are also important for viral clearance. Effective killing/apoptosis of infected cells occurs, promoting viral clearance and resolution of inflammation. **B:** Respiratory epithelial cells from asthmatics produce less IFN-β and TLR 3. Inflammatory cell stimulation is different with infiltration of eosinophils, a Th2 response with less IFN-γ, longer survival of infected cells, and delayed viral clearance.

TABLE 61.3

Viral Infections Associated with Autoimmune Diseases

AUTOIMMUNE DISEASE	VIRUS
Type 1 diabetes mellitus	Coxsackie B4, enteroviruses, rotavirus
Multiple sclerosis	Measles, EBV, HHV-6
Rheumatoid arthritis	CMV, parvovirus B19
Sjögren syndrome	EBV, CMV, HHV-6, hepatitis C
Systemic lupus erythematosus	CMV, EBV, hepatitis C, parvovirus B19
Inflammatory bowel disease	CMV, EBV, measles

Adapted from Osawa R, Singh N. Cytomegalovirus infection in critically ill patients: A systematic review [Review]. *Crit Care* 2009;13(3):R68.

damage. Since viral infections also potently induce IFN-α, it is possible that the presence of IFN-α (administered exogenously or produced endogenously) is responsible for the association of viral infections with autoimmune exacerbations. There are implications to critical illness caused by autoimmune disease if viral infection can precipitate exacerbations. It may be prudent to evaluate the host fully for new or reactivated viral infection by serum polymerase chain reaction when an autoimmune exacerbation occurs. This would guide and define a potential role for antiviral treatment during autoimmune exacerbations requiring augmentation of immunosuppressive regimens.

POTENTIAL THERAPEUTIC AND DIAGNOSTIC STRATEGIES

Unfortunately, the paucity of successful antiviral therapies makes specific treatment of many viral infections impossible with the exception of the herpes family viruses. One important therapeutic strategy for the treatment of influenza is the use of neuraminidase inhibitors (NIs). Multiple large studies have demonstrated reduction in length of illness by 1–4 days if an NI is begun within the first several hours of influenza symptoms. In addition, prophylactic use has also been effective for high-risk populations and recently exposed individuals. NI treatment reduces the incidence of otitis media by 44%, lower respiratory tract complications requiring antibiotics by 55%, and hospitalizations for any cause by 59%. Improvement is seen even when the NI is administered as late as 5 days after the onset of influenza. NI treatment does not reduce viral titers but does reduce bacterial adherence. These data suggest that inhibition of NA decreases NA-mediated changes in respiratory epithelium permissive for bacterial colonization and establishment of pneumonia. **Figure 61.2** depicts a schematic diagram of hypothetical impact of NI on bacterial adherence/infection. These data support the use of NI agents not only to reduce the morbidity from influenza but also to reduce secondary bacterial infection in high-risk children. These drugs are not yet approved for use in infants.

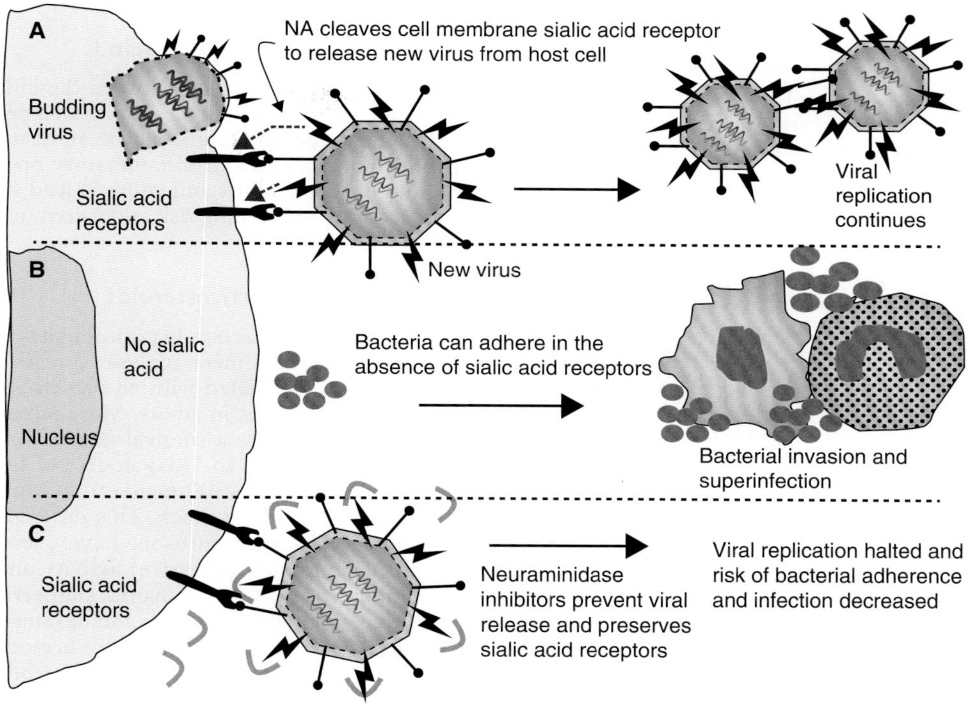

FIGURE 61.2. Mechanism of action of neuraminidase inhibitors. **A:** New virus is released from the cell surface by neuraminidase cleavage of hemagglutinin bound to sialic acid cell receptors. New virus continues to replicate leading to destruction of infected tissue clinical symptomatology. **B:** Bacteria such as pneumococcus can adhere to cell surfaces in the absence of sialic acid residues leading to bacterial superinfection. **C:** Neuraminidase inhibitors block the release of new viruses limiting viral replication and spread to other cells. Also by limiting neuraminidase activity, protective sialic acid residues are preserved decreasing bacterial adherence and invasion. Neuraminidase (⚡); hemagglutinin (⚲); neuraminidase inhibitor (⌒); neuraminidase activity (--►).

CHAPTER 62 ■ IMMUNE MODULATION AND IMMUNOTHERAPY IN CRITICAL ILLNESS

MARK W. HALL AND JENNIFER A. MUSZYNSKI

The immune response and its regulation are critical for defending against pathogens and for healing of injured tissues. Unfortunately, patient morbidity is often a result of abnormal regulation of this immune response.

TARGETING PROINFLAMMATION

Tumor necrosis factor (TNF)-α, interleukin (IL)-1β, and interferon (IFN)-γ are proinflammatory cytokines released by innate immune cells (TNF-α, IL-1β) and lymphocytes (IFN-γ) in response to an inflammatory stimulus. The cytokine that is consistently associated with adverse outcomes in proinflammatory disease is IL-6, likely because IL-6 is released in response to more potent proinflammatory cytokines and, therefore, serves as a *marker* for inflammation. IL-6, while an inducer of the acute-phase response, has significant anti-inflammatory properties of its own. More potent anti-inflammatory cytokines, produced by both innate and adaptive immune cells, include IL-10 and transforming growth factor (TGF)-β. Innate immune cells include neutrophils, monocytes, macrophages, and dendritic cells, whereas adaptive immune cells include T and B lymphocytes.

Severe Sepsis and Septic Shock

The signs and symptoms of severe sepsis (fever, altered vascular tone, and increased capillary permeability) are largely the result of the effects of proinflammatory cytokines rather than the offending pathogen.

Anti-endotoxin Strategies

Studies in this area initially focused on gram-negative lipopolysaccharide (LPS). Unfortunately, a trial of anti-LPS therapy demonstrated *higher* mortality in treated patients. Recombinant bactericidal/permeability-increasing protein (BPI), an endogenous antimicrobial peptide capable of neutralizing endotoxin, evaluated in children with meningococcemia conferred no improvement in survival but improved functional outcome.

Anti-cytokine Strategies

Recombinant IL-1 receptor antagonist (IL-1ra), a naturally occurring IL-1β antagonist, failed to improve adult sepsis survival. TNF-α has been similarly targeted with neutralizing monoclonal antibody therapy. Findings that patients with plasma IL-6 levels of >1000 pg/mL have better survival suggest that the most profoundly inflamed patients might benefit from TNF-α depletion.

Activated Protein C

Significant overlap occurs between the inflammatory and hemostatic pathways. Activated protein C (APC) is an endogenous protein with antithrombotic, profibrinolytic, and anti-inflammatory properties. Studies in septic adults and children lead to safety concerns due to bleeding risk and its removal from the market.

Corticosteroids

The role of corticosteroids in critical illness remains controversial. Early meta-analyses concluded that their use was associated with an *increased* risk of mortality from sepsis in adults. More recent meta-analyses demonstrate a survival *benefit* associated with the use of a 5- to 7-day course of low-dose hydrocortisone (200–300 mg/day) in adults with severe sepsis or septic shock. This difference may be explained by hydrocortisone having less glucocorticoid (immunosuppressive) activity and more mineralocorticoid (hemodynamic supporting) activity than methylprednisolone and dexamethasone (**Table 62.1**). Hydrocortisone use for hemodynamic support in septic children has yet to be studied in a randomized, controlled trial.

Extracorporeal Therapies

Another approach to the restoration of immunologic homeostasis is the bulk removal of inflammatory mediators through hemofiltration, membrane adsorption, plasmapheresis, or plasma exchange. Plasmapheresis and plasma exchange have shown the most promise, perhaps because the replacement of patient plasma with donor plasma both removes unwanted mediators and replaces deficient ones. In particular, restoration of plasma activity of von Willebrand factor–cleaving protease, ADAMTS13, via plasma exchange has been reported to improve outcomes in the setting of pediatric thrombocytopenia-associated multiple organ failure (TAMOF).

TABLE 62.1

Relative Potencies of Corticosteroids

DRUG	ANTI-INFLAMMATORY (IMMUNOSUPPRESSIVE)	MINERALOCORTICOID
Dexamethasone	30	0
Methylprednisolone	5	1
Hydrocortisone	1	5

Acute Respiratory Distress Syndrome

Reduction of inflammation and inhibition of the fibroproliferative phase seem a reasonable goal in the management of ARDS. In adults, methylprednisolone started >14 days after the onset of ARDS failed to show a survival benefit and, in fact, showed *increased* mortality rates. Using lower doses and earlier initiation of methylprednisolone demonstrated improvements in morbidity and mortality. No pediatric studies exist.

Cardiopulmonary Bypass

Exposure of leukocytes and complement to the tubing and membranes associated with extracorporeal procedures, including cardiopulmonary bypass (CPB), induces a potent proinflammatory response. The administration of glucocorticoids reduces neutrophil activation and proinflammatory cytokine release. Bulk removal of proinflammatory cytokines through modified ultrafiltration during CPB yields variable results.

IMMUNOPARALYSIS

Severe depression of innate immune function has been associated with adverse outcomes following trauma, sepsis, and transplantation. This phenomenon, *immunoparalysis*, has been quantified in two ways. First, surface expression of the class II major histocompatibility complex molecule HLA-DR, important in antigen presentation, is reduced in circulating monocytes from patients with compensatory anti-inflammatory response syndrome. Severe reduction in HLA-DR expression (<30% of circulating monocytes are strongly HLA-DR$^+$ by flow cytometry) is characteristic of immunoparalysis. A more functional measure of innate immune capability is the ex vivo LPS-induced TNF-α production assay. In this test, whole blood is incubated with a standard concentration of LPS, and TNF-α production is measured in the supernatant. Patients with immunoparalysis demonstrate a severe reduction in their ability to make TNF-α ex vivo. Patients with this syndrome exhibit skewing toward a T_H2-like immune phenotype with high levels of circulating IL-10. The adaptive arm of the immune system is also involved in the compensatory anti-inflammatory response syndrome. Lymphocyte depletion, in the form of widespread apoptosis in lymphoid organs as well as circulating lymphopenia, has been associated with mortality and secondary infection in critically ill adults and children. Lymphocyte-mediated responses are thought to take place over a longer time frame than innate immune responses due to the requirement for antigen presentation and clonal expansion.

The laboratory measures of immunoparalysis represent evidence that a patient's compensatory anti-inflammatory response, initially an adaptive attempt to restore immunologic homeostasis, can progress to a maladaptive state that can be thought of as a type of secondary immunodeficiency. Mounting evidence suggests that immunoparalysis is reversible, with a beneficial effect on clinical outcomes, through the use of immunostimulatory agents or through the tapering of exogenous immunosuppression. The drugs IFN-g, granulocyte–macrophage colony-stimulating factor (GM-CSF), and fms-related tyrosine kinase 3 ligand reverse experimental immunoparalysis. Trials, in which GM-CSF was given to subjects who demonstrated immunoparalysis, have shown prompt reversal of immunoparalysis and improved outcomes in critically ill adults and children. It is critically important that assays of innate immune function be standardized to survey for immunoparalysis and target patients who may benefit from inclusion in prospective trials of immunostimulatory agents.

PATIENTS WITH OVERT IMMUNOSUPPRESSION

Immunosuppressive medications are the mainstay of pediatric treatment of cancer, transplantation, autoimmunity, and other chronic inflammatory diseases (**Table 62.2**). Antibody-based or recombinant therapies target highly specific aspects of immune function, but are still immunosuppressive (**Table 62.3**). Accordingly, these patients are at high risk for morbidity and mortality due to infectious complications.

The Neutropenic Patient

Severe, prolonged neutropenia most commonly results from the administration of myelosuppressive

TABLE 62.2

Commonly Used Non–Antibody-Based Immunosuppressive Agents

CLASS	DRUG	TARGET	NONIMMUNE TOXICITIES
Glucocorticoids	Methylprednisolone Dexamethasone Prednisone	Inhibition of proinflammatory and cell-proliferation gene transcription in lymphocytes and other immune cells	Hypertension, hyperglycemia, impaired wound healing, neuromuscular weakness, growth impairment
Calcineurin inhibitors	Tacrolimus (FK506) Cyclosporine A (CsA)	Inhibition of T cell signaling pathways	Nephrotoxicity, CNS toxicity (including seizures), tremor, hypertension, hyperglycemia (FK506), hirsutism (CsA)
TOR protein kinase inhibitor	Sirolimus	Inhibition of T and B cell proliferation	Hyperlipidemia, hypertension, thrombocytopenia, rash
Antimetabolite	Azathioprine Mycophenolate mofetil	Purine synthesis inhibition	Bone marrow suppression, diarrhea, cholestasis

CNS, central nervous system; TOR, target of rapamycin.

TABLE 62.3

Antibody-Based and Recombinant Immunosuppressive Agents

THERAPY	EXAMPLE	POTENTIAL USES
Anti-TNF-α	Infliximab, Etanercept	IBD, autoimmune arthritis
Anti-CD20	Rituximab	B cell leukemia/lymphoma, multiple sclerosis, autoimmune arthritis
Anti-IL-2Rα	Basiliximab, Daclizumab	Transplant rejection
Anti-T cell (polyclonal)	Anti-thymocyte globulin	Transplant rejection
Anti-IL-6R	Toclizumab	Autoimmune arthritis
Recombinant IL-1 RA	Anakinra	Autoimmune arthritis, NOMID

RA, receptor antagonist; IBD, inflammatory bowel disease; NOMID, neonatal onset multisystem inflammatory disease.

chemotherapy in the context of cancer treatment, but can also be seen with infection-induced marrow failure and as a side effect of drugs, including antibiotics. It is understood that an absolute neutrophil count (ANC) of <500 cells/mm^3 is associated with increased incidence of sepsis and death in patients with malignancy. Prophylaxis against pneumocystis pneumonia and candidal infections with trimethoprim/sulfamethoxazole and fluconazole should be considered population when these patients are critically ill. Use of granulocyte colony-stimulating factor (GCSF) has become standard in the treatment of cancer patients with fever and neutropenia. Administration of GCSF results in increased myelopoiesis and neutrophil maturation. Another therapeutic option for severely neutropenic children with life-threatening infection is granulocyte transfusion. Importantly, donor leukocytes can induce a potent proinflammatory response following infusion. Evidence to support or contraindicate the use of granulocyte transfusion therapy is inconclusive, but patients who received $>1 \times 10^{10}$ cells per dose fared better than those receiving lower doses.

The Lymphopenic Patient

Lymphopenia frequently accompanies critical illness and has been associated with increased risk of death and secondary infection. It is especially important to note that the definition of lymphopenia varies by age, with infants and toddlers requiring more robust lymphocyte numbers to remain immunocompetent (**Table 62.4**).

CDC recommendations include the administration of trimethoprim/sulfamethoxazole, dapsone, or pentamidine for pneumocystis pneumonia prophylaxis in children with severe reductions in CD4$^+$ T cell count. A potential consequence of lymphocyte depletion is a lack of antibody production by B cells. Assessment of quantitative immunoglobulin levels can identify patients with hypogammaglobulinemia

TABLE 62.4

Centers for Disease Control Definitions of Severe Reductions in $CD4^+$ Count in Children

AGE (YEARS)	$CD4^+$ COUNT (Cells/mm^3)
<1	<750
1–5	<500
6–12	<200

Adapted from National Pediatric and Family HIV Resource Center; National Center for Infectious Diseases; Centers for Disease Control and Prevention. 1995 revised guidelines for prophylaxis against *Pneumocystis carinii* pneumonia for children infected with or perinatally exposed to human immunodeficiency virus. *MMWR Recomm Rep*1995;44(RR-4):1–11.

who may benefit from replacement with IVIG. Glucocorticoids are potent inducers of lymphocyte apoptosis. Dopamine use has also been associated with the development of lymphopenia, presumably through its inhibitory effect on the neuroendocrine axes, most notably prolactin, which is known to be a necessary growth factor for lymphocytes.

The Transplant Patient

Multidrug regimens that include calcineurin inhibitors, corticosteroids, and other immunosuppressives (e.g., mycophenolate or azathioprine) are employed in transplant patients to shut down the adaptive immune response against the transplanted organ, often with significant systemic toxicities. The suppressive effects of these regimens are not limited to the adaptive immune response and inhibit the innate response causing reductions in monocyte function associated directly or indirectly with calcineurin inhibition. The most comprehensive set of recommendations for antimicrobial prophylaxis comes from the Centers for Disease Control Guidelines for Preventing Opportunistic Infection in Hematopoietic Stem Cell Transplant Recipients (**Table 62.5**). While not generalizable to all transplant populations, they highlight the scope of the problem and identify a rational approach to prophylaxis. Also, the use of antibody-based immunosuppressive regimens, including anti–IL-2 receptor antibodies, has been an effective antirejection strategy without the systemic toxicity profiles of drugs such as cyclosporine and tacrolimus. Lastly, the ICU practitioner can rapidly taper the exogenous immunosuppression to allow for a more robust immune response in the setting of suspected or proven infection. Rapid tapering of immunosuppression in immunoparalyzed adult transplant patients with sepsis provides 90% patient survival (with 98% graft survival) compared with an 8% survival for those who do not get rapid tapering. While plasma tacrolimus levels of <10 ng/mL and cyclosporine A levels of <200 ng/mL can be generally thought of as mildly-to-moderately immunosuppressive, functional assays of the immune response, such as ex vivo LPS-induced TNF-α production capacity, have the potential to serve as more relevant targets for titration of these potent drugs.

INTRAVENOUS IMMUNOGLOBULIN

Polyclonal IVIG has been administered to adults and children with sepsis (*without* preexisting hypogammaglobulinemia) with mixed results. A meta-analysis of IVIG treatment of proven infection in critically ill neonates showed a lowered mortality risk. In children <2 years of age with sepsis, 3 days of polyclonal IVIG treatment improved survival to discharge and shortened durations of pediatric intensive care unit. Interestingly, IVIG may be of particular benefit in the setting of severe invasive group A strep infection. Evidence suggests that IgM-enriched IVIG may be beneficial in postoperative sepsis in adult patients, though a multicentered trial failed to show benefit in the setting of chemotherapy-induced neutropenic sepsis.

IMMUNONUTRITION

With immunonutrition, patients are provided nutritional supplementation that, in the course of metabolism, has an effect on the immune response. The two substrates that have been the focus of the most investigation are the n-3 polyunsaturated fatty acids (PUFAs) and the amino acid arginine. The n-3 PUFAs, including docosahexaenoic, eicosapentaenoic, and α-linoleic acid, promote an anti-inflammatory immune state through at least two mechanisms. By incorporating into the cell's phospholipid membrane, n-3 PUFAs compete with arachidonic acid precursors, resulting in lower arachidonic acid production. In addition, n-3 PUFAs directly inhibit nuclear receptors, including peroxisome proliferator-activated receptor (PPAR-g), which impairs propagation of the inflammatory response. No mortality benefit has been shown. Arginine, by contrast, is thought to promote a more vigorous immune response through augmentation of intracellular killing and lymphocyte function. Significant impact on clinical outcomes has yet to be demonstrated. Routine use of immunonutrition is not currently recommended.

THE IMPACT OF CRITICAL ILLNESS ON INFLAMMATION

The ICU practitioner must be aware of the profound immunologic effects of many of the therapies routinely used in the ICU. Catecholamines enhance (α receptors) or inhibit (β receptors) the immune response. Bactericidal antibiotics transiently exacerbate the

TABLE 62.5

Routine Preventive Regimens for Pediatric Hematopoietic Stem Cell Transplant Recipients

INFECTION	INDICATION	FIRST-LINE DRUG
Bacterial infections	Severe hypogammaglobulinemia (serum IgG level <400 mg/dL) at <100 d after transplant	IVIG 400 mg/kg/mo (or as needed to keep IgG level >400 mg/dL)
Candida species	Allogeneic recipients or high-risk autologous recipients from transplant to engraftment or until 7 d after ANC >1000 cells/mm³	Fluconazole 3–6 mg/kg/d PO or IV (6 mo–13 y); or 400 mg PO or IV daily (>13 y). Max dose 600 mg/d
Cytomegalovirus	All patients from engraftment through day 100	Ganciclovir 5 mg/kg/dose IV every 12 h for 5–7 d, followed by 5 mg/kg/dose IV daily for 5 d/wk
Pneumocystis jirovecii pneumonia	Allogeneic recipients or high-risk autologous recipients until 6 mo posttransplant (longer if immunosuppression continued or GVHD)	Trimethoprim/sulfamethoxazole (TMP/SMX; 150 mg TMP/750 mg SMX) PO twice daily 3 times weekly[a]
Herpes simplex virus	Seropositive patients from the beginning of conditioning therapy until engraftment	Acyclovir 250 mg/m²/dose IV every 8 h or 125 mg/m²/dose IV every 6 h
Varicella-zoster virus	Postexposure prophylaxis in actively immunosuppressed patients	Varicella-zoster immunoglobulin 125 units/10 kg body weight IM (max dose 625 units)
Methicillin-resistant *Staphylococcus aureus*	Known MRSA carriers	Mupirocin calcium ointment 2% to nares twice daily for 5 d or to wounds daily for 2 wk

[a]Adapted from Centers for Disease Control and Prevention; Infectious Disease Society of America; American Society of Blood and Marrow Transplantation. Guidelines for preventing opportunistic infections among hematopoietic stem cell transplant recipients. *MMWR Recomm Rep* 2000;49(RR-10):1–128.

Recommendations include vaccination against influenza, respiratory syncytial virus, *Streptococcus pneumoniae*, and *Haemophilus influenzae* type b.

ANC, absolute neutrophil count; GVHD, graft-versus-host disease; IM, intramuscularly; MRSA, methicillin-resistant *Staphylococcus aureus*; IVIG, intravenous immunoglobulin; PO, orally.

inflammatory response due to release of bacterial components at the time of cell death. Conversely, β-lactams lead to immunodeficiency through bone marrow suppression, while macrolides impair proinflammatory cytokine production. Opioids induce lymphocyte and macrophage apoptosis and can induce the anti-inflammatory cytokine TGF-β. Insulin has significant anti-inflammatory properties both through reduction of hyperglycemia-induced proinflammatory cytokine production and through direct inhibition of the NF-κB pathway. Even furosemide is immunologically active, resulting in attenuation of the inflammatory response in mononuclear cells. Red blood cell transfusion may be immunosuppressive as well, particularly in relation to long RBC storage times.

Concomitant organ failure and other conditions associated with critical illness further complicate the picture. Hepatic failure, with its associated impairment of cytokine clearance, is frequently associated with a proinflammatory state. Uremic plasma from patients with renal failure has been shown to induce apoptosis in innate and adaptive immune cells. As noted earlier, extracorporeal therapies, including hemodialysis and continuous venovenous hemofiltration, can promote the inflammatory state through immune reactions to plastic tubing and membranes.

CHAPTER 63 ■ IMMUNE DEFICIENCY DISORDERS

TRACY B. FAUSNIGHT, E. SCOTT HALSTEAD, SACHIN S. JOGAL, AND JENNIFER A. MCARTHUR

The intensivist should recognize the need of an immunologic workup for a child presenting with a second invasive bacterial infection, an opportunistic infection, or an infection poorly responsive to therapy. The pathogen and host response may indicate a cellular, phagocytic, or innate immune defect (**Table 63.1**).

DISORDERS PREDOMINANTLY AFFECTING IMMUNOGLOBULINS

Defects of antibody production and function comprise 65% of the congenital immunodeficiencies. Children with severe pneumonia poorly responsive to therapy deserve examination of immunoglobulin (IG) levels.

X-linked agammaglobulinemia (XLA) usually presents beyond 6 months of life due to persistent maternal IG. Presentation is typically at 2–5 years with recurrent and refractory sinopulmonary infections involving extracellular pyogenic bacteria (pneumococci, streptococci, meningococci, *Haemophilus influenzae*, and *Pseudomonas aeruginosa*). Fungal pathogens and *Pneumocystis jirovecii* are reported, and there is a unique susceptibility to enteroviral infections. Neutropenia is present at diagnosis in 25%. Mature B cells, plasma cells, and IGs are absent in the circulation or lymphoid tissue. IG levels are <10% of normal, and antigen-specific responses are absent. An early clue is a low total protein in the presence of a normal albumin level (gammaglobulin is the largest fraction of the total protein measurement). The diagnosis is supported by genotyping, but the absence of mature B cells with normal T-cell numbers is virtually diagnostic in a male. Therapy is intravenous immunoglobulin (IVIG) replacement, which helps control and clear severe infections. Despite IgG replacement, XLA patients can progress to bronchiectasis (prevented by chronic antibiotic therapy).

Common variable immunodeficiency (CVID) usually presents in the second decade, but ~20% present during childhood. Total IgG levels in CVID are <2 standard deviations below the mean for age, but not as low as in XLA. Like XLA, they present with recurrent sinopulmonary disease by encapsulated organisms. Malabsorptive symptoms suggest *Giardia lamblia* infection and autoimmune enteritis. Autoimmune cytopenia and other autoimmune manifestations are reported. Nearly half manifest mild cellular immune deficiency characterized by chronic viral and fungal infections. Impaired cellular immunity underlies the increase in malignancies. Mature B cells are detected by flow cytometry. Impaired vaccine responses (e.g., diphtheria and tetanus toxoid) are helpful in diagnosis. Treatment involves IVIG replacement. IgA-depleted products are required in IgA-deficient patients because of risk of anaphylaxis from anti-IgA antibodies. Patients with granulomatous disease have been treated with corticosteroids and etanercept after consideration of malignant and infectious etiologies.

Transient hypogammaglobulinemia of infancy can present in premature and, occasionally, term infants as an exaggerated hypogammaglobulinemia at the normal nadir of maternal IG at 6–9 months. Normal antigen responses are present. Normalization of IgG levels occurs between 2 and 4 years of age. Upper respiratory infections are common, and IVIG is rarely used to treat more invasive infections.

Hyper-IgM syndrome (HIGM) presents as hypogammaglobulinemia with normal to high IgM. The X-linked form accounts for 70% of cases. These males present in infancy with respiratory tract infections (interstitial pneumonitis from *P. jirovecii* in 40%). Diarrhea from *cryptosporidium* is common. Cytopenias, lymphoid hyperplasia, inflammatory bowel disease, and seronegative arthritis result from autoimmune T-cell dysfunction. Mortality from chronic liver disease and malignancy has justified trials of stem cell transplantation.

DISORDERS PREDOMINANTLY AFFECTING CELLULAR FUNCTION

T-cell defects affect either maturation of T cells or specific T-cell function. Dysgammaglobulinemia, as in the HIGM syndrome, results from T-cell dysfunction in the role of T-cell signaling in IG class switching and affinity maturation. The cardinal features of T-cell dysfunction are fungal infections, chronic viral infections, opportunistic infections, autoimmune disorders, and malignancies.

The *DiGeorge syndrome* (DGS) and *velocardiofacial syndrome* have a 22q11.2 deletion and manifest T-cell deficiency due to lack of thymic development. Genes

TABLE 63.1

Summary of Primary Immune Deficiency Disorders

CATEGORY	NAME	TYPE OF DEFICIENCY	GENE	PRIMARY ORGANISMS	USUAL SITES	TREATMENT	ASSOCIATED FINDINGS
Humoral	1. X-linked agammaglobulinemias	Absent or low levels of all immunoglobulins	BTK	Encapsulated bacteria, enteroviruses	Sinopulmonary, GI	IVIG/SCIG, antibiotics as needed	Respiratory failure, bronchiectasis, sepsis, diarrhea
	2. Common variable immunodeficiency	Low levels of IgG, ± low IgA, IgM	ICOS, TACI	Encapsulated bacteria	Sinopulmonary, GI	IVIG, antibiotics as needed	T-cell dysfunction, autoimmunity
	3. Transient hypogammaglobulinemia	Low levels of immunoglobulins until age 4 years	Unknown	Encapsulated bacteria	Sinopulmonary	None	None
	4. Hyper-IgM syndrome	Low levels of IgG and IgA, neutropenia	CD154, CD40, AICDA, UNG, NEMO	Encapsulated bacteria, PJP, *Cryptosporidium*	Sinopulmonary, lymph nodes, GI, liver	IVIG, antibiotics as needed, TMP-SMX	PJP, autoimmunity, chronic liver disease, cancer
Cellular	1. 22q11.2 deletion syndrome (DGS/velocardiofacial syndrome)	Thymic hypoplasia, absence of mature T cells	TBX 1	*Candida*, viruses, PJP	MM, skin, lung	Antifungals as needed, TMP–SMX, thymic transplant/HSCT?	Congenital heart disease, hypoparathyroidism, hypocalcemia
	2. IFN-γ–IL-12 axis	Decreased or absent IFN-γreceptor	IFNGR1, IFNGR2, IL12RB1	Mycobacteria, *Salmonella*, *Listeria*	Pulmonary, bone, lymph nodes	SC IFN-γ, antibiotics as needed, HSCT	None
Cytotoxic defects	1. Hemophagocytic lymphohistiocytosis	NK-cell and cytotoxic T-cell dysfunction	IL12B, PFR, MLNC13-4, STX 11	EBV, protozoa, bacteria	Blood/bone marrow, liver, CNS	Corticosteroids, cyclosporine A, etoposide, HSCT?	Fever, ↑triglycerides, ↓fibrinogen, ferritin
	2. Macrophage activation syndrome	IL-1 dysregulation?	MUNC13-4?	Nonspecific viruses or bacteria	Blood, liver, CNS	Corticosteroids, cyclosporine A, FFP	Juvenile idiopathic arthritis, systemic lupus erythematosus
Combined disorders	1. Severe combined immunodeficiency	Dysplastic thymus, low or absent levels of immunoglobulins, lymphopenia	IL2R gamma, JAK3, RAG1/2, ZAP-70, PNP, ADA, IL-7	Encapsulated bacteria, *Candida*, viruses, PJP	Sinopulmonary, MM, skin, liver, GI, blood	IVIG, TMP–SMX, antibiotics, antivirals, antifungals, HSCT, gene therapy?	Fatal without HSCT, enzyme replacement, or gene therapy
	2. Bare lymphocyte syndrome	Partial or complete absence of MHC class I or MHC class II on T cells	MHC Class I: unknown; MHC Class II: RFXANK, MHC2TA, RFX5, RFXAP	Encapsulated bacteria, *Candida*, viruses	Sinopulmonary, skin, GI	Antibiotics, HSCT?	Eczema, autoimmunity, lymphadenopathy

	3. Autoimmune lymphoproliferative syndrome	Elevated *a*/*b* double negative T cells	FAS, FASLG, CASPIO	None	Lymph nodes	Mycophenolate, sirolimus	Autoimmunity, malignancy
	4. Immune deficiency, polyendocrinopathy, X-linked	T-regulatory cell dysfunction	FoxP3	*Staphylococcus*, gram-negative bacteria, PJP, *Candida*, CMV	Sinopulmonary, MM, skin, GI	Steroids, sirolimus, antibiotics as needed, HSCT?	Growth failure, IDDM, eczema, rash, autoimmunity
	5. Autoimmune polyendocrinopathy–candidiasis–ectodermal dystrophy	T-cell anergy to candida antigen stimulation, variable B-cell defects	AIRE	*Candida*	MM, skin	Antifungals	Autoimmunity, hypoparathyroidism, Addison disease
	6. Wiskott–Aldrich syndrome	Low levels of IgM, elevated IgA, B- and T-cell dysfunction	WASP	Encapsulated bacteria, PJP, *Candida*, viruses	Sinopulmonary, MM, skin	IVIG, antibiotics as needed, HSCT	Eczema, bleeding, thrombocytopenia, HSM, malignancy, autoimmunity
	7. X-linked lymphoproliferative disorder	T- and B-cell dysfunction, low immunoglobulins	SH2D1A	EBV	Sinopulmonary, lymph nodes, liver	Rituximab or etoposide, acutely IVIG, HSCT	Lymphadenopathy, hepatic necrosis, HLH, malignancy
	8. Ataxia telangiectasia	Low levels of IgA and IgG_2, cutaneous anergy	ATM	Encapsulated bacteria	Sinopulmonary	IVIG, antibiotics as needed	Muscle weakness, ataxia, malignancy, telangiectasias
	9. Dedicator of cytokinesis 8 deficiency	Dysfunctional T-cell expansion, lymphopenia, B-cell dysfunction, elevated IgE	DOCK 8	*Staphylococcus aureus*, viruses (esp. herpes, HPV, molluscum)	Sinopulmonary, skin	Antibiotics, HSCT?	Eczema, severe allergies, asthma, malignancy
Neutropenia	1. Severe congenital neutropenia	Neutrophil maturation defect	ELANE?HAX1	Pyogenic bacteria	Skin, MM, lymph node, blood	GCSF	Agranulocytosis, MDS/AML
	2. Cyclic neutropenia	Neutrophil maturation defect	ELANE?	Pyogenic bacteria	Skin, MM, lymph node	GCSF	Periodic fevers, aphthous ulcers
	3. Primary autoimmune neutropenia	Antibody directed against neutrophil	Unknown	Pyogenic bacteria	Sinopulmonary, skin	Antibiotics, TMP–SMX, GCSF	URI, may resolve by age 3
	4. Shwachman–Diamond syndrome	Neutropenia, T-, B-, and NK-cell abnormalities	SBDS	Pyogenic bacteria	Sinopulmonary	GCSF, antibiotics as needed	Pancreatic insufficiency, leukemia, skeletal anomalies, pancytopenia, MDS
Neutrophil dysfunction	1. Neutrophil adhesion defects, LAD-1/LAD-2/LAD-3	Abnormal neutrophil migration	CD18/Sialyl-Lewis X, FERMT3	*Staphylococcus* species, gram-negative bacteria, fungi	Skin, lymph node, MM, liver, bone	Antimicrobials, HSCT, oral fucose—LAD-2	Gingivitis, impaired wound healing, UC separation delayed

(*continued*)

TABLE 63.1

Summary of Primary Immune Deficiency Disorders (*continued*)

CATEGORY	NAME	TYPE OF DEFICIENCY	GENE	PRIMARY ORGANISMS	USUAL SITES	TREATMENT	ASSOCIATED FINDINGS
	2. Hyper-IgE syndrome	Impaired chemotaxis, T- and B-cell dysfunction	Unknown	*Staphylococcus* species, *Streptococcus* species	Skin, lung (abscesses with pneumatoceles)	*Staphylococcus* prophylaxis, antibiotics as needed, IVIG?	Skeletal/connective tissue abnormalities, eczema, ↑eosinophils
	3. Chronic granulomatous disease	Oxidative burst and bactericidal activity impaired	gp91^{phox}, P22^{phox}, p47^{phox}	*Staphylococcus* species, catalase-positive bacteria, fungi	Sinopulmonary, lung, bone, liver, GI, skin, MM	Antifungal prophylaxis, TMP–SMX, IFN-γ, HSCT	Intestinal and bladder obstruction Osteomyelitis, liver abscesses
	4. Chediak–Higashi syndrome	Abnormal degranulation	LYST	Pyogenic bacteria	Sinopulmonary, Skin	Ascorbic acid, folate, antibiotics as needed	Bleeding, albinism, HLH, peripheral neuropathy
Complement	1. C1, C2, C3, C4	Low component levels	C1, C2, C3, C4	Encapsulated organisms	Skin, blood	Antibiotics as needed	Lupus-like syndrome
	2. C5–9	Absent membrane attack complex	C5–9	Meningococci	Blood, meninges	Vaccination, early antibiotic therapy	Recurrent meningitis
	3. Properdin deficiency	Unstable C3 and C5 convertases	PFC	Meningococci	Blood, meninges	Vaccination, early antibiotic therapy	Recurrent meningitis
	4. Mannan-binding lectin deficiency	Impaired MASP activation	MBL	Various bacteria	Sinopulmonary, meninges, blood	Antibiotics as needed	Autoimmunity, ↑SIRS/severity, Kawasaki disease?
	5. Mannan-binding lectin-associated serine protease 2 deficiency	Decreased MASP-2 levels	MASP-2	Various bacteria	Sinopulmonary, meninges, blood	Antibiotics as needed	↑Risk febrile neutropenia in cancer patients
	6. Hereditary angioedema	Low C4 and C1-INH	C1-INH	None	GI, upper respiratory tract, extremities	C1-INH replacement, kinin-pathway modulators, FFP	Abdominal crises, airway obstruction
Toll-like receptors	MYD88 serineprotease deficiency, IRAK-4 deficiency	Impaired TLR signaling	NEMO, IRAK-4	Gram-positive bacteria	Sinopulmonary, Blood	Antibiotics as needed	Recurrent sepsis

GI, gastrointestinal; SC, subcutaneous; NEMO, nuclear factor-κB essential modulator; PJP, *Pneumocystis jirovecii* pneumonia; MM, mucous membrane; TMP–SMX, trimethoprim–sulfamethoxazole; FFP, fresh frozen plasma; PNP, polynucleotide phosphorylase; HSM, hepatosplenomegaly; IDDM, insulin-dependent diabetes mellitus; SBDS, Shwachman–Bodian–Diamond syndrome; URI, upper respiratory infections; UC, umbilical cord.

within the deletion direct neural crest migration, and their absence results in conotruncal cardiac defects, parathyroid hypoplasia, and thymic hypoplasia. DGS occurs in patients with interrupted aortic arch type B (80%), persistent truncus arteriosus (35%), and tetralogy of Fallot (10%). The characteristic deletion is present in 90% of infants with the DiGeorge phenotype and a smaller percentage with the velocardiofacial phenotype. Most DGS infants are recognized as neonates due to heart defects or hypocalcemia. The clinical syndrome of cardiac defects, hypocalcemia, facial dysmorphology, and complete thymic absence (complete DiGeorge) occurs in no more than 5% of affected infants. The remainder has variable degrees of thymic hypoplasia, altered T-cell kinetics, and occasional increased susceptibility to infection. Minimal difficulties with bacterial infections are typical while a significant incidence of autoimmune disease is reported. Absolute CD3 counts <50 predict poor T-cell function and the need for immune reconstitution with either a thymic or hematopoietic stem cell transplant (HSCT). Spontaneous improvement in T-cell numbers and function has been documented, and serial T-cell counts are needed to distinguish complete DGS from delayed T-cell maturation. Infants with absolute CD3 counts <1500 at birth should receive *P. jirovecii* prophylaxis. Cytomegalovirus (CMV)-negative and irradiated blood products should be transfused to avoid risks of infection and graft-versus-host disease (GVHD). Perioperative corticosteroids may confound the diagnosis in infants requiring cardiac surgery, and flow cytometry should be repeated at 1 month of age.

IMMUNODEFICIENCY WITH CYTOTOXIC DEFECTS

Hemophagocytic lymphohistiocytosis (HLH) and *macrophage activation syndrome* (MAS) are disorders related to defective natural killer (NK) or cytotoxic T cells. They share diagnostic criteria, and their pathophysiology is characterized by uncontrolled inflammation. MAS is typically seen in patients with autoimmune disease and resolves with treatment of the autoimmune disorder. HLH requires more aggressive therapy, often including HSCT. HLH is divided into familial and acquired HLH, which are often indistinguishable. The familial form presents at <1 year of age in 70% of the cases, while the acquired form presents at any age. Familial forms of HLH may be associated with an immunodeficiency, most notably Chediak–Higashi syndrome, Griscelli syndrome type 2, and X-linked lymphoproliferative disease (XLP). Acquired HLH is associated with infection, malignancy, inborn errors of metabolism, and after HSCT. In HLH, the ongoing stimulation of NK cells and cytotoxic T lymphocytes produces high levels of inflammatory cytokines that activate the histiocytes that infiltrate tissues and cause clinical findings. Patients present with high, prolonged fevers and hepatosplenomegaly. Neurologic symptoms, a rash, and lymphadenopathy may occur. Infectious sources may or may not be found. Infections associated with HLH are viruses, especially Epstein–Barr virus (EBV). Bacteria and protozoa have also been described as triggers. Patients often rapidly deteriorate into a life-threatening illness if HLH is not diagnosed and treated promptly. The diagnosis of HLH can be made by a molecular diagnosis consistent with HLH or having 5 of 8 criteria that include fever, splenomegaly, cytopenia affecting ≥ 2 cell lines, hypertriglyceridemia and/or hypofibrinoginemia, hemophagocytosis, low or absent NK-cell activity, hyperferritinemia, or elevated soluble CD25 (IL-2R α chain). Patients with the most severe forms of HLH will not improve until treatment is initiated. Corticosteroids help decrease cytokine and chemokine production. Dexamethasone crosses the blood–brain barrier in patients with central nervous system (CNS) involvement. Cyclosporine A inhibits activation of T lymphocytes. Etoposide is toxic to monocytes and histiocytes. These three medications are the mainstay of therapy.

IMMUNODEFICIENCY WITH COMBINED ANTIBODY AND CELLULAR DEFECTS

Patients affected by combined immunodeficiencies (CIDs) manifest failure to thrive and recurrent infections with opportunistic pathogens, such as CMV, *Candida albicans* (thrush), and *P. jirovecii* pneumonia. *P. jirovecii* infection in an infant nearly always indicates a CID. Other common findings include chronic diarrhea, recurrent bacterial infections, and failure to clear adequately treated infections. Maternal–fetal or transfusion-acquired GVHD is an important concern in infants with CID.

Severe combined immunodeficiency (SCID) is the most severe in the spectrum of CIDs. Infants with SCID present in the first month of life with refractory oral candidiasis and persistent viral infections. *P. jirovecii* is a frequent cause of morbidity and mortality. Absolute lymphopenia <2000 cells/mm^3 is common, even on cord blood. Flow cytometry will indicate very low absolute CD3 or T-cell numbers. Maternal T-cell engraftment may affect the fetal T-cell population. T-cell–deficient, B-cell–present (T–B+) SCID is the largest subtype of SCID. *Omenn syndrome* is characterized by erythroderma, eosinophilia, lymphoid hyperplasia, and hypogammaglobulinemia. Metabolic defects in the purine salvage pathway do not spare NK cells, and thus, patients who present with *adenosine deaminase (ADA) deficiency* often have the most profound lymphopenia. In addition to ADA deficiency, several other immune-osseous syndromes combine skeletal abnormalities with variable degrees of CID, including short-limbed dwarfism with and without ectodermal dysplasia, cartilage hair hypoplasia, CID with metaphyseal dysplasia, and Schimke immune-osseous dysplasia. The intensive care of an infant suspected or known to have SCID should include strict isolation and the use of only irradiated, CMV-negative, and leukocyte-depleted blood products. The intensivist should maintain a high index of suspicion for *P. jirovecii* infection. Respiratory secretions and stool should be tested for a variety of pathogens. Infants with SCID may benefit from antiviral therapies in addition to antibiotics and IVIG. An immunologist or hematologist should be involved to facilitate HSCT, the most successful therapy for SCID. Survival rates of >90% are possible with HLA-matched sibling transplants, and haploidentical parent transplants are 75% successful.

Deficiencies in Apoptosis and Tolerance

Immune deficiency, polyendocrinopathy, X-linked syndrome (IPEX) is characterized by enteropathy, eczematoid rash, and early endocrinopathy (diabetes mellitus). Half the patients present prior to diagnosis with a serious infection (*Staphylococcus*, *Candida*, or CMV). Autoimmune cytopenias and splenomegaly are common. Sirolimus therapy is effective for the autoimmune manifestations. Survival beyond age 2 is unusual, although milder phenotypes have been reported. The value of HSCT for this disorder remains unclear.

Deficiencies in Activation and Differentiation

Wiskott–Aldrich syndrome (WAS) is an X-linked disorder with the classic triad of eczema, thrombocytopenia, and immunodeficiency. Boys present with bleeding in the first year of life, often bloody diarrhea or oozing from a circumcision. Platelets are small and defective in contrast to the large, functionally normal platelets in immune thrombocytopenic purpura. The intensivist must be cognizant of both the bleeding and infection risks. Infections involve encapsulated organisms related to the inability to produce antibodies in response to polysaccharide antigens. IgM levels are typically low. B-cell dysfunction is apparent early; T-cell dysfunction is progressive over time. Autoimmune phenomena are common due to T-cell dysfunction. IVIG therapy and splenectomy help maintain platelet counts and minimize infections but HSCT offers the best long-term survival.

XLP (Duncan disease) represents an abnormal immune response to EBV infection. Patients present with massive lymphadenopathy, hepatic necrosis, and bone marrow failure, like posttransplant lymphoproliferative disease. This presentation is responsible for the 70% mortality by age 10. The remaining 30% present late with varying degrees of immune deficiency. One-third of long-term survivors develop a lymphoreticular malignancy. Diagnosis is facilitated by positive EBV serology and blood or tissue polymerase chain reaction assays. Bone marrow indicates hemophagocytosis. Rapid diagnosis is made by flow cytometry. Etoposide and rituximab are useful in acute lymphoproliferation diagnosed prior to EBV exposure.

Ataxia telangiectasia presents with delayed ambulation and speech with deterioration of gross and fine motor skills. Cerebellar ataxia and oculocutaneous telangiectasias are evident around 7 years. Frequent pulmonary infections are related to subtle antibody defects or swallowing dysfunction and aspiration. Deficiencies in humoral and cellular immunity are reported. Median survival is 25 years, and mortality is frequently attributed to malignancy. The 10%–30% prevalence of malignancies is attributable to a defective DNA repair mechanism.

DISORDERS AFFECTING PHAGOCYTE FUNCTION

Neutrophil Disorders

Disorders of polymorphonuclear leukocytes, neutrophils, are uncommon. Neutrophils proliferate and mature in the bone marrow. During maturation they form granules containing bactericidal and hydrolytic proteins for killing pathogens. Once mature, they emigrate into the circulation where they undergo several complex processes. *Rolling* involves rolling loosely along the endothelial surface until they approximate a target. There, they flatten and bind tightly to the endothelial surface by *adhesion*. Finally, they migrate across the endothelium via *diapedesis*. For these processes to occur, the neutrophil must communicate with the endothelial surface through cell-surface proteins (e.g., selectins, integrin, intercellular adhesion molecule (ICAM)-1, and platelet endothelial cell adhesion molecule (PECAM)-1). Once through the endothelial membrane, the neutrophil is attracted to the pathogen by chemotactic factors (e.g., lipopolysaccharide (LPS), IL-1, TNF-α, and IFN-γ) via *chemotaxis*. The neutrophil then digests the pathogen through *opsonization* and *phagocytosis*. In opsonization, opsonins (such as IgG or C3b) bind to the pathogen and to receptors on the neutrophil (Fc receptors and complement receptors) allowing the neutrophil to phagocytose the pathogen. Neutrophil disorders present as either decreased numbers of neutrophils (neutropenia) or impaired neutrophil function. Neutrophil disorders are common with (a) positive family history, (b) young age, (c) deep-seated infections, (d) multiorgan involvement, (e) opportunistic infections, or (f) tissue granulomas of unknown etiology.

Disorders Associated with Primary Neutropenia

Severe congenital neutropenia (SCN) and *cyclic neutropenia* are inherited neutropenic disorders. Myeloid precursor cells in these conditions have an impaired response to hematopoietic growth factors but respond to granulocyte colony-stimulating factor (GCSF). This response to GCSF decreases the degree of neutropenia and the rate of serious infection.

Patients with SCN have profound neutropenia (an absolute neutrophil count [ANC] <500 neutrophils/m^3), and experience recurrent bacterial infections in the first year of life (commonly *Staphylococcus aureus* and *P. aeruginosa)*. SCN is characterized by a maturational failure of promyelocytes to myelocytes. The risk of death from sepsis is 0.9% per year and there is a significant risk of malignant transformation to MDS/AML. In patients at high risk of malignant transformation HSCT should be considered. *Cyclic neutropenia* is a rare AD disorder. Patients with cyclic neutropenia have recurrent episodes of severe neutropenia (lasting 3–6 days) in cycles of 14–36 days. These patients develop aphthous ulcers, gingivitis, stomatitis, and cellulitis and are at increased risk of mortality from serious infection. In contrast to severe SCN, these patients do not appear to be at increased risk for MDS/AML.

Autoimmune neutropenia may be primary or secondary. *Secondary autoimmune neutropenias* are associated with rheumatoid arthritis (Felty syndrome) and systemic lupus erythematosus (SLE). Often, these patients have thrombocytopenia and hemolytic anemia. Successful treatment of the underlying disease is the most effective therapy. *Primary autoimmune neutropenia* is diagnosed within the first months of life. Infants present with significant neutropenia, an ANC often <500–1000 neutrophils/m^3. Severe infections are uncommon (~10%), most infants present with otitis media, upper respiratory infections, and dermatitis. This disease resolves by 2–3 years of age. Testing for antibodies against neutrophils is often falsely negative, and repeat testing may be indicated. A direct granulocyte immunofluorescence test (D-GIFT) is more sensitive and may decrease the need for repeated testing. Treatment for a benign form is antibiotics as needed or antibiotic prophylaxis. For patients with serious infections, GCSF is first-line therapy. Corticosteroids and IVIG are not as beneficial as GCSF.

Disorders of Neutrophil Function

Leukocyte adhesion disorders exhibit neutrophils that are unable to bind to the endothelial surface, complete diapedesis, and migrate to the infection. Leukocyte adhesion deficiency type 1 (LAD-1) is an AR disorder in which neutrophils are unable to adhere and migrate to infection. Patients present with recurrent, severe infections (enteric gram-negative bacteria, *S. aureus*, *Candida*, and *Aspergillus* species) and may have delayed umbilical cord separation. These patients exhibit impaired wound healing. They have elevated neutrophil counts in the blood because their neutrophils are not able to marginate. LAD-2 patients have impaired fucose metabolism that interferes with leukocyte rolling along the vessel walls. Patients with this disorder are characterized by immunologic deficiencies as well as mental retardation, short stature, and distinctive facies. These patients may benefit from oral fucose therapy. LAD-3 patients have impaired activation of β-integrins. They have severe recurrent infections, bleeding tendency, leukocytosis, and occasionally bony defects similar to osteopetrosis. Treatment includes prophylactic antibiotics, blood transfusions, and HSCT.

Hyper-IgE syndrome (HIES, or *Job syndrome*) is characterized by recurrent staphylococcal infections, eczema, recurrent respiratory infections with pneumatoceles, elevated IgE levels, eosinophilia, abnormal cytokine and chemokine expression, and T-cell dysfunction. Neutrophil chemotaxis may be impaired. Treatment is antibiotic prophylaxis against staphylococcal infections; IVIG may benefit individual patients.

Defects of phagocytic function are associated with increased risk of infection. Neutrophils have Fcg receptors on their surface that bind IgG and signal the cell to phagocytose invading pathogens. Impaired phagocytosis has been detected in patients with severe meningococcal disease and may have implications for genetic screening and prophylactic immunization of family members of patients with severe meningococcal disease.

Chronic granulomatous disease (CGD) is a defect in intracellular killing caused by a mutation of the nicotinamide adenine dinucleotide phosphate (NADPH) oxidase apparatus. The defect in NADPH oxidase causes an inability to produce superoxide and impairs the killing of ingested microorganisms. It is inherited in an X-linked recessive or AR manner. The disease is characterized by recurrent infections of the skin, lungs, and liver and by excessive granuloma formation that can obstruct the gastrointestinal or genitourinary tract. Most infections are caused by *S. aureus*, *Burkholderia cepacia*, *Aspergillus* species, *Nocardia* species, and *Serratia marcescens*. *S. aureus* liver abscesses are highly indicative of CGD. Patients are most susceptible to catalase-positive microorganisms. This diagnosis is made by analyzing superoxide formation with nitroblue tetrazolium or by flow cytometry with dihydrorhodamine dye. Patients with CGD are commonly treated with prophylactic trimethoprim–sulfamethoxazole and itraconazole to prevent bacterial and fungal infections. IFN-γ therapy has also been found to be effective. HSCT has been curative; however, transplant-related complications require careful consideration. Two disorders in the differential include severe glucose-6-phosphate dehydrogenase deficiency and myeloperoxidase deficiency.

Disorders of neutrophil granules include *Chediak–Higashi syndrome*, an AR disorder of a protein involved with the formation and function of vacuoles. Their neutrophils have impaired chemotaxis and are characterized by large perinuclear granules. Elastase and cathepsin G may be absent from their neutrophil granules. Clinical features include recurrent bacterial infections, peripheral nerve disorders, mental retardation, autonomic dysfunction, partial albinism, silvery colored hair, and platelet dysfunction. Patients often die in the first decade of a lymphoproliferative process similar to HLH. Although HSCT prevents the lymphoproliferation, it does not prevent the neurologic sequelae. *Neutrophil-specific granular deficiency* is a rare autosomal disorder characterized by the absence of neutrophil granules. Patients have recurrent severe infections, particularly with *Staphylococcus aureus, Staphylococcus epidermidis,* and enteric bacteria. The neutrophils of these patients are not able to migrate to the site of infection and create suppuration and inflammation. Aggressive treatment with antibiotics and early surgical management are indicated. HSCT has been used successfully.

COMPLEMENT DEFICIENCY

The complement system is a key component of innate immunity. It may be activated by three pathways, all of which require activation of the complement protein C3 (**Fig. 63.1**). The *classical complement pathway* is activated by antigen–antibody complexes derived from acquired immunity. The *alternative complement pathway* is triggered by the recognition of pathogen-associated molecular patterns (PAMPs) on the surface of bacteria. Complement may also be activated by the *lectin pathway* beginning with the detection of bacterial surface carbohydrates (i.e., mannose) by mannan-binding lectin (MBL) protein, which induces MBL-activated serine proteases (MASPs) and activates the complement cascade. Complement C1, a complex macromolecule, initiates activation of the classical pathway and plays a significant role in host defense against pathogens. The C1q recognition protein mediates the binding of C1 to a target cell or molecule. The binding of C1 results in the subsequent activation of C4, C2, and ultimately C3. Of note, all three pathways of complement activation converge at C3 and lead to the formation of C3a and C5a and the *terminal membrane attack complex*, C5b–C9. Activated C3 is critical to opsonization. Activated C5 has numerous effects important in the pathogenesis of sepsis with C5b initiating formation of the terminal membrane attack complex. The terminal membrane attack complex lyses the cell membrane of the target cell. The classical pathway may be initiated without antigen–antibody complexes by the direct binding of bacteria, viruses, and apoptotic cells to C1q and subsequent activation of the cascade. The alternative complement pathway is critical to innate immunity and activates complement in the absence of antibody. C3 is again the pivotal component. Under normal physiologic conditions, C3 in the plasma is activated via slow hydrolysis and interaction with alternative pathway proteins. Once C3 is activated, the pathway progresses identical to the classical pathway (**Fig. 63.1**). Of note, the alternative pathway C3 convertase is highly unstable and requires properdin for stability. MBL initiates the lectin pathway. MBL recognizes specific carbohydrate sequences on the surface of microbes. Once bound to these surfaces, MBL activates two proteases: MASP-2 triggers the complement cascade by activating C4, while MASP-1 activates C3 directly.

Strict control of the complement system is essential to prevent complement-mediated destruction of host tissues. Many regulatory proteins function in this role. C1 esterase inhibitor (C1-INH) is a glycoprotein that recognizes and inactivates activated C1r and C1s. Because it is consumed during the process of inactivation, high levels of C1 inhibitor must be produced. Deficiency of C1-INH results in hereditary angioedema (HAE) (described later).

An increased susceptibility to invasive infection is a prominent feature of inherited complement deficiencies. The type of infection is associated with the deficient component. C3 deficiency increases the risk for encapsulated organisms: C3 is important for opsonization, a critical component of defense against encapsulated organisms. The terminal components, C5 through C9—the membrane attack complex, are responsible for bacterial lysis and death. Because C3 is not deficient, opsonization remains intact, and

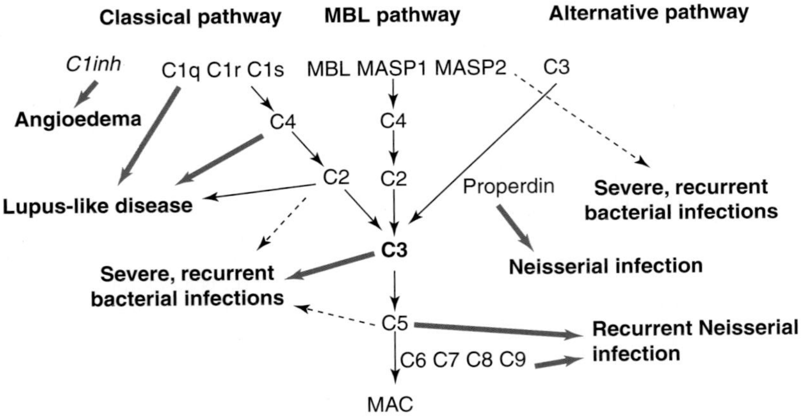

FIGURE 63.1. The figure depicts the complement components involved in activation of the three pathways of the complement cascade and consequences of specific deficiencies. MAC, membrane attack complex. (From Paul WE, ed. *Fundamental Immunology*, 7th ed. Philadelphia, PA: Lippincott Williams & Wilkins, 2013.)

terminal component deficient patients are not excessively susceptible to encapsulated bacteria. Instead, they display increased susceptibility to *Neisseria* infections in which bactericidal activity is critical. *Neisseria meningitides* is also the most common pathogen with *X-linked properdin deficiency*, the most common complement deficiency of the alternative pathway. These children may also present with unusual patterns of infection; meningococci considered avirulent may cause fulminant sepsis or meningitis. Infections from *Neisseria* serogroups W-135 and Y have been reported with increased frequency among patients deficient in the terminal components of the complement cascade. Vaccination against meningococcal disease may be important for these patients. These patients mount normal antibody responses to the tetravalent meningococcal vaccine.

Among critically ill patients, MBL deficiency not only appears to increase susceptibility to sepsis and septic shock but also may be associated with worse outcomes. In addition to sepsis, there are data suggesting that low MBL levels, as well as MBL variant genotypes, may be related to autoimmune disorders, such as SLE, rheumatoid arthritis, celiac disease, and inflammatory bowel disease. MBL deficiency has been associated with rejection among heart transplant recipients, atherosclerosis, myocardial infarction, recurrent spontaneous abortions, and other obstetric and gynecologic complications. Treatment for MBL deficiency is being investigated. The safety of infusing MBL, purified from donor plasma as well as clinical grade recombinant MBL, has been established in phase I trials. Clinical trials testing MBL reconstitution remain to be performed.

HAE is a rare AD disorder producing edema of skin, abdomen, or upper airway that can cause limb swelling, painful abdominal crises, and life-threatening airway obstruction. The edema may persist for up to 4 days. Approximately 50% of HAE patients have throat swelling; however, the edema involves the intestines more frequently than the larynx. HAE result from a deficiency in the C1 esterase inhibitor protein (C1-INH) due to a deletion, duplication, or mutation. HAE type I patients have a reduced level of C1-INH and type II have a dysfunctional C1-INH. Both also have a very low C4 level. Type I accounts for 80% of patients. Without treatment, the disease has a high mortality. Diagnosis may be delayed in the absence of a family history. A high index of suspicion is needed. A C4 level is the appropriate screening test. Analysis of both C1-INH level and function is used to establish the diagnosis. The critical care provider encounters HAE in the setting of laryngeal edema causing upper airway obstruction or with intestinal obstruction. Treatment options include plasma-derived C1-INH concentrate, kinin-pathway modulators, and fresh frozen plasma if C1-INH is not available. C1-INH concentrate infusion is the treatment of choice. In children with suspected HAE, *any* upper airway symptom merits treatment with C1-INH concentrate. When treating intestinal obstruction from HAE, failure of clinical improvement following C1-INH infusion warrants consideration of alternative diagnoses for the abdominal symptomatology.

INNATE IMMUNE SIGNALING DEFECTS

The innate immune system uses pattern recognition receptors (PRRs), such as toll-like receptors (TLRs), to detect microbial pathogens. TLRs are cell surface and intracellular PRRs that identify microbial invasion by recognizing PAMPs. The TLR–PAMP interaction triggers a complex signaling cascade that ultimately activates NF-κB and activated protein-1 (AP-1) and produces proinflammatory cytokines critical to the innate host defense. Many of the TLRs and IL-1Rs contain the intracellular Toll-IL-1R domain (TIR). This TIR domain recruits adaptor proteins, including MyD88 and TRIF proteins, which recruit cytosolic kinases, such as IL-1R–associated kinases (IRAKs). The canonical TIR pathway depends on MyD88. The IRAKs form a complex and activate both NF-κB and mitogen-activated protein kinases (MAPKs). Four primary immunodeficiencies associated with the canonical TIR MyD88-dependent pathway have been described. Two separate AR immunodeficiencies are caused by mutations in the *IRAK4* and *MyD88* genes. Neither mutation leads to any developmental abnormalities, and these children have increased susceptibility to infection, but primarily only to pyogenic, encapsulated, gram-positive bacteria (e.g., *Streptococcus pneumoniae* and *Staphylococcus aureus*). Their infections occur early in life, and the condition appears to improve with age, presumably because with age adaptive immunity maturation compensates for the innate immunodeficiency. *X-linked anhidrotic ectodermal dysplasia with immunodeficiency* presents with absent or conical teeth, decreased numbers of sweat glands and hypohidrosis, and sparse scalp and eyebrow hair due to abnormal ectoderm development. These children have increased susceptibility to a variety of severe infections and half die of overwhelming infection during childhood. An AD form has been reported that is caused by mutation of IκBα. This condition is phenotypically similar to the X-linked form but is more severe and include severe T-cell dysfunction. HSCT successfully treats the immunodeficiency but does not prevent the ectodermal dysplasia of the AD form.

IMMUNOLOGIC EFFECTS OF CANCER AND ITS TREATMENT

Most cancer patients are immunocompromised as a result of their disease or therapy. Many present with immunocompromise prior to receiving cytotoxic therapy. Acute leukemia often presents with pancytopenia, and leukemia and lymphoma patients have impaired neutrophil function. Sarcoma and lymphoma patients have reduced peripheral blood B and T-cell populations. Antineoplastic therapy further compromises immune function and increases the risk of severe infection. Neutropenia, loss of mucosal integrity, and T-cell dysfunction contribute to an increased susceptibility of invasive infections in pediatric cancer patients. Treatment-induced neutropenia is one of the most significant risk factors for severe infection among cancer patients. The more severe the neutropenia, both in number (ANC is <100 cells/mm^3) and duration (>1 week), the greater the risk of infection. The prompt return of neutrophils following cytotoxic therapy portends a favorable outcome even in the setting of a documented infection.

The impact of antineoplastic therapy on T-cell dysfunction is particularly detrimental. The regeneration of T cells is prolonged and incomplete. This means cancer patients are susceptible to viral, fungal, and parasitic infections long after the end of their therapy and neutrophil recovery. $CD4^+$ T-cell subpopulations are more severely depleted (relative to $CD8^+$) after receiving intensive chemotherapy regimens rendering these patients more susceptible to opportunistic infection. In addition, these patients have increased susceptibility to bacterial infections, including *Legionella, Listeria, Salmonella, Mycobacterium tuberculosis*, and atypical mycobacteria. T-cell dysfunction also increases the risk of EBV-associated lymphoproliferative disorder and posttransfusion GVHD. Protracted intensive chemotherapy or allogeneic HSCT have the highest risk of complications related to T-cell deficiency states.

IMMUNE DYSFUNCTION ASSOCIATED WITH HEMATOPOIETIC STEM CELL TRANSPLANT

Immunosuppression is severe during allogeneic HSCT. The near-complete replacement of the host lymphohematopoietic system requires intense immunosuppression. HSCT patients remain profoundly immunocompromised until effective immune reconstitution occurs. Complete immune reconstitution is a complex and prolonged process that may require years despite early neutrophil engraftment. Children differ from adults in that the thymus enhances the kinetic and functional recovery of adaptive immunity in the pediatric transplant patient. This results in improved recovery of $CD4^+$ T-cell levels, which is associated with a decreased risk of opportunistic infection following HSCT engraftment. Children also have a lower incidence of GVHD compared to adults. GVHD impedes immune restoration and requires further immunosuppressive therapy. Immune reconstitution following HSCT is influenced by patient-, disease-, and transplant-related factors. These factors include patient age, underlying disease, disease status, transplant type (autologous vs. allogeneic), preparative regimen, the presence of infection, HLA compatibility, GVHD, and the stem cell source, mobilization, and manipulation techniques.

Innate Immunity Recovery

NK cells are one of the initial lymphoid cells to recover following HSCT. They play crucial roles in direct and antibody-dependent cytotoxicity of infected and tumor cells. They protect against viral infections (particularly CMV) and GVHD, as well as increasing the graft-versus-leukemia (GVL) effect. Functional recovery occurs simultaneously with the return of NK cellularity.

Granulocytes and monocytes also recover early in the posttransplant period with neutrophil recovery preceding that of monocytes and tissue macrophages. Grafts with more differentiated precursors allow quicker recovery of these subsets. Recovery in cellularity does not correspond with functional recovery, and impaired bactericidal activity for 2 months following allogeneic HSCT places the child at risk of pyogenic infection.

Dendritic cells play an important part in immune function after allogeneic bone marrow transplantation. Dendritic cells reconstitute to pretransplant levels within 2 months but take up to 1 year to recover to levels of healthy individuals. Like neutrophil recovery, manipulations in the stem cell source appear to influence the speed of dendritic cell recovery. Early dendritic cell recovery may protect the transplant recipient against infection. Low levels of dendritic cells are associated with an increased risk of relapse, acute GVHD, and death.

Adaptive Immunity Recovery

Early post-HSCT, host plasma cells that survive the preparative regimen produce IgG. Progenitor cells from the allograft produce naïve B cells yielding IgM 4–6 months after transplant. Isotype switching for production of IgG requires $CD4^+$ T-helper cells and occurs later. IgG levels may remain abnormal for up to 1 year. Severe acute GVHD and chronic extensive GVHD are associated with reduced B cells and $CD4^+$ T-helper cells. In general, B-cell recovery tends to occur before T-cell reconstitution. The type of transplant may affect reconstitution of cells. Lymphocyte subset populations are higher after allogeneic peripheral blood stem cell transplant (PBSCT) than bone marrow transplant. There is a decreased risk of severe infections (especially fungal) in patients receiving PBSCT.

T-cell reconstitution occurs via two pathways. A thymic-independent pathway termed homeostatic peripheral expansion (HPE) involves the expansion of mature T cells that either survived preparative regimens, were contained within the allograft, or were given via donor lymphocyte infusion. These T cells are quantitatively and qualitatively deficient and are not active for antigens absent at expansion. This impedes responses against microbes and tumor cells. Recovery of thymic function provides the optimal pathway for T-cell reconstitution. Unfortunately, thymic recovery takes several months following allogeneic HSCT. Thymic recovery is hampered by age-related decrements in thymic function, as well as by cytotoxic-, radiation-, and GVHD-induced thymic injury. GVHD is particularly detrimental to immune reconstitution. It is directly toxic to the thymic microenvironment and impairs negative selection of T cells that react to host antigens. This combination not only decreases thymic function and recovery, but fosters further GVHD. By causing widespread apoptosis, GVHD limits the effectiveness of HPE, thereby hindering thymic-independent immune restoration. Both GHVD and the immunosuppression used to treat it impede immune reconstitution after HSCT.

CHAPTER 64 ■ BACTERIAL SEPSIS

NEAL J. THOMAS, ROBERT F. TAMBURRO, SURENDER RAJASEKARAN, JULIE C. FITZGERALD, SCOTT L. WEISS, AND MARK W. HALL

Bacterial sepsis is a common reason for children to require intensive care, and worldwide, sepsis-related illnesses are the most common cause of death in infants. In developed countries, great progress has been made and the majority of children survive sepsis. An International Consensus has provided pediatric-specific definitions for SIRS, sepsis, severe sepsis, and septic shock (**Table 64.1**).

Upper and lower limits of these four systemic inflammatory response syndrome (SIRS) criteria for the six specific age groups were also established (**Table 64.2**).

Bacterial sepsis is a worldwide problem, with mortality at ~6%–10% for all age groups. The most common sites of infection in children are respiratory, blood, genitourinary, abdominal, device-related, soft tissue, and central nervous system (CNS). The bacterial pathogens that cause severe sepsis vary by age, institution, and presence of underlying risk factors (e.g., immune compromise, vascular catheter, and immunization status). Gram-positive bacteria (*Staphylococcus* and *Streptococcus* species) are the most prevalent organisms, while gram-negative bacteria (*Escherichia coli*, *Klebsiella* species, and *Pseudomonas*

TABLE 64.1

Definitions of Systemic Inflammatory Response Syndrome, Infection, Sepsis, Severe Sepsis, and Septic Shock in Children

SIRS
The presence of at least two of the following four criteria (one must be abnormal temperature or leukocyte count): 1. Core temperature of >38.5°C or <36°C 2. Tachycardia (mean heart rate > 2 SD above normal for age) in the absence of external stimulus, chronic drugs, or painful stimuli; OR otherwise unexplained persistent elevation over a 0.5- to 4-h period; OR for children <1 y old: bradycardia (mean heart rate < 10th percentile for age) (in the absence of external vagal stimulus, β-blocker drugs, or congenital heart disease or otherwise unexplained persistent depression) over a 0.5-h period 3. Mean respiratory rate > 2 SD above normal for age or mechanical ventilation for an acute process (not related to underlying neuromuscular disease or the receipt of general anesthesia) 4. Leukocyte count elevated or depressed for age (not secondary to chemotherapy-induced leukopenia) or >10% immature neutrophils
Infection
A suspected or proven (by positive culture, tissue stain, or polymerase chain reaction test) infection caused by any pathogen OR a clinical syndrome associated with a high probability of infection. Evidence of infection includes positive findings on clinical exam, imaging, or laboratory tests (e.g., white blood cells in a normally sterile body fluid, perforated viscus, chest X-ray consistent with pneumonia, petechial or purpuric rash, or purpura fulminans)
Sepsis
SIRS in the presence of, or as a result of, suspected or proven infection
Severe Sepsis
Sepsis plus one of the following: cardiovascular organ dysfunction OR acute respiratory distress syndrome OR two or more other organ dysfunctions
Septic Shock
Sepsis and cardiovascular organ dysfunction

From Goldstein B, Giroir B, Randolph A; International Consensus Conference on Pediatric Sepsis. International pediatric sepsis consensus conference: Definitions for sepsis and organ dysfunction in pediatrics. *Pediatr Crit Care Med* 2005;6:2–8, with permission.

TABLE 64.2

Age-Specific Vital Signs and Laboratory Variables

AGE GROUP	HEART RATE, (Beats/min) TACHYCARDIA	HEART RATE, (Beats/min) BRADYCARDIA	RESPIRATORY RATE, (Breaths/min)	LEUKOCYTE COUNT × (10^3/mm)	SYSTOLIC BLOOD PRESSURE (mm HG)
0 d–1 wk	>180	<100	>50	>34	<59
1 wk–1 mo	>180	<100	>40	>19.5 or <5	<79
1 mo–1 y	>180	<90	>34	>17.5 or <5	<75
2–5 y	>140	NA	>22	>15.5 or <6	<74
6–12 y	>130	NA	>18	>13.5 or <4.5	<83
13 to <18 y	>110	NA	>14	>11 or <4.5	<90

Lower values for heart rate, leukocyte count, and systolic blood pressure are for the 5th and upper values for heart rate, respiration rate, or leukocyte count are for the 95th percentile.
From Goldstein B, Giroir B, Randolph A; International Consensus Conference on Pediatric Sepsis. International pediatric sepsis consensus conference: Definitions for sepsis and organ dysfunction in pediatrics. Pediatr Crit Care Med 2005;6:2–8, with permission.

aeruginosa) are also common (especially in neonates, neutropenic patients, and hospital-acquired sepsis). A microbial pathogen is not isolated in up to 75% of children with sepsis. This "culture-negative" sepsis may indicate a host response to bacterial components, insufficient sensitivity of diagnostic testing, or antibiotic treatment before obtaining cultures.

Streptococcus agalactiae (group B *Streptococcus*), *E. coli*, *Listeria monocytogenes*, *Enterococcus*, non–group D α-hemolytic streptococci, and nontypeable *Haemophilus influenzae* are associated with neonatal sepsis. *Staphylococcus* is currently the most common infecting organism among neonates (90% due to coagulase-negative *Staphylococcus*, *S. aureus*—10%). *P. aeruginosa*, gram-negative enteric bacteria, and environmental bacilli cause neonatal hospital-acquired sepsis. Low birth weight is a risk factor for sepsis, and respiratory and cardiovascular diseases are common underlying conditions in newborns.

In older children, *S. aureus* and *Streptococcus* species are most common. Sepsis associated with a thrombophlebitis occurs with *Fusobacterium necrophorum*. Primary bacteremia without a focal source is uncommon in older children. Sepsis due to *H. influenzae* type b (Hib), *Streptococcus pneumoniae*, and *Neisseria meningitidis* has decreased due to the vaccines for these bacteria. Rickettsial infections can also manifest as sepsis (*Rickettsia rickettsiae* causes Rocky Mountain spotted fever and may resemble meningococcemia). Human ehrlichioses can be mistaken for Rocky Mountain spotted fever.

Comorbidities that depress immunity (e.g., malignancies, renal failure, hepatic failure, HIV/AIDS, and immunosuppression) are common among patients with severe sepsis or septic shock. Certain conditions predispose to specific bacterial infections (**Table 64.3**). Patients with febrile neutropenia get typical gram-positive and gram-negative infections, but unusual pathogens include *Streptococcus viridians*, *P. aeruginosa*, *Enterobacter*, *Citrobacter*, and *Acinetobacter* species, and *Stenotrophomonas maltophilia*. In sickle cell disease and functional asplenia, *S. pneumoniae* and other encapsulated bacteria (*Salmonella*) are commonly identified. In catheter-associated bloodstream infections, coagulase-negative *Staphylococcus*, *P. aeruginosa*, *E. coli*, *Klebsiella* species, and *Enterobacter* are commonly isolated. Lastly, certain foods are linked with pathogens (**Table 64.4**).

TABLE 64.3

Clinical Conditions That Predispose the Host to Specific Bacteria

CONDITION	BACTERIA
Asplenia, polysplenia	*Streptococcus pneumoniae* *Salmonella*
Sickle cell disease	*Streptococcus pneumoniae* *Salmonella*
Nephrotic syndrome	*Streptococcus pneumoniae*
HIV/AIDS	*Streptococcus pneumoniae* *Haemophilus influenzae* type b *Staphylococcus aureus* *Pseudomonas aeruginosa*
Complement deficiencies (C5, C6, C7, C8, C9)	*Neisseria meningitidis* *Neisseria gonorrhoeae*
Iron overload	*Yersinia enterocolitica* *Listeria monocytogenes* *Vibrio vulnificus*
Neutropenia	*Streptococcus viridans*

HIV, human immunodeficiency virus; AIDS, acquired immune deficiency syndrome.

TABLE 64.4

Environmental Conditions That Predispose the Host to Specific Bacteria

■ ORGANISM	■ ENVIRONMENTAL SOURCE
Listeria monocytogenes	Food, especially dairy and pork products
Enterococcus faecium	Commercial chicken and meat products
Clostridium perfringens	Soil
Salmonella	Poultry, pork, beef, egg, and dairy products
Yersinia	Pork, chitterlings (pork intestines), and dairy products
Vibrio vulnificus	Seawater and undercooked seafood (clams, oysters, and mussels)

Viruses (e.g., influenza, adenovirus, and dengue) may cause sepsis syndrome. The presence of bacterial coinfection (particularly methicillin-resistant *Staphylococcus aureus* [MRSA]) should be suspected in a viral infection and severe sepsis. Secondary bacterial pneumonia due to *Staphylococcus aureus*, *Streptococcus pneumoniae*, nontypeable *H. influenzae*, and *Moraxella catarrhalis* can follow infection with respiratory syncytial virus (RSV) or other respiratory viruses.

The prevalence of antibiotic resistance is increasing. Multidrug-resistant organisms include MRSA, β-lactam-resistant and multidrug-resistant *pneumococci*, vancomycin-resistant *enterococci*, extended-spectrum β-lactamase-producing gram-negative enteric pathogens, and carbapenem-resistant *Pseudomonas*. Local resistance patterns need to be considered when selecting empiric therapy.

MECHANISM OF DISEASE: CORE PATHOPHYSIOLOGY

Host Risk Factors

Genetic Predisposition

Genetic composition influences the risk of developing sepsis and outcome. Death from infection has a stronger heritable component than death from cancer or cardiovascular disease. The effects of polymorphisms and epigenetic changes on the inflammatory response to infection are complex and multifactorial. Translating these findings into clinically relevant information remains a challenge.

Race/Ethnicity/Gender/Age Differences

Race, ethnicity, gender, and age may influence the incidence and outcomes from sepsis. African-American adults are more likely to be hospitalized for severe sepsis than are Caucasians. The racial influence on mortality is less clear. Less is known about this in pediatrics, but a worse sepsis outcome occurs among African-American newborns.

A higher incidence of severe sepsis is seen in males. Potential explanations in postpubertal males and females include differences in hormones, comorbidities, the infectious etiology, and health-related behaviors (including time to seek medical care). Humoral and cell-mediated immune responses to antigen challenge are enhanced in females. Hormones of the endocrine system, including sex steroids, contribute to the difference in immunologic response between the genders.

Age influences the incidence and outcome of sepsis. Infants demonstrate the highest sepsis-related mortality, with a case-fatality rate twice that of children over 1 year. Very-low-birth-weight infants have the highest sepsis-related case-fatality rate of all age groups.

Comorbidities

An underlying comorbidity is reported in ~40% of septic children (>60% if prematurity is included). In infants, chronic lung disease and congenital heart disease are the most common comorbidities. Neuromuscular disorders and neoplasms are the most common in children >1 year of age. Case-fatality rates among septic children with a comorbid condition are higher.

Environmental Risk Factors

Sepsis can result from exposures from the environment, medical devices, and procedures. Healthcare-associated infections (HAIs) are a large source of morbidity and create a high cost.

Central Venous Lines

Central line-associated bloodstream infections (CLABSIs) are preventable rather than inevitable. Approximately half are due to coagulase-negative *Staphylococcus* and *Enterococcus* species, followed by *Candida*, *S. aureus*, and then gram-negative organisms (*K. pneumoniae*, *Enterobacter* species, *P. aeruginosa*, *E. coli*, and others). Factors that increase risk include the very young, the chronically ill, poor nutritional status, loss of skin integrity, and neutropenia. Specific risk factors for CLABSI in the pediatric intensive care unit (PICU) include parenteral nutrition, presence of a gastrostomy tube, duration of central venous access, use of alteplase, and repair of broken catheters. Use of chlorhexidine skin baths, antibiotic-impregnated catheters, regular assessment of catheter need, and compliance audits can help decrease CLABSI rates.

Urosepsis

Longer duration of urinary catheterization is the largest risk for catheter-associated urinary tract infection (CAUTI) in critically ill children. Closed-system urinary catheters are colonized within 30 days, and open systems much sooner. Higher rates of infection are associated with diarrhea, low urine flow, and urinary stasis. The most common bacteria are *E. coli*, other gram-negative bacilli, *Enterococcus*, and *Candida*.

Hemodialysis

Arteriovenous fistulas are at risk for contamination with each dialysis run. *S. aureus* causes most dialysis graft infections. Tunneled catheters carry a higher risk of infection than arteriovenous fistula.

Surgical-Site Infections

Surgical-site infections (SSIs) account for ~15% of all nosocomial infections. Risk factors include younger age, contaminated procedure, surgery > 2 hours, an abdominal or thoracic procedure, and presence of a urinary catheter. The frequency and microbiology differ by procedure. *S. aureus* and coagulase-negative *Staphylococcus* account for a majority of pediatric SSIs.

Osteomyelitis

Nonhematogenous osteomyelitis is uncommon but associated with open fractures, fascial infections, implanted devices, and chronic open ulcers. *S. aureus* is the typical pathogen, but enteric gram-negative organisms and anaerobic bacteria can infect exposed bone. Osteomyelitis is a rare complication of intraosseous line use. Bone biopsy with culture is the definitive method for diagnosis of osteomyelitis.

Endocarditis

Preexisting congenital heart disease is the most common risk factor for endocarditis. Endocarditis within 2 months of cardiac surgery is a consequence of thrombi forming at a surgical site. Sites can become infected with bacteria introduced via the bypass pump, from a surgical wound infection, secondary to a catheter-associated infection, or from an exposed pacemaker wire. *S. aureus* and viridans *Streptococci* are responsible for the majority of cases. Fungi are increasingly important.

CLINICAL PRESENTATION AND DIFFERENTIAL DIAGNOSIS

Clinical Presentation

Severe sepsis denotes decreased tissue and organ perfusion on physical examination. The clinical presentation depends on the timing of infection, the organism responsible, and the patient's previous state of health. The classic signs include change in temperature (hyperthermia or hypothermia), tachypnea, tachycardia, and change in mental status. Children can have severe sepsis or septic shock without hypotension, as compensatory vasoconstrictive mechanisms are potent (often at the expense of cardiac function and distal perfusion).

Septic shock is usually a combination of distributive, hypovolemic, and cardiogenic shock. Septic shock includes manifestations of decreased organ perfusion (change in mental status, decreased urine output, delayed capillary refill, increased base deficit, or increased serum lactate). Usually, a compensatory respiratory alkalosis occurs in the face of metabolic acidosis unless pulmonary edema, pneumonia, or acute respiratory distress syndrome interferes. Altered mental status may be accompanied by seizures if the decrease in cerebral perfusion is severe. Renal and hepatic injury may occur. Hematologic failure includes disseminated intravascular coagulation (DIC), thrombocytopenia (purpura or petechiae), or bone marrow failure.

Hemodynamic Data

Abnormal vital signs are defined by age (**Table 64.2**). Tachycardia is common and maintained variability is encouraging. Bradycardia may signify severe infection and be a near-terminal event. Hypotension is not required (due to compensation). Decreased central venous oxyhemoglobin saturation ($Scvo_2$) can be due to decreased cardiac output or increased metabolism. Increased $Scvo_2$ can be due to mitochondrial dysfunction (tissue dysoxia) and decreased oxygen consumption. Sepsis presentation in children is different than in adults. Children may present with the classic adult picture of "warm," vasodilated shock (increased cardiac output and decreased systemic vascular resistance) but most present with "cold" shock (decreased cardiac output and increased systemic vascular resistance). The phenotype may change during their course of sepsis, and therapies may have to be adjusted.

Laboratory Abnormalities

Sepsis induced accelerated energy use can lead to increased free fatty acids, hyperglycemia, and protein catabolism. An elevated lactate indicates cellular injury or transition to anaerobic metabolism. Leukocytosis occurs due to demargination, increased production, and release from bone marrow of polymorphonuclear cells (PMNs). Neutropenia can develop from bone marrow failure or peripheral consumption of PMNs attached to endothelial cells and ensnared in capillaries. Platelet count can be decreased due to peripheral consumption or increased as a result of reactive thrombocytosis. Serum levels of albumin, prealbumin, transferrin, and retinol-binding protein may fall, as a result of decreased production or capillary leak. Anemia can be due to underproduction of red blood cells, hemolysis from endothelial damage and microcirculatory changes, or resuscitation-related hemodilution. Coagulation abnormalities include decreased fibrinogen, factors V or VIII, protein C, and antithrombin levels, while tissue factor is increased. Patients with DIC will have prolonged prothrombin and partial thromboplastin times, fibrin degradation products present, elevated D-dimer (most specific) and microangiopathic changes on peripheral smear.

Differential Diagnosis

Other Infectious Diseases

Candidemia in premature infants is associated with immunocompromised status, receipt of parenteral nutrition, presence of central venous catheter, and exposure to broad-spectrum antibiotics. Viruses can be indistinguishable from a bacterial process in young infants, especially herpes simplex and the TORCH complex (toxoplasma, rubella, cytomegalovirus, and herpes simplex virus) agents. Varicella, primary herpes simplex, adenovirus, influenza, and respiratory syncytial virus can cause life-threatening infections in children (especially if immunocompromised or history of extreme prematurity).

Noninfectious Diseases

Severe Kawasaki disease, Stevens–Johnson syndrome, drug reactions, juvenile rheumatoid arthritis, pancreatitis, hemophagocytic lymphohistiocytosis, myocarditis, systemic lupus erythematosus, and antibody or cytokine treatment for malignancy can all masquerade as sepsis or be complicated by superimposed bacterial sepsis.

Diagnosis

Procurement of bacterial cultures should include blood, and potentially cerebrospinal fluid (CSF), urine, respiratory secretions, pleural fluid, skin lesions, vaginal specimens, synovial fluid, or peritoneal fluid. Blood cultures should be obtained from all lumens of indwelling central venous catheters as well as percutaneously. It is preferable to obtain cultures prior to antimicrobial agents, but treatment should not be delayed for a critically ill child while waiting to obtain cultures. Empiric broad-spectrum antibiotics should be administered within 1 hour of presentation. Obtaining the recommended amount of blood per culture is important (1–2 mL in neonates, 2–3 mL in infants, 3–5 mL in children, and 10–20 mL in adolescents).

For nonbacterial pathogens, other diagnostic testing (e.g., viral culture, polymerase chain reaction [PCR], rapid immunoassay antigen test, or direct immunofluorescent antibody staining) may help establish the source. Viral cultures can be obtained from conjunctiva, nasopharynx, urethra, vagina, and vesicles or ulcers on skin and mucous membranes. Blood and CSF can be sent for viral culture, but specific PCR assays are more sensitive. PCR-based tests are particularly useful to detect herpes simplex, enteroviruses, Epstein–Barr virus, cytomegalovirus, and respiratory viruses (e.g., influenza, RSV, adenovirus, parainfluenza, human metapneumovirus). Ordinary blood cultures are often sufficient for the detection of fungemia (alert your microbiology laboratory for concern of fungal infection as special media or incubation conditions can improve recovery). Adjunctive tests for fungal disease include galactomannan and β-D-glucan. Galactomannan is recommended when concern for invasive aspergillosis is high.

White blood cell count, immature PMNs ("bands"), and C-reactive protein may be informative but are neither sensitive nor specific for bacterial sepsis. Procalcitonin, a precursor to calcitonin, is upregulated in the presence of bacterial and fungal disease to a greater degree than in viral or noninfectious inflammatory states. There is potential for procalcitonin detection to be used to determine length of therapy.

CLINICAL MANAGEMENT/ TREATMENT

Importance of Early Intervention

The first hours represent the opportunity to reverse shock and prevent or attenuate organ dysfunction. Fluid resuscitation with >40 mL/kg (average 60 mL/kg) in the first hour confers a survival advantage to children with septic shock. Administration of antibiotics should not take precedence over resuscitation, but shorter time to correct empiric antibiotics improves outcome. A de-escalating use of empiric antimicrobial agents should be adopted, with broad-spectrum agents used initially. Empiric antibiotic therapy must cover community-acquired or nosocomial pathogens and account for regional, hospital, and unit-specific resistance patterns.

Guidelines for Early Clinical Management

A detailed algorithm with a rigorous timeline for the clinical practice parameters for hemodynamic support of pediatric and neonatal patients in septic shock is provided (**Fig. 64.1**). Within the first 5 minutes, the airway and breathing should be maintained and IV access established. Continuous and frequent vital sign assessment is necessary. Isotonic fluid boluses should be administered IV in 20 mL/kg aliquots up to and over 60 mL/kg in the next *15 minutes* if the shock state is not reversed. If shock persists despite fluid, then arterial and central venous access is obtained and a dopamine infusion initiated. Initiation of inotropic support should be via peripheral IV access until central access is obtained. If shock is not reversed, the transition is to an epinephrine infusion for vasoconstrictive (cold) shock or central norepinephrine for vasodilatory (warm) shock. Titration of inotropic or vasopressor support should be based upon frequent reassessment of the child's hemodynamic state.

Should either type of shock state persist despite vasoactive therapy, hydrocortisone is used for empiric treatment of adrenal insufficiency. Adrenal insufficiency can develop due to inhibitory effects of proinflammatory cytokines. A short course of low-dose hydrocortisone may improve mortality and rapidly reverse shock. Hydrocortisone has less glucocorticoid effect and more mineralocorticoid effect than methylprednisolone or dexamethasone. Risk factors that favor the use of hydrocortisone include prior corticosteroid use, purpura fulminans, HIV infection, chronic pituitary

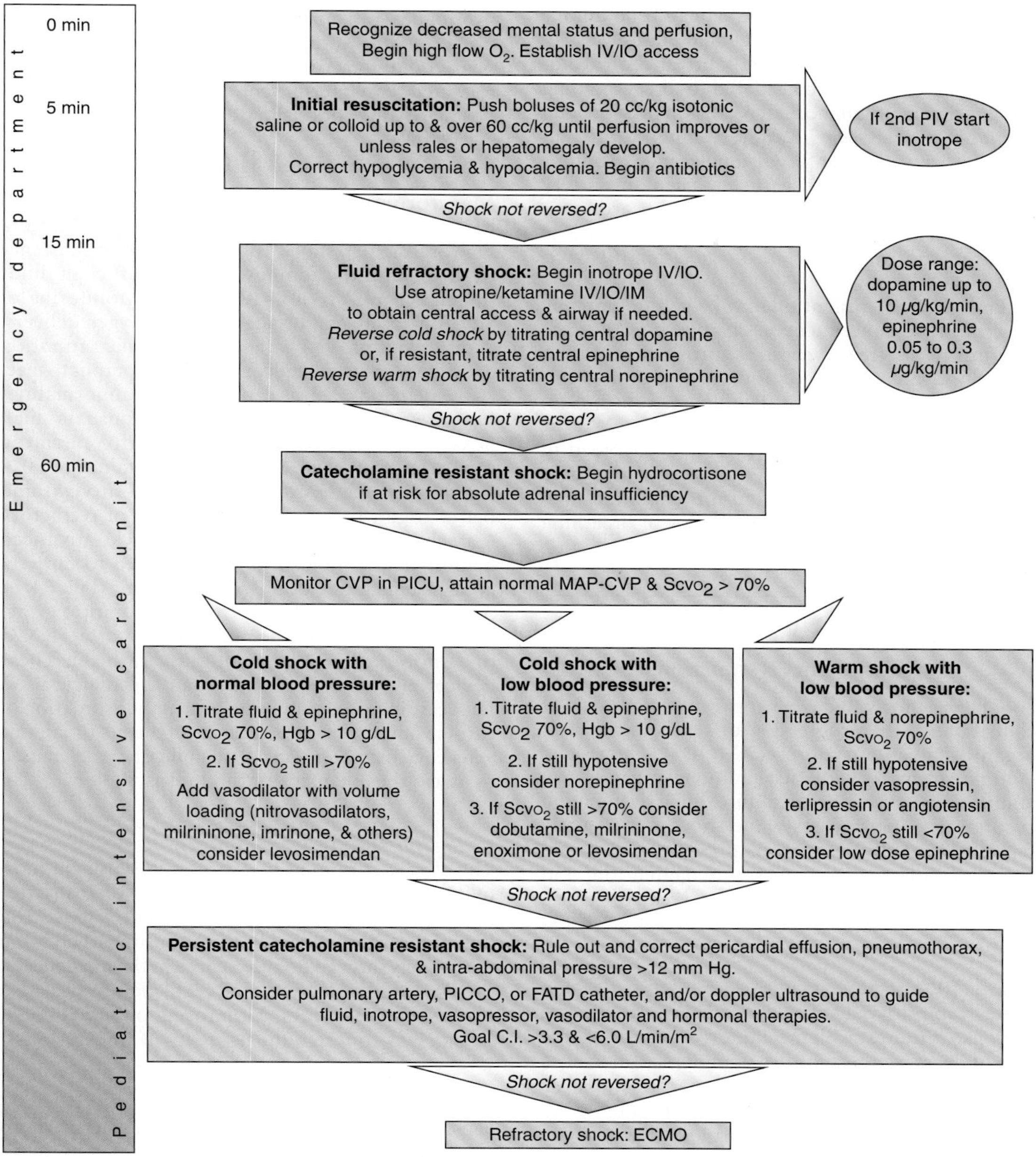

FIGURE 64.1. Algorithm for time-sensitive, goal-directed stepwise management of hemodynamic support in infants and children. (Reproduced from Brierley J, Carcillo J, Choong K, et al. Clinical practice parameters for hemodynamic support of pediatric and neonatal septic shock: 2007 update from the American College of Critical Care Medicine. *Crit Care Med* 2009;37:666–88.)

or adrenal abnormalities, a basal cortisol level of <18 μg/dL, a peak ACTH-stimulated cortisol concentration of <18 μg/dL, or catecholamine-resistant shock. A loading dose of 2 mg/kg is followed by maintenance dosing, either every 6 hours or as a continuous infusion, with a total daily dose of 2 mg/kg reached *within 60 minutes* of the diagnosis of shock.

Should shock continue in the second hour of resuscitation, patients with normal blood pressure, cold shock, and $Svo_2 < 70\%$ should be treated with afterload reduction with careful attention to preservation of preload. Children with low blood pressure, cold shock, and $Svo_2 < 70\%$ should be treated with titration of epinephrine and ongoing optimization of volume status. Refractory shock despite volume loading and first-line cardiovascular medications may require a second-line agent (milrinone in the volume-loaded cold shock, and vasopressin in the warm shock patient). Levosimendan and enoximone represent options outside the United States.

Should these maneuvers fail, advanced cardiovascular monitoring is considered to direct ongoing therapy and maintain normal perfusion pressure and cardiac index between 3.3 and 6 L/min/m^2 (e.g., pulmonary artery catheter [PAC], a pulse index contour cardiac output [PiCCO] catheter, a femoral artery thermodilution catheter, or Doppler echocardiography). A final recommendation is to consider the use of extracorporeal membrane oxygenation (ECMO) as a rescue therapy.

Endotracheal intubation may be helpful but may have negative consequences. Positive intrathoracic pressure may decrease venous return, cardiac output, and blood pressure. Sedation for intubation can cause vasodilation and cardiac depression. Etomidate impairs cortisol production with a single dose, increases mortality risk, and should be avoided in favor of ketamine. Supplemental oxygen will help reverse oxygen supply–demand mismatch and mechanical ventilation can offload work of breathing and redirect cardiac output to vital organs.

Subacute Management

Multiorgan Dysfunction

Poor perfusion, hypoxia, hyperglycemia, and acidosis contribute to the progression of sepsis to multiple organ dysfunction syndrome (MODS). The risk of mortality increases with each additional organ system failure and severity of each failure. Lung dysfunction occurs early and persists while shock occurs early but either rapidly resolves or progresses to death. Abnormalities of liver function, coagulation, and CNS function occur within hours and tend to persist.

Ventilation Strategies

Nearly 50% of patients with severe sepsis develop acute respiratory distress syndrome (ARDS). The response requires a high minute ventilation in the face of decreased respiratory compliance, increased airway resistance, decreased diffusion, and impaired muscle efficiency. There is a benefit of a high positive end-expiratory pressure and low-tidal-volume (lung protective) approach. The goal is to maintain oxygenation with an inspired gas (FIO_2) below 0.6, and allow hypercapnia with pH > 7.25.

Renal Replacement Therapy

Acute kidney injury (AKI) during severe sepsis portends a poor prognosis and mortality. Sepsis, with MODS and fluid overload $> 20\%$ at the time of continuous renal replacement therapy (CRRT) initiation has increased mortality. Hemofiltration can clear mediators of inflammation, treat fluid overload, and may be beneficial in sepsis even without AKI. CRRT should be considered for fluid removal after shock resuscitation for patients who are $>10\%$ fluid overloaded and unable to achieve fluid balance with urine output. In the hemodynamically unstable patient, continuous venovenous hemofiltration is better tolerated than intermittent hemodialysis. On CRRT dosing of antibiotics should be reassessed.

Cardiac Monitoring

Monitoring the central venous pressure (CVP) helps assess the adequacy of fluid resuscitation. Fluid-refractory shock is defined as the persistence of shock after the administration of sufficient fluids to achieve a CVP of 8–12 mm Hg. Monitoring of $ScvO_2$ helps assess the adequacy of oxygen delivery. A difference of $>30\%$ between systemic saturation and $ScvO_2$ suggests inadequate cardiac output to meet tissue demands. Sepsis can also cause abnormalities in oxygen utilization that result in unusually high $ScvO_2$. Early goal-directed therapy for pediatric septic shock in which $ScvO_2$ was maintained at 70% for the first 72 hours had improved survival and better organ function. In the setting of refractory (catecholamine-resistant) septic shock, advanced hemodynamic monitoring can be used to target a goal cardiac index of 3.3–6.0 L/min/m^2 (**Fig. 64.1**). Alternatives to the PAC for the quantitation of hemodynamic variables include the use of a PiCCO or femoral artery thermodilution catheter. These devices are potentially safer than a pediatric PAC. Echocardiography can be helpful in the estimation of cardiac output. Ultrasound measurements of inferior vena cava diameter and collapsibility have been used to assess the adequacy of fluid resuscitation.

Transfusion

The efficacy of blood transfusion in sepsis on mortality is controversial. A comparison of a restrictive transfusion threshold of hemoglobin 7 g/dL to a liberal threshold of 9 g/dL in a subgroup of children with sepsis showed no differences in the incidence of MODS, duration of mechanical ventilation, oxygenation indices, and ICU days. Monitoring of $ScvO_2$ might be one way to weigh the necessity of transfusions.

Nutrition

Sepsis promotes a catabolic state and negative nitrogen balance (accentuated by exogenous steroids). Enteral nutrition reduces villous atrophy, intestinal permeability, gut translocation, and septic complications. Early enteral feeding of critically ill children on vasoactive drugs and mechanical ventilation is feasible and may be well tolerated. Patients with sepsis on vasopressors and narcotics often have gastroparesis and may benefit from transpyloric feeding (a shorter time interval to full-strength feeds and a decreased incidence of nosocomial pneumonia). If critically ill patients are not expected to be feeding by mouth within 3 days, enteral nutrition should be commenced. Enteral feeding advantages include gastric pH buffering, avoidance of parenteral-nutrition catheters, a physiologic pattern of enteric hormone secretion, administration of a complete nutritional mixture (including fiber), and lower costs.

Glycemic Control

Hyperglycemia during sepsis may be related to hypoinsulinemia or insulin resistance. Tight glycemic control may improve white blood cell function, phagocytosis, and suppress the acute-phase response. The utility of tight glycemic control is unclear in septic children. Children are more prone to hypoglycemia so insulin therapy should be used cautiously.

Source Control of Infection

Source control includes the drainage of infected fluid collections, debridement of infected tissue, and removal of infected devices or foreign bodies. The length of time to bacterial growth and colony count often determine if a catheter is the infectious source. If bacteremia persists with appropriate antibiotics, the catheter should be removed. Deep abscesses can be drained surgically or using interventional radiology services. Necrotizing soft-tissue infections require immediate surgical debridement.

Other Therapies for Acute Management of Sepsis

Treatments aimed at attenuating the inflammatory response have been studied as adjunctive therapy. Activated protein C (APC) and anti-cytokine therapy failed to show benefit. Extracorporeal therapies (e.g., hemofiltration, plasmapheresis, and plasma exchange) represent another approach to restore inflammatory homeostasis. Plasma exchange offers the advantage of replacement of depleted plasma proteins. Data from small trials suggest a survival benefit in the setting of thrombocytopenia-associated multiple organ failure. The benefit of IVIG is unclear and it is not a part of pediatric sepsis treatment, with the exception of toxic shock syndrome.

PREVENTION OF SEPSIS

Healthcare-Associated Infections

Healthcare-associated infections (HAI) occur during a hospitalization when no evidence for that infection was present at admission. HAIs include bloodstream infections (e.g., CLABSI), ventilator-associated pneumonia and tracheitis (VAP and VAT), urinary tract infections (e.g., CAUTI), and SSI. Prevention of HAI is discussed in Chapter 69.

High-Risk Patient Populations

Burns

Improved resuscitation of burn victims has reduced early death from shock but with an increase in late mortality from infection. Burn patients are predisposed to sepsis due to: (a) global decrease in cellular immune function; (b) neutropenia, depressed neutrophil function, and altered T-cell transcription; (c) increased gut permeability; and (d) bacteremia with wound manipulations.

Trauma

Traumatically injured children are at risk for nosocomial and injury-related infections (wound, intra-abdominal, and CNS).

Human Immunodeficiency Virus

HIV-infected children are at increased risk of viral, bacterial, and fungal sepsis, with increased mortality. The use of highly active antiretroviral therapy (HAART) has decreased the progression to acquired immune deficiency syndrome, prevalence of complications (sepsis), and mortality.

Asplenia

Congenital or acquired (e.g., sickle cell disease or splenectomy) asplenia increases the risk of bacterial sepsis (particularly due to encapsulated organisms). Vaccination and prophylactic antibiotics are used to prevent pneumococcal, meningococcal, and Hib disease.

Cancer and Hematopoietic Stem-Cell Transplantation

Children with neoplasia account for nearly 13%–17% of severe sepsis cases. However, oncology patients should not be considered a homogeneous group. Leukemia/lymphoma patients receive more intensive myeloablative therapy than patients with solid tumors. Neutropenia and bone marrow transplantation increase the incidence of (and risk of death from) sepsis.

Prophylaxis

The use of prophylactic antibiotics has been categorized into three major indications: (a) postexposure, (b) periprocedure, and (c) prevention in high-risk populations. Postexposure antibiotics are recommended for specific pathogens (*N. meningitidis*) or following a procedure (when the period of risk is defined and brief, the expected pathogens have predictable antimicrobial susceptibilities, and the site is accessible to antimicrobial agents). The use of antibiotics to prevent bacterial endocarditis is an example of periprocedure prophylaxis. The third category prevents infection in specific high-risk patient populations (asplenic child). *Selective decontamination* to alter oral or gut flora to reduce nosocomial infections remains controversial.

CHAPTER 65 ■ PRINCIPLES OF ANTIMICROBIAL THERAPY

CHERYL L. SARGEL, TODD J. KARSIES, LULU JIN, AND KEVIN B. SPICER

Appropriate empiric antibiotic use is essential in critically ill patients with infection. Inappropriate or delayed empiric antibiotic administration for bacteremia or septic shock is associated with increased mortality. Antimicrobials also account for many commonly seen drug-associated adverse events (rash, anaphylaxis, organ injury [renal or hepatic impairment], and drug–drug interactions). Other complications include antibiotic-associated diarrhea/colitis, superinfection with drug-resistant bacteria or fungi, perturbation of the resident microbiome that impacts susceptibility to later infections, and antimicrobial resistance. Antibiotic-resistance has made empiric antibiotic selection more challenging. Risk factors for antibiotic resistance include recent hospitalization, antibiotic exposure, immunosuppression (due to disease or medications), and chronic structural lung disease. To decrease emergence of antibiotic resistance, some centers use broad coverage in high-risk patients and narrow coverage for low-risk patients.

Knowledge of unit and community microbiology is needed to develop an empiric strategy. Initial combination antibiotic therapy is one strategy to prevent the emergence of resistance. To ensure coverage of resistant gram-negative organisms, an antipseudomonal β-lactam or carbapenem is combined with an aminoglycoside (AG) rather than fluoroquinolone. Once a pathogen is identified, de-escalation to monotherapy appears safe, provided there is clinical improvement. Another strategy is antibiotic heterogeneity (e.g., cycling), the rotation of empiric antibiotics where it is either restricted or preferred. A final strategy focuses on the use of shorter antibiotic courses for infections (e.g., using biomarkers to shorten treatment courses).

Another important question is whether antibiotics can be de-escalated after identification of a viral pathogen. In critically ill children with respiratory syncytial virus (RSV) bronchiolitis requiring mechanical ventilation, coinfection with bacterial pathogens occurs in 40%–50% of cases. *S. aureus* is also frequently seen in patients with influenza requiring ICU admission. For children requiring intubation, culturing the lower respiratory tract and providing empiric coverage until culture results are available is a reasonable strategy.

Once the pathogen and susceptibilities are known, antimicrobials should be targeted with a spectrum as narrow as possible. If cultures remain negative at 48–72 hours, the patient who has improved could have therapy de-escalated with observation for worsening. Rapid improvement in inflammatory markers (e.g., procalcitonin, C-reactive protein [CRP]) supports de-escalation. A short duration of therapy (e.g., 5 days) may be sufficient, although for sepsis and septic shock, duration of 7–10 days may be appropriate. The culture-negative patient whose condition is not improved is problematic. One should consider de-escalation in a stepwise approach and limiting the duration of therapy. Consideration of noninfectious etiologies should also occur. In the patient showing deterioration, repeat cultures, expand laboratory or radiographic work-up, engage consultants, review trends of inflammatory markers, and consider escalation of antimicrobial therapy or starting empiric antifungal therapy. It is vital to suspect new nosocomial infection, remember source control (e.g., drainable abscess), and ensure appropriate dosing.

Laboratory markers of infection have shown promise in guiding decisions. CRP shows overlap in bacterial, viral, and fungal infections. Absolute values are less helpful than trends. Decreasing CRP levels allows more confidence in discontinuation of antimicrobial therapy. Procalcitonin may be elevated in bacterial infection and in noninfectious conditions, but levels have been shown to safely reduce antibiotic use.

PHYSIOLOGIC CHANGES IN CRITICALLY ILL PATIENTS—IMPACT ON DOSING

Drug metabolism and elimination are affected by large fluid volume administration, extracorporeal support, drains, plasmapheresis, renal replacement therapies, end-organ dysfunction, and obesity. Changes in volume of distribution (Vd) and clearance (CL) alter the plasma concentration of antimicrobials. Capillary leak lowers plasma levels of hydrophilic drugs (e.g., AGs, β-lactams, glycopeptides, lipopeptides, echinocandins, fluconazole, acyclovir, ganciclovir). Extracorporeal circuits (e.g., ECMO) alter pharmacokinetics by circuit binding, increased Vd, and decreased drug elimination. Lipophilic and highly protein-bound drugs (e.g., voriconazole, fluoroquinolones) are sequestered in the circuit, while hydrophilic drugs (e.g., β-lactams, AGs) are affected by hemodilution.

Drug levels should be monitored, if available. Plasmapheresis removes drugs that are in the plasma and not sequestered within cells or tissues. The amount of drug removed is influenced by the duration of the procedure, the volume of plasma removed, and the frequency of plasmapheresis. Drugs with a low Vd (<0.2 L/kg) and/or a high degree of protein binding (>80%) are likely to be removed and include ampicillin, ceftriaxone (variable), AGs, vancomycin (variable), and teicoplanin. Postsurgical drains lead to antimicrobial loss and may require increased dosing and frequent drug levels.

Renal Function

Renal function assessment involves using serum creatinine as an indirect measure of glomerular filtration rate (GFR). Patients with lower-than-expected muscle mass are at risk for overestimation of GFR using creatinine. Cystatin C may be superior because production is independent of sex, body size, or age; however, laboratory assays have not been standardized. Direct measurement of GFR involves administering a known quantity of a marker that is filtered by the kidney and using levels to calculate the elimination rate. For patients requiring renal replacement therapy (RRT), any residual kidney function may contribute to drug clearance. Serum creatinine is unsuitable as a marker as it will be cleared by RRT. Patients on intermittent hemodialysis (IHD) should have drug doses timed at the end of their IHD sessions or have a supplemental dose given after IHD. With peritoneal dialysis (PD), changes in dwell time, number of cycles per day, and dextrose concentration may all affect drug removal rate. For an AG or vancomycin, frequent drug levels may be helpful. Reference manuals and literature searches may offer some guidance for specific drugs.

Liver Function

Hepatic metabolism occurs in as many as 70% of current antibiotics. Patients on potentially hepatotoxic medications should have liver function test (LFT) screening. Vd can be affected due to diminished protein synthesis. Bilirubin has a high affinity for albumin, may displace protein-bound drugs, may increase free (active) fractions, and has an increased risk of toxicity. Ascites and third-spacing will increase the Vd for water-soluble drugs. The more severe the liver injury, the more it affects drug metabolism. Phase I reactions (oxidation [i.e., P450 reactions], reduction, hydrolysis) are affected more than phase II reactions (glucuronidation, sulfation, glutathione conjugation, acetylation, methylation).

Obesity

Obesity can alter both the Vd and CL of antimicrobials. Drug absorption is not modified by obesity, but drug distribution into tissue is dependent on body composition, blood flow, drug lipophilicity, and plasma protein binding. For weight-based antimicrobials, the maximum dose for children should not exceed maximum adult dosing. Acyclovir dosing is based on ideal body weight (IBW). AGs are dosed by adjusted body weight in patients weighing >120% of their IBW or >95% body mass index. Liposomal amphotericin distributes into fat more readily than other formulations. Adjusting doses based on serum levels is optimal when possible.

APPLICATION OF PHARMACOKINETICS–PHARMACODYNAMICS TO ANTIBIOTIC THERAPEUTICS

Antibiotic treatment requires integration of the disposition characteristics (i.e., pharmacokinetics [PK]) with an understanding of the clinical activity (i.e., pharmacodynamics [PD]). Crucial pharmacodynamic variables that are linked to microbiologic effect are time-dependent versus concentration-dependent and bacteriostatic versus bactericidal activities of different antibiotics (**Fig. 65.1A**).

Time Dependency

The activity of time-dependent antibiotics is driven by the relationship between the concentration achieved at the site of the infection relative to the minimum inhibitory concentration (MIC). The MIC is the lowest concentration of antibiotic that hinders the growth of bacteria. There are two groups of time-dependent antibiotics: those that lack a postantibiotic effect (PAE) and those that display a moderate PAE. The PAE prevents bacterial growth for a short time when antibiotic concentrations fall below the MIC. In time-dependent antibiotics with no PAE, the target PK/PD parameter is maximizing time > MIC. Antibiotics in this group include penicillins, carbapenems, cephalosporins, erythromycin, and linezolid. Increased drug concentration beyond the MIC does not increase killing; however, maximizing the duration of time above the MIC will. For time-dependent drugs with a moderate PAE, the target PK/PD goal is to maximize the daily area under the curve (AUC)/MIC. This represents the ratio of the integral of the drug concentration over time above MIC. A larger AUC can be achieved with an increased peak concentration (C_{max}) or longer time above MIC. Antibiotics in this group include azithromycin, clindamycin, vancomycin, and tetracyclines.

Concentration Dependency

The activity of concentration-dependent antibiotics is also driven by the relationship between the

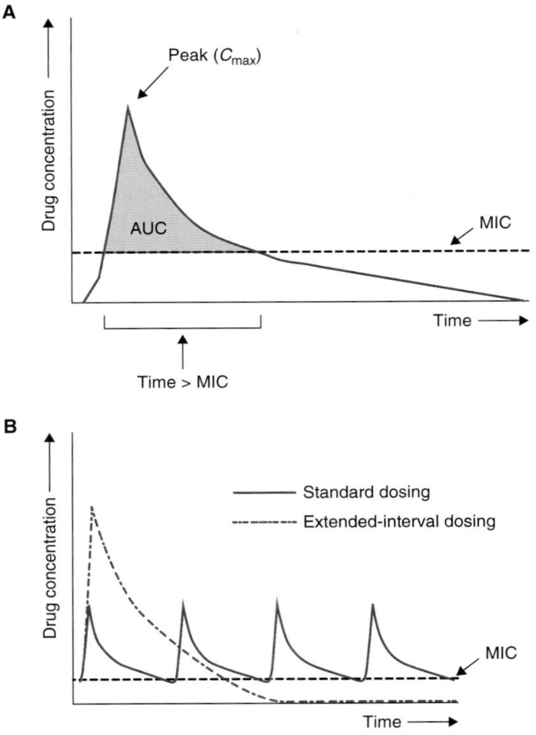

FIGURE 65.1. Pharmacokinetic/pharmacodynamic factors affecting antibiotic potency. **A:** Bacterial killing may be time-dependent (time with drug concentration > MIC), concentration-dependent (C_{max}/MIC), or both (AUC/MIC). **B:** Extended-interval dosing can be used with some antibiotics, though prolonged periods of time without detectable drug levels (>8 hours) should be avoided.

concentration achieved at the site of infection relative to the MIC. Antimicrobials in this group include the AGs, fluoroquinolones, daptomycin, ketolides, and amphotericin. In some, killing correlates with peak serum concentration (C_{max})/MIC (e.g., AGs); in others (e.g., fluoroquinolones and azithromycin), the effect is correlated with AUC/MIC. All concentration-dependent antibiotics are slowly bactericidal and demonstrate a PAE.

Bacteriostatic/Bactericidal Properties

Antibiotics are bactericidal if they kill bacteria, or bacteriostatic if they slow the growth or reproduction of bacteria. At high concentrations, bacteriostatic agents are often bactericidal against some organisms.

Continuous Infusion versus Standard/Bolus Dosing

Continuous infusion of time-dependent antibiotics allows consistent steady-state concentrations and maximizes time > MIC. Some β-lactams are not stable at room conditions for long enough to allow for extended infusion, and additional vascular access may be needed for incompatibilities with other drugs. There is no advantage of infusions of β-lactams. Bolus dosing prior to the start of the infusion is important to achieve target concentrations early.

Extended-Interval Aminoglycoside Dosing

AGs display concentration-dependent killing and a reliable PAE. Giving a larger dose increases the C_{max} and optimizes the C_{max}/MIC ratio and the bactericidal activity (**Fig. 65.1B**). Longer intervals between doses allow greater time for drug elimination and decrease the risk of toxicity (associated with elevated trough concentrations). Extended-interval aminoglycoside dosing (EIAD) (giving total daily dose every 24 hours) improves the efficacy and safety of AGs. It is recommended to not exceed an 8-hour duration without detectable drug levels. EIAD may not be appropriate with renal failure, extensive burns, obesity, ascites, or in meningitis, osteomyelitis, persistent bacteremia, or endocarditis.

ANTIBACTERIAL AGENTS

β-Lactams

The β-lactams include penicillins, cephalosporins, monobactams, and carbapenems. They inhibit bacterial cell wall synthesis using the penicillin-binding protein (PBP). PBPs are expressed during cell division; so they only affect dividing bacteria. Resistance mechanisms include β-lactamases, alterations in PBPs, and changes in cell membrane permeability. *Group 1* ("AmpC") β-lactamases hydrolyze all β-lactams except carbapenems and are resistant to clavulanate. They are encoded on the *amp*C sequence in *P. aeruginosa*, *Enterobacter cloacae*, *Serratia marcescens*, *Citrobacter freundii*, and *Morganella morganii*. *Group 2 β-lactamases* are encoded on plasmids, include extended-spectrum β-lactamases (ESBLs), and are prevalent in *Klebsiella* and *E. coli*. Both β-lactamases are promoted by, and resistant to, third-generation cephalosporins, and reliable treatment is with a carbapenem. *Alteration of PBPs* occurs on penicillin-resistant *Streptococcus pneumoniae*, MRSA, and hospital-acquired coagulase-negative staphylococci. In mildly penicillin-resistant pneumococcus, cure is achieved with high doses of β-lactam (plus vancomycin in meningitis). The β-lactam resistance in MRSA and coagulase-negative staphylococci is high grade and requires an alternative class of drug. Transport across the outer membrane in gram-negative bacteria is necessary for β-lactams to reach the target PBP and occurs through channels created by porins. A change in porin channels infers β-lactam resistance in *Pseudomonas* spp.

β-Lactams have a broad range of antimicrobial activity, are bactericidal in dividing cells (in *Enterococcus* spp., they are bacteriostatic), and display time-dependent killing. Most β-lactams undergo little metabolism and are renally excreted (except oxacillin and nafcillin). Dose adjustment in renal insufficiency and during dialysis is likely to be needed. Drug level monitoring is not available.

Penicillins

Penicillins contain β-lactam and thiazolidine rings with various side chains are attached. The penicillins bind to PBP on the bacterial cell wall, inhibit synthesis of the bacterial peptidoglycan, and cause cell wall breakdown and cell death. The emergence of penicillin resistance among *S. aureus* due to β-lactamase (a penicillinase) stimulated development of the penicillinase-resistant penicillins (e.g., nafcillin).

Penicillin G has a narrow spectrum, covering most *Streptococcus* species. Drug modifications have led to the aminopenicillins with enhanced gram-negative coverage (e.g., ampicillin), antistaphylococcal penicillins (e.g., nafcillin), and antipseudomonal penicillins (e.g., ticarcillin, piperacillin). The combination of these drugs with a β-lactamase inhibitor (e.g., sulbactam or clavulanate) allows for enhanced coverage of anaerobes and some staphylococci.

The penicillins vary markedly in biodisposition. Many are not well absorbed and are administered parenterally. Protein binding varies markedly from 17% for ampicillin to >90% for nafcillin. Few undergo significant metabolism, although some display hepatic elimination. Most excretion is renal, employing both glomerular filtration and tubular secretion. Significant developmental changes occur in elimination during the first year of life, and doses need to be adjusted according to the patient's age or renal function. Virtually all of the parenteral penicillins penetrate into the CSF in concentrations that are adequate to treat meningitis when meningeal inflammation is present. In the absence of inflammation, very little penetration occurs.

Adverse events are rare and varied. Allergy to penicillins is manifest by maculopapular rash, urticarial rash, fever, bronchospasm, vasculitis, serum sickness, exfoliative dermatitis, Stevens–Johnson syndrome, or anaphylaxis. Other β-lactam agents can often be substituted for penicillin with a low risk of cross-reactivity. If allergy is potentially severe or life-threatening or susceptibility patterns do not permit substitution, desensitization can be performed. Other adverse events are rare and include thrombocytopenia, eosinophilia, and a positive Coombs reaction. Inhibition of platelet aggregation can occur, although clinically significant bleeding is rare. Additional adverse effects include interstitial nephritis; electrolyte abnormalities (especially sodium and potassium); and bone marrow suppression, particularly neutropenia, observed with prolonged use. Seizures are a possibility with massive overdoses or accumulation due to renal insufficiency. Changes in GI flora can lead to diarrhea, pseudomembranous colitis, and *C. difficile* infection.

Few drug–drug interactions are reported with penicillins. Probenecid competes with penicillins for renal tubular secretion, and prolongs the elimination half-life of penicillin or ampicillin. Antipseudomonal and extended-spectrum penicillins interact in vitro with AGs, causing AG degradation (resulting in falsely low drug levels).

Cephalosporins

The cephalosporins also bind to PBP on the bacterial cell wall. They contain modifications that make them more resistant to penicillinases, create modified pharmacokinetic properties, and alter antimicrobial activity. Bacterial resistance to cephalosporins has been described by the same three mechanisms as penicillins.

Cephalosporins are classified by generation. Earlier generations have better gram-positive coverage, with improving gram-negative coverage, loss of some gram-positive coverage, and less susceptibility to β-lactamases as generations escalate. Cefepime (fourth generation) has excellent gram-negative, and antipseudomonal coverage, and regains gram-positive coverage. Ceftaroline (fifth generation) extends cefepime's coverage, by including MRSA and *Enterococcus* spp. coverage. Currently available cephalosporins do not have reliable activity against enterococci, coagulase-negative staphylococci, MRSA (with the exception of ceftaroline), *Listeria monocytogenes*, and *S. maltophilia*.

The cephalosporins vary in biodisposition with patient age and agent. Dosage must be adjusted on the basis of renal function. Only third- and fourth-generation agents penetrate into CSF enough to treat bacterial meningitis. Ceftriaxone is not recommended in neonates due to protein binding and bilirubin displacement. Few cephalosporins undergo significant metabolism, and most are renally excreted. Several third-generation agents have biliary excretion and are used to treat hepatobiliary infections (e.g., cefoperazone and ceftriaxone).

Gastrointestinal conditions are the most common adverse side effects. Allergic reactions occur in 1%–3% of patients, less frequently than with penicillins. The cross-reactivity in patients with documented penicillin allergy is higher than the general population, but is likely to be safe. Less common adverse reactions include positive Coombs reactions, hemolytic anemia, bone marrow suppression, thrombocytosis, acute tubular necrosis, inhibition of platelet aggregation, and mild transaminase elevations. Ceftriaxone has been associated with biliary sludge that leads to cholecystitis. The concomitant administration of ceftriaxone and intravenous calcium can form precipitates and cause death in neonates. New onset seizures have been described when using cefepime, particularly in renal impairment.

First-generation cephalosporins are used for treatment and perioperative prophylaxis of skin and skin structure infections (SSSIs). In neonates, ampicillin plus cefotaxime is a standard regimen for the treatment of sepsis and meningitis (ceftriaxone after 1 month of life). Ceftazidime or cefepime have become standard agents for empiric therapy in critically ill children, those with fever and neutropenia, and those with nosocomial infections in the ICU. Additional empiric gram-positive coverage (to cover MRSA or penicillin-resistant pneumococcus) may be indicated in the critically ill child.

Aztreonam

Aztreonam is a bactericidal monobactam whose spectrum is limited to aerobic gram-negative bacteria (e.g., the Enterobacteriaceae family and *P. aeruginosa*). It is devoid of gram-positive or anaerobic activity. Aztreonam can act synergistically with AGs. Aztreonam is well distributed into most body fluids and tissues, including CSF. Approximately 30%–50% of the drug is bound to plasma proteins. It is eliminated primarily via the kidney and also by hepatic mechanism and is removed by dialysis. Aztreonam should not be used as empiric monotherapy, given its limited spectrum. It can be useful with a documented β-lactam allergy or in situations in which nephrotoxicity is a concern. Aztreonam can also be administered via inhalation for the treatment of *P. aeruginosa* infections in patients with CF.

Carbapenems

Carbapenems share the basic β-lactam, but a structural alteration confers stability in the presence of β-lactamases. Carbapenems bind to all of the PBPs, having the greatest affinity for PBP1 and PBP2, and are bactericidal. The carbapenems are highly resistant to β-lactamases, although bacteria expressing carbapenemases have emerged. *Pseudomonas* spp., in particular, may acquire resistance to the carbapenems through multiple outer membrane mutations or development of an efflux pump after sustained exposure. *Stenotrophomonas* isolates usually are intrinsically resistant. Carbapenems possess a broader spectrum of antibacterial activity against aerobic and anaerobic gram-positive and gram-negative pathogens. The ability to exert a PAE varies by bacterial isolate.

Carbapenems are not absorbed enterally. Meropenem, imipenem/cilastatin, and doripenem are well distributed including the CNS. Protein binding is low (except ertapenem which does not penetrate the CNS). Excretion of unchanged drug is renal, and dosing adjustment is necessary. Imipenem is degraded by a proximal tubular brush border enzyme and ineffective in treating serious urinary tract infections and is administered along with a competitive inhibitor of dehydropeptidase I, cilastatin.

The adverse effect profile is similar to other β-lactams. Seizures are reported in reduced renal function with high-dose therapy with imipenem. Patients with an underlying seizure disorder should receive carbapenems with caution. There are few serious drug interactions reported with the carbapenems. A notable exception is a very serious drug interaction with valproic acid, resulting in subtherapeutic valproic acid levels. This interaction can persist after the carbapenem has been discontinued and can be resistant to increases in valproic acid dosing. Probenecid reduces renal clearance of carbapenems, resulting in increased concentrations.

The carbapenems are very broad-spectrum and provide effective empiric antimicrobial coverage for serious infections, particularly healthcare-acquired infections or infections in the immunocompromised patient. Concerns of resistance make de-escalation strategies paramount.

Aminoglycosides

AG antibiotics inhibit bacterial protein synthesis by irreversibly binding to the 30S ribosomal subunit and are bactericidal. AGs are used to treat aerobic gram-negative bacteria. Cellular uptake of AGs is oxygen-dependent and anaerobic bacteria are resistant. While not useful single agents against gram-positive bacteria, AGs exhibit synergistic activity with other antimicrobial agents against staphylococci, streptococci, and enterococci. Resistance is derived from enzymes that inactivate AGs, from decreased transport into the cell, or from mutations affecting proteins in the bacterial ribosome. The genes encoding these enzymes are transferred on plasmids; thus, there can be cross-resistance between members of the class. Amikacin is the most stable AG against these enzymes and can often be used in cases of gentamicin or tobramycin resistance.

AGs are poorly absorbed and administered parenterally. The AGs are not metabolized and are excreted unchanged via glomerular filtration. Hepatic disease does not interfere with AG elimination. AGs are large, hydrophilic, cationic molecules, do not cross the blood–brain barrier well, and should not be used as single agents to treat meningitis.

The most common adverse effects are ototoxicity and nephrotoxicity. Ototoxicity can be vestibulotoxicity or cochleotoxicity. Ototoxicity is bilateral, symmetrical, nonreversible, and may be delayed or immediate. Complaints of tinnitus should be taken seriously. AG-associated nephrotoxicity can be reversible, resulting from proximal tubular necrosis and due to elevated trough levels. Close monitoring of renal function is vital. Allergic reactions (rash, fever, and eosinophilia) are uncommon. AG-associated neuromuscular weakness is rare. The mechanism, competitive antagonism of acetylcholine activity at the neuromuscular junction results in risk in those with myasthenia gravis, severe hypocalcemia, infantile botulism, or who have recently received neuromuscular-blocking agents or steroids.

AGs are sensitive to changes in extracellular body water composition and the Vd varies by age. AG pharmacokinetics are altered in renal dysfunction, CF, burns, meningitis, and an abnormal body habitus.

Doses should be individualized using drug levels early, to direct AG dosing and to interpret culture data. Peak serum concentrations are related to drug efficacy and trough concentrations to toxicity. Volume overload, unstable renal function, and prolonged courses warrant close monitoring. Patients utilizing extracorporeal circuits should have therapeutic drug monitoring performed with changes in devices or fluid removal strategy. Care should be taken with other medications that cause ototoxicity or nephrotoxicity (e.g., nonsteroidal anti-inflammatory medications, IV contrast, amphotericin, and diuretics). Penicillins, at very high dose or during renal failure, may interact and cause degradation of AGs.

AGs exhibit concentration-dependent killing, a pronounced PAE, with PK/PD targets for maximizing peak/MIC and AUC/MIC ratios. AGs are used initially as empiric combination therapy for serious aerobic gram-negative infections (5 days of initial double coverage). Antimicrobial synergy between antipseudomonal β-lactams and AGs has been described with *P. aeruginosa*, *Serratia*, *Acinetobacter*, *Citrobacter*, and *Enterobacter* spp. Data in the immunocompromised host with pseudomonal infections show a better survival and cure rate with this combination. Combination therapy increases the likelihood of receiving an appropriate antibiotic, may reduce the induction of resistance, but may increase the incidence of adverse effects (nephrotoxicity). AGs also are indicated in the treatment of serious enterococcal infections, as susceptible enterococci are killed synergistically when given with penicillin or ampicillin. The levels necessary for gram-positive synergy are lower than for gram-negative infections, and dosing is lower. Synergy between AGs and β-lactams or glycopeptides can also be exploited in the treatment of serious infections due to viridans streptococci, group B streptococci, *S. aureus*, and coagulase-negative staphylococci.

Glycopeptides

The glycopeptides (e.g., vancomycin) inhibit cell wall synthesis in replicating bacteria by binding to cell wall precursors and inhibiting transpeptidation. The rise of vancomycin-resistant enterococci (VRE) is due to a readily transferable plasmid that profoundly reduces affinity for vancomycin. There are also intermediate and resistant *S. aureus* and *Staphylococcus epidermidis* isolates, related to thickened cell walls (*S. aureus*) and production of biofilm (*S. epidermidis*). *S. aureus* MIC > 2 should prompt alternative antibiotic therapy. These drugs are bactericidal against gram-positive bacteria except the enterococci (bacteriostatic). Vancomycin cannot pass across the membrane and has no utility in the treatment of gram-negative infections.

The glycopeptides are not absorbed enterally. Vancomycin has erratic IM absorption and must be given IV for systemic use. Teicoplanin may be given IM or IV. Approximately 55% of vancomycin and 90% of teicoplanin are protein bound. The Vd varies based on age. Vancomycin distributes to most body fluids, but because of its large molecular size, penetration into some infected spaces is poor. Vancomycin does not penetrate well into the CNS unless the meninges are inflamed. The glycopeptides are not metabolized and most drug elimination occurs via glomerular filtration. Renal function should be closely monitored and dosing intervals extended to allow for adequate clearance of drug. Most children require dosing intervals of every 6 hours, whereas many adult patients will need 8–12 hours. Vancomycin dosing should be based on actual body weight, even for obese patients.

"Red man syndrome," (flushing, pruritus, tachycardia, and erythema) is due to the rapid IV administration of vancomycin (due to histamine release) and not seen with teicoplanin. Pretreatment with an antihistamine and slowing the infusion rate reduce frequency and severity. The incidence of vancomycin-associated ototoxicity and nephrotoxicity approximates 2% and 5%, respectively. Their occurrences are dependent on concurrent ototoxic and nephrotoxic drugs, patient age, and severity of disease. Nephrotoxicity tends to be reversible. There is also a potential to increase the effect of neuromuscular blockers.

Vancomycin exhibits time-dependent killing, and an AUC/MIC ratio of $\geq$400 has been established as a pharmacodynamic target. Trough serum concentrations should be $>$10 mg/L to minimize development of resistance. Trough concentrations of 15–20 mg/L are recommended for treatment of bacteremia, endocarditis, osteomyelitis, meningitis, and hospital-acquired pneumonia caused by *S. aureus*. Peak vancomycin concentrations are unlikely to be helpful. Patients with changing renal function, volume status, or extracorporeal therapies require frequent levels.

Therapy is indicated for the empiric or definitive treatment of MRSA, other resistant gram-positive organism, or as an alternative in children with a β-lactam allergy. β-Lactams have superior penetration into most body spaces and are the preferred agent if the organism is susceptible. The empiric use of vancomycin remains controversial, and local resistance patterns should be considered to determine if it is warranted.

Oxazolidinones (Linezolid)

Linezolid binds to the P site of the 50S ribosomal subunit, preventing protein synthesis. Linezolid is active against gram-positive organisms, including staphylococci, streptococci, enterococci, gram-positive anaerobic cocci, and gram-positive bacilli, such as *Corynebacterium* spp. and *L. monocytogenes*, and devoid of activity against gram-negative bacteria. It is bacteriostatic against enterococci and staphylococci, and bactericidal against streptococci. Linezolid is available in both parenteral and oral preparations. Linezolid is not nephrotoxic, does not require adjustment in renal dysfunction, but does undergo hepatic metabolism via oxidation. Adverse effects include myelosuppression, elevations in hepatic function tests, and (when therapy extends for >8 weeks) with peripheral neuropathy, optic neuritis, and lactic acidosis. Drug interactions are rare, but its MAOI–like structure means combination with serotonergic agents may result in serotonin syndrome.

Lipopeptides

Daptomycin is a bactericidal, parenteral agent that binds to bacterial cell membranes leading to depolarization, loss of membrane potential, and cell death. Daptomycin has activity against virtually all isolates of *S. aureus*, coagulase-negative staphylococci, and enterococci (including VRE), but experience in children is limited. Resistance is rare. The most significant toxicity is musculoskeletal damage and elevation in creatine kinase. Daptomycin is indicated for complicated skin and soft-tissue infections, complicated bacteremia, and right-sided endocarditis. It cannot be used for pneumonia owing to inactivation by surfactant.

Quinupristin/Dalfopristin

Quinupristin/dalfopristin (Q/D) inhibits protein synthesis by binding to the 50S ribosomal subunit, similar to macrolides. Q/D is active against gram-positive cocci, including *S. pneumoniae*, *Enterococcus faecium* (but not *Enterococcus faecalis*), and coagulase-positive and coagulase-negative staphylococci. Q/D is also active against *Mycoplasma pneumoniae, Legionella* spp., *Chlamydia pneumoniae,* and gram-negative organisms *Moraxella catarrhalis* and *Neisseria* spp. It is bactericidal against streptococci and many staphylococci but bacteriostatic against *E. faecium.* Resistance occurs by changes on the binding site, production of inactivating enzymes, and development of efflux pumps. Q/D should be reserved for treatment of serious infections caused by multiple-drug-resistant gram-positive organisms, such as VRE. Adverse effects are rare and consist mostly of myalgias.

Clindamycin

Clindamycin binds to the 50S subunit of bacterial ribosomes, suppressing protein synthesis. It is active against susceptible strains of pneumococci, *Streptococcus pyogenes*, viridans streptococci, methicillin-sensitive *S. aureus* (MSSA), some MRSA, and most anaerobic gram-positive bacteria. Aerobic gram-negative bacilli are resistant. Clindamycin is distributed in fluids, tissues, and bone, but not CSF (not even with inflamed meninges). In critical care, clindamycin is useful for treatment of abscesses, anaerobic infections, as an alternative for susceptible MRSA infections, as an adjunct in toxic shock (inhibits toxin production by both *S. aureus* and *S. pyogenes*). Clindamycin use has been associated with the development of *C. difficile* colitis.

Fluoroquinolones

Concern for arthropathy and tendon injury has limited use of fluoroquinolones in children. Pediatric indications have been added for ciprofloxacin and levofloxacin. Fluoroquinolones are bactericidal, inhibiting bacterial DNA-topoisomerase (gram-positive organisms)/DNA-gyrase (gram-negative organisms). Resistance to fluoroquinolones is a result of mutations that alter drug binding or the expression of multidrug efflux pumps. Fluoroquinolones are effective against many gram-negative pathogens, including *P. aeruginosa* (the newer agents, levofloxacin, gatifloxacin, and moxifloxacin, have improved pneumococcus coverage). They also have activity against atypical respiratory pathogens (*M. pneumoniae, C. pneumoniae,* and *Legionella*) and thus are good choices for community and hospital-acquired respiratory infections.

Oral bioavailability approaches 100%, offering an enteral option in the patient who lacks IV access, but food–drug interactions, particularly with ciprofloxacin, need to be addressed. They undergo hepatic metabolism, and dosage adjustments may be necessary in liver disease. Dose adjustments are necessary in renal disease only if it is severe.

Nausea, diarrhea, headache, and dizziness are common adverse events. Less common effects include skin rash, photosensitivity reactions, CNS manifestations (headache, confusion, and dizziness), hepatotoxicity, and prolongation of the QT interval. Joint complaints are reported in teenagers with CF, but the incidence of arthropathy in young children is unknown. Enteral administration of fluoroquinolones with antacids, sucralfate, iron, and food or feeds containing these elements results in chelation and reduces absorption. Concomitant use of corticosteroids may increase the risk of arthropathy and tendon rupture. The risk of QTc prolongation increases when fluoroquinolones, particularly moxifloxacin, are used in combination with other QT-prolonging medications (e.g., methadone, ondansetron, and haloperidol). Ciprofloxacin in combination with theophylline, decrease its metabolism resulting in toxicity.

The use of fluoroquinolones in pediatrics may be justified when infection is caused by a multidrug-resistant pathogen for which there is no safe and effective alternative. The newer agents, with enhanced *S. pneumoniae* coverage, are excellent monotherapy in adult CAP and HCAP (not recommended for first-line therapy in children). Fluoroquinolones may also be useful as combination therapy with an antipseudomonal β-lactam to avoid AG nephrotoxic effects for high-risk patients.

Macrolides and Related Drugs

Macrolides are bacteriostatic compounds that competitively bind to the 50S ribosomal subunit, antagonizing bacterial protein synthesis. Resistance to macrolides develops by changes to the 23S ribosomal subunit, an efflux pump, or enzymatic inactivation. Macrolides are active against atypical pathogens (*Mycoplasma*, *Legionella*, and *Chlamydia*) as well as pneumococcus, MSSA, and *S. pyogenes*. They have less activity against *Haemophilus influenzae* and are the drugs of choice for eradication of *Bordetella pertussis*.

Erythromycin is degraded by the acidic environment of the stomach, clarithromycin and telithromycin undergo significant first-pass metabolism. Macrolides are widely distributed throughout the body, with the exception of CNS. Serum protein binding is modest and variable. Macrolides have significant intracellular but relatively low extracellular concentrations, thus are less effective against extracellular organisms (e.g., *H. influenzae*) and more effective against intracellular pathogens (e.g., *Chlamydia* and *Legionella*). Elimination of macrolide antibiotics (exception azithromycin) is through hepatic metabolism and biliary excretion. Dose adjustment is not necessary in renal or hepatic impairment, except for clarithromycin and telithromycin where dose reduction is recommended in severe renal impairment.

The common adverse effects are abdominal pain and diarrhea; more serious adverse effects include hepatic toxicity, ototoxicity, and cardiac toxicity. Hepatotoxicity may be delayed by 14 days after discontinuation. Ototoxicity is reversible. Prolonged QT interval and ventricular tachyarrhythmias are the cardiac toxicities (erythromycin > clarithromycin > azithromycin), and caution should be utilized when combining other QT-prolonging medications. Telithromycin is contraindicated in patients with myasthenia gravis; hepatotoxicity has also limited its use. Many drug interactions exist via the CYP3A4 enzyme including carbamazepine, corticosteroids, cyclosporine, warfarin, digoxin, benzodiazepines, and theophylline. Sudden cardiac death occurred in an adult taking concomitant methadone. The 50S ribosome subunit binding site is the same target of other antibiotics (clindamycin and Q/D) and could result in antibacterial antagonism if coadministered.

Erythromycin has largely been replaced by azithromycin, commonly used as part of a combination regimen for the treatment of infections of the respiratory tract or for *B. pertussis*.

Tetracyclines and Related Drugs

Tetracyclines are bacteriostatic and inhibit protein synthesis by binding reversibly to the 30S subunit of the bacterial ribosome. Resistance develops by impaired intracellular entry, efflux pump out of the cell, impaired binding to the ribosome, and enzymatic inactivation. Resistance is plasmid mediated and inducible. Tetracyclines have broad activity for many aerobic and anaerobic gram-positive and gram-negative bacteria, and for microorganisms resistant to cell wall–active agents (*Rickettsia, Coxiella burnetii, M. pneumoniae, Chlamydia* spp., *Legionella* spp., *Ureaplasma*, and *Plasmodium* spp.). Tetracyclines are active against spirochetes such as *Borrelia burgdorferi* (Lyme disease) and nontuberculosis strains of mycobacteria (e.g., *Mycobacterium marinum*). Tetracyclines are not active against *Pseudomonas, Proteus*, and *Providencia* spp.

Tetracyclines are widely distributed including low levels within the CSF. They accumulate in reticuloendothelial cells of the liver, spleen, and bone marrow, and in bone, dentine, and enamel of unerupted teeth. Tetracyclines are excreted in bile and urine, and undergo enterohepatic circulation. Adjustment in renal impairment may be necessary (except for doxycycline and tigecycline, they are eliminated nonrenally).

Children may develop permanent discoloration of teeth. Thrombophlebitis frequently follows intravenous administration. Common are nausea, vomiting, diarrhea, and photosensitivity. Hepatotoxicity, pancreatitis, and azotemia are uncommon. Reversible pseudotumor cerebri may develop in infants. Tetracyclines form chelation complexes and should not be administered enterally with dairy products, antacids, multivitamins, or iron supplements. The anticoagulant effects of warfarin may be enhanced. Carbamazepine, (fos)phenytoin, and barbiturates increase metabolism, leading to lower antibiotic levels.

Extensive use in animal farming has led to increased resistance. Availability of better tolerated, easier to administer antimicrobials has left tetracyclines reserved for rickettsial diseases, *Mycoplasma* and *Chlamydia*.

ANTIFUNGAL DRUGS

Most serious fungal infections occur in immunocompromised patients. Drug targets for fungi are different because they are eukaryotes with unique cell wall structures. Combination therapy utilizing different classes may be considered for patients who fail single-agent therapy; this strategy remains poorly investigated.

Polyenes

Amphotericin B is the gold-standard treatment for critical fungal infections. There are four formulations: conventional amphotericin B (C-AMB), liposomal amphotericin B (L-AMB), amphotericin B lipid complex (ABLC), and amphotericin B colloidal dispersion (ABCD). Toxicity of C-AMB led to other formulations. Amphotericin B binds to ergosterol (principal sterol of the fungal cell membrane) leading to cell death. Oxidative species are generated that damage fungal mitochondria. It is rare for resistance to develop.

Amphotericin has concentration-dependent killing, with a prolonged PAE. Susceptible pathogens include *Candida*, *Aspergillus*, non-*Aspergillus* molds, *Cryptococcus*, endemic fungal pathogens (*Histoplasma*, *Blastomyces*, *Coccidioides*, and *Sporothrix*), and the agents of mucormycosis. *Candida lusitaniae*, *Aspergillus terreus*, *Fusarium*, and *Pseudallescheria boydii*, display intrinsic amphotericin B resistance. Amphotericin B must be given intravenously. Its highest concentrations are in liver, kidney, and lung, and lowest in bronchial secretions and CNS. It has been used for CNS infections, particularly *Cryptococcus* and

Coccidioides, although intraventricular administration may also be required. The mechanisms of elimination are unknown. Blood levels are not influenced by renal or hepatic insufficiency. Children < 20 kg may require higher dosing of L-AMB.

Amphotericin B toxicity can be infusion related (fever, chills, rigors, nausea, vomiting, arthralgias, myalgias, respiratory distress, and hypotension) or dose related (nephrotoxicity, hypokalemia, hypomagnesemia, bicarbonate wasting, and anemia). Every-other-day dosing after the patient has stabilized or a sodium load may decrease nephrotoxicity. The lipid-complexed amphotericins decrease toxicity. Concomitant nephrotoxic medications increase nephrotoxicity. Corticosteroids may enhance the associated hypokalemia. There is a concern of antagonism if used in combination with the azole class, which inhibit ergosterol synthesis.

Amphotericin is used with systemic mycoses, primary invasive aspergillosis, and empirically for neutropenic patients with persistent fever.

Azoles

Azoles consist of imidazoles and triazoles. Triazoles have less effect on human sterol synthesis and are better tolerated. The azoles inhibit lanosterol 14α-demethylase, necessary for the synthesis of ergosterol. Azole resistance has been documented (particularly in *Candida* spp.). The mechanisms include multidrug efflux pumps, alteration of the synthetic pathway for ergosterol, upregulation of the enzymes, and replacement of ergosterol. Resistance to one azole does not imply resistance to others. Azoles are active against *Candida* spp., *Cryptococcus neoformans*, *Blastomyces dermatitidis*, *Histoplasma capsulatum*, *Coccidioides* spp., and *Paracoccidioides brasiliensis*. Variably susceptible are *Aspergillus* spp. and *Fusarium*. *Candida krusei* and the agents of mucormycosis are intrinsically resistant. Posaconazole is active against the agents of mucormycosis.

Itraconazole, voriconazole, and posaconazole are mainly hepatically cleared. Enteral voriconazole is preferred if GFR is <50 mL/min as the IV vehicle accumulates. Fluconazole has a wide distribution, excellent CNS penetration, and is cleared by the kidneys (dose adjustment needed in renal failure/dialysis). Itraconazole, ketoconazole, and posaconazole are highly protein bound, not dialyzed, and not reliable for CNS infections. Voriconazole exhibits nonlinear pharmacokinetics (20% of non-Indian Asians achieve fourfold higher voriconazole levels because of genetic polymorphisms).

Fluconazole is first-line for suspected *Candida albicans* without shock, for treatment or prophylaxis of cryptococcal meningitis, and prophylaxis in severely immunosuppressed patients. Some *Candida* spp. are becoming resistant (*C. krusei* and some *Candida glabrata* are resistant). Fluconazole has no activity against *Aspergillus* or other molds. Itraconazole is the azole of choice for dimorphic fungi (*Histoplasma, Blastomyces*, and *Sporothrix*). Effectiveness and use can be limited by poor bioavailability, drug–drug interactions, and lack of CNS penetration. Voriconazole has excellent activity against *Candida* spp. (including fluconazole-resistant species, such as *C. krusei*), the dimorphic fungi, and is the treatment of choice for invasive aspergillosis. Several reports suggest that it is useful for CNS infections. It is not active against Zygomycetes. Therapeutic drug monitoring is available. Posaconazole possesses the broadest activity, including virtually all *Candida* spp., *Cryptococcus*, nearly all *Aspergillus* spp., and non-*Aspergillus* molds, including many *Fusarium* spp. and *P. boydii*. It is the only azole active against Zygomycetes, including *Rhizopus* and *Mucor*. Posaconazole is only available enterally; absorption is enhanced with high-fat meals and an acidic environment. Absorption may be inadequate for patients not being fed or on medications to increase gastric pH.

The common adverse effects include nausea, abdominal pain, headache, and elevation of transaminases (significant transaminase elevations is unusual and fulminant hepatitis is rare). Voriconazole has several distinct side effects, temporary visual disturbance (blurred vision, photophobia, and optic neuritis), hallucinations and rash, sometimes severe, are rare. Drug–drug interactions with benzodiazepines, barbiturates, phenytoin, carbamazepine, tacrolimus, sirolimus, cyclosporine, warfarin, rifampin, omeprazole, and calcium-channel blockers are common. Azoles may contribute to QT prolongation directly or through drug–drug interactions.

Echinocandins

Echinocandins (caspofungin, micafungin, and anidulafungin) share a favorable safety profile with lack of significant drug–drug interactions. Echinocandins inhibit 1,3-β-D-glucan synthase, the enzyme responsible for the production of the fungal cell wall. Echinocandins are fungicidal against *Candida* spp., but fungistatic against *Aspergillus*. Mutations in the gene encoding for the 1,3-β-D-glucan synthase complex are associated with *Candida* resistance. Echinocandins are effective against *Candida* and *Aspergillus* spp., including *C. krusei, C. glabrata*, and *C. lusitaniae*. They have no activity against *Cryptococcus*, Zygomycetes, *Fusarium*, and *Pseudallescheria* and its asexual form *Scedosporium*, or *Trichosporon*.

Echinocandins must be administered IV, are highly protein bound, and poorly penetrate the CNS. Caspofungin and micafungin are metabolized in the liver and dose adjustment is suggested for hepatic insufficiency, but not renal insufficiency. Anidulafungin slowly degrades in plasma and not affected by renal or hepatic insufficiency. Children require larger doses than adults. Echinocandins are indicated for suspected or proven disease caused by *Candida* or *Aspergillus*, especially those failing more conventional therapy, have sepsis, or septic shock. They are noninferior to L-AMB as antifungal therapy in febrile neutropenia.

The most frequent adverse effects are pain and phlebitis at injection site. Increases in liver transaminases and histamine-like reaction during infusion occur. Cyclosporine increases caspofungin levels, and caspofungin decreases tacrolimus levels.

ANTIVIRAL AGENTS (NON-HIV)

Viruses are obligate intracellular organisms, dependent on host cells for replication. Antiviral agents must either block viral entry or exit from the cell or be active inside the host cell. Antiviral drugs are static against replicating viruses. Antiviral therapy is currently available for herpesviruses, hepatitis C virus (HCV), hepatitis B virus (HBV), papillomavirus, influenza, and HIV.

The noninfluenza antivirals share a common final pathway; they inhibit viral DNA synthesis. Acyclovir, ganciclovir, cidofovir, and ribavirin are nucleoside/nucleotide analogs which are preferentially incorporated into viral DNA resulting in chain termination. Foscarnet inhibits viral nucleic acid synthesis by interacting directly with herpesvirus DNA polymerase or HIV reverse transcriptase. Ribavirin's mechanism relates to alteration of cellular nucleotide pools and inhibition of viral messenger RNA synthesis. Resistance to acyclovir and ganciclovir results from intracellular drug inactivation or altered viral DNA polymerase. Cidofovir and foscarnet resistant viruses are infrequent, but due to mutations in viral DNA polymerase. Cidofovir resistance may be higher with prior prolonged exposure to ganciclovir or with CMV strains displaying high-level resistance. Resistance to ribavirin has not been reported for RSV infections.

Acyclovir is active against herpes simplex virus type 1 (HSV-1), HSV type 2 (HSV-2), weaker against varicella-zoster virus (VZV), and very weak against Epstein–Barr virus (EBV), cytomegalovirus (CMV), and human herpesvirus 6 (HHV-6). Ganciclovir is active against all herpesviruses, but most notably against CMV and HHV-6. Cidofovir has in vitro activity against all of the HHVs, adenovirus, human papilloma and polyoma viruses, and poxviruses (e.g., monkeypox, smallpox, and vaccinia). Foscarnet is active against HSV-1 and HSV-2, VZV, CMV, and HHV-6, as well as HBV. Ribavirin has broad spectrum activity against RNA viruses, including RSV, HCV, measles, hantaviruses, and Lassa viruses.

Intensivists use acyclovir for neonatal herpes, HSV encephalitis, HSV, and VZV infections in immunocompromised patients, and prophylactically to suppress reactivation of HSV. *Ganciclovir* is used in CMV as well as disseminated HHV-6 infections. Severe cases of CMV pneumonitis may benefit from combined therapy with intravenous immunoglobulin or CMV immunoglobulin. Ganciclovir or valganciclovir is used for CMV prophylaxis in transplant recipients. *Cidofovir* is used for adenovirus in immunocompromised patients and is second-line therapy for herpetic or CMV infections. Probenecid and aggressive fluid hydration are given to prevent nephrotoxicity. *Foscarnet* is used in HHV disease unresponsive to less-toxic drugs. It is first line in CMV infection in the already neutropenic host when trying to avoid the bone marrow suppressive effects of ganciclovir. Aerosolized *ribavirin* for treatment of RSV bronchiolitis is generally not recommended since treatment has not consistently improved outcomes.

Combination with intravenous immunoglobulin may reduce mortality from RSV infection in immunocompromised patients. Ribavirin use has been reported for severe influenza, adenovirus, vaccinia, parainfluenza, measles virus infections, and hemorrhagic fevers. Pregnant women should not directly care for patients receiving ribavirin aerosol.

ANTIVIRAL AGENTS (INFLUENZA)

Children at high risk for influenza complications and recommended to receive antiviral treatment for suspected or confirmed influenza include: children aged <2 years; children with chronic pulmonary, cardiovascular, renal, hepatic, hematologic, neurologic/neurodevelopmental, and metabolic disorders; immunosuppressed children; children who take long-term aspirin therapy; American Indians/Alaska Natives; morbidly obese children; and children who reside in chronic care facilities.

Two classes of antiviral agents are available for influenza: *neuraminidase inhibitors* (NIs) (oseltamivir and zanamivir) and the *adamantanes* (amantadine and rimantadine). Neuraminidase is responsible for detachment of virions from the infected cell's membrane and for viral penetration through respiratory secretions. Adamantanes block the uncoating of influenza A virus preventing penetration of virus into the host and assembly of progeny virions. The NIs are active against influenza A and B, the adamantanes are active only against influenza A. Oseltamivir and zanamivir are recommended first-line empiric agents as >99% of strains are sensitive.

ANTI-INFECTIVES FOR MYCOBACTERIUM TUBERCULOSIS

Mycobacteria are difficult to treat, owing to their thick lipid dense cell wall, a high concentration of drug efflux pumps, and a propensity to exist intracellularly. Multidrug regimens must be used to limit resistant strains. Therapy is typically initiated with a four-drug regimen of isoniazid, a rifamycin, and pyrazinamide plus either ethambutol or streptomycin. Isoniazid–rifampin combination therapy will cure the majority of *Mycobacterium tuberculosis* (TB). Adding pyrazinamide for the first 2 months decreases duration of therapy from 9 months to 6 months. Ethambutol and streptomycin provide additional coverage in the case of resistance.

Isoniazid enters the cell by passive diffusion and is converted to an active form. It inhibits synthesis of the mycobacterial cell wall. Resistance is often due to mutations in the enzyme that activates the drug. It is well absorbed from the GI tract and widely distributed into all body fluids, including the CSF. Metabolism is via acetylation by liver *N*-acetyltransferase and can vary genetically (affecting dosing regimens and hepatotoxicity). Dose adjustments are not necessary in renal or hepatic insufficiency. A symptomatic, potentially fatal, hepatitis requiring cessation of drug occurs in 1%. CNS side effects occur (peripheral neuropathy, memory loss, and seizures). Pyridoxine can reverse or prevent the CNS side effects. Other reactions include anemia, a lupus-like syndrome, tinnitus, and GI upset. Isoniazid inhibits the metabolism of phenytoin, carbamazepine, anticoagulants, benzodiazepines, and vitamin D.

Rifamycins (rifampin, rifapentine, and rifabutin) inhibit bacterial RNA synthesis by blocking RNA transcription. Rifampin, the most commonly used, is bactericidal for mycobacteria. Resistance develops when the target binding site is altered. Rifampin has activity to *Mycobacterium*, most gram-positive bacteria (including MRSA), and some gram-negatives (*Neisseria meningitidis* and *H. influenzae*). *Rifampin* is highly lipophilic and widely distributed into body fluids, but CSF penetration is poor if meninges are not inflamed. Drug metabolism occurs in the liver to an active metabolite, and then excretion in the bile (60%–70%) and urine (~30%). Drug interactions include benzodiazepines, antimicrobials (use with voriconazole is contraindicated), and many others. The most common adverse reactions are rash, fever, nausea, and vomiting. For patients with preexisting liver disease or on other hepatotoxic medications, hepatitis and liver failure can occur.

Pyrazinamide is activated in an acidic environment (pH of 5.5) and is converted to active pyrazinoic acid by mycobacterial pyrazinamidase. The mechanism of action likely involves disruption of the cell membrane and alterations in transport. Resistance may be due to impaired uptake or mutations in the gene that encodes for conversion of pyrazinamide to its active form. Pyrazinamide is well absorbed, widely distributed throughout the body, including the CSF, and concentrates in the epithelial fluid of the lungs. Drug metabolism occurs in the liver with metabolites excreted by the kidney. Drug clearance and Vd increase with patient mass. Dosing should be reduced if patients have a GFR < 30 mL/min. Hemodialysis removes pyrazinamide. It may increase the risk of rifampin induced liver injury, and may increase cyclosporine levels. Major adverse effects include hepatotoxicity (in 1%–5% of patients), nausea, vomiting, drug fever, and hyperuricemia.

Streptomycin is an AG antibiotic. It is mostly active against extracellular TB, as it has poor intracellular penetration. *Ethambutol* inhibits an essential polymerization component of the mycobacterial cell wall. Resistance arises due to a mutation in the target enzyme or by enhanced efflux pumps. Ethambutol has activity against most mycobacteria. Children have reduced absorption so that good peak concentrations of drug are often not achieved with standard dosing. Distribution is extensive with high concentrations in kidneys, lungs, saliva, and red blood cells, but low in the CSF. About 20% of drug is metabolized in the liver and ~50% of drug is eliminated unchanged by the kidneys. Renal adjustment is needed and 5%–20% of drug is removed by dialysis. Hyperuricemia is common but not always symptomatic. Paresthesias, GI upset, increase in liver aminotransferases, and drug fever/rash can be seen. Reversible, dose-related visual disturbances, such as loss of red/green differentiation and optic neuritis, may necessitate drug discontinuation.

ANTIMALARIAL DRUGS

Most cases of malaria can be treated with oral therapy. Treatment for children with severe disease includes quinidine gluconate plus either: doxycycline, tetracycline, or clindamycin. An alternative, investigational, regimen is artesunate followed by atovaquone–proguanil, clindamycin, or mefloquine. *Artesunate* is first-line therapy for treatment of severe malaria in African children (reduced mortality compared to quinine). *Quinidine gluconate* is the only first-line agent for severe malaria in the United States. It acts as an intraerythrocytic schizonticide, with little effect on sporozoites. Quinidine is cidal to *Plasmodium vivax* and *malariae*, but not *falciparum*. Resistance is increasing, and artemisinin derivatives should be considered if disease is contracted within a highly resistant region. Quinidine is metabolized in the liver to inactive substances but has many drug interactions. Dose adjustments should be made if GFR is <10 mL/min or if on hemodialysis. Patients with severe liver disease have a larger Vd and impaired CL so larger loading doses and reduced maintenance doses are indicated. Dose-related toxicities include cinchonism (tinnitus, high-tone deafness, visual disturbances, headache, dysphoria, nausea, vomiting, and postural hypotension), hypoglycemia (due to hyperinsulinemia), and hypotension. QTc prolongation and arrhythmias have been reported. Rarely, severe hematologic effects as a result of a hypersensitivity reaction may occur. "Blackwater fever" (massive hemolysis, hemoglobinemia, and hemoglobinuria) leads to anuria, renal failure, and death and requires immediate discontinuation. In people with Glucose-6-Phosphate Dehydrogenase deficiency, hemolysis is also a concern, but tends to be milder.

Artesunate is an artemisinin derivative. The mechanisms of action are not understood. Resistance is limited, but is emerging in Cambodia and Thailand. Artemisinins have action against all erythrocytic stages, results in rapid clinical benefit, and decreased transmission of malaria. Artemisinins have short half-lives and recurrence can occur if not used in combination with a longer-acting agent. Artesunate should be administered IV. Dose adjustment is not needed in renal or hepatic failure. It is rapidly hydrolyzed to an active metabolite, dihydroartemisinin. Dihydroartemisinin undergoes hepatic metabolism to inactive metabolites. There are no known interactions between artesunate and other drugs. The most common adverse reactions are nausea, vomiting, anorexia, and dizziness. More serious adverse effects include neutropenia, anemia, hemolysis, and elevated levels of liver enzymes, neurotoxicity, and embryotoxicity.

CHAPTER 66 ■ DENGUE AND OTHER HEMORRHAGIC VIRAL INFECTIONS

SIRIPEN KALAYANAROOJ AND RAKESH LODHA

DENGUE INFECTIONS

Dengue viral infections present with a spectrum of clinical illnesses from the common *dengue fever (DF)* to the more severe presentations of *dengue hemorrhagic fever (DHF)* and *dengue shock syndrome (DSS)*. Unusual presentations have led to a classification of *expanded dengue syndrome (EDS)*, which includes severe CNS, liver, myocardial, or abdominal dysfunction.

Epidemiology

Since the 1980s, the incidence of dengue has increased dramatically. An estimated 100 million symptomatic cases occur worldwide every year. Without early diagnosis and proper management, the case-fatality rate (CFR) may be 10%–30%. With modern supportive therapy, the CFR can be reduced to less than 1%.

Virus

Dengue viruses are small (50 nm), single-stranded RNA viruses, belonging to the family Flaviviridae. Infection with any one of five serotypes confers lifelong immunity to that serotype and temporary cross-protection (months) to *secondary infection* with one of the other serotypes.

Transmission

Aedes aegypti and *Aedes albopictus* mosquitoes are the most important vectors of dengue viruses. Dengue can also be transmitted by blood transfusion and vertical transmission. The typical incubation period after a mosquito bite is 4–6 days (range 3–14 days). Dengue is unlikely when symptoms arise in a traveler >14 days after return from an endemic area.

PATHOGENESIS AND PATHOPHYSIOLOGY

After a mosquito bite, viruses spread to lymph nodes and reticulo-endothelial organs, where they multiply and ultimately enter the bloodstream. Immune activation during the secondary dengue infection leads to an exaggerated cytokine response, resulting in increased vascular permeability. Capillary leak is predominantly in pleural and peritoneal spaces and usually lasts 24–48 hours.

Sequential infection with any two serotypes of dengue virus results in DHF/DSS in endemic areas. Cross-reactive antibodies bind to the virions but are unable to neutralize them; this results in a more rapid activation and proliferation of memory T cells. Cytokines are implicated in the pathogenesis of the vascular compromise and hemorrhage. Complement activation also contributes to vascular leakage. Antibodies against dengue virus proteins cross-react with platelet surface proteins and cause thrombocytopenia. Dengue virus infection also activates blood clotting and fibrinolytic pathways. Mild disseminated intravascular coagulation (DIC), liver injury, and thrombocytopenia all contribute to the hemorrhagic tendency. Central nervous system (CNS) involvement is attributed to a direct neurotropic effect of dengue virus.

Risk factors for DHF/DSS include the virus strain (DENV-2 highest risk), preexisting antidengue antibody, age (younger children at increased risk), genetic predisposition, and hyperendemicity (two or more virus serotypes circulating simultaneously at high level).

Pathology

Most fatalities in DHF/DSS occur within 24 hours after shock onset. Autopsy reveals hemorrhage in the skin and subcutaneous tissue. The heart typically shows flame-shaped subendocardial hemorrhage in the left ventricular septum and occasionally over papillary muscles. Hemorrhage may be present in nasal mucosa, gums, gastrointestinal tract, and liver (subcapsular). Frank bleeding in serous cavities is rare. The meninges and brain show only petechial hemorrhage. Serous effusion with high protein content is common in the pleural, abdominal, and pericardial spaces. Analysis of the plasma reveals low levels of protein, especially albumin.

The majority of dengue presentations (up to 80%–90% of symptomatic cases) are DF, which is a mild illness and rarely leads to death. Minor bleeding manifestations, petechiae, epistaxis, and gum bleeding are found in all dengue-infected patients, but significant bleeding occurs in DHF, DSS, and EDS patients. EDS is increasing, especially in countries with new outbreaks and in adult patients. The majority of EDS cases result from prolonged shock with multiple organ failure, comorbidities, and coinfections in dengue-infected hosts.

CLINICAL MANIFESTATIONS AND NATURAL COURSE

Early manifestations are nonspecific with high fever for 2–7 days, poor appetite, nausea, vomiting, and abdominal pain. Some patients have associated upper respiratory tract symptoms or diarrhea. Bleeding manifestations are a more specific sign of dengue. Petechiae, epistaxis, and gum bleeding are common. More severe bleeding (hematemesis, melena, hematuria, and hypermenorrhea) is uncommon early in the febrile phase except in patients taking aspirin, NSAIDs, or steroids. Hemoglobinuria is common in patients with underlying hemoglobinopathy or G-6-PD deficiency. Severe muscle and joint pain is common (*breakbone fever*). The *tourniquet test* is 70%–80% specific for dengue, when >10 petechiae/square inch appear on an extremity after inflating a blood pressure cuff between systolic and diastolic pressure for 5 minutes. Symptoms of DF disappear as fever subsides in children. Prolonged fatigue for a few weeks is common in adult patients. Depression and psychosis have been reported in adult cases.

The natural course of DHF/DSS patients is divided into the febrile, critical or leakage, and convalescence phases (**Fig. 66.1**). The *febrile phase* lasts for 2–7 days. The *critical phase* usually occurs over 24–48 hours and coincides with the onset of defervescence and thrombocytopenia. Plasma leakage in the form of pleural effusions and ascites is the most specific manifestation of DHF/DSS during the critical phase. Hemoconcentration (a 20% increase above baseline in hematocrit) is another sign of plasma leakage. Hypoalbuminemia is indirect evidence of plasma leakage. In cases with massive plasma leakage, the patients develop shock (DSS). Those patients with shock usually present with a narrow pulse pressure and postural hypotension. They may have coexistent bleeding that aggravates the cardiovascular compromise. The *convalescence phase* follows the critical phase. About 30% of DH/DHF patients have the typical convalescent rash (a confluent macular or maculopapular rash with small islands of hypopigmentation) especially on both lower extremities, but also often involving face and trunk. Some patients have itching. Reabsorption of effusions may begin as early as 12 hours after leakage ceases. Patients may develop acute pulmonary edema or heart failure. Sinus bradycardia can occur.

The most common EDS presentations involve liver failure and encephalopathy. There have been

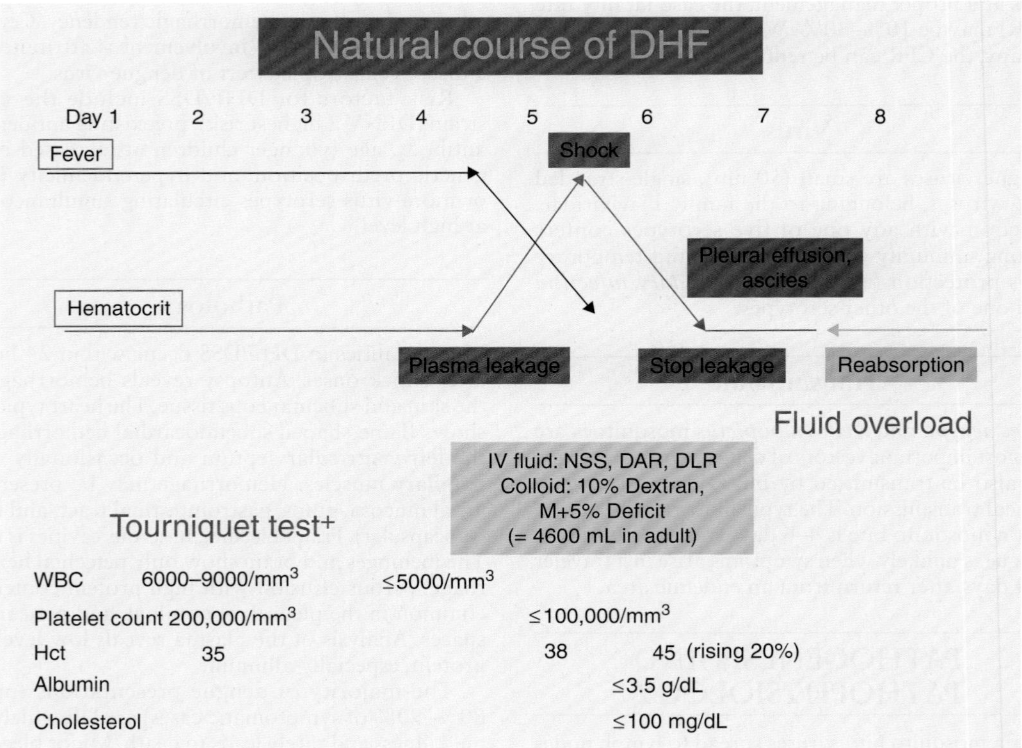

FIGURE 66.1. Natural course of DHF.

reports of EDS with gastrointestinal tract involvement (cholecystitis, pancreatitis), renal involvement (renal failure, hemolytic uremic syndrome), cardiac involvement (myocarditis, pericarditis, conduction abnormalities), respiratory tract involvement (pulmonary hemorrhage, acute respiratory distress syndrome), musculoskeletal involvement (myositis, rhabdomyolysis), lymphoreticular/bone marrow involvement (infection associated hemophagocytic syndrome, idiopathic thrombocytopenic purpura), eye involvement (macular hemorrhage, optic neuritis, impaired visual acuity), postinfectious fatigue syndrome, depression, psychosis, and alopecia.

DIAGNOSIS AND DIFFERENTIAL DIAGNOSIS

Diseases that mimic DF/DHF/DSS include those that cause influenza-like illnesses followed by severe manifestations. These include gram-negative infections such as *Neisseria meningitidis* (meningococcemia), *Salmonella typhi* (typhoid, enteric fever), and *Yersinia pestis* (plague). Malaria caused by *Plasmodium falciparum* may manifest with fever and bleeding but is distinguished by the presence of splenomegaly and significant pallor. Chikungunya, Rift Valley fever, sandfly fever, hepatitis, and rickettsial diseases may be difficult to distinguish. Common acute febrile/viral illness, upper respiratory tract illness (pharyngitis, tonsillitis), acute gastritis, and acute gastroenteritis are included in the differential diagnosis in the first few days of fever.

Diagnosis of DHF

The World Health Organization (WHO) case definition for DHF includes *clinical criteria*: (a) acute onset high fever, (b) hemorrhagic manifestations (at least a positive tourniquet test), (c) hepatomegaly, and (d) shock. Laboratory criteria include thrombocytopenia and evidence of plasma leakage (hemoconcentration, effusions, or hypoalbuminemia).

Laboratory Investigations

During the early febrile phase, hematocrit (Hct), WBC, differential, and platelet counts may be normal. Toward the end of febrile phase, leukopenia (WBC $\leq$ 5000 cells/mm^3), lymphocytosis, increased numbers of atypical lymphocytes, and thrombocytopenia ($\leq$100,000 cells/mm^3) are present. A rising Hct occurs in DHF patients without significant bleeding. Hct is normal or decreased in cases with bleeding (usually concealed in the upper GI tract). As the disease progresses, a leukocytosis with predominant polymorphonuclear cells (PMN) may be found. The mean platelet count in DHF patients is <50,000 and <10,000 cells/mm^3 in fatal cases. Microscopic hematuria is found in 40%–50% of DHF/DSS cases and may be detected in the early febrile period. Hemoglobinuria is common in patients with underlying hemoglobinopathy or G-6-PD deficiency. Mild elevations of aspartate aminotransferase (AST) and alanine aminotransferase (ALT) are observed early in the febrile phase in 80%–90% of all dengue patients. In cases with shock or prolonged shock, AST and ALT elevation may be >5000–10,000 Unit/L, which indicates a worsening prognosis. Hypoglycemia is usually due to poor intake and vomiting. Dengue patients with liver failure may also present with hypoglycemia. Hyponatremia and hypocalcemia are common. Most DHF patients have normal or transient elevations of blood urea nitrogen (BUN) and creatinine. Severe/complicated cases may progress to oliguria with persistent elevations of BUN and creatinine, portending a grave prognosis. A prolonged partial thromboplastin time (PTT) is observed in 50% of DHF/DSS patients and 10%–20% also have a prolonged thrombin time (TT). Prolonged prothrombin time (PT) is observed in patients with prolonged shock and liver failure. Erythrocyte sedimentation rate (ESR) is normal throughout the course of dengue illness in both DF and DHF and may be used to differentiate DSS from septic shock.

Chest X-ray

The right lateral decubitus chest X-ray better demonstrates right pleural effusion. The chest X-ray is not necessary in most dengue cases; it is highly recommended in cases of suspected internal bleeding, where the absence of a rising Hct might cause the clinician to miss the diagnosis.

TESTS FOR DENGUE CONFIRMATION

Demonstration of dengue virus on culture, detection of dengue nucleic acid by polymerase chain reaction (PCR), detection of dengue antigen (NS1 Ag), or demonstration of antibodies against dengue virus is required for confirming dengue infection. Serologic methods are used if blood samples are taken after 5 days or during convalescence. PCR is not used routinely because it is costly and often only available in the research laboratories. A commercial NS1 Ag kit yields test results in 5–10 minutes, but is expensive in most endemic countries. This NS1 Ag has a good specificity (>95%) but low sensitivity (40%–70%). Commonly used serologic tests to detect antibodies include IgM or IgG antibody-capture enzyme-linked immunosorbent assay tests. These tests can differentiate primary and secondary dengue infections.

MANAGEMENT

Febrile Phase

Management in the febrile phase is mostly supportive. Acetaminophen/paracetamol is recommended for fever. Aspirin and NSAIDs are contraindicated because they may cause gastritis (massive bleeding) or Reye syndrome. Other symptomatic medicines may be given according to clinical symptoms (e.g., anticonvulsants, antihypertensive drugs, H2-blocker or proton pump inhibitors). Antibiotics are not indicated if there are no associated bacterial infections. Steroids have no benefit. Oral electrolyte solutions are used in cases of severe anorexia, nausea, or vomiting. Red, black, or brown foods are avoided so that stool discoloration is not misinterpreted as blood. Some patients with moderate-to-severe dehydration may need IV fluids. The rate of IV fluid administration is reduced as soon as possible to prevent fluid overload during the reabsorption phase after plasma leakage.

Critical Phase (Leakage Phase)

Detection of early plasma leakage (rising Hct, CXR, ultrasonography, or hypoalbuminemia) is important to diagnose DHF. Leukopenia and thrombocytopenia usually precede plasma leakage and serve as an indicator of impending plasma leakage. Hospitalized patients are admitted to a mosquito-free environment to prevent nosocomial transmission. The absence of fever for >1 day indicates resolution of viremia and no further risk of viral dissemination from mosquito bites.

VOLUME REPLACEMENT

General Principles

DHF/DSS patients should receive the minimum amount of fluid required to maintain effective circulatory volume. The IV fluid should be isotonic (e.g., normal saline [NS], lactate Ringer [LR], or acetate Ringer [AR] solution). Randomized controlled trials failed to reveal an advantage of colloid solutions. Inadequate fluid resuscitation risks prolonged shock and excessive fluid administration risks fluid overload, respiratory failure, and multiple organs failure.

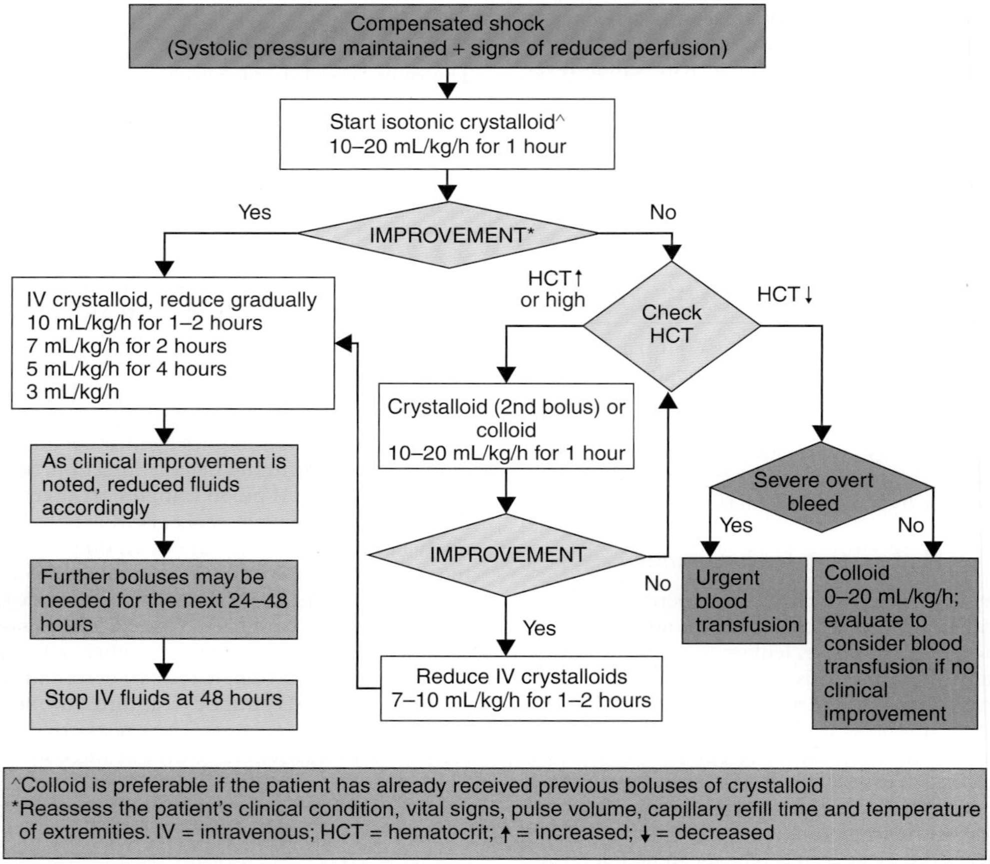

FIGURE 66.2. Algorithm for fluid management in dengue-compensated shock (grade III). (Reproduced with permission from World Health Organization. *Handbook for Clinical Management of Dengue*. Geneva, Switzerland: WHO, 2012. http://apps.who.int/iris/bitstream/10665/76887/1/9789241504713_eng.pdf.)

IV fluid with addition of 5% dextrose is preferred because these DHF/DSS patients usually have poor appetites and marginal levels of blood sugar. Plain water without electrolytes is avoided, as it may aggravate hyponatremia and contribute to plasma leakage or convulsions.

Fluid Administration for Shock Patients (Grade III)

The amount and rate of IV fluid resuscitation for DSS is much less compared with other kinds of shock (septic, anaphylactic, or hypovolemic shock). **Figure 66.2** displays the fluid management protocol for grade III patients (compensated shock), who should receive LR or NS at a rate of 10 mL/kg/h for children (500 mL/h in the adult) for 1–2 hours. Fluid administration is reduced to 7 mL/kg/h for the child (250 mL/h in the adult) for another 1–2 hours and further reduced to 5 mL/kg/h (child) or 100–120 mL/h (adult) for 4–6 hours. After 12 hours of shock, IV fluid should be at maintenance rates for 4–6 hours before reducing to minimal rates. The total duration of IV fluid should not exceed 24–36 hours.

Fluid Administration for Profound Shock Patients (Grade IV)

For patients in severe shock (**Fig. 66.3**), isotonic crystalloid is given rapidly at 20 mL/kg/h until the blood pressure (BP) is restored. If the BP cannot be restored within 15–30 minutes, additional laboratory investigations may identify causes of prolonged shock. *The common abnormalities/complications associated with prolonged DSS are massive internal bleeding, hypoglycemia, hypocalcemia, and acidosis.* Liver and renal injuries are also common.

Indication for Colloidal Solutions

Colloidal solutions are used for DHF/DSS patients with clinical signs of fluid overload, with persistently

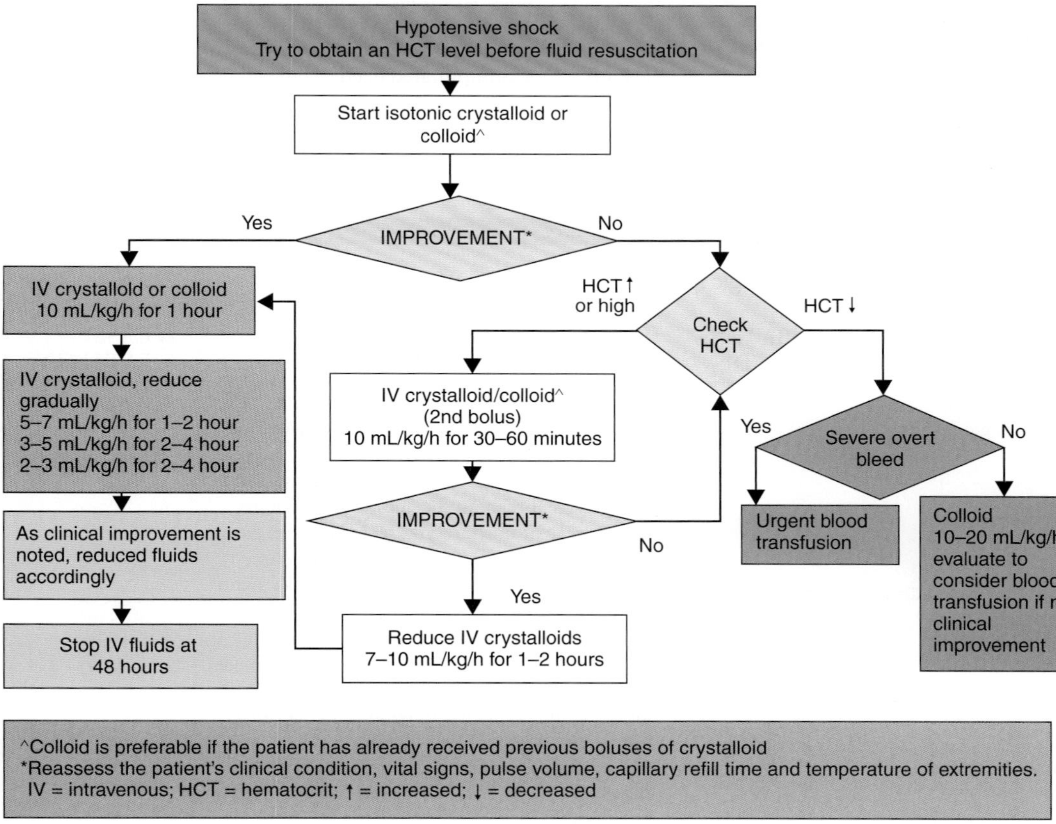

FIGURE 66.3. Algorithm for fluid management in hypotensive shock (grade IV). (Reproduced with permission from World Health Organization. *Handbook for Clinical Management of Dengue*. Geneva, Switzerland: WHO, 2012. http://apps.who.int/iris/bitstream/10665/76887/1/9789241504713_eng.pdf.)

elevated Hct despite IV fluid administration, and with a history of hypotonic solutions administration before shock. Colloidal solutions should be *plasma expanders* such as *10% Dextran-40* or 6% heta-starch. An Hct reduction > 10%, after hydration with dextran-40, may indicate bleeding. Patients should be monitored closely during the first few minutes of the dextran infusion because severe anaphylactoid reactions have been reported.

Blood/Blood Component Transfusion

When transfusing for hemorrhage, whole blood (WB) is preferred. Fresh frozen plasma is usually not needed in uncomplicated DHF/DSS. An abnormal coagulation profile is usually self-corrected within a few days. Indications and relative indications for blood transfusion include (1) significant bleeding (>10% of total blood volume; >6–8 mL/kg in children), (2) no significant rise of Hct in DSS patients, (3) fall in Hct without clinical or vital signs improvement, and (4) patients with refractory shock despite IV fluid hydration. Prophylactic platelet transfusion in the absence of clinical bleeding is not used regardless of the degree of thrombocytopenia unless the patient had previously received antiplatelet or anticoagulant medications. Patients with fluid overload are at greater risk of pulmonary edema or heart failure with platelet transfusion.

Prevention and Vaccines

Dengue vaccines are under active development. Recently, a tetravalent dengue vaccine has been launched and has been approved by the regulatory bodies of some countries.

VIRAL HEMORRHAGIC FEVERS

Viral hemorrhagic fevers (VHF) compose a group of clinical syndromes characterized by hemorrhagic manifestations. DIC appears to be the common mechanism. The viruses are from the *Flaviviridae* family (Kyasanur forest disease, Omsk, dengue, and yellow fever viruses), *Bunyaviridae* family (Congo, Hantaan, and Rift Valley fever viruses), the *Arenaviridae* family (Junin, Machupo, Guanarito, and Lassa viruses), and the *Filoviridae* family (Ebola and Marburg viruses). The dengue viruses, Rift Valley fever virus, and yellow fever virus are transmitted by mosquitoes. Ticks are responsible for transmission of Omsk, Kyasanur forest disease, and Congo viruses. Human infection may occur from infected animals or materials in case of Junin, Lassa, Marburg, Ebola, and Hanta viruses. Some viruses that cause hemorrhagic fever, such as Ebola, Marburg, Lassa, and Crimean-Congo hemorrhagic fever viruses, can spread from one person to another through close contact or body fluids. Contaminated needles have played a role in outbreaks. The clinical features of viral hemorrhagic fevers are summarized in **Table 66.1**.

TABLE 66.1

Clinical Features of Viral Hemorrhagic Fevers

DISEASE	INCUBATION PERIOD (D)	CLINICAL FEATURES	CASE FATALITY
Crimean-Congo hemorrhagic fever	3–12	Fever, severe headache, myalgia, abdominal pain, anorexia, nausea, and vomiting; erythematous facial or truncal flush and injected conjunctivae; hemorrhagic enanthem on the soft palate and a fine petechial rash on the chest and abdomen. Large areas of purpura and bleeding from gums, nose, intestine, lungs, or uterus may be seen. Hepatomegaly in absence of icterus. CNS symptoms and signs in severe illness.	2%–50%
Kyasanur forest disease	3–8	Severe myalgia, prostration, and bronchiolar involvement. Often presents without hemorrhage (occasionally with severe gastrointestinal bleeding), pneumonia, acute renal failure, and focal liver damage, meningoencephalitis.	3%–10%
Omsk hemorrhagic fever	3–8	Moderate epistaxis, hematemesis, and a hemorrhagic enanthem (but no profuse hemorrhage), pneumonia.	1%–10%
Rift Valley fever	3–6	Fever, headache, prostration, myalgia, anorexia, nausea, vomiting, conjunctivitis, lymphadenopathy, purpura, epistaxis, hematemesis, and melena	~1%

TABLE 66.1

Clinical Features of Viral Hemorrhagic Fevers (*continued*)

■ DISEASE	■ INCUBATION PERIOD (D)	■ CLINICAL FEATURES	■ CASE FATALITY
Argentine, Venezuelan, and Bolivian hemorrhagic fever and Lassa fever	~7–14	Fever, headache, diffuse myalgia, anorexia, sore throat, dysphagia, cough, oropharyngeal ulcers, nausea, vomiting, diarrhea, pains in chest or abdomen, pleuritic chest pain. Tourniquet test may be positive. Hypovolemic shock may be accompanied by pleural effusion and renal failure; respiratory distress (airway obstruction, pleural effusion, or congestive heart failure), neurologic symptoms, seizures.	10%–40%
Marburg disease and Ebola hemorrhagic fever	4–7	Headache, malaise, drowsiness, lumbar myalgia, vomiting, nausea, and diarrhea. Maculopapular eruption, hemorrhagic, dark red enanthem on the hard palate, conjunctivitis, and scrotal or labial edema. Gastrointestinal hemorrhage in severe illness. Hypotension and coma in severe cases. DIC and thrombocytopenia are seen in most patients.	Marburg disease: 25% Ebola hemorrhagic fever: 50%–90%
Hemorrhagic fever with renal syndrome (Hanta, Puumala)	9–35	Fever, petechiae, mild hemorrhagic phenomena, mild proteinuria. Thrombocytopenia, petechiae, proteinuria. Hypotension may follow defervescence. Hemoconcentration, ecchymoses, oliguria. Confusion, extreme restlessness. Fatal cases may manifest retroperitoneal edema and hemorrhagic necrosis of the renal medulla	5%–10%
Yellow fever	3–6	Abrupt onset. Fever, headache, severe myalgias, diarrhea, vomiting, severe prostration, conjunctival suffusion, photophobia, cervical and axillary adenopathy. Rarely, splenomegaly or hepatosplenomegaly. Papulovesicular lesions involving the soft palate and pulmonary manifestations during the first stage. The second stage of the illness is associated with neurologic involvement. Hemorrhagic manifestations are similar to those observed with other viral hemorrhagic fevers.	<10%

CNS, central nervous system; DIC, disseminated intravascular coagulopathy.

Diagnosis

In VHF, virus can be recovered during the early febrile stage. Specific complement-fixing and immunofluorescent antibodies appear during convalescence. Antibody tests using viral subunits are available. Serologic diagnosis depends on demonstrating seroconversion in acute and convalescent serum samples taken 3–4 weeks apart. Viral RNA may also be detected in blood or tissues, using reverse-transcriptase PCRs. Handling blood and other biologic specimens requires special training. Healthcare providers need training and protective equipment.

Treatment

Ribavirin administered IV reduces mortality in Lassa fever and hemorrhagic fever with renal syndrome (HFRS). The management of these diseases requires reversal of dehydration, hemoconcentration, renal failure, and protein, electrolyte, or blood losses. The management of hemorrhage should be individualized. Transfusions of fresh blood and platelets are common. Good results have been reported after the administration of clotting factor concentrates. The efficacy of corticosteroids, ε-aminocaproic acid, pressor amines, or α-adrenergic blocking agents has not been established. Sedatives should be selected with regard to the possibility of kidney or liver damage. The successful management of HFRS may require renal dialysis. No vaccines are currently available for most of these diseases. A novel synthetic adenosine analogue, BCX4430, has been shown to protect against Ebola and Marburg virus disease in animal models.

CHAPTER 67 ■ CRITICAL VIRAL INFECTIONS

RAKESH LODHA, SUNIT C. SINGHI, AND JAMES D. CAMPBELL

SEVERE INFLUENZA INFECTIONS

Influenza type A and type B viruses are important in human infection, and both types have surface glycoproteins hemagglutinin (HA) and neuraminidase (NA). Influenza A is subtyped into 16 H and 9 N types based on HA and NA antigens. New strains emerge due to point mutations leading to "antigenic drift" that helps the virus evade host defenses. Another characteristic of influenza A (not shared by type B) is a genome with eight single-stranded RNA segments. When the host cell is infected with more than one influenza virus, these genes can get reassorted and produce a very different strain. This "antigenic shift" is responsible for pandemics of influenza.

The common mode of influenza transmission is inhalation of airborne particles produced by coughing and sneezing (microdroplet method). It is also spread by direct contact and large-particle aerosols. Influenza predominantly infects ciliated columnar epithelial cells in the respiratory tract. The receptor on the viral HA attaches to a sialic acid moiety on the cell membrane, inducing endocytosis. The ion channel activity of the M2 protein and activity of the HA create an acid environment that leads to fusion of the lipid coat with the cell membrane and the entry of the viral RNA into the cytoplasm. Cytopathic effects cause necrosis of the ciliated epithelial cells (evident early in the clinical course). Immunocompetent hosts control influenza infection by innate and adaptive immune responses and limit the effects to mild illness. Some of the reassorted influenza viruses evade immune responses and infect the lung, causing pneumonia.

Many of the symptoms of influenza are due to cytokine release. Cytokine storm may play an important role in causing tissue injury and mortality from influenza virus infection. Patients who die have higher cytokine/chemokine levels but equivalent viral titers in pulmonary samples compared to patients with milder infection. Reassorted influenza viruses can infect lung tissue and induce an exaggerated immune response that leads to a severe and often fatal pneumonia.

Pneumonia from influenza infection may result from primary viral infection, bacterial superinfection, or combined bacterial–viral infection. Severe influenza pneumonia is characterized by diffuse hemorrhagic alveolar exudates, necrosis of bronchiolar epithelium, peribronchial lymphocytic infiltration, and marked lymphocytic infiltration of the alveolar walls and interstitial lung tissue. In severe cases, the effects on other organ systems include focal and diffuse myocarditis, mediastinal lymph node enlargement and necrosis, encephalopathy, encephalitis, and cerebral edema. Reye syndrome is associated with influenza B and the use of salicylates in children. The pathogenesis of influenza-related encephalopathy is not clear; it is hypothesized that viral invasion of the central nervous system (CNS), proinflammatory cytokines, metabolic disorders, or genetic susceptibility may have a role.

Clinical features of influenza infection seen more commonly in children include sudden onset symptoms, anorexia, abdominal pain, vomiting, nausea, cervical adenopathy, and temperature > 38.9°C. Influenza B may cause an epidemic in which children have typical symptoms of influenza but adults have only mild symptoms because antigenic changes in influenza B viruses are less frequent and adults are more likely to have protective immunity. Young children may present with febrile seizures. In uncomplicated illness, the fever usually persists for 2–3 days. A biphasic temperature pattern may occur. Respiratory tract symptoms become prominent by days 2–4, and systemic complaints subside. Dry and hacking cough usually persists for 4–7 days. Nasal and eye complaints are more prominent with influenza B virus, and dizziness and prostration are more common with influenza A infection.

Pandemic H1N1 influenza infection features include fever (79%), cough (73%), dyspnea (54%), vomiting (30%), diarrhea (12%), and seizures (10%) with the onset 3 days before PICU admission. At presentation, 10% require vasopressors for shock, 1.3% have cardiac arrest, and 3.5% have CNS complications. On the day of admission to the PICU, 57.5% received assisted breathing and 8.9% died. Independent risk factors for mortality are female gender, presence of a chronic neurologic condition or immune compromise, diagnosis of acute myocarditis or encephalitis, and methicillin-resistant *Staphylococcus aureus* (MRSA) coinfection of the lung. For children who were previously healthy, MRSA coinfection of the lung increased the risk of death eightfold. Of children needing hospitalization, ~15% need ICU care. The mortality in hospitalized children is ~0.5%. In addition to respiratory illness, influenza may present as encephalopathy, myocarditis, myositis, or with bacterial (particularly *S. aureus*) coinfection.

Risk factors for severe disease include age (<2 years, especially <6 months), comorbidity, chronic lung diseases (asthma), neurologic or neuromuscular disorders (cerebral palsy), immunosuppression, diabetes mellitus, and morbid obesity.

Influenza should be considered in children admitted with lower respiratory tract infections, myocarditis, or encephalopathy. Diagnosis is made by detection of antigen, isolation of virus from respiratory secretions, or demonstrating a rise in serum antibody during convalescence. *Reverse transcription polymerase chain reaction (RT-PCR)* has >90% sensitivity versus a 70% sensitivity of antigen-detecting techniques that use *fluorescent antibodies*. RT-PCR results require 2 days so therapeutic decision making proceeds on clinical criteria. A rapid antigen result is available within 10–30 minutes, but a negative rapid antigen test does not rule out influenza.

The management of influenza includes supportive care of critical illness and antiviral therapy. Antiviral drugs include M2 protein inhibitors (amantadine and rimantadine) and NA inhibitors (oseltamivir and zanamivir). Zanamivir is approved for children 5 years and older and oseltamivir for children >2 weeks of age. Oseltamivir and zanamivir modestly reduce duration of illness. Amantadine–rimantadine resistance is increasing, and they are not used. New and more effective antiviral drugs such as peramivir, laninamivir, and favipiravir are not yet approved. Treatment is recommended for suspected or confirmed influenza in children at high risk for complications, children hospitalized with influenza regardless of immunization status, and children with suspected influenza experiencing a severe or complicated course. Treatment should not be delayed while waiting for confirmatory tests. Discretion is exercised in the use of antiviral therapy for healthy children to prevent resistance and maintain drug supplies.

The prognosis of uncomplicated influenza is good. Complications such as primary influenza pneumonia, staphylococcal pneumonia, encephalitis, and Reye syndrome have a guarded prognosis. Children with underlying chronic diseases have a poorer prognosis.

HIV INFECTION IN THE CRITICALLY ILL CHILD

HIV-1 and HIV-2 are members of the Retroviridae family and belong to the *Lentivirus* genus. Transmission of HIV-1 occurs via sexual contact, parenteral exposure to blood, or vertical transmission. Vertical transmission is the major mode of transmission in children. Vertical transmission rates in untreated women are up to 30% in developed countries and 50% in undeveloped countries. Perinatal treatment of infected mothers with antiretroviral drugs dramatically decreases this rate. The risk factors for vertical transmission include preterm delivery (<34 weeks gestation), a low maternal antenatal CD4 count, use of illicit drugs during pregnancy, >4 hour duration of ruptured membranes, and birth weight < 2500 g. Blood donor screening has dramatically reduced the risk of transfusion-associated HIV infection. HIV-2 is a rare cause of infection in children. It is most prevalent in Western and Southern Africa. If HIV-2 is suspected, a specific test that detects antibody to HIV-2 peptides should be used.

When HIV enters the mucosa, it first infects dendritic cells, which process antigens and transport them to the lymphoid tissue. In the lymph node, HIV binds to CD4 molecules on the surface of helper T lymphocytes (CD4 cells), monocytes, and macrophages. The CD4 lymphocytes activate and proliferate, contributing to the lymphadenopathy characteristic of acute retroviral syndrome in adults and adolescents. HIV preferentially infects the cells that respond to it (i.e., HIV-specific memory CD4 cells), causing loss of response by these cells and loss of control of HIV replication. Within 3–6 weeks of infection, a burst of viremia occurs. A cellular and humoral immune response is established within the next 4 months, and the viremia declines, symptoms diminish, and CD4 cells return to moderately decreased levels. Unlike adults, early HIV-1 replication in children has no apparent clinical manifestations. Almost all HIV-infected infants have detectable HIV-1 in blood by 4 months of age.

HIV-infected children have immune system changes similar to adults. CD4 cell depletion may be reduced because infants have a relative lymphocytosis. Lymphopenia, rare in perinatally infected children, is seen in older children or end-stage disease. B-cell activation occurs early, evidenced by high levels of anti-HIV-1 antibody, reflecting dysregulation of T-cell suppression of B-cell antibody synthesis or CD4 enhancement of B-lymphocyte humoral responses. CD4 depletion and inadequate antibody responses lead to increased susceptibility to various infections that varies with the severity of immunodeficiency.

Three patterns of disease are described in children without highly active antiretroviral therapy (HAART) administration. Up to 20% of HIV-infected newborns in developed countries and >85% in resource-poor countries present with a rapid onset of symptoms in their first few months and, if untreated, die by age 4 years. Their intrauterine infection coincides with a period of expansion of CD4 cells in the fetus infecting the majority of immunocompetent cells. They have a positive HIV-1 culture or detectable virus in plasma in the first 48 hours of life, suggesting in utero infection. The majority of infected newborns (60%–80%) present with a slower progression of disease and survive to 6 years. This group has a negative viral culture or PCR in the first week of life and is considered to be infected intrapartum. The viral load rapidly increases by 3 months of age due to the immaturity of the immune system and then declines over 24 months. The third perinatal infection pattern (i.e., long-term survivors) occurs in a small percentage (<5%). They have minimal progression of disease with relatively normal CD4 counts and low viral loads for >8 years.

The clinical manifestations of HIV infection vary with age. Physical examination at birth is usually normal. Symptoms found in children more often than in adults include recurrent bacterial infections, chronic parotid swelling, lymphoid interstitial pneumonitis (LIP), and early onset of progressive neurologic deterioration. The most common HIV-related diseases that lead to PICU admission are respiratory infection, respiratory failure, septic shock, and disorders of the CNS. As antiretroviral therapy use increases, complications of therapy may cause PICU admissions. Acute respiratory failure (due to *Pneumocystis jirovecii* or bacterial infection) is the most important cause of PICU admission.

Pneumocystis jirovecii pneumonia (PCP) is a common AIDS-defining illness, with most cases occurring between 3 and 6 months of life (see Chapter 72). If PCP develops on prophylaxis, trimethoprim/sulfamethoxazole is still used as poor compliance or unusual pharmacokinetics may have occurred. If drug resistance is the cause, an alternative drug is recommended. Untreated, PCP is universally fatal. With therapy, mortality is <10%. Mortality is associated with the severity of disease and the immunosuppression.

Recurrent bacterial infections in the lung occur in 90% of HIV-infected children. The initial pneumonia often occurs before significant immunocompromise develops and pneumonia frequency increases as immunocompromise increases. The common pathogens are *Streptococcus pneumoniae*, *Haemophilus influenzae*, and *Staphylococcus aureus*. In severe immunosuppression or hospital-acquired infections, gram-negative organisms, such as *Pseudomonas aeruginosa*, gain importance. Severe immunocompromise may diminish the signs of infection. Response to therapy is slow, and relapse rates are high. Bacteremia is common (up to 50%). Attempts to isolate the causative organism should not delay empirical parenteral antibiotics. Choice of antibiotics is based on patterns of etiologies and susceptibilities. If *P. jirovecii* pneumonia cannot be excluded in a severe respiratory infection, co-trimoxazole should be added.

Tuberculosis (TB) is increasing with the spread of the HIV infection. Coexistent TB and HIV accelerates the progression of both diseases. HIV-infected children are more likely to have active TB (5–10 times more likely), extrapulmonary TB, disseminated TB, and a more rapid course (see Chapter 72). HIV-infected children with active TB should receive long-duration therapy (9–12 months) and close follow-up to diagnose nonresponse/drug resistance early.

Mycobacterium avium-intracellulare (MAI) pulmonary disease is unusual in children with HIV. Symptoms include fever, failure to thrive, night sweats, lymphadenopathy, organomegaly, and refractory anemia. Pulmonary findings are lymphadenopathy and localized parenchymal lesions. Diagnosis of disseminated disease requires isolation of the organism from blood. Therapy for disseminated MAI involves clarithromycin or azithromycin with ethambutol.

Viral infections in the lung caused by RSV, influenza, and parainfluenza viruses are more likely to be symptomatic in HIV-infected children. Infections with adenovirus and measles virus lead to serious sequelae. Cytomegalovirus (CMV) is a known opportunistic pathogen, but CMV pneumonia is rare in HIV. Diagnosis and treatment of these infections are similar to those in non–HIV-infected children.

Fungal infections in the lung are usually secondary to disseminated disease in immune compromised children (Chapter 72). Pulmonary candidiasis should be suspected in HIV-infected children not responding to therapy. Invasive candidiasis is diagnosed by blood culture.

LIP is a distinctive marker for pediatric HIV. Without antiretroviral therapy, nearly 20% of HIV-infected children develop LIP. Suggested etiologies include an immunologic response to inhaled or circulating antigens and primary infection of the lung with HIV, Epstein–Barr virus, or both. LIP is characterized by diffuse infiltration of the alveolar septae by lymphocytes, plasmacytoid lymphocytes, plasma cells, and immunoblasts. No involvement of the blood vessels or destruction of the lung tissue occurs. LIP is diagnosed in perinatally acquired HIV infection after 1 year of age, unlike with PCP. Most children with LIP are asymptomatic; tachypnea, cough, wheezing, and hypoxemia may be seen; and crepitations are uncommon. Clubbing is present in advanced disease. Chronic LIP is associated with bronchiectasis. A reticulonodular pattern that persists on chest X-ray for 2 months and is unresponsive to antimicrobial therapy is presumptive evidence of LIP. A definitive diagnosis requires histopathology. Management is conservative; antiretrovirals have limited effect. Steroids are indicated for symptoms of chronic pulmonary disease, clubbing, and/or hypoxemia. A 4–12-week course of prednisolone is followed by a taper and then by chronic low-dose prednisolone.

Gastrointestinal involvement can be clinically significant. Causes include bacteria (*Salmonella, Campylobacter, M. avium-intracellulare* complex [MAC]), protozoa (*Giardia, Cryptosporidium, Isospora*, microsporidia), viruses (cytomegalovirus, herpes simplex virus [HSV], rotavirus), and fungi (*Candida*). The protozoal infections are most severe and can be protracted. Children with cryptosporidium infestation can have severe diarrhea that leads to hypovolemic shock. AIDS enteropathy (malabsorption, partial villous atrophy, and no specific pathogen) is probably a direct HIV infection of the gut. Chronic liver inflammation is common. Hepatitis caused by cytomegalovirus, hepatitis B or C viruses, or MAC may lead to liver failure and portal hypertension. Pancreatitis is uncommon and may result from drug therapy (e.g., didanosine, lamivudine, nevirapine, or pentamidine) or opportunistic infections (e.g., MAC or cytomegalovirus). Management of these conditions is similar to non–HIV-infected children.

Neurologic involvement occurs in >50% of perinatally infected children in developing countries (less in developed countries) with onset around 1.5 years of age. It commonly presents as progressive encephalopathy with loss or plateau of developmental milestones, cognitive deterioration, microcephaly, and symmetric motor dysfunction. CNS infections (meningitis due to bacterial pathogens, fungi, such as *Cryptococcus*, and a number of viruses) may be indications for PICU admission. CNS toxoplasmosis is rare in young infants but occurs in HIV-infected adolescents. They usually have serum IgG anti-toxoplasma antibodies. The management of these conditions is similar to non–HIV-infected children but with poorer response rates and outcomes.

Cardiac involvement is common, persistent, and often progressive, but most abnormalities are subclinical. Left ventricular (LV) structure and function progressively deteriorate in the first 3 years of life, resulting in persistent mild LV dysfunction, increased LV mass, and higher mortality. Resting sinus tachycardia has been reported in up to two-thirds, and marked sinus arrhythmia in one-fifth of HIV-infected children. Gallop rhythm with tachypnea and hepatosplenomegaly are the best clinical indicators of congestive heart failure in HIV-infected children. Anticongestive therapy is effective when initiated early. Electro- and echocardiography are helpful in assessing cardiac function before the onset of clinical symptoms.

Renal involvement can present as a nephrotic syndrome (edema, hypoalbuminemia, proteinuria, and azotemia). Polyuria, oliguria, and hematuria have also been observed but hypertension is unusual. Nephropathy is unusual and more commonly occurs in older symptomatic children.

Diagnosis of HIV requires appropriate testing. Infants may be antibody positive at birth because of maternal HIV antibody transfer across the placenta. Uninfected infants usually lose maternal antibody by 6 to 12 months. Because some uninfected infants have persistent maternal antibody, IgG antibody tests cannot make a definitive diagnosis until after 18 months of age. HIV DNA or RNA PCR assays, HIV culture, or HIV p24 antigen immune-dissociated p24 (ICD-p24) are essential for diagnosis of infants born to HIV-infected mothers. By 6 months of age, HIV culture and/or PCR identifies all infected infants not having continued exposure from breast-feeding.

Decisions about antiretroviral therapy for children with HIV are based on the viral load, CD4 lymphocyte count, and clinical condition. In the developed world, the decision to initiate HAART is based on clinical, immunologic, and virologic parameters. In settings without access to laboratory tests, the decision to treat may be based only on clinical symptoms. Antiretroviral therapy has transformed HIV infection from a fatal condition to a chronic infection with a near-normal life. The three main groups of drugs are nucleoside reverse transcriptase inhibitors (NRTIs), non-NRTIs (NNRTIs), and protease inhibitors (PIs). HAART is a combination of two NRTIs with a PI or an NNRTI. Some complications of antiretroviral therapy, such as lactic acidosis, severe pancreatitis, and Stevens–Johnson syndrome, may require discontinuing the drug, supportive care, and possibly PICU admission.

Outcome data are limited regarding antiretroviral treatment in critically ill HIV-infected children. Without access to antiretroviral therapy, 20% of children infected by their mothers (vertical transmission) progress to AIDS or death during their first year of life, and >50% of HIV-infected children die before their fifth birthday. Limitation of intervention decisions, usually made in the PICU, directly influences short-term survival and the opportunity to commence HAART. Although few critically ill HIV-infected children in developing countries survived to become established on HAART, the long-term outcome of children on HAART remains encouraging.

Prevention of transmission of HIV in the PICU requires adherence to universal precautions, regardless of suspected HIV status. In case of exposure, the staff should follow the standard guidelines for postexposure prophylaxis (PEP). The US Public Health Service now recommends that expanded PEP regimens be PI based. PEP should be initiated as soon as possible, preferably within hours of exposure. If a question exists concerning which antiretroviral drugs to use or whether to use a basic or expanded regimen, the basic regimen should be started immediately rather than delaying PEP administration. PEP should be administered for 4 weeks, if tolerated.

MEASLES

Measles remains common in developing countries, where >95% of measles deaths occur. More than 30 million people are affected each year by measles. Cases imported from other countries are the most important source of infection in countries where measles has been eliminated. Unimmunized children remain at risk of acquiring the infection and can suffer a severe course.

The measles virus is spread by aerosolized droplets of respiratory secretions, facilitated by close person-to-person contact. There is no animal reservoir, and asymptomatic carriers are unknown. Measles is highly contagious with a 90% infection rate in unimmunized contacts. The initial infection site is the respiratory epithelium of the nasopharynx. The virus spreads to the regional lymphoid tissue followed by a primary viremia (day 2–3 after infection), that seeds the reticuloendothelial system. Between the days 8 and 10, a secondary viremia occurs and infection in the skin, conjunctivae, and the respiratory tract is established and produces the clinical syndrome. The maximum viral burden occurs between days 11 and 14 and then rapidly declines. Immunologically compromised patients have defective clearing of the virus and increased severity of organ involvement. Malnourished children experience more severe measles infection.

The incubation period of measles is 8–12 days followed by high fever that lasts 1–7 days. During the initial stage, the child develops cough, coryza (runny nose), conjunctivitis (the 3 Cs), and an enanthem. *Koplik spots,* small white spots on a reddened background, appear on the buccal mucosa near the molars. Children are very irritable. After several days of fever, a rash develops on the face (often in the hairline) and upper neck. The rash is initially erythematous and maculopapular with a typical coexistence of discrete and confluent red maculopapules. Microvesicles may be seen on the top of the erythematous base. Over a 3-day period, the rash extends downward, eventually reaching the hands and feet. The rash lasts for 5–6 days. Pharyngitis, cervical lymphadenopathy, diarrhea, vomiting, laryngitis, and croup may also occur.

Measles pneumonia is common. It is characterized by hyperinflation and fluffy perihilar infiltrates. Infants may present with features of bronchiolitis. Extensive infection leads to hypoxemia. Children with defects in cell-mediated immunity are prone to develop severe pneumonia. Secondary bacterial pneumonias are responsible for measles-related complications and deaths. The bacterial pneumonias are usually due to *H. influenzae*, *S. pneumoniae*, and *S. aureus*. Coinfection with other viruses (parainfluenza and adenovirus) has been reported. Acute respiratory distress syndrome and air leaks are common respiratory complications. Other complications include otitis media, mastoiditis, laryngitis, and laryngotracheobronchitis.

Measles encephalitis occurs in 1 per 1000 measles cases. The three forms of CNS infections are acute progressive infectious encephalitis (inclusion body encephalitis), acute postinfectious encephalitis, and subacute sclerosing panencephalitis (SSPE). The acute progressive form reflects a direct viral attack that overpowers cell-mediated immunity. The postinfectious acute disease reflects an autoimmune reaction. SSPE is a rare, progressive degenerative loss of intelligence, behavioral difficulties, and seizures. Symptoms of encephalitis develop in the second week of illness. Rapid deterioration with increased intracranial pressure and herniation may occur. Cerebellar ataxia, myelitis, and motor deficits have been reported. Sequelae include seizures, deafness, and motor deficits. Non-CNS complications of measles include myocarditis, pericarditis, bleeding related to thrombocytopenia, and DIC in severe disease.

Diagnosis of measles is clinical in endemic areas. Confirmatory studies include antimeasles IgM antibody in serum, a rise in IgG antibodies to measles (acute and convalescent sera), and isolation of the virus from urine, blood, throat, or nasopharyngeal secretions. The identification of prodromal signs (Koplik spots, 3 Cs) may help with earlier isolation of infectious individuals.

Treatment for mild infections is supportive. A reduction in morbidity and mortality in severe measles with vitamin A has led to the recommendation of vitamin A for children with measles in regions where vitamin A deficiency is a problem or the case-fatality ratio is >1%. Successful use of inhaled or IV ribavirin in severe infections has been anecdotally reported. Associated bacterial infections are managed with appropriate antimicrobials. Supportive care and monitoring are important in severe infections, as multiple organ systems may be affected. Complication rates are higher in malnourished children, immunocompromised children, and in those with vitamin A deficiency. A 26% mortality was reported in children with measles admitted to the PICU.

NONPOLIO ENTEROVIRAL INFECTIONS

Enteroviruses cause 55%–65% of hospitalizations for suspected sepsis in infants during the summer and fall (25% year-round). Severe CNS or cardiopulmonary disease is associated with outbreaks of hand-foot-mouth disease (enterovirus 71) and enterovirus meningitis. Factors associated with severity include young age (infants), male sex, poor hygiene, overcrowding, and low socioeconomic status. Breast-feeding reduces the risk of infection.

Within 24 hours of contact with oral or respiratory mucosa, the infection spreads to lymphoid tissue. Minor viremia occurs on day 3, leading to infection at secondary sites and coinciding with onset of clinical symptoms. Viral multiplication at secondary sites leads to viremia, which lasts until day 7. When antibody appears in the blood, viremia ceases and secondary infection sites decrease. However, virus may replicate in the gastrointestinal tract for weeks.

Mild enteroviral infections include nonspecific febrile illness, common cold, pharyngitis, croup, herpangina, stomatitis, and parotitis. Bronchitis, bronchiolitis, or pneumonia can be caused by coxsackie and echovirus infections. Epidemic pleurodynia is caused by coxsackie B3 and B5. Gastrointestinal manifestations are common in coxsackie and echoviral infections; manifestations other than diarrhea and vomiting include peritonitis, mesenteric adenitis, appendicitis, hepatitis, and pancreatitis. Pericarditis and myocarditis can be caused by coxsackie or echoviruses. Neurologic illness is common, usually aseptic meningitis. Encephalitis, paralytic disease due to anterior horn cell infection, Guillain–Barré syndrome, transverse myelitis, and cerebellar ataxia may occur. Genitourinary manifestations include nephritis, orchitis, and epididymitis. Arthritis and myositis may be caused by coxsackie virus. Skin rashes are common with enterovirus and may be maculopapular, morbilliform, petechial, or vesicles. A common distribution is in the palms, soles, and oral mucosa (hand-foot-mouth syndrome).

The diagnosis of enterovirus infection is confirmed by virus isolation and detection. Samples may be collected from the nasopharynx, throat, stool, rectal swab, blood, urine, and cerebrospinal fluid (CSF). Viral isolation in culture takes less than a week. The virus may be detected in body fluids by cDNA or RNA probes and PCR. Serology is not used for diagnosis.

Treatment is supportive. IV immunoglobulin has been used in neonates with severe disseminated infection and children with persistent CNS infection due to immune deficiency–associated hypogammaglobulinemia. Pleconaril may have limited benefit for treatment of neurologic infections, myocarditis, and infections in immunodeficient patients. In absence of any evidence indicating benefit, corticosteroids should be avoided. Children with enteroviral infections require universal and contact precautions.

SEVERE VARICELLA INFECTIONS

Primary infection with varicella-zoster virus (VZV) presents as varicella (chickenpox) and reactivation as zoster (shingles). VZV produces cytopathic effects indistinguishable from HSV. Transmission occurs by airborne droplets, secretions, or infected vesicular fluid. The incubation period is 2 weeks (range of 10–21 days). Chickenpox is characterized by rash, low-grade fever, and malaise. Patients have constitutional symptoms 1–2 days before onset of rash. The rash evolves from maculopapules to pruritic vesicles to crusts. It initially appears on the trunk or face and spreads to involve the entire body. Skin lesions (250–500 in unvaccinated children) often appear as crops (groups). Simultaneous lesions in various stages is a hallmark of chickenpox. Most patients uneventfully recover after 1 week. Severe manifestations such as pneumonia, hepatitis, encephalitis, and DIC are more likely in neonates, pregnant women, adolescents, adults, and the immunocompromised. Up to 3.5% of children have a complicated course. Deaths are uncommon (<2 deaths per 100,000) in children.

Secondary bacterial complications can occur in skin, soft tissues, and other sites. They are often caused by group A *Streptococcus* (GAS) and *S. aureus*. Varicella is an important risk factor for severe invasive GAS infections in children. A GAS infection should be considered in varicella cases with localized findings of erythema, warmth, swelling, or induration, with fever after having been afebrile, a temperature > 39°C beyond day 3 of illness, or fever beyond day 4 of illness. GAS infections are usually painful out of proportion to the clinical findings.

Varicella-zoster pneumonia is the most serious complication of disseminated VZV infection. Its prevalence is 4%–50% of adult varicella infections with a 9%–50% mortality. Most cases of VZV pneumonia occur in patients with immunocompromise or chronic lung disease. It presents 1–6 days after onset of the rash with tachypnea, chest tightness, cough, dyspnea, fever, and occasionally pleuritic chest pain and hemoptysis. Chest symptoms may start before the skin rash. Physical findings are often minimal, and chest X-ray reveals nodular or interstitial pneumonitis. Hilar lymphadenopathy and pleural effusion are unusual. The nodules usually resolve within a week after disappearance of skin lesions but may calcify and persist for months. High-resolution CT usually shows 1- to 10-mm nodules throughout both lungs. Nodules with a surrounding halo of ground-glass opacity, patchy ground-glass opacity, and coalescence of nodules are also seen.

Varicella-zoster encephalitis, another serious complication, is discussed in Chapters 68 and 72. *Disseminated varicella-zoster* with multivisceral involvement occurs in immunocompromised patients, particularly with deficient cell-mediated immunity, bone marrow and renal transplant recipients, and AIDS. Even with treatment, the disease carries a high mortality. Less common complications include transverse myelitis, Guillain–Barré syndrome, purpura fulminans, myocarditis, arthritis, and hepatic failure (see Chapter 68 for diagnosis and management).

SEVERE HERPES SIMPLEX VIRUS INFECTIONS

HSV-1causes orolabial, ocular, and CNS infection and is more prevalent than HSV-2, which predominantly causes genital infections, neonatal infections, and aseptic meningitis. HSV infections commonly involve oral and genital skin and mucosa. Visceral involvement is uncommon and carries high morbidity and mortality.

Herpes simplex encephalitis (HSE) is the most commonly identified cause of sporadic viral encephalitis beyond 6 months of age. Although HSE is rare, mortality is 70% without therapy and a minority returns to normal function. This dreaded manifestation can occur within weeks after birth (neonatal HSV disease) or in childhood or adulthood (HSE). Most neonatal cases are caused by HSV-2 and non-neonatal cases by HSV-1. The majority of cases of HSE are due to reactivated virus from dorsal root ganglia, but virus can also reach the CNS via olfactory bulbs during viremia of primary infection. Evidence also suggests persistence of HSV genome in the CNS of asymptomatic individuals. HSV encephalitis is discussed in detail in Chapter 68.

HSV pneumonia is seen in immunocompromised patients and carries a high mortality. The diagnoses of this and other herpes infections are made difficult by the phenomenon of latency.

Disseminated HSV (cutaneous and visceral) is most common in children with immune deficiencies (particularly those affecting T lymphocytes), severe malnourishment, organ transplants, malignancy, immunosuppression, high-dose steroid therapy, AIDS, or burns. Disseminated disease may manifest as a sepsis-like syndrome with fever or hypothermia, leukopenia, hepatitis, DIC, and shock and often results in death. This form of herpes has a high mortality, even with appropriate therapy.

Neonatal HSV infection (caused by HSV-2 in 70% of cases) occurs in 1 in 4000 newborns in the United States. Neonatal infection is usually acquired during the intrapartum period. Primary infection in the mother, rupture of membranes >6 hours, and fetal invasive monitoring appear to increase the risk. Neonatal herpes may manifest in three ways. The least severe form is limited to skin, eyes, and mucous membranes (*SEM disease*) and has onset between 5 and 19 days of life. Disseminated HSV is rapidly progressive, usually fatal, and has onset before the third week of life. Localized CNS HSV is usually diagnosed late because of a lack of cutaneous findings. Most survivors of disseminated or CNS disease have neurologic sequelae, and a mortality without therapy of 80%.

Cutaneous HSV infection can be rapidly diagnosed by microscopic findings of giant cells with intranuclear inclusions (Tzanck smear). HSV PCR has been found to be as sensitive as viral culture for cutaneous HSV infection and provides rapid diagnosis. PCR of the CSF is the method of choice for diagnosis of HSE, but CSF PCR results can be negative in the first 72 hours. CSF virus culture is of little value. For details of the role of neuroimaging, see Chapter 68. Neonatal herpes may occur in the absence of skin lesions and, if suspected, swabs of the mouth, nasopharynx, conjunctiva, rectum, skin lesions, mucosal lesions, and urine should be submitted for virus culture. Evidence of disseminated or CNS infection should be sought using liver function tests, complete blood cell count, CSF analysis, and chest X-ray, if respiratory abnormalities are present. Microscopic examination, culture, and PCR assay of bronchoalveolar lavage fluid may help in the diagnosis of HSV pneumonia.

Serious HSV infections require IV acyclovir treatment for 21 days. SEM disease requires treatment for 14 days. Neonates require higher dosing than older children. Dosing should be adjusted for renal impairment. Patients with HSE should undergo a CSF HSV PCR after 14 days to document elimination of replicating virus. Acyclovir-resistant strains have been reported in immunocompromised patients. The drug of choice for acyclovir-resistance is IV foscarnet.

With therapy, most infants with SEM HSV infection improve. For HSV infection limited to the skin, eyes, or mouth, $\geq$3 recurrences of vesicles is associated with neurologic impairment. The mortality rate is significantly higher in the neonates with disseminated infection and encephalitis. The risk of death increases in neonates with coma, DIC, or prematurity. In babies with disseminated disease, HSV pneumonitis is associated with greater mortality.

CHAPTER 68 ■ CENTRAL NERVOUS SYSTEM INFECTIONS

PRATIBHA D. SINGHI, AND SUNIT C. SINGHI

To cause central nervous system (CNS) infections, pathogens must gain access to the subarachnoid space to cause meningitis or to the brain parenchyma and spinal cord to cause encephalitis, CNS abscess, or myelitis. Most infections spread to the CNS from the bloodstream. Direct spread may come from a focus adjacent to the brain (otitis media, sinusitis, dental abscess), a cerebrospinal fluid (CSF) shunt, or a skull fracture.

BACTERIAL MENINGITIS

Etiology

Haemophilus influenzae, *Neisseria meningitidis*, and *Streptococcus pneumoniae* cause the majority of cases of bacterial meningitis. *Haemophilus* spp. are small, gram-negative, pleomorphic coccobacilli that are either encapsulated or unencapsulated. Nearly all invasive *H. influenzae* infections are caused by serotype b (Hib). *Neisseria* spp. are nonmotile gram-negative cocci that often appear in pairs (diplococci). Most disease is caused by organisms in serogroups A, B, C, Y, and W135. *Pneumococci* are gram-positive streptococci generally seen in pairs or chains. The serotypes that cause meningitis have a strong correlation with those that cause pneumonia and bacteremia. Neonatal meningitis may be caused by *Escherichia coli*, group B streptococci, or *Listeria monocytogenes*. Gram-negative bacterial meningitis in children beyond the neonatal period is generally nosocomial or may be associated with other conditions, such as gut infections, head trauma, neurosurgical procedures, and immunodeficiency. A decrease in the incidence of neonatal invasive group B streptococcal disease has been seen in developed countries, secondary to treatment of colonized pregnant women at delivery. *Staphylococcus aureus* infections are generally seen in malnourished children with staphylococcal skin lesions, dermal sinuses, CSF shunts, or following trauma or surgical procedures. Anaerobic pathogens are seen with extension from localized infections, surgical hardware, anatomic abnormalities, or immunosuppression.

Epidemiology

Hib remains the leading cause of bacterial meningitis in countries where Hib vaccine is not available. Hib meningitis in the first 2 months of life is rare because of placental transfer of protective antibodies. *Meningococcal meningitis* occurs primarily in children and young adults. In developed countries, most cases are due to serogroups B and C. However, serogroup A is responsible for large-scale epidemics in many developing countries. Neisserial infections have been associated with defects of late complement components (C5, C6, C7, or C8, and perhaps C9). *Pneumococcal meningitis* occurs in all age groups, but maximum incidence rates are seen at the extremes of age. Common predisposing factors include pneumonia, otitis media, sinusitis, CSF fistulas or leaks, head injury, sickle cell disease, and thalassemia major. Vaccines against Hib, *S. pneumoniae*, and *N. meningitidis* have decreased the disease burden by 99%, 94%, and 90% where vaccines are available.

Pathogenesis and Pathophysiology

Most organisms that cause bacterial meningitis are transmitted by the respiratory route. Pathogens must overcome host defenses of circulating antibodies, complement-mediated bacterial killing, and neutrophil phagocytosis. The blood–brain barrier (BBB) normally protects against meningeal invasion. Penetration of BBB depends on capsule characteristics, fimbriae, surface proteins of bacteria, and a critical magnitude of bacteremia. After penetrating the meninges, the bacteria multiply in the CSF, which has diminished host defense mechanisms. The release of bacterial cell wall fragments and lipopolysaccharide trigger a strong inflammatory response in the subarachnoid space. The increase in cytokines enhances permeability of the BBB and recruits leukocytes from the blood into CSF, leading to CSF pleocytosis. These mediators also affect cerebral blood flow (CBF) and metabolism. An increase in CBF is seen in early meningitis followed by a progressive decline, most likely as a result of vasospasm. Loss of autoregulation makes cerebral perfusion dependent on the systemic blood pressure. Focal hypoperfusion can occur due to vasculitis of large and small arteries crossing the inflamed subarachnoid space.

Cerebral edema in bacterial meningitis may be vasogenic, cytotoxic, or interstitial. Vasogenic cerebral edema occurs as a result of increased BBB permeability. Cytotoxic edema occurs because of an increase in intracellular water secondary to alterations of the cell membrane permeability. Interstitial edema occurs due to increased production or decreased reabsorption of CSF. Death from meningitis may occur because of elevated intracranial pressure (ICP), cerebral infarction, disseminated intravascular coagulation (DIC), circulatory failure from septic shock, or refractory status epilepticus (SE).

Clinical Presentation

The presentation in neonates and infants is generally nonspecific with fever, poor feeding, vomiting, lethargy, irritability, high-pitched cry, and seizures. Fever may be absent. The anterior fontanel is often full or bulging. Older children present with fever, headache, vomiting, anorexia, photophobia, and altered sensorium. A preceding upper respiratory or gastrointestinal infection is often present. Examination shows signs of meningeal irritation (stiffness and pain on flexion of the neck), a Kernig sign, and Brudzinski sign. Papilledema is uncommon. Focal signs are seen in ~14% cases and suggest subdural collection, cortical infarction, or cerebritis. A fulminant picture with sepsis, shock, and rapid progression to death is typical of meningococcemia, a syndrome distinct from meningococcal meningitis. Patients with meningococcemia present with a maculopapular rash that rapidly progresses to a petechiae or purpura. Rashes can occasionally be seen in *H. influenzae* or pneumococcal meningitis.

Laboratory Diagnosis

The diagnosis of meningitis is often missed on initial evaluation. A high index of suspicion is essential. Definitive diagnosis is made by analysis and culture of the CSF (**Table 68.1**). Lumbar puncture (LP) should be performed in all infants <6 months of age with febrile seizures and in all children with suspected meningitis unless there is concern for raised ICP (unequal pupils, blood pressure/heart rate changes, abnormal respiratory pattern, deep coma/deteriorating consciousness), focal neurologic symptoms or signs (obtain a CT to exclude space-occupying lesion), shock/cardiorespiratory instability, thrombocytopenia (platelet count <40,000/mm^{3} or coagulation disorder), or local infection at LP site.

Antibiotics should be administered in all cases of suspected meningitis even if the LP is delayed. A CT scan before LP should be obtained only in select cases in which focal neurologic symptoms or signs, clinical evidence of critically elevated ICP, or papilledema are observed, or when doubt exists regarding the diagnosis. The characteristic CSF findings are increased opening pressure, polymorphonuclear pleocytosis, decreased glucose, and increased protein concentration. Normal CSF in children has 0–5 mononuclear cells/mm^3 (lymphocyte and monocytes); polymorphonuclear cells are very rarely seen; in neonates, the upper limit of normal extends to a WBC count of 20–30 WBC/mm^3. The CSF glucose is <40 mg/dL in 50%–60% cases. The CSF may occasionally be completely normal in early stages of bacterial meningitis.

A grossly traumatic LP can be used for CSF culture alone, and the WBC and RBC counts in blood and CSF can sometimes be used to predict the absence of culture-positive meningitis. Most cases of viral meningitis have a lymphocytic response, but an initial polymorphic response may occur. The CSF glucose is rarely below 30 mg/dL in viral meningitis. Although tubercular meningitis (TBM) may occasionally have an acute presentation, generally the symptoms are more prolonged.

Rapid diagnostic tests that detect the pathogen by countercurrent immunoelectrophoresis, enzyme-linked immunosorbent assay (ELISA), and latex agglutination may be useful in providing early diagnosis and in suspected cases of partially treated bacterial meningitis. PCR assays detect the nucleic acids of the common organisms that cause meningitis and are very specific. These tests are expensive and not easily available. To prove tubercular, herpetic, or cryptococcal infection, special staining techniques/tests may be required.

Complications

Subdural effusions are a common complication of meningitis. They often resolve spontaneously. Persistent or recurrent fever or focal signs suggest subdural empyema. Cerebritis and infarction present

TABLE 68.1

Cerebrospinal Fluid Characteristics in Meningitis

CHARACTERISTICS	VIRAL	BACTERIAL	TUBERCULAR
WBC/mm^3	N (<5) or raised to 10–100	Raised 100 to >1000	Raised 100–1000
Predominant cell type	Lymphocytes	Neutrophils	Lymphocytes
Glucose (CSF: serum)	N (~0.6) or decreased (<0.4)	Decreased (<0.4 or much lower)	Decreased (<0.4 or lower)
Protein (mg/dL)	N (<50) or up to 100	Raised 100 to >500	Raised 100–500

WBC, white blood cells; CSF, cerebrospinal fluid; N, normal.

with new focal features and are caused by inflammatory involvement of the blood vessels or direct spread of infection from the subarachnoid space. Sensorineural deafness occurs in 5%–30% cases, especially with pneumococcal meningitis. Spread of infection to cause pneumonia, pericarditis, arthritis, and osteomyelitis is rare.

Treatment

CSF, blood, and pertinent cultures are ideally taken before starting antibiotics. If specimens are difficult to obtain, therapy should be started and specimens obtained later. Initial empiric antibiotic therapy should be broad and based on epidemiologic patterns of organisms and resistance. In babies up to3months of age, ampicillin along with cefotaxime or an aminoglycoside is generally used; in older children, a third-generation cephalosporin is used. In the United States and countries where pneumococcal resistance to third-generation cephalosporins has emerged, vancomycin is added to the empiric regimen. In developing countries, ampicillin and chloramphenicol may be used if financial constraints prevent cephalosporin use, but resistance is increasing. Gatifloxacin, moxifloxacin, and trovafloxacin have been found to be as effective as cephalosporins for bacterial meningitis, but are not usually first line. Meropenem has better CSF penetration than imipenem.

Steroid therapy reduces cerebral edema, elevated ICP, and CSF outflow obstruction in experimental models of meningitis. Dexamethasone use in *H. influenzae* meningitis reduces the incidence of hearing loss among survivors. The use of steroids for pneumococcal or meningococcal meningitis is controversial. Benefit of steroids has not been established in neonatal meningitis and in children with meningitis in developing countries.

Mortality rates of meningitis are 15%–20%. Neurologic sequelae include hydrocephalous, spasticity, visual and hearing loss, cognitive deficits, and developmental delay. For *H. influenzae* meningitis, rifampin prophylaxis is recommended for household contacts if at least one unvaccinated contact is <4 years old. With meningococcal disease, rifampin prophylaxis is recommended for household and day care contacts. A single intramuscular dose of ceftriaxone or a single oral dose of ciprofloxacin or azithromycin are sometimes alternatives. *H. influenzae* vaccination has wiped out *H. influenzae* meningitis from developed countries.

ASEPTIC MENINGITIS

Most cases of aseptic meningitis are caused by viral infections. Other causes include fungi, unusual bacteria, mycoplasma, autoimmune diseases, malignancies, and drug reactions. Aseptic meningitis from mumps virus, lymphocytic choriomeningitis virus, and poliovirus are uncommon today. Enteroviruses are the most common agents and have a benign course in immunocompetent individuals. Other viruses, including arboviruses, herpesviruses, paramyxoviruses, and orthomyxoviruses, are discussed in detail in the encephalitis section.

TUBERCULAR MENINGITIS

CNS TB may take a number of forms, including tubercular meningitis (TBM), tuberculomas, tubercular abscesses, and, rarely, myeloradiculopathy. TBM is the most common. It is caused by *Mycobacterium tuberculosis*; meningitis due to *Mycobacterium bovis* or atypical *Mycobacteria*, such as *Mycobacterium avium-intracellulare*, is extremely rare. Involvement of the CNS mostly occurs during a primary infection in children, whereas in adults it occurs during reactivation. Infection can cause inflammation, obstruction of vessels, and subsequent infarction of the cerebral cortex. The brainstem and various cranial nerves, particularly nerves III, VI, and VII, are surrounded by exudates. Interference with the flow of CSF leads to hydrocephalus.

Onset is insidious, with low-grade fever, poor feeding, irritability, headache, and vomiting, followed by neck rigidity and altered sensorium. Infants and young children may experience symptoms for only a few days before the onset of acute hydrocephalus, seizures, and cerebral edema. The main presenting clinical symptoms and signs in children include alteration in consciousness (79%), focal neurologic signs (66%), fever (66%), and seizures (53%). Contact with an infected adult can be found in approximately half of cases.

In TBM, the CSF generally has a cell count of 10–500 cells/mm^3, predominantly lymphocytes, although polymorphonuclear leukocytes may be present. The CSF glucose is <40 mg/dL, and the protein is elevated (generally 150–200 mg/dL but may increase to 1000–2000 mg/dL). Identification or isolation of *Mycobacterium* on smear or culture is the gold standard. The rare "serous" or sterile TBM with a CSF that resembles aseptic meningitis is considered an immunologic reaction to tuberculoprotein. The CSF is often normal in children with tuberculomas.

Neuroimaging is extremely valuable in the diagnosis of TBM, because isolation of acid-fast bacilli is not possible in many cases. CT characteristically shows thick basilar enhancement, parenchymal enhancement, hydrocephalus, cerebral edema, early focal ischemia, or infarcts- particularly in basal ganglia, and, sometimes, silent tuberculomas. MRI may detect posterior fossa lesions. Both may be normal during early stages of disease. Corroborative evidence of TB elsewhere in the body, especially pulmonary involvement on chest X-ray, choroid tubercles on fundoscopy, gastric aspirates for acid-fast bacilli, and family screening for contacts may aid in the diagnosis. The tuberculin skin test is positive in 30%–50% of cases.

Initial treatment regimens vary, using either three or four drugs. All regimens include isoniazid and rifampicin. The third drug used is generally pyrazinamide, but sometimes it is ethambutol or streptomycin. In the four-drug regimen, isoniazid + rifampicin + pyrazinamide + either ethambutol or streptomycin are used. The initial regimen is given for 2 months, followed by a continuation phase generally with two or three drugs. A total duration of at least 12 months therapy is recommended. Resistant strains are being reported from both developed and developing countries, particularly in association with HIV and malnutrition. The duration of treatment of multidrug-resistant TB is at least 18–24 months.

Corticosteroids improve survival and intellectual outcome of children with TBM, especially when administered early. External ventricular drainage may be necessary emergently for raised ICP. Clinical improvement may take weeks and the CSF may take months to normalize. Most patients who present late have permanent disabilities, including blindness, deafness, paraplegia, epilepsy, or developmental disabilities.

ENCEPHALITIS AND MYELITIS

Encephalitis denotes inflammation of brain parenchyma. Acute inflammatory demyelination following a systemic viral infection or immunization but without direct viral invasion in the CNS is called *postinfectious encephalitis* or*acute disseminated encephalomyelitis* (ADEM) when the spinal cord is also involved.

Epidemiology

The most common cause of neonatal encephalitis is HSV, most often HSV type 2 (HSV-2). Other viruses (enterovirus or adenovirus) may cause encephalitis in the neonate. In childhood, the most common causes of epidemic encephalitis are arthropod-borne viruses (arboviruses) and enteroviruses. Eastern equine encephalitis (EEE) and western equine encephalitis are caused by Alphaviridae. HSV-1 is common, often caused by reactivation of latent infection. St. Louis encephalitis, West Nile virus encephalitis, and Japanese encephalitis (JE) are caused by Flaviviridae. Colorado tick fever is caused by an orbivirus. Enteroviruses are viruses that infect primarily the enteric tract and include polio, echo, and coxsackie viruses. Adenovirus, Epstein–Barr virus (EBV), measles, mumps, varicella, and the bacterium *Bartonella henselae* also cause sporadic cases. Subacute sclerosing panencephalitis is a chronic, persistent infection of the measles virus, quite rare due to use of measles vaccine. Tick-borne bacterial diseases, such as borreliosis, rickettsial diseases, and ehrlichiosis, may also cause encephalitis. In many cases, the etiologic agent may not be identified.

In neonates, encephalitis generally presents with nonspecific symptoms and signs of systemic sepsis, including fever, poor feeding, irritability, lethargy, seizures, or apnea. An HSV PCR should be considered for any neonate with suspected sepsis from whom CSF is obtained. Older children usually have acute-onset fever, headache, seizures, behavioral changes, and rapid alteration in sensorium, progressing to coma. Seizures are common. Associated spinal cord involvement (myelitis) may cause flaccid paraplegia with abnormalities of the deep tendon reflexes. A history of recent travel, exposure to persons with infections, and insects or animal bites should be obtained. A history of focal seizures, personality changes, and aphasia suggests herpes. Fever with severe pharyngitis and fatigue may indicate EBV. Fever, parotitis, and dysphagia suggest mumps. Fever, conjunctivitis, and the characteristic rash may indicate measles. Dog bites or bat exposure raise the possibility of rabies. Exposure to kittens suggests *B. henselae* (cat-scratch) encephalitis. Rocky Mountain spotted fever, enteroviruses, arboviruses, and Lyme disease occur in summer.

CSF findings in encephalitis are nonspecific. The opening pressure may be high, and CSF cell count and protein are generally slightly elevated or normal. RBCs in the CSF may be seen in late stages of HSV encephalitis. Confirmatory diagnosis is performed by culture, rapid diagnostic tests (including antigen detection and PCR), demonstration of rise in specific antibody titer, and direct visualization of the organism. Serology may be helpful if high titers are identified acutely or a fourfold rise is noted when measured 3–4 weeks later. EEG may distinguish generalized from focal encephalitis. The EEG is particularly helpful in HSV encephalitis, wherein characteristic *periodic lateralized epileptiform discharges (PLEDs)* may be seen. MRI detects brain inflammation and edema in the cerebral cortex, the gray–white matter junction, the basal ganglia, or the cerebellum. MRI is the diagnostic modality of choice in differentiating acute infectious encephalitis from ADEM.

Bacterial, fungal, and parasitic etiologies of encephalitis require specific antimicrobial therapy. Antiviral therapy is important for HSV encephalitis. Acyclovir is not effective for CMV encephalitis and ganciclovir or foscarnet must be used. Amantadine and rimantadine are effective against influenza A, whereas oseltamivir and zanamivir are effective against influenzas A and B. Highly active antiretroviral therapy (HAART) is available for HIV infection. No specific antiviral therapy is available for enteroviral and arboviral encephalitis. Passive immunity in the form of IV immune globulin may help immunocompromised individuals who cannot mount an effective immune response. The role of high-dose steroid therapy has not been established.

Most arboviral encephalitides except EEE and JE have a good prognosis in children. The prognosis of HSV encephalitis has improved significantly with use of early acyclovir therapy. Children with severe encephalitis and/or delayed therapy may be left with permanent neurologic deficits.

ACUTE DISSEMINATED ENCEPHALOMYELITIS

ADEM is an inflammatory demyelinating disorder of the CNS that follows infections or, less frequently, immunization. The common preceding infections are respiratory and gastrointestinal viral illnesses. Typically, the subcortical white matter is affected; sometimes additional gray matter lesions are seen. ADEM is increasingly being reported, possibly due to increased availability of MRI. It is more common in the winter months. The incidence of severe forms of ADEM (e.g., hemorrhagic encephalomyelitis) that may follow measles has diminished in developed countries because of widespread immunization. Most cases have fever, headache, and irritability, progressing rapidly to altered sensorium and an abrupt multifocal neurologic deficit. Seizures occur in ~25%–33% of cases. Hemiparesis or quadriparesis may be present. Ataxia is predominant in some cases and extrapyramidal symptoms, such as choreoathetosis or dystonia, may occur in others. Predominant brainstem involvement may be seen. Simultaneous involvement of the spinal cord presents with a transverse myelitis-like presentation. Mental or psychiatric disturbances have been reported.

A clinical definition of ADEM has recently been put forth (https://brightoncollaboration.org/public/what-we-do/setting-standards/case-definitions/available-definitions.html). CSF cell counts are not helpful in making a diagnosis. CSF myelin basic protein concentration, reflecting demyelination, may be elevated. Elevation of WBC, platelet, CRP, and sedimentation rates may be seen occasionally. The CT scan is less sensitive than MRI. Multiple, large confluent centrifugal white matter lesions seen generally at the junction of deep cortical gray and subcortical white matter are characteristic. Lesions may also be seen in deep gray matter, basal ganglia, and thalami in a third of cases. The brainstem, optic nerves, cerebellum, and spinal cord may also be involved. In fulminant cases, areas of hemorrhage may be seen. Rarely, the MRI may be normal on initial presentation.

The mainstay of treatment is high-dose IV methylprednisolone. Improvement may be observed within hours but usually takes several days. Generally, a taper of oral steroids for 3–6 weeks is used. Plasmapheresis and IV immune globulin have also been used. Most children with a mild-to-moderate illness who receive appropriate therapy show good recovery. Residual deficits are seen in one-third of cases and include motor, visual, autonomic, and intellectual deficits, as well as epilepsy. Children with transverse myelitis may have residual bladder and bowel dysfunction and motor deficits. A small number of children may have recurrent ADEM during the taper of corticosteroid therapy.

BRAIN AND SPINAL CORD ABSCESS

Abscesses in the brain and spinal cord can occur as a primary event or as a complication of bacterial meningitis. Common pathogens include anaerobic bacteria, gram-negative organisms, streptococci, and staphylococci. In neonates, gram-negative organisms are more common. In children with cyanotic heart disease, the most common organisms are the α-hemolytic streptococci. Streptococci and *S. aureus* are seen with endocarditis. In children with direct spread from otitis or sinusitis, anaerobic or aerobic streptococci, *B. fragilis*, *Proteus* spp., *Pseudomonas*, or *H. influenzae* may be isolated. Congenital defects such as dermal sinuses, epidermoid cysts, and encephaloceles, may become infected and lead to brain or spinal cord abscess.

The presentation is generally subacute, with fever, headache, vomiting, altered sensorium, seizures, and focal neurologic deficits. A bulging fontanelle and increasing head size may be seen in infants, and neck rigidity in older children. Papilledema, sixth-nerve palsy, and cerebral herniation syndromes may occur. Hydrocephalus may develop due to mass effect. Symptom onset may be abrupt if the abscess ruptures into the ventricles or if hemorrhage occurs in the abscess cavity.

An LP is often contraindicated because of the risk of cerebral herniation and may not show pleocytosis or a positive culture unless the abscess has ruptured into the ventricles. Confirmation of the etiologic organism is achieved by culture from an aspirate of the abscess, blood, or sinuses or mastoids. Contrast-enhanced CT scan shows a characteristic ring-enhancing lesion with central hypodensity and surrounding edema in a mature abscess (**Fig. 68.1**). Mass effect with midline shift may be seen. Tubercular

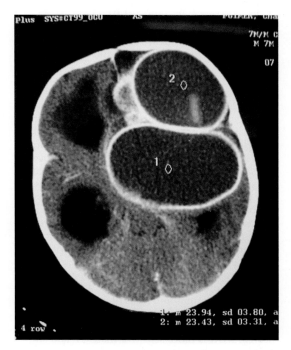

FIGURE 68.1. Contrast-enhanced CT showing multiple staphylococcal brain abscesses with ring enhancement and midline shift.

abscesses are generally seen at the base of the brain, especially in the cerebellum. MR spectroscopy may sometimes be necessary to differentiate an abscess from a neoplasm.

Surgical excision is undertaken if no improvement ensues despite aspiration and antibiotics. Corticosteroids given IV at presentation may help to reduce cerebral edema and ICP. The fear that steroids reduce penetration of antibiotics in the abscess cavity has not been substantiated. Early decompression improves outcome.

SUBDURAL EMPYEMA

Subdural empyema is a suppurative collection in the subdural space. It may occur as a complication of meningitis or by direct spread from infected sinuses, otitis media, osteomyelitis of skull bones, or head trauma. The onset is subacute, with fever, headache, vomiting, and, often, seizures. Neck rigidity and focal signs may be present. Infants present with poor feeding, irritability, fever, full fontanelle, and an enlarging head. Persistent or recurrent fever in a child with recent bacterial meningitis, focal seizures or other focal neurologic signs suggests a subdural empyema. MRI is more sensitive than CT for detecting small collections and for differentiating from cerebritis and thrombosis. A contrast-enhanced, crescent-shaped, hypodense lesion with loculations is characteristic. Organism identification can be performed by Gram stain and culture of fluid obtained surgically. Removal of the purulent collection and IV administration of appropriate antibiotics in high doses for 3–6 weeks are warranted. Surgical removal of an adjacent source of infection, such as chronic otitis media or osteomyelitis, is also necessary.

EPIDURAL ABSCESS

Causative organisms for epidural abscess include staphylococci, streptococci, and some anaerobic organisms, such as *B. fragilis*. Pneumococci, streptococci, and salmonellae, may be responsible in some cases. The spread of infection is usually hematogenous but may occur by local spread of an adjacent infection or from spinal trauma. Progression of inflammation can lead to spinal cord ischemia and even infarction. Inflammation of blood vessels causes vasculitis and venothrombophlebitis. Children present with fever, headache, vomiting, neck rigidity, focal seizures, and focal neurologic deficits, including hemiparesis. Those with spinal epidural abscess present with fever, back pain, and symptoms and signs of cord compression, localized tenderness, bladder and bowel involvement or a sensory level. An LP is usually contraindicated. MRI is more sensitive than CT and shows an enhancing lenticular collection between the dura and the cranium or the cord. Treatment involves surgical drainage, appropriate antibiotics, and supportive management. No evidence supports the use of corticosteroids. Paralysis for >36 hours before intervention is associated with a poor prognosis.

FUNGAL INFECTIONS OF THE CENTRAL NERVOUS SYSTEM

Most patients with a fungal infection of the CNS have an immunodeficiency. Fungi that can infect the CNS can be divided into those that can cause disease in healthy hosts (*Histoplasma*, *Blastomyces*, *Coccidioides immitis*, *Sporothrix* spp., etc.) and those that cause opportunistic infection in immunocompromised hosts (*Aspergillus* spp., Zygomycetes, and *Trichosporon* spp.). *Cryptococcus* and *Candida* spp. can infect both healthy and immunocompromised hosts.

Fungal meningitis is most commonly caused by *Cryptococcus neoformans*, *Coccidioides immitis*, *Candida*, and *Aspergillus*. Patients usually present with some combination of fever, headache, lethargy, nausea, vomiting, neck rigidity, impaired mental status, convulsion, and focal neurologic deficits. Raised ICP may develop acutely or during progression of the disease. *Rhino-orbital-cerebral mucormycosis* is due to zygomycosis (*Rhizopus* and *Mucor* spp.), often in patients with poorly controlled diabetes. It presents with orbital pain, nasal discharge, and facial edema. Proptosis and visual loss may occur. Carotid involvement may cause hemiparesis. Blackish necrotic areas are seen in the palate and nasal turbinates. Aspergillosis or mucormycosis may produce sudden onset of neurologic deficit due to vasculitis. Rarely, subarachnoid hemorrhage occurs due to mycotic aneurysmal bleed. *Fungal brain abscess* is the most common presenting feature of CNS aspergillosis, which presents as single or multiple brain abscesses with focal neurologic deficits. It can also be caused by yeast (*Candida*, *Cryptococcus* spp.) and dimorphic fungi (*Histoplasma*, *Coccidioides*, *Blastomyces* spp.) in immunocompromised patients.

CSF examination in fungal disease usually reveals high protein, low glucose, and mononuclear leukocytosis ranging between 20 and 500 cells/mm^3. Cell count may be normal in patients with HIV infection or those on corticosteroid therapy. India ink staining may identify encapsulated cryptococci in >50% cases. Methenamine silver stain of a direct aspirate or biopsy may identify *Aspergillus* and Zygomycetes. CSF cultures are frequently negative. Latex agglutination or complement fixating antibody titers of CSF can be useful. Serum or CSF galactomannan may help diagnose *Aspergillus*. Neuroimaging may be nonspecific and may underestimate the extent of disease. Clusters of round-to-oval low-density cystic lesions in basal ganglia and thalamic region on CT strongly suggest cryptococcal infection. Intracranial findings may include thrombosis of cavernous sinus and infarct involving internal carotid artery territory.

Optimal treatment includes specific antifungal therapy, measures to control ICP, supportive treatment, surgical intervention, and management of underlying risk factors such as hyperglycemia, acidosis, and reversal of immunosuppression. Amphotericin B remains the most used drug, with potential advantages of using lipid formulations. Corticosteroids should be discontinued when possible with cryptococcal infections. *Aspergillus* infections of the CNS are very difficult to eradicate. In patients with Zygomycetes (*Rhizopus*, *Mucor*) or *Aspergillus* infection, direct surgical removal of infected tissue should be undertaken if lesions are accessible. CNS neurosurgical devices should be removed if possible. The outcome of cryptococcal CNS infection is usually better than that of other forms of fungal meningitis. The mortality with *Candida* meningitis is 10%–20%. Mortality is improving with *Aspergillus*, although when disseminated it approaches 100%. CNS zygomycosis has a very high mortality.

PARASITIC INFECTIONS

Malaria, amebiasis, toxoplasmosis, helminth infections (e.g., neurocysticercosis, echinococcus), and nematode infections (*Trichinella, Strongyloides, Ascaris*) can all present with CNS involvement. Symptoms of acute meningitis or meningoencephalitis are most typical, with fever, headache, vomiting, photophobia, neck stiffness, altered sensorium, and seizures. Cystic echinococcal infection may present insidiously over years with a slowly enlarging cyst. Characteristic neuroimaging findings include a scolex within a cyst in neurocysticercosis or a round, thin-walled fluid-filled cyst in *Echinococcus*. Small, ring-enhancing lesions (particularly in deep gray matter) in a child with HIV suggest toxoplasmosis.

Neurocysticercosis (NCC) is an important cause of epilepsy in the tropics. Presentation with focal neurologic deficits, obstructive hydrocephalus, stroke, eye involvement, or spinal involvement is also possible. NCC is caused by larvae of *Taenia solium* and is acquired by ingestion of undercooked pork infected with *T. solium* followed by autoingestion of eggs or human-to-human transmission via the fecal–oral route. Cysticerci may live within host tissues for years without causing any inflammation or disease. Diagnosis is usually by pathology or characteristic neuroimaging findings (small, low-density, ring- or disc-enhancing lesions, with perilesional edema and calcifications). Cysticidal therapy, if used early, is effective for both live and enhancing lesions. In cases with severe cerebral edema, it should be used after edema subsides with steroid therapy. Albendazole is preferred over Praziquantel as it is safe and cheap and its bioavailability is increased with co-administration of steroids. Seizures due to NCC are usually well controlled with a single anticonvulsant.

CHAPTER 69 ■ NOSOCOMIAL INFECTIONS

JASON W. CUSTER, JILL S. THOMAS, AND JOHN P. STRAUMANIS

A *nosocomial infection* is an infection that is acquired in the hospital setting and was not present at admission. *Community-acquired infections* are present at admission even if they do not cause symptoms at the time of admission. *Surgical site infections* are associated with a surgical wound or procedure. *Colonization* is the presence of potentially infectious organisms without a host reaction, clinically adverse event, or disease.

OVERVIEW AND EPIDEMIOLOGY

In the United States, there are 2 million hospital-acquired infections annually. These nosocomial infections are associated with increased mortality, and at least one-third are preventable. The highest rates occur in the ICU. The common pediatric nosocomial infections are bloodstream infections (BSIs), pneumonia, and urinary tract infections (UTIs). Younger children, particularly neonates, have the highest risk. The use of parenteral nutrition with a high glucose concentration and lipids is an additional risk factor. Severity of illness, understaffing, and red blood cell transfusion increase the risk of nosocomial infections in the PICU.

Isolation precautions are divided into two categories: standard and transmission-based precautions. *Standard precautions* should be in use at all times. They prevent the practitioner from contact with potentially infectious bodily fluids. The most important standard precaution is hand hygiene. Soap and water hand washing is the gold standard. Waterless antiseptic agent use is appropriate unless there is visible dirt, proteinaceous bodily fluid contact (blood), or likely contamination with spores. Hand hygiene must be done both before and after patient contact even if gloves are worn. Barriers such as gloves, masks, eye protection, and nonsterile gowns should be worn when contact with bodily fluids or secretions is likely.

Transmission-based precautions are aimed at protection against transmission of infectious organisms from patients. *Contact precautions* are used for organisms that spread by direct contact with the patient or indirect contact via fomites such as toys, stethoscopes, and unwashed hands. *Droplet precautions* are used for organisms that spread short distances (<3 feet) from the patient via coughing or sneezing. The use of a mask with an eye shield is added to standard precautions. *Airborne precautions* include additional safeguards for organisms transmitted by air currents (e.g., tuberculosis, measles, and varicella). Patients should be in private rooms with negative air flow. For measles and varicella isolation, susceptible healthcare providers should avoid contact. For airborne precautions, a fitted respirator should be worn while in the patient's room. Disposable N95 respirators (filter at least 95% of particles with a median diameter of 0.3 mm or greater) are commonly used. Specialized devices may be necessary for individuals with facial hair.

Surveillance cultures are used in areas with a high level of resistant organisms to screen for colonization at admission. This approach has been used for methicillin-resistant *Staphylococcus aureus* (MRSA). Discussions with infection-control personnel can determine the frequency of screening. Routine screening of medical staff is not recommended. Cohorting patients with the same organism and their staff may be beneficial.

CATHETER-RELATED BLOODSTREAM INFECTIONS

Central venous catheter (CVC) use in ICUs approaches 15 million days per year. Catheter-related infections are associated with increased morbidity and healthcare costs and occur in ICU patients at a rate of 80,000 annually. CDC guidelines provide criteria for diagnosing bloodstream infections (BSIs) involving intravascular catheters. A catheter-related bloodstream infection (CRBSI) is a clinical definition that requires testing to pinpoint the central line as the source of the infection. Clinical evidence of an infection, including a host response, must be present and not attributable to any source other than the catheter. A catheter-associated bloodstream infection (CABSI) has less rigorous criteria; it requires a central line be in place during the 48 hours prior to obtaining a positive blood culture and compelling evidence that the infection is related to the line. This definition is helpful for surveillance but can overestimate the true incidence of bloodstream infections.

Coagulase-negative staphylococci are the most common cause of pediatric nosocomial BSIs, accounting for 20%–50% of isolates. Gram-negative bacteria account for 25% of PICU nosocomial BSIs. *S. aureus* and *Candida* species are responsible for ~10% each in children. *β*-hemolytic streptococci are more prevalent in the neonatal population. *Enterococcus* accounts for <10% of infections in infants and adolescents.

Diagnosis and Treatment of Catheter-Related Infections

To aid in the diagnosis of a CRBSI, it is recommended that paired central and peripheral cultures be either quantitative cultures or qualitative cultures with continuously monitored *differential time to positivity.* A differential time to positivity of at least 2 hours earlier for the central line than the peripheral culture indicates a central-line infection.

Exchanging the catheter over a guidewire avoids the risks associated with needle puncture at a new site but does not lower the risk of infection. For those patients with suspected line infections and mild to moderate symptoms (in addition to fever), a change over a guidewire may be an alternative to removing the line while awaiting blood and catheter tip cultures. Nontunneled catheters may be replaced once appropriate antibiotic therapy has been instituted. Antibiotic therapy is indicated even when catheter removal is not (**Fig. 69.1**). Persistent bacteremia or lack of clinical improvement should prompt evaluation for infective endocarditis, septic thrombosis, and other sites of seeding, especially if symptoms persist more than 3 days after catheter removal.

Successful treatment of central-line infection without removal of the device as long as the patient is not worsening has been reported. Initial therapy is usually vancomycin along with a third-generation cephalosporin or aminoglycoside. Extended-spectrum gram-negative coverage (e.g., drugs with anti-pseudomonal activity) may be appropriate depending on the clinical situation. For severe infections in immunosuppressed patients, the addition of antifungal coverage is appropriate. Once an isolate's sensitivities are known, the antibiotic regimen should be appropriately adjusted. Infections caused by fungi or gram-negative organisms are extremely resistant to treatment if the catheter is left in place. Regardless of the culture results, if the child does not respond or worsens within the first 3 days of antibiotic therapy, the line should be removed.

Prevention of Catheter-Related Infections

Mandatory education of physicians and nurses as well as the establishment of a unit-based infection-control nurse position can reduce the rate of CRBSI. Real-time feedback to the staff about rates of infection raises awareness. A daily discussion of the continued need for central access should be incorporated to aid in timely line removal.

Hand Washing: Strong emphasis should be placed on thorough hand washing prior to insertion. Aseptic technique should be maintained throughout insertion.

Skin Preparation: Skin preparation with 2% aqueous chlorhexidine gluconate reduces catheter-related infections compared with either 10% povidone–iodine or 70% alcohol. When chlorhexidine is not available or contraindicated, povidone–iodine or 70% alcohol should be used. Chlorhexidine preparations should not be used on infants younger than 2 months of age.

Maximal Barrier Precautions: Full barrier precautions (a large sterile or full-body drape, long-sleeved sterile gown, cap, mask, and sterile gloves) reduce infection risk compared with small drape and sterile gloves.

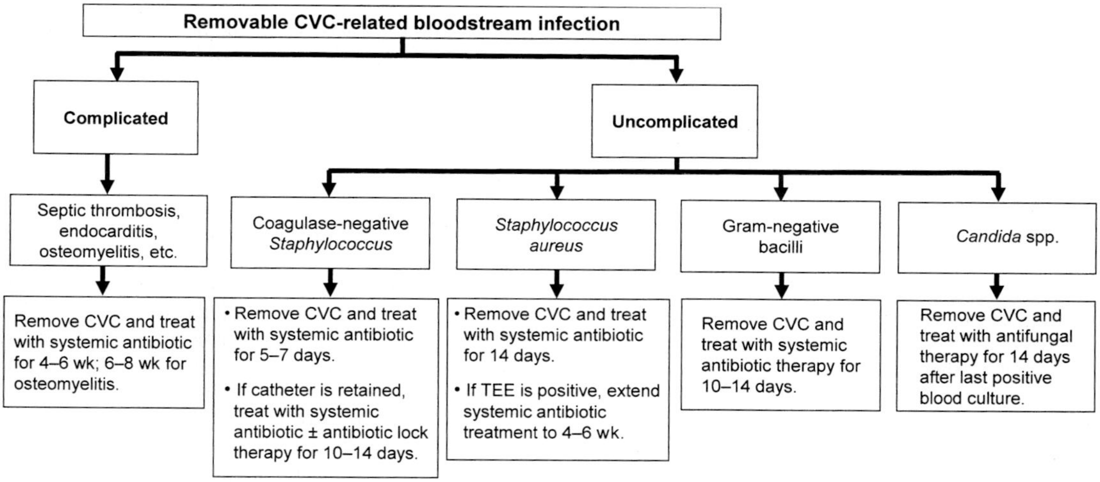

FIGURE 69.1. Approach to the management of patients with nontunneled CVC-related bloodstream infection. Duration of treatment will depend on whether the infection is complicated or uncomplicated. The catheter should be removed, and systemic antimicrobial therapy should be initiated, except in some cases of uncomplicated catheter-related infection due to coagulase-negative staphylococci. For infections due to *S. aureus*, transesophageal echocardiography (TEE) may reveal the presence of endocarditis and help to determine the duration of treatment. (From Mermel LA, Farr BM, Sherertz RJ, et al. Guidelines for the management of intravascular catheter-related infections. *Clin Infect Dis* 2001;32(9):1249–72, with permission.)

Catheter Site Dressing: The use of transparent, semipermeable polyurethane dressings further secures the device and allows for visual inspection of the catheter and insertion site. Proper dressings can allow for bathing, reduce skin irritation, reduce frequency of dressing changes, save time, and reduce the risk of introducing infection. Regardless of the type of dressing utilized, it should be replaced when damp, soiled, loosened, or visual inspection of the site is needed. Chlorhexidine-impregnated sponge dressings at the site of catheter insertion reduce bacterial colonization with a reduction in catheter-related infections in critically ill adults. Antibiotic ointments should not be used at the insertion site, as they risk development of resistance as well as colonization with *Candida* species. A catheter hub containing 3% iodinated alcohol in an antiseptic chamber has shown a fourfold reduction in catheter infections. The use of antibiotic lock prophylaxis and systemic antibiotic prophylaxis is not recommended owing to the risk of creating resistance.

Central-Line Choice and Antimicrobial/Antiseptic-Impregnated Catheters

Prompt removal of the catheter once it is no longer needed is one of the most effective means to reduce catheter-related infections. Placing lines with only the number of lumens required for care decreases the risk of developing a catheter-related infection. In adults, there is a lower infection risk of the subclavian site compared with internal jugular or femoral sites. In children, femoral sites are associated with fewer mechanical complications and have an equivalent infection rate compared with other sites. Polyvinyl chloride and polyethylene catheters do not impede bacterial adherence to the catheter and are not usually available in the United States. Teflon and polyurethane catheters are associated with fewer line-related infections. Infection risk can be further reduced by coating or impregnating CVCs with antiseptics or antibiotics.

Central-Line Replacement

In adults the need for central-line replacement every few days due to the higher cumulative risk of catheter infection has been disproved. Replacement at a new site carries all the risks associated with insertion and does not lower the cumulative risk of infection. Routine replacement of tubing and infusion sets does decrease the risk of catheter infection. It is recommended that a 15-second friction scrub with either 70% alcohol or 3/15% chlorhexidine/70% alcohol be used to sterilize entry ports every time they are accessed. Instituting and enforcing care and maintenance "bundles" along with continuing education reduces infection rates in multiple populations and settings. Assigning a multidisciplinary team including physicians, nurses, and infection-control personnel aids in maintaining vigilance and increasing awareness.

Extracorporeal Membrane Oxygenation

The risk factors identified for nosocomial infections associated with extracorporeal membrane oxygenation (ECMO) are prolonged ECMO support, support for cardiac disease, undergoing a major surgical procedure immediately prior to or while on ECMO, and having an open chest while on ECMO. The reported nosocomial infection rate for children on ECMO is 11%. Infections associated with ECMO include wound infections of the neck and chest, BSIs, UTIs, and respiratory infections. Yeast infections are noted and believed to be due to the use of broad-spectrum antibiotics.

NOSOCOMIAL RESPIRATORY INFECTIONS

Contamination of the patient's respiratory tract can occur from devices in direct contact with the patient, including laryngoscopes blades, endotracheal tubes (ETTs), nasoenteric tubes, suction catheters, and bronchoscopes, as well as those with indirect contact, including mechanical ventilators, ventilator tubing, nebulizers, and oxygen delivery devices. Cross-contamination between devices such as rigid laryngoscope blades and handles can occur, highlighting the need for standardized decontamination, sterilization, and maintenance of respiratory equipment. The human vector most likely to transmit infection to the patient is the hospital staff. Poor hand hygiene and improper isolation practices are the most common risk factors. Family members and other patients can also transmit infection.

Ventilator-Associated Pneumonia

Nosocomial pneumonia is one of the most common hospital-acquired infections. Inoculation of the sterile lower respiratory tract can occur in part because the vocal cords are held open by the ETT, increasing secretion aspiration and colonization of the trachea. The risk of nosocomial pneumonia is increased in patients who require mechanical ventilation. Independent risk factors for ventilator-associated pneumonia (VAP) in children are immunodeficiency, immunosuppression, neuromuscular blockade, neuromuscular weakness, burns, steroid administration, and use of total parenteral nutrition. As in adults, children are at higher risk for VAP with prior antibiotic use, longer ICU lengths of stay, use of indwelling catheters, use of H_2-antagonist therapy, tracheal reintubation, and transport out of the ICU while intubated. The presence of a nasoenteric tube increases risk because it provides a direct route from the upper gastrointestinal tract to the oropharynx. VAP is associated with an increase in the length of ventilation and PICU length of stay. Underlying illness, preterm age, time of onset of VAP, and causative organism may be important determinants of morbidity. Bacterial organisms most often identified in VAP are gram-negative; *Pseudomonas aeruginosa* is the most common followed by *Escherichia coli*, *Klebsiella pneumoniae*, and *Enterobacter* species. *S. aureus* and coagulase-negative staphylococci are the common gram-positive isolates and have a lower mortality than with the gram-negative organisms. Anaerobic nosocomial pneumonia is rare in the pediatric population. Viruses, predominantly respiratory syncytial virus (RSV), are the most common cause of nosocomial respiratory infections. Fungal infections are exceedingly rare but may occur in children who are immunosuppressed. The incidence of polymicrobial infections is high.

Diagnosis

Pediatric VAP is classified based on the time of onset. Early onset pneumonia occurs within the first 4 days of mechanical ventilation and subsequent diagnoses are classified as late onset pneumonia. The diagnosis of VAP in infants and children can be made on clinical grounds without microbiologic evidence. Determination of the causative organism is necessary to direct antibiotic therapy. For adults and older children, bronchoalveolar lavage and protected-specimen brush collection have been used with success. Tracheal aspiration can be used to culture tracheal secretions but has low specificity due to colonization of the ETT and upper airway. Recognized methods to determine the causative organism include positive blood cultures that cannot be attributed to another source, positive cultures from pleural fluid, a positive bronchoalveolar lavage or protected brush specimen quantitative culture, a direct microscopic exam showing ≥5% of cells from a bronchoalveolar lavage sample containing intracellular bacteria, a histopathologic exam demonstrating evidence of fungal hyphae, abscess formation in the bronchioles and alveoli or a positive quantitative culture of lung parenchyma, and a positive detection of viral antigen or antibody from respiratory secretions.

Prevention

Healthcare personnel should receive education regarding VAP risk factors, evidence-based practice recommendations, unit-based VAP rates, and patient outcomes. Hand hygiene, along with universal precautions and appropriate isolation are the most effective infection-control practices. Ventilator bundle interventions include elevation of the head of bed 30–45 degrees, daily oral care with chlorhexidine and a daily readiness-for-extubation assessment. The application of such a bundle can reduce the incidence of VAP. Subglottic drainage of secretions with specialized ETTs and noninvasive ventilation diminish the risk of VAP. If condensation should occur in the ventilator circuit, it should be removed from the circuit through the use of a trap. Ventilatory circuits should be changed when visibly soiled or malfunctioning. Constant, high-dose sedation should be avoided, and appropriate sedation scales should be used. If neuromuscular blockade is being used, it is reasonable to intermittently hold the muscle-relaxing agents if clinically appropriate. The use of acid suppressive therapy may increase colonization of the aerodigestive tract and increase VAP risk. The risk of developing a stress ulcer or gastritis should be balanced against the risk of developing VAP, and there is controversy regarding when stress ulcer prophylaxis is appropriate.

Sinusitis

Sinusitis is a risk factor for the development of pneumonia. Patients in intensive care are at risk for developing a nosocomial sinus infection because of supine positioning, decreased sinus drainage due to positive-pressure ventilation, and nasal placement of therapeutic devices that obstruct sinus drainage. Additional risk factors include nasal colonization with gram-negative bacilli, sedative usage, and a Glasgow Coma Scale score < 7. Infection is often polymicrobial with *Pseudomonas* and *Streptococcus* species isolated most frequently.

Respiratory Syncytial Virus

RSV is the most common nosocomial infection on pediatric wards. The risk factors for contracting an RSV nosocomial infection are young age (especially neonates), underlying chronic illness (cardiac or pulmonary disease), a long hospitalization, overcrowding, staff shortages, and hospitalization during the RSV endemic season (most important). Infections can be severe in immunosuppressed patients, who can also have prolonged shedding. The most common modes of transmission of RSV from person to person are via large droplet aerosols and adherence to fomites. RSV can survive and remain infectious on nonporous surfaces for 6–12 hours. Studies of transmission in multi-bed rooms have found a 3% transmission rate from infected to uninfected patients. Transmission rates can be lowered with efforts to educate the healthcare team about the modes of RSV transmission, prospective surveillance for RSV infection, early diagnosis, strict cohorting and isolation policy, and daily disinfectant of surfaces in the isolation rooms.

Influenza and Other Respiratory Viruses

Most respiratory viruses are transmitted and contained as described for RSV. An effective method of preventing the nosocomial transmission of influenza is through the annual immunization of healthcare workers.

Severe Acute Respiratory Syndrome

Personal protective equipment appeared effective in preventing acquisition of severe acute respiratory syndrome (SARS). The N95 respirator, separation of patients, methods to decrease infectious aerosols during at-risk therapies, and environmental decontamination and containment were used to prevent large droplet transmission. Intubation, continuous positive-airway pressure, and nebulization therapy seemed to increase transmission of SARS. It is postulated that these procedures provided smaller droplets, which can travel further distances.

NOSOCOMIAL URINARY TRACT INFECTIONS

The rate of catheter-associated UTIs (CAUTIs) in ICUs ranges from 3.1 to 7.4 per 1000 catheter days, with higher incidences in burn and neurologic units. Secondary urosepsis is uncommon in the PICU population. Most infections are caused by a single organism, with 82% identified as gram-negative bacteria or yeast species. Twenty percent of nosocomial UTIs have antibiotic resistance. The acquisition of a CAUTI by a critically ill patient is associated with increased morbidity, prolonged hospital length of stay, bacterial resistance, and greater healthcare expenditures. Strategies to prevent or decrease nosocomial UTIs include minimizing exposure to urinary catheters, using a sterile insertion technique, maintaining uninterrupted use of a closed collection system, and removing the device as soon as possible (ideally in <3 days). Automatic urinary catheter reminder and stop orders are effective. Portable ultrasound devices can be used in patients with low urine output to reduce unnecessary catheter insertion. The usage of antimicrobial/antiseptic-impregnated catheters can be considered if the CAUTI rate is not decreasing after implementation of a comprehensive strategy to decrease nosocomial UTIs.

NOSOCOMIAL GASTROINTESTINAL INFECTIONS

Nosocomial diarrhea is defined as loose stools occurring >48 hours after admission, a stool frequency of at least two per 12 hours, and no identified noninfectious cause. The reported PICU rate is 4%–5%. Viral etiologies predominate (as a group) and are usually similar to organisms in the community (rotavirus, adenovirus, and Norwalk virus). The single most common organism isolated in the PICU is *Clostridium difficile*. *C. difficile* is almost exclusively isolated as a cause of diarrhea in children over 1 year of age. Although present in the gastrointestinal tract of newborns, *C. difficile* does not typically cause disease in neonates and young infants. Good hand hygiene and contact precautions are key to prevention. Soap and water hand cleansing is necessary since alcohol-based solutions do not kill the spore. Viruses that cause diarrheal illnesses can survive on fomites and other surfaces for hours, and spores of *C. difficile* can survive over a day on inanimate surfaces.

SURGICAL SITE INFECTIONS

Pediatric surgical site infections are most commonly caused by *S. aureus* (20%). Coagulase-negative staphylococci and *P. aeruginosa* account for ~14% each. Chlorhexidine bathing decreases surgical site infections in adults. Pediatric studies are lacking, but such bathing may be considered in high-risk patients.

CHAPTER 70 ■ INTERNATIONAL AND EMERGING INFECTIONS

TROY E. DOMINGUEZ, CHITRA RAVISHANKAR, MIRIAM K. LAUFER, AND MARK W. HALL

INTERNATIONAL INFECTIONS

Malaria

Malaria is the most significant parasitic disease in humans. Malaria is transmitted by the female anopheline mosquito. The areas of highest transmission are sub-Saharan Africa, South Asia, Southeast Asia, the South Pacific, and Central and South America. Repeated exposure to malaria infection, in individuals who live in malaria-endemic areas, causes "semi-immunity." Patients are still at risk for infection, but their immune system controls the level of parasitemia, and severe disease is rare. In the areas of highest transmission, semi-immunity occurs around the age of 5 years. In areas of lower transmission, it is delayed or absent. Semi-immunity is lost within 6 months of leaving an endemic area, a problem for returning natives. Hemoglobinopathies (hemoglobins S, C, and E, glucose-6-phosphate dehydrogenase deficiency, pyruvate kinase deficiency, and α-thalassemia) are associated with decreased risk of severe malaria. The Duffy antigen on the red blood cell is necessary for invasion by *Plasmodium vivax*. Most Africans lack this antigen, and as result, *P. vivax* is rare in Africa.

All human *Plasmodia* species have a similar life cycle. Sporozoites are injected by a mosquito and travel to the liver. In the *hepatic stage* (1–2 weeks), the parasites reproduce and become schizonts; no symptoms occur in this exo-erythrocytic stage. When the hepatic schizonts rupture, merozoites emerge into the bloodstream and begin the *erythrocytic stage*. Merozoites infect erythrocytes, mature into trophozoites, and become schizonts, which rupture and produce more merozoites that invade more red blood cells. The cycle of multiplication, infection, and rupture results in the clinical manifestations. The parasite burden multiplies 12- to 15-fold with each erythrocytic cycle. With *Plasmodium falciparum*, these cycles last ~48 hours. Some merozoites differentiate into gametocytes that are taken up by an *Anopheles* mosquito and reproduce in the mosquito midgut. Severe *P. falciparum* disease occurs when infected cells adhere to vessel walls in the microvasculature (*sequestration*), causing end-organ damage. Sequestration in the brain microcirculation causes the dreaded complication—cerebral malaria. In endemic areas, sequestration is prominent in the gastrointestinal tract and the skin.

The presentation of uncomplicated malaria is a febrile illness with chills, headache, and diaphoresis. Paroxysmal fevers reflect the replicating cycle of parasites. Other symptoms include nausea, vomiting, diarrhea, malaise, myalgias, dizziness, diarrhea, and dry cough. Patients without sufficient immunity can rapidly deteriorate and develop severe disease, or present with severe disease. Clinical features that identify a high risk of death include prostration, impaired consciousness, acidotic breathing, multiple convulsions, circulatory collapse, pulmonary edema, abnormal bleeding, jaundice, and hemoglobinuria. Laboratory results associated with severe disease include severe anemia, hypoglycemia, acidosis, renal impairment, hyperlactatemia, and hyperparasitemia. The classic syndrome of severe disease among children is cerebral malaria (discussed in detail in Chapter 68). Coma in cerebral malaria is due to sludging in the cerebral microcirculation along with central nervous system (CNS) inflammation. Cerebral edema, seizures, intracranial hypertension, and cranial nerve abnormalities are typical. Prompt use of IV antimalarial drugs, seizure control, and supportive care are essential. Patients with impaired consciousness should be treated as cerebral malaria. Cerebral malaria is fatal if untreated, but survival is 80%–85%with IV antimalarial drugs. Residual CNS deficits are common in survivors.

Most severe infections and deaths occur in children <5 years of age. An important marker of severity is metabolic acidosis. The acidosis is common with cerebral malaria, anemia, hypoglycemia, or hypovolemia. Plasma lactate is elevated. Hypovolemia, hypoperfusion, severe anemia, and low oxygen-carrying capacity contribute to the acidosis. Hypoglycemia occurs in 10%–30% of severe disease. Parasite consumption of glucose, increased host demand for glucose, and impaired gluconeogenesis contribute. Treatment with quinine stimulates insulin secretion. In children, hypoglycemia is frequently seen on presentation and is usually associated with appropriately low insulin levels. Hypoglycemia can occur in the absence of high–parasite-density parasitemia because nonvisualized intracellular parasites consume large quantities of glucose.

Severe malarial anemia presents with profound pallor. It frequently occurs in highly endemic areas due to repeated malarial infections. Lung and renal disease can be seen in children with severe malaria. The progression to acute lung injury or acute respiratory distress syndrome (ARDS) may be rapid, and may happen even after treatment and parasite clearance. The etiology of renal failure in severe malaria is not well understood. Other severe complications include shock, splenic rupture, and disseminated intravascular coagulation (DIC). Hypersplenism, known as *hyper-reactive malarial splenomegaly* or *tropical splenomegaly syndrome*, is an abnormal immune response that leads to stimulation of B lymphocytes. Rhabdomyolysis has rarely been reported. Blackwater fever (hemoglobinuria, hemolysis, and renal failure) and algid malaria (cardiovascular collapse, shock, and hypothermia) are rare in children. Laboratory findings in severe malaria include thrombocytopenia, hyperbilirubinemia, anemia, elevated hepatic transaminases, C-reactive protein, and erythrocyte sedimentation rate. Coagulation abnormalities may be due to DIC. Hypokalemia occurs in ~40% of patients and is caused by renal potassium loss. For travelers returning from tropical countries, the differential diagnosis includes typhoid fever, dengue, leptospirosis, rickettsial diseases, and bacterial sepsis.

The diagnosis is established by thick and thin blood smears stained with a 3% Giemsa stain. Parasite identification after lysis of red blood cells is more sensitive. In a thin smear, the parasites are visualized within the erythrocytes, which is useful for determination of species. A negative set of malaria smears does not rule out malaria, as parasites move between the bloodstream and sequestration within organs. Three sets of thick and thin smears 12–24 hours apart are recommended. Rapid testing with dipstick immunoassays can be used.

For uncomplicated malaria, the decision for specific antimicrobial therapies depends on the infecting species and the geographic source. The appropriate therapies for uncomplicated disease are listed in **Table 70.1**. Although medication can be administered orally, it is recommended that patients remain in the hospital until parasite clearance can be documented, ensuring compliance and monitoring for deterioration in clinical status.

Patients with severe disease should be treated with IV therapy. Quinine is the main therapy in endemic areas, but is not available in the United States. Quinidine is recommended in the United States. Treatment with quinidine is based on dosing of quinine. A loading dose of quinidine is given if the patient did not receive mefloquine in the previous 12 hours or over 40 mg/kg of quinidine in the previous 48 hours. The treatment regimen is listed in **Table 70.1**. Once the level of parasitemia is <1% and oral intake started, oral quinidine is administered at the same dose to complete a total 3- to 7-day course. Clindamycin, tetracycline, or doxycycline is administered at the same time as the quinidine. These drugs can be administered orally and should be continued for 7 days. Cardiac monitoring is essential during IV quinidine administration due to the risk of prolonged QT, widening of the QRS, and hypotension. A baseline ECG should be obtained before beginning the medication. The quinidine infusion should be decreased if the QRS complex increases >50%, the QTc prolongs to >0.6 seconds or >25%, or hypotension develops. Malaria smears should be repeated every 8 hours in severe disease. Quinine and quinidine are slow-acting, and parasites may increase in the blood for the first 24 hours. Once the patient has a good response and a parasite density <1%, smears can be obtained once or twice daily. Artemisinin-based therapies are more rapid-acting and have fewer adverse effects, and resistance has not been detected. Artemisinin derivatives are being used to treat severe disease in the United States and abroad. Artemether–lumefantrine is dosed by weight in children. The parenteral drug artesunate is available on an emergency basis through the CDC.

Adequate supportive care is essential. Hypoglycemia increases morbidity and mortality and should be corrected with dextrose infusions. Metabolic acidosis can be corrected with volume replacement. In patients with impaired consciousness or suspicion of cerebral malaria, volume resuscitation should proceed cautiously, as cerebral edema is common. Rapid fluid resuscitation in severe malaria-related anemia (hemoglobin < 5 g/dL) is associated with increased mortality regardless of the use of crystalloid or colloid. In the absence of renal disease, renal output is a good measure of fluid status. Children who remain oliguric after 40 mL/kg bolus of saline should have a central catheter placed to monitor intravascular status. Potassium levels may fall during treatment due to improved acid–base status and rise in pH. The oliguric renal failure can be treated using hemodialysis/hemofiltration or peritoneal dialysis. Hemofiltration results in a more rapid resolution of acidosis, shorter duration of renal replacement therapy, and lower mortality than peritoneal dialysis. Packed red blood cell transfusions are indicated for symptomatic anemia. The role of exchange transfusion is controversial. Anecdotal experience suggests that exchange transfusion may be of benefit. An analysis of exchange transfusions for severe malaria showed no survival benefit. The mortality rate for severe malaria in endemic areas is 15%–30%, with most deaths occurring within 24 hours of admission. Impaired consciousness and respiratory distress are associated with death. Among returned travelers, the mortality rate was 5%–10%. *P. falciparum* infection has no chronic phase. Once the infection has resolved, it does not emerge again. Neurologic impairment following cerebral malaria is well described.

Typhoid

Typhoid fever is caused by *Salmonella enterica* (serotypes Typhi or Paratyphi), a gram-negative rod in the family Enterobacteriaceae. This organism is carried only by humans, and transmission occurs via contaminated food or water (usually from poor water sanitation). The highest burden is in Asia, Latin America, and Africa. In the United States, >50% of travelers with typhoid fever visited the Indian subcontinent. The

TABLE 70.1

Treatment of Uncomplicated and Severe Malaria

■ DIAGNOSIS	■ THERAPY
Uncomplicated malaria with *P. falciparum* or unknown species: chloroquine sensitive (*only* Central America west of the Panama Canal, Haiti, Dominican Republic)	**Chloroquine phosphate** 10 mg base/kg initial dose, followed by 5 mg base/kg at 6, 24, and 48 h Total dose 25 mg base/kg Maximum adult dose: 1500 mg base
Uncomplicated malaria with *P. falciparum* or unknown species: chloroquine resistant or unknown resistance (all regions except for those mentioned above)	**Atovaquone-proguanil** Adult tabs: 250 mg atovaquone/100 mg proguanil Pediatric tablets: 62.5 mg atovaquone/25 mg proguanil Doses given once per day for 3 d: 5–8 kg: 2 pediatric tabs 9–10 kg: 3 pediatric tabs 11–20 kg: 1 adult tab 21–30 kg: 2 adult tab 31–40 kg: 3 adult tabs >40 kg: 4 adult tabs **Artemether–lumefantrine** 1 tab = 20 mg artemether and 120 mg lumefantrine A total of 6 doses given over 3 d with the second dose following the first by 8 h, then 1 dose PO bid for the next 2 d 5–<15 kg: 1 tab per dose 15–<25 kg: 2 tabs per dose 25–<35 kg: 3 tabs per dose ≥35 kg: 4 tabs per dose **Quinine sulfate** 8.3 mg base/kg PO TID for 3–7 d Maximum adult dose: 542 mg base/dose *PLUS* one of the following for 7 d **Doxycycline** 2.2 mg/kg PO BID Maximum adult dose: 100 mg/dose **Tetracycline** 25 mg/kg/d divided QID Maximum adult dose 250 mg/dose **Clindamycin** 20 mg/kg/d divided TID **Mefloquine** 15 mg salt/kg PO initial dose, followed by 10 mg salt/kg PO 6–12 h after initial dose Total dose: 25 mg salt/kg Maximum adult dose: 1250 mg salt
Complicated/severe malaria	**Quinidine gluconate** *Continuous infusion*: 6.25 mg base/kg IV over 1–2 h, followed by 0.0125 mg base/kg/min continuous infusion for at least 24 h *Every 8-h dosing*: 15 mg base/kg over 4 h, followed by 7.5 mg base/kg every 8 h Switch to oral therapy when parasite density is <1% Complete 3–7 d of quinidine therapy *plus* **doxycycline, tetracycline, or clindamycin** as above. If patient cannot tolerate oral medication, doxycycline or clindamycin may be administered intravenously

Refer www.cdc.gov for additional region- or species-specific modifications to this table and/or call the CDC Malaria Hotline at (855) 856-4713, (770) 488-7788, or (770) 488-7100.

organism is ingested, passes into the mesenteric lymph nodes, liver, and spleen where it replicates for 7–14 days, and then enters the bloodstream. The symptoms of typhoid fever begin with the bacteremic phase. Although *S. typhi* produces exotoxin, typhoid fever has a case-fatality rate of <1%. Mortality is a result of unusual complications. Children <5 years of age are more likely to develop severe illness.

The typical presentation is fever, chills, vomiting, anorexia, myalgia, and nonfocal abdominal pain. The fever is sustained, unlike the paroxysms of malaria. Diarrhea occurs in 8%–35%, more common in children, although constipation may be a presenting complaint. Physical examination often reveals hepatosplenomegaly and abdominal pain. *Rose spots*, the typical rash, are 2–4 mm blanching erythematous papules on the trunk. They are transient and difficult to see on dark skin. Relative bradycardia in the face of high fever is typical. CNS manifestations are variable. An "apathetic affect" is common, and episodes of confusion can occur in the absence of CNS infection. Altered mental status is a manifestation of typhoid encephalopathy, a severe complication, usually accompanied by shock and carries a high mortality rate. Seizures may occur in young children. Complications usually occur late, 1–2 weeks after the onset of symptoms. Gastrointestinal bleeding is common, but rarely requires transfusion or surgery. Intestinal perforation can occur, usually in the ileum, the site of the greatest bacterial replication. Laboratory findings are nonspecific. The white blood cell count is often low (young children may have leukocytosis). Mild increases in liver function tests are common. In severe disease, coagulopathy may be present, with thrombocytopenia and signs of DIC. The differential diagnosis depends on the travel and exposure history. Malaria is frequently considered because typhoid and malaria coexist in many regions. The pattern of fever may distinguish the two diseases. However, treatment for both infections may be indicated as evaluation is under way. Other diseases to consider include bacterial sepsis, leptospirosis, rickettsial disease, dengue, hepatitis, Epstein–Barr virus, typhus, brucellosis, and tularemia.

The diagnosis of typhoid fever is challenging. Blood culture sensitivity is 40%, which can go up to 80% when repeat cultures are obtained. The best sensitivity is achieved by large-volume specimens during the first week of illness. Bone marrow culture is more sensitive. It remains positive beyond the first week of illness, even after initiation of antimicrobial therapy. In endemic areas, the Widal serologic test is used. The test is neither reliable nor specific and not used where other options are available. No rapid tests exist.

Fluoroquinolones and third-generation cephalosporins are the medications of choice for empiric therapy. If cultures are positive and the susceptibility patterns are known, treatment may be tailored. The advantage of completing therapy with a fluoroquinolone is a decreased incidence of chronic intestinal carriage. For fluoroquinolone-susceptible infections, 5-day duration is sufficient for therapy of uncomplicated disease. The emergence of fluoroquinolone-resistant *S. typhi* has complicated the treatment of typhoid fever. Recommended therapies are listed in **Table 70.2.**

Hospitalization is typical for young children (high risk for complication) and patients with complicated disease, persistent vomiting, or severe diarrhea. Severe disease requires parenteral therapy for at least 10 days. Dexamethasone is beneficial for severe typhoid with delirium, obtundation, or shock but may mask further intestinal complications. Severe intestinal bleeding or perforation requires hemodynamic stabilization and surgery. Relapse occurs in 5%–10% of appropriately treated infections with the identical organism, and the treatment can be repeated. Relapse is more common with fluoroquinolone-resistant infections. Chronic carriage is excretion for >3 months (rarely occurs in children). If it occurs, prolonged ciprofloxacin or combined amoxicillin and probenecid is recommended for eradication.

Chagas Disease

Trypanosoma cruzi causes Chagas disease, a parasite that infects 7–8 million people throughout Mexico,

TABLE 70.2

Treatment of Typhoid Fever

	DRUG	DOSE (mg/kg/d)	DURATION (d)
Empiric	Ceftriaxone	60	7–14
Fully susceptible	Ciprofloxacin or ofloxacin	15	5–7
	Amoxicillin (second line)	75–100	14
	Trimethoprim/sulfamethoxazole (second line)	8/40	14
Multidrug resistant	Ceftriaxone	60	10–14
	Azithromycin	8–10	7
	Ciprofloxacin or ofloxacin (nalidixic acid–*susceptible* infection)	15	5–7
	Ciprofloxacin or ofloxacin (nalidixic acid–*resistant* infection)	20	10–14

Central America, and South America. The reduviid bug (kissing bug) transmits the disease via feces contamination after a bite or through feces contamination of conjunctiva or mucosa. Reduviid bugs live in the walls of mud and straw houses. Transfusion is another mode of transmission in high-prevalence countries (Brazil).

The initial symptoms are nonspecific and often unrecognized. General malaise begins 6–10 days after exposure and lasts up to 2 months. Other findings include hepatosplenomegaly, lymphadenopathy, rash, and edema. Reduviid bugs bite exposed areas during sleep, often in the periorbital or perioral areas, producing swelling of the eyelid and face called *Romaña sign*. Cardiac abnormalities can develop during the acute illness. ECG and chest X-ray changes are common (but generally not symptomatic) and due to inflammatory response to parasites that have a tropism for cardiac muscle. Life-threatening illness is rare during the *acute phase*, although meningitis and myocarditis can occur. After acute infection, most patients enter a prolonged asymptomatic *indeterminate phase,* usually for the rest of their lives. Some patients (15%–30%) develop end-organ damage, typically decades after the initial infection. Chronic infection occurs in the myocardium or esophagus and colon. Chagas cardiomyopathy is a diffuse process presenting with chest pain, dizziness, and peripheral edema. Chest X-rays show cardiomegaly in all heart chambers and the ECG typically has a right-bundle-branch block. *Megaviscera syndrome* is neuronal loss in the gastrointestinal tract causing megaesophagus and megacolon. Megaesophagus presents with dysphagia, occurs late in the disease, and is diagnosed by upper gastrointestinal contrast study. Megacolon presents with constipation, fecaloma on examination and is confirmed by barium enema. Reactivation of *T. cruzi* infection can occur in immunocompromised patients and in children infected before 2 years of age. The CNS is the most common site of reactivation. Trypanosome invasion of the brain forms chagoma masses, causing headache, fever, cognitive changes, focal neurologic impairment, and seizures. The heart is also commonly affected during reactivation presenting as acute myocarditis or cardiomyopathy. Reactivation of cardiac disease may occur with or without neurologic disease.

During the acute phase, parasitemia can be detected on stained blood smears or buffy coat, in infected organs, lymph nodes, bone marrow, and pericardial fluid. Xenodiagnosis and blood culture in specific medium may be more sensitive, but the tests are rarely available and require 2–8 weeks for diagnosis. During the indeterminate and chronic phase, the diagnosis can be made by serology. A positive IgM does not differentiate acute from chronic infections. A serologic diagnosis can be made using an anti-*T. cruzi* IgG ELISA test, complement fixation, hemagglutination, or indirect immunofluorescence. Because of poor specificity, two serologic tests are needed. Polymerase chain reaction (PCR) can detect low-level chronic infection but is not widely available.

Treatment is most beneficial during the acute infection. For those with end-organ damage due to chronic infection, treatment does not improve outcome. The two effective treatment regimens are nifurtimox for 90–120 days or benznidazole for 30–90 days. Patients <40 kg require higher treatment doses. Hypersensitivity, bone marrow suppression, and peripheral neuropathy may require suspension of treatment with benznidazole. Weight loss, gastrointestinal distress, and psychiatric disturbance result from treatment with nifurtimox. Treatment is successful when parasitemia is cleared and serology is negative. During the acute illness, patients may require intensive care for treatment of pancarditis. Thromboembolism is common, and anticoagulants are used for thrombogenic arrhythmias. Clinically significant pericardial effusions can occur. Chronic sequelae (cardiomyopathy, megaesophagus, and megacolon) are rare among children. Symptomatic management is required. For patients with *T. cruzi* reactivation, specific antitrypanosomal treatment is indicated, although survival is uniformly poor. The restoration of the immune system is important to control the infection.

Patients treated during the acute phase are cured (disappearance of IgG) in 30%–80% of cases. Severe cardiac disease may require heart transplantation. Reactivation of chronic infection may occur due to transplant immunosuppression. Sudden death occurs in 38% of patients with cardiomyopathy (without a recognized change in cardiac status). Risk factors for death include heart failure, cardiomegaly, and left ventricular dysfunction. Immunocompromised individuals with reactivation CNS infection rarely survive 3 months.

Human African Trypanosomiasis

Trypanosoma are parasitic protozoa transmitted by biting insect vectors. The life cycle involves both a vector stage and a host stage when the infective trypomastigote reaches the CNS. Human African trypanosomiasis (HAT) is an important regional health problem with two forms. West African sleeping sickness and East African sleeping sickness are caused by infection with *T. brucei gambiense* and *T. brucei rhodesiense*, respectively. Areas with high infection rates include The Congo and Uganda. East African HAT is endemic at a very low rate in Kenya, Mozambique, Zambia, Tanzania, and Malawi. HAT is extremely rare in travelers. Transmission occurs after a bite from the tsetse fly contaminated by infected saliva. Other mechanisms of transmission include blood transfusions, contaminated needles, and congenital transmission.

HAT has an early, *hemolymphatic stage* and a late, *encephalitic stage* that differ by CNS involvement. In West African HAT a prolonged asymptomatic period occurs followed by fever when trypanosomes are found in blood and lymphatic systems. Myalgias, malaise, lymphadenopathy and fatigue develop. Pruritus and facial edema are rare but clues to diagnosis. The late-stage West African HAT occurs months later (progression to CNS disease is more rapid in children) with headaches, somnolence, and night-time insomnia. Developmental delay is more common than somnolence in children. Extrapyramidal signs, cerebellar ataxia, and hemiparesis may occur. East African HAT has a more acute presentation. A chancre occurs 5–15 days after the bite, with cellulitis or regional adenopathy. Myocarditis is rare, but patients may die due to dysrhythmia or cardiac failure before the neurologic disease becomes clinically apparent.

Cerebrospinal fluid (CSF) shows increased monocytes and elevated protein. A white cell count > 5 cells/mm^3 is positive for CNS disease. Foamy plasma cells, the pathognomonic *Mott morula cells*, are seen. Elevated CSF total IgM levels help establish the diagnosis. Brain imaging may show basal ganglia involvement (similar to Parkinson disease), ventriculomegaly, and asymmetric white matter abnormalities. Electroencephalography in encephalopathic patients may be abnormal, but findings are not pathognomonic. The differential diagnosis includes malaria, tuberculosis, HIV, leishmaniasis, toxoplasmosis, typhoid, and viral encephalitis.

Diagnosis is made by visualizing trypomastigotes in blood or tissue. Aspiration of lymph nodes has a high yield. Thick and thin blood smears are prepared with Giemsa stains, similar to malaria. If parasitemia is low, repeated specimens should be examined. Serological testing (*T. b. gambiense* only) can help. In advanced cases, trypanosomes may be easier to visualize in the CSF. To maximize CSF examination, 6–8 mL of CSF should be centrifuged and the sediment examined.

Treatment varies based on the infecting organism and stage of illness. *T. b. gambiense* can be distinguished from *T. brucei rhodesiense* based on travel or exposure history. Any patient with evidence of trypanosomiasis and a CSF white blood cell count > 5 cells/mm^3 is considered to have late disease. First-line treatment of the hemolymphatic stage is parenteral pentamidine for *T. brucei gambiense* and IV suramin for *T. brucei rhodesiense*. Suramin has a risk of anaphylaxis and a test dose must be given. Eflornithine is only useful for late *T. brucei gambiense* disease and has adverse effects, convulsions (6%–7%) and bone marrow toxicity (common). For CNS disease, IV melarsoprol is effective for both varieties of HAT. The treatment is effective but toxic, with death rates of 4%–6%. Encephalopathy, generalized seizures, coma, and neurogenic pulmonary edema complicate therapy. Prednisone can decrease adverse effects without impairment of efficacy. Polyneuropathy may lead to permanent weakness unless thiamine is administered and treatment is suspended until symptoms resolve. Combination treatment with nifurtimox and eflornithine is effective in the treatment of severe disease due to *T. brucei gambiense*, but not *T. brucei rhodesiense*.

HAT is fatal if untreated. Patients are followed up to 2 years with periodic lumbar punctures to evaluate recurrence of CNS disease. Recurrences require different treatment regimens or higher doses. Long-term prognosis depends on the stage of disease when treatment is initiated and the recurrence of disease, as significant CNS injury occurs with disease progression. Significant CNS disease leads to demyelination, cortical and subcortical atrophy, and multifocal deep white matter lesions.

Leptospirosis

Leptospirosis is caused by the anaerobic spirochete, *Leptospira interrogans*. Infections range from asymptomatic to hemorrhage, renal failure, and death. Leptospires are carried by asymptomatic rodents, dogs, and livestock that shed the organisms in urine. Excreted leptospires survive for months in moist, warm conditions. Transmission occurs by contact with infected water or soil (commonly spread by flooding). The clinical presentation is often attributed to other causes. In Southeast Asia, leptospirosis causes up to 13% of nonmalarial fever, and is frequently confused for dengue. Leptospires cell wall lipopolysaccharide antigens are the target of natural immunity and the basis for serovar grouping. *Leptospira* cause disease through direct infection and the host immune response. The organisms penetrate and infect the liver, kidney, lungs, brain, and eyes. A disseminated vasculitis occurs with endothelial damage and inflammatory infiltrates.

Most infections by *Leptospira* are asymptomatic. The clinical course is biphasic. The *acute* (septicemic) *phase* lasts 1 week and involves fever, chills, headache, conjunctival suffusion, myalgia, nausea, and vomiting. Myalgias can be severe. Mild changes in mental status may occur without meningitis. A pretibial papular rash may develop. Jaundice occurs in <50%. In the *immune phase* symptoms resolve, antibodies are produced, and leptospires are excreted in the urine. Manifestations of the immune phase are aseptic meningitis and anterior uveitis. CSF reveals lymphocytic pleocytosis and a high opening pressure. Focal neurologic findings are rare. A severe icteric form, *Weil disease*, is characterized by jaundice, renal failure, and hemorrhage. Serum bilirubin levels are elevated out of proportion to transaminase levels. Renal failure occurs during the second week of illness. Pulmonary symptoms may take the form of dyspnea or cough or may be severe with hemorrhage and ARDS. Thrombocytopenia is common but is not usually associated with DIC. Hemorrhagic complications can occur in severe disease. Purpura, petechiae, epistaxis, and mild hemoptysis are the frequent manifestations. The pathognomonic sign, conjunctival suffusion, is due to conjunctival hemorrhage and scleral icterus. In anicteric disease, the white blood cell count has a neutrophil predominance, while lymphocytosis is a hallmark of Weil disease. Elevations in serum muscle enzymes are common. Patchy infiltrates on chest X-ray represent intra-alveolar and interstitial hemorrhage, usually bilateral at the lung bases and periphery. Histologic findings represent endothelial damage and hemorrhage, not inflammatory exudate. Disease can progress to diffuse alveolar infiltrates and radiographic evidence of ARDS.

The differential diagnosis includes influenza, Epstein–Barr virus, hepatitis viruses, and community-acquired pneumonia. Other vector-borne infections include malaria, dengue, hantavirus, typhoid fever, rickettsial infections, and arbovirus disease. Toxic shock syndrome may also mimic leptospirosis. Diagnosis can be made by direct visualization of the organism or serologic evaluation. The gold standard for diagnosis is serology using the microscopic agglutination test. A fourfold increase in antibody titers or conversion from seronegative to a titer > 1:100 is considered diagnostic. Culture of the organism from the CSF, blood, or urine is not dependable. Real-time PCR is a rapid and reliable strategy where available and offers a quantitative assessment of the bacterial load, which may be prognostic.

Antibiotic therapy decreases the duration of illness, thrombocytopenia, and extent of renal failure. Treatment of severe disease is recommended. Penicillin, doxycycline, ceftriaxone, and cefotaxime are effective. In areas endemic for both leptospirosis and rickettsiosis, cephalosporin or doxycycline are preferred. Empiric therapy with an IV cephalosporin should be closely monitored as the Jarisch–Herxheimer reaction (release of endotoxin from large-scale death of bacteria) can occur with β-lactam therapy. Aside from antibiotic therapy, management is supportive. The oliguria usually responds to fluid treatment. In acute, intrinsic renal failure, prompt treatment with renal replacement therapy can reduce mortality. Peritoneal dialysis is inferior to veno-venous hemofiltration. Extracorporeal membrane oxygenation (ECMO) has been successful in some severe cases.

Case fatality for severe disease ranges from 5% to 40%. Death is due to acute renal failure and pulmonary hemorrhage. Hemodialysis improves mortality rates. Among survivors, normalization of glomerular filtration rate occurs by 6 months, some hyposthenuria may persist. Hepatic function returns to normal, elevated bilirubin levels may persist for weeks. Chronic visual disturbances and anterior uveitis may persist for weeks.

Hantavirus

Hantaviruses are of the Bunyavirus family. "Old World" viruses (Europe and Asia) cause *hemorrhagic fever with renal syndrome* (HFRS). "New World" viruses (Americas) cause *hantavirus pulmonary syndrome* (HPS). The viruses have asymptomatic rodent reservoirs that excrete virus in urine, feces, and saliva. Transmission occurs by inhalation of aerosols from rodent feces. Hantavirus in the US is carried by a deer mouse. Infection is rare and children account for <10%. The states with highest incidence are New Mexico, Montana, Utah, Nevada, Arizona, and Colorado. Cases are also reported in Canada and Mexico. The Andes virus is common in South America HPS. In Latin America, disease occurs in family clusters and involves children. The most severe forms of HFRS are cases of Hantaan virus (Korean peninsula) and Dobrava virus (Balkans). A milder disease is caused by Seoul virus (Southeast Asia). The Puumala virus (Scandinavia, Western Europe, and Russia) causes benign *nephropathia epidemica*, an interstitial nephritis associated with HFRS.

HFRS is characterized by fever, renal failure, and hemorrhage. Symptoms begin 2–3 weeks after exposure; incubation is 2 days to 6 weeks. There are five phases. The *febrile phase* lasts 5 days and includes sudden fever, headache, back pain, abdominal pain, vomiting, myalgias, weakness, chills, flushing, and dermatographism. In the *hypotensive phase,* shock develops as does capillary leak, proteinuria, leukocytosis, thrombocytopenia, hypotension, petechiae, hemorrhage, hepatosplenomegaly, conjunctivitis, and visual changes. The *oliguric phase* includes normalization of blood pressure or hypertension for 3–7 days before urine output improves. It has the highest risk of death (due to hemorrhage). The *diuretic phase* lasts weeks. The *convalescent phase* may be asymptomatic or associated with polyuria or hyposthenuria. Permanent renal damage is a long-term sequela. Laboratory results show thrombocytopenia and leukocytosis in the febrile and hypotensive phases, followed by proteinuria, renal insufficiency, and electrolyte imbalance during the oliguric phase. Symptomatic patients have enlarged kidneys, ascites, or pleural effusion on ultrasound. The differential diagnosis includes rickettsial disease, Dengue virus, leptospirosis, renal disease, and renal vein thrombosis.

HPS has a 1–2-week incubation and three phases. The *prodromal phase* (3–6 days) includes fever, myalgia, headache, sore throat, abdominal pain, and diarrhea. The *cardiorespiratory phase* (7–10 days) develops rapidly, with cough, shortness of breath, tachypnea, tachycardia, hypotension, and hypoxemia. Renal insufficiency, bleeding, and petechiae (not seen in the United States) are common with Andes virus. The *convalescence phase* is marked by thrombocytopenia, leukocytosis, hemoconcentration (South America), myelocytosis, lack of neutrophil granulation, and lymphocytosis. DIC may develop. Renal impairment is common in South American HPS and may require dialysis. Chest X-ray demonstrates interstitial edema, airspace disease, and pleural effusions. The differential diagnosis includes pneumonia, septic shock, ARDS, acute gastroenteritis, leptospirosis, plague, Colorado tick fever, tularemia, relapsing fever, Rocky Mountain fever, Legionnaire disease, ehrlichiosis, Q fever, coccidioidomycosis, and histoplasmosis. A history of contact with rodent-infested structures is usually present. Severe HFRS resembles hemolytic uremic syndrome, but lacks a microangiopathic, hemolytic anemia.

Diagnosis is based on antibody to the nucleocapsid. IgM is present during clinical symptoms. IgG peaks during the first week. A fourfold rise in IgG distinguishes previous exposure from acute infection. Diagnosis may require a reverse-transcriptase PCR in regions with high seroprevalence. Viral isolation is unusual.

Treatment is supportive. Severe HFRS or HPS may require mechanical ventilation and renal replacement therapy. ECMO criteria include a cardiac index < 2.3 L/min/mm^2, PaO_2/FIO_2 < 50 or unresponsive to conventional support. Early ECMO is begun because of rapid decompensation. Ribavirin for HPS is not active in vivo. Administration of ribavirin within 4 days reduced incidence of renal failure in HFRS in China. End-organ damage is due to the inflammatory response but steroids have not been studied. Outcome for HFRS depends on the infecting virus. Dobrava and Hantaan viruses have a mortality rate of 5%–10%, Seoul1%–2%, and Puumala virus < 0.2%. In severe cases, 15%–20% of the children require renal replacement therapy. Renal insufficiency resolves in most cases. The case fatality for HPS in the US is 33%–35%. An elevated prothrombin time was associated with mortality. Mortality rates are high with Andes virus (47%) related to hemorrhage or renal insufficiency. Most deaths with HPS result from hypoxemia, ventricular dysfunction, and arrhythmias.

Poliomyelitis

Polioviruses are enteroviruses in the family Picornaviridae. In the US, wild-type poliomyelitis disappeared in 1986 and vaccine-associated poliomyelitis in 1999. Endemic cases occur in Africa, India, Pakistan, and Afghanistan. The peak incidence is summer and fall in temperate climates. Humans are the only hosts. Infection is spread via fecal–oral and oral–oral routes. The virus enters the alimentary tract and replicates (alimentary phase), spreads to lymph tissue, multiplies, produces a minor viremia seeding other organs (lymphatic phase), replicates, and produces major viremia and CNS infection (viremic phase). Antibody formation clears the viremia by day 7 (intestinal shedding continues for weeks). Replication in the CNS damages anterior and dorsal horn cells of the spinal cord and medulla producing paralysis. Other affected areas include the midbrain, hypothalamus, thalamus, and cerebellum. The white matter of the cerebral cortex and spinal cord are spared. CNS lesions are more widespread than the clinical manifestations.

The four types of infection are inapparent (90%), abortive (4%), nonparalytic (1%), and paralytic (<1%). In endemic areas, children <5 years account for the majority of paralytic cases. Risk factors for paralytic disease include older age, pregnancy, recent vaccination, and physical exercise or trauma at time of infection. Tonsillectomy is a risk factor for bulbar poliomyelitis. Immunodeficiency and recent IM injection increase the risk for vaccine-associated paralytic poliomyelitis. Nonparalytic cases can have CNS injury including meningismus, muscle spasms, and CSF values that suggest aseptic meningitis. Paralytic polio is life-threatening due to respiratory failure. The incubation period is 3–5 days for minor illness, 1–2 weeks for CNS involvement, and 1 month for paralysis. In children, the disease progresses in a *minor phase* with prodromal symptoms (sore throat, fever, nausea, vomiting, abdominal discomfort, rash, constipation, and flu-like symptoms) followed days later by *CNS disease*. Irritability, high fever, anxiousness, and diminished superficial reflexes herald paralysis. Weakness progresses to flaccid paralysis with loss of tendon reflexes. The lower extremities are more commonly affected. Transient fasciculations and muscle spasm may be present prior to paralysis. Brainstem disease causes bulbar symptoms (pharyngeal hypotonia, hoarseness, deviation of the soft palate, diminished swallowing, increased secretions, aphonia, and "rope" sign [hypotonia of hyoid muscles]) and autonomic dysfunction (paralytic ileus, bladder paralysis, cardiac arrhythmias, and systemic hypertension).

Paralytic poliomyelitis has three forms. *Pure spinal poliomyelitis* (79%) has muscular weakness without cranial nerve involvement. Respiratory failure is due to paralysis of thoracic muscles and diaphragm. *Pure bulbar poliomyelitis* (2%) has weakness of cranial nerves IX, X, or XII. Patients have agitation or delirium, cardiac dysrhythmias, hypertension, hypothermia, and disordered breathing. Respiratory failure is due to extrathoracic airway obstruction or aspiration. *Bulbospinal disease* (19%) has a combination of features. Encephalitic poliomyelitis (rare) has fever, mental status changes, spasticity, seizures, and bulbar signs.

Diagnosis is confirmed by virus recovery from stool, oropharynx, or CSF. Typing rules out a vaccine strain. The presence of IgM antibodies suggests acute infection. The differential diagnosis includes Guillain–Barré, other enterovirus infections, acute disseminating encephalomyelitis, rabies, botulism, WNV, Ebstein–Barr virus, aseptic meningitis, and encephalitis. Flaccid paralysis and lack of sensory changes helps rule out other diseases.

Treatment is primarily supportive. Bulbar or bulbospinal poliomyelitis requires maintenance of airway patency with suctioning and positioning. Gas exchange is closely assessed. Airway obstruction, risk of aspiration, and significant weakness or paralysis require intubation and ventilation. Respiratory failure is frequent with bulbar poliomyelitis. Given the prolonged time to recovery, tracheostomy may be necessary. No antiviral therapy is available. Pleconaril treatment has been reported, but efficacy is unknown. Analgesia is needed for myalgia or headaches and laxatives for constipation. Physical and occupational therapy can facilitate recovery. Patients with mild weakness may have complete recovery. Patients with flaccid paralysis usually have persistent weakness. Recovery is 60% by 3 months, 80% by 6 months, and plateaus at 18 months. The mortality rate (4%) is higher in adults and patients with bulbar disease (25%–75%). Post-poliomyelitis syndrome (exacerbation or new weakness and muscle pain) occurs in ~25%–40% 30 to 40-years after infection.

EMERGING INFECTIONS

West Nile Virus

West Nile virus (WNV) is a single-stranded RNA virus similar to other Flaviviruses in the Japanese encephalitis virus complex. WNV is sustained through an enzootic cycle between birds and mosquitoes. Mosquitoes of the order Culex are vectors for transmitting WNV and most infections occur during July to December. Humans are "dead-end" hosts who develop insufficient viremia to infect feeding mosquitoes. Other modes of transmission include blood transfusion, breast-feeding, organ transplantation, and transplacental infection (no adverse effects of transmission to neonates documented). Blood components are screened using WNV nucleic acid amplification tests. In the US >4000 cases occur annually in 45 states. Increasing incidence and severity may be related to increasing virulence, changes in host factors, or predisposing chronic disease.

After inoculation WNV replicates in dendritic cells, ascends to regional lymph nodes, and disseminates to the blood and organs. The incubation period is 2–6 days, up to 14 days. Prolonged incubation (up to 3 weeks) occurs in immunocompromised patients. WNV is present in the blood 2 days before the onset of symptoms and viremia clears after 4 days. In immunocompromised hosts, the viremia can be prolonged up to 1 month.

Symptomatic infection with WNV is categorized as West Nile fever or West Nile neuroinvasive disease (WNND). West Nile fever develops in 20% of infected patients and presents as fever, headache, myalgia, nausea, vomiting, abdominal pain, or diarrhea. Sore throat, cough, and maculopapular rash may occur. Most symptoms resolve within 1 week, malaise and fatigue may persist for several weeks. WNND develops in <1% of infected patients. In children, ~50% have meningitis. They present with headache, nuchal rigidity, fever, rash (50%) and muscle weakness (33%). Patients with encephalitis have fever, headache, nuchal rigidity, and alteration in consciousness. Muscle weakness is seen in 80% of patients with encephalitis and none have a rash. Patients with encephalitis may have bulbar findings and hyperreflexia. Rare extraneurologic complications include myocarditis, pancreatitis, and hepatitis. The risk factors for the development of WNND and death are advanced age (>70 years), disruption of the blood–brain barrier, and immunosuppression. WNND occurs less in children than adults and children have more asymptomatic infections or milder disease.

WNV nucleic acid can be detected using reverse-transcriptase PCR however it often cannot be detected after the viremia has resolved (3–5 days after the symptoms appear). IgM ELISA can be performed on the serum or CSF. IgM is detectable 3–5 days into illness. WNV IgM cross-reacts with other Flaviviruses. IgM antibody has been detectable in patients up to 1 year after WNV infection. Laboratory evaluation reveals a mild leukopenia or leukocytosis. Hyponatremia and CSF findings of mild lymphocytic pleocytosis, mild-to-moderate protein level elevation, and normal glucose levels can occur in patients with WNND. CT and MRI imaging of the brain may be normal or show only mild leptomeningeal enhancement despite significant neurologic findings. Follow-up neuroimaging with MRI may show gray matter abnormalities. Electromyography and nerve conduction studies may be consistent with a motor axonal polyneuropathy and demonstrate evidence of anterior horn cell injury. Other causes of aseptic meningitis should be considered, including infections with enterovirus and other viruses in the *Flavivirus* family. The acute muscle weakness resembles Guillain–Barré syndrome. Treatable infections (herpesvirus or bacterial meningoencephalitis), should be considered.

Treatment is mainly supportive. Endotracheal intubation may be necessary for airway protection. Seizures occur rarely but should be treated aggressively. Ribavirin and interferon-α inhibit WNV replication and cytopathogenicity but clear benefit has not been demonstrated in patients. Adult mortality with WNV meningoencephalitis is 4%–14%. Deaths occur in patients with encephalitis. Cases in children are rarely fatal. Half of the adults report that they have not recovered physically, functionally, or cognitively at 12 months postillness. Details regarding the course of pediatric recovery are lacking.

Avian Influenza

Influenza A viruses belong to the Orthomyxoviridae family. Antigenic subtypes are defined by two major surface glycoproteins: hemagglutinin (HA) and neuraminidase (NA). *Antigenic drift*, change within the same viral subtype, is responsible for the annual epidemics. *Antigenic shift*, causes circulation of a new subtype and leads to pandemics. The reservoir for influenza type A is wild waterfowl. In birds, influenza A viruses cause asymptomatic gastrointestinal infection with fecal–oral transmission. Avian influenza virus strains H5N1 and H7N9 have spread to humans from exposure to infected poultry. Humans are primarily infected by contact with poultry through handling diseased birds or consumption of uncooked poultry. The spread of avian influenza to humans is limited. Avian influenza viruses bind to intestinal epithelium and human influenza viruses bind respiratory epithelium. With few of the appropriate receptors available in human lungs, replication and propagation of the avian virus is reduced. Human-to-human transmission has been suspected but not documented. Nosocomial transmission to health-care workers has not occurred.

Presenting symptoms depend on the type of avian influenza viral infection. The incubation period ranges from 2 to 8 days for the avian influenza viruses. The early symptoms are high fever, influenza-like illness, and lower respiratory involvement. Upper respiratory symptoms occur occasionally. Gastrointestinal symptoms, including diarrhea (with or without blood), vomiting, and abdominal pain, are common and may precede the respiratory illness. Most patients have symptoms of pneumonia (dyspnea, tachypnea, and rales) that may progress to ARDS multiorgan failure, cardiac dysfunction, pulmonary hemorrhage, pancytopenia, and systemic inflammatory response syndrome without bacteremia.

Diagnosis begins with a history of potential exposure—travel to an endemic area and contact with poultry, ill birds, or an individual with avian influenza. The geographic distribution of human and bird infections is available at (http://www.who.int/csr/disease/avian_influenza/en/). Other considerations for patients with severe pneumonia and travel to Southeast Asia include leptospirosis and melioidosis (for unvaccinated children: measles and *Haemophilus influenzae* B).

Leukopenia (especially lymphopenia), thrombocytopenia, elevated aminotransferases, and elevated creatinine can occur. The chest X-ray shows multifocal consolidation that takes on a ground-glass appearance as respiratory failure and ARDS developed. The preferred method for diagnosis is oropharyngeal and respiratory tract specimens for reverse-transcriptase PCR testing. Throat swabs have higher yield than nasal swabs. Viral antigen testing may also be useful. The common test for influenza A may detect avian strains. If avian influenza is suspected, the laboratory must be informed that a specimen is being submitted.

H5N1 and H7N9 are sensitive to the NA inhibitors oseltamivir and zanamivir. Administration within 48 hours improves survival. Nausea and vomiting are common while anaphylaxis and severe dermatologic reactions are rare adverse events. In mild cases, standard dose is administered for 5 days, in severe cases the standard dose can be doubled. Oseltamivir prophylaxis is recommended for 7–10 days after a high- to moderate-risk exposure. A case of oseltamivir-resistant H5N1 raises concern that wide scale postexposure prophylaxis during a threatened epidemic would select drug-resistant strains. Oseltamivir is preferred over zanamivir because it is easier to administer. Other antivirals, such as the amantadane derivatives and ribavirin, are not currently recommended but may be considered for combination therapy. Both NA inhibitor drug dosages must be adjusted for renal failure. Oseltamivir also undergoes significant hepatic metabolism. Infection control should be addressed immediately. Standard, contact, airborne, and eye infection-control measures should be instituted. Intensive care is essential for severe disease. Respiratory failure requiring intubation occurs in most hospitalized patients. Renal dysfunction occurs commonly (etiology unknown). Inotropic support may be necessary. Mortality is high for patients with H5N1 (50%) and H7N9 (30%). Death usually occurs due to progressive respiratory failure and multiple organ dysfunction 9–10 days after onset of illness.

Novel Coronavirus Infections (SARS and MERS)

The SARS coronavirus (SARS-CoV) and MERS coronavirus (MERS-CoV) cause severe acute respiratory syndrome (SARS) and Middle East respiratory syndrome (MERS). The first SARS case occurred in 2003 in Hong Kong and infected >8000 people in multiple countries, and with a high mortality rate in adults. No cases have been reported since 2004.

The disease appears to be transmitted through droplet contact with the mucosa of the respiratory system. The large number of nosocomial cases is generated by respiratory equipment that amplifies transmission. Disease in children occurs through household or hospital contacts, with no major spread through schools. Infection-control procedures effectively control the spread of SARS. Quarantine measures are effective; no transmission is reported prior to the onset of symptoms. Factors that contribute to rapid spread include a long incubation period (usually 4–7, up to 14 days), insidious onset of symptoms, and infectivity that increases as symptoms progress.

The disease course is triphasic, patients present with myalgia, fever, malaise, and rigors. Rhinorrhea and sore throat are less common. Phase 1 is associated with viral replication, is transient, and resolution occurs in one-third. Two-thirds develop persistent fever, cough, oxygen desaturation, chest pain, tachypnea, dyspnea, and bronchopneumonia (phase 2). This phase represents an exaggerated immunologic response and viral load is decreasing. Some patients have watery diarrhea. Between symptom onset and hospital admission is 3–5 days.

Laboratory data reveal lymphopenia (56%–90%), thrombocytopenia (13%–41%), and elevated transaminases. Chest radiographs are abnormal in 60%–100% with a ground-glass appearance or focal consolidation. CT scans are abnormal in 67% with normal chest X-rays. Pneumomediastinum can develop without positive-pressure ventilation. Some patients progress to ARDS with diffuse alveolar damage and pulmonary fibrosis (phase III). Children usually have mild disease, with severe cases occurring in adolescents.

The diagnosis for pediatric cases requires a positive test for SARS-CoV. RT-PCR analyses of nasopharyngeal or stool specimens have 50% sensitivity in children. Higher sensitivity and faster turnaround are possible using one-step, real-time RT-PCR to detect viral RNA in plasma. Acute and convalescent serology for SARS-CoV is useful for confirmation of infection but not for triage. In addition to specific testing for SARS-CoV, testing for other viral and/or bacterial etiologies should be performed, as coinfection (human metapneumovirus and Chlamydia have been reported) could be present.

A key component of treatment is the use of infection-control procedures to control spread of disease. Effective control also involves successful triage of suspected cases. Antimicrobial therapy should be administered for bacterial etiologies in the differential diagnosis. A temporal relationship has been seen between the administration of corticosteroids and clinical improvement in seriously ill children. Immunomodulation during this phase of illness (phase II) is thought to have theoretic benefit. SARS-CoV has not been found to be sensitive to ribavirin.

Approximately 30% of adults with SARS require ICU admission and the mortality rate is up to 50%

in older patients. Terminal events in adult are associated with progressive respiratory failure, multiple organ dysfunction, or intercurrent illness (myocardial infarction). Children make up <10% of SARS cases. Children <12 years of age have a less severe course, 5% require PICU admission, 1% require mechanical ventilation, and no deaths have been reported. Abnormal biochemical markers and lymphopenia persist longer in children with severe disease. Sore throat and peak neutrophil count predict severity. Most children treated with steroids were adolescents. Six months after SARS diagnosis, symptomatic lung disease has resolved but mild lung abnormalities are still seen on high-resolution CT in 34% (residual ground-glass changes and/or air trapping).

Ebola Virus Disease

Hemorrhagic fevers are reviewed in Chapter 66. In 2014, there were more than 10,000 cases of laboratory-confirmed ebola virus disease (EVD) with nearly 6000 deaths in West Africa (Sierra Leone, Liberia, Guinea, Senegal, Nigeria, and Mali). This outbreak was notable for its scale and for the spread of EVD via infected international travelers or health workers, with cases reported in Spain and the US. Health-care workers in both countries became infected.

EVD is caused by exposure to blood, urine, vomit, feces, sweat, tears, breast milk, or semen from infected individuals. Infection with ebola virus causes fever and nonspecific flu-like symptoms after an incubation period of 2–21 days. Humans are not infectious until they develop symptoms. Patients with EVD usually have vomiting, diarrhea, and rash: some will experience clinically significant internal and external bleeding.

It is important to distinguish EVD from other sources of fever in West African travelers (malaria and typhoid fever). Blood tests such as antigen-capture ELISA, IgM ELISA, PCR, and viral culture can be diagnostic within days of onset of symptoms. IgM and IgG titers can be helpful in later stages.

Treatment includes aggressive hydration and replacement of massive volumes of gastrointestinal fluid output (up to 10 L a day in adults). The remainder of treatment is supportive, potentially including mechanical ventilation, renal replacement therapy, and management of secondary infections. Patients have been successfully treated with convalescent plasma from ebola survivors and chimeric monoclonal antibodies against ebola. The experimental antiviral brincidofovir has activity against ebola, but efficacy is unclear.

Appropriate isolation and use of personal protective equipment (PPE) are. While EVD is thought to not be transmissible through the air, airborne infection isolation (including negative pressure rooms) is recommended given the possibility of the generation of aerosols in the course of caring for patients. The global case-fatality rate for EVD is ~50%. With early and aggressive supportive care, it is likely that the mortality rate from EVD is much lower.

CHAPTER 71 ■ TOXIN-RELATED DISEASES

SUNIT C. SINGHI, M. JAYASHREE, JOHN P. STRAUMANIS, AND KAREN L. KOTLOFF

TETANUS

Tetanus is a potentially fatal disease characterized by hypertonia, muscle spasms, and autonomic instability. It is caused by the action of tetanospasmin (commonly called *tetanus toxin*), a potent neurotoxin elaborated by the organism *Clostridium tetani*, an anaerobic, gram-positive bacillus that forms endospores on maturation. The spores are widely distributed (soil, house and operating room dust, freshwater, saltwater, and animal feces) and may survive for years. The World Health Organization (WHO) estimated in 2011 that the number of tetanus-related deaths globally in children <5 years of age was 72,600. Newborns account for half of all cases. In industrialized nations, tetanus is a disease of the elderly—those either born before immunization was implemented or who have an age-related decline in antitoxin levels.

Pathogenesis

Disease typically occurs after acute soft-tissue injury, particularly deep puncture wounds and lacerations, in which anaerobic bacterial growth is facilitated. Tetanus also occurs as a result of animal bites, use of dirty medication needles, dental abscesses, body piercing, drug abuse (notably skin popping), burns, and surgical procedures. It also occurs in patients with chronic infections, such as otitis media or decubitus ulcers. After entering the body, tetanospasmin spreads via lymphatics and blood vessels to enter the nervous system at the neuromuscular junction of the lower motor neurons. The toxin spreads through the central nervous system (CNS) by retrograde axonal transport. It inhibits the release of neurotransmitters, predominantly glycine, in the spinal cord and γ-aminobutyric acid (GABA) in the brainstem, causing sustained, uninhibited contraction of muscles (tetany). Excitatory transmission is also disrupted, causing weakness. Autonomic dysfunction is caused by toxin effects on the neurologic system and the myocardium and by adrenal inhibition. Acetylcholine release may be impaired, and tetanospasmin probably has an angiotensin-converting enzyme–like effect that contributes to hypertension.

Clinical Features

The incubation period varies from 2 days to months (average 2 weeks). The most common form of tetanus is *generalized tetanus*, which manifests with classical trismus or "lockjaw," followed by *risus sardonicus* (a facial grimace that results from hypertonia of the orbicularis oris), generalized muscle rigidity, hyper-reflexia, dysphagia, opisthotonos, and spasms. The muscle spasms are very painful. If prolonged, spasms may lead to rhabdomyolysis, laryngeal obstruction, respiratory failure, and cardiac arrest. Sympathetic overactivity, associated with elevated plasma norepinephrine and epinephrine concentrations, causes fluctuating heart rate, peripheral pallor, labile hypertension, and fever with profound sweating. These may be accompanied by hypotension and cardiac arrhythmias. Parasympathetic involvement may manifest as excessive salivation and increased bronchial secretions as well as bradycardia and sudden cardiac arrest. Recovery usually begins after 3 weeks and takes about 4 weeks.

With *localized tetanus*, rigidity may occur only at the site of spore inoculation. Symptoms may be mild and self-limited or progress to generalized tetanus. *Neonatal tetanus* develops through contamination of the umbilical stump in infants born to inadequately immunized mothers. The contamination may be caused by the use of unsterile instruments to cut the cord or by cord care practices. The first signs are poor sucking and excessive crying, followed by variable degrees of trismus, risus sardonicus, and repeated generalized muscle spasms. Apnea may occur. *Cephalic tetanus* is uncommon and is often associated with otitis media or head injuries. Facial paresis is usually present. Rarely, extraocular movements are affected, causing "ophthalmologic tetanus."

Diagnosis

The diagnosis of tetanus is made entirely on clinical grounds. There is no serologic test to determine the presence of toxin in serum or cerebrospinal fluid (CSF). A history of full immunization almost excludes tetanus. Culture of *C. tetani* from a suspicious wound is not useful.

Management

Neutralization of the Unbound Toxin

Passive immunization to neutralize circulating (unbound) toxin by using antitoxin shortens the course and reduces the severity of tetanus. Human tetanus immunoglobulin (HTIG) consists of immunoglobulin G and has a half-life of 25 days. Where HTIG is unavailable, equine anti-tetanus serum may be used after testing for hypersensitivity. Whether antitoxin should also be infiltrated locally at the portal of entry is unclear. Intrathecal administration of antitoxin has variable results.

Removal of the Source of Toxin

Toxin production may continue in suppurated wounds, wounds with retained foreign bodies, persistent otitis, untreated dental abscess, etc. The portal of entry should be identified and treated with IV antibiotics and wound debridement.

Antibiotic Therapy

Antibiotic therapy should be given to eradicate toxin-producing *C. tetani*. Benzyl penicillin, benzathine penicillin (single IM injection), and metronidazole are equally effective.

Control of Rigidity and Spasms

Stimulation (noise or touch) can trigger muscle spasms. It is essential to keep the patient's surroundings quiet and dark. No single drug or group of drugs is consistently effective in controlling rigidity and spasms in severe tetanus. Benzodiazepines are commonly used for control of rigidity and spasms, as they are GABAA agonists and antagonize the effect of toxin on inhibitory receptors. Initial control is achieved with IV diazepam; enteral administration through a feeding tube may start once spasms are under control. Neuromuscular blockade is required when sedatives do not fully control rigidity and spasms. Vecuronium and atracurium are preferred; pancuronium can worsen autonomic instability. Intrathecal administration of baclofen has been useful. Dantrolene may be useful in select cases.

Control of Autonomic Dysfunction

Propranolol, a β-adrenergic blocking agent, is commonly used for quick control of sympathetic dysfunction. It should be used in small doses, as it may produce serious side effects. Enteral administration may be dangerous as absorption and response may be erratic. *Labetalol* may be preferred for its combined α- and β-adrenergic effect. *Esmolol* is also attractive as a short-acting agent. *Morphine* acts centrally to reduce sympathetic tone, reducing heart rate and blood pressure. The sedative effect is an added advantage. *Magnesium* inhibits the release of humoral and neuronal catecholamines, and reduces the sensitivity of α-adrenergic receptors. Magnesium infusions reduce the need for neuromuscular blocking agents and sedatives in adults but do not improve mortality or ICU needs. *Clonidine* inhibits sympathetic outflow and potentiates parasympathetic activity, but further investigation in tetanus is needed. Anecdotal reports exist of using *atropine* for parasympathetic autonomic dysfunction, *valproate* for sedation, *angiotensin-converting enzyme inhibitors* for hypertension, and *adenosine* for arrhythmias. The role of pyridoxine is controversial, and corticosteroids are not advised.

Supportive Treatment

Endotracheal intubation should be performed in all patients who have generalized rigidity on arrival as the disease is likely to progress in severity for 10–14 days after onset. Strict asepsis, meticulous mouth care, chest physiotherapy, and regular endotracheal tube care are essential to prevent atelectasis, lobar collapse, and pneumonia. Adequate sedation is mandatory when interventions are performed to minimize the risk of uncontrolled spasms. Energy demand is high in patients with tetanus, and adequate caloric intake should be ensured early; enteral feeding is preferred. Special mattresses to allow turning the patient with minimal stimulation and to prevent pressure ulcers are preferred. Passive range-of-motion exercises must be instituted early to maintain muscle strength, prevent deformities, and stimulate circulation.

Outcome and Prognosis

Mortality rates are <10% in mild generalized disease but are as high as 50% in severe disease, and up to 90% in neonates. Autonomic disturbances that appear later in the course of the illness and intensive care-related complications are now major causes of death. Generally, the longer the incubation period, the milder the illness and better the prognosis.

Prevention

The vaccine confers protective antibody levels in 81%–95% of previously unimmunized people after two doses and in 100% after three doses. A booster dose of tetanus toxoid is recommended every 10 years. All pregnant women should receive Tdap, which contains a reduced diphtheria toxoid and acellular pertussis vaccine. Postinjury prophylaxis is not required in people who have received a tetanus toxoid booster dose within the previous 5 years. Children who have received partial immunization need only the remaining doses from the schedule, rather than to restart from the first dose. A semiquantitative bedside test, Tetanus Quick Stick (TQS), can be used to check seroprotection against tetanus in patients with "tetanus-prone" wounds and no clear history of vaccination. If the test is not available, individuals with a tetanus-prone wound and an uncertain history of vaccination or the last dose of tetanus toxoid >5 years before injury should receive one dose of HTIG and one dose of tetanus toxoid *at separate sites with separate syringes*. HTIG should also be given to immunodeficient patients with a tetanus-prone wound.

DIPHTHERIA

Diphtheria is an acute localized infection of skin or respiratory mucous membranes caused by toxin-producing strains of *Corynebacterium diphtheriae*. In 2011, diphtheria caused 5000 cases and 2500 deaths globally. Disease is characterized by a pseudomembrane in the throat and a systemic illness that results from absorption of toxin. Transmission of the organism occurs by exposure to respiratory secretions or exudates from skin lesions. Carriers can transmit the disease, but patients with active infection are more likely to do so. *C. diphtheriae* can survive for weeks in floor dust.

Pathogenesis

Both toxigenic and nontoxigenic strains can cause localized mucocutaneous infection, bacteremia, and seeding of distant sites. The toxin inhibits cellular protein synthesis, and while all human cells are susceptible to the effects, there is a predilection for myocardium, peripheral nerves, and kidneys. The toxin also causes local destruction of the respiratory mucosa at the site of infection, facilitating formation of a dense coagulum of organism, necrotic epithelial cells, fibrin, and pus cells over the mucosa, the so-called *pseudomembrane*. Immunization does not prevent carriage or infection with toxigenic *C. diphtheriae*, but antitoxic immunity decreases local tissue spread and necrosis (and therefore ameliorates the incidence and severity of disease). It is estimated that 70%–80% of a population must be immunized to prevent epidemic spread.

Clinical Manifestations

Onset of symptoms follows an incubation period of 2–5 days. Sore throat and fever are almost universal. Cough, stridor, hoarseness, and dysphagia are frequent. Cervical lymphadenopathy with a brawny edema of the cervical region, described as "bull-neck," is common in severe cases. Unilateral, purulent to blood-tinged nasal discharge is characteristic of nasal diphtheria. Nausea, vomiting, malaise, and headache may be present. The characteristic thick, adherent fibrinous pseudomembrane looks dull and grayish and bleeds easily on touch. It may be found on the palate, pharynx, tonsils, epiglottis, and larynx, or may extend to the tracheobronchial tree. Isolated laryngeal membrane, nasal diphtheria, or tracheal membrane without pharyngeal involvement is rare. *Cutaneous diphtheria* infection typically presents as a chronic nonhealing ulcer with a gray membrane. Infection is most often found in the tropics and in hosts subjected to inadequate hygiene. Clusters of invasive disease (endocarditis, septic arthritis, and osteomyelitis) have been reported in similar populations.

Complications

Upper airway obstruction occurs in nearly 75% of patients with severe disease. The airway should be secured early, as rapid progression of the membrane may preclude a later opportunity. Myocarditis is one of the most serious complications. Electrocardiographic changes occur in 68% of cases and symptomatic myocarditis in 10%–25%. Myocarditis usually occurs at the end of the second week but may be seen as early as 5 days after the onset of respiratory symptoms. Prolonged PR interval is frequent. Bradyarrhythmias in the form of bundle-branch blocks progressing to complete heart blocks are more common than tachyarrhythmias. Polyneuropathy occurs 3–16 weeks after onset in a minority of patients. The neuropathy involves the cranial and peripheral nerves with predominantly motor findings. In severe cases, respiratory and abdominal muscles are involved. Weakness begins proximally and spreads distally. Autonomic disturbances (tachycardia, hypotension, hypertension, and hyperhidrosis) may be seen. CSF may show pleocytosis and elevated protein levels. Renal failure may be secondary to acute tubular necrosis or a consequence of decreased cardiac output due to myocarditis and cardiogenic shock. Thrombocytopenia and bleeding are considered rare manifestations.

Diagnosis and Differential Diagnosis

The diagnosis of diphtheria and indication for antitoxin therapy are based on clinical findings. Diphtheria should be suspected in any patient with membranous tonsillopharyngitis (especially if extending to the uvula and soft palate) or if bull-neck, hoarseness, stridor, unilateral bloody nasal discharge, and palatal palsy are observed. Other conditions that cause a membranous tonsillopharyngitis include acute streptococcal pharyngitis, candidiasis, Vincent angina, infectious mononucleosis, and agranulocytosis (mucositis). Coinfection with group A streptococci is common, so identification of streptococcal infection does not exclude diphtheria.

Laboratory Diagnosis

Presumptive rapid diagnosis is obtained with methylene blue and Gram stain of pharyngeal smear. *C. diphtheriae* is seen as club-shaped, gram-positive, pleomorphic bacillus, arranged in a Chinese letter pattern. Diphtheroids that are normal commensals in the throat may cause a false-positive test. A four-fold or greater rise in serum antibody confirms the diagnosis. The laboratory must be alerted to the suspicion of diphtheria, as routine cultures are not likely to identify the organism. Prior antibiotic use may substantially reduce the yield.

Management

Antitoxin therapy must be initiated immediately after taking appropriate cultures. Endotracheal intubation may be difficult because of friable mucosa and carries a high risk of dislodgement of the membrane. Tracheostomy may be a better form of airway. Strict isolation should be maintained until therapy has been completed, and two cultures obtained 24 hours apart (after completion of antibiotic therapy) are negative. Diphtheria equine antitoxin neutralizes unbound toxin and prevents its binding to the cell membrane surface receptors. Antitoxin may provoke severe hypersensitivity reactions, and a test dose is recommended. Treatment with antitoxin at the onset of respiratory illness decreases mortality by ≥80%. It may also prevent spread to susceptible contacts. Antibiotics are adjuncts and not a substitute for antitoxin. Only penicillin and erythromycin are currently recommended. Carnitine supplementation has been studied for the treatment and prevention of diphtheria myocarditis, with some trials suggesting benefit. Temporary pacing is also of possible benefit.

Outcome and Prognosis

Overall, case-fatality rate is 5%–10%. Mortality rates are higher at extremes of age, in severe form of disease, in unimmunized patients, and if antitoxin administration is delayed. Mortality in diphtheritic myocarditis may be 60%–70%. Generally, patients who survive diphtheria make a complete recovery.

Prevention and Treatment for Contacts and Carriers

Patients who recover from diphtheria should begin or complete active immunization with diphtheria toxoid during convalescence. Contacts, regardless of immunization status, and carriers should receive oral erythromycin for 7–10 days or IM benzathine penicillin. Booster doses or primary series should be administered as needed. Carriers should be placed in strict isolation until two cultures taken 24 hours apart 2 weeks after cessation of therapy are negative. If cultures remain positive, a course of erythromycin should be repeated.

BOTULISM

Human botulism is caused by the neurotoxin produced by *Clostridium botulinum* and, rarely, by *C. baratii, C. butyricum, C. novyi*, and *C. bifermentans*. These organisms are ubiquitous, anaerobic, spore-forming, gram-positive bacilli. The organism and its spores are found in all types of soil.

Toxin Mechanism

Botulinum toxin blocks the release of acetylcholine from nerve endings. The toxin affects the neuromuscular junction, parasympathetic nerve endings, autonomic ganglia, and acetylcholine sympathetic nerve endings. The toxin enters the body through a wound or mucosal surface with rapid absorption from the gastrointestinal tract. The light chain of the toxin cleaves one of the soluble *N*-ethylmaleimide-sensitive factor attachment protein receptor (SNARE) proteins. Without it, presynaptic vesicles cannot bind and release acetylcholine into the synaptic cleft, causing paralysis. The nerve cell itself is uninjured by the toxin. Recovery may take months through sprouting of new presynaptic axons with the formation of a new neuromuscular junction.

Infant Botulism

Infant botulism occurs when infants ingest *C. botulinum* spores. Once in the digestive tract, the spores germinate and bacteria multiply. The infant digestive tract lacks the normal intestinal flora to compete with and prevent the growth of *C. botulinum*. Older children and adults routinely ingest *C. botulinum* spores without developing disease. Infant botulism averages 2.1 cases per 100,000 live births annually in the United States. Approximately 94% of patients are <6 months of age. The source of the spore exposure is not identified in the majority of cases, but reported exposures include soil, honey, and household dust.

Clinical Features

Most cases have an insidious onset. The most common symptom is constipation, often identified after presentation with more severe symptoms. No evidence of infection, such as fever, leukocytosis, or positive cultures is observed. The frequency of signs noted at admission are: weakness/floppiness (88%), poor feeding (79%), constipation (65%), lethargy or decreased activity (60%), poor cry, (18%), irritability (18%), respiratory difficulties (11%), and seizures (2%). The classic presentation is an infant with normal sensorium and cranial nerve palsies associated with symmetric, descending weakness. Fatigue can be elicited by repeated examination of the pupillary light reflex, with slowing of the pupil's constriction over 2–3 minutes. Deep tendon reflexes diminish as the paralysis worsens. Autonomic effects are responsible for the constipation and may occasionally cause hypertension. Affected infants have a characteristic appearance (**Fig. 71.1**). The peak incidence of infant botulism and SIDS overlap. Infant botulism as an etiology has been further established by the isolation of botulinum toxin in the stool of children who died of SIDS.

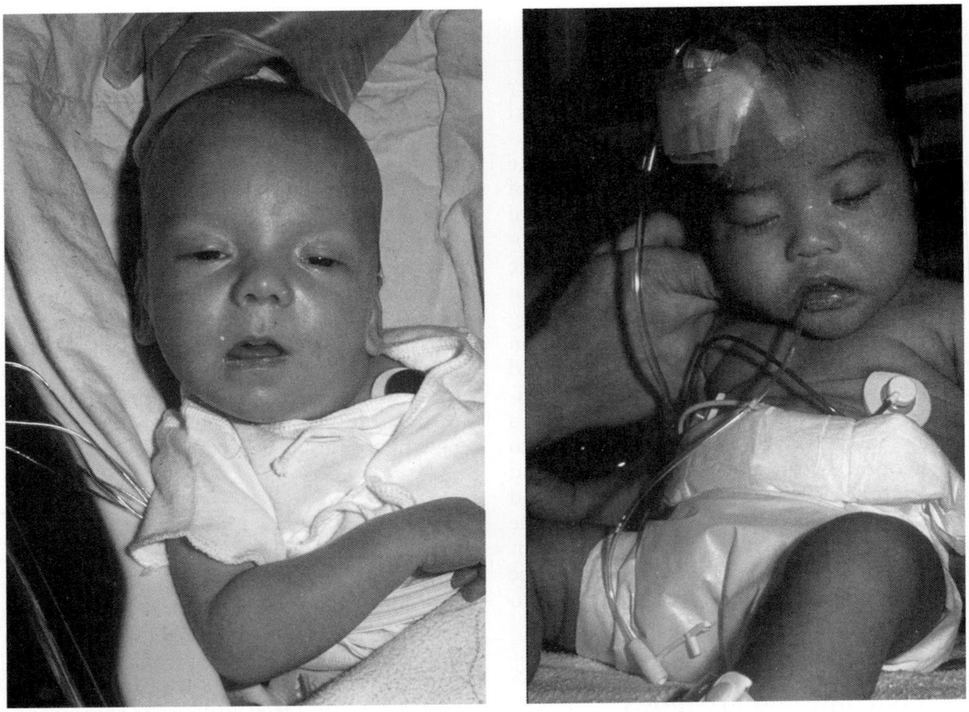

FIGURE 71.1. Photographs showing characteristic appearance of infants affected with botulism. Note the floppy appearance, poor head control, expressionless faces, and ptosis. (Left photo is courtesy of Johnson RO, Clay SA, Arnon SS. Diagnosis and management of infant botulism. *Am J Dis Child* 1979;133:586–93. Right photo is courtesy of Infant Botulism Treatment and Prevention Program, California Department of Public Health.)

Diagnosis and Differential Diagnosis

EMG may be equivocal or negative at presentation. A negative EMG should not prevent treatment if the clinical symptoms are compatible. In most patients, stool samples are eventually confirmatory. CSF studies are not always necessary but can evaluate for meningitis, encephalitis, Guillain–Barré syndrome, and poliomyelitis. A normal electroencephalogram is expected. Thyroid function testing rules out hypothyroidism. Spinal muscular atrophy can be differentiated by EMG findings, the presence of tongue fasciculation, and by genetic testing.

Treatment

Human botulism immune globulin should be given as soon as the diagnosis is strongly suspected. Treatment in the first 3 days decreases hospitalization costs and length of stay (2 vs. 5.7 weeks). Information on how to obtain botulism immune globulin can be obtained from the California Department of Health Services' Infant Botulism Treatment and Prevention Program at www.infantbotulism.org or calling 510-231-7600. The overall goal of supportive treatment is to prevent hospital-acquired infections, skin breakdown, malnutrition, and airway complications until recovery of the neuromuscular junction is complete. Antibiotics are not indicated. Aminoglycosides in particular should be avoided owing to the risk of worsening the weakness. Monitoring of vital capacity and negative inspiratory force can determine the need for mechanical ventilation. Most children can be managed without tracheotomy. Nutrition should be given enterally. Children hospitalized with access to intensive care have an excellent prognosis for full recovery.

Food-Borne Botulism

Unlike infant botulism, food-borne botulism is caused by the ingestion of food contaminated with preformed botulinum toxin. Large outbreaks are usually associated with restaurants, whereas small outbreaks or single cases are usually related to home-prepared foods, such as home-canned vegetables, fruits, and fish products. Abdominal pain, nausea, vomiting, and diarrhea occur shortly after ingestion of toxin. Constipation and neurologic symptoms occur 1–5 days after consumption of the toxin. The first symptoms to occur are dry mouth, diplopia, and dilated pupils. These bulbar palsies progress to ptosis, facial droop, depressed gag reflex, dysphagia, dysarthria, and dysphonia. The paralysis continues to descend in a proximal-to-distal pattern, with diaphragmatic involvement typically prior to that of the lower extremities. CNS and sensory function are not impaired. Antitoxin (equine cleaved immunoglobulin) is the most important treatment modality. The respiratory status should be closely monitored for deterioration, even after administration of the antitoxin. Paralysis associated with botulism can be lengthy, and tracheotomy may be considered.

TOXIC SHOCK SYNDROME

Toxic shock syndrome (TSS) is an acute toxin-mediated, multisystem, febrile illness caused by *S. aureus*, *S. pyogenes* (group A β-hemolytic *Streptococcus*), and other bacteria (rarely). It is characterized by high fever, hypotension, vomiting, and erythematous rash that can rapidly progress to multiorgan system failure with serious morbidity and mortality. The toxins that cause the disease have been labeled "superantigens" (SAgs) due to their ability to bypass usual steps in the antigen-mediated immune response in activating the immune system. They bind directly to the major histocompatibility complex (Class II) to trigger a massive expansion of T cells displaying T-cell receptor-specific β-chain variable regions. Superantigens can stimulate over 20% of all T cells (conventional antigens stimulate 1 in 10,000 T cells).

Staphylococcal Toxic Shock Syndrome

Staphylococcal TSS has two forms: menstrual and nonmenstrual. Nonmenstrual TSS is associated with *S. aureus* colonization of nasal packing or focal infections such as wound infection, soft-tissue infections, lymphadenitis, sinusitis, tracheitis, empyema, abscesses, infected burn, abortion, animal and insect bites, or osteomyelitis. Most patients are merely colonized with the offending bacteria, though some have evidence of bacteremia or deep tissue infection. The major toxins responsible are TSS toxin 1 (TSST-1) and enterotoxins A, B, and C. The superantigens stimulate the release of cytokines that cause capillary leak, massive vasodilatation with extravasations of fluids and serum, severe hypotension, and multiple-organ dysfunction.

Clinical Features

The onset of disease is abrupt, with high fever (≥39°C), headache, vomiting, diarrhea, and myalgia, rapidly progressing to hypotension and shock. A diffuse erythematous rash that resembles sunburn appears within 24 hours and may be associated with hyperemia of pharyngeal, conjunctival, and vaginal mucous membranes. Mental status changes, diarrhea, and diffuse abdominal pain can occur. Renal involvement manifests with pyuria, hematuria, and oliguria. Recovery from TSS starts within 7–10 days. It is associated with desquamation particularly of palms and soles. Hair and nail loss may occur after 1–2 months. Complications include acute renal failure, acute respiratory distress syndrome (ARDS), disseminated intravascular coagulation, electrolyte imbalance (hypocalcemia, hypophosphatemia, and hypomagnesemia), rhabdomyolysis, cardiomyopathy, and encephalopathy. Nonmenstrual TSS is more likely to cause renal and CNS complications.

Diagnosis and Differential Diagnosis

The CDC has established diagnostic criteria based on clinical and laboratory findings (**Table 71.1**). When the illness lacks one of the defining criteria, the term "probable TSS" is used.

Treatment

Volume replacement with appropriate crystalloids and colloids as well as vasoactive therapy may be required. Infected wounds and necrotizing skin lesions should be debrided immediately. All packings and foreign objects, including retained tampons, should be removed. Abscesses should be drained and irrigated. Cloxacillin, oxacillin, or nafcillin in combination with aminoglycosides are the first-line agents. Clindamycin and vancomycin can be used in patients who are allergic to penicillin or if methicillin-resistant *S. aureus* (MRSA) is suspected. Clindamycin can be used in combination with a β-lactamase-resistant antistaphylococcal antibiotic for the first few days to decrease the synthesis of TSST-1. Antibiotics do not shorten the duration of acute illness but are useful in decreasing the organism load, the risk of bacteremia, and the rate of relapse. Combination therapy with rifampicin or mupirocin may help eliminate carriage. Intravenous immunoglobulin (IVIG), 1 g/kg for 2 days, is suggested for severe cases, although its efficacy has not been confirmed. Plasma exchange reduces circulating toxins. Corticosteroids are not effective.

Streptococcal Toxic Shock Syndrome

Streptococcal TSS (STSS) is a severe, potentially fatal infection caused by invasive group A *Streptococcus* (GAS). GAS TSS most often accompanies invasive GAS infection rather than colonization. GAS is a gram-positive organism classified by the presence of surface proteins, primarily M and T antigens. Most of the strains responsible for STSS have M protein types 1 and 3. Extracellular products of GAS include the hemolysins; streptolysins O and S; and pyrogenic exotoxins A, B, C, and F. The streptococcal exotoxins possess superantigenic properties and trigger massive T-cell proliferation and cytokine release in the same way as staphylococcal superantigens. In children, STSS commonly occurs following varicella, during the use of nonsteroidal anti-inflammatories, or pharyngitis. Presentation is similar to that of staphylococcal TSS, although erythroderma is less common. Eight

TABLE 71.1

Centers for Disease Control and Prevention: Case Definition of Staphylococcal Toxic Shock Syndrome 2010

Clinical criteria: An illness with the following clinical manifestations:

1. Fever—temperature ≥ 38.9°C (102°F)
2. Rash—diffuse macular erythroderma
3. Desquamation—1–2 wk after onset of illness, particularly palms and soles
4. Hypotension—systolic blood pressure ≤ 90 mm Hg for adults or less than 5th percentile by age for children <16 years of age; orthostatic drop in diastolic blood pressure ≥15 mm Hg from lying to sitting, orthostatic syncope, or orthostatic dizziness
5. Multisystem involvement—three or more of the following:
   Gastrointestinal: vomiting or diarrhea at onset of illness
   Muscular: severe myalgia or creatine phosphokinase level at least twice the upper limit of normal
   Mucous membrane: vaginal, oropharyngeal, or conjunctival hyperemia
   Renal: blood urea nitrogen or creatinine at least twice the upper limit of normal or urinary sediment with pyuria (≥5 leukocytes per high-power field) in the absence of urinary tract infection
   Hepatic: total bilirubin, serum alanine aminotransferase (ALT), or serum aspartate aminotransferase (AST), at least twice the upper limit of normal
   Hematologic: platelets < 100,000/mm^3
   CNS: disorientation or alterations in consciousness without focal neurologic signs when fever and hypotension are absent

Laboratory criteria

Negative results on the following tests, if obtained:

1. Blood, throat, or CSF cultures (blood culture may be positive for *S. aureus*)
2. Rise in titer to Rocky Mountain spotted fever, leptospirosis, or measles

Case classification

Probable: A case which meets laboratory criteria and four of five clinical criteria

Confirmed: A case which meets laboratory criteria and all five clinical criteria described above, including desquamation, unless the patient dies before desquamation occurs

Adapted from Centers for Disease Control and Prevention. CSTE position statement 10-ID-14 (page last reviewed and updated on January 17, 2014).

percent of patients have clinical signs of soft-tissue infection, which may require surgical debridement, fasciotomy, or amputation. Endophthalmitis, myositis, perihepatitis, peritonitis, myocarditis, or overwhelming sepsis can be seen.

Diagnosis

CDC criteria also exist for streptococcal TSS (see full text edition or CDC website). Hemoglobinuria may be present and serum creatinine values are usually >2.5 times normal. Creatine kinase elevation may detect deep soft-tissue infections (necrotizing fasciitis). Mild leukocytosis may be seen with a striking left shift. Hypocalcemia, hypoalbuminemia, and elevated liver transaminases are common at admission. Bacteremia is common in STSS (60%). Cultures from sites of infection, including tissue taken at surgery, CSF, pleural fluid, and synovial fluid, yield organism in up to 95% of cases.

Treatment

The goals of management are removing the source of toxin (appropriate antibiotic therapy and surgical debridement of necrotic tissues), neutralization of toxin (IVIG therapy), and aggressive supportive therapy for shock (fluids and vasopressors) and multiorgan failure. An antibiotic combination of high-dose penicillin and clindamycin should be given when concomitant invasive GAS infection is suspected. IVIG did not improve outcome in STSS in children. The role of hyperbaric oxygen in STSS remains uncertain. Prognosis of STSS is worse than staphylococcal TSS. Mortality from STSS is 5%–10% in children and 30%–70% in adults.

CHAPTER 72 OPPORTUNISTIC INFECTIONS

SUSHIL K. KABRA AND MATTHEW B. LAURENS

DEFECTS IN THE IMMUNE SYSTEM AND OPPORTUNISTIC PATHOGENS

Defects in the immune system may occur due to primary or secondary immune deficiency disorders. Other causes include irradiation, removal of thymus, and administration of biologic agents. Various immune defects and risk for development of infections are given in **Table 72.1**.

OPPORTUNISTIC INFECTIONS DUE TO VIRUSES

Cytomegalovirus Infection

Cytomegalovirus (CMV) is in the herpes virus group. It is a common infection but can have devastating effects in the immunocompromised. The organism can be transmitted congenitally or by breast milk, saliva, urine, and blood transfusion. Immunosuppressed individuals who acquire the virus are at risk for severe CMV disease, and "reactivation" pneumonia is also possible in those previously infected. CMV as an opportunistic infection can affect all organ systems.

CMV pulmonary involvement is a major cause of interstitial pneumonia in children with congenital immunodeficiency, AIDS, organ or hematopoietic stem-cell transplant (HSCT), malignancy, or on chemotherapy. *CMV pneumonitis* usually occurs 1–3 months following transplantation and begins with symptoms of fever, a dry, nonproductive cough, and progressive dyspnea that may require ventilatory support. Coinfection occurs with other pathogens, especially gram-negative enteric bacteria, fungal pathogens in transplant recipients, and *P. jiroveci* in patients with AIDS.

Mononucleosis syndrome may occur in immunocompetent as well as immunosuppressed patients. The clinical course is subacute and includes fever, malaise, headache, myalgia, abdominal pain, and loose stools. There may be enlargement of liver, spleen, and peripheral lymph nodes. Investigations may show peripheral lymphocytosis with atypical lymphocytes and mildly elevated liver enzymes.

CMV retinitis has emerged as a common manifestation of CMV disease in patients with severe immunosuppression, especially in HSCT recipients and patients with AIDS. CMV produces characteristic white perivascular infiltrates and hemorrhage, with a necrotic, rapidly progressive retinitis. At an advanced stage, it can cause blurred vision, decreased visual acuity, visual field defects, and blindness. CMV may also produce conjunctivitis, corneal epithelial keratitis, and disk neovascularization.

CMV hepatitis manifests as fever, thrombocytopenia, and lymphopenia or lymphocytosis with mild hepatomegaly. Other hepatic manifestations include vanishing bile duct syndrome, cholangitis, and chronic rejection (in liver transplant recipients). Gastrointestinal manifestations include esophagitis, gastritis, gastroenteritis, pyloric and small bowel obstruction, duodenitis, colitis, proctitis, pancreatitis, hemorrhage, and acalculous cholecystitis.

CMV myocarditis has been documented in children who have undergone renal and heart transplant. These patients may manifest with congestive cardiac failure, cardiomegaly, ST-segment and/or T-wave changes, and poor left ventricular ejection fraction. Diagnosis involves documenting CMV inclusion bodies on biopsy and CMV DNA in tissue.

Diagnosis

CMV is diagnosed by serology, polymerase chain reaction (PCR), antigenemia, and viral culture. For CNS infections, PCR of cerebrospinal fluid (CSF) is the most sensitive diagnostic method.

Management

In the immunocompetent host, treatment is indicated only in severe or life-threatening disease. Among the immunocompromised, 85% of patients with AIDS and CMV retinitis improve or show stabilization of lesions after induction therapy with ganciclovir, valganciclovir, foscarnet, or cidofovir. Combination therapy with ganciclovir and foscarnet is associated with longer time to recurrence, compared with monotherapy. For solid organ transplant recipients, most regimens include prophylaxis for CMV disease with intravenous immune globulin (IVIG) or CMV-specific IVIG, antiviral agents, or some combination before and during the period of highest risk. Preemptive therapy is an alternative in allogeneic HSCT recipients, using regular lab screening with antigenemia or PCR. Autologous and stem-cell HSCT recipients have lower risk of CMV disease and might not warrant prophylaxis.

TABLE 72.1

Conditions Predisposing an Individual to Opportunistic Infections

■ MAJOR DEFECTS IN IMMUNE SYSTEM	■ CLINICAL CONDITIONS	■ INFECTIONS/CLINICAL MANIFESTATIONS
B-cell defects (humoral deficiencies)	Agammaglobulinemia, hypogammaglobulinemia, selective IgA deficiency, IgG subclass deficiencies, common variable immune deficiency, hyper-IgM syndrome	Infections with *S. aureus*; encapsulated organisms, such as *S. pneumoniae, H. influenzae*; and gram-negative organisms, such as *Pseudomonas* species Arthritis due to echoviruses, coxsackieviruses, adenoviruses, and *U. urealyticum* Infections due to *P. jiroveci* pneumonitis, and *Cryptosporidium*
T-cell defects (cell-mediated immunity)	Thymic dysplasia (DiGeorge syndrome), defective T-cell receptor, defective cytokine production, T-cell activation defects, CD8 lymphocytopenia	Disseminated viral infections due to herpes simplex, varicella zoster, and CMV Progressive pneumonia caused by parainfluenza, respiratory syncytial virus, cytomegalovirus, varicella, and *P. jiroveci* Superficial and systemic fungal infections and parasitic infections. Severe mucocutaneous candidiasis; disseminated BCG disease after BCG vaccination
Combined B- and T-cell defects	Severe combined immunodeficiency, Omenn syndrome, Wiskott–Aldrich syndrome, ataxia telangiectasia, hyper-IgE syndrome	Infections caused by bacteria, fungi, or viruses Chronic diarrhea, mucocutaneous or systemic candidiasis, *P. jiroveci* pneumonitis, and CMV early in life Infections with *S. pneumoniae* or *H. influenzae* type b, *P. jiroveci* Late-onset recurrent sinopulmonary infections from bacteria and respiratory viruses Recurrent episodes of *S. aureus* abscesses of the skin, lungs, and musculoskeletal system
Abnormalities in phagocytic system	Inadequate numbers (congenital or acquired), Chronic granulomatous disease, leukocyte adhesion deficiency, Chédiak-Higashi syndrome	Recurrent pyogenic and fungal infections due to *Pseudomonas, S. marcescens*, and *S. aureus*, and fungi such as *Aspergillus* and *Candida* present as cellulitis, perirectal abscesses, or stomatitis Pulmonary infection, suppurative adenitis, subcutaneous abscess, liver abscess, osteomyelitis, and sepsis due to fungi or bacteria (*Staphylococcus*) Gastric outlet obstruction, urinary tract obstruction, and enteritis or colitis History of delayed cord separation and recurrent infections of the skin, oral mucosa, and genital tract, Predisposed to development of ecthyma gangrenosum and pyoderma gangrenosum
Disorders of the complement system	Disorders involving any one of the complement components, asplenia, splenic dysfunction due to hemoglobinopathies, splenectomy	Infections due to *Salmonella* spp. and encapsulated bacteria including *S. pneumoniae* and *H. influenzae*. These agents can cause sepsis, pneumonia, meningitis, and osteomyelitis
Infections occurring with acquired immunodeficiencies	HIV and other virus infections, cancer chemotherapy, immunosuppressive therapy after organ transplant, diabetes mellitus, sickle cell disease, severe malnutrition	Similar to cell-mediated immune deficiency Neutropenic patients: infections due to gram-positive cocci and gram-negative organisms, such as *P. aeruginosa, E. coli*, and *Klebsiella* Fungal infections due to *Candida* and *Aspergillus* in prolonged neutropenia

CMV, cytomegalovirus; BCG, Bacille Calmette–Guérin.

For those who acquire CMV pneumonia post-transplant, combined therapy with IV ganciclovir and IVIG or CMV-IVIG is indicated. In recipients of renal transplant, prophylactic antiviral therapy is recommended when the donor or recipient is seropositive and antilymphocyte treatment is part of the immunosuppressive regimen and for seronegative recipients of grafts from seropositive donors.

Varicella Zoster Virus Infection

Varicella zoster virus (VZV) is a DNA virus that typically causes benign infections of the skin and mucous membranes. It may cause both varicella and zoster in the normal host. In immunocompromised patients, VZV can lead to visceral dissemination and pneumonia.

Varicella pneumonia is a serious manifestation that can present with fever, cough, dyspnea, chest pain, cyanosis, and hemoptysis. The chest X-ray reveals a diffuse nodular or miliary pattern. Varicella pneumonia may be complicated by acute respiratory distress syndrome, rhabdomyolysis, acute hepatitis, and disseminated intravascular coagulation.

CNS complications of VZV include cerebellar ataxia and encephalitis. Patients with varicella may develop ischemic strokes and radiologic and histopathologic evidence of CNS vasculitis. Ocular manifestations include conjunctivitis, keratitis, iridocyclitis, panuveitis, and acute retinal necrosis. Liver and heart involvement are uncommon.

Diagnosis

Varicella can be diagnosed on the basis of physical findings, vesicle scrapings, serology, or PCR. The direct fluorescent antibody test is rapid and can differentiate HSV from VZV. The *Tzanck smear* of vesicle scrapings will show multinucleated giant cells but is not specific for VZV.

Management

Management of VZV Exposure. Susceptible persons exposed to varicella should be given immune globulin (either varicella zoster immune globulin [VZIG] or IVIG) as soon as possible. Exposure to varicella merits airborne and contact precautions from 8 until 21 days after the onset of rash in the index case, and for 28 days after exposure to the index case in those treated with VZIG or IVIG.

Management of VZV Disease. Patients at risk for moderate-to-severe varicella should be considered candidates for oral therapy with acyclovir or valacyclovir. Those at increased risk include people >12 years of age, those with chronic cutaneous or pulmonary disorders, those receiving long-term salicylate therapy, and those receiving short, intermittent, or aerosolized courses of corticosteroids. Salicylates should be avoided in children with varicella, as they increase the risk of Reye syndrome. Immunocompromised patients should receive IV acyclovir. Oral, high-dose acyclovir can be considered in patients who are mildly immunosuppressed and at lower risk for developing severe varicella. Experience with efficacy of famciclovir and valacyclovir in children is limited.

Management of Herpes Zoster Disease. In immunocompromised patients, IV acyclovir is the therapy of choice for acute herpes zoster. Treatment should be initiated as soon as vesicles are recognized to prevent progression to disseminated disease.

Herpes Virus Type 6

Human herpes virus 6 (HHV-6) is a DNA virus that is the etiologic agent for most cases of roseola. The virus remains latent in the body after primary infection and reactivates in immunocompromised patients. In immunocompetent children, HHV-6 causes exanthem subitum, febrile episodes without skin rash, and non-EBV and non-CMV infectious mononucleosis. The clinical features in immunocompromised children may result in fever, skin rash, pneumonia, bone marrow suppression, encephalitis, and rejection.

Diagnosis

Testing for HHV-6 includes serology, culture, immunohistochemistry, and nucleic acid assays. Serology testing is usually reserved for the immunocompetent. Plasma PCR and reverse transcriptase (RT) PCR detect circulating virus and are thought to be indicative of active infection. However, the best method for detection of active HHV-6 is quantitative RT-PCR analysis of body secretions.

Management

Treatment is not indicated in healthy children. Antiviral therapies have not been evaluated in randomized clinical trials in immunocompromised children. Drugs used include ganciclovir, cidofovir, and foscarnet. Patients may also benefit from a reduction in immunosuppression. Adoptive T-cell immunotherapy is currently being explored.

FUNGAL INFECTIONS

Candidiasis

Candida spp. are recognized as a leading contributor to morbidity and mortality in patients with oncohematologic malignancies, HIV infection, primary immunodeficiencies, prolonged neutropenia, diabetes, corticosteroid administration, broad-spectrum antibiotic treatment, IV hyperalimentation, and presence of central venous lines.

Disseminated candidiasis may affect lungs, kidneys, liver, spleen, and brain. The clinical manifestations are often similar to sepsis caused by other organisms. Presence of endophthalmitis and maculopapular rash suggest the diagnosis. The skin lesions consist of generalized rashes or discrete, firm papules with a nodular center often surrounded by an erythematous halo. Candidiasis may involve bones, joints, heart, and CNS.

Oral candidiasis can be an early sign of illness. Esophageal candidiasis may present with concurrent oropharyngeal candidiasis, odynophagia, retrosternal pain, fever, nausea/vomiting, drooling, dehydration, hoarseness, and upper gastrointestinal bleeding. *Candida* infection may also manifest as epiglottitis. The airway, from pharynx to bronchi, may be involved. A child may present with hoarseness of voice, low-grade fever, tachypnea, or nonspecific physical examination findings. Candida peritonitis may occur secondary to bowel perforation, peritoneal dialysis, or intestinal surgery. Pulmonary infection may be complicated by development of abscess and empyema. Renal involvement can include renal microabscesses, papillary necrosis, calyceal distortion, and obstruction due to fungal ball or perinephric abscesses.

Diagnosis

Mucocutaneous candidiasis is diagnosed clinically and confirmed with demonstration of budding yeast from scrapings of skin or mucosal lesions. Diagnosis of invasive infection can be made by demonstration of fungal elements beyond stratum corneum in skin biopsy. Endoscopy is useful for diagnosis of esophageal candidiasis. The addition of potassium hydroxide to specimens may help to identify yeast and pseudohyphae. For retinal infections, ophthalmologic examination identifies characteristic findings. In contrast-enhanced computed tomography (CT), fungal microabscesses usually appear as multiple, round, discrete areas of low attenuation but may appear late in disease. In situ hybridization techniques can diagnose *Candida* spp. in a matter of hours. Serologic techniques are being developed. The (1,3) β-D-glucan assay shows high sensitivity and specificity.

Management

Oropharyngeal candidiasis is treated with topical clotrimazole, nystatin, or amphotericin B suspensions or by systemic therapy with fluconazole or other azoles. Esophageal disease should be treated by systemic therapy for 2–3 weeks. For neonatal invasive candidiasis, amphotericin B is the drug of choice, and combination therapy with flucytosine for those with CNS disease. For immunocompromised patients with suspected systemic candidemia, first-line therapies include lipid formulation amphotericin B, caspofungin, or voriconazole. For yeast specimens identified as *C. albicans* and for isolates that are susceptible, fluconazole therapy should be used. In addition to treatment, infected vascular lines and hardware should be removed.

Pneumocystis jiroveci

P. jiroveci (*P. carinii*) is a eukaryotic microorganism of uncertain taxonomy. Patients with AIDS typically have a long duration of symptoms and an insidious presentation. Physical findings may reveal tachypnea, nasal flaring, retractions, and cyanosis. High-grade fever generally precedes the nonproductive cough, tachypnea, and severe dyspnea. Disease often occurs after discontinuance or a reduction in the dose of corticosteroid therapy. Extrapulmonary pneumocystosis represents <1% of infections with *P. jiroveci*. Several organs may be involved, and the most common sites are lymph nodes, spleen, liver, and bone marrow. Mortality is very high with disseminated disease.

Diagnosis

Diagnosis is by identification of organisms from lung tissue or sputum. PCR testing increases diagnostic yield. A positive PCR in immunocompetent patients may indicate colonization.

Management

First-line treatment is IV trimethoprim-sulfamethoxazole (TMP-SMZ). Second-line treatments include IV pentamidine, oral dapsone with oral or IV TMP-SMZ, or oral atovaquone. For patients with moderate-to-severe disease, early corticosteroid administration is also indicated. Prophylaxis with TMP-SMZ or second-line therapies should be used, including dapsone, dapsone and pyrimethamine, atovaquone, or aerosolized pentamidine.

Invasive Aspergillosis

Aspergillus is a ubiquitous fungal organism, including the hospital environment. Aspergillosis of the lung is often accompanied by invasion of the nose and paranasal sinuses in susceptible hosts. Invasiveness depends on the genetic and immune status of the host and on the extent and duration of exposure to spores. Invasive pulmonary aspergillosis manifests as necrotizing bronchopneumonia or hemorrhagic infarction, although single or multiple abscesses, granulomata, or lobar infiltrates are occasionally present. Patients may present with fever, dyspnea, nonproductive cough, mild hemoptysis, and pleuritic chest pain. Coexisting sinusitis is common. Invasive sinusitis can occur with profound neutropenia and lead to direct extension to the orbit and anterior cranial fossa, widespread dissemination, and a high mortality rate. In children with chronic granulomatous disease, direct extension from the lungs to the chest wall may occur. Otomycosis may occur in immunosuppressed children. Occasionally, otitis externa and mastoiditis may occur in malnourished children. Cutaneous lesions progress from erythematous or violaceous papules or plaques through a hemorrhagic bullous stage to a purpuric ulcer with central necrosis and eschar formation, called *ecthyma gangrenosum*. Endophthalmitis may be an important finding. CNS aspergillosis is rare but has a very high fatality rate. *Aspergillus* endocarditis may occur following open-heart surgery or as part of disseminated disease. Abscesses may develop in the liver, thyroid, testis, spleen, kidney, and adrenal glands.

Diagnosis

Chest X-ray findings are nonspecific. CT of the chest may show a characteristic halo sign or air-crescent sign, though this is not diagnostic. Bronchoalveolar lavage (BAL), transthoracic percutaneous needle aspiration, or video-assisted thoracoscopic biopsy may be helpful. The galactomannan assay, commonly used in adults, is difficult to interpret in children. Identification from tissue culture renders a definitive diagnosis. If allergic aspergillosis is suspected clinically, results of *Aspergillus*-specific IgE serology, eosinophilia, and a positive skin test can provide evidence for the diagnosis.

Management

Voriconazole is first-line treatment for invasive aspergillosis. Children metabolize voriconazole at greater rates. Trough concentrations should be monitored. Amphotericin B or caspofungin are second-line therapy. Eye infection requires intraocular amphotericin B and vitrectomy.

Mucormycosis

Mucormycosis is an acute and often fatal infection caused by fungus. Infections typically arise in patients with substantial immunosuppression. Disease may involve lungs, brain, sinuses, kidneys, and skin. Pulmonary involvement may present with persistent fever, chest pain, hemoptysis, and weight loss. Cavitation may occur. Sudden death may occur due to massive pulmonary hemorrhage, mediastinitis, or airway obstruction. *Rhinocerebral mucormycosis* is uncommon but often fatal. Sinusitis may occur in children with an underlying disease (e.g., malignancy) and may progress to involve orbits and brain. Primary cutaneous mucormycosis is an uncommon, deep, and aggressive fungal infection that occurs mainly in immunosuppressed or diabetic patients. Skin involvement may begin as a vascular, hemorrhagic, erythematous plaque and rapidly progress to a dark, necrotic, painful ulcer with erythematous border.

Diagnosis

Diagnosis of zygomycosis is achieved through aggressive pursuit of tissue culture. While wet mounts of sputum, sinus secretions, or BAL fluid are often negative, positivity denotes invasive zygomycosis that should be treated. Cultures of blood or urine are rarely positive. Tissue samples yield higher results. PCR assays are beginning to be used.

Management

Treatment includes reduction of immunosuppression combined with antifungal therapy and surgical debridement. Hyperglycemia and metabolic acidosis may predispose and should be corrected. Outcome is related to neutrophil recovery; antifungal therapy may be ineffective in patients with persistent neutropenia. Granulocyte colony-stimulating factor and granulocyte-macrophage colony-stimulating factor should be considered. Lipid formulation of amphotericin B is first-line therapy, usually at high doses. An option in refractory cases is the concomitant use of an echinocandin. Hyperbaric oxygen therapy can be considered where available. Surgical debridement results in increased survival compared with patients treated medically.

Cryptococcosis

Cryptococcus neoformans is a yeast-like encapsulated fungus. Disease usually presents as subacute or chronic meningitis but liver, spleen, skin, lymph node, eye, bones, adrenals, and ears may also be involved. Pulmonary illness is rare in children. Cases of cryptococcosis that presents as acute abdomen or mimic pulmonary metastasis in Wilms tumor have been reported.

Diagnosis

Diagnosis is based on demonstration of organisms in body fluids using India ink stain. Serologic tests exist. Chest X-ray findings of diffuse infiltrations with hilar adenopathy may be seen. The organism is slow-growing in culture, requiring a week to proliferate.

Management

Patients who are immunosuppressed should be evaluated for disseminated disease as well as treated with a combination of amphotericin B and flucytosine. A regimen of high-dose fluconazole and flucytosine may also be considered.

Histoplasmosis

Histoplasmosis is a systemic disease caused by the dimorphic fungus *Histoplasma capsulatum*, which exists as a soil saprophyte. Manifestations of disseminated histoplasmosis include fever, cough, respiratory difficulty, abdominal pain, weight loss, and diarrhea. Liver, spleen, and lymph nodes may be enlarged. Skin may show mucocutaneous lesions, maculopapular rash, papules, nodules, pustules, and ulcerative lesions. Children may present with meningitis or encephalitis and focal brain lesions.

Diagnosis

Diagnosis is via culture, fungal stain, antigen detection, and serologic tests for antibodies. Rapid antigen testing is sensitive for disseminated disease. Fungal silver or Wright stain can be used on peripheral blood or tissue culture.

Management

For complicated disease or in immunocompromised children, amphotericin B is the standard therapy, followed by itraconazole for long-term suppressive therapy. Second-line therapies include voriconazole and posaconazole. For isolated pericarditis, drainage of pericardial fluid and nonsteroidal anti-inflammatory drugs are the mainstays of therapy.

MYCOBACTERIAL INFECTIONS

Nontuberculous Mycobacteria

Lymphadenitis is the most common manifestation of infection due to nontuberculous mycobacteria. Other findings include prolonged fever, weight loss, lymphadenopathy, hepatosplenomegaly, diarrhea, anemia, and leucopenia. Diagnosis is established by cultures from body fluids and PCR testing. If surgical excision is not possible or incomplete, therapy with clarithromycin or azithromycin should be considered. For pulmonary disease due to *M. avium* complex, treatment includes clarithromycin and ethambutol, with rifabutin added for severe disease. Alternative therapies include azithromycin, ciprofloxacin, levofloxacin, or amikacin.

Mycobacterium tuberculosis

Children with disseminated TB may have fever, respiratory difficulty, lymphadenopathy, hepatosplenomegaly, and skin lesions. The diagnosis of TB in an immunocompromised patient requires a heightened suspicion and diagnostic modalities beyond the purified protein derivative (PPD) skin test. Evaluation for pulmonary TB should include a chest X-ray or CT scan. An early-morning gastric aspirate may be useful. AFB smear and culture of suspected sterile body sites and PCR testing can also be performed.

Management

Latent TB infection is managed with 6–9 months of isoniazid. In cases with isoniazid resistance, rifampin may be given once daily for 6 months. In immunosuppressed children, an initial intensive phase with isoniazid, rifampin, pyrazinamide, and ethambutol for 8 weeks is followed by a daily regimen of isoniazid plus rifampin or an intermittent regimen of isoniazid and rifampin thrice weekly for 9–12 months. Treatment of TB should be based on drug resistance in the index case, in the local geographic area, or in the country of origin for imported cases.

CHAPTER 73 ■ PRINCIPLES OF GASTROINTESTINAL PHYSIOLOGY, NUTRITION, AND METABOLISM

PATRICK O'NEAL MAYNORD AND Z. LEAH HARRIS

GI TRACT ANATOMY AND PHYSIOLOGY

The Stomach

Parietal cells secrete gastric acid via a hydrogen–potassium pump that transports protons into the gastric lumen and potassium into the cell. Muscarinic (M_3), type B cholecystokinin (CCKb), and histamine (H_2) receptors on the parietal cell activate the proton pump when stimulated by acetylcholine, gastrin, and histamine. Protein is the major stimulant for gastrin release. Postprandial acid hypersecretion is prevented by somatostatin. When the stomach pH falls below 3, somatostatin release suppresses gastrin and histamine and inhibits acid secretion from parietal cells. Pepsinogen, secreted by chief cells, in the presence of acid is cleaved into pepsin, a protease that begins protein digestion. Mucus production by mucous cells helps prevent acid injury. Stimuli for mucus production include acetylcholine and prostaglandins. Mucus cannot be broken down by gastric acid but is damaged by bile salts, ethanol, and nonsteroidal anti-inflammatory drugs. H^+ cannot pass through the apical membrane of the mucosa but can diffuse between cell junctions to reach the basolateral surface. Parietal cells possess a bicarbonate/chloride anti-porter that secretes bicarbonate to the basolateral membrane for every proton transferred out of the cell. This anti-porter is activated by prostaglandins. H_2 blockers (ranitidine) or proton pump inhibitors (omeprazole) are used to limit gastric acid secretion and promote mucosal healing.

Parietal cells secrete intrinsic factor (IF), an essential cofactor in absorption of vitamin B_{12}. In addition, gastric acid promotes Ca^{2+} and Fe^{2+} absorption in the duodenum. The stomach also helps regulate osmolarity; it can handle extremely hypotonic and hypertonic fluids and solids and deliver an isosmotic chyme to the duodenum. During critical illness, transpyloric feeds may be used when gastric motility is decreased. The loss of osmoregulation during transpyloric feeds particularly during advancement of caloric density can lead to malabsorption, diarrhea, and electrolyte derangements.

The Small Intestine

The small intestine breaks down chyme into micronutrients for absorption. In the duodenum, acidic chyme mixes with pancreatic chymotrypsin and trypsinogen, which are activated by enterokinase to the proteolytic enzymes trypsin and chymotrypsin to digest proteins into peptides. Bile salts, secreted into the duodenum, emulsify fats, and pancreatic lipases initiate triglyceride breakdown to monoglycerides and free fatty acids (FAs). Pancreatic amylase breaks down starch into maltose, dextrins, and maltotriose. Pancreatic secretions are rich in bicarbonate and buffer acidic chyme. The small intestine surface area contact with lumen substrate is maximized, and 95% of nutrients are absorbed in the small intestine. Enterocytes absorb macronutrients (carbohydrate, fat, and protein). Goblet cells secrete mucins and trefoil factors. Mucins form the glycocalyx mucous barrier that limits bacterial contact with the epithelium. Trefoil stimulates epithelial regrowth and repair. Enteroendocrine cell lines secrete peptides and hormones that act on neighboring cells (paracrine function), local neural networks (neuronal function), or the lamina propria (endocrine function). The epithelium turns over every 4–5 days. Paneth cells secrete antimicrobial peptides and trophic factors for stem cell maintenance and growth. Intestinal barrier dysfunction occurs in intestinal hypersensitivity, irritable bowel syndrome, and permeability associated with multiple organ dysfunction syndrome. The secretion and absorption of electrolytes and fluids are essential functions of the small intestine. The adult GI tract secretes 8–10 L of fluid per day combined with 1.5–2 L of oral input, but the net flow across the ileocecal junction is only 2 L/d. The proximal duodenum absorbs water by osmosis, but the distal jejunum and colon absorb water against an osmotic gradient. Cl^-/HCO_3^- exchangers facilitate secretion of HCO_3^- into the lumen while Cl^- moves into the enterocyte. Duodenal bicarbonate secretion regulates the pH of chyme entering from the stomach.

The Large Intestine

The colon recovers electrolytes, water, and energy. In the adult, 10 L a day of fluid enter the small intestine, it absorbs 7.5 L, and 1.5 L are absorbed in the colon. The epithelial layer of the colon is a single sheet of predominately (95%) columnar and goblets cells; the remaining 5% are enterochromaffin cells. Columnar cells secrete and absorb liquids and electrolytes. Goblet cells secrete mucus to provide lubrication to feces. Water and ion transport is similar to the small intestine. Basolateral Na^+/K^+ ATPase pumps establish low intracellular sodium content. Apical Na^+/H^+ exchange pumps bring sodium into the cell and H^+ out. Cl^-/HCO_3^- exchangers bring Cl^- in and secrete HCO_3^-. Water is absorbed due to net movement of NaCl by the transcellular or paracellular pathways. Aldosterone increases the absorption in the proximal intestine (Na^+H^+) and the distal colon (epithelial Na^+ channel). The paracellular pathway allows for the efflux of water in response to shifts in the osmolarity. Bacterial colonization occurs during the birth process. The bacterial content has been implicated in inflammatory bowel disease, obesity, and development of the innate immune system. In the small intestine, aerobic bacteria transition to anaerobes in the large intestine occurs. The colonic bacteria ferment starch, unabsorbed sugars, and cellulosic and noncellulosic polysaccharides into short-chain fatty acids (SCFAs) and gases. Absorbed SCFAs are used as an energy source by enterocytes and are transported into peripheral tissue. Microbes are also responsible for the production of vitamin K as evident at birth when the GI tract is sterile.

The Physiology of Absorption

Carbohydrates account for >50% of calories in the Western diet. Oligo- and polysaccharides are the majority of these starches and are not appreciably absorbed by the small intestine. Starch is first cleaved by α-amylase and hydrolyzed into maltose and maltotriose and amylopectin into dextrins, which interact with the disaccharidases of enterocytes. Factors that affect carbohydrate absorption include gastric emptying, small intestine contact time, pancreatic amylase function, and thickness and contents. In general, slowed motility facilitates nutrient absorption. Protein absorption occurs in the luminal, brush border, and cytoplasmic phases. The luminal phase begins in the stomach with acidic degradation and pepsin digestion that release free amino acids. In the upper jejunum and the proximal ileum, protein is absorbed via the brush border. Na^+/amino acid cotransport occurs via the gradient developed by Na^+K^+ ATPase pump. Peptide carriers transport dipeptides and tripeptides into enterocytes where tripeptidases and dipeptidases hydrolyze them into amino acids. The basolateral membrane also has transporters that move amino acids into the lamina propria, where they are absorbed for transport to the portal vein. The gut accounts for 12% of energy used but only 5% of total body mass. Luminal glutamine, glutamate, and aspartate are major enterocyte fuel sources in addition to glucose. Lysine and threonine are important in neonates during rapid growth. The function of glutamine as a fuel source and precursor for nucleotides forms the basis for its use in immunonutrition. Ingested fat consists of triglycerides (90%), phospholipids, cholesterol, and FAs. In addition to energy, fat provides the essential n-6 and n-3 series (linoleic and α-linolenic acid [ALA]) FAs essential for gray matter health and retinal development. Triglyceride digestion is initiated in the stomach by gastric lipase (HGL). Emulsification takes place in the stomach without bile salts. As fat particles enter the duodenum, pancreatic colipase-dependent triglyceride lipase (PTL) and bile salts begin hydrolysis and emulsification of fat, respectively. The acidic contents trigger the release of secretin, which stimulates the pancreas to secrete bicarbonate and water. The increased pH aids lipase function and draws FAs to the surface of the lipid droplet. The key enzyme in phospholipid breakdown, pancreatic phospholipase A2 (PLA2), hydrolyzes phospholipids. Lipases are activated by colipase, and bile salt lipases hydrolyze the lipids into FAs, monoglycerides, cholesterol, and lysophospholipids. Large multilamellar droplets are emulsified further by bile salts to the mixed micelle. Mixed micelles and unilamellar vesicles can be absorbed from the intestinal lumen. FA absorption occurs via a carrier-mediated transport. Monoglyceride absorption occurs via passive diffusion. Absorption begins in the distal duodenum and is finished in the distal jejunum. Bile salts are reabsorbed in the terminal ileum and undergo enterohepatic circulation. After penetration through the membrane, long-chain FAs are formed into chylomicrons for transport to the lymphatic system where, as medium-chain FAs, they are transported into the liver via the portal vein.

Neural Control of the GI Tract

The enteric nervous system (ENS) integrates with local reflexes triggered by muscle, chemosensory, and mucosal level information. The major plexuses of the ENS are the myenteric plexus regulating muscle activity and the submucosal plexus regulating mucosal function. The prevertebral sympathetic ganglia integrate the peripheral reflex pathways and preganglionic sympathetic fibers from the spinal cord. Brain centers supply sympathetic and parasympathetic outflow to the gut via the autonomic nervous system, and the gut sends sympathetic and parasympathetic outflow to the central nervous system. Neural control of the stomach involves vagal reflexes responsible for passive relaxation (allows food bolus to enter) and regulation of lower esophageal sphincter tone (prevents reflux). In the stomach and small and large intestine, pacemaker activity within the muscle layers controls rhythmic, phasic contractions. Peristalsis involves rapid orthograde movement of contents toward the anus. The migrating myoelectric complex (MMC) is a slow orthograde propulsive movement that occurs every 90 minutes in the fasted state and prevents bacterial overgrowth in the small intestine by sweeping contents into the colon. Retropulsion is the expulsion of noxious substances from the small intestine back into the stomach followed by vomiting. Nerve fibers from sympathetic nervous system innervate gut lymphoid tissue and control inflammatory and anti-inflammatory functions. In response to stimuli (i.e., shock or injury), intestinal macrophages are activated and cytokines released. Inflammatory signals stimulate vagal afferents, which feed into brain nuclei and return efferent signals back to the gut via the vagus, releasing acetylcholine, which inhibits macrophage activity and cytokine release. Anti-inflammatory cytokines IL-10 and transforming growth factor-10 are activated by this cholinergic pathway. These mechanisms maintain the beneficial interaction between normal bacterial flora, the gut epithelium, and its immune function.

GI Perfusion

Arterial blood is supplied by the superior mesenteric, celiac, and inferior mesenteric arteries. The celiac and superior mesenteric arteries feed the small intestine and liver, the body's most metabolically active organs. Oxygen diffusion is flow rated, and as flow increases, more oxygen is delivered to the distal villi. During fasting, 20%–25% of total cardiac output goes to the hepatosplanchnic circulation. Following a meal, this percentage doubles. Splanchnic blood flow is regulated locally by chemical mediators, ENS responses, and sympathetic nervous system responses and globally by circulating vasoactive substances, systemic perfusion, and systemic sympathetic responses. Alpha agonists (predominantly norepinephrine), angiotensin II, and endothelin-1 (ET-1) produce vasoconstriction in the gut. The predominant local vasoconstrictor during shock is ET-1. Endothelial cells of the splanchnic vasculature contain endothelin-converting enzyme and produce ET-1, which functions as a paracrine hormone. ET-1_A receptor (vascular smooth muscle in the muscularis, submucosa, and mucosa) stimulation leads to vasoconstriction in shock from hypovolemia. During low-flow states, vasoconstriction is mediated by the renin–angiotensin system, endothelin system, sympathetic nervous system, and vasopressin. The main local vasodilators are prostacyclin (PGI_2), endothelial-derived hyperpolarizing factor, and nitrous oxide (NO). Prostaglandins are locally produced and vasodilate during low-flow states and after mucosal injury. Low-level NO production becomes unregulated during circulatory shock and results in shunting of blood through the vascular bed without adequate time for oxygen extraction. Systemic catecholamines induce local vasodilation via β_2 and dopamine receptors. During feeding, splanchnic blood flow increases by 40%–60% ("intestinal hyperemia"). The degree of hyperemia varies with nutritional content, and fat induces the highest blood flow. The hyperemic response links oxygen delivery to metabolic activity (digestion). During circulatory shock, splanchnic vasoconstriction preserves cardiac output and gut epithelium can become hypoxic. Restoration of blood flow generates oxygen radicals and *intestinal reperfusion injury*. Feeding during hypotension can lead to demand–supply mismatch and increased mucosal permeability.

Neuroendocrine Control of the GI Tract and Metabolism

Ghrelin is secreted by the stomach and proximal intestine and stimulates appetite, stomach acid secretion, gastric and small intestine motility, and release of growth hormone (GH). During cachexia of chronic illness (e.g., COPD, chronic heart failure, or renal failure), ghrelin levels are significantly elevated. Ghrelin infusion induces positive energy balance, stimulates food intake, induces adiposity, improves cardiovascular function, decreases proinflammatory cytokines IL-1β, IL-6, and TNF-α, and increases anti-inflammatory IL-10. *Motilin* promotes motility in the interdigestive phase. Erythromycin binds motilin receptors and promotes motility. Tachyphylaxis occurs in 60% of patients after 7 days, due to downregulation of motilin receptors. *Cholecystokinin* secretion is stimulated by luminal fat and protein. CCK secretion leads to gallbladder contraction, increases pancreatic fluid secretion, slows gastric emptying, and accelerates small intestine transit. Its actions promote absorption of fat and protein. During critical illness, elevated CCK delays gastric emptying. *Peptide YY* (PYY) inhibits motility and promotes satiety (opposite of ghrelin). PYY is secreted by the colon, and fat and protein stimulate its release. Short-chain FAs produced by commensal bacteria in the stomach also stimulate PYY release, slowing local motility to allow more energy harvesting. Elevated PYY levels in critical illness correlate with poor motility and early satiety. *Glucagon-like peptide-1* (GLP-1) and -2 (GLP-2) are secreted by the small intestine and colon in response to luminal nutrients. GLP-1 slows gastric emptying and blunts the hyperglycemic response to glucose via increasing insulin secretion and decreasing glucagon secretion. GLP-2 stimulates intestinal growth and absorptive function, and promotes intestinal mesenteric perfusion.

THE GUT AS AN IMMUNE SYSTEM

Immunonutrition

Enteral nutrition (EN) may decrease infectious complications and reduce hospital costs. Nutrition provided to the gut protects the mucosal barrier and delivers nutrients critical for immune function. Nutritional deficiencies are associated with immunodeficiencies. Protein calorie malnutrition is associated with leukotriene reduction and impaired microbial ingestion and killing. Cellular immunity is very sensitive to protein calorie malnutrition. Thymus function deteriorates and T-cell memory response to antigen is reduced. Targets for specific nutritional manipulation include the mucosal barrier, cellular immunity, and the inflammatory response. The mucous coat acts as a filter, allows small nutrients to pass, and blocks large molecules (antigens, pathogens). The cell surface is a barrier; microvilli density, rhythmic movement, and negative charge repel macromolecules, antigens, and microorganisms. Disease processes that result in altered charge, decreased microvilli number, or microvilli atrophy increase susceptibility to disease and infiltration by antigens and microorganisms. Antigens pass into the enterocyte and are either taken up via endocytosis and degraded by lysosomes (major pathway), or pass through the cell untouched into the systemic circulation (minor pathway). Processed antigens are presented to T lymphocytes within or beneath the enterocyte epithelium by the major histocompatibility complex class I and class II molecules on the enterocyte surface. The role of antigen presentation in the development of tolerance is critical. During infection and inflammation, costimulatory cytokine production in conjunction with antigen presentation by the enterocyte on its cell surface generates a significant immune response.

Glutamine supplementation is associated with heat shock protein induction, reduced heat shock–induced cell death, restoration of mucosal immunoglobulin (IgA), enhanced bacterial clearance in peritonitis, and enhanced intestinal and hepatic glutathione stores. Neither conclusive benefit nor adverse outcome of glutamine supplementation during critical illness has been shown. *Arginine*, a precursor for multiple proteins and signaling molecules, can enter the body as arginine or as citrulline. Arginine is a unique substrate for NO, formed by the oxidation of L-arginine by NO synthase. NO plays a significant role as an immunomodulator. Wound healing results improved with arginine supplementation. Unfortunately, clinical studies suggest that NO potentiates systemic inflammatory response in sepsis and is associated with worse outcomes. Clinical trials studying oral citrulline in children who underwent cardiopulmonary bypass and were at risk to develop pulmonary hypertension showed promising results. *Nucleotide* biosynthesis is severely impaired during catabolic stress or protein malnutrition. Rapidly dividing cells are the most sensitive to this loss, and immune cells are exceptionally susceptible. T-helper cells are selectively lost, and IL-2 production is impaired with selective dietary loss of urines and pyrimidines. *Omega-3 polyunsaturated fatty acids* (PUFAs) are metabolized to the 3-series of prostanoids and the 5-series of leukotrienes. As compared to metabolites of the omega-6 subclass of long-chain omega FAs, these prostanoids and leukotrienes lack inflammatory and immunosuppressive characteristics, notably vasoconstriction, induced platelet aggregation, impaired cytokine secretion, defective leukocyte migration, and abnormal macrophage function. Nutritional intervention with omega-3 PUFAs downregulates inflammatory eicosanoids and prostaglandin E_1 production. Deficiencies of these PUFAs have been associated with delayed growth, skin lesions, decreased visual acuity, delayed learning ability, and neuropathology. PUFAs have been shown to be safe in reversing parenteral nutrition–associated liver failure. Immunomodulating enteral formulas are appropriate in most critically ill patients but should be used cautiously in patients with sepsis. A meta-analysis found that continuous infusion of PUFAs for patients with acute respiratory distress syndrome reduced organ dysfunction and adult mortality. The *branched-chain amino acids* (BCAA) include leucine, isoleucine, and valine. Leucine promotes protein synthesis and inhibits protein degradation via a leucine-specific signaling of the mechanistic target for rapamycin. Current consensus reports recommend early EN with an immuno-enhancing diet for moderately or severely malnourished patients who undergo elective GI surgery, severely malnourished patients who undergo colonic or rectal surgery, and patients who have suffered blunt and penetrating torso trauma. A clear position on the effectiveness and safety of immuno-enhanced diets for both children and adults has yet to be determined.

Probiotics are live microorganisms that confer a health benefit by maintaining or repopulating a damaged microbiome. Theories for this conferred cytoprotection include enhanced intestinal barrier function, improved mucus production, and upregulation of protective cytokines and innate and cellular immune responses. A trial of probiotics in PICU was halted early due to an association between administration of *Lactobacillus rhamnosus* and nosocomial illness. Large-scale, well-designed trials are needed to determine the future of probiotic use in critically ill individuals.

ENERGY EXPENDITURE AND METABOLISM

The metabolic response in critically illness is characterized by an increase in *resting energy expenditure* (REE). REE is the amount of calories required during a nonactive, 24-hour period and represents 70%–80% of the calories used per day. The REE is synonymous to the *resting metabolic rate*. The *basal metabolic rate* is the energy expended at rest in a neutral temperature under fasting conditions (12-hour fast). The REE is used to optimize nutrition management. The Harris–Benedict equations are two of many equations available to calculate REE (**Table 73.1**). The Harris–Benedict equations overestimate energy expenditure measured by *indirect calorimetry* (IC) by 6%–15%. The Harris–Benedict equation is the most accurate for adult critical care when an activity factor is used to predict energy expenditure. For any of the calculations, a large variation between individuals should be considered when their measured energy expenditure is compared to the calculated amount.

TABLE 73.1

Equations for Calculating Resting Energy Expenditure

Harris–Benedict Equations (cal/d)
Male: 66.5 + [13.8 × weight (kg)] + [5.0 × height (cm)] − [6.8 × age (y)]
Female: 655.1 + [9.6 × weight (kg)] + [1.8 × height (cm)] − [4.7 × age (y)]
FAO/WHO/UNU (cal/d)
Male (3–10 y): REE = [22.7 × weight (kg)] + 495
Female (3–10 y): REE = [22.5 × weight (kg)] + 499
Male (10–18 y): REE = [12.2 × weight (kg)] + 746
Female (10–18 y): REE = [17.5 × weight (kg)] + 651
Schofield-HW (cal/d)
Male (3–10 y): REE = [19.6 × weight (kg)] + [1.033 × height (cm)] + 414.9
Female (3–10 y): REE = [16.97 × weight (kg)] + [1.618 × height (cm)] + 371.2
Male (10–18 y): REE = [16.25 × weight (kg)] + [1.372 × height (cm)] + 515.5
Female (10–18 y): REE = [8.365 × weight (kg)] + [4.65 × height (cm)] + 200

FAO, Food and Agriculture Organization; WHO, World Health Organization; UNU, United Nations University; REE, resting energy expenditure; HW, height–weight.

Large variations in critically ill children lead to inaccurate predictions using these equations. IC using a metabolic cart that allows gas exchange measurements is a more accurate method to determine REE. IC measures volumetric oxygen consumption ($\dot{V}O_2$) and carbon dioxide production ($\dot{V}CO_2$) and derives the REE using the modified Weir equation (REE = 3.94 ($\dot{V}O_2$) + 1.11 ($\dot{V}CO_2$) × 1.44). The ratio of $\dot{V}CO_2$ to $\dot{V}O_2$ is the *respiratory quotient* (RQ). In the Krebs cycle, energy is derived from catabolism of fats, carbohydrate, and protein to produce ATP. This process consumes oxygen and produces carbon dioxide. The physiologic range of RQ is 0.67–1.3. An RQ >1.0 indicates a greater oxidation of carbohydrate and might indicate the need to decrease calorie intake or decrease the carbohydrate-to-fat ratio. An RQ of <0.81 represents a greater oxidation of fat, which may indicate a need to increase the total calorie intake or increase the carbohydrate-to-fat ratio. IC or metabolic carts are not routinely used in PICUs because of technical difficulties in performing the technique on mechanically ventilated children, lack of experience in handling expired gases, limitations on its use for patients requiring high-inspired oxygen, and lack of resources. To improve accuracy, infused feeds should be constant for 12 hours and intermittent feeds held for 4 hours, ventilator settings must remain constant for 6 hours, and no procedures (including dialysis) performed for 2 hours before testing. In critically ill children, the ability to accurately predict energy expenditure helps prevent underfeeding (nutrient depletion, protein-energy malnutrition, decreased immunocompetence, and increased morbidity and mortality) and overfeeding (thermogenesis, hepatic fat deposition, and increased CO_2 production).

KEY NUTRIENTS

Macronutrients

Macronutrients (carbohydrates, fats, and protein) are metabolized to meet energy demands. Carbohydrates undergo oxidation through glycolysis, pyruvate oxidation to acetyl-CoA, followed by the tricarboxylic acid (TCA) cycle, in which acetyl-CoA is converted to energy, carbon dioxide, and water. β-Oxidation of FAs produces acetyl-CoA that enters the TCA cycle. Acetyl-CoA produced by fat β-oxidation during decreased glucose intake is converted to ketones in the liver and converted by the brain back to acetyl-CoA for entry into the TCA cycle. Proteins enter either as precursors for acetyl-CoA or as other intermediaries of the TCA cycle. Energy produced per gram of the substrate metabolized is as follows:

- Carbohydrate 4–5 kcal/g
- Protein 4–5 kcal/g
- Fat 9 kcal/g

Body composition over age groups reveals that carbohydrate as a percentage of total body weight is constant (0.4%), but there are differences in fat composition (infant, 14%; child, 17%; adult, 19%) and protein (infant, 11%; child, 15%; adult, 18%). Recommendations for protein and energy requirements in healthy individuals are (requirements in critically ill children are varied):

- Infants 2.2 g/kg/d protein, 120 kcal/kg/d total cal
- Children 1.0 g/kg/d protein, 70 kcal/kg/d total cal
- Adults 0.8 g/kg/d protein, 35 kcal/kg/d total cal

Glucose production is critical to meet energy demands, especially during illness. It is imperative to provide adequate carbohydrate calories to minimize autocatabolism. Glucose is the preferred energy substrate for the brain, red blood cells, and renal medulla. Without adequate carbohydrate replacement, catabolism of the diaphragm and intercostal muscles additionally compromises respiratory function in an already ill child.

Fats are categorized as total fat, saturated FA, monounsaturated FA, polyunsaturated FA, trans-FA, and dietary cholesterol. Saturated FAs require more energy to burn than do unsaturated FAs. Free FAs, released from glycerol in the hydrolysis of triglycerides, are the primary lipid source for energy. The glycerol released is converted to pyruvate and shuttled into glucose metabolism as a gluconeogenic precursor. Critically ill children who do not receive lipids develop essential FA deficiencies within a week. To prevent FA deficiency, administration of linoleic acid (4.5% total calories), and linolenic acid (0.5% total calories) is recommended. Free FAs interfere with leukocyte function, and hyperlipidemia decreases oxygenation in premature infants receiving IV fat infusions. Neonates have a theoretical risk of IV lipid displacing unconjugated bilirubin and causing kernicterus. Restricting the infusion of lipid to 2–3 g/kg/d protects against bilirubin displacement.

Unlike fat, the body has no storage depots of protein; 98% of the amino acids are incorporated in proteins. Protein recycling represents the major pathway for amino acid/protein utilization. Newborns have a protein turnover of 6.7 g/kg/d versus adults' 3.5 g/kg/d. Burns, trauma, and ECMO increase protein turnover. Urinary nitrogen excretion increases 100% in infants with bacterial sepsis or requiring ECMO support. To provide adequate amino acids for wound healing, protein synthesis, and preservation of skeletal muscle mass, the recommended protein requirements during critical illness are:

- Low-birth-weight infants 3–4 g/kg/d
- Term neonates 2–3 g/kg/d
- Children 1.5 g/kg/d

Protein administration >6 g/kg/d is associated with toxicity to the liver and kidneys. Infants should receive 43% of protein as essential amino acids (children, 36%). Infants should receive a minimum of 30% of their calories from fat. Children should receive a maximum of 30% of total calories from fat and no more than 10% of calories from saturated or unsaturated fats.

Micronutrients

Micronutrients are classified as *vitamins* (A [retinol], B_1 [thiamin], B_2 [riboflavin], B_3 [niacin], B_5 [pantothenic acid], B_6 [pyridoxine], B_7 [biotin], B_9 [folate], B_{12} [cobalamin or cyanocobalamin], C, D, E [tocopherol], and K), *trace elements/minerals* (zinc, iron, copper, selenium, fluoride, iodine, chromium, molybdenum, cobalt, and manganese), and *amino acids* (glutamine, arginine, homocysteine).

Vitamin A (retinol) is a member of the family of *retinoids*. *β*-Carotene and carotenoids that are converted into retinoids are referred to as *provitamin A carotenoids*. These compounds are critical for cellular differentiation, embryonic limb development, cardiac development, ocular and otic development, GH expression, development and differentiation of T lymphocytes, and stem cell differentiation into red blood cell precursors. Retinol plays an essential role in the formation of the visual pigment rhodopsin. Vitamin A deficiency leads to decreased retinal function and is the leading cause of blindness in developing nations.

Thiamin (thiamine, B_1) is a water-soluble B vitamin required for the coenzyme thiamin pyrophosphate, a critical component of multiple dehydrogenase enzymes located in the mitochondria and required for ATP generation. A deficiency of B_1 results in dry beriberi (characterized by peripheral neuropathy), wet beriberi (characterized by neurologic and cardiovascular abnormalities—congestive heart failure), and cerebral beriberi (Wernicke disease). Thiamine disease is associated with inadequate intake (malnutrition) and alcoholism or loss (hemodialysis). The cardiac disease is somewhat reversible, while the neurologic injury remains fixed.

Riboflavin (B_2) is a water-soluble B vitamin essential for cofactors FAD and FMN. Deficiency is caused by inadequate intake or impaired absorption and can result in cataracts and migraine headaches.

Niacin (B_3) is an essential ligand for the enzymes NAD and NADP. Niacin deficiency is secondary to inadequate intake, administration of isoniazid, inadequate absorption of tryptophan (Hartnup disease), or inadequate synthesis of niacin from tryptophan (carcinoid syndrome). The late stage of severe niacin deficiency, known as *pellagra,* results in dermatitis, diarrhea, dementia, and death if untreated. Niacin can be synthesized from tryptophan and severe tryptophan deficiency may also present as pellagra.

Pantothenic acid (B_5) is found in every living cell in the form of CoA, an enzyme critical for glucose metabolism, fat metabolism, protein homeostasis, cholesterol synthesis, steroid synthesis, neurotransmitter synthesis, and heme synthesis. Deficiency is unknown.

Vitamin B_6 exists as pyridoxine and pyridoxal 5′-phosphate. Humans cannot synthesize B_6. Infant seizures are associated with pyridoxine deficiency. Irritability, depression, and confusion frequently occur with this disorder. Pyridoxal phosphate is linked to nucleic acid synthesis, steroid hormone synthesis, heme-oxygen–carrying capacity, red blood cell formation, and neurotransmitter synthesis and secretion. Homocysteine, an intermediate in the metabolism of methionine, can be metabolized by either a folate/B_{12} pathway or a B_6 pathway. Deficiency can be due to inborn enzyme abnormalities, inadequate intake, or as a complication of administration of either isoniazid or estro-progestational hormones.

Biotin (B_7) (the vitamin formerly known as vitamin H) is essential for FA metabolism, gluconeogenesis, leucine metabolism, and histone biotinylation/DNA replication and transcription. Biotin is the cofactor for the carboxylase reactions required for FA metabolism: Acetyl-CoA carboxylase catalyzes the formation of malonyl-CoA, methylcrotonyl-CoA carboxylase catalyzes leucine metabolism, propionyl-CoA carboxylase catalyzes cholesterol and FA metabolism, and pyruvate carboxylase is critical for gluconeogenesis. Once the carboxylase reaction has occurred, biotin is recycled by a biotinidase. Biotin deficiency may result from either a biotinidase mutation or severe dietary restriction. Despite being required by all organisms, biotin is synthesized exclusively by bacteria, yeasts, molds, and select plant species. The signs of biotin deficiency include an erythematous, scaly skin eruption distributed around the eyes, nose, mouth, and perineum, as well as alopecia, conjunctivitis, and neurologic abnormalities. Because biotin requirements are low and it is readily available, deficiency is rare. One cause is prolonged consumption of raw egg whites. Other causes of biotin deficiency include genetic inborn errors, extended parenteral nutrition, pregnancy, or long-term anticonvulsant therapy.

Folic acid (B_9) and folate coenzymes are required for methionine synthesis, homocysteine regulation, rapidly dividing cell growth, and DNA methylation. Folate deficiency manifests with bone marrow abnormalities, megaloblastic or macrocytic anemia, and hypersegmented neutrophils, and disrupted homocysteine metabolism. The link with homocysteine metabolism (folate lowers elevated homocysteine levels) suggests that a folate-rich diet is associated with decreased heart disease. Folates also appear to reduce colorectal cancer risk, Alzheimer disease, and cognitive impairment. Folate deficiency can be caused by inadequate intake, malabsorption (celiac disease, alcoholism), pregnancy and lactation, hemodialysis, and medications (methotrexate, phenytoin, primidone, sulfasalazine, triamterene, and trimethoprim-sulfamethoxazole).

Vitamin B_{12} (cobalamin or cyanocobalamin) is the largest and most complex vitamin, and is unique in that it contains cobalt. Cyanocobalamin and methylcobalamin are required for the function of the folate-dependent enzyme methionine synthase (also known as tetrahydrofolate-methyl-transferase or 5′-tetrahydrofolate-homocysteine methyltransferase), which produces methionine from homocysteine. In the acid stomach, B_{12} is released from food stuffs and binds to *R-proteins* or *R-binders*. In the alkaline duodenum, the R-proteins are degraded by pancreatic enzymes and B_{12} binds to IF. The B_{12}–IF complex traffics through the enterocyte. Deficiency can cause anemia (macrocytic megaloblastic anemia) or demyelination (numbness, tingling, ataxia). Deficiency can be seen with stomach abnormalities (intact stomach needed for acid environment and R-protein), pancreas (proteolytic enzymes cleave R-protein), gastric parietal cells (release IF), and terminal ileum (cyanocobalamin absorption). The causes of B_{12} deficiency are inadequate intake, autoantibodies against gastric parietal cells (pernicious anemia), malabsorption, and metformin administration.

Vitamin C (L-ascorbate) is an antioxidant and reductant that must be obtained from the diet. It is required for collagen synthesis, neurotransmitter release, carnitine synthesis, and redox stability. Scurvy is seen in vitamin C deficiency and is fatal if untreated. Vitamin C cannot be stored and ascorbic acid deficiency occurs soon after supply becomes inadequate.

Vitamin D is a group of fat-soluble vitamins essential for maintaining calcium homeostasis. Vitamin D_3 (cholecalciferol) is synthesized in the skin after it is consumed in the diet or after exposure to ultraviolet light. It is then transported to the liver, where it is hydroxylated to 25-hydroxycholeclaciferol (calcidiol). An additional hydroxylation in the kidneys produces 1,25-dihydroxycholecalciferol (calcitriol), which is the active form. The biologic effects are mediated through a nuclear transcription factor, the vitamin D receptor (VDR). The activation of the VDR is responsible for maintenance of blood levels of calcium and phosphorus and of bone mineral content. VDR activation on the surface of T cells and antigen-presenting cells leads to cell proliferation and differentiation. Severe vitamin D deficiency is seen as rickets, osteopenia, or osteoporosis. The main cause of vitamin D deficiency is inadequate intake; rarely, it is secondary to inadequate exposure to ultraviolet light. Lower 25(OH)D levels have been associated with higher PICU illness severity on day of admission. Postoperative cardiac surgery patients had lower vitamin D levels than counterparts in the PICU. Levels did not correlate with length of stay or mortality but was associated with a higher inotrope requirement.

Vitamin E covers eight forms of this fat-soluble antioxidant vitamin. α-Tocopherol, the most active form, is an antioxidant that prevents lipid peroxidation and cell membrane destruction. Vitamin E deficiency is seen in children with fat malabsorption syndromes (cystic fibrosis, pancreatic insufficiency, gastrectomy, Crohn disease, and cholestatic liver disease), very low–birth-weight neonates, and abetalipoproteinemia. Vitamin E deficiency presents with ataxia, peripheral neuropathy, myopathy, and a pigmented retinopathy.

Vitamin K represents a group of fat-soluble vitamins that are essential for clotting factor function. This fat-soluble vitamin is responsible for the γ-carboxylation of glutamic acid such that calcium binding occurs and a signaling pathway generates a clot. Vitamin K-dependent coagulation factors are synthesized in the liver.

Trace Elements and Minerals

The trace elements and minerals are compounds found in minute quantities in the body. A micronutrient is considered "essential" if the body maintains homeostatic control over its uptake (into bloodstream or tissue) and elimination. The *essential micronutrients* are cobalt, copper, chromium, fluorine, iron, iodine, manganese, molybdenum, selenium, and zinc. Nickel, tin, vanadium, silicon, and boron are *important micronutrients*. Trace elements that support antioxidant function are the most advantageous. Selenium is a trace element that functions as a cofactor for reduction of antioxidant enzymes such as glutathione peroxidases and thioredoxin reductase. Selenium supplementation may reduce 28-day mortality following sepsis. Coenzyme Q_{10} is a vitamin-like substance present in mitochondria and essential for generating ATP. Studies in children with idiopathic dilated cardiomyopathy reveal an increase in ejection fraction after 8 months of treatment.

Refeeding Syndrome

To prevent refeeding syndrome, it is important to slowly initiate enteral feeds and vigilantly monitor electrolytes and trace elements (particularly for hypophosphatemia, hypomagnesemia, and hypokalemia). Insulin concentrations decrease while glucagon levels increase during starvation, resulting in the rapid conversion of glycogen stores to glucose. Many parallel pathways are activated, and the body shifts from carbohydrate to fat metabolism and catabolizes fat and muscle to provide energy. Gluconeogenesis results in glucose synthesis via lipid and protein breakdown products, adipose stores release large quantities of FAs and glycerol, muscle releases amino acids, and ketone bodies and free FAs replace glucose as the major energy source. During refeeding, insulin secretion resumes and results in increased glycogen, fat, and protein synthesis. This process requires phosphates, magnesium, and potassium (already depleted secondary to starvation). Thiamine deficiency results in cellular oxidative failure, a shunting of pyruvate into an anaerobic path and manifests as a lactic acidosis. Refeeding syndrome in the PICU is seen in children not receiving adequate nutrition for >10 days, chronically ill children on parenteral nutrition that is inadequate, athletes practicing starvation for competition, patients with liver failure, patients with excessive vomiting or diarrhea that has limited oral intake, and oncology patients. Prevention includes slowly increased early hypocaloric feeding coupled with micronutrient supplementation prior to the initiation of a robust caloric challenge.

BODY COMPOSITION

Body mass index (BMI), a proxy for body fat percentage, is calculated by dividing weight by height. A routine anthropometric assessment includes weight, length, head circumference, abdominal circumferences, and skinfold thickness. Other methods to follow body composition include underwater weighing, whole-body air displacement plethysmography, bioelectric impedance analysis, near-infrared interactance, body average density measurements, and dual-energy X-ray absorptiometry (DXA) scans. Anthropometric measurements may be inaccurate in critical illness due to fluid shifts and edema, as well as being age- and disease-specific. DXA scans measure bone mineral, lean soft tissue, and adipose tissue compartments. The lean soft-tissue compartment is composed of the metabolically active body cell mass and any extracellular fluid and is really a subtraction of fat and bone mineral mass from the total DXA measurement. Childhood obesity may be a risk factor for higher mortality in hospitalized children who are critical ill, carry an oncologic diagnosis, or are transplant candidates.

ENTERAL VERSUS PARENTERAL NUTRITION

Markers of nutritional sufficiency are lacking. Vitamin levels are variable, and micronutrient pools are rapidly depleted. Macronutrient values appear to provide the most accurate serum markers of nutrition status. Albumin, prealbumin, transferrin, and retinol-binding proteins represent the four proteins most commonly measured to assess protein malnutrition and extrapolated to reflect total body nutrient needs. The serum protein half-lives of these proteins are:

Albumin (3.5–5.5 g/dL)	20 days
Transferrin (200–400 mg/dL)	8 days
Prealbumin (16–35 mg/dL)	2 days
Retinol-binding protein (2.6–7.6 mg/dL)	10 hours

Even small-volume feeds can maintain normal gut flora, minimize bacterial overgrowth, decrease the rate of drug-resistant bacteria emergence, and reduce bacterial translocation. Despite providing caloric and substrate support, parenteral nutrition is associated with increased incidence of central-line infections, wound infections, and secondary hepatobiliary dysfunction. Parenteral nutrition does not confer the gastric-stimulated gut peristalsis or neutralization of gastric acid that protects from both ulcer development and bacterial translocation that are accomplished with enteral feeds. Hence, EN is the mode of choice for nutrient delivery in the ICU.

CHAPTER 74 ■ NUTRITIONAL SUPPORT

WERTHER BRUNOW DE CARVALHO, ARTUR F. DELGADO, AND HEITOR P. LEITE

ANTHROPOMETRIC EXAMINATION

Despite limitations in critically ill children, anthropometric measurements allow an objective assessment, enable the detection of undernutrition, and aid in the planning and monitoring of nutritional support. The established criteria for the nutritional assessment of a child without associated comorbidities assume a predictable sequence of events during nutritional deprivation beginning with weight loss and followed by linear stunting. WHO criteria compare the weight–height ratio against a population median; if the weight–height ratio is >2 standard deviations below median, the child is moderately undernourished. Using *Waterlow criteria*, acute malnourishment is determined by the ratio of the child's *actual* weight as a percentage of the *expected* weight for height. Children whose actual weight is <90%, 80%, or 70% of their expected weight for height have mild, moderate, or severe acute undernutrition, respectively.

NUTRITIONAL STATES

Undernutrition

Undernutrition is common at admission and often worsens during hospitalization. Undernutrition is associated with impaired wound healing and respiratory, immune, and gastrointestinal dysfunctions. Undernutrition may reduce cardiac output, glomerular filtration rate, renal blood flow, and renal solute excretion. Intracellular K^+ and Na^+ pump activity is lowered.

Starvation

The physiologic changes of severe malnutrition and starvation may result from inadequate intake of energy and nutrients (simple starvation) or from increased energy expenditure (EE) unmatched by adequate intake (stress starvation). Stress starvation often develops more quickly than simple starvation (**Table 74.1**). The starvation response may be divided into three phases (despite overlapping biochemical events) that depend on baseline nutritional status, comorbidities, and the extent of the nutrient restriction. During phase I, glucose remains the primary source of energy and is produced by breakdown of absorbed carbohydrates and from glycogen stored in muscle and liver. Phase I begins after the consumed meal has been digested and the body has entered the postabsorptive phase. Glycogen stores are usually exhausted within 24 hours in young children. During phase II, fats become the primary source of energy after glycogen stores have been depleted. Lipolysis mobilizes fat stores to release free fatty acids (FAs), which are oxidized to ketone bodies (aceto-acetate and β-hydroxybutyrate). These ketone bodies are an alternative energy source for the brain during limited glucose supply. Proteolysis liberates amino acids from muscle to support gluconeogenesis and mitigate the risk of hypoglycemia. Hormonal changes include decreasing insulin levels and increasing glucagon (and other counterregulatory hormone) levels and contribute to maintenance of serum glucose levels. If starvation continues, fat stores become exhausted and the body enters phase III. During this phase, proteins become the major source of energy. This phase is characterized by further breakdown of muscle (including cardiac muscle) to support gluconeogenesis, a process known

TABLE 74.1

Simple versus Stress Starvation

	■ SIMPLE STARVATION (>72 h)	■ STRESS STARVATION
Metabolic rate	↓	↑
Protein catabolism (relatively)	↓	↑
Protein synthesis (relatively)	↓	↑
Protein turnover	↓	↑
Nitrogen balance	↓	↓↓
Gluconeogenesis	↓	↑
Ketosis	↑↑	None
Glucose turnover	↓	↑
Blood glucose	↓	↑
Salt and water retention	?	↑↑↑
Plasma albumin	None	↓↓

as "protein wasting." Adaption to starvation involves reducing EE by suppressing metabolic rate and body temperature, and delaying growth/reproduction. During stress starvation, the adaptative responses of simple starvation (that conserve body protein) are overridden by the neuroendocrine and cytokine effects of injury. Metabolic rate rises rather than falls, ketosis is minimal, protein catabolism increases to meet the demands for tissue repair and gluconeogenesis, and there is hyperglycemia and glucose intolerance. Salt and water retention is exacerbated and may result in a kwashiorkor-like state with hypoalbuminemia and edema.

Refeeding Syndrome

Refeeding syndrome (nutritional recovery syndrome) is a potentially lethal condition that occurs within 1–3 days after reinstitution of nutrition following 5–10 days of fasting. Patients at risk include those with severe undernutrition and anorexia nervosa. The major manifestations of refeeding syndrome include hypophosphatemia, hypokalemia, hypomagnesemia, fluid overload, and thiamine deficiency. The pathophysiology of refeeding syndrome begins with a contraction of intracellular spaces and depletion of major intracellular ions (phosphorus, potassium, and magnesium) during starvation despite normal serum levels. Refeeding of carbohydrates increases glucose levels, stimulates insulin release, and induces protein, glycogen, and fat synthesis. Elevated insulin levels shift phosphorus, potassium, magnesium, and thiamine to the intracellular space. Cardiovascular manifestations include heart failure and dysrhythmias. Because severely undernourished patients are usually bradycardic, the restoration of a "normal" heart rate may indicate impending heart failure. Pulmonary complications include respiratory muscle weakness. Hypophosphatemia may lead to ventilatory failure. Neurologic complications include seizures, delirium, and frank encephalopathy from thiamine deficiency (Wernicke encephalopathy). Prevention is the key to management of refeeding syndrome. Electrolytes abnormalities should be anticipated and corrected when discovered. Nutritional supplementation (especially carbohydrate intake) should be advanced gradually. Excess fluid and sodium administration are avoided. Observation for cardiac arrhythmias is important (the major cause of fatalities). Vitamin supplementation (especially thiamine) should be implemented and continued for at least 10 days.

Hypercatabolism

Hypercatabolic states occur in many clinical conditions (sepsis, trauma, burns, etc.) and include insulin resistance, increased circulating catabolic hormones, and increased inflammatory cytokines. The systemic inflammatory response activates the sympathetic nervous system and the hypothalamic–pituitary–adrenal axis. These responses change glucose and lipid metabolism and increase protein turnover, which results in increased EE, a negative nitrogen balance, and muscle protein loss. Levels of catecholamines, cortisol, glucagon, growth hormone, aldosterone, and antidiuretic hormone are increased. Insulin is elevated but not enough to impede hyperglycemia. Insulin secretion, initially suppressed by the α-adrenergic mechanism, is later increased together with glucagon levels. Peripheral resistance to growth hormone occurs, with a reduction in insulin-like growth factor (IGF)-1 secretion, while hyperglycemia and lipolysis remain. Increased counterregulatory hormone concentrations induce insulin- and growth hormone-resistant states (a sign of stress), which results in protein catabolism and the utilization of carbohydrate and fat stores to meet the increased basal metabolic rate. An additional pathophysiologic process is the synthesis and release of inflammatory and metabolic response mediators by monocytes (primarily Kupffer cells and alveolar macrophages). These mediators include cytokines, products of arachidonic acid metabolism, and platelet activation factors.

Obesity

Severe childhood obesity is defined as a body mass index (BMI) > 35 kg/m^2. Pseudotumor cerebri, slipped capital femoral epiphysis, steatohepatitis, cholelithiasis, and sleep apnea represent some of the major comorbidities associated with severe obesity. Special problems for morbidly obese patients in the PICU include difficult airway, gastroesophageal reflux and acid aspiration, obstructive sleep apnea and obstructive hypoventilation, rapid desaturation during intubation (decreased functional residual capacity and increased O_2 consumption), and drug dosing based on lean, or ideal, body weight rather than total body weight.

NUTRITIONAL MANAGEMENT

Component Requirements

Fluid Intake

Daily assessment of weight, urinary osmolality, and fluid balance is used to estimate hydration status. Fluid retention from the endothelial permeability that occurs with the systemic inflammatory response may require fluid restriction. Once the systemic inflammatory response and other reasons for fluid restriction resolve, an increase of up to 50% over basal fluid requirements can be made to improve nutrient intake and promote anabolism.

Energy Intake

Excessive amounts of energy, particularly glucose, can be deleterious and result in lipogenesis, increased respiratory quotient, increased carbon dioxide production, hepatic steatosis, and liver dysfunction. Calorie administration to sedated infants in intensive care during acute metabolic stress is limited to that needed to reach basal metabolic rate plus a stress factor (between 1.1 and 1.2). The basal metabolic rate in newborns and infants is ~50–55 kcal/kg/day and falls (until adolescence) to 25 kcal/kg/day. This calculation represents an estimate; the rules tend to overestimate EE and vary up to 30% over a 24-hour period.

Electrolyte Intake

Undernutrition leads to losses in intracellular potassium, magnesium, and phosphorus and increases in sodium and water. The demand for phosphorus is greater in children because it is needed for the formation of new tissues. The recommended amounts of electrolytes by parenteral route are shown in **Table 74.2.**

Carbohydrate

Hydrated glucose supplies 3.4 kcal/g and is vital to the central nervous system, red blood cells, leukocytes, and renal medulla. The maximum rate of glucose that can be oxidized by adults and adolescents is 5 mg/kg/min. Glucose intake exceeding 18 g/kg/day (12.5 mg/kg/min) in neonates can lead to lowered energy benefit, hepatic lipogenesis, and increased CO_2 production. The glucose infusion rate in full-term newborns to prevent hypoglycemia is between 3 and 4 mg/kg/min (higher in extreme prematurity). Acute stress and corticosteroid therapy call for reduced glucose intake. Hyperglycemia may trigger glycosuria (with osmotic diuresis), hamper immunologic function and healing, and may be associated with intracranial hemorrhage. Current evidence favors conventional glycemic control with careful monitoring of serum glucose levels to avoid hypoglycemia. The severely burned child is an exception and tight glycemic control with insulin administration appears to decrease infection, sepsis, and organ dysfunction associated with the intense catabolic and inflammatory response to a burn.

Lipids

Lipids are the primary energy source for infants and young children. In addition to providing energy, they supply essential FAs and lipid-soluble vitamins required for growth and development of tissues, including the brain. Medium-chain FAs are a rapid source of energy. They are spontaneously hydrolyzed in the intestinal lumen, independent of pancreatic lipase and bile salts for absorption, and are not dependent on plasma binding with albumin or carnitine for use in mitochondria. FAs from the ω-6 and ω-3 families and their derivatives originate from linoleic acids and α-linolenic acids, respectively, and are considered vital. Endogenous production is insufficient to ensure suitable concentrations of polyunsaturated FAs (PUFAs). The series 6 PUFAs are involved in inflammation, modulation of the immune system, regulation of vascular tone, and platelet aggregation. An excess of ω-6 PUFA may elevate the synthesis of proinflammatory eicosanoids, depress immune defense, and increase the systemic inflammatory response. The series 3 PUFAs play a key role during pregnancy and in growth and development in the first years of life. The ω-3 PUFAs inhibit production of inflammatory eicosanoids and decrease production of inflammatory cytokines, providing potential benefit in chronic disease and during the acute stress response. Infant diets should supply 30% of energy in lipid form, where 1%–2% of energy intake is from linoleic acid and 0.5% is from α-linolenic acid.

Amino Acids

The hypercatabolic state of injury or sepsis is characterized by a marked negative nitrogen balance. Estimates of protein requirements should be made on an individual basis; they may differ according to the child's age, clinical condition, intake of energy and other nutrients, and quality of the protein given. Protein needs using the parenteral route are lower than through the enteral route. A positive nitrogen balance is needed to enable return to anabolism.

TABLE 74.2

Daily Electrolyte Requirements by Parenteral Route

ELECTROLYTE	NEONATES (mEq/kg)	INFANTS/CHILDREN	ADOLESCENTS
Sodium	2–5	2–6 mEq/kg	Individualized
Chloride	1–5	2–5 mEq/kg	Individualized
Potassium	1–4	2–3 mEq/kg	Individualized
Calcium	3–4	1–2.5 mEq/kg	10–20 mEq
Phosphorus	1–2	0.5–1 mmol/kg	10–40 mmol
Magnesium	0.3–0.5	0.3–0.5 mEq/kg	10–30 mEq

Adapted from ASPEN. Board of Directors and the Clinical Guidelines Task Force. Guidelines for the use of parenteral and enteral nutrition in adult and pediatric patients. *JPEN J Parenter Enteral Nutr* 2002;26(1):97SA–128SA.

Parenteral protein needs also vary according to age. Recommended intakes are 2.5–3 g/kg/day for neonates, 2–2.5 g/kg/day for infants, 1–1.2 g/kg/day for older children, and 0.8–1 g/kg/day for adolescents. The proportion of protein as caloric source should represent 8%–15% of total energy intake, attaining 20% or more in hypercatabolic states. To promote anabolism, the nitrogen:nonprotein calorie ratio must lie between 1:150 and 1:250 (between 1:90 and 1:150 in hypercatabolism). One gram of protein provides 4 kcal; 1 g of protein corresponds to 0.16 g of nitrogen, or 1 g nitrogen is contained in 6.25 g of protein.

Micronutrient Intake

Micronutrients act as cofactors in metabolic processes and in the elimination of oxygen-free radicals. Besides increasing utilization of micronutrients, critical illness may affect micronutrient metabolism through reduced intestinal absorption, loss of water-soluble micronutrients (diarrhea, tubes, fistula, dialysis) and increased utilization (marked losses in zinc, copper, and selenium), and intracellular release and excretion in urine (especially zinc, secondary to increased protein turnover that occurs in the acute-phase response). Plasma zinc concentrations are low in critically ill children and correlate with measures of inflammation (C-reactive protein and interleukin-6) and with the degree of organ failure.

NUTRITIONAL THERAPY

Enteral Nutrition

In critically ill children, enteral nutrition is preferable as it prevents intestinal atrophy, reduces infectious complications, and is less expensive compared with parenteral nutrition. It is reasonable to recommend that critically ill children not be kept fasting for more than 24–48 hours. Parameters that indicate adequate intestinal function are the presence of bowel sounds, absent abdominal distension or vomiting, and a small quantity of gastric residue. The use of vasopressor agents and neuromuscular blockers are not an obstacle to use enteral nutrition in the majority of the patients in the PICU. Selection of the most suitable diet requires knowledge of the formula composition and the possible alterations in the processes of digestion and absorption secondary to the disease. High-osmolarity formulas may cause diarrhea when administered through duodenal or jejunal routes. The osmolarity of infant formulas for oral or intragastric administration should be <460 mOsm/kg and 300–310 mOsm/kg for duodenal or jejunal administration. *Human milk* is indicated as the exclusive food source in infants up to 6 months of age. After 6 months, solid foods can be introduced, and breast milk is continued up to 12 months or older. Contraindications of breast-feeding are maternal infections caused by microorganisms transmittable through maternal milk, inborn errors of metabolism or conditions that cause intolerance to the components of human milk (e.g., galactosemia or tyrosinemia), and maternal exposure to foods, drugs, or environmental agents that, when excreted in milk, can harm the infant. *Cow's milk–based formulas* fulfill the nutrient needs of healthy children when used exclusively up to the age of 4–6 months. Their main carbohydrate source, as in maternal milk, is lactose and the caloric density of infant formula is 0.67 kcal/mL (the same as human milk). Protein levels in infant formula are 1.5 times maternal milk, but the ratio of whey protein to casein is 60:40 (similar to human milk). The main whey protein in formulas is β-lactoglobulin, whereas in human milk, it is α-lactalbumin. *Soy-based formulas* are indicated for children with cow's-milk protein or lactose intolerance. They are milk free and have sucrose and hydrolyzed starch carbohydrates. They contain minerals and vitamins in greater quantities than milk-based formulas to compensate for possible mineral absorption antagonists such as soy phytates. *Protein hydrolysate formulas* consist of free amino acids, dipeptides, and tripeptides that do not require additional digestion. These formulas are lactose free. Fats are provided by a blend of medium- and long-chain triglycerides. Protein hydrolysates are recommended for children who are intolerant to whole-milk formulas because of decreased intestinal length, absorptive capacity, or pancreatic or hepatobiliary diseases. These formulas might be considered during the systemic inflammatory response, when alterations in permeability and reduction of the absorptive surface of the intestinal epithelium take place. *Amino acid–based formulas* (elemental formulas) are indicated for patients who have protein hypersensitivity unresponsive to hydrolyzed protein formulas.

Immune-Enhancing Formulas

Immunonutrition and pharmaconutrition refer to the concept that nutrition provides energy substrates and substances lacking in the critically ill or that modify inflammatory and immune responses. Studies demonstrate immunostimulating properties of glutamine, arginine, ω-3 chain fatty acids, probiotics, nucleic acids, and antioxidants in critically ill patients. Given the potential risk reported and that these formulas are not designed to pediatric standards, their use is not recommended in critically ill children.

Method of Enteral Feeding

Gastric feeding is more physiologic than *postpyloric feeding* (duodenal or jejunal) and easier to access, but may be limited by intolerance due to gastric dysfunction and excessive residual volumes. Postpyloric feeding may overcome these problems, avoid feeding interruptions, and reduce aspiration risks (**Fig. 74.1**).

Enteral Nutrition for Premature Newborns

Enteral tube feeding using breast milk has benefits over formula and a lower risk of necrotizing enteritis and death. Supplements to maternal milk are

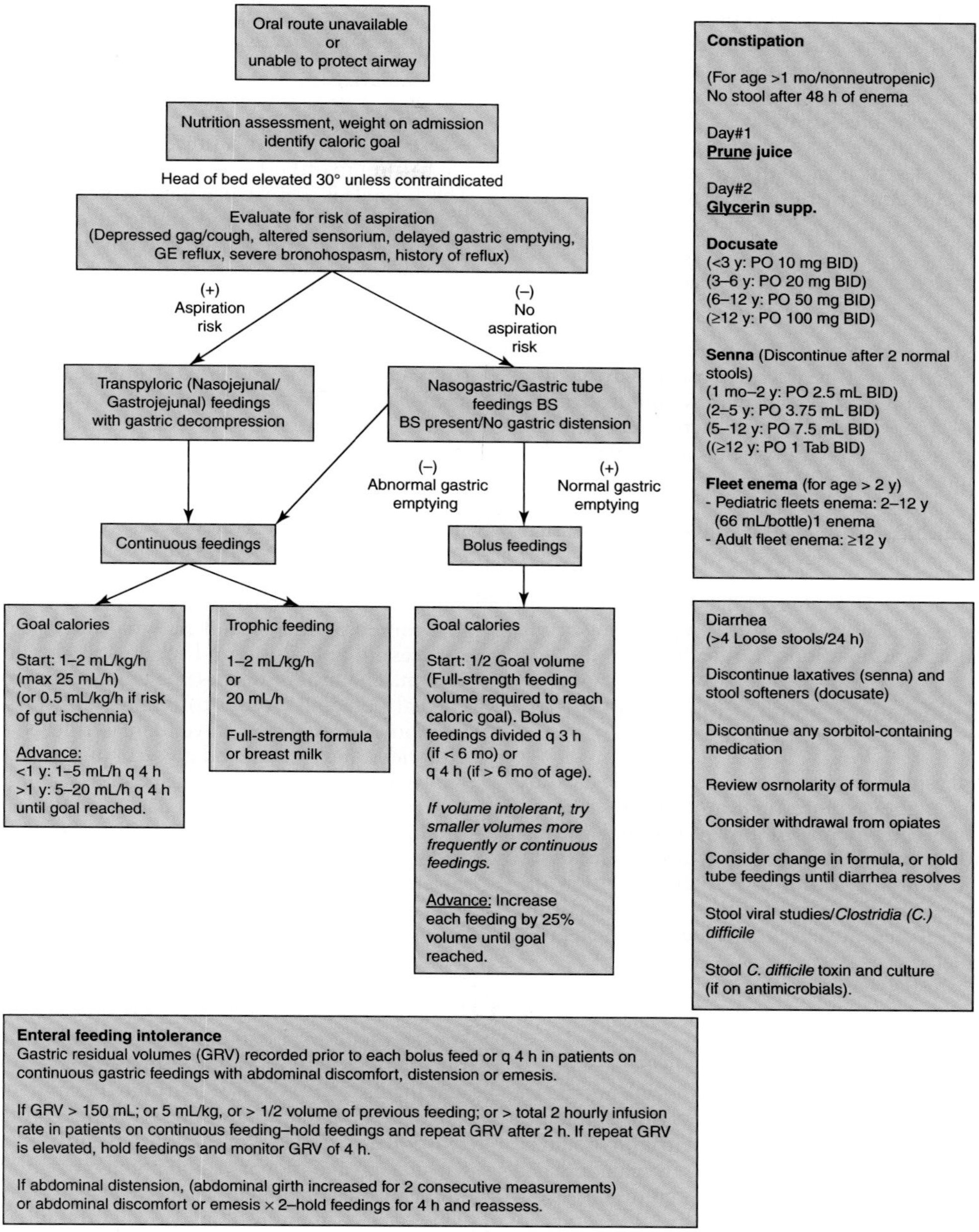

FIGURE 74.1. Enteral nutrition support algorithm. GE, gastroesophageal; BS, bowel sounds; EN, enteral nutrition; PO, per oral; BID, twice daily; q, every. (From Mehta NM. Approach to enteral feeding in the PICU. *Nutr Clin Pract* 2009;24(3):377–87.)

recommended in very-low-birth-weight (VLBW) premature newborns. Increased calcium, phosphorus, protein, and caloric content allows for greater weight gain. Early trophic feeding, during the first week after birth, may promote intestinal maturation, enhance feeding tolerance, and decrease time to reach full enteral feeding. Low duodenal lipase and biliary acid activities in premature neonates reduce absorption of fats to 65%–70%. Maternal milk is advantageous because it contains lipase, which aids triglyceride digestion. Medium-chain triglycerides (MCTs) are added to formulas for premature infants to improve fat absorption. Formulas for premature infants contain greater protein levels, specifically higher amounts of cysteine because they are enzymatically immature and poorly convert methionine into cysteine (conditionally essential). Premature infants run the risk of uremia, metabolic acidosis, and neurologic disturbances if protein intake exceeds metabolic capacity. Increased calcium, phosphorus, and vitamin D concentrations are needed to make bone incorporation and mineralization rates similar to intra-uterine life. Formulas for premature infants yield higher calorie (0.81 kcal/mL), protein, vitamin, and mineral levels, along with lower lactose levels than for term children. Use of these formulas is indicated up to the postnatal age of 9 months.

Enteral Nutrition for Children Aged 1–10 Years

With energy density of 1 kcal/mL, formulas for children aged 1–10 years vary in osmolarity from 300 to 650 mOsm/L (transpyloric administration use 300–310 mOsm/kg) and are lactose free. Vitamin and trace elements' requirement can be met with a total intake of 950–2000 mL.

Enteral Nutrition for Children Older than 10 Years

These patients can be fed adult formulas. Children with severe trauma or burns need high-nitrogen and high-calorie formulations (1.5 kcal/mL).

Difficulties and Complications with Enteral Nutrition

The total aspirated gastric volume is a simple measure for assessing gastrointestinal motility in critically ill patients, but increased gastric residual volume may not accurately express low gastric emptying. Complications may occur with enteral nutrition and medication use. Some medications are incompatible with enteral diets or cause tube blockage when given in parallel.

Parenteral Nutrition

Previously well-nourished patients who will not receive effective enteral nutrition for 5–7 days are candidates for parenteral nutrition. Parenteral nutrition should be commenced within 48 hours in severely malnourished patients or neonates not receiving enteral nutrition, provided they are hemodynamically and metabolically stable. Nutritional need is the main factor that determines access route; the peripheral venous route is preferred when use will be <2 weeks. In parenteral nutrition solutions, amino acids, electrolytes, and glucose contribute to the final osmolarity. Concentrations of glucose higher than 8% generally have osmolarity > 600 mOsm/L, independent of amino acid concentration. In the case of intermediate concentrations between 6% and 8%, raised osmolarity is found when amino acid concentration is ≥10%. Notably, even solutions with osmolarity of ~600 mOsm/L have been associated with thrombophlebitis in peripheral veins. Infusion time is another factor to be considered; vein tolerance of increased osmolarity lessens with increased infusion time. Parenteral nutrition osmolarity in children can be estimated using

$$\text{Osmolarity (mOsm/L)} = (A \times 8) + (G \times 7) + (Na \times 2) + (P \times 0.2) - 50$$

where A = amino acids (mg/L), G = glucose (g/L), Na = sodium (mEq/L), and P = phosphorus (mg/L). This formula is useful when the glucose concentration is >7% or it is <7% and amino acids are >10% (conditions when osmolarity may not be <600 mOsm/L). To lower the risk of phlebitis, solutions with osmolarity > 600 mOsm/L should be administered in a central vein.

Conventional lipid emulsions are composed of soybean oil and phospholipids from egg yolk and are available in 10% and 20% concentrations. Emulsions of 20% concentrations are more easily cleared in patients receiving high doses of lipids, an advantage over lower-concentration emulsions. An olive oil– and soy oil–based emulsion is now available that is less subject to lipid peroxidation. Also new is a soy oil and olive oil mix that is enriched with α-tocopherol to inhibit lipid peroxidation in cell membranes due to high levels of long-chain PUFAs. This lipid emulsion is a source of energy and essential fatty acids and reduces inflammation and modulates the immune system. The benefit of these new lipid emulsions on clinical outcome has yet to be proven. Children in metabolic stress states have increased levels of triglycerides, fatty acids, and glycerol due to increased lipolysis. Elevated plasma triglycerides (>200 mg/dL) saturate the lipoprotein lipase system, resulting in clearance through phagocytosis by the liver's endothelial-reticular system and the lungs and possible depression in immunologic function. Infusion of lipid emulsions in high doses may cause inflammatory changes, edema, and surfactant alterations in adults with acute lung injury. In newborn infants who cannot receive sufficient enteral feeding, IV lipid emulsions should be started before day 3 of life, but may be started on day 1. Lipid emulsions in newborns may impair oxygenation, reduce immunologic function, and increase levels of free bilirubin. IV lipid infusion can reduce arterial Po_2 through eicosanoid production (vasodilates vessels around poorly ventilated alveoli causing intrapulmonary shunt and hypoxemia) or by the deposition of fat in the capillary-alveoli membrane. This effect is minimized by slowing the infusion of lipid emulsion over 20–24 hours.

Hyperlipidemia in the premature infant with jaundice increases the risk of kernicterus, as fatty acids compete with bilirubin for binding sites on albumin. Icteric premature newborns should be started on 0.5 g/kg/day doses, increasing after bilirubin levels fall or on determination of free fatty acid levels. Liver function tests should be monitored when lipid emulsions are given. If progressive hepatic dysfunction or cholestasis develops, lipid administration should be decreased, especially if other concurrent morbidities (e.g., sepsis, thrombocytopenia) are present. In patients with severe thrombocytopenia, lipid administration can activate mechanisms that contribute to platelet aggregation, reduced lifespan, and promote hemophagocytosis. In these patients, serum triglyceride concentrations should be monitored and a reduction of parenteral lipid dose considered. Lipid emulsions should be protected by light-protected tubing during phototherapy to decrease the formation of hydroperoxides. Carnitine facilitates transport of long-chain fatty acids through the mitochondrial membrane for oxidation and energy production. Given the low serum and tissue levels of carnitine in newborns, its administration is recommended with persistent hypertriglyceridemia or in infants who are exclusively on parenteral nutrition for >4 weeks.

Additional Considerations

Manganese should be included in parenteral nutrition solutions in sufficient quantities to meet daily requirements. Manganese intoxication may provoke parkinsonian-like symptoms. Several parenteral component–nutrition solutions contain aluminum. Additional supply of aluminum raises risk of toxicity in children on TPN, owing to the element's tendency to become incorporated into body tissues. If prolonged TPN is predicted (>2 weeks), hepatic function tests should be performed, particularly in VLBW neonates. Increased bilirubin and transaminase are late indicators of cholestasis. The earliest indicator is γ-glutamyl transpeptidase, and its specificity increases when it is used in conjunction with alkaline phosphatase. Cholestasis-associated risk factors include absence of enteral feeding, immaturity, infection, hypoxia, excessive glucose and caloric intake, and toxicity of amino acids (such as methionine) or trace elements (including copper, chromium, and manganese).

Underfeeding

Hyponatremia occurs with sodium depletion or water intoxication. Hypokalemia may result from insufficient intake or increased losses of potassium (vomiting, diarrhea, digestive fistula, malnutrition). Hypophosphatemia is the result of inadequate phosphorus intake or an increase in phosphorus intracellular shift and uptake during the anabolic protein phase. Hypocalcemia occurs due to insufficient intake, excessive losses, poor intestinal absorption, or concomitant with hypomagnesemia (chronic diarrhea, digestive fistula, or malnutrition). Osteopenia occurs in newborns who weigh <1500 g and undergo prolonged TPN or those with fluid or protein restrictions treated chronically with diuretics. Alkaline phosphatase levels are high and phosphorus levels are low in children with osteopenia. Hypoglycemia is a serious TPN complication, given its neurologic consequences. Patients on TPN at risk of iron deficiency include premature newborns, those with low enteral intake, and those with poor absorption or fluid loss. Zinc deficiency is seen in patients with severe diarrhea, poor absorption, digestive fistula, and insufficient zinc intake. Children with zinc deficiency present with enteropathic acrodermatitis. Low selenium causes cardiomyopathy, whereas excessive selenium leads to alopecia, headache, nausea, and garlic-like breath odor.

Overfeeding Syndrome

Overfeeding is associated with fatty infiltration of the liver, hypertriglyceridemia, hyperglycemia, increased metabolic rate, and electrolyte disturbances. Excessive caloric intake may increase oxygen uptake, carbon dioxide (CO_2) production, and CO_2 retention in children with pulmonary or cardiac insufficiency. Overfeeding with glucose may increase the risk of infectious complications. Intolerance to lipid use may occur in children who are preterm, septic, or malnourished, have hepatic or renal insufficiency, or in those who are receiving steroids. The use of medicines that contain lipids (e.g., propofol and amphotericin B) may increase the possibility of hyperlipidemia. Triglyceride levels must be measured 4 hours after initiation of fat infusion or 4 hours after increased infusion rate, given that hypertriglyceridemia tends to occur within this time frame. High levels of triglycerides are also attributed to carnitine deficiency (premature newborns < 34 weeks have limited stores of carnitine).

NUTRITIONAL MONITORING

Nutritional Biomarkers

Serum levels of electrolytes, urea, lactate, ammonia, proteins, arterial blood gas, glucose, triglycerides, and nitrogen balance are parameters for monitoring. *Nitrogen balance* is the difference between nitrogen intake and nitrogen excreted. It assesses the suitability of protein intake and degree of hypercatabolism. It is expressed by:

$$\frac{\text{ingested protein (g/24 h)}}{6.25} - \frac{\text{urinary urea (g/24 h)}}{2.14} + 4^{*}$$

A positive nitrogen balance is a reflection of anabolism. A negative balance could be due to insufficient protein ingestion or hypercatabolism. Unmeasured losses (burns, renal disease, diarrhea, and protein-losing enteropathy) contribute to a negative nitrogen balance not reflected by the calculation. Nitrogen excretion is related to the degree of injury and the metabolic state; urinary urea nitrogen is reported between 170 and 254 mg/kg/day in critically ill children.

Serum Proteins

The principal nutritional proteins are albumin, prealbumin, apolipoprotein A1, retinol-binding protein,

*Estimated value of extraurinary nitrogen losses, used in adolescents and adults only (the Wilmore nomogram is used in younger children.

transferrin, and fibronectin. Prealbumin, due to its short half-life and being affected by malnutrition, is the most relevant as a plasma protein pool marker. It is synthesized by the liver and has a half-life of 2 days. Its concentration falls rapidly when calorie and protein intake is below normal, but rises soon after the initiation of nutritional support and is useful in detecting acute malnutrition. It should be assessed together with C-reactive protein to provide a reference for the magnitude of inflammatory response. Serum albumin, given its long half-life and redistribution from the extravascular pool, may not reflect protein-calorie malnutrition. In critically ill patients, hypoalbuminemia is indicative of the degree of metabolic stress more than alterations in nutritional state. Interleukin 6 (IL-6), a proinflammatory cytokine, levels have been associated with patients with nutritional risk.

Plasma Triglyceride Concentrations

No data define the triglyceride level at which adverse effects occur. In children with mild hypertriglyceridemia (175–225 mg/dL), steady increases in infusion rates are recommended. At moderately elevated concentrations (225–275 mg/dL), infusion rates should be reassessed without further increase until levels have normalized. At concentrations that exceed 400 mg/dL, it is recommended that infusion be halted for 12–24 hours and then resumed at 0.02–0.04 g/kg/h.

Measured EE (Indirect Calorimetry)

Indirect calorimetry (IC) has technical limitations (requires trained personnel with available time, costly equipment, an inspired oxygen fraction of less than 60%, hemodynamic stability, no air leaks around the endotracheal tube, adequate sedation, no fever, and no anaerobic metabolism). In a clinical setting, total daily EE is usually estimated with a 1- to 2-hour measurement, while EE can change throughout the day. When it is not possible to perform IC, EE can be calculated using a predictive formula (see Chapter 73), but a disparity can be observed between equation-estimated EE, measured resting EE, and total energy intake.

CHAPTER 75 ■ SECRETORY AND MOTILITY ISSUES OF THE GASTROINTESTINAL TRACT

EITAN RUBINSTEIN AND SAMUEL NURKO

Gastrointestinal (GI) complications are commonly encountered in the intensive care unit (ICU). Intestinal function and the ability to tolerate nutrition affect outcomes, morbidity, and mortality.

DIARRHEA

Diarrhea is the most common GI complication encountered in the ICU, with a prevalence of 14%–78%. Severe diarrhea can lead to dehydration, malnutrition, electrolyte imbalances, skin breakdown, and hemodynamic instability. In children, stool output greater than 10 cc/kg/day is consistent with diarrhea.

Etiologies of Diarrhea that Develops in the ICU

Factors associated with developing diarrhea in the ICU (**Table 75.1**) include severity of illness, oxygen saturation, glucose control, albumin concentration, white blood cell count, and mechanical ventilation. Other factors include nosocomial infections (e.g., *Clostridium difficile*) and diarrhea associated with antibiotic use.

Diarrhea is a frequently reported complication of enteral feedings, even in the absence of GI dysfunction. Enteral feeding–related diarrhea is associated

TABLE 75.1

Causes of Diarrhea Developing in the PICU

Infectious
Bacteria—*C. difficile* (±*pseudomembranous colitis in severe cases)*
Other bacteria (*Salmonella* spp., *Shigella* spp., *Campylobacter jejuni, Yersinia enterocolitica, Vibrio cholerae, Escherichia coli*— enteropathogenic, enterotoxigenic, enteroinvasive, enteroaggregative, and enterohemorrhagic)
Viruses (rotavirus, norovirus, sapovirus, adenovirus, astrovirus)
Other (*Giardia, Cryptosporidium, Entamoeba*)
Noninfectious
Enteral nutrition
Malabsorption
Prolonged fasting > 5 d
Hyperosmolar formula
Medication related
Contrast dye
Antibiotic use
Opioid or benzodiazepine withdrawal
Other
Intestinal ischemia
Toxic megacolon (secondary to bacterial infection, Hirschsprung disease, or inflammatory bowel disease)
Hypoalbuminemia (<2.5 g/dL), especially chronic severe hypoalbuminemia
Fecal impaction
Psychological stress
Tumor (hormone secreting—carcinoid, gastrinoma, VIPoma, mastocytosis)
Endocrine disorder (adrenal insufficiency, hyperthyroidism)
Inflammatory bowel disease exacerbation
Overuse of stool softeners

with intolerance to enteral nutrients during illness (or after fasting), decreased absorptive capacity of the enteral mucosa, or the effect of osmolar load from the enteral formula. A short period of enteral fasting is associated with duodenal mucosal atrophy in critically ill patients. The role that formula osmolarity plays in the development of diarrhea is not clear. Higher osmolality may result in excessive intraluminal volume and subsequent diarrhea. A randomized controlled study showed no difference in diarrhea when feeds were delivered into the stomach versus postpyloric. The jejunum is more reliant on isosmotic feeds, and so hyperosmotic feeds and bolus feeds (bolus feeds cause *dumping syndrome*) into the jejunum have been associated with diarrhea. A decrease in the absorptive ability of the bowel can significantly interfere with nutrient uptake and lead to an *osmotic diarrhea* (fluid is drawn into the intestine by the increase in osmotically active contents). Patients with chronic hypoalbuminemia have a greater incidence of diarrhea than those with acute hypoalbuminemia, suggesting that chronicity of malnutrition is more important than disease severity for diarrhea. Malabsorption of nonabsorbable solutes in the GI tract (e.g., carbohydrates) causes osmotic diarrhea. In addition, bacterial fermentation of nonabsorbed carbohydrate reaching the colon results in the formation of short-chain fatty acids contributing to the osmotic load presented to the colon and limits water reabsorption. In addition, short-chain fatty acids stimulate peristalsis. Bile acid malabsorption has been associated with diarrhea in the critically ill.

Antibiotic use is associated with diarrhea, either via direct effect on the GI tract or in association with the development of *C. difficile*. Antibiotic use may directly increase intestinal motility or reduce bacterial fermentation of carbohydrates. Factors that put ICU patients at risk of *C. difficile* and other infections include antibiotic use, immune compromise, and acid blockade. In children, while much of the focus is on *C. difficile*, it is estimated that 91%–94% of hospital-acquired infectious diarrhea is due to virus, especially rotavirus. The occurrence of *C. difficile* is increasing. The antibiotics most frequently implicated in *C. difficile* infection in children are ampicillin, penicillin, cephalosporins, amoxicillin, and clindamycin. Although diarrhea is the hallmark of *C. difficile*, it can also present with abdominal pain or severe ileus. *C. difficile* is diagnosed by testing the stool for specific toxins or by PCR. If toxin assays are used, there are two toxins associated with *C. difficile* infections (A and B) and not all commercially available assays measure both.

Another type of diarrhea that can develop in the ICU patient is *secretory diarrhea*. This type of diarrhea is voluminous and, unlike osmotic diarrhea, does not stop when the patient is fasted. It usually occurs from active intestinal secretion (e.g., secondary to cholera toxin), and it results in major shifts in fluid and electrolytes. It can occur in the setting of critical illness or systemic processes that affect the GI tract. Osmotic diarrhea typically has less stool volume per day, a lower Na content, and a pH of <5; tests positive for reducing/nonreducing sugars; and usually responds to fasting.

Evaluation and Management

A thorough history will help detect triggers that could be discontinued (like medications) or treated (infections, malabsorption, and underlying inflammatory bowel disease). Physical examination will help determine the presence of impaction. Gross stool examination can detect blood, leukocytes, mucus, ova, and parasites. Presence of leukocytes suggests presence of invasive or toxin-producing microorganism in the gut. The pH and presence of reducing substances indicate the presence of carbohydrate malabsorption. The discontinuation of enteral feeds during diarrhea is not always justified. Feedings may need to be adjusted to decrease osmolar load by reducing infusion rate, repositioning feeding tube, or dilution of formula. When there is severe osmotic diarrhea from malabsorption, it is likely that there is damage to the absorptive surface of the intestine, and it may be necessary to change to more predigested formulas. The replacement of fluids and electrolytes and the establishment of hemodynamic stability are the major goals in diarrhea management. The role of probiotics in the ICU is controversial. The addition of soluble fiber to feeds has also been suggested to prolong transit time and decrease diarrhea. Specific treatment needs to be administered in the case of infections like *C. difficile*. The most common treatments are oral metronidazole and vancomycin, and rifaximin. The enteral route is preferred, but parenteral metronidazole may also be effective. In cases of secretory diarrheas, it may be necessary to slow down intestinal secretions with the use of loperamide, or similar agents, although they must be used with caution in the critically ill. Loperamide is not indicated in children <3 years old or who may suffer overgrowth of invasive infectious organisms associated with dysentery.

INTESTINAL HYPOMOTILITY (ILEUS)

Several conditions resulting in critical illness are associated with GI motility dysfunction. These include respiratory failure (particularly with mechanical ventilation), increased intracranial pressure, sepsis, trauma, postoperative conditions, burns, and cardiac injury. Some of the common terms used to describe motility dysfunction include feeding intolerance, abdominal distension, and the absence of bowel sounds. *Ileus* is defined as transient impairment of GI motility, clinically characterized by delayed passage of stool and flatus, absent bowel sounds, nausea, vomiting, abdominal distension, and accumulation of gas and fluid in the bowel. Bowel sounds have been used as a marker of intestinal motility, but there is little evidence that the absence of bowel sounds indicates that enteral nutrition should be withheld in the critically ill. The drainage of liquid and air from the stomach may reduce the components that create bowel sounds. Gastric hypomotility is one of the most frequently encountered complications in critically ill children receiving gastric feeds. Reduced GI motility has been noted in 50% of critically ill children with delay in gastric emptying.

The pathophysiology of GI hypomotility is not well understood. Mechanical ventilation, increased intracranial pressure, infections, sepsis, volume overload with intestinal wall edema, hypotension, vasoactive drugs reducing splanchnic blood flow, direct catecholamine-induced inhibition of intestinal motility, and electrolyte disorders have all been associated with hypomotility. Altered proximal gut motility has been associated with such factors as increased intra-abdominal pressure, and metabolic abnormalities (such as hyponatremia, hypernatremia, hypokalemia, hyperkalemia, hypomagnesemia, and hyperglycemia). *Mechanical ventilation* is associated with abnormal proximal gastric motor responses to small intestinal nutrients that include less-frequent and lower-amplitude fundic volume waves. Mechanical ventilation can also contribute to splanchnic hypoperfusion via increased intrathoracic pressure, increased plasma–renin–angiotensin–aldosterone activity, and elevated catecholamines in the setting of high levels of positive end-expiratory pressure. Cytokine production during mechanical ventilation can also lead to splanchnic hypoperfusion and impaired intestinal smooth muscle function. *Shock* can result in elevated proinflammatory mediators and reduced splanchnic perfusion inducing functional and structural changes in the GI tract, which can alter the tolerance to enteral nutrition. *The gastric and duodenal reflexes* appear to be abnormal in the critically ill. It is suggested that duodenal feedback is pathologically increased in the critically ill and the presence of smaller than usual amounts of nutrients in the duodenum can activate a reflex that inhibits gastric emptying. Elevated levels of proinflammatory cytokines such as IL-2 and IL-6 and tumor necrosis factor lead to increased leukocyte migration and inflammation in the muscularis of the intestinal wall, which can have inhibitory effects on contractility. Tachykinins (such as substance P and neurokinin) have been shown to be elevated in critical illness and associated with intestinal hypomotility. Elevation of plasma cholecystokinin both in fasting and nutrient-stimulated states in critical illness has been associated with delayed gastric emptying. *Postoperative ileus* is considered an expected occurrence. The stomach and duodenum tend to return to function in the first 24–48 hours and the colon within 72 hours after abdominal surgery. Ileus is secondary to disturbances of intestinal motility (in particular of the migrating motor complex, which is the intrinsic motor activity of the small bowel) that result in reduced flushing of luminal contents to the colon. This stagnation of luminal contents can lead to microbial overgrowth and bacterial translocation. The most significant complication of ileus might be secondary to increased luminal pressure, which can lead to gut wall ischemia and increased intra-abdominal pressure. *Medications* used in the ICU for cardiovascular support and pain management (especially opioids) are also likely to contribute to GI dysfunction. Most sedatives (e.g., benzodiazepines, barbiturates) decrease gastric motility and can also interfere with feeding tolerance. There is little evidence regarding the effect of the sedative dexmedetomidine on intestinal motility. The use of high doses of catecholamines may reduce intestinal perfusion. However, the effect of catecholamine infusions on feeding tolerance is unclear.

Management

The focus of management is to eliminate the underlying condition (if possible) and provide supportive care to minimize the effects of hypomotility and its complications (**Fig. 75.1**). Medications that inhibit GI motility such as catecholamines, sedatives, and opioids should be decreased or withdrawn, and conditions impairing motility such as electrolyte imbalance and hypovolemia should be corrected.

Nutrition is an important factor in the management of hypomotility. In burn patients, early enteral feeds (in <18 hours after injury) lower the rate of gastroparesis and the need for parenteral nutrition. If gastric feeds are not tolerated due to gastroparesis, postpyloric feeds might be a suitable option. Postpyloric feeds should be considered when prokinetic therapy is not effective. The reason to try prokinetics first is the risks of severe small bowel dilatation, intussusception, minor GI hemorrhage, or perforation in rare cases. In pediatrics, the use of transpyloric tubes is very common and for the most part tolerated well. *Erythromycin* can increase upper GI tract motility in critically ill and mechanically ventilated patients. It activates motilin receptors on smooth muscle cells and enteric neurons to facilitate neurotransmitter release stimulating high-amplitude, antral, migrating myenteric complex III contractions, which propagate across the pylorus into the duodenum. Along with an increased amplitude of antral contractions, it can also improve antroduodenal coordination. At low doses, it exhibits prokinetic effects; at higher doses, it can induce strong antral contraction, which could slow duodenal-to-cecal transit. Aside from dose, duration of administration should be considered. Prolonged administration (greater than 3 or 4 days) has been associated with reduced efficacy. *Metoclopramide* is also used as a prokinetic agent though its effects seem limited to the proximal gut. It increases gastric motility and has a moderate stimulant effect on the small bowel. It improves antroduodenal coordination and reverses the inhibitory effects of dopamine on GI motility. It is a dopamine D_2 receptor antagonist, 5-HT_3 receptor antagonist, and 5-HT_4 receptor agonist. It exerts its prokinetic effects by facilitating acetylcholine release from enteric cholinergic neurons (5-HT_4 receptors), dopamine D_2 receptor antagonism

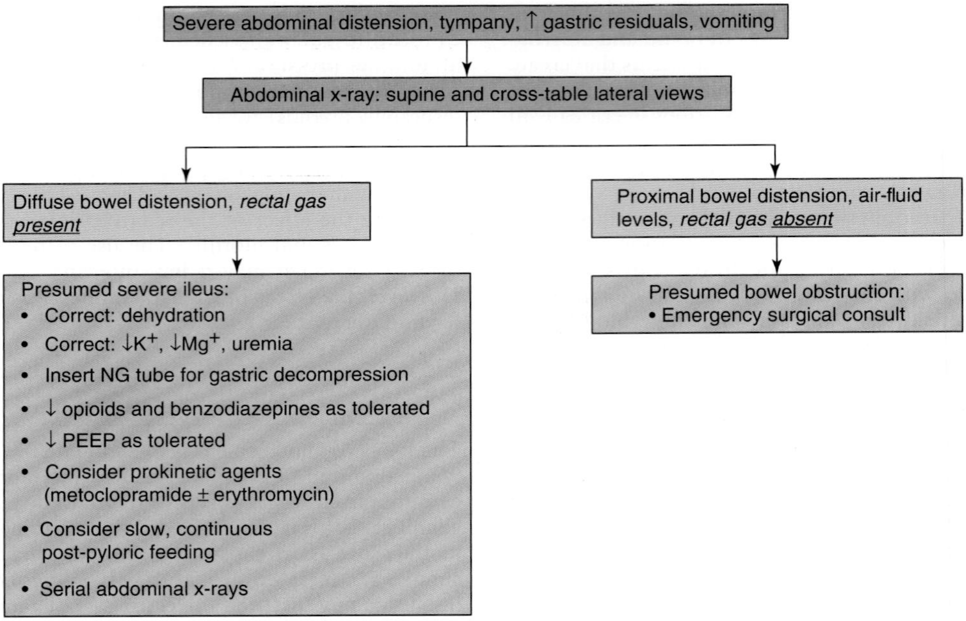

FIGURE 75.1. Management algorithm for severe ileus. ↑, increased; ↓, decreased; NG, nasogastric; K^+, potassium; Mg^+, magnesium; PEEP, positive end-expiratory pressure.

in the myenteric plexus, and direct smooth muscle contraction via muscarinic receptor sensitization. Unfortunately, it can cross the blood–brain barrier and lead to side effects in 10%–20% of patients. The most significant side effect is irreversible tardive dyskinesia associated with long-term use or high doses. Due to its side-effect profile, the Food and Drug Administration (FDA) has placed a black box warning on its use. As with erythromycin, prokinetic effects of the drug also diminish rapidly over time. Using both agents together may be more successful than erythromycin alone in allowing gastric feed tolerance. *Domperidone* and *cisapride* are not routinely available in the United States, but have been used in other countries. Domperidone acts as an antagonist at the peripheral dopamine D_2 receptor. Its antidopamine effects can stimulate gastric motility, resulting in improved emptying of solids and liquid. Cisapride is a 5-HT_4 receptor agonist that stimulates antral and duodenal contractions, improves antroduodenal coordination, and accelerates gastric emptying and small bowl transit. It acts by stimulating myenteric cholinergic nerves with subsequent increase in acetylcholine release. However, cisapride has been associated with Q–T prolongation, torsades de pointes, ventricular tachyarrhythmias, and sudden death and thus it has been withdrawn from the US market. *Octreotide* has prokinetic properties; at low doses, it stimulates motility via induction of migrating motor complexes. However, at higher doses, it has antisecretory effects, which may inhibit motility. Octreotide can have inhibitory effects on antral function, so it is often necessary to administer a prokinetic when it is being used. *Neostigmine* works as a cholinergic agonist by its actions as a cholinesterase inhibitor. Its prokinetic effects are more significant in the distal intestinal tract (especially the colon) where it stimulates contractility. It does, however, carry potentially significant side effects due to its cholinergic properties such as increased secretions, bradycardia, abdominal cramping, blurred vision, bladder cramps, increased micturition, and stimulation of acid secretion. It can be used in cases of acute colonic pseudobstruction, like Ogilvie syndrome (acute colonic obstruction and dilation without mechanical blockage). Opioid antagonists have been developed to counteract the GI motility impairment but preserve the opiate's analgesic function. *Methylnaltrexone* is a pure μ-opioid antagonist that has peripheral effects. Because of its poor lipid solubility, it does not cross the blood–brain barrier and does not interfere with the central analgesic effect of opioids. It has been shown to prevent the delayed gut transit time induced by methadone. *Alvimopan* is a different peripherally acting μ-opioid receptor antagonist. It is orally effective and, as with methylnaltrexone, does not cross the blood–brain barrier, so it does not compromise analgesia. Its use has been shown to speed recovery of bowel function. It is currently approved for management of postoperative ileus after bowel resection in adults. *Laxatives* can improve colonic transit and have been recommended to avoid bowel dysfunction. Due to delayed onset of action, laxative drugs should be given prophylactically. If necessary, rectal administration of laxatives may be an option. If patients remain unable to tolerate enteral nutrition despite all efforts, the use of parenteral nutrition should be instituted.

Prognosis

GI hypomotility has been associated with a worse outcome in the ICU patient. Ileus is identified as a clinical factor that increases the risk for aspiration, nutritional deficiencies, sepsis, and prolonged ventilation. Along with feeding difficulty and undernutrition, ileus can affect volume status and circulation, as well as the hepatic, pulmonary, renal, and neurologic systems.

GASTROESOPHAGEAL REFLUX

In children, particularly infants, gastroesophageal reflux (GER) is common and usually benign. In the setting of critical illness, particularly with intubation and ventilation, the condition can be serious and potentially life-threatening related to aspiration or ventilator-associated pneumonia (VAP).

Etiologies

Children with chronic lung disease, structural tracheal and esophageal anomalies, or neurologic impairment are at increased risk for GER. Prolonged supine positioning, esophageal dysmotility, increased intra-abdominal pressure (secondary to seizures and hypertonicity), central vomiting, and lower esophageal sphincter immaturity also increase the risk of GER. The combination of lower esophageal hypotension, esophageal body dysmotility, and gastroparesis places patients at a very high risk for GER and subsequent aspiration. Along with dysmotility, the presence of nasogastric tube also contributes to GER. The use of a proton-pump inhibitor (PPI) for stress ulcer prophylaxis is common and is associated with the development of respiratory infection in children that use them chronically. The role of acid blockade in the development of VAP is controversial. Pediatric data are limited with contradictory results.

Management

The management of GERD includes efforts to improve dysmotility and gastric emptying and to avoid complications (aspiration and malnutrition). The use of acid inhibition is usually achieved with the administration of PPIs. ICU patients are at increased risk of stress ulcers, and the use of acid inhibition with PPIs has been found to be protective. Given the possible complications associated with gastric feedings, it is common to use postpyloric feedings in the ICU setting. Aside from the possible reduction of VAP, no difference was noted in GERD, feeding intolerance, and pulmonary aspiration in a study with groups that had postpyloric feeds during endotracheal extubation compared to those made NPO 4 hours before and 4 hours after. Postpyloric feeds may be useful if gastric feeds have been tried and failed or if significant risk factors for aspiration or history of aspiration exist.

CHAPTER 76 ■ GASTROINTESTINAL BLEEDING

SABINA MIR AND DOUGLAS S. FISHMAN

The reported incidence of GI bleeding in the pediatric ICU (PICU) is 6%–25%. Fortunately, the risk of life-threatening bleeding in children admitted in the PICU with upper GI bleeding is only 0.4%.

ANATOMICAL LOCATION

GI bleeding is divided into upper and lower GI tract bleeding, depending on the anatomical origin. The ligament of Treitz (junction at the end of duodenum and beginning of jejunum) provides the division between the upper and lower GI tracts; upper bleeding originates proximal to the ligament, and lower bleeding originates distally. Upper GI bleeding is further characterized into variceal and nonvariceal bleeding. It is essential to exclude other, non-GI, sites where bleeding may originate, such as from the nose or lungs, as different management is required.

DEFINITIONS AND CLINICAL PRESENTATION

Hematemesis is vomiting fresh blood and indicates a rapidly bleeding lesion. *Coffee ground emesis* is vomit with a dark brown color due to the effects of gastric acid on the blood. *Melena* is a dark-, black-, or tar-colored stool, secondary to bleeding from above the ileocecal valve or, if colonic transit time is slow, from proximal large bowel. A small volume of blood in the stomach can cause melena for 3–5 days and may not indicate ongoing bleeding. *Hematochezia* is the passage of bright red blood per rectum or maroon-colored stools, resulting from a colonic source or massive upper GI bleeding. *Obscure GI bleeding (OGIB)* is blood loss that occurs with a negative upper endoscopy and colonoscopy or obvious source from basic imaging.

ETIOLOGY

There are numerous causes of GI bleeding, and they vary with the age of the child. **Tables 76.1–76.3** summarize the etiology of GI bleeding in children.

DIAGNOSTIC EVALUATION

A detailed history, including medications that may potentiate GI bleeding (e.g., antiplatelet agents and nonsteroidal anti-inflammatory drugs [NSAIDs]), and physical examination are important to elucidate the cause and source of bleeding. Physical findings characteristic of underlying disease help establish the diagnosis (bruising, jaundice, ascites, hepatosplenomegaly, etc.). There are a number of interventions

TABLE 76.1

Causes of Nonvariceal Upper Gastrointestinal Bleeding in Children

■ NEWBORN	■ INFANT	■ CHILD–ADOLESCENT
Swallowed maternal blood	Esophagitis	Esophagitis
Maternal breast milk irritation	Maternal breast milk irritation	*H. pylori* (gastritis)
Stress gastritis, ulcers	Duodenitis	Salicylates, NSAIDs
Vitamin K deficiency	Peptic ulcer disease	Mallory–Weiss tear
Vascular malformation	Mallory–Weiss tear	Duodenal Crohn
Milk protein sensitivity	Gastric esophageal duplication	Vascular malformation
Necrotizing enterocolitis	Salicylates, NSAIDs	Dieulafoy lesion
Hemophilia	Foreign body	Coagulopathy (DIC, ITP)
Gastric esophageal duplication	Coagulopathy (DIC, ITP)	
Maternal ITP	Vascular malformation	
	Dieulafoy lesion	

NSAIDs, nonsteroidal anti-inflammatory drugs; DIC, disseminated intravascular coagulopathy; ITP, idiopathic thrombocytopenic purpura.

TABLE 76.2

Causes of Variceal Gastrointestinal Bleeding in Children

PREHEPATIC	POSTHEPATIC	INTRAHEPATIC
Portal vein thrombosis	Budd–Chiari syndrome	Biliary atresia
Splenic vein thrombosis	Congestive heart failure	Autoimmune hepatitis
Arteriovenous fistula	Inferior vena cava obstruction	Metabolic liver disease (Wilson disease, hemachromatosis)
	Constrictive pericarditis	Toxins
		Sinusoidal obstruction syndrome (veno-occlusive disease)
		Infectious hepatitis

TABLE 76.3

Causes of Lower Gastrointestinal Bleeding in Children

NEONATE	INFANT	CHILD–ADOLESCENT
Hemorrhagic disease of newborn	Anal fissure	Anal fissure
Coagulopathy	Infectious colitis	Infectious colitis
Milk protein sensitivity	Intussusception	Polyp
Necrotizing enterocolitis	Meckel diverticulum	Vascular malformation
Volvulus	Volvulus	Inflammatory bowel disease
Vascular malformation	Vascular malformation	Vasculitis (Henoch–Schönlein purpura)
Hirschsprung disease enterocolitis	Intestinal duplication	Intestinal duplication

available for diagnostic evaluation and intervention (described in the following sections and summarized in **Figure 76.1**).

The Nasogastric Tube

An assessment for active bleeding (and gastric decompression) can be accomplished by nasogastric (NG) tube placement, although the role of tube placement is controversial. A clear NG aspirate does not exclude a bleeding source proximal to the ligament of Treitz. Conversely, the presence of blood in the NG aspirate confirms UGI bleeding in a consistent clinical context. Potential complications of NG tube insertion should be considered in patients with basil skull fracture, severe facial trauma, clotting disorders, esophageal varices, esophageal tumors, or esophageal surgery.

Laboratory Tests

Hemodynamic changes (e.g., tachycardia, hypotension) are signs of hypovolemic shock and require immediate resuscitation measures prior to further evaluation. Initial laboratory investigations (complete blood count and coagulation profile) should be instituted during resuscitation. Once the child is hemodynamically stable, additional laboratory testing (**Table 76.4**) to investigate the cause and to direct therapy includes liver panel, metabolic panel, erythrocyte sedimentation rate (ESR), C-reactive protein (CRP), and stool cultures. Fecal and gastric contents can be tested for hemoglobin using a guaiac-based test to detect occult bleeding. False-positive guaiac reactions occur with intake of red meat, raw fruits or vegetables, and foods with peroxidase activity.

Radiologic and Nuclear Medicine Imaging

Plain X-ray film may be useful for suspected GI perforation or intestinal obstruction presenting with bleeding. Ultrasonography with Doppler flow is useful for portal hypertension, liver disease, large vascular anomalies (arteriovenous malformations, hemangiomas), and intussusception. Air contrast or barium contrast enema can confirm the diagnosis and treat colonic intussusception. Regular and angiographic CT and MRI are noninvasive and useful in detecting mass lesions and vascular malformations. Technetium 99m pertechnetate (TPT) rapidly binds to gastric mucosa and is useful in detecting ectopic gastric mucosa, particularly Meckel diverticulum. Pretreatment with pentagastrin, histamine H_2 blockers, or glucagon enhances the sensitivity of the Meckel scan. Bleeding sites can be visualized by a tagged red blood cell (RBC) scan if the rate of bleeding is greater than 0.5 mL/min. Angiography (interventional or CT) is an alternative in massive bleeding (greater than 0.5 mL/min) or when endoscopic evaluation and therapy are difficult. These modalities provide an approach for both diagnosis and the potential for therapeutic embolization or coiling (**Fig. 76.1**).

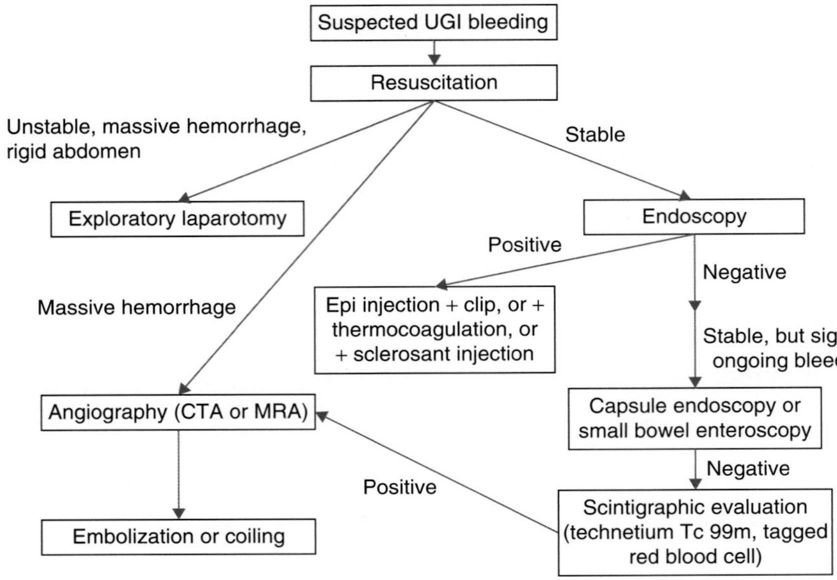

FIGURE 76.1. Diagnostic algorithm for severe upper GI hemorrhage. Epi, epinephrine.

TABLE 76.4

Investigation

■ INVESTIGATION	■ INDICATION
Laboratory	
Complete blood count	Assess severity of bleeding (anemia and thrombocytopenia)
PT/INR and PTT	Coagulopathy (liver dysfunction, DIC)
BUN/Cr	High ratio (>30) suggestive of UGI bleed (in adults)
Stool culture	Infectious colitis (*Shigella, Salmonella, Yersinia, Campylobacter,* and enteropathic *E. coli*)
	Stool PCR for *C. difficile*
ESR/CRP	Infectious and inflammatory disorders
Guaiac-based tests	Detection of hemoglobin in gastric or fecal content
Imaging	
X-ray	Foreign body, bowel perforation, or obstruction
Abdominal ultrasound	Portal hypertension, vascular malformation, intussusception
Radionuclide scanning	TPT (Meckel scan), detection of heterotopic gastric mucosa
CT/MRI abdomen	Mass, vascular malformation, intestinal duplication
Angiography	In massive UGI bleed (bleeding must be at least 0.5 mL/min to be detected)
Endoscopy	
Esophagogastroduodenoscopy	For assessing acute UGI bleeding requiring transfusion or unexplained recurrent bleeding
Colonoscopy	Polyps, colitis, vascular malformations
Enteroscopy	Small bowel polyps, ulcers, colitis, vascular malformations
Wireless capsule study	Small bowel polyps, ulcers, colitis, vascular malformations

PT, prothrombin time, INR, international normalized ratio; PTT, Pediatric Triage Tape, BUN, blood urea nitrogen; ESR, erythrocyte sedimentation rate; DIC, disseminated intravascular coagulopathy; UGI, upper gastrointestinal; TPT, technetium 99m pertechnetate.

Endoscopic Evaluation

GI endoscopy is indicated in GI bleed requiring blood product transfusions, recurrent bleeding, or if additional diagnostic information is needed. Urgent endoscopy with surgical backup may be required in variceal and nonvariceal bleeding refractory to medical therapy. Urgent endoscopy performed within 24 hours is recommended in adults with Hb <8 g/dL and hypovolemic shock after initial resuscitation. Administration of PPIs allows for platelet aggregation and clot formation by inhibiting gastric acid production. The use of high-dose IV PPI after endoscopy in patients with bleeding ulcers has shown to reduce the risk of rebleeding. High-dose IV PPI (omeprazole or esomeprazole, 80-mg bolus followed by 8 mg/h for 72 hours) reduces rebleeding compared with standard dose for adults with bleeding peptic ulcers. A decreased rate of repeat endoscopy in UGI bleed has been reported with administration of IV prokinetic (erythromycin: 3–5 mg/kg to max of 250 mg IV; or metoclopramide: 0.1–0.2 mg/kg to max of 10 mg IV) 20–120 minutes prior to procedure. Various modalities are available to provide effective endoscopic hemostasis in patients with GI bleeding. Sclerotherapy with injection of several available sclerosants (e.g., sodium morrhuate, ethanol, ethanolamine, fibrin, and cyanoacrylate glue) is frequently used. Hemostasis of bleeding sites may also be achieved endoscopically by using clips, band ligation, and several types of cautery. Available cautery devices include mono-, bi-, or multipolar electrocautery, argon plasma coagulation, and heater probes. Small bowel visualization for GI bleeding is indicated in suspected Crohn disease (CD), hereditary polyposis syndrome, OGIB, and evaluation of abdominal pain. In wireless capsule endoscopy, the patient swallows a video capsule made of biocompatible gastric acid-resistant material that allows noninvasive visualization of the entire small bowel by taking multiple pictures. This method does not allow mucosal biopsy or therapeutic interventions. Capsule endoscopy has been safely used in children as young as 10 months of age. The diagnostic yield of capsule endoscopy has been shown to be significantly higher than angiography (53.3% vs. 20%). Enteroscopy allows visualization of the entire small intestine with the benefit of therapeutic interventions (polypectomy, biopsies, and cautery). Colonoscopy allows direct visualization of the entire colon, making it useful for diagnosis and treatment of a variety of lower GI bleeding disorders (colitis, polyps, and vascular malformations). Therapeutic interventions to achieve hemostasis during colonoscopy include epinephrine injection therapy, clipping, electrocoagulation, and argon plasma coagulation. To optimize visualization, a proper bowel cleanout is important. Certain conditions (e.g., fulminant colitis, suspicion of toxic megacolon, GI obstruction, and perforation) are relative contraindications.

MANAGEMENT

Immediate management for GI bleeding may require airway protection and insertion of two large bore IV catheters for hemodynamic resuscitation by volume replacement (**Fig. 76.2**). Packed RBCs or whole blood is transfused to a goal of Hb 7–8 g/dL. While Hb 7 g/dL is a typical goal for a stable patient, the transfusion plan and goal Hb are tailored to the patient depending on factors such as decompensated shock, ongoing blood loss, and the presence of underlying disease (e.g., cyanotic heart disease and portal hypertension).

Coagulopathy secondary to liver failure is a complex phenomenon involving decrease in procoagulants and anticoagulants (protein C, protein S, and antithrombin III), vitamin K deficiency from cholestasis (resulting in decreased synthesis of factors II, V, VII, IX, and X, protein C, and protein S), hypofibrinogemia, increased platelet destruction, and impaired platelet function. The INR is unreliable in liver failure patients and does not indicate risk of bleeding. It is unrealistic to aim for complete correction of coagulopathy and thrombocytopenia, as this may result in volume overload that increases the risk of variceal rebleeding, raised intracranial pressure, and pulmonary edema. Administration of vitamin K, cryoprecipitate, FFP, and platelets is recommended in patients with active bleeding and prior to an invasive procedure. A platelet count of 50,000/μL is the goal for patients who are actively bleeding and prior to invasive procedures. FFP in the absence of bleeding is typically not recommended as it does not appear to reduce the risk of GI bleeding. Recombinant activated factor VII is not recommended for variceal bleeding based on randomized control trials.

Acid blockers may have a beneficial role in management of GI bleed. One explanation is that increasing the gastric pH indirectly stabilizes clot formation. Available pharmacologic drugs (**Table 76.5**) target acid suppression (intravenous PPI, histamine [H_2] blockers). Vasoactive medications (vasopressin, somatostatin, and octreotide) are used in acute management of bleeding from portal hypertension. Vasopressin increases splanchnic vascular tone, causing a decrease in arterial splanchnic flow and portal venous pressure. Due to the vasoconstriction, side effects include organ ischemic injury. Octreotide and somatostatin decrease azygos blood flow, resulting in decreased variceal flow. Octreotide has a longer half-life than somatostatin and is therefore more commonly used.

SPECIFIC CONDITIONS

Neonatal GI Bleeding

Swallowed maternal blood during birth or nursing from cracked nipples can present with hematemesis in neonates within the first few days of life. Hemorrhagic disease of the newborn is a rare entity in

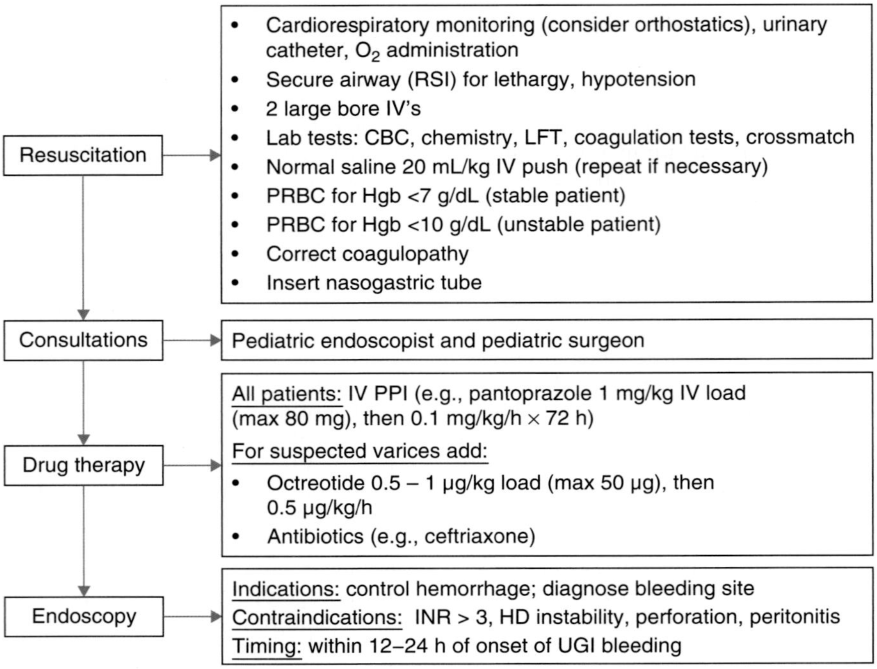

FIGURE 76.2. Emergency management for severe UGI bleeding. A goal-directed approach involving a multidisciplinary team (intensivist, endoscopist, and surgeon) is indicated. The management proceeds from resuscitation to emergency consultation, drug therapy, and endoscopy. For esophageal varices, alternative management includes balloon tamponade (Sengstaken Blakemore tube), surgical shunt, and transjugular intrahepatic portosystemic shunt (TIPS). CBC, complete blood count; EST, endoscopic sclerotherapy; EVL, endoscopic variceal ligation.

TABLE 76.5

Pharmacologic Therapies

DRUGS	DOSE
Vasoconstriction (for acute management of bleeding secondary to portal hypertension)	
Vasopressin	0.002–0.005 units/kg/min, maximum 0.01 units/kg/min (continuous IV)
Octreotide	0.5–2 μg/kg bolus (max 100 μg), then 0.5–1 μg/kg/h (continuous IV)
Acid Suppression	
Ranitidine	2–4 mg/kg/d divided 6–8 h, maximum 200 mg/d (IV)
Lansoprazole	0.6–1.8 mg/kg daily (IV)
Omeprazole	40 mg/1.72 m^2 daily (IV)
Esomeprazole	1 mo–1 y: 0.5 mg/kg daily; 1–17 y (less than 55 kg): 10 mg daily; > 55 kg: 20 mg daily (IV)
Pantoprazole	1 mg/kg/d, maximum 40 mg (IV)
Cytoprotection	
Sucralfate	40–80 mg/kg/d divided 6 h, maximum 1 g/d (oral)
Misoprostol	100–200 μg every 6–8 h (oral)

IV, intravenous.

the developed world (incidence of 0.01%–0.44%). Neonatal food allergies to cow's milk or soy protein represent a spectrum of disorders from sensitivity to severe enterocolitis presenting with hematemesis and/or hematochezia. Other causes of neonatal GI bleeding include necrotizing enterocolitis, liver disease, and hemorrhagic gastropathy. Preterm infants exposed to indomethacin, dexamethasone, mechanical ventilation, and *nil per os* status may benefit with stress-ulcer prophylaxis. High-pressure mechanical ventilation is an independent risk factor for UGI bleed in children. A decrease in cardiac output from high positive end-expiratory pressure, which compromises splanchnic blood, can contribute to GI complications.

Ulcers and Gastritis

Gastroduodenal ulcers are rare in children. *Helicobacter pylori* is a well-recognized cause of gastric and duodenal ulcers (more prevalent in underdeveloped countries). It is the primary cause of duodenal ulcers in children. There are several pharmacologic regimens for eradication of *H. pylori*, mostly using a combination of two antibiotics plus a PPI. The most commonly used regimen is "triple therapy" with amoxicillin, clarithromycin, and a PPI. Metronidazole may be substituted for amoxicillin in patients allergic to penicillin. The duration of therapy is usually 7–14 days. "Quadruple therapy" should be attempted in geographic regions with known resistance to triple therapy antibiotics or in patients who have recently received triple therapy antibiotics. The quadruple therapy is defined by the addition of bismuth to a PPI and two antibiotics to which helicobacter is sensitive (e.g., metronidazole or tetracycline). Secondary etiologies of PUD include stress (shock, sepsis, trauma, burns, multiorgan failure, and surgery) and medications (typically NSAIDs and steroids). Impaired blood flow to the gut mucosa, dysmotility, loss of mucosal protective layer from impaired prostaglandin production, decreased gastric pH, and ischemia are implicated in the pathogenesis of stress ulcers in critically ill patients. Prophylactic therapy against stress ulcers and gastritis (omeprazole, ranitidine, sucralfate, or almagate) in critically ill children is more likely to prevent UGI bleeding compared to no treatment. In critically ill adults, PPI administration is more effective compared to histamine H_2 receptor antagonists for preventing UGI bleed. Patients in critical care units are at high risk of GI bleeding from stress-related mucosal ulcers and may benefit from prophylactic antisecretory therapy.

Hematopoietic Stem-cell Transplant/ Immunosuppressed Patients

GI complications are a major cause of mortality and morbidity of hematopoietic stem-cell transplantation (HSCT) recipients. Etiologies of GI bleeding include infectious enteritis (mainly cytomegalovirus [CMV] and *Clostridium difficile*) and noninfectious causes (graft-versus-host disease [GVHD], typhlitis, and autoimmune and radiation-induced colitis). High-dose chemotherapy is also associated with GI bleeding. Immunosuppressed individuals (secondary to disease or medications) are at a high risk for *C. difficile infection* and require early recognition and treatment. The clinical presentation can include diarrhea, hematochezia, toxic megacolon, and perforation. Fecal enzyme immunoassay for *C. difficile* toxins is a commonly available diagnostic test with a sensitivity of 63%–94% and specificity of 75%–100%. Real-time PCR of toxins A and B has a sensitivity of 90%–95% and specificity of 95%–96%. Available antibiotics for treatment include metronidazole, oral vancomycin, rifaximin, and fidaxomicin. Fecal bacteriotherapy, or fecal transplant, is a strategy for recurrent *C. difficile* infections, but is not widely available. Patients with fulminant *C. difficile* colitis may benefit from surgical intervention. *CMV enteritis* is a less common presentation of CMV infection after HSCT. It is usually observed relatively late in the postengraftment period (2–3 months). Many centers avoid prophylactic ganciclovir, but start it preemptively (i.e., in the absence of symptoms) as soon as a surveillance test (serology, quantitative PCR, or culture) suggests CMV infection. Histologic examination of intestinal tissue after endoscopy or colonoscopy may aid in making the diagnosis. *Typhlitis* (neutropenic enterocolitis) is an inflammation of the colon with or without involvement of the small bowel. It occurs in 5% of patients with chemotherapy-induced neutropenia (lower incidence in children). Typhlitis classically presents as abdominal pain, fever, vomiting, and diarrhea, rapidly progressing to hemorrhage and perforation. In neutropenic patients, these classical signs and symptoms may be absent, due to inability to mount an effective inflammatory response. Treatment is supportive with bowel rest, parenteral nutrition, and broad-spectrum antibiotic coverage for gram-positive and gram-negative organisms, including *Pseudomonas*, *C. difficile*, and fungus. Surgical management should be considered for persistent GI bleeding, perforation, and obstruction failing supportive therapy with decompression of the bowel. Colonoscopy in this setting carries a very high risk of perforation. Patients with severe neutropenia have a high risk of bacteremia with GI procedures. Antibiotic prophylaxis is recommended prior to GI procedures (variceal sclerotherapy, esophageal dilation, laser therapy, and endoscopic retrograde cholangiopancreatography) in patients with a neutrophil count $<500/\mu L$ ($0.5 \times 10^9/L$).

Inflammatory Bowel Disease

Inflammatory bowel disease is broadly categorized as ulcerative colitis (UC) and CD, both of which can manifest with GI bleeding. Although up to 60% of children with CD may present with hematochezia, life-threatening GI hemorrhage is rare. Conversely, severe acute UC is a life-threatening condition with 1%–2% mortality, and approximately 20%–25% of patients require colectomy within 5 years of disease onset. IV corticosteroids are the first line of treatment for moderate-to-severe disease, and rescue therapy with tacrolimus, infliximab, or cyclosporine is recommended for failure to respond to steroids in 3–5 days. Uncontrolled lower GI hemorrhage is an indication for colectomy in UC. Other indications for colectomy include failure of rescue therapy by days 6–10, toxic megacolon, or bowel perforation.

Variceal Bleeding

Gastroesophageal varices develop secondary to portal hypertension. Causes of portal hypertension (**Table 76.2**) can be prehepatic, hepatic, or extrahepatic. Portal hypertension is defined as an increase in venous pressure greater than 10 mm Hg (normal: 5–10 mm Hg) in the vessels that bring blood from the GI tract and spleen to the liver. Variceal hemorrhage may occur at pressure greater than 12 mm Hg. Splanchnic vasodilatation increases portal vein flow and maintains portal hypertension, leading to the formation of porto-systemic collaterals in the esophageal, gastric, and colonic vessels. Approximately two-thirds of children with varices present with hematemesis or melena. Hematochezia may indicate anorectal varices or portal colopathy. Mortality in children from first bleeding episode is approximately 5%–15%. In children, cirrhosis is often secondary to biliary atresia (BA).

After immediate resuscitation (**Fig. 76.2**), the management of portal hypertension in patients with intrahepatic disease (cirrhosis) can be broadly classified into reduction of portal pressure (vasoconstriction and shunts) and obliteration of varices (endoscopic band ligation, sclerotherapy, and glue). Available pharmacologic drugs (**Table 76.5**) target acid suppression and portal vasoconstriction (lower portal pressure by decreasing the splanchnic flow). Cirrhotic patients are prone to bacterial infections as a result of multiple factors that increase gut permeability. Antibiotic prophylaxis in individuals with cirrhosis and UGI bleed should be considered and has been shown to decrease mortality. Fluoroquinolones or IV ceftriaxone have been suggested. In the presence of severe hemorrhage, balloon tamponade (Sengstaken–Blakemore or Linton tubes) may serve as a temporary measure for uncontrolled bleeding from esophageal or gastric varices. Effective prophylactic sclerotherapy has been reported in infants with BA (mean age: 13 months; mean weight: 8.2 kg). Successful obliteration of varices by sclerotherapy was achieved in 92%–95% of patients. Another option of treatment for life-threatening variceal bleeding while waiting for a liver transplant is transjugular intrahepatic portosystemic shunt (TIPS). The TIPS procedure creates a portacaval shunt (stent placement between intrahepatic portal vein and hepatic vein) that results in decreased portal venous pressure. TIPS is reserved for cases that have failed pharmacologic and endoscopic interventions to control bleeding. Complications of the TIPS procedure include hepatic encephalopathy, shunt stenosis, liver failure, and hepatic perforation during placement.

CHAPTER 77 ■ ABDOMINAL COMPARTMENT SYNDROME

MUDIT MATHUR AND JANETH C. EJIKE

Abdominal compartment syndrome (ACS) results from a sustained pathologic increase in intra-abdominal pressure (IAP) leading to organ dysfunction and failure. Recent efforts have led to consensus for the diagnosis and management of ACS in adults and children.

CONSENSUS DEFINITIONS

Intra-abdominal pressure (IAP) is the steady-state pressure concealed within the abdominal cavity. IAP in critically ill children is approximately 4–10 mm Hg. *Intra-abdominal hypertension (IAH) in children* is a sustained or repeated pathologic elevation in IAP >10 mm Hg (>12 mm Hg in adults). IAH can be classified by severity on the basis of the IAP reading: Grade I (12–15 mm Hg), Grade II (16–20 mm Hg), Grade III (IAP 21–25 mm Hg), or Grade IV (IAP > 25 mm Hg). *Abdominal compartment syndrome (ACS) in children* is defined as a sustained elevation in IAP greater than 10 mm Hg associated with new or worsening organ dysfunction that can be attributed to elevated IAP. *Primary ACS* is associated with an injury or disease in the abdomen or pelvis (e.g., abdominal trauma or peritonitis). *Secondary ACS* originates from outside the abdomino-pelvic region (e.g., massive fluid resuscitation for septic shock). *Tertiary ACS* occurs when ACS redevelops after medical or surgical treatment of primary or secondary ACS. *Abdominal perfusion pressure (APP)* is the mathematical difference between the mean arterial pressure (MAP) and the IAP (APP = MAP − IAP). Normative data for APP are not available for children. The threshold APP below which organ dysfunction ensues is likely lower in children than the 60 mm Hg value used in adults because normal MAP values are lower in children.

Clinical Interpretation of IAP Values

Early recognition and management of IAH and ACS are important to prevent progression to multisystem organ dysfunction and death (**Fig. 77.1**). The increase in IAP is exponential beyond a "critical IAP" threshold

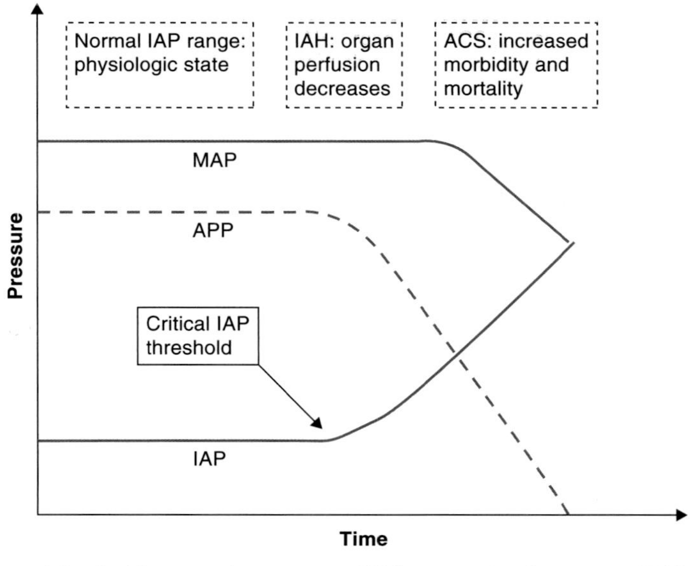

FIGURE 77.1. The intra-abdominal hypertension spectrum: With progression from normal IAP to IAH, APP falls and organ perfusion is compromised. If untreated, IAH may lead to ACS, increasing morbidity, and mortality. MAP, mean arterial pressure; APP, abdominal perfusion pressure; IAP, intra-abdominal pressure; IAH, intra-abdominal hypertension; ACS, abdominal compartment syndrome.

and leads to reduced APP, decreased organ perfusion, and end-organ injury. Serial IAP monitoring and comprehensive medical and surgical management, using goal-directed optimization of APP, systemic perfusion, and organ function, improve survival in adults with IAH/ACS. Optimal APP in the pediatric population is unknown. In 585 neonates and children undergoing laparoscopy, cardiopulmonary function was affected at IAP as low as 6 mm Hg in newborns and at 12 mm Hg in older children. Elevated IAP in the 9–13 mm Hg range has been associated with exacerbation of necrotizing enterocolitis in newborns.

TECHNIQUES FOR MEASURING IAP

IAP is measured with the patient supine, in the absence of abdominal muscle contraction, and recorded in mm Hg at end-expiration using a closed, de-bubbled system with the pressure transducer zeroed at the mid-axillary line.

Indirect Methods

The indirect method most commonly used is the *intravesical method* performed via a urinary catheter. When the bladder is drained or has a minimal volume, the IAP is transmitted through the bladder's compliant wall and is measured by transducing the urinary catheter. A minimum volume of 3 mL or 1 mL/kg up to 25 mL saline is instilled into the Foley catheter to establish a continuous fluid column, with the pressure transducer and the IAP recorded. IAP may be measured using a fluid column, in which case the reading is in cmH_2O, and should be converted to mm Hg by dividing by 1.36. Bladder detrusor muscle spasm may occur during saline instillation; thus, allowing time (30 seconds to 1 minute) for equilibration of pressures permits an accurate steady-state IAP to be measured. Instilling a standard volume of 3 mL appears as reliable as the 1 mL/kg volume for IAP measurements in children weighing less than 50 kg.

Direct Method

The direct method measures IAP in the peritoneal space using a pressure transducer or a fluid column. Direct measurement involves placement of a needle or catheter into the peritoneum; it is more invasive, and generally less preferred than indirect measurement. If a preexisting catheter (a peritoneal dialysis catheter) is in place, the direct method can be used with equal ease.

Variables Affecting IAP Readings

In children, elevation of the head of the bed significantly increases the IAP. An elevation from 0 to 30 degrees increases the IAP reading by 2 mm Hg. If the head of the bed cannot be lowered briefly for IAP measurement, subsequent IAP readings should be measured at the same elevation for consistency of comparison. Inappropriately large instillation volume, transducer location, prone positioning, inadequate sedation, coughing, or agitation may falsely raise measured IAP. Air bubbles or a "vapor lock" in the transducer tubing may also lead to erroneous measurements.

ANATOMY AND PATHOPHYSIOLOGY

Anatomy

Increase in IAP first leads to anterolateral abdominal distension and upward displacement of the diaphragm, but then compromises the perfusion, viability, and function of various intra-abdominal and extra-abdominal organ systems as IAH progresses to ACS.

Pathophysiology

Abdominal Vasculature

Even with mild induced IAH in volunteers (median IAP 12–15 mm Hg, Grade I IAH), compression and distortion of the inferior vena cava (IVC) and portal vein are demonstrated by sonography. Progressive increase in IAP further affects IVC flow and patency. The resistive index in renal arteries also increases, suggesting direct compression of renal parenchyma and microvasculature.

Kidneys

The use of an external pressure of 70–80 mm Hg applied to the abdomen to raise the IAP measured in the IVC to 20 mm Hg decreases renal plasma flow and glomerular filtration rate by 25%. Urine volume declines dramatically while IAP is high and recovers upon release of the pressure. In adults, an IAP of 12 mm Hg is the best cutoff for acute kidney injury (AKI) using the Risk Injury Failure Loss and End-stage renal disease (RIFLE) criteria for acute renal dysfunction. There are no pediatric data to define an IAP threshold predictive of kidney injury.

Gastrointestinal Tract and Liver

Gastric mucosal oxygen saturation during elective laparoscopic surgery in adults measured by reflectance spectrophotometry decreases significantly with progressive elevation of IAP to 8 and 12 mm Hg. Reduced hepatic arterial flow, portal venous flow, and IVC compression due to elevated IAP may further exacerbate hepatic congestion.

Respiratory System

Elevation of the diaphragm from IAH can lead to lower lobe atelectasis, reduced functional residual capacity, increased ventilation–perfusion mismatch, hypoxia, and hypercarbia. Lung neutrophil activation and increase in extravascular lung water may further worsen lung injury. IAP elevation also decreases chest wall compliance and results in flattening and rightward shift of the pressure–volume curve. As the lung and chest wall compliance decreases, higher positive airway pressures are needed to deliver the same tidal volume. In ARDS resulting from extrapulmonary pathology, IAP elevation above 16 cmH_2O (12 mm Hg) was associated with a significant increase in chest wall elastance.

Cardiovascular System

MAP rises initially as systemic vascular resistance (SVR) increases. Pulmonary vascular resistance and pulmonary artery pressure are also increased. At first, cardiac output is maintained, but decreasing venous return soon results in a fall in cardiac output. With progressive IAP elevation, the pulmonary capillary wedge pressure (PCWP) increases and cardiac index decreases further. Acute rises in IAP cause decreased LV compliance and regional wall motion abnormalities due to increased LV afterload.

Central Nervous System

Decompressive laparotomy (DL) has been utilized as a management tool for refractory elevation in ICP in patients with "multiple compartment syndrome" (increased ICP, IAP, and intrathoracic pressure after severe brain injury).

Multisystem Organ Failure

Fluid resuscitation aimed at restoring preload and MAP may result in "third-spaced" peritoneal fluid, bowel wall edema, and contribute to incremental IAP elevation. As IAH progresses, it initiates a vicious cycle, IVC compression reduces venous return, and the resulting decrease in cardiac output further reduces organ perfusion and function.

EPIDEMIOLOGY

ACS has been seen in 0.6%–1% of PICU patients with 40%–60% associated mortality. In a prospective study, in one-third of mechanically ventilated infants and children admitted to the PICU, both the IAP and a PRISM score greater than 17 were predictive of developing ACS. Other conditions associated with a risk for developing ACS in adult studies include abdominal surgery, major trauma, burns, high-volume crystalloid resuscitation, polytransfusion, positive fluid balance, oliguria, prone positioning, increased head of bed angle, intra-abdominal infection or abscess, laparoscopy with excessive insufflation pressures, damage-control laparotomy, anemia, acidosis, coagulopathy, hypothermia, bacteremia, increased APACHE-II or SOFA score, and high gastric regional to end-tidal carbon dioxide differences.

COMMON ETIOLOGIES

Though IAH and ACS can occur in any critically ill child, certain PICU patient populations are at greater risk (**Table 77.1**).

CLINICAL PRESENTATION AND RECOGNITION OF IAH AND ACS

IAH can only be determined by objective IAP measurement. When clinical manifestations resulting from sustained IAH become evident, ACS is present. The common features seen in ACS are a distended

TABLE 77.1

Pediatric Populations at Risk for ACS

Primary ACS
Decreased abdominal compliance/reduced abdominal domain
Gastroschisis
Pentalogy of Cantrell
Increased intraluminal contents
Small intestine intussusception
Ileus
Hirschprung disease
Increased abdominal contents
Intra-abdominal trauma (edematous viscera)
Intestinal transplantation
Intra-abdominal bleeding/retroperitoneal bleeding
Gastrointestinal bleeding
Extracorporeal life support
Nonpancreatic pseudocyst
Abdominal tumors
Burkitt lymphoma
Pyonephrosis/obstruction megaureter
Pancreatitis
Tension pneumoperitoneum/intestinal perforation
Peritonitis/intra-abdominal infection
Infectious enterocolitis
Postsurgical complication (abdominal surgery)
Bowel obstruction or perforation
Secondary ACS
Capillary leak/fluid resuscitation
Sepsis/septic shock
Toxic shock syndrome
Dengue shock syndrome
Trauma shock
Cardiogenic shock/cardiac arrest
Burns

ACS, abdominal compartment syndrome.
From Ejike JC, Mathur M, Moores DC. Abdominal compartment syndrome: Focus on the children. *Am Surg* 2011;77(suppl 1):S72–7.

abdomen associated with hemodynamic instability, oliguria or anuria, metabolic acidosis, and respiratory deterioration. Morbidity and mortality related to IAH and ACS can be prevented by using serial IAP measurements performed in at-risk patients (**Table 77.1**) to identify those with progressive IAH and guide early management. Infants and children with catecholamine refractory shock should have IAP measured to rule out IAP >12 mm. Evolving physiologic changes such as rising serum lactate, worsening metabolic acidosis, decreasing urine output, worsening pulmonary compliance with elevated peak and plateau pressures, hypercapnia, hypoxemia, and decreasing cardiac output in the setting of IAH may be better triggers for initiating management targeted at lowering IAP.

MEDICAL MANAGEMENT

Medical management is based on the principles of treating the underlying conditions that led to the development of IAH, supporting organ function, and lowering the IAP.

1. Improving abdominal wall compliance: Adequate sedation and neuromuscular blockade (when necessary) may be used to improve abdominal wall compliance. Several studies have demonstrated a prompt drop in IAP (4–12 mm Hg) with the use of neuromuscular blocking agents. Removal of constrictive abdominal dressings, eschars, or intra-abdominal packing may need to be considered.
2. Evacuation of intraluminal contents: Strategies include using naso-gastric, oro-gastric, and/or rectal tubes; administering enemas or prokinetic agents when appropriate, to help evacuate intestinal contents; and minimizing or stopping enteral feeds to decrease gastric contents. Rectal and colonic decompression using endoscopy may also be useful.
3. Identification and evacuation of space occupying abdominal lesions: Free intraperitoneal fluid or air can be evacuated by paracentesis or percutaneous catheter drainage. In some cases, placement of drains using ultrasound or CT guidance may avoid the need for laparotomy. Space occupying lesions may need to be removed surgically or embolized using interventional radiology techniques.
4. Optimizing fluid balance: Excessive resuscitation fluids (especially crystalloids) may lead to the development of IAH and ACS with associated increases in mortality and should be avoided. Judicious use of diuretics, ultrafiltration via continuous renal replacement therapy, or hemodialysis (if tolerated) may be considered.
5. Optimizing systemic and regional perfusion, and organ function: Development or worsening of multi–organ system dysfunction is an integral part of the definition of ACS. Therapies to achieve an adequate APP should be the overarching goal for effective organ support in the presence of respiratory, cardiovascular, and renal failure.

Adult recommendations consider surgical decompression for IAP over 25 mm Hg refractory to medical management with onset of organ dysfunction or failure. In children, a suitable trigger for surgical decompression may be progression of IAH to ACS with early detection of new and progressive organ dysfunction despite medical management, rather than a specific IAP threshold.

SURGICAL MANAGEMENT

Surgical management options include decompression using paracentesis, a percutaneously or surgically placed drain, or DL. A percutaneously placed catheter can be used to drain free peritoneal fluid and relieve ACS in children receiving ECMO and to minimize the risk of bleeding. DL is the specific treatment of choice for patients with ACS refractory to medical management. Surgical exploration of the abdomen is an essential part of DL to identify occult primary causes of ACS or identify and treat consequences of ACS such as bowel ischemia or necrosis. Abdominal decompression should be performed before irreversible organ damage occurs, for improved outcomes. Surgical decompression in the ICU at the bedside may help prevent unnecessary delays in trying to secure an operating room (OR) and decrease inherent risks in transporting an unstable patient. Patients without primary intra-abdominal pathology who develop secondary ACS may be better candidates for DL in the PICU. Patients with suspected primary intra-abdominal pathology may be best dealt with in the OR where specific surgical resources are more easily accessible if unexpected pathology is discovered. DL is associated with significantly improved patient survival in ACS.

Clinical Consequences of Surgical Decompression

ICU clinicians should be prepared to manage sudden hypovolemia that may occur as venous capacitance is reestablished following surgical decompression for ACS. Acute changes in respiratory dynamics occur as the chest wall compliance dramatically improves, and PEEP and peak inspiratory pressure (or HFOV mean airway pressure) may need to be rapidly weaned. Electrolyte abnormalities resulting from reperfusion of compromised tissues (hyperkalemia, acidosis, hyperphosphatemia, or hypocalcemia) may precipitate an acute decompensation, though the patient should stabilize quickly once these issues are promptly addressed.

Open Abdomen Management

This strategy involves electively leaving the abdomen open after laparotomy in patients at risk for developing ACS postoperatively. The fascia and skin are left unopposed following laparotomy, and a temporary abdominal closure (TAC) dressing is applied. This may also be necessary after operations in which edematous viscera preclude easy fascial closure, when adult-sized organs are transplanted in small children, or when second-look surgery is anticipated. This practice has increased survival in patients with abdominal wall defects, trauma, intestinal and liver transplantation, and ACS.

CHAPTER 78 THE ACUTE ABDOMEN

EDUARDO J. SCHNITZLER, TOMAS IÖLSTER, AND RICARDO D. RUSSO

Acute abdomen is a clinical syndrome with a rapid onset of signs and symptoms indicating intra-abdominal pathology and requiring prompt decision making and often emergent surgical intervention. Accurate and timely assessment is essential to make a diagnosis and begin appropriate medical or surgical treatment.

CLINICAL ASSESSMENT

Causes of acute abdomen appear in **Table 78.1** and are divided into three diagnostic groups: primary abdominal pathology (originating from the gastrointestinal tract), abdominal pathology as a consequence of critical illness (secondary), and abdominal manifestations in some systemic diseases that may present as acute abdomen.

Primary Evaluation and Stabilization

It is essential to determine whether the patient requires an urgent laparotomy or laparoscopy for diagnosis and treatment. The presence of severe abdominal distension, board-like rigidity, abdominal ecchymoses, or discoloration may be signs of a severe abdominal condition. Monitoring of pulse oximetry, heart rate, electrocardiogram, and noninvasive blood pressure is essential to guide therapy. Two large-bore peripheral venous catheters should be established for vascular access. Samples should be obtained for complete blood count, coagulation profile, chemistries, blood typing and cross-matching, blood cultures, and urine studies. Fluid boluses should be administered until perfusion is improved, and broad-spectrum intravenous antibiotic treatment should be considered. If perforation, peritonitis, or ischemic bowel compromise is suspected, immediate surgical intervention is necessary. A systematic review noted that opioid administration may alter the physical examination findings but does not result in management errors.

History

The presence of fever, vomiting, diarrhea, constipation, urinary symptoms, and pelvic symptoms (in female teenagers) aids the diagnosis. Localization and radiation of the pain should be determined. History should include previous medical pathologies, previous surgery, chronic drug therapy, recent trauma, and possibility of accidental ingestion of harmful substances in young children.

Physical Examination

Inspection may reveal distension, masses, hernias, surgical scars, or other alterations in the skin. The presence of petechiae, purpura, or rash suggests a systemic disease. Auscultation should precede palpation to avoid modification of the peristalsis by external stimulation. Bowel sounds are typically altered but may be absent in mild diseases or present even during intra-abdominal catastrophes. Abdominal percussion

TABLE 78.1

Causes of Acute Abdomen

Primary Abdominal Pathology
Mechanical obstruction
Intussusception, peritoneal adhesion, others
Acute intestinal ischemia
Malrotation, volvulus, others
Infection/inflammation
Peritonitis, intra-abdominal abscess, fistula
Enteritis, neutropenic enterocolitis
Acute pancreatitis
Acute cholecystitis[a]
Hollow viscera perforation
Abdominal trauma
Diseases linked to the reproductive organs
Abdominal Pathology of the Critical Patient
Gastrointestinal hemorrhage
Ileus
Pseudomembranous colitis
Toxic megacolon
Abdominal compartment syndrome
Abdominal Manifestations of Systemic Diseases
Diabetic ketoacidosis
Acute intermittent porphyria
Henoch–Schönlein purpura
Kawasaki disease
Sickle cell crisis

[a]Cholecystitis can also present as an abdominal pathology of the critical patients.

helps to differentiate between gaseous distension (tympanic) and distension due to masses or ascites (dull). Palpation should be systematic, beginning with a superficial examination in the most distant quadrant from the site of maximum pain and moving toward the painful area. Abdominal X-ray and/or ultrasound are indicated when abdominal pathology is suspected and the diagnosis is not obvious. Examination of the inguinal and scrotal regions is essential to detect hernias. Digital rectal examination is not routine in the evaluation of abdominal pain or acute abdomen. Pelvic examination is only indicated for adolescents in whom the pain is suggestive of gynecologic pathology. Pregnancy tests should be done on all postpubertal females. Children with immunocompromise or low white blood cell counts may not mount an inflammatory response or manifest signs of acute abdomen.

Diagnostic Imaging

The plain abdominal X-ray is useful to diagnose bowel obstruction, renal lithiasis, pneumoperitoneum, and pneumatosis intestinalis. In bowel obstruction, the distribution of air may show a few localized loops (sentinel loops) of small intestine or cecum, distended loops of small bowel in an organized, obstructive pattern, or in the upright view, numerous air–fluid levels.

PRIMARY ABDOMINAL PATHOLOGY

Bowel Obstruction

Bowel obstruction is a mechanical blockage to the transit of intestinal contents that may be intrinsic (intraluminal or from the bowel wall) or due to extrinsic compression. Intrinsic obstruction may be secondary to *Ascaris lumbricoides* (still existent in developing countries) or intussusception; extrinsic compression may be due to postsurgical adhesions or incarcerated hernia. Congenital causes of small bowel obstruction include annular pancreas, malrotation-volvulus, malrotation-Ladd bands, Meckel diverticulum with volvulus or intussusception, and inguinal hernia. Other congenital anomalies such as intestinal duplication, remnant omphalomesenteric duct, or mesenteric cyst cause intestinal obstruction by means of internal hernia or volvulus. Duodenal or ileal atresia, Hirschsprung disease, pseudo-obstruction, imperforate anus, or colonic atresia may be diagnosed. The most frequent causes of acquired obstructions are postsurgical adhesions and intussusception. Crohn disease (CD) may also cause small bowel obstruction. In patients with cystic fibrosis, obstructive syndromes in the distal ileum or in the colon may be present. Less frequent causes include duodenal hematoma and superior mesenteric artery syndrome.

Bowel obstruction may present with cramping abdominal pain, nausea, bilious vomiting, and absence of intestinal transit. Abdominal pain becomes continuous when intestinal ischemia begins. In ileus, symptoms are less intense and have a slower progression. Bowel sounds are usually increased. Signs of peritoneal irritation, such as rebound tenderness or abdominal rigidity, suggest ischemia and perforation. No clinical or laboratory findings clearly predict the presence of intestinal ischemia. Plain abdominal X-rays may reveal air–fluid levels in the small bowel, dilated small bowel, or colon loops, as well as intestinal wall edema or minimal intestinal gas distal to obstruction. The upright or lateral position is necessary to visualize air–fluid levels. Abdominal CT identifies less clear causes of obstruction or evaluates the presence of ischemia. Imaging studies should never delay exploratory laparotomy when an urgent indication is clear. Abdominal ultrasound is useful to diagnose intussusception, and the presence of free fluid suggests a collection secondary to bowel perforation. Surgical resolution of complete obstruction is a priority.

Intussusception

Intussusception is the most common cause of acute abdomen in infants and preschoolers, with a peak incidence between 5 and 9 months of age. It occurs when one segment of the intestine (proximal) is telescoped into the adjacent segment (distal). Usually, no lead point is identified; possible links are swollen Peyer patches (lymphoid tissue) in the terminal ileum. Meckel diverticulum, mesenteric lymph nodes, intestinal polyps, hemangioma, mucosal hemorrhage, and lymphoma can be lead points. The most frequent form of intussusception is ileocolic, where the terminal ileum telescopes into the colon. During intussusception, mesenteric venous drainage of the intussuscepted segment is obstructed, resulting in increased volume of the segment, edema, and mucosal bleeding. The apex of the intussusception may extend and displace itself through the interior of the colon. After 24 hours, the risk of severe ischemia and gangrene increases progressively.

The typical presentation is severe paroxysmal colicky pain accompanied by drawing up the legs. Initially, the child recovers between episodes; however, if diagnosis is delayed, progressive lethargy occurs. Emesis is usually present, and initially, normal stools may be present. Passage of (red) currant jelly stool or presence of blood on rectal examination may be seen. A slightly tender, sausage-shaped mass may be palpable in the subhepatic region. Ultrasound is a very sensitive test. Pneumatic enema or saline-solution enema under ultrasound guidance reduces the intussusception in 70%–90% when performed within the first 48 hours. Perforation during pneumatic reduction has been reported in 0.1%–0.2% of cases. Nonsurgical reduction is contraindicated when symptoms have been present for >48 hours or in the presence of shock, peritoneal irritation, perforation, pneumatosis, or ultrasound findings suggestive of a lead point. The need for surgical reduction or bowel resection and the risk of complications are related to the time between onset of symptoms and laparotomy. Intussusception may recur within 6 months and is more frequent on the first day after reduction.

Peritoneal Adhesions

Fibrous adhesions following abdominal surgery are a frequent cause of bowel obstruction. Postsurgical adhesions may produce folding or strangling of bowel loops or predispose to intestinal volvulus secondary to loop distension and peritoneal shortening. Usual treatment includes NG tube placement, hydration, and antibiotic therapy. Surgical intervention is often necessary.

Other Causes of Intestinal Obstruction

Other causes of intestinal obstruction include incarcerated hernia, intestinal strictures related to CD, Meckel diverticulum, and, rarely, neoplastic pathology (intestinal lymphoma, Wilms tumor, or neuroblastoma). *Hirschsprung disease* (congenital aganglionic colon) is usually diagnosed during the neonatal period due to the failure to pass meconium within 24 hours after birth. Enterocolitis is the principal cause of morbidity and mortality. Hirschsprung disease is diagnosed by anorectal manometry and rectal mucosal biopsy. Colonic contrast study shows an area of transition between the normal colon and the distal aganglionic, narrowed segment. Children with chronic intestinal *pseudo-obstruction* present with abdominal distension, vomiting, chronic constipation, failure to thrive, diarrheal episodes, and abdominal pain. The diagnosis is suspected due to the absence of anatomical causes of obstruction. Diagnosis is confirmed by manometric studies and bowel biopsy, which reveals muscular fiber involvement or compromise of the enteric nervous system.

Intestinal Ischemia

Bowel ischemia may arise from malrotation, intestinal volvulus, delayed management of abdominal pathology, such as intussusception, incarcerated hernia, or any complete mechanical obstruction, following repair of coarctation of the aorta or other cardiac surgery, and, less frequently, arterial mesenteric thrombosis or venous occlusive thrombosis. Colonic ischemia may be secondary to vasculitic processes as the hemolytic uremic syndrome. Patients with severe bowel ischemia progress from mucosal ischemia to transmural necrosis and bowel perforation. Combined sepsis and multiorgan failure are frequently present. The presence of abdominal distension, severe hypovolemia, hemoconcentration, refractory metabolic acidosis, or hematochezia may lead to the diagnosis. In patients with no obvious surgical pathology, useful diagnostic tests include sigmoidoscopy, colonoscopy, and multidetector CT. When signs of perforation are present, surgery must not be delayed.

Midgut volvulus secondary to malrotation may cause one of the most severe forms of bowel ischemia. An abnormal orientation of the intestine in which the ascending colon is not fixed to the right side of the abdomen allows Ladd's bands to kink the duodenum, predisposing to volvulus generation. The mesenteric vessels and bowel are twisted in the volvulus, which leads to intestinal ischemia and necrosis. This diagnosis should be suspected in infants and children with severe abdominal pain and bilious vomiting. Hematochezia is a late sign. The presence of diarrhea does not exclude the diagnosis. The classic radiologic finding is the double-bubble sign (**Fig. 78.1**) that shows an abdomen with scarce intestinal air with two air bubbles—one in the stomach and one in the duodenum—air–fluid levels, abnormal position of the cecum, and absence of distal air. Although ultrasound or abdominal CT may yield the diagnosis, contrast studies under fluoroscopic control (upper gastrointestinal series) remain the diagnostic gold standard. Treatment is always surgical.

Peritonitis

Peritonitis is inflammation of the peritoneal lining of the abdominal cavity that results from infection, perforation, or chemical processes. Perforation of the appendix is the most frequent cause. In young children, the diagnosis may be difficult. Primary peritonitis occurs when the source of infection is outside the abdomen and reaches the peritoneal cavity via hematogenous or lymphatic dissemination.

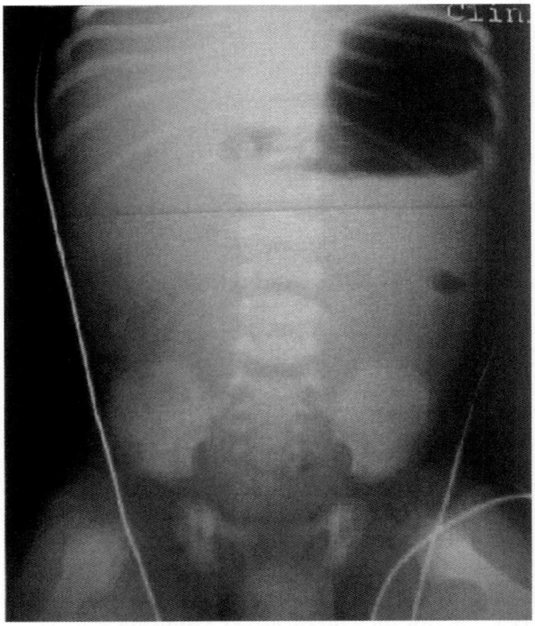

FIGURE 78.1. Abdominal X-ray showing a double-bubble (stomach and duodenum) image.

Secondary peritonitis originates from the rupture or extension of an intra-abdominal viscus or abscess. Tertiary peritonitis occurs when surgical procedures fail to control an intra-abdominal infectious process.

Primary Peritonitis

Spontaneous bacterial peritonitis (SBP) is a rare peritoneal infection with no intra-abdominal pathology. It is usually caused by a single organism, most frequently *Streptococcus pneumoniae*, group A streptococci, *Escherichia coli*, or other enteric bacteria. Children who have undergone splenectomy are especially susceptible to SBP caused by encapsulated organisms. In children with ascites, primary peritonitis should be suspected in the presence of fever, increased ascites, or worsening clinical condition. The most frequent causative agents are *Enterococcus*, *Streptococcus*, *Staphylococcus*, or enteric bacteria (e.g., *E. coli* or *Klebsiella pneumoniae*). In children with ascites caused by cirrhosis or nephrotic syndrome, the disease may have an insidious progression without significant clinical findings or may present with severe hypovolemic shock. Diagnostic paracentesis should be undertaken when spontaneous peritonitis is suspected. A neutrophil count >250 cells/m^3 in the ascitic fluid confirms the diagnosis. Gram-stain and culture may be negative. Empiric antibiotic treatment includes ceftriaxone or cefotaxime in combination with aminoglycosides.

Peritoneal dialysis-related peritonitis (PDRP) should be suspected among patients receiving peritoneal dialysis in the presence of fever, local signs at the entry site of the cannula, or changes in the characteristics of the dialysate. Cytologic analysis of the dialysate after a dwell time of approximately 40 minutes usually shows >100 white blood cells/μL (polymorphonuclear > 50%). The empiric antibiotic treatment depends on the predominant infections in each center.

Secondary Peritonitis

Secondary peritonitis occurs when bacteria enter the peritoneal cavity through a perforation of the intestinal wall, other viscus, surgical site, or abscess. Perforation may result from inflammatory diseases (such as CD), gangrenous cholecystitis, typhlitis, or peripancreatic abscess. In postpubertal females, *Neisseria gonorrhoeae* and *Chlamydia trachomatis* may invade the pelvic cavity through the fallopian tubes. Symptoms include high fever, diffuse abdominal pain, and vomiting. Physical findings include rebound tenderness, abdominal wall rigidity, and diminished or absent bowel sounds. Leukocytosis is usually present. Upright abdominal X-ray may show free air in the abdominal cavity, ileus, and signs of obstruction or obliteration of the psoas shadow.

Tertiary Peritonitis

Tertiary peritonitis is the appearance of peritonitis following the failure of one or more surgical procedures undertaken to control an intra-abdominal focus of infection. It is characterized by nosocomial polymicrobial flora, such as coagulase-negative *Staphylococcus*, *Candida*, *Enterococcus*, *Pseudomonas*, or *Enterobacter*.

Intra-abdominal Abscesses

Abscesses may develop in abdominal viscera, such as liver, spleen, kidneys, pancreas, or uterine adnexa, as well as in the interintestinal, periappendiceal, subhepatic, pelvic, and retroperitoneal spaces. Intra-abdominal abscesses may be caused by community-acquired infections (e.g., secondary to appendicular infection) or they may be the consequence of complications related to surgical procedures. Pelvic abscesses may present symptoms such as rectal tenesmus and dysuria. Abdominal ultrasound is useful for diagnosis and to guide percutaneous drainage of fluid collections. CT is the best diagnostic tool, and oral and intravenous contrasts significantly improve diagnostic sensitivity. A combination of an aminoglycoside or third- or fourth-generation cephalosporin with an antianaerobic antimicrobial (clindamycin or metronidazole) is most frequently used. Single antibiotic regimens with imipenem, meropenem, or piperacillin-tazobactam are not superior and are more expensive. Adequate source control is usually needed (i.e., surgical removal or drainage of the primary cause). Percutaneous drainage may be possible for a well-circumscribed, accessible abscess that is not loculated.

Necrotizing Enterocolitis

Necrotizing enterocolitis (NEC) occurs between 0.3 and 2.4 per 1000 live births. It is more frequent among younger preterm neonates. It is characterized by bowel necrosis and multisystem organ failure. NEC usually occurs during the second week of life after initiation of enteral feeds. Diagnosis is based on physical examination, laboratory studies, and abdominal radiographies. Up to 25%–50% of patients with NEC require surgical intervention. Significant bowel resection is one of the most severe complications of NEC and is the major cause of short-bowel syndrome in pediatric patients. Mortality is 20%–30% for infants that require surgery.

Prenatal glucocorticoids act as an intestinal maturation factor and help to prevent NEC. Risk factors for NEC are: (a) preterm birth, (b) enteral feedings, (c) dysfunctional motility, (d) reduced intestinal blood flow, (e) microbe-induced proinflammatory epithelial signaling, and (f) enteroinvasive infection. NEC is rare in term infants and is usually associated with congenital cardiovascular disease, intestinal atresia, sepsis, hypotension, premature rupture of membranes, chorioamnionitis, and exchange transfusion. There are reports of institutional outbreaks. Exposure to antibiotics may delay beneficial colonization by normal gastrointestinal flora and promote development of pathogens. The role of probiotic and prebiotic agents is currently being evaluated.

Clinical signs of NEC are feeding intolerance, abdominal distention, tenderness, and gross blood in stools. The abdominal wall can present with reddish or bluish discoloration and is painful at palpation. The NG tube may retrieve variable volumes of gastric and later bilious residuals. General clinical signs include temperature instability, alterations in the glucose levels, lethargy, apnea, bradycardia, or hypotension. Abdominal radiographic views can show irregular gas distribution with intestinal distension, pneumoperitoneum, pneumatosis, portal venous gas, or a fixed loop. The presence of gas in the portal venous tree is due to the passage of gas from the bowel wall in patients with pneumatosis and suggests a poor prognosis. There is no specific laboratory study that confirms NEC diagnosis.

Medical treatment consists of gut rest, antibiotic therapy against enteropathogenic bacteria, and clinical stabilization of the septic syndrome (hemodynamic support, respiratory assistance, and correction of hematologic, hydroelectrolytic, and metabolic alterations). Gastric decompression via orogastric tube minimizes gut distention. Discontinuation of enteral feeds is usually indicated for ~7–10 days. Total parenteral nutrition should be used until enteral alimentation can deliver adequate calories. Surgical priorities are control of sepsis by removal of necrotic bowel and preservation of intestine to avoid short-bowel syndrome. Defining the best moment for surgery can be difficult. Some advocate peritoneal drainage instead of surgery, but a recent meta-analysis showed a 50% increase in mortality with peritoneal drainage compared to laparotomy.

Neutropenic Enterocolitis

Typhlitis, also known as neutropenic enterocolitis, is an acute life-threatening condition characterized by transmural necrotizing inflammation of the cecum with possible extension to terminal ileum and ascending colon. It occurs in children receiving chemotherapy for lymphomas, leukemias, and solid tumors or after conditioning for bone marrow transplantation, but can also present in children receiving immunosuppressive therapy for solid-organ transplants or with acquired immunodeficiency syndrome. The most common symptoms are abdominal pain and fever, but nausea, vomiting, and diarrhea are frequently present. Pain may be localized in the right iliac fossa or may be diffuse. Abdominal distension and peritoneal signs are associated with more severe disease. Neutropenia (absolute neutrophil count < 500 cells/μL) is found in most patients. The diagnosis is confirmed by ultrasound or CT showing thickening of the walls of the cecum or other involved areas. Other findings may include mucosal edema, fat or mesenteric infiltration, pneumatosis, hepatic portal venous gas, and free cavity fluid. Treatment is with broad-spectrum antibiotics and intestinal rest. Parenteral nutrition should be given until enteral feeds can be started. Placement of an NG tube is usually necessary. Recombinant granulocyte colony-stimulating factor may improve the neutrophil count. Conservative medical treatment may be preferred due to the risks of surgery in patients with frequent pancytopenia. Signs of perforation, persistent bleeding, or progressive worsening that require hemodynamic or respiratory support indicate the need of surgery.

Acute Pancreatitis

Inflammation of the pancreas can cause an acute abdomen and life-threatening disease when severe or with local complications (necrosis, pseudocyst formation, or pancreatic abscesses). These cases may develop systemic inflammatory manifestations or multiorgan failure. Approximately 30% of pediatric cases have no identifiable cause, and the remainder are obstructive (e.g., choledochal cysts, pancreatic duct stricture, or stones) or nonobstructive (e.g., trauma, hemorrhage, infection, or medications). Hereditary forms may arise from mutations in the trypsinogen gene or in the cystic fibrosis transmembrane regulator gene. Genetic assays can detect alterations and explain some cases of recurrent pancreatitis, previously categorized as idiopathic. Milder inflammation with only moderate increase of amylase and lipase is usually the consequence of viral infection or systemic diseases. Pancreatitis is rare in the previously healthy child.

Children usually present as acutely ill with nausea, vomiting, and abdominal pain. The pain is usually epigastric and may radiate toward the back. Abdominal distension and muscular guarding are frequent features. Hemodynamic compromise, fever, jaundice, ascites, hypocalcemia, and pleural effusion may be present. The diagnosis is confirmed by increased amylase and lipase levels of at least three times the normal value. Lipase elevation is more specific in adults; this has not been validated in pediatrics. Pancreatic enzymes may be elevated in other situations, including perforated gastroduodenal ulcers, intestinal perforation or occlusion, peritonitis, acidosis, and renal failure. Ultrasound and CT scan can confirm the diagnosis, evaluate the etiology, and search for complications. Ultrasound helps locate gall stones. In 20% of pediatric cases, the initial ultrasound is normal. The CT scan is the most useful study to confirm the diagnosis and contrast allows the identification of necrotic areas. When contrast cannot be used, MRI is an alternative. MR cholangiopancreatography and endoscopic ultrasonography have been incorporated as diagnostic tools in pediatric care. Endoscopic retrograde cholangiopancreatography can be used in patients with recurrent pancreatitis and in selected case of AP or choledocholithiasis.

Management includes early fluid resuscitation, NG tube insertion, and parenteral nutrition while enteral feedings are withheld. Opioids should be used with caution because of biliary spasm. Hypocalcemia and hyperglycemia may require treatment. Gastric acid should be suppressed using antacids. No clear evidence supports prophylactic antibiotic treatment in preventing infection of the necrotic areas. When the area of necrosis exceeds 30% of the parenchyma, the risk of infection is increased and antibiotics may be considered. Enteral feeding can be started once symptoms subside and pancreatic enzymes decrease; however, ~20% of patients will not tolerate feeding. A meta-analysis in adults shows a lower risk of infection, reduced need for surgery, and reduced length of stay in an early enteral nutrition group.

A frequent complication is the formation of pseudocysts, named for the capsule that is formed by granulation tissue without an epithelial layer. These are diagnosed by ultrasound, are usually asymptomatic, and often resolve spontaneously. With persistent vomiting, pain, ileus, and elevated enzymes, percutaneous drainage or laparotomy should be considered. Local infection should be suspected in the presence of fever, leukocytosis, pain, or abdominal guarding. Patients with infected necrosis require surgical debridement or percutaneous drainage of necrotic material. The mortality in children is lower than adults; however, it can be as high as 10%.

Inflammatory Bowel Disease

Inflammatory bowel disease includes two important entities, ulcerative colitis (UC) and CD. Clinical manifestations include abdominal pain, diarrhea, vomiting, lethargy, dehydration, weight loss, anemia, hypoalbuminemia, or signs of systemic toxicity. Manifestations of severe abdominal disease are acute bloody diarrhea, acute ileitis, and acute abdomen. Fistulas, abscesses, perforations, and intestinal obstruction are possible causes of acute abdomen in CD, whereas UC can present with toxic dilatation of the colon, potentially resulting in toxic megacolon with high risk of perforation or severe bleeding. Abdominal CT and MRI may help to identify transmural lesions and bowel dilations and to exclude strictures. Endoscopy shows patchy lesions and granulomas and is used for initial diagnosis. Biopsies should be obtained to confirm the diagnosis.

Treatment is with steroids or other immunosuppressive agents as rescue therapy. Severe hemorrhage may require surgical intervention. Intra-abdominal abscesses are usually localized in the terminal ileum. Percutaneous drainage in combination with antibiotic treatment is frequently effective. Bowel obstruction is most frequent in ileal CD. Obstruction is usually not complete and improves with medical treatment that includes enteral rest, gastric drainage, adequate fluid replacement, and frequent radiologic evaluation. If obstruction is complete, surgical treatment is indicated.

Pelvic Inflammatory Disease

Pelvic inflammatory disease (PID) is an infection of the upper genital tract that frequently involves the endometrium and fallopian tubes. It can be the cause of acute lower abdominal pain in sexually active female adolescents. The clinical presentation is variable, and the most frequent symptoms in mild disease are dyspareunia (pain during sexual activity), lower abdominal pain, and vaginal discharge. Patients with severe PID are ill-appearing and often have intense pain, fever, or vomiting. Abdominal complications include tubo-ovarian abscess, ectopic pregnancy, and chronic pain.

ABDOMINAL PATHOLOGY OF THE CRITICAL PATIENT

Ileus

Ileus is intestinal dysmotility in the absence of a mechanical obstruction. Symptoms include diminished or absent bowel sounds, failure to pass stools or flatus, abdominal distension, vomiting or increased drainage through the NG tube, and increased gastric residual volume during enteral feeds. The three types of ileus are adynamic, spastic, and ischemic. The latter is observed in hemodynamically unstable patients or in patients with nonocclusive mesenteric ischemia. Abdominal CT has a high sensitivity and specificity to differentiate ileus from mechanical obstruction. The causes of ileus are multiple, the most frequent being intestinal manipulation during abdominal surgery. Severe sepsis can cause ileus by diminishing visceral muscle contractility. Narcotic administration is another contributing factor for ileus. Severe hypokalemia, exogenous catecholamines, general anesthetics, and medications, such as benzodiazepines, calcium-channel blocking agents, and anticholinergics, may be involved in the development of ileus. The primary treatment for ileus is gastric decompression with an NG tube to reduce the risk of vomiting and aspiration pneumonia. The use of promotility drugs should be undertaken with caution, only after ruling out other causes of an acute abdomen.

Pseudomembranous Colitis

Clostridium difficile is a gram-positive, anaerobic, spore-forming rod that can cause colitis. The spores germinate in the anaerobic environment of the colon before toxin is released. The incidence of *C. difficile* infection among hospitalized children is increasing. Manifestations of disease range from mild diarrhea to pseudomembranous colitis or toxic megacolon. Severe *C. difficile* infection is suspected in the presence of fever, rigors, abdominal pain, leukocytosis, increased serum creatinine, endoscopic findings consistent with pseudomembranous colitis, or evidence of colitis on CT scan. *C. difficile* usually affects patients who are receiving or have received antibiotics during the previous 3 weeks. The diagnosis is confirmed by stool culture, stool assay for toxin, cytotoxin test in tissue cultures (to detect toxin B), or polymerase chain reaction. Treatment with metronidazole is used for mild-to-moderate cases. Severe infection is treated with oral vancomycin. In the presence of systemic compromise, ileus or toxic megacolon, oral vancomycin plus IV metronidazole is recommended. Broad-spectrum antibiotics should be stopped to stimulate recovery of endogenous flora.

Toxic Megacolon

Toxic megacolon can develop as a consequence of inflammatory bowel disease and present as an acute abdomen characterized by colonic dilation with systemic toxicity. It can also be seen with infections such as *C. difficile*, *Salmonella*, *Shigella*, *Yersinia*, *C. jejuni*, *E. coli*, cytomegalovirus, rotavirus, and others. Examination of the abdomen may show distension, tenderness, and reduced bowel sounds or signs of peritonitis that may indicate colonic perforation. The most severe cases can progress to septic shock and multiorgan failure. Plain abdominal X-ray shows dilatation of the colon usually in the ascending and transverse portions. Fluid–air levels and alteration of the normal haustration can also be evident. CT scan shows colonic dilation, submucosal edema, areas of wall thickening, or areas of wall thinning, and is useful to detect intra-abdominal complications. Ultrasound may aid in the diagnosis also by demonstrating the colonic dilatation.

Electrolyte abnormalities that deteriorate the tone of the colon, especially hypokalemia and dehydration, should be corrected. Severe anemia and hypoglycemia need to be corrected. The use of drugs that inhibit colonic movement should be avoided. Bowel rest with parenteral nutrition is necessary during the acute phase. NG suction has no effect on colonic dilatation and is usually not necessary. For UC, steroid therapy should be started rapidly. If an infectious cause is suspected, appropriate antimicrobial treatment should be started. Enteral probiotics that stimulate the immune response are being evaluated. Surgical resection by subtotal colectomy may be necessary.

ACUTE ABDOMINAL MANIFESTATION OF SYSTEMIC DISEASES

Some children present with symptoms of an abdominal surgical emergency in the context of systemic diseases. Recognizing these situations may avoid unnecessary surgical interventions. *Diabetic ketoacidosis* may present with abdominal pain, vomiting, a tense abdomen, guarding, and absent bowel sounds, simulating an acute abdomen. *Porphyrias* are both hereditary and acquired diseases in which the activity of the enzymes responsible for the heme biosynthesis pathways is deficient. *Acute intermittent porphyria* may present with nausea, vomiting, abdominal pain, diarrhea, constipation, or ileus and may occasionally be confused with an acute surgical abdomen. *Rheumatologic diseases* may cause abdominal complications that include ischemic lesions due to mesenteric vascular compromise. *Henoch–Schönlein purpura* is a vasculitis that affects small vessels and is the most frequent cause of nonthrombocytopenic purpura in children. The association of colicky abdominal pain, arthralgia or arthritis, edema in dependent or distensible areas, palpable nonthrombocytopenic purpura, and proteinuria is the basis of the diagnosis. *Kawasaki disease* is occasionally associated with severe abdominal symptoms. *Sickle cell disease* can have severe abdominal pain as one of the clinical manifestations.

CHAPTER 79 ■ DIAGNOSTIC IMAGING OF THE ABDOMEN

SWAPNIL S. BAGADE AND REBECCA HULETT BOWLING

PLAIN RADIOGRAPHS

The plain abdominal radiograph is an indispensable tool for both suspected abdominal pathology and the placement of tubes and catheters in children. Low-dose techniques using increased tube potential (kVp) between 60 and 70 and a low milliampere-second (mAs) of 2–4 significantly decrease the radiation dose. Assessment of the abdomen can include supine, decubitus, and cross-table lateral views. The left lateral decubitus view is preferred over the right lateral decubitus view for detection of a pneumoperitoneum because gas is easily seen between liver and abdominal wall. The bowel gas pattern should show symmetric loops that often have a polygonal pattern ("chicken wire") on the supine image (**Fig. 79.1**). Free intraperitoneal fluid may be seen on a plain film if the amount is sufficient; it will cause the bowel loops to move centrally, with increased opacity in the flanks (**Fig. 79.2**). Abdominal radiographs may also reveal a lower lobe pneumonia or pleural effusion.

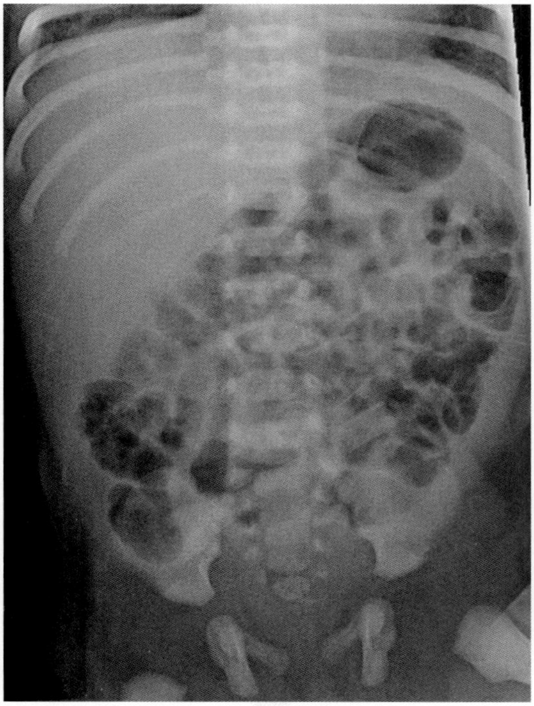

FIGURE 79.1. Normal abdominal bowel gas pattern.

Abnormal Plain Film Findings

Bowel Obstruction

Differentiation between large and small bowel on plain film in neonates and very young children can be difficult. The radiologic findings in obstruction differ depending on the level of pathology. Air may be only in the stomach in cases of gastric outlet obstruction such as in pyloric stenosis, antral dyskinesia, or antral

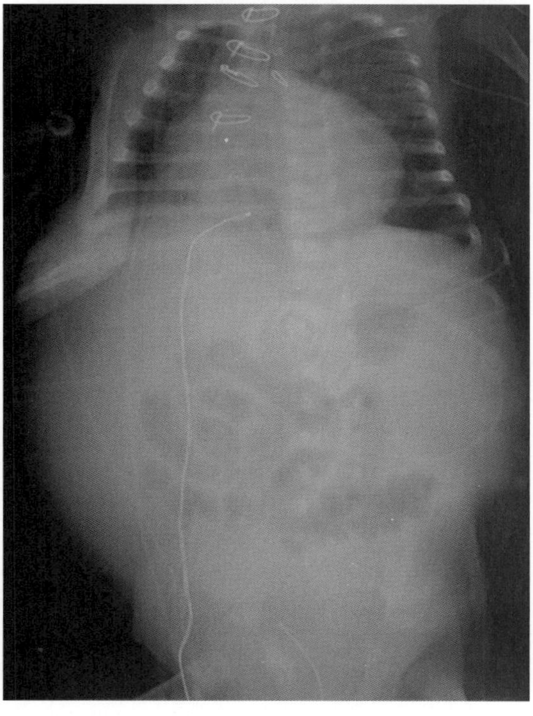

FIGURE 79.2. Increased soft-tissue density in the periphery of the abdomen (from ascitic fluid) with centrally located (floating) bowel loops.

web. Two dilated bowel loops (double bubble) are seen with duodenal atresia (DA), annular pancreas, or duodenal web. A low bowel obstruction shows multiple loops of dilated bowel. Contrast enemas are helpful in determining whether the colon or distal small bowel is the cause of low intestinal obstruction.

Pneumoperitoneum

Causes of pneumoperitoneum include necrotizing enterocolitis (NEC), spontaneous perforation, ruptured Meckel diverticulum, dissection from pneumomediastinum, gastric perforation (e.g., from a nasogastric tube, mechanical ventilation, indomethacin administration, or child abuse), colonic perforation (possibly secondary to an enema or a rectal thermometer), peritoneal dialysis, paracentesis, recent surgery, and abdominal trauma. Locations of gas in the abdomen include intraluminal, extraluminal, intramural, and intraparenchymal. Free intraperitoneal air (extraluminal) is seen in nondependent areas (subdiaphragmatic along the liver dome, or along the lateral margin of the liver in a left lateral decubitus view) (**Fig. 79.3A and B**). Portal venous gas can be seen as branching linear lucencies along the periphery of the liver (**Fig. 79.4**).

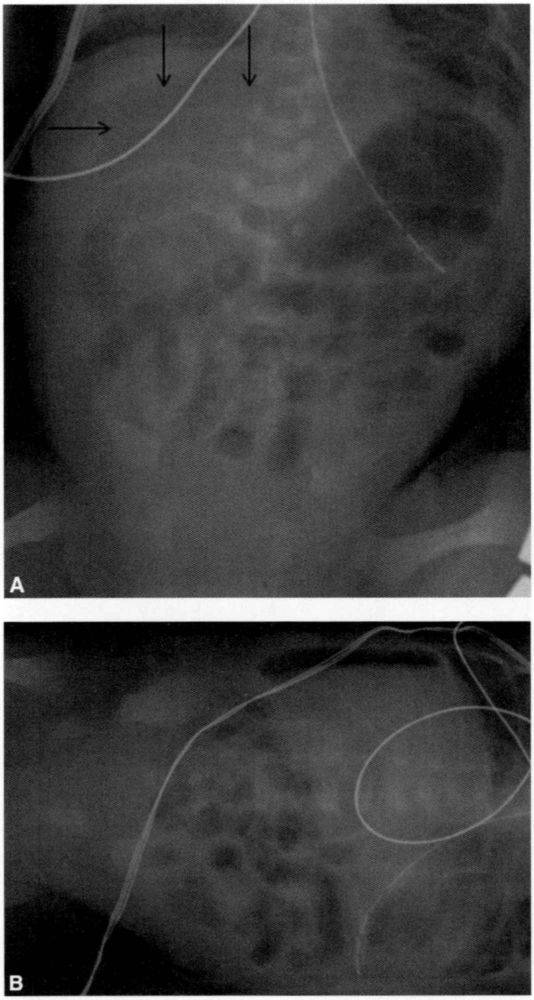

FIGURE 79.3. Pneumoperitoneum. **A:** Large amount of free intraperitoneal air causing lucency (*arrows*) over upper abdomen and liver. No definite pneumatosis or portal venous gas identified. **B:** Free air is seen bordering the edge of the liver on lateral decubitus view. Patient had bowel perforation.

Pneumatosis Intestinalis

Pneumatosis intestinalis (PI) is when air accumulates within the bowel wall. In cases of NEC, it portends bowel infarction. PI can also appear in intestinal ischemia, bowel obstruction, graft-versus-host disease, short-bowel syndrome, infection with rotavirus, decompensated cardiac disease, and nonischemic colitis. A more benign occurrence of pneumatosis can be seen in chronic steroid use, immunodeficiency, nutritional deficiencies, bronchopulmonary dysplasia (BPD), or pneumomediastinum. On radiographs, pneumatosis may appear as small linear or bubbly lucencies within the bowel wall (**Fig. 79.5**).

Abdominal Masses

Plain abdominal radiographs are the initial imaging performed in the evaluation of a suspected abdominal mass and may help determine the location of the mass, associated bowel obstruction, and whether calcifications are present. Sonography is a useful adjunct in the workup of abdominal masses.

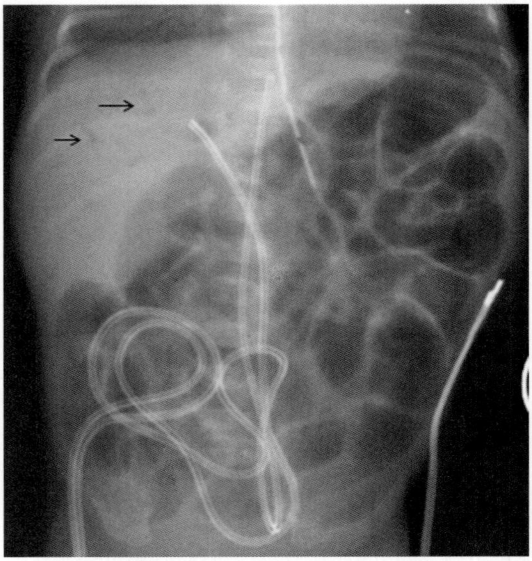

FIGURE 79.4. Portal venous gas. Abdominal radiograph showing branching linear lucencies (*arrows*) along the periphery of the liver owing to portal venous gas.

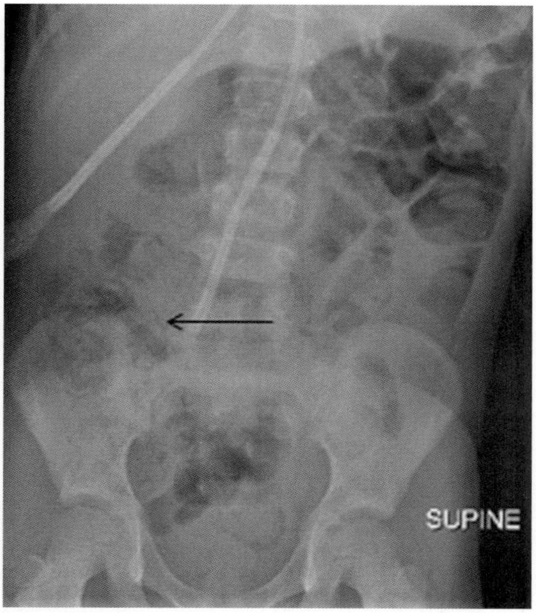

FIGURE 79.5. Pneumatosis intestinalis. Intramural air in the right-sided bowel is seen as streaky lucencies in the right abdomen (*arrow*). This patient was a 7-year-old with inflammation of the ileocecal area who developed PI.

CONTRAST STUDIES

An upper gastrointestinal (UGI) study includes the esophagus, stomach, and duodenum to the duodenojejunal junction and is adequate to assess malrotation. A small-bowel follow-through (SBFT) is used to assess the small bowel beyond the duodenum to the cecum, using serial imaging over several hours.

ULTRASOUND

Ultrasonography (US) is usually the first investigation in a child with a palpable abdominal mass after a plain film. US can also be used to evaluate the relationship of the superior mesenteric artery (SMA) with the superior mesenteric vein (SMV) in cases of malrotation. High-resolution US can be used to evaluate the bowel wall and to detect pneumatosis and portal venous gas. US is the modality of choice to confirm the presence or absence of intussusception. US is also an excellent tool to assess for ascites and can be used to guide paracentesis. US is the first approach in suspected post–liver transplant complications including hepatic artery thrombosis, hepatic necrosis, perihepatic fluid collections, and biliary obstructions. Doppler also reliably determines the portal vein flow direction and velocity. The lack of ionizing radiation, easy portability, and availability makes it an ideal modality for use in children.

COMPUTED TOMOGRAPHY

Computed tomography (CT) is performed only when radiographs or US does not diagnose the condition. CT is more useful than US in trauma and to delineate the extent of visceral and intraperitoneal abscesses. When ordering CT imaging, one should consider alternative imaging modalities not involving ionizing radiation such as US or magnetic resonance imaging (MRI). Development is underway of CT scanner algorithms that decrease radiation dose while maintaining images of diagnostic quality.

MAGNETIC RESONANCE IMAGING

Improved detail due to better soft-tissue contrast and lack of ionizing radiation make MRI an important tool. The limitations for MRI are its cost, availability, and motion artifacts due to long scanning time. Various fast imaging techniques can reduce motion artifact. Techniques such as MR cholangiopancreatography to evaluate biliary and pancreatic abnormalities, MR enterography for gastrointestinal pathologies, and MR urography for evaluation of renal collecting system abnormalities and renal function are available. Diffusion-weighted sequences are used widely for imaging of neoplasms.

Differential Diagnosis and Imaging of Abdominal Pathology

Esophageal atresia with Tracheoesophageal Fistula (TEF)

Esophageal atresia (EA) is the most common congenital abnormality of the esophagus. A dilated esophageal pouch in the neck with absent abdominal bowel gas may be seen in EA without a distal fistula (**Fig. 79.6A**). The most suggestive finding on the radiograph in a newborn is coiling of the nasogastric tube in the proximal esophagus (**Fig. 79.6B**).

Diaphragmatic (Bochdalek) Hernia

On the chest radiograph, bowel loops are seen within the thoracic cavity with contralateral mediastinal shift (**Fig. 79.7**). The position of the tip of the nasogastric tube localizes the stomach.

Hypertrophic Pyloric Stenosis

The caterpillar sign (markedly dilated stomach with exaggerated incisura) may be seen on plain film and represents a distended, peristalsing stomach. US is the imaging gold standard and the method of choice for both diagnosis and exclusion of hypertrophic pyloric stenosis (HPS) with a sensitivity and specificity of close to 100%.

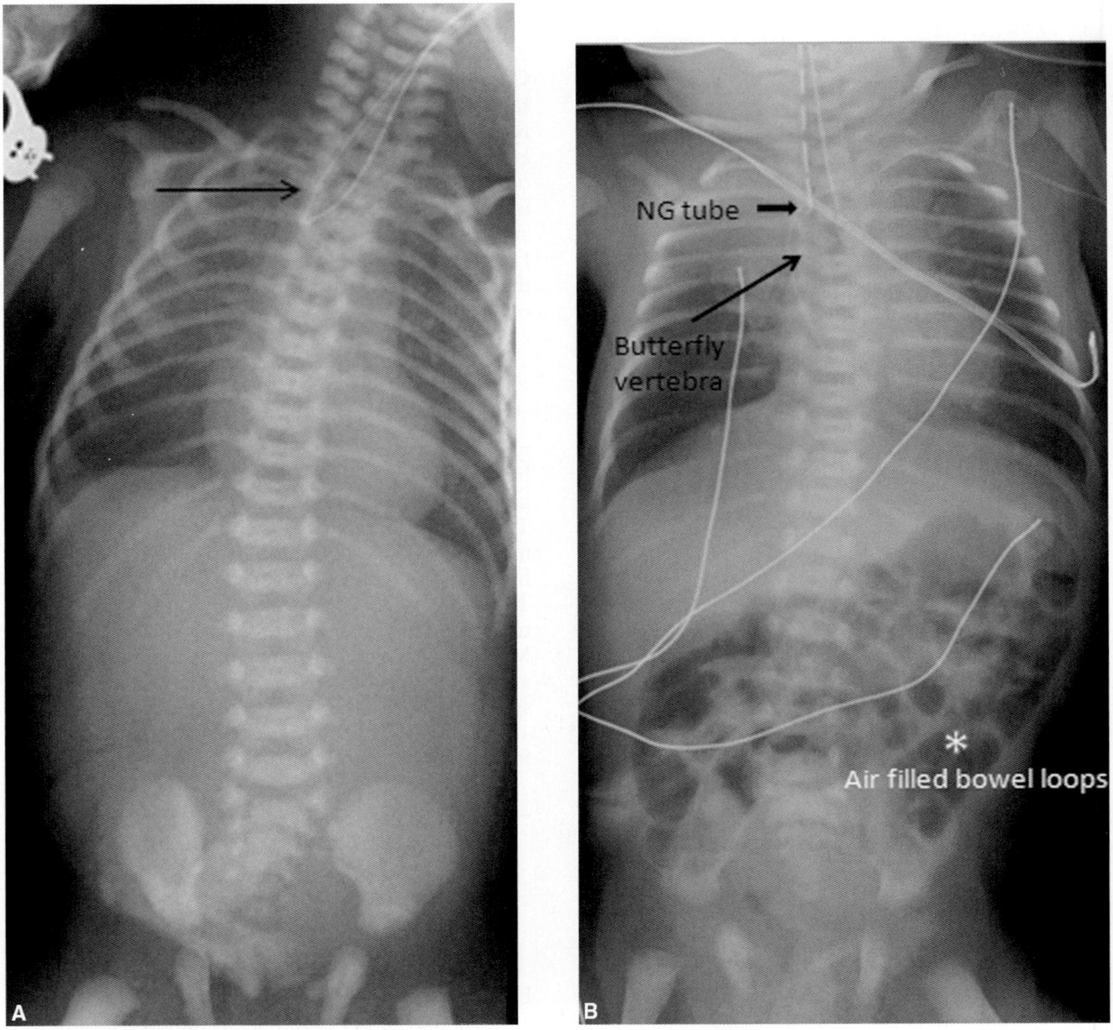

FIGURE 79.6. Esophageal atresia. **A:** The tip of the nasogastric tube is doubled back on itself in the upper esophagus (*arrow*) and is positioned in the region of the pharynx. Gasless abdomen suggests absence of distal TEF. **B:** Known case of EA with TEF in which the NG tube terminates high in the thorax (*short arrow*). Air-filled bowel loops are seen (*asterisk*). Patient also had 13 ribs with a butterfly T4 vertebra (*long arrow*). EA plus TEF can occur as a part of VACTERL association.

Congenital Gastric/Duodenal Obstruction

DA is the most common cause of high intestinal obstruction in a child, and the diagnostic plain radiograph finding is a *double bubble*, with air present in the distended stomach and duodenal bulb.

Malrotation and Volvulus

Malrotation of the intestines results when the intestinal rotation and fixation fail to occur during fetal life. Fibrous adhesive (Ladd's) bands are usually present. Plain radiographs often fail to provide convincing evidence of malrotation. An UGI contrast series is the gold standard for diagnosis. Radiographic findings of malrotation include displacement of the duodenojejunal junction from its normal left upper quadrant location to the right side and inferiorly with a relative anterior position of the duodenum on the lateral view. The third part of the duodenum does not cross the midline, and the proximal small bowel is seen on the right side of the abdomen. If volvulus occurs, there is spiraling of the small bowel downward, often to the right of midline.

Meconium Ileus

This usually occurs in patients with cystic fibrosis as they produce thick, tenacious meconium in utero.

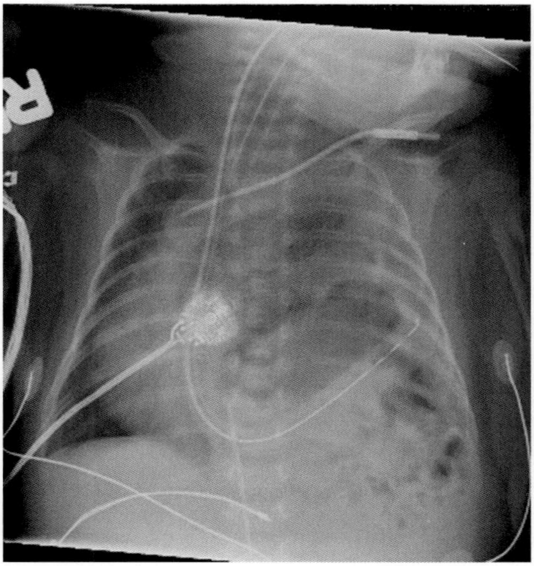

FIGURE 79.7. Diaphragmatic hernia. Newborn with left diaphragmatic hernia with bowel loops in the lower left chest and contralateral mediastinal shift. Tip of the NG tube indicates intrathoracic position of the stomach.

On imaging, low intestinal obstruction is noted with a bubbly appearance in the right lower quadrant owing to air mixed with meconium (**Fig. 79.8A**). A water-soluble contrast enema typically shows a microcolon and multiple filling defects in the terminal ileum (**Fig. 79.8B**). An attempt is made to reflux the contrast into the terminal ileum in order to relieve the obstruction. Serial enemas can be performed as long as the patient remains stable.

Hirschsprung Disease

Hirschsprung disease (HD) is a functional low intestinal obstruction resulting from absence of ganglion cells in the myenteric plexus of the distal bowel. There may be ultrashort segment disease involving the internal sphincter, short segment disease involving the rectum and a portion of the sigmoid, long segment disease involving a variable portion of colon, or total aganglionosis involving the entire colon and variable portion of small bowel. On contrast enema, the transition zone is visualized at the site of absent ganglion cells. An abnormal rectosigmoid index is seen with the diameter of the rectum appearing narrower than the diameter of the sigmoid (**Fig. 79.9A** and **B**). Toxic megacolon appears as mucosal irregularity, colonic dilation, and possibly a colon cut-off sign in the rectosigmoid region with absence of air distally. These patients should not undergo enema, as the risk for perforation is high.

Gastroenteritis

In gastroenteritis, diffuse bowel distension without evidence of focal obstruction is seen on abdominal

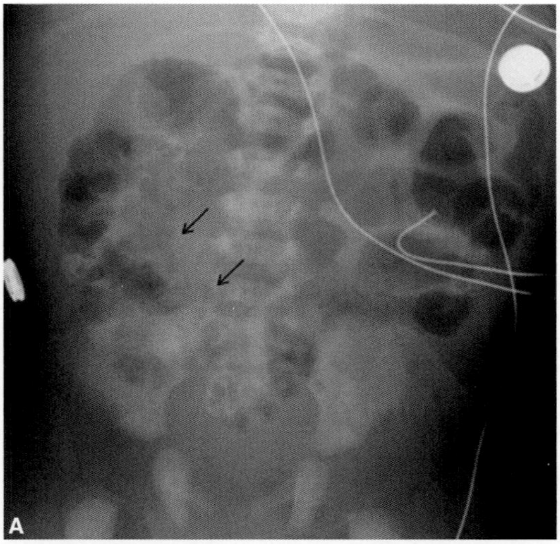

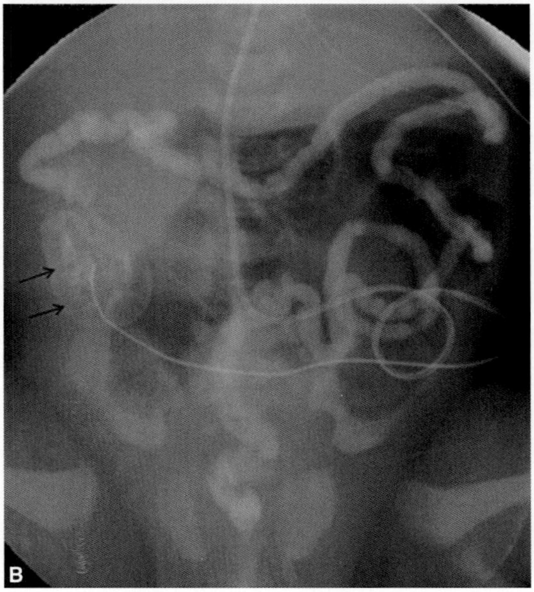

FIGURE 79.8. Newborn with delayed passage of meconium. **A:** Bubbly lucencies are seen within the right lower quadrant (*arrows*) in a patient with meconium ileus. **B:** Lower GI study in a newborn with delayed passage of meconium shows microcolon with multiple filling defects (*arrows*) in the terminal ileum, compatible with meconium ileus.

radiographs (**Fig. 79.10**). US may be successful in demonstrating thickened bowel wall, particularly in the ileocecal region with or without free peritoneal fluid. Bowel wall thickening with enhancement is a nonspecific feature on CT scan.

Meconium Peritonitis

Meconium when leaked into peritoneum, either by obstruction or by malformation, causes chemical

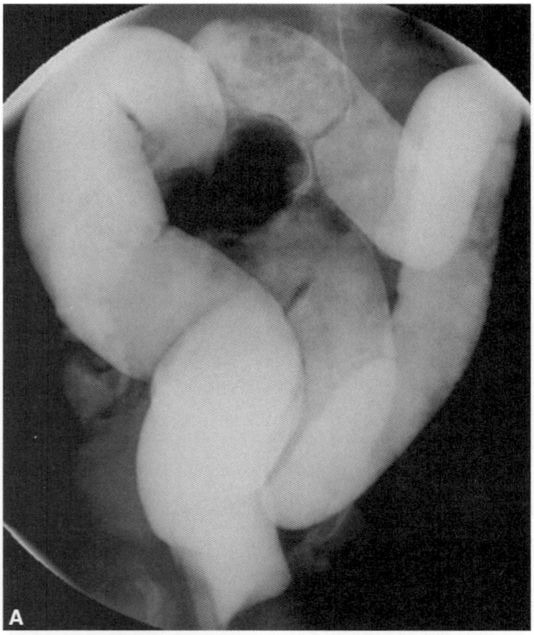

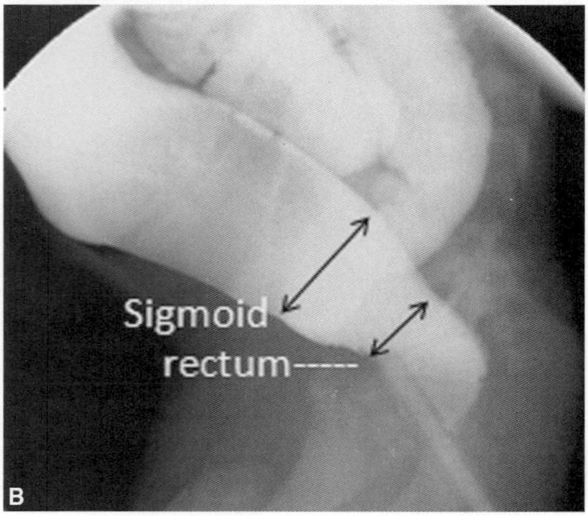

FIGURE 79.9. Hirschsprung disease. **A** and **B:** Four-week-old boy with constipation and poor feeding. Lower GI study with ionic contrast instilled in usual retrograde fashion in the rectum by gravity filling the colon up to the cecum. There is no presacral mass. There is no definite transition zone identified. The diameter of the sigmoid is larger than that of the rectum (rectosigmoid ratio < 1, consistent with HD at the rectosigmoid level).

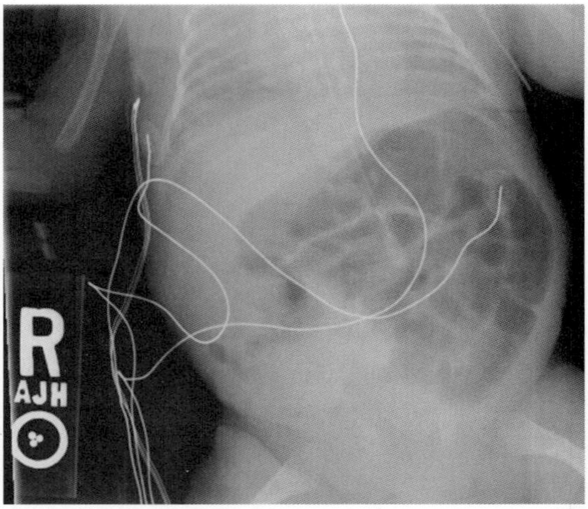

FIGURE 79.10. Gastroenteritis. Four-week-old boy with abdominal distension and diarrhea. Radiograph shows diffuse bowel dilation with a paucity of bowel gas in the right lower quadrants.

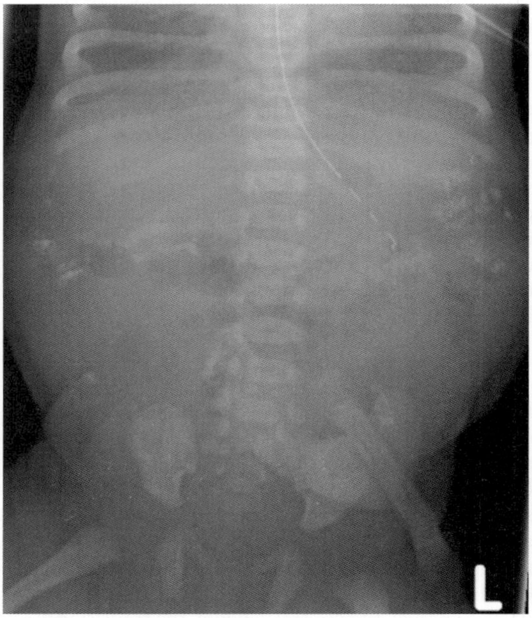

FIGURE 79.11. Meconium peritonitis. Diffuse coarse abdominal calcification. The meconium in the peritoneum secondary to bowel perforation tends to result in scattered intra-abdominal calcifications.

peritonitis. The resulting diffuse peritoneal inflammation results in calcifications scattered throughout the abdomen often seen well on plain films (**Fig. 79.11**).

Hepatitis and Hepatic Abscess

US in hepatitis shows heterogeneous echogenicity of the liver with or without periportal thickening. The gallbladder and the biliary tree are normal. Often, the US may not show any findings. With hepatic abscess, US shows a hypoechoic center with irregular margin in a pyogenic abscess. Peripheral heterogenous wall enhancement with a necrotic nonenhancing center on CT is suggestive of abscess in the correct clinical setting. Internal gas may also be seen.

Appendicitis

Acute appendicitis is an important differential in children with acute abdominal pain, and it is the most common cause of a pediatric acute abdomen requiring surgery. US is the first diagnostic study in children for whom an experienced surgeon has determined the findings for appendicitis to be equivocal. If the US is nondiagnostic and urgent diagnosis is indicated, the patient should undergo contrast-enhanced CT. The US usually shows a dilated appendix (diameter 7 mm or more) with thickened walls with hyperemia seen on Doppler. Surrounding anechoic fluid and an echogenic appendicolith are other findings sometimes seen on US (**Fig. 79.12A** and **B**). CT may also detect peritoneal abscess in the case of perforated appendicitis, which might track away to a location other than the right lower quadrant.

Meckel Diverticulitis and Bleeding

Meckel diverticulum is the most common embryologic remnant of the omphalomesenteric duct (OMD), seen in 2% of the population. Technetium-99m pertechnetate scintigraphy is the investigation of choice in evaluation of pediatric patients with suspected bleeding from a Meckel diverticulum (**Fig. 79.13**). US has a limited role in imaging of remnants of the OMD.

Typhlitis or Neutropenic Colitis

Typhlitis or neutropenic colitis is inflammation in neutropenic patients involving the cecum, which may also involve the ascending colon or terminal ileum. Bowel wall thickening is the most notable finding on imaging, which is accurately measured by US and correlates with the duration of neutropenia. CT scan will show a thickened cecal wall with or without involvement of the terminal ileum.

Masses

MRI is the investigation of choice in patients with liver lesions, but US may provide preliminary information. In neonates, the most frequent primary tumors are infantile hemangioendothelioma, cavernous hemangioma, mesenchymal hamartoma, hepatoblastoma, and, less commonly, benign or malignant germ cell tumors. In older children, benign hepatic lesions, including infantile hemangioendothelioma (commonest), hepatic cysts, adenoma, and focal nodular hyperplasia, can occur. Other malignant tumors in this age group include hepatocellular carcinoma, fibrolamellar carcinoma, angiosarcoma, or lymphoma. Most hepatic masses are metastatic lesions, with the commonest metastases from Wilms tumor and neuroblastoma. Lymphoproliferative masses of the liver are increasingly seen. Choledochal cyst is a benign congenital anomaly of the biliary tree characterized by cystic dilatation of the extrahepatic and/or intrahepatic bile ducts. US demonstrates a cystic structure in the hepatic hilum. Magnetic resonance cholangiopancreatography (MRCP) may be useful in diagnosing biliary tract disease.

Renal masses can include hydronephrosis, multicystic dysplastic kidney, and obstructed upper pole of a duplicated collecting system. Wilms tumor (nephroblastoma) is the most common solid renal mass of childhood. Mesoblastic nephroma is the most common solid renal neoplasm in neonates and infants. Renal cell carcinoma is rare before the second decade. Neuroblastoma is a solid tumor that often arises from the adrenal gland and may be difficult to differentiate from nephroblastoma. Polycystic kidney, nephroblastomatosis, and renal vein thrombosis are other common renal masses that are detected radiographically. On abdominal radiographs, a soft-tissue renal mass may cause displacement of bowel

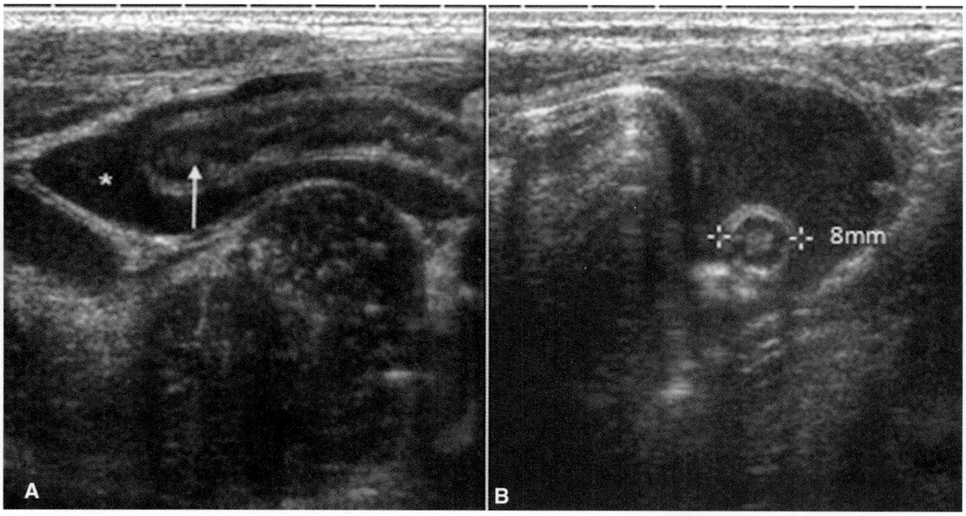

FIGURE 79.12. Appendicitis. **A** and **B**: Longitudinal and transverse US images of an inflamed appendix with a diameter of 8 mm in the right lower quadrant (*arrow*) with surrounding free fluid (*asterisk*).

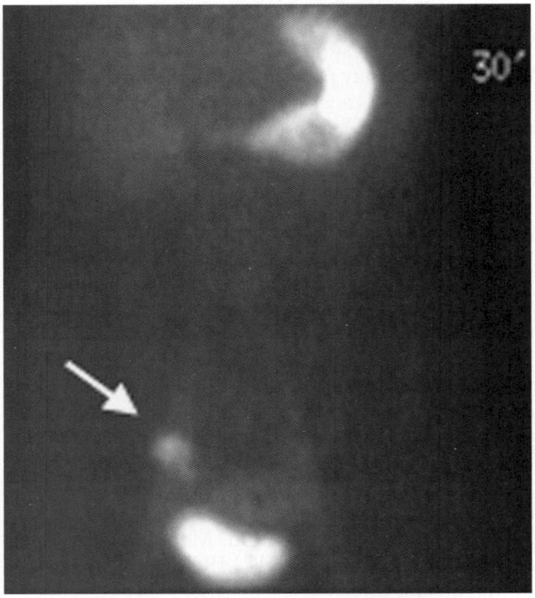

FIGURE 79.13. Meckel diverticular bleeding. Technetium-99m pertechnate scan shows a focus of gastric mucosa in the right lower abdomen (*arrow*), suggestive of Meckel diverticulum (the cause of gastrointestinal bleeding).

loops. US followed by CT scan or MRI is helpful in determining the origin as well as etiology of the mass.

The differential diagnoses of an intra-abdominal cystic lesion in the newborn (excluding renal, hepatobiliary, and retroperitoneal origin) include ovarian cyst, enteric duplication cyst, mesenteric cyst (abdominal lymphatic malformations), and meconium pseudocyst. Most gastrointestinal masses are enteric duplication cysts, occurring more commonly in the ileocecal region. The recognition of the "rim" sign of the cyst wall on US is considered virtually diagnostic of enteric duplication cysts. This comprises the echogenic inner rim of the mucosa and the hypoechoic outer rim of the muscle layer, giving a double layer.

Intussusception usually occurs in the age group of 3 months to 3 years. The classic clinical triad consists of acute colicky abdominal pain, "currant jelly" or frankly bloody stools, and either a palpable mass or vomiting. The presence of a curvilinear intraluminal mass in the right upper quadrant on plain film is highly specific for intussusception (**Fig. 79.14A**). US is a highly sensitive and specific test for intussusception and the imaging modality of choice for diagnosis. When viewed transversely, the alternating concentric hypoechoic and echogenic layers of an intussusception have an appearance referred to as the "target" or "donut" sign (**Fig. 79.14B**). Reduction of the intussusception can be performed with air or water-soluble contrast enema, and surgical intervention can be avoided in most cases.

Trauma

Focused abdominal sonography for trauma (FAST) can be employed in trauma, where the right and left upper quadrants and the pelvis are evaluated for the presence of free fluid or hemoperitoneum. US is fast and easily available and can be particularly helpful in the evaluation of a hemodynamically unstable patient. CT is the more definitive imaging modality and is useful for evaluating the injured bowel and bladder, as well as vascular injury. Because of the necessity for evaluating these patients urgently, oral contrast is generally not used. The liver is frequently injured in pediatric abdominal trauma, with the posterior segment of the right lobe the most commonly involved (**Fig. 79.15**). Splenic injury is usually associated with

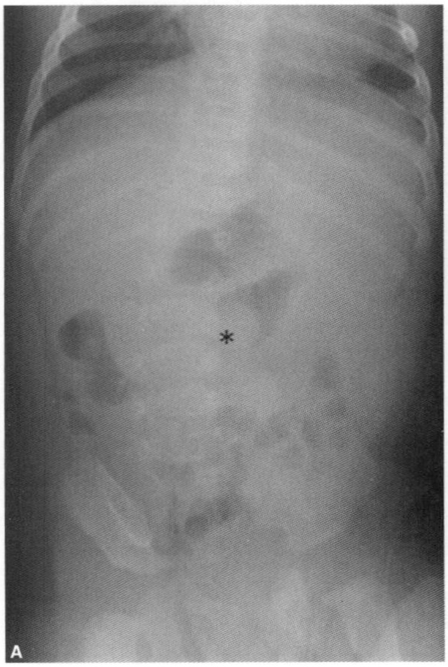

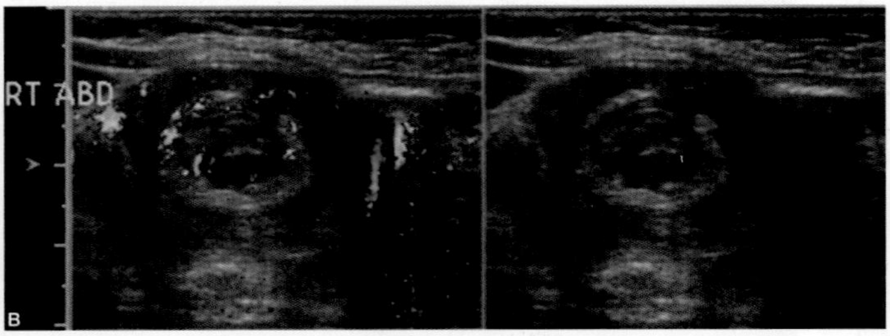

FIGURE 79.14. Intussusception. **A:** Three-month-old female with abdominal pain, vomiting, and lethargy. There is clinical concern for intussusception with an abnormal bowel gas pattern with a soft-tissue mass (*asterisk*) in the center of the abdomen seen on the obstructive series. There was no pneumoperitoneum. **B:** Targeted survey sonogram of the abdomen demonstrates the right upper quadrant ileocolic intussusception. In transverse US images, echogenic serosa of the intussusceptum is seen inside the lumen of intussuscipiens, giving rise to a target sign or donut sign through the intussusception. Color Doppler blood flow is demonstrated within the walls of bowel loops.

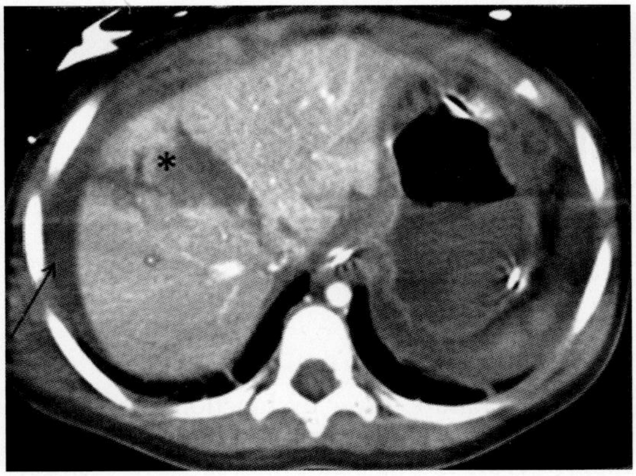

FIGURE 79.15. Liver laceration. Infant with blunt abdominal trauma. CT scan shows irregular hypoattenuation through the right hepatic lobe in keeping with a laceration (*asterisk*). Free abdominal fluid is also noted (*arrow*).

hemoperitoneum with the blood tracking along the splenorenal ligament into the anterior pararenal space around the pancreas, although 25% cases of splenic injury may not have free blood or fluid in the peritoneum. CT in the venous phase, that is, approximately 70-minute postintravenous contrast, can diagnose splenic lacerations (**Fig. 79.16**). Bowel injury can occur in the form of intramural hematoma or bowel rupture. CT scan without contrast would show a hyperdense mass in the peripancreatic region related to the duodenum with or without mass effect. In the case of rupture of the bowel wall, wall thickening, mesenteric fat infiltration, bowel wall discontinuity, or extraluminal air can be seen. Hemoperitoneum on US appears as free fluid with internal echoes. On CT, measurement of density of the peritoneal fluid helps detect the presence of blood.

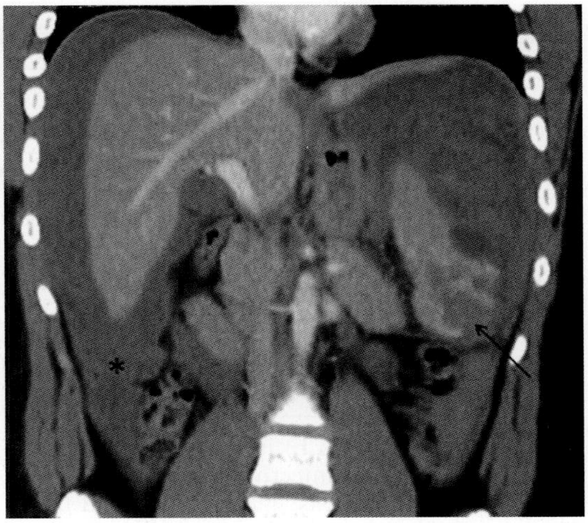

FIGURE 79.16. Splenic injury. CT with contrast of a 17-year-old with blunt abdominal injury following a football game shows splenic lacerations along the inferior pole (*arrow*) with an extensive perisplenic/subcapsular hematoma. CT scan with contrast can also help in detecting areas concerning for active extravasation as described. High-density ascites (*asterisk*) is suggestive of hemoperitoneum.

CHAPTER 80 ■ ACUTE LIVER FAILURE AND LIVER TRANSPLANTATION

PIERRE TISSIERES AND DENIS J. DEVICTOR

ACUTE LIVER FAILURE

Acute liver failure (ALF) is classified into seven categories: metabolic, infective, toxic, autoimmune, malignancy-induced, vascular-induced, and undetermined (18%–47% of cases). Early identification is important for etiologies that can be reversed with specific therapy (e.g., metabolic diseases, Wilson disease, autoimmune hepatitis, and acetaminophen-induced). Determining etiology also guides decision to transplant.

Etiologies in Neonates and Infants

Viral Infections

Enteroviruses (particularly echovirus 11) frequently cause ALF in neonates. Treatment with the anti-picornaviral drug, pleconaril, may improve outcome. Liver failure may also occur with neonatal herpes simplex virus (HSV 1 and 2) infection. Treatment is with acyclovir, but prognosis is poor. Human herpes virus 6 (HHV6), adenovirus, parvovirus B19, and paramyxovirus are other viral causes of neonatal ALF.

Inborn Metabolic Disorders

Congenital galactosemia is a recessive disorder due to deficiency of galactose-1-phosphate uridyltransferase (GALT). Elimination of dietary lactose/galactose resolves liver failure. Galactosemia should be considered in neonates with cataracts and/or *Escherichia coli* sepsis. *Hereditary fructose intolerance* (HFI) is a recessive disorder due to deficiency of fructose-1-phosphate aldolase. Symptoms develop after fructose is introduced in the diet. Elimination of fructose results in dramatic improvement. *Hereditary tyrosinemia type 1* (HT-1) is a recessive disorder caused by deficiency of fumarylacetoacetate hydrolase. The accumulation of toxic metabolites causes liver and proximal renal tubular dysfunction and porphyria-like crises. Infants present with coagulopathy soon after birth and liver failure between 1 and 6 months of age. Management includes nitisinone (NTBC [2-(2-nitro-4-trifluoromethylbenzoil)-1,3 cyclohexanedione]) therapy and a tyrosine- and phenylalanine-restricted diet. *Mitochondrial respiratory chain disorders* (e.g., inborn errors of oxidative phosphorylation) can also cause liver failure. Liver dysfunction may precede neurologic involvement by weeks, months, or years. *Inborn errors in bile acid synthesis* have been recognized as a cause of ALF associated with neonatal cholestasis. Oral administration of chenodeoxycholic acid and/or cholic acid may be curative. *Neonatal hemochromatosis* is a rare disorder of abnormal iron storage. Liver injury has been identified as early as 28 weeks of gestation. High-dose IV immunoglobulin G combined with exchange transfusion provides 75% survival without liver transplantation (LT).

Other Causes

Familial hemophagocytic lymphohistiocytosis is a rare disorder involving inappropriate activation of macrophages that can present as ALF. Initial management includes chemotherapy, but long-term survival requires a bone marrow transplant. LT is contraindicated due to recurrence in the graft.

Etiologies in Older Children

Drug- or Toxin-Induced

Acetaminophen is the most common toxic cause of ALF in the West. Toxicity results from conversion of acetaminophen to the reactive metabolite, *N*-acetyl-p-benzoquinone imine (NAPQI) by the cytochrome P450 system. NAPQI is detoxified by hepatic glutathione until depleted, and then NAPQI binds to cysteine groups, forming hepatotoxic protein adducts. Therapy is the immediate start of *N*-acetylcysteine. Volatile anesthetics (halothane, enflurane, isoflurane, and sevoflurane) cause ALF in children. Sodium valproate, carbamazepine, sulfasalazine, antituberculosis drugs, and recreational drugs (ecstasy, cocaine) can lead to drug-induced ALF. Amanita toxin (found in wild mushrooms, Amanita phalloides, Lepiota species), phosphorus, and carbon tetrachloride intoxication are other potential causes of ALF.

Immune Dysregulation

Autoimmune hepatitis is an immune reaction to liver cell antigens. Patients present with progressive jaundice, encephalopathy, and coagulopathy over 1–6 weeks. Corticosteroid treatment prior to the onset of hepatic encephalopathy (HE) may preclude the need for LT. Macrophage activation syndrome can also be associated with ALF and is frequently secondary to a viral infection (Parvovirus B19, HHV6).

Virus-Induced and Infective ALF

Hepatitis virus (A, B, and E), adenovirus, HHV6, parvovirus B19, and Epstein–Barr virus (EBV) can cause pediatric ALF. In rare cases, congenital syphilis could cause ALF in infants. Leptospirosis, brucellosis, Q fever, and dengue fever have been reported to cause ALF.

Metabolic Causes

Wilson disease is the most common metabolic disease cause of ALF in children >7 years. They have Coombs-negative hemolytic anemia, coagulopathy, increased serum aminotransferase levels, low alkaline phosphatase, and elevated bilirubin. Serum and urine copper levels are increased. Serum ceruloplasmin is decreased. The diagnosis is confirmed if Kayser–Fleischer rings are seen on slit lamp examination. Renal function is frequently impaired. If initiated early, chelating agents may preclude the need for LT.

Vascular Causes

Veno-occlusive disease, Budd–Chiari syndrome, or congested liver secondary to right heart failure can cause ALF. Reversible hepatic insufficiency also occurs after significant hypoperfusion.

Diagnosis

ALF must be considered in any neonate with coagulopathy. Hypoglycemia and hyperammonemia are common, but may be caused by the underlying disease. High transaminases result from hepatocyte necrosis associated with acute viral infection, toxin, or ischemic injury. There is often a prodromal phase of malaise, nausea, and anorexia. Jaundice is usually a late development. Hemorrhage is usually spontaneous, involving the digestive tract. Hypoglycemia is frequent. In older children, symptoms are similar to adults' but asterixis, tremors, and fetor hepaticus are often absent.

Hepatic encephalopathy is a complex neuropsychiatric syndrome that occurs when liver function is altered. As opposed to chronic liver disease, HE that occurs during ALF is often associated with cerebral edema and intracranial hypertension. In the newborn, HE may have nonspecific behavior changes, agitation, and a high-pitched cry. Subsequently, the patient may develop brisk reflexes, clonus, and coma with hypertonia, agitation, and pupillary abnormalities (sluggish, then fixed), followed by deeper coma with hypotonia and brainstem coning. EEG pattern may correlate with prognosis. Status epilepticus may complicate HE.

The diagnostic workup of ALF should establish a diagnosis and characterize severity (**Table 80.1**). Cholestasis is usually present in viral-induced ALF. The absence of hyperbilirubinemia suggests Reye syndrome. Elevation of liver enzymes >3000 IU/L usually indicates hepatic necrosis; however, normal liver levels could represent end-stage necrosis. Hemostasis abnormalities correlate with severity of ALF. A factor V activity <30% indicates severe liver injury. Respiratory alkalosis may indicate neurogenic hyperventilation, renal failure may indicate hepatorenal syndrome, and lactic acidosis may indicate tissue hypoxia and severe liver failure.

Abdominal sonography can assess hepatic size, condition of the parenchyma, ascites, and the vascular supply. Liver biopsy may be deferred or the transjugular approach considered due to risk of bleeding. CT scan is not a sensitive modality for detection of cerebral edema. ALF etiology remains undetermined in ~30% of cases. Decompensated, previously unrecognized chronic liver disease may appear similar to viral ALF (e.g., fulminant Wilson disease, tyrosinemia, or chronic active autoimmune hepatitis).

Complications of ALF

Cerebral Edema and Intracranial Hypertension

Cerebral edema causes 40% of deaths following ALF. The pathophysiology involves cytotoxic and vasogenic edema, increased blood–brain barrier permeability, increased cerebral blood flow, loss of vascular cerebral autoregulation, and alteration in cerebral metabolism.

Hemorrhage

In ALF, hemorrhage may occur spontaneously (<10%). Procoagulant (e.g., factors V, VII, X, and fibrinogen) and anticoagulant proteins (e.g., antithrombin, protein C, and protein S) are reduced. The balanced reduction in pro- and anticoagulant proteins may account for the infrequency of bleeding in the absence of invasive procedures.

Renal Failure

Renal failure may be secondary to hypovolemia, acute tubular necrosis, or functional renal failure (hepatorenal syndrome). Hepatorenal syndrome is thought to result from the activation of vasoconstrictor systems (i.e., renin–angiotensin system, sympathetic nervous system, and arginine vasopressin) as a homeostatic response to improve extreme underfilling of the splanchnic circulation. Renal perfusion and glomerular filtration rate are greatly reduced, but tubular function is preserved. Nephrotoxic drugs such as aminoglycosides should be avoided. Renal wasting of phosphate, magnesium, and potassium can occur.

Cardiovascular and Pulmonary Complications

Pulmonary edema occurs in <35% of patients and may be related to the development of central

TABLE 80.1

Diagnostic Workup of Acute Liver Failure

General Workup	
Na, K, Cl, Mg, Ca, BUN, creatinine, LDH, lactate, ammonia, blood gas, complete blood count, Coombs test, cultures from blood, urine, and CSF, blood group determination, AST, ALT, alkaline phosphatase, γ-glutamyl transferase, total and conjugated bilirubin, α-fetoprotein, prothrombin time, international normalized ratio, partial thrombin time, fibrinogen, factors II, V, VII, IX, X activity, D-dimer.	
Metabolic Workup	
Hereditary tyrosinemia type 1	Urine succinylacetone, wrist X-ray, plasma tyrosine, phenylalanine, methionine
Galactosemia	Red blood cell galactose-1-phosphate uridyltransferase activity (spot test) and GALT activity
Hereditary fructose intolerance	Mutations by PCR amplification of genomic DNA
Neonatal hemochromatosis	Ferritin level, extrahepatic iron deposition, i.e., salivary gland (biopsy, NMR)
Wilson disease	Serum ceruloplasmin, serum, and urinary copper, Kayser–Fleisher ring
Reye syndrome and fatty-acid oxidation disorders	Urinary and blood organic acid chromatography, carnitine and fatty-acid level
Mitochondrial cytopathy	Blood lactate/pyruvate. 3-OH-butyrate/acetoacetate; organic acids in urine. Mitochondrial DNA, muscle and liver biopsy for quantitative respiratory chain enzyme determination. CSF lactate, creatine kinase, echocardiography
Inborn errors of bile acid synthesis	Serum total bile acids, FAB-MS and GC-MS urine analysis
Urea cycle disorders	Plasma amino acids, urinary orotic acid
Congenital disorder of glycosylation syndrome	Transferrin isoelectric focusing
Infectious Workup	
Hepatitis A, B; HHV-1, 2, 6; CMV; EBV; VZV; echovirus; adenovirus; enterovirus; parovirus B19; paramyxovirus	Viral serology (mother and infant), keep frozen serum, PCR (blood, CSF), stool culture
Treponema pallidum (syphilis)	VDRL (maternal if newborn)
Other	
Familial lymphohistiocytosis and macrophage activating syndrome	Blood triglycerides, cholesterol, ferritin, bone marrow analysis and phenotyping
Autoimmune	Coombs test, autoantibodies, biopsy
Leukemia	Bone marrow study
Neonatal lupus	Maternal autoantibodies
Intoxication	Acetaminophen level, salicylate level, keep frozen urine and blood
Vascular/hypoxic–ischemic	Echocardiography

BUN, blood urea nitrogen; LDH, lactate dehydrogenase; CSF, cerebrospinal fluid; AST, aspartate aminotransferase; ALT, alanine aminotransferase; GALT, galactose-1-phosphate uridylyltransferase; NMR, nuclear magnetic resonance, FAB-MS, fast atom bombardment—mass spectrometry; GC-MS, gas chromatography—mass spectrometry; HHV, human herpes virus; CMV, cytomegalovirus; EBV, Epstein–Barr virus; VZV, varicella-zoster virus; VDRL, Venereal Disease Research Laboratory test.

neurogenic pulmonary edema and fluid overload. Ventilation–perfusion mismatch due to circulating vasodilatory substances occurs and can result in hypoxemia. Hemodynamically, there is cardiac hyperkinesia with elevated cardiac index and low systemic vascular resistance. Dysrhythmias are less frequent in children than in adults and are usually associated with electrolyte abnormalities.

Metabolic Complications

Hypoglycemia frequently occurs due to impaired glycogen storage, decreased gluconeogenesis, hyperinsulinism, and increased glucose use. Hyponatremia, hypokalemia, hypophosphatemia, and hypomagnesemia can occur. Kernicterus may precipitate HE if direct bilirubin is >26 mg/dL.

Management of ALF

Pharmacodynamic processes and drug kinetics are modified during ALF, and toxic effects (neurologic and hemodynamic) can occur. Some causes of ALF (e.g., galactosemia, fructosemia, tyrosinemia, hemochromatosis, ornithine transcarbamylase [OTC] defect, Wilson disease, herpetic ALF, acetaminophen or mushroom intoxications, and autoimmune FHF) may respond to specific therapy.

Cerebral Edema Management

Cerebral edema and intracranial hypertension should be aggressively treated. *Hyperammonemia* should be avoided. Treatment includes lowering endogenous nitrogen intake (limit GI bleeding and infection and prevent slowed intestinal transit) or exogenous nitrogen intake (keep protein delivery below 0.5 g/kg/day and limit fresh frozen plasma [FFP] administration). Lactulose is not recommended; it can increase bowel distension during a subsequent transplant procedure. Neomycin is also not recommended; it may precipitate renal failure. Rifaximin is used for HE associated with chronic liver failure but is of unproven benefit in ALF. Hemofiltration remains the main treatment of acute hyperammonemia. No consensus exists on invasive ICP monitoring. Management of elevated ICP in ALF is similar to other causes. Corticosteroids and flumazenil are not recommended.

Hemorrhage and Digestive Tract Bleeding

In the absence of bleeding or an imminent surgical procedure, routine correction of abnormal coagulation values in ALF is not indicated. The volume load from FFP may worsen ascites and the protein load may worsen encephalopathy. IV Vitamin K should be administered. Profound thrombocytopenia ($<$10,000/mm^3) and hypofibrinogenemia ($<$0.5 g/L) should be corrected and FFP administration considered if an invasive procedure (central venous catheter) is planned. Sucralfate is preferred for prophylaxis against GI hemorrhage. Histamine-2 receptor blockers should be avoided because of their effect on the central nervous system. No study has evaluated proton-pump inhibitors for GI bleeding prophylaxis in ALF patients. Activated recombinant factor VII has been used to treat life-threatening hemorrhage. It has been shown to correct coagulopathy, but has not been shown to alter long-term outcomes.

Renal Failure

Adequate renal perfusion should be maintained and nephrotoxic drugs avoided. If renal failure occurs, dialysis should not be delayed. Hepatorenal syndrome usually reverses after LT.

Cardiopulmonary Failure

Vasoplegia generally responds to α-adrenergic agents. Adrenal insufficiency can occur in ALF, and hydrocortisone may be beneficial if hemodynamic instability occurs. Patients may require intubation for severe hypoxemia or grade III or IV encephalopathy.

Metabolic Disorders

Glucose requirements may require central venous delivery of high-concentration dextrose in small volumes. Phosphate, magnesium, and potassium supplementation is often needed. Enteral nutrition is preferred.

Liver Support Devices

Liver support techniques can be divided into ex vivo whole-organ perfusion, bioartificial liver support using hepatocytes, “detoxification” methods, or a combination of techniques. The principal detoxification systems involve hemodiafiltration, high-volume plasma exchange, and albumin dialysis. The molecular absorbent recirculating system (MARS) is currently the most widely used. MARS improves liver function and HE in patients with acute decompensation of chronic liver disease and improves renal function in patients with hepatorenal syndrome, but fails to impact survival. Liver support may serve as a bridge to LT or provide time to evaluate the recovery capacity of the failing liver.

Emergency LT for ALF

The decision to list a child for LT depends on the cause and severity of ALF, the potential for spontaneous liver regeneration, the availability of a specific therapy to reverse ALF, and comorbidities (especially the risk of permanent neurologic damage). Criteria predicting outcome in children, either mortality or liver transplant–free survival, include coagulation parameters (PT, INR, factor V), bilirubin, HE, age, and ALF etiology. Emergency LT should be considered if HE is greater than grade II, cofactor V activity is below 20%, or prothrombin index is below 20% (PT $>$ 60 seconds) or INR $\geq$ 2. Other criteria include a rapid decrease in liver size, seizures, ascites, hepatorenal syndrome, a fibrinogen level $<$1 g/L, bilirubinemia $>$ 400 μmol/L, worsening lactic acidosis, and hyperammonemia $>$ 150 mmol/L. LT may be contraindicated in 11%–20% of cases. Diseases not cured with LT such as malignant disease (i.e., leukemia, lymphoproliferative syndrome, and lymphohistiocytosis), Reye syndrome and mitochondrial, respiratory chain, and disorders with neurologic involvement may be contraindications. Uncontrolled intracranial hypertension or uncontrolled multiorgan failure may be contraindications due to the poor prognosis.

LIVER TRANSPLANTATION

Pediatric LT is one of the most successful solid organ transplantations. The 1-year actuarial survival rate is >90% in elective patients and >70% in children with ALF. Long-term survival is >80% with excellent health-related quality of life.

Cholestatic Liver Disease: Biliary atresia is the most common cause of chronic cholestasis in infants and accounts for ~50% of pediatric LT. These children often have had a Kasai procedure (hepatoportoenterostomy) that failed to reestablish effective biliary flow. Consequently, they develop secondary biliary cirrhosis leading to chronic end-stage liver failure. Indications for LT in children with biliary atresia are cholangitis or progressive jaundice (35%), portal hypertension or hepatorenal syndrome (41%), and decreased liver synthetic functions. Intrahepatic cholestasis such as sclerosing cholangitis, Alagille syndrome, nonsyndromic paucity of intrahepatic bile ducts, and progressive familial intrahepatic cholestasis represent ~15% of all transplantations.

Metabolic Diseases: Metabolic diseases are the second most common indication for pediatric LT. They include primary hepatic diseases (e.g., Wilson disease, α-1-antitrypsin deficiency, and cystic fibrosis) and nonhepatic diseases (e.g., OTC deficiency, Crigler–Najjar syndrome type 1, primary hyperoxaluria type 1, and organic acidemia). In primary hyperoxaluria type 1, combined liver and kidney transplantation is considered.

Liver Tumors: Tumor resection or LT for hepatoblastoma is considered after chemotherapy. Hepatocellular carcinoma in children is rare and is usually associated with preexisting liver or metabolic disease.

Prioritization of Potential Candidates for LT

The pediatric end-stage liver disease (PELD) score was introduced to stratify the degree of illness in children competing for pediatric liver grafts. This formula includes total bilirubin, INR, serum albumin, age, and growth failure. Additional points may be awarded for hepatopulmonary syndrome, metabolic diseases, and liver tumors. Since the use of the PELD score, fewer children are now dying on waiting lists.

Intraoperative Care of Children Undergoing LT

Donor Selection: Attention is paid to donor's age, cause of death, intensive care hospitalization time, infections, hemodynamic stability, and use of vasopressors. The development of techniques for transplantation of portions of a liver from adult donors has expanded the donor pool, and reduced the waiting period, and improved the survival rates. Reduced-liver grafts to the left lateral segments and split livers provide the majority of grafts in infants, whereas left or right lobes are used in older recipients.

Whole-Liver Transplantation: Donor weight should range 15% above or below the recipient weight for whole-liver grafts. Bigger grafts result in difficult abdominal closure and risk abdominal compartment syndrome. Undersized grafts are associated with hemorrhagic necrosis due to excessive portal flow.

Split-Liver Transplantation: Split-LT doubles the number of recipients and allows two functional allografts. The left lateral segment is transplanted in a child and the right liver into an adult. Split-LT may require a longer ischemic period, so selection of donors is crucial. This procedure has comparable results to conventional techniques and decreases waiting times for children.

Living-Related LT: Living-related LT is a substantial percentage of pediatric LT. The procedure involves a left lobectomy with separation of segments 2 and 3 from the remaining liver. The controversy of living-related LT involves the ethics of performing major surgery on a healthy person. Donor mortality and morbidity are estimated at ~0.2% and 10%, respectively. Infants and small children do better than older children with living donor transplantation. Living-related transplant allows transplantation before the child's condition deteriorates.

Graft Implantation

The surgical procedure follows three phases. First is the recipient hepatectomy, which may be difficult secondary to portal hypertension, coagulopathy, or adhesions from prior surgery. Second, the anhepatic phase involves placing the graft, beginning with the vascular outflow anastomosis, followed by the vascular inflow of the portal vein, and finally the hepatic artery. Blood circulated from the graft is cold, acidotic, and hyperkalemic and can result in significant cardiovascular instability. The biliary anastomosis is performed in the third, postimplantation phase. A Roux-en-Y anastomosis (hepaticojejunostomy) is necessary in patients undergoing LT for biliary atresia. This approach is also used in young children receiving a segmental graft, those with an abnormal native biliary tree (as in sclerosing cholangitis), or if the donor or recipient duct is very small.

Postoperative Care of Children after LT

General Postoperative Management

Mechanical ventilation may be necessary because of fluid overload, increased abdominal pressure, malnutrition, postoperative pain, or complications (sepsis, liver dysfunction, refractory ascites, or right phrenic nerve paresis). Pleural effusions secondary to ascites passing across the diaphragm are common and can be treated with diuretic therapy and pleural puncture. Excessive abdominal hemorrhage may warrant hemostasis laparotomy. Restrictive or obstructive cardiomyopathy and pulmonary hypertension may be encountered. Postoperative vasoplegia may require vasopressor support. Hypertension may be a side effect of immunosuppressive agents, volume overload, or pain, but warrants a careful neurologic evaluation for raised ICP.

It is crucial to immediately assess synthetic, metabolic, and excretory function of the graft. Improvement in coagulation abnormalities is the best indicator of synthetic function. Adequate metabolic function is reflected in normalizing lactate levels and awakening within several hours following the transplant procedure. After 48 hours, the total bilirubin, coagulations tests, and transaminases are reliable indicators of liver function. The transaminase levels may rise dramatically within 2 days but should be near normal after 7 days.

Primary Nonfunction and Subfunction of the Graft. Primary nonfunction of the graft is a rare but catastrophic event. It usually occurs within 48 hours of the procedure, and diagnosis is based on absence of neurologic awakening, HE, bleeding, increasing liver enzymes, lactic acidosis, and persisting vasoplegic shock. The only therapy is emergency retransplantation. The cause is presumed to be the result of donor (rather than recipient) factors probably related to ischemia/reperfusion injury of the graft.

Vascular Complications. Vascular thrombosis is the main postoperative complication that causes graft loss. Hepatic artery thrombosis occurs in children (5%–15%) three times more frequently than adults, usually within 30 days after transplantation. This complication is related to size of the vessels and is prevented by anticoagulation, antiplatelet aggregation therapy, and avoiding hemoconcentration. Suspected hepatic artery thrombosis requires prompt evaluation with duplex sonography, magnetic resonance angiography, or angiogram. Successful thrombectomy is possible if the diagnosis is made before graft necrosis occurs. Hepatic artery thrombosis can also cause biliary complications because the hepatic artery supplies the vasculature of the bile duct. Early portal vein thrombosis occurs within the first week after transplantation and requires emergency thrombectomy in most cases. Refractory ascites may indicate a portal thrombosis or stenosis of suprahepatic veins.

Biliary Complications. Bile duct complications (bile leaks, stenosis, and strictures) usually result from technical problems or ischemic injury of the donor duct. Early leaks are diagnosed by the appearance of bile in the drains. Many leaks resolve with decompression by transhepatic tube drainage. Surgical revision of the anastomosis should be performed for patients with bile peritonitis and those with persistent leaks. Biliary strictures can occur later, even years after transplant.

Infections. Because of immunosuppression, patients are at risk for nosocomial and opportunistic infections. Bacterial sepsis in the immediate posttransplant period is most frequently due to gram-negative enteric organisms, Enterococcus and Staphylococcus species. Fungal sepsis (*Candida* and *Aspergillus* spp.) may occur in the early posttransplant period. Postoperative prophylactic regimens include acyclovir, an antifungal agent, a β-lactam antibiotic, and trimethoprim-sulfamethoxazole. The risk of EBV or CMV infection is greatest in seronegative recipients of seropositive donor organs. The use of ganciclovir or valganciclovir has improved mortality from CMV but morbidity remains high. Quantitative PCR for EBV has helped prevent progressive disease and posttransplant lymphoproliferative disease (PTLD) by allowing reduction of immunosuppression in response to rinsing EBV titers.

Acute Rejection. About 20%–50% of patients develop acute rejection in the first few weeks after LT. It can occur later, often associated with immunosuppressant noncompliance. The presentation includes fever, ascites, and jaundice. Diagnosis usually includes increasing liver enzymes, γ-glutamyl transferase level, and liver biopsy. High-dose methylprednisolone is effective in treating rejection in 80% of cases.

Other Complications and Retransplantation. Early second-look reoperation may be used for bile leakage, hemorrhage, bowel injury, and sepsis. GI perforation occurs in 20% of children with biliary atresia. Acute pancreatitis occurs in <2% of children who undergo LT but is associated with high mortality. PTLDs are a heterogeneous group of diseases, ranging from benign lymphatic hyperplasia to lymphomas. It is more likely with intense immunosuppression, an EBV-seronegative host, and an EBV-seropositive donor. Treatment requires an immediate decrease or withdrawal of immunosuppression. If tissue expresses the B-cell marker CD20, the anti-CD20 monoclonal antibody rituximab is indicated. Recurrence of the primary liver disease in the graft is uncommon in children, but can occur with primary sclerosing cholangitis. Autoimmune hepatitis can occur in any graft, regardless of the original disease, and is therefore considered a new entity. It may be associated with the use of steroid-free regimens. Chronic hepatitis has been recently recognized as a problem in late allograft dysfunction.

Immunosuppression

Corticosteroids. Corticosteroids are effective in prevention and treatment of rejection. They inhibit IL-2, reduce the proliferation of T cells (helper and suppressor T cells, cytotoxic T cells), and decrease migration and activity of neutrophils. Their use is associated with risk for infection (bacterial, viral, and fungal), malignancy, and detrimental metabolic effects (bone marrow suppression, hypertension, diabetes mellitus, polyphagia, obesity, gastric ulcers, and sodium and water retention). Long-term use may result in osteoporosis, growth retardation, avascular necrosis of joints, and depression. Many pediatric centers use steroid-free protocols, combining calcineurin inhibitors and antibody to the IL-2 receptors of T cells (basiliximab).

Calcineurin Inhibitors. Calcineurin inhibitors inhibit T-cell response and bind to intracellular immunophilins. Side effects include nephrotoxicity, neurotoxicity, and hypertension. Tacrolimus is preferred over cyclosporine. It is 100 times more potent and associated with less hyperlipidemia and cardiovascular risk. Tacrolimus can be given as an IV infusion or orally. Daily determination of levels is essential.

IL-2 Receptor Antibodies. Anti-IL-2 receptor antibodies (basiliximab) combined with calcineurin inhibitors have drastically improved graft survival. Basiliximab is a chimeric (mouse and human) monoclonal antibody. Combination with calcineurin inhibitors allows steroid-free immunosuppression to reduce hypertension, growth retardation, and the cosmetic effects of steroid therapy.

Other Immunosuppressive Drugs. Mycophenolate mofetil, a selective inhibitor of the inosine monophosphate dehydrogenase (necessary for B-cell and T-cell growth), has been successfully used as an alternative immunosuppressive agent in patients with chronic rejection, refractory rejection, or severe calcineurin inhibitor toxicity. Large interindividual variations indicate the need for therapeutic drug monitoring and individualized dosing. Sirolimus (rapamycin) is a macrolide antibiotic with immunosuppressive properties that acts by blocking T-cell activation by way of IL-2R post–receptor signal transduction. It has been used as a rescue treatment in chronic rejection and calcineurin inhibitor toxicity.

Results and Outcome for Pediatric LT

Early postoperative death is related to sepsis, graft failure, multiorgan failure, and cardiopulmonary and neurologic complications. Late mortality is related to sepsis. Overall survival of children after LT is 70%–80%, and 15-year graft survival is 52%–65%. Ten years after transplant, 79% of children attend normal school and 69% without school performance delay. Clinical factors associated with improved post-LT health-related quality of life are younger age at LT, allograft longevity, and strong social support. Seventy-three per cent of long-term survivors have abnormal liver histology due to chronic rejection. Linear growth impairment is common. Renal dysfunction is present in >30% of long-term survivors. Current immunosuppressive agents are associated with increased risk for diabetes, dyslipidemia, and obesity. Lifestyle modification and minimization of immune suppressants can reduce these risks.

CHAPTER 81 ■ PEDIATRIC INTESTINAL AND MULTIVISCERAL TRANSPLANTATIONS

GEOFFREY J. BOND, KATHRYN A. FELMET, RONALD JAFFE, KYLE A. SOLTYS, JEFFREY A. RUDOLPH, DOLLY MARTIN, RAKESH SINDHI, AND GEORGE V. MAZARIEGOS

Diseases associated with loss of intestinal function have either surgical or nonsurgical etiologies. Patients with surgical causes generally suffer from loss of bowel length after resection due to ischemia or obstruction or from strictures and fistulas (as with Crohn disease). Nonsurgical causes of intestinal failure include motility disorders (e.g., intestinal pseudo-obstruction, Hirschsprung disease) and disorders of enterocyte function (e.g., microvillus inclusion disease). The management of intestinal failure should provide a medical focus to optimize nutritional status and minimize cholestatic liver injury from parenteral nutrition (PN) and a surgical focus to provide options (such as stoma closure or bowel lengthening) that reduce the need for transplantation. When transplant becomes necessary, the best options are based on the anatomic and functional integrity of the remaining gut and abdominal organs as well as their vascular supplies. Liver replacement in intestinal transplant candidates may be required. Hypercoagulable patients deficient in proteins S or C or antithrombin III may develop splanchnic thromboses and undergo transplantation for mesenteric venous hypertension rather than for intestinal failure. Extensive portomesenteric thrombosis can make transplant unfeasible.

CLINICAL MANAGEMENT OF THE PRETRANSPLANT CHILD IN THE PICU

Liver disease develops in 40%–60% of infants who require long-term PN for intestinal failure. Wait times until transplant are long, often 6 months to 1 year. The success of the intestinal or multivisceral transplantation depends in large measure on the health and nutritional status of the transplant recipient. Even if the child does not ultimately require a transplant, early referral to a center experienced in the management of intestinal failure can dramatically impact outcomes.

Parenteral Nutrition Dependence

PN-dependent patients have chronic problems with venous access because of infection and thrombosis. The central lines of patients with short gut syndrome become infected by external contamination of the line or by translocation of bacteria across a gut with inadequate barrier function. The risk of fungal infections is also increased compared to the general population. Enteric feedings may help preserve the intestinal mucosal barrier function and decrease infectious complications. Patients with liver failure also have impaired immune responses. Patients with severe liver failure may have a hyperdynamic state at baseline, but a blunted contractile response to stress. Both systolic and diastolic ventricular functions may be impaired. Resuscitation should be appropriately aggressive, but with careful attention to signs of intravascular volume overload as well as vigilance for concomitant hepatopulmonary or hepatorenal syndrome. Echocardiogram can be used in difficult cases to assess cardiac filling and function. In patients with advanced liver disease, albumin may be preferable to crystalloid as a resuscitation fluid to avoid worsening anasarca. High salt loads (e.g., normal saline) should be avoided. Low diastolic blood pressures may be present in association with advanced liver disease. Early septic shock in these children follows a vasodilatory pattern commonly seen in adults and may respond to vasopressor agents. In patients with catecholamine unresponsive septic shock, adrenal function should be evaluated with a cortisol level and/or adrenocorticotropic hormone (ACTH) stimulation test. Empiric treatment may be needed.

When infections cannot be cleared, it may be necessary to remove and replace lines. Intestinal transplant candidates are at high risk for forming clots around central lines that can become occlusive and persist after line removal. An inadequate synthesis of both coagulation factors and anticoagulation factors is common. Clotting in most or all of the available sites for central venous catheterization can make transplantation technically challenging or impossible. The development of liver disease may be influenced by nutritional and metabolic parameters. Healing after a major operation is dependent on preoperative nutritional status. A nutritional specialist should be involved in the care of all prospective intestinal transplant patients. When possible, delivery of some enteral calories may preserve intestinal epithelial barrier function, decrease the risk or severity of intestinal failure–associated liver disease, and improve hospital mortality.

Liver Failure

Isolated intestinal transplant candidates may have mild, reversible liver disease. Patients awaiting combined liver and small intestinal or multivisceral transplants struggle with the problems seen in hepatic failure but over a longer waiting period compared to isolated liver candidates. Coagulopathy, portal hypertension with ascites and hepatomegaly, variceal bleeding, hypoalbuminemia, hyperbilirubinemia, hyperammonemia with hepatic encephalopathy, and hepatorenal and hepatopulmonary syndrome are seen in this patient population.

Intestinal transplant candidates with cirrhosis and liver failure have increased abdominal girth due to organomegaly and ascites. The enlarged liver and other abdominal contents may impinge on lung volumes and impede respiration. If ascites predominates over organomegaly as a cause of increased abdominal girth, drainage of ascitic fluid may relieve symptoms. Relief is usually temporary, as the circumstances leading to the fluid collection persist. The indications for peritoneal drainage must be weighed against the risk of infection. Additionally, rapid drainage of large volumes of peritoneal fluid may lead to intravascular hypovolemia and shock. Patients often have some degree of renal dysfunction that renders them sensitive to fluid overload. They are typically exposed to multiple nephrotoxic agents. Additionally, episodes of septic shock can expose the kidney to low-flow states, causing acute tubular necrosis. Hepatorenal syndrome is a very late finding in liver failure.

Persistent coagulopathy is a significant complication. Clinical evidence of bleeding should guide therapy. Intracranial hemorrhage can occur. Correction of disordered coagulation with large volumes of clotting factors can lead to fluid overload. In cases of severe or recurrent bleeding, plasma exchange (plasmapheresis) and judicious use of recombinant factor 7 have been used successfully to correct coagulopathy without fluid overload. Plasma exchange may also have a role as a liver support therapy. Extracorporeal liver support attempts to mimic the liver's detoxifying function relying on diffusion of molecules across a membrane (dialysis with or without albumin-enriched dialysate), absorption (by charcoal, albumin), or dilution (exchange of plasma volumes). Studies in adults have documented clinical improvement, but it has been difficult to demonstrate survival benefit.

THE TRANSPLANT OPERATION

Abdominal Visceral Procurement

Optimal donor selection is imperative to a successful transplant. Size disparity is an issue, especially in the very young where size-matched donors are infrequent. Both allograft reductions and efforts to provide increased abdominal domain (e.g., abdominal wall

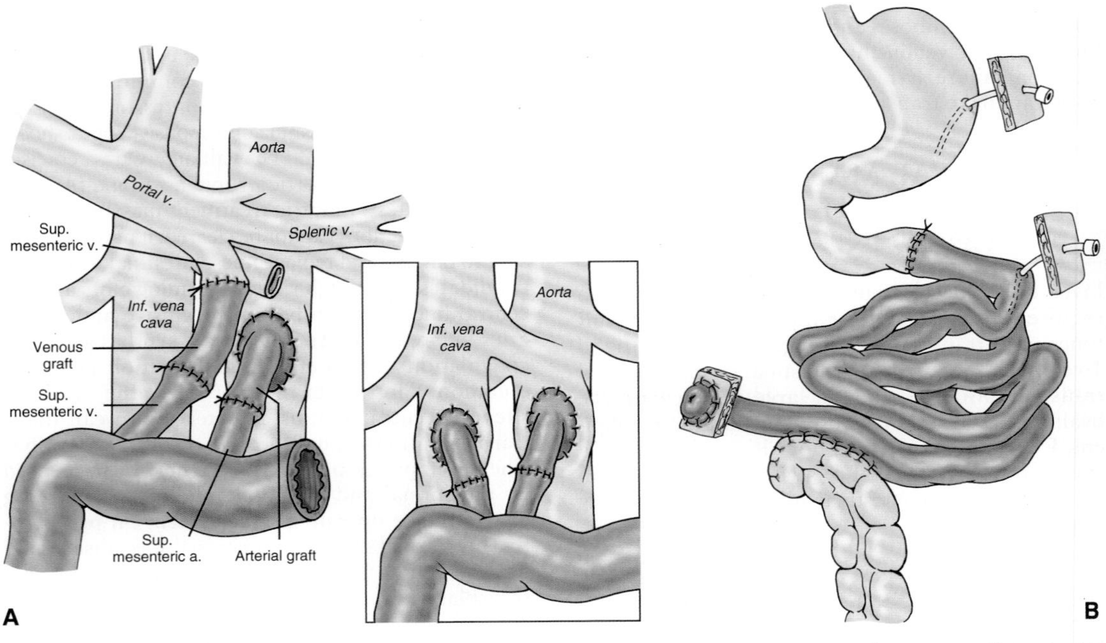

FIGURE 81.1. Arterialization and potential venous drainage options of the isolated small intestine allograft (**A**). Illustration of an isolated small bowel graft; the distal ileal chimney allows easy access to bowel mucosa (**B**).

transplant or delayed closure) have been attempted to expand the donor pool.

Recipient Operations

Obtaining vascular access, especially when the liver requires transplantation, can be problematic in patients who have multiple thrombosed veins. The recipient operation consists of removal of the failed organs after exposure of the vascular anatomy, followed by allograft implantation.

Isolated Small Bowel

In cases of surgical short gut, the recipient's diseased small intestine is removed and the superior mesenteric artery (SMA) of the donor bowel is sewn to the infrarenal aorta (or occasionally the native SMA), and the donor superior mesenteric vein is anastomosed to the recipient superior mesenteric vein or inferior vena cava (**Fig. 81.1A**). Intestinal continuity is completed with proximal and distal gastrointestinal anastomoses, and access to the ileum for endoscopic examination is provided by a temporary chimney ileostomy (**Fig. 81.1B**), except in the case of a permanent end ileostomy.

Liver–Small Bowel

The diseased liver is removed, with the retrohepatic vena cava preserved in situ ("piggyback"), and a permanent portacaval shunt draining the native stomach and pancreas is performed (**Fig. 81.2A**). Prior to implantation of the allograft (**Fig. 81.2B**), the double arterial stem of the celiac and superior mesenteric arteries is connected to the infrarenal aorta using a donor aortic conduit homograft. A proximal jejunojejunostomy, ileocolostomy, and a temporary distal ileostomy complete the operation.

Multivisceral Transplantation

After removal of the native liver, distal stomach, duodenum, pancreas, and intestine, the retroperitoneal aorta is exposed and the multivisceral graft is connected to its vascular inflow and outflow. No portal vein anastomosis is required in this procedure as the recipient's portal vein and its inflow native organs (gastrointestinal tract, pancreas, and liver) are removed with the enterectomy. Patients with a normal native liver receive a modified multivisceral procedure where allograft portal venous return is directed into the recipient's native portal vein, preserving the native liver.

In all types of intestinal recipients, the ileostomy is primarily placed to allow for ease of allograft monitoring via ileoscopy and ileal allograft biopsies. Takedown of the ileostomy can be performed once oral nutrition is consistently adequate and a stable immunosuppressant regimen has been achieved with less need for frequent endoscopic surveillance.

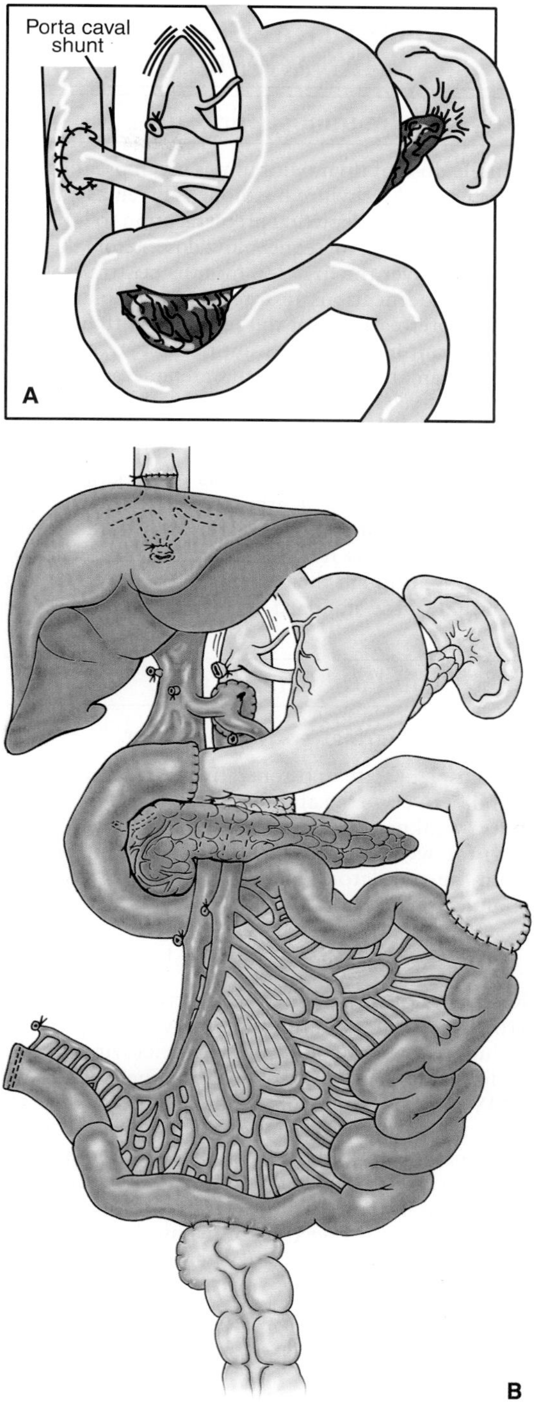

FIGURE 81.2. Combined liver and small intestinal allograft. Systemic portacaval shunt allows venous outflow of retained pancreas and stomach from recipient (**A**). Composite liver and intestine graft with preservation of the duodenum in continuity with the graft jejunum and hepatobiliary system (**B**).

POSTTRANSPLANT MANAGEMENT

Immunosuppression

A single dose of thymoglobulin is given preallograft reperfusion. Methylprednisolone is given as a bolus as a lymphocyte-depleting premedication to limit the cytokine reaction; subsequent low-dose steroid therapy is weaned over the first 3–6 months posttransplant. Recent modifications in intestinal transplantation include pretreatment of the recipient with antilymphocyte antibody such as antithymocyte antibody or basiliximab to eliminate maintenance steroid use postoperatively. Rejection is treated with optimization of tacrolimus levels, supplemental corticosteroids, and monoclonal or polyclonal antibody if necessary. Additional or alternative agents have occasionally been used, including azathioprine, rapamycin, and mycophenolate mofetil, especially in the face of complications such as renal dysfunction and recurrent rejection, although their efficacy appears to be less than that of the standard agents.

Postoperative Care

Ventilatory Management

Pretransplant status, postoperative graft status, sepsis, inability to close the abdominal wall, and diaphragmatic weakness or paralysis are considered in the plan for weaning the intestinal transplant patient from the ventilator. Pain management is a serious complicating factor.

Infection Control

Recipients of intestinal grafts receive prophylactic, broad-spectrum IV antibiotics. Antiviral prophylaxis includes a 2-week course of IV ganciclovir, with the addition of CMV-specific hyperimmune globulin for CMV-negative recipients who receive an allograft from a CMV-positive donor. Oral administration of trimethoprim–sulfamethoxazole is used as prophylaxis against *Pneumocystis jirovecii* pneumonia. Bacterial translocation most commonly occurs during episodes of acute rejection, or in enteritis associated with Epstein–Barr virus (EBV) infection.

Gastrointestinal Function and Assessment

Postoperative changes in the ileal stoma should be promptly investigated and vascular, technical, or immunologic causes ruled out. Routine endoscopic surveillance is used to assess graft integrity and for the diagnosis of intestinal rejection. Zoom endoscopy has been used in some centers to try to establish a prompt visual tool to diagnose rejection. Normal stomal output is 40–60 mL/kg/day. No reliable serum tests exist for monitoring the function of intestinal grafts. Enteral nutrition is introduced once integrity of the gastrointestinal tract has been demonstrated by contrast study, usually at 1 week posttransplant.

Management of Complications

Graft Rejection

Intestinal allograft rejection may be clinically asymptomatic or present with fever, abdominal pain, distention, nausea, vomiting, or a sudden change (increase or decrease) in stomal output. The stoma may be normal in appearance or lose its normal velvety appearance and become friable or ulcerated. Histologically, the rejection is graded by the degree of epithelial damage. In mild rejection, apoptosis leads to epithelial cell loss within the deep crypts. In moderate rejection, there is more severe crypt damage with focal crypt loss. Severe rejection leads to denuded mucosa. Regeneration occurs by reepithelialization over the surface of a lamina propria devoid of crypts. Chronic rejection is observed in ~15% of isolated small bowel recipients. The presentation may include weight loss, chronic diarrhea, intermittent fever, or gastrointestinal bleeding. Acute rejection occurs in ~50% of patients with the use of a preconditioning protocol. Reduction in immunosuppression has resulted in a concomitant decrease in CMV and EBV disease, especially in pediatric recipients. Mild graft rejection in most cases responds to intravenous methylprednisolone combined with optimization of tacrolimus levels to 15 ng/mL. Antibody therapy with OKT3 is used when rejection has progressed despite steroids, or as the initial therapeutic agent in cases of severe mucosal injury and crypt damage.

Biliary Complications

Biliary and pancreatic complications from leaks and strictures at anastomoses are avoided through modification in donor technique to preserve the donor duodenum and pancreas and to maintain the hepato-pancreato-biliary system. Obstruction can occur months to years posttransplantation and is managed via percutaneous transhepatic cholangiography (PTC) with balloon dilatation or endoscopic retrograde cholangiopancreatogram (ERCP) and stenting or incising the ampulla. In modified multivisceral grafts, continuity of the biliary axis is surgically reestablished, via either a Roux-en-Y enteric loop or duct-to-duct in bigger donors and recipients. Correspondingly, these grafts can develop biliary system–related surgical complications (i.e., leaks and obstructions). Alternatively, the native spleen, pancreas, and duodenum are preserved and gastrointestinal/biliary continuity restored by a duodeno-duodenostomy.

Infection

Infectious complications are responsible for significant morbidity and mortality after intestinal transplantation.

Sepsis following intestinal transplantation should prompt a rapid search for technical complications (intra-abdominal abscess, anastomotic dehiscence, etc.) and immunologic causes (rejection may lead to bacterial translocation, over-immunosuppression places the recipient at risk of infection). Immunosuppression modifications have decreased the incidence of life-threatening bacterial complications so that fungal and viral infections are the main source of morbidity in current transplant series.

Posttransplantation lymphoproliferative disease (PTLD) may present as asymptomatic findings at routine endoscopy, EBV enteritis, systemic symptoms, bleeding, lymphadenopathy, or tumors. PTLD has decreased in incidence to 10% under current immunosuppression. Therapy includes reduction of immunosuppression; antiviral therapy using ganciclovir, acyclovir, and/or hyperimmunoglobulin; rituximab; and chemotherapy.

Graft-versus-Host Disease

Graft-versus-host disease is a risk from donor cell chimerism in peripheral blood. Cases have been treated with optimization of immunosuppression and limited steroid therapy if necessary.

OUTCOMES

Current overall patient actuarial survival at 1 and 5 years is 90% and 78%, respectively, and full nutritional support has been achieved in 91% of surviving patients.

CHAPTER 82 ■ ADRENAL DYSFUNCTION

ABEER HASSOUN AND SHARON E. OBERFIELD

BIOLOGY OF ADRENAL FUNCTION

The adrenal glands can be considered as two unique endocrine organs: the adrenal cortex and the adrenal medulla. The adrenal cortex consists of the outermost zona glomerulosa (15%), the middle zona fasciculata (75%), and the inner zona reticularis (10%). The zona glomerulosa is the primary site of mineralocorticoid synthesis. The zona fasciculata is involved in the production of cortisol. The zona reticularis produces androgens. The adrenal medulla should be considered part of the sympathetic nervous system and is composed of chromaffin cells arranged in nests and cords with sympathetic ganglion cells. In adults, epinephrine is the major catecholamine synthesized and stored in the adrenal medulla; at birth, it is norepinephrine. In cord blood and in newborns, the concentrations of cortisol and cortisone are low and about equal (4–10 µg/100 mL). After 4 weeks of life, the cortisol concentration increases in relation to cortisone. There is little diurnal variation of glucocorticoid concentration until about 4–6 months of age. Cortisol secretion rates, corrected for body surface area, remain constant during childhood, puberty, and adulthood, and maintain a diurnal variation. In parallel with cortisol, ACTH peaks between 6 a.m. and 9 a.m., declines to nadir between 11 p.m. and 2 a.m., and then starts to rise between 2 a.m. and 3 a.m. Aldosterone is secreted at a constant rate during infancy, childhood, and adulthood, albeit the concentrations of aldosterone in infancy tend to be relatively higher than those observed later on in childhood for specific levels of sodium. Adrenal androgen secretion is low during childhood. Prior to puberty with onset of adrenarche (physically noted as the onset of pubic hair), there is an increase in the secretion of dehydroepiandrosterone (DHEA), dehydroepiandrosterone sulfate (DHEA-S), and androstenedione.

Adrenal Cortex

Three classes of hormones are produced by the adrenal cortex: glucocorticoids (e.g., cortisol), mineralocorticoids (e.g., aldosterone), and sex steroids (e.g., testosterone, DHEA, and androstenedione).

Regulation of the Adrenal Cortex (Hypothalamic–Pituitary–Adrenal Axis)

The major regulator of glucocorticoid secretion is adrenocorticotropic hormone (ACTH). ACTH is released from the anterior pituitary in bursts that vary in amplitude throughout the 24-hour cycle. The diurnal rhythm of cortisol secretion is established after infancy. The pulses of ACTH and cortisol are highest in the early morning hours, become lower in late afternoon, and reach their nadir 1 or 2 hours after sleep begins. ACTH secretion from the anterior pituitary is stimulated mainly by corticotropin-releasing hormone (CRH). This hormone is synthesized in the hypothalamic paraventricular nucleus. The secretion of ACTH and CRH is predominantly regulated by cortisol through a negative feedback effect. ACTH can also inhibit its own secretion. Aldosterone secretion is regulated mainly by the renin–angiotensin system and serum potassium levels. ACTH plays a small role in the regulation of its synthesis. Predominantly, in response to decreased intravascular volume, renin is secreted by the juxtaglomerular apparatus of the kidney. Renin cleaves angiotensinogen and results in the formation of angiotensin I, which is cleaved further by angiotensin-converting enzyme (ACE) in the lungs and other tissues yielding the biologically active angiotensin II. Angiotensin II is cleaved further to produce the angiotensin III. Angiotensin II and III are potent stimulators of aldosterone secretion.

Adrenal Steroid Action

Glucocorticoids increase hepatic gluconeogenesis, glycolysis, proteolysis, and lipolysis. Glucocorticoids can increase insulin levels, which inhibits peripheral tissue glucose uptake, leading to hyperglycemia. In addition, glucocorticoids work in parallel to insulin by stimulating glycogen deposition and production in the liver, providing protection against starvation. An increase in free fatty acid levels associated with glucocorticoid administration results from enhancement of lipolysis, decrease of cellular glucose uptake, and decrease in glycerol production. In addition, there is an increase of amino acid substrates that are used in gluconeogenesis due to proteolysis in fat, skeletal muscle, bone, lymphoid, and connective tissues. In the fetus and neonate, they accelerate the differentiation and development of various tissues, such as the development of the hepatic and gastrointestinal systems, as well as the production of surfactant in the fetal lung. Glucocorticoids also play a major role in immune regulation. They suppress the inflammatory process. Depletion of monocytes, eosinophils, and lymphocytes (T lymphocytes) is observed with the administration of high doses of glucocorticoids. T lymphocytes are reduced more than the B lymphocytes, leading to a predominantly humoral immune response. Glucocorticoids also inhibit immunoglobulin synthesis and stimulation of lymphocyte apoptosis. In addition, they block other anti-inflammatory effects, such as histamine and proinflammatory cytokine secretion (e.g., tumor necrosis factor-α, interleukin-1, and interleukin-6).

Glucocorticoids have a positive inotropic effect that leads to an increase in left ventricular output. In the vascular smooth muscles and the heart, glucocorticoids have a permissive effect on the actions of epinephrine and norepinephrine. They increase the sensitivity to vasopressor agents, such as catecholamines and angiotensin II, while reducing nitric oxide–mediated endothelial dilatation. Hypertension is observed in patients with glucocorticoid excess due to the activation of mineralocorticoid receptor. Glucocorticoids induce a negative calcium balance by increasing renal calcium excretion and inhibition of calcium absorption by the intestine. Long-term use of glucocorticoid can lead to osteopenia and osteoporosis as they inhibit the osteoblastic activity. Glucocorticoids also have effects on brain metabolism and mood changes such as emotional liability with irritability, euphoria, as well as appetite stimulation, and insomnia can occur. The major role of mineralocorticoids is to maintain intravascular volume. The main target tissues for the action of mineralocorticoids are the kidney, gut, and salivary and sweat glands. Mineralocorticoids act mainly on the distal convoluted tubules and cortical collecting ducts of the kidney. They stimulate the reabsorption of sodium and the secretion of potassium in the distal convoluted tubules. The mineralocorticoid receptor has a similar affinity for cortisol and aldosterone, yet glucocorticoids have limited mineralocorticoid activity.

The Effects of Stress on Adrenocortical Function

Physical and emotional stress can lead to the increased secretion of ACTH. This involves an immune-endocrine cascade, which results in the activation of the hypothalamic–pituitary–adrenal (HPA) axis. IL-1 is secreted by macrophages in response to immunologic and inflammatory reactions and triggers a proinflammatory response that leads to antibody production. The CRH–ACTH–cortisol axis activation leads to increased plasma cortisol concentration, which results in a negative feedback on the macrophages. IL-6, tumor necrosis factor-α, and IL-1 also stimulate CRH release and are also inhibited by cortisol. A low cortisol level during stress or illness may indicate adrenal insufficiency or inadequate central nervous system activation of the adrenal axis. Impaired cortisol metabolism and decreased protein binding can occur in chronic liver disease. Such patients may show increased sensitivity to steroid therapy, while cortisol secretion usually remains normal. Renal failure results in a reduced excretion of steroid metabolites despite the normal secretion of cortisol. It is important to note that aldosterone secretion is increased in hyperkalemia that is associated with renal failure. In patients with heart failure, renin–angiotensin–aldosterone is secreted in response to inadequate systemic perfusion.

Adrenal Medulla

The catecholamines, such as dopamine, norepinephrine, and epinephrine, are produced by the adrenal medulla. Catecholamine metabolites are excreted in the urine. They include 3-methoxy-4-hydroxymandelic acid (VMA), metanephrine, and normetanephrine. Epinephrine and norepinephrine levels in the adrenal gland vary with age. Norepinephrine is detected in fetal stages; at birth, it is the principle catecholamine, and in adults, it constitutes up to one-third of the pressor amines in the medulla. In stress, high levels of glucocorticoids are released in the venous drainage of the adrenal cortex; this exposure is required for the release of epinephrine from the medulla.

ADRENOCORTICAL INSUFFICIENCY

Primary Adrenal Insufficiency

Primary adrenal insufficiency (**Table 82.1**) can result from congenital or acquired lesions of the adrenal cortex and cause reduced production of cortisol and occasionally aldosterone. Lesions in the anterior pituitary or hypothalamus may cause a deficiency of ACTH (secondary adrenal insufficiency) or CRH (tertiary adrenal insufficiency), and lead to insufficient production of cortisol by the adrenal cortex. The signs and symptoms of adrenocortical insufficiency (**Table 82.2**) vary, determined by the hormones that are deficient and the specific steroids that are oversecreted (as in cases of inborn errors of biosynthesis of cortisol and aldosterone).

Adrenal Crisis Overview

Adrenal crisis may occur in patients with primary adrenal insufficiency, hypopituitarism, after a stressful insult (infection, trauma, or dehydration), and abrupt discontinuation of chronic steroid treatment. The patient may complain of abdominal pain, confusion, fever, and fatigue. Hypotension, tachycardia, and dehydration are common signs. Laboratory evaluation shows hyponatremia, hyperkalemia, acidosis, hypoglycemia, and low cortisol level. Treatment includes hydration with normal saline and intravenous glucocorticoid administration.

TABLE 82.1

Etiology of Adrenal Insufficiency

1. Primary Adrenal Insufficiency
   A. Adrenal hypoplasia or aplasia
      i. X-linked
         a. Duchenne muscular dystrophy and glycerol kinase deficiency (Xp21 deletion)
         b. Hypogonadotropic hypogonadism (DAX1 mutation)
      ii. Familial glucocorticoid deficiency
         a. Corticotropin-receptor mutations/ACTH unresponsiveness
         b. Alacrima, achalasia, and neurologic disorders (triple A syndrome)
   B. Defects of steroid biosynthesis
      i. Lipoid adrenal hyperplasia (StAR mutation)
      ii. 3 β-Hydroxysteroid dehydrogenase deficiency
      iii. 21-Hydroxylase (P450C21) deficiency
      iv. Isolated aldosterone (P450C18) deficiency
      v. P450 Oxidoreductase deficiency
   C. Pseudohypoaldosteronism (aldosterone unresponsiveness)
   D. Adrenoleukodystrophy (peroxisomal membrane protein defect)
   E. Acid lipase deficiency
      i. Wolman disease
   F. Destructive lesions of adrenal cortex
      i. Granulomatous lesions (e.g., tuberculosis)
   G. Autoimmune adrenalitis (idiopathic Addison disease)
      i. Isolated
      ii. Associated with hypoparathyroidism or mucocutaneous candidiasis (type I autoimmune polyglandular syndrome/AIRE gene mutation), or both
      iii. Associated with autoimmune thyroid disease and insulin dependent diabetes (type II autoimmune polyglandular syndrome)
   H. Neonatal hemorrhage
   I. Acute infection (Waterhouse–Friderichsen syndrome)
   J. Mitochondrial disorders
   K. Acquired immunodeficiency syndrome
2. Secondary Adrenal Insufficiency (ACTH deficiency)
   A. Isolated
   B. Autosomal recessive
   C. Multiple deficiencies
      i. Pituitary hypoplasia or aplasia
      ii. Destructive lesions (e.g., craniopharyngioma)
      iii. Autoimmune hypophysitis
3. Tertiary Adrenal Insufficiency
   A. Isolated
   B. Multiple deficiencies
      i. Congenital defects (e.g., anencephaly, septo-optic dysplasia)
      ii. Destructive lesions (e.g., tumor)
      iii. Idiopathic (e.g., idiopathic hypopituitarism)
4. Secondary or Tertiary, or Combined Forms of Adrenal Insufficiency
   A. Iatrogenic
      i. Abrupt cessation of exogenous corticosteroids or corticotropin
      ii. Removal of functioning adrenal tumor
      iii. Adrenalectomy for Cushing disease
      iv. Drug administration: aminoglutethimide, mitotane (o, p´-DDD), metyrapone, ketoconazole
   B. Fetal adrenal suppression—maternal hypercortisolism

Congenital Causes

Congenital Adrenal Hyperplasia. In infancy, the salt-wasting forms of congenital adrenal hyperplasia are the most common cause. These patients commonly have deficiency of P450c21 (21-hydroxylase) or of 3 β-hydroxysteroid dehydrogenase. Inability to synthesize cortisol or aldosterone can lead to salt wasting (shock and vascular collapse) with hyponatremia, hyperkalemia, and acidosis in newborns. Patients with salt-wasting crisis usually present in the first week

TABLE 82.2

Signs and Symptoms of Adrenal Insufficiency

■ GLUCOCORTICOID DEFICIENCY	■ MINERALOCORTICOID DEFICIENCY	■ ADRENAL ANDROGEN DEFICIENCY
Fasting hypoglycemia	Weight loss	Decreased pubic and axillary hair
Increased insulin sensitivity	Fatigue	Increased β-lipotropin levels
Nausea	Nausea	Hyperpigmentation
Vomiting	Vomiting	
Fatigue	Salt-craving	
Muscle weakness	Hypotension	
	Hyperkalemia, hyponatremia, metabolic acidosis (normal anion gap)	

of life. Females with 21-hydroxylase deficiency are easier to diagnose due to virilization of the external genitalia, which results from extra-adrenal androgen production in utero.

Adrenal Hypoplasia Congenita. Adrenal hypoplasia congenita with adrenal insufficiency also presents with a salt-wasting crisis in the first few weeks of life. However, the presentation can be more delayed into later childhood and adulthood. This disorder is caused by a mutation of the *DAX1* gene. It affects primarily boys who can also present with cryptorchidism and hypogonadotropic hypogonadism, and who do not undergo puberty. This disorder also occurs as part of a syndrome together with Duchenne muscular dystrophy, glycerol kinase deficiency, and mental retardation.

Other Congenital Causes of Adrenal Insufficiency. Familial glucocorticoid deficiency is another form of inherited adrenal insufficiency. Hypoglycemia, seizures, and increased pigmentation are the presenting symptoms in such patients. These symptoms commonly present in the first decade of life, and patients usually have an isolated deficiency of glucocorticoid, elevated levels of ACTH, and normal aldosterone production. The disorder has an autosomal recessive mode of inheritance. Smith–Lemli–Optiz syndrome (SLOS), an autosomal recessive disorder, results from a defect in the *DHCR7* gene that leads to cholesterol biosynthesis defect. Patients present with multiple congenital anomalies and sometimes with adrenal insufficiency. Wolman disease is a rare disorder, from a mutation in the LIPA gene, that results in lysosomal acid lipase defect and intralysosomal accumulation of cholesterol esters in different body organs; this can lead to hepatosplenomegaly, steatorrhea, abdominal distention, bilateral adrenal calcification with adrenal insufficiency, and failure to thrive.

Acquired Causes

Addison disease is currently used to describe primary adrenal insufficiency that is mainly due to autoimmune adrenalitis.

Autoimmune Adrenalitis. Autoimmune adrenalitis is the most common cause (90% of the cases) of acquired adrenal insufficiency. The medulla is preserved while the cortex is markedly infiltrated with lymphocytes. Antiadrenal cytoplasmic antibodies and anti-21-hydroxylase (CYP21) are the most frequently reported antibodies. Clinically, Addison disease has also been described in association with two syndromes: type I autoimmune polyendocrinopathy (APS-1), known as the autoimmune polyendocrinopathy candidiasis ectodermal dystrophy (APECED) syndrome, and type II autoimmune polyendocrinopathy (APS-2), which consists of Addison disease associated with autoimmune thyroid disease (Schmidt syndrome) or type 1 diabetes (Carpenter syndrome).

Adrenoleukodystrophy. Patients have demyelination of the central nervous system due to the accumulation of high levels of very long–chain fatty acids in tissues, including the adrenal gland, as a result of a mutation in the gene encoding the protein ALDP that leads to impaired β-oxidation in the peroxisomes. The diagnosis should be considered in patients with Addison disease of unknown etiology, and screening for very long–chain fatty acids is advisable.

Other Acquired Causes. Tuberculosis was considered a common cause of adrenal destruction but is much less prevalent now. Meningococcemia is the most common infection that causes adrenal insufficiency. It can present as adrenal crisis and is referred to as the Waterhouse–Friderichsen syndrome. Although frank adrenal insufficiency is rare, AIDS patients may show different subclinical abnormalities in the HPA axis. Adrenal hemorrhage in pediatrics can lead to hypoadrenalism in the neonatal period. It is observed after breech presentation or difficult labor. These patients may present with an abdominal mass, anemia, unexplained jaundice, or scrotal hematoma. Medications, including rifampin and anticonvulsants (phenytoin, phenobarbital), induce steroid-metabolizing enzymes (cytochrome P450 superfamily) in the liver and reduce the effectiveness and bioavailability of corticosteroid replacement therapy. Ketoconazole, by inhibiting adrenal enzymes, can cause adrenal insufficiency. Mitotane is cytotoxic to the adrenal cortex. It is used in the treatment of refractory Cushing syndrome and in the treatment of adrenal carcinoma.

Clinical Features of Primary Adrenal Insufficiency

In primary adrenal failure, there is decreased or absent production of one or all three groups of adrenal steroid hormones. Usually the signs and symptoms develop slowly. Most of the patients present with fatigue, muscle pain, and weight loss. Gastrointestinal and orthostatic symptoms are common. Children may present with anorexia, nausea, vomiting, diarrhea, and growth failure. Hyperpigmentation is present in >90% of the patients. The typical distribution of hyperpigmentation is over the extensor surfaces of the extremities, particularly in sun-exposed areas. The mucous membranes (vaginal mucosa, gingival borders), axillae, and palmar creases are involved, and hyperpigmentation of these areas is the hallmark of Addison disease. In early infancy, the most common cause of adrenal insufficiency is sepsis, inborn errors of steroid biosynthesis, adrenal hypoplasia congenita, and adrenal hemorrhage.

Laboratory Findings

Hypoglycemia, hyponatremia, hyperkalemia, and ketosis are common. Hyperkalemia may not manifest in patients who also have significant vomiting and diarrhea, and it can be detected by EKG in critically ill children. In primary adrenal insufficiency, ACTH levels are high. Hypercalcemia is also associated with Addison disease. Biochemically, adrenal insufficiency is diagnosed by measuring serum cortisol before and 60 minutes after the administration (IV or IM) of cosyntropin (synthetic ACTH). The patient is considered to have a normal response if the 60-minute cortisol measures ≥18 μg/dL.

Treatment

A blood sample should be obtained before therapy for determination of electrolytes, glucose, ACTH, cortisol, aldosterone, and plasma renin activity to establish the etiology of adrenal insufficiency. If it is possible, specifically in infants, 17 α-hydroxyprogesterone (steroid precursor) level should be obtained. An ACTH stimulation test can be performed while initial fluid resuscitation is underway. Stress doses of hydrocortisone, preferably a water-soluble form, such as hydrocortisone sodium succinate, should be given intravenously. Acute doses of 10 mg for infants, 25 mg for toddlers, 50 mg for older children, and 100 mg for adolescents should be administered immediately and then every 6 hours for the first 24 hours. These doses may be tapered during the next 24 hours if the patient has a satisfactory progress. Most of the patients require chronic replacement therapy for their cortisol and aldosterone deficiencies. Hydrocortisone may be given orally in doses of 10 mg/m^2/day in three divided doses. During stress, such as infection or minor operative procedures, the dose of hydrocortisone should be increased two- to threefold. Major surgery under general anesthesia requires high IV doses of hydrocortisone similar to those used for acute adrenal insufficiency. If aldosterone deficiency is present, fludrocortisone (Florinef), a mineralocorticoid, is given orally in doses of 0.05–0.3 mg daily, since there is no IV or intramuscular preparation available. IV sodium chloride is administered to help correct sodium levels.

Mineralocorticoid Deficiency

CYP11B2 Deficiencies. A genetic defect in the CYP11B2 gene impairs the production of mineralocorticoids without compromising glucocorticoid production. Deficiency of corticosterone methyloxidase I (CMO I) deficiency or corticosterone methyloxidase II (CMO II) causes elevated renin activity and aldosterone deficiency, with the accumulation of steroid precursors prior to the biosynthetic block. These precursors have some mineralocorticoid activity, which compensate partially for the aldosterone deficiency. Thus, partial salt loss is the usual presentation rather than the typical salt-losing crisis of complete mineralocorticoid deficiency. The diagnosis is accomplished by laboratory evaluation, which reveals a low aldosterone level and elevated DOC and corticosterone in CMO I deficiency. Laboratory evaluation in CMO II deficiency reveals an increased corticosterone concentration and 18-hydroxycorticosterone. Treatment consists of giving fludrocortisone (0.05–0.3 mg daily), sodium chloride, or both in order to achieve normal plasma renin activity.

Pseudohypoaldosteronism. In this condition, the kidneys do not respond to aldosterone. The infant presents with dehydration, hyponatremia, and hyperkalemia despite marked elevation of aldosterone and renin levels. The mutations are either in the gene encoding the mineralocorticoid receptor (autosomal dominant and mild) or in the genes encoding the amiloride-sensitive epithelial sodium channel (autosomal recessive and severe). Treatment with mineralocorticoid is ineffective; the only effective treatment is sodium chloride.

Acquired Hypoaldosteronism. As in hyporeninemic hypoaldosteronism, there is damage to the juxtaglomerular apparatus and hence renin deficiency. Patients have hyponatremia, hyperkalemia, and normal or elevated blood pressure with both low aldosterone and plasma renin activity. Patients usually have impaired renal function, as seen in diabetes, SLE, myeloma, amyloid, AIDS, and use of nonsteroidal anti-inflammatory drugs. Many patients are asymptomatic, with only mild hyperkalemia. Administration of heparin may exacerbate relative hypoaldosteronism by inhibiting its synthesis and precipitate salt wasting and volume loss.

Pituitary Disease and ACTH Deficiency (Secondary Adrenal Insufficiency)

Pituitary or hypothalamic dysfunction can cause ACTH deficiency, usually associated with deficiencies of other pituitary hormones (growth hormone and thyrotropin). Craniopharyngioma and germinoma are the most common causes of corticotropin deficiency. Surgical removal or radiotherapy of tumors in the midbrain can lead to damage of the pituitary or hypothalamus with resultant secondary adrenal insufficiency. Congenital lesions of pituitary, alone or with additional midline structure defect, may be involved (septo-optic dysplasia). Severe developmental anomalies of the brain (anencephaly and holoprosencephaly) can also affect the pituitary.

Hypothalamic Disease and Corticotropin-Releasing Hormone Deficiency (Tertiary Adrenal Insufficiency)

By definition, this implies a hypothalamic decrease in CRH secretion or production. This commonly occurs when the HPA axis is suppressed by prolonged administration of high doses of a potent glucocorticoid and then that agent is withdrawn suddenly or tapered too rapidly. Patients at risk are those undergoing treatment for leukemia, asthma, collagen vascular disease, or autoimmune conditions that require massive doses of potent glucocorticoids and those who have undergone tissue transplants or neurosurgical procedures. The maximum duration and dose of glucocorticoid that can be administered before encountering this problem is not known, but when high doses of dexamethasone are given to children with leukemia, it can take more than a month after therapy is stopped before the return of the integrity of the HPA axis. These patients, when subsequently subjected to stress should be presumed adrenally incompetent for up to 1 year unless documented to have a normal cortisol response to provocative stimulation (e.g., ACTH stimulation test).

Secondary and Tertiary Adrenal Insufficiency

The signs of secondary and tertiary adrenal insufficiency are hypoglycemia, orthostatic hypotension, or weakness. Electrolytes are usually normal. Hyponatremia may be due to decreased glomerular filtration and free water clearance associated with cortisol deficiency. When secondary adrenal insufficiency is due to an inborn or acquired anatomic defect involving the pituitary, there may be signs of deficiencies of other pituitary hormones. When the patient is thought to be at risk, tapering the steroid dose rapidly to a level equivalent to or slightly less than physiologic replacement (~10 mg/m^2/24 h) and further tapering over several weeks may allow the adrenal cortex to recover without signs of adrenal insufficiency. Patients with anatomic lesions of the pituitary should be treated indefinitely with glucocorticoids. Mineralocorticoid replacement is not required. In cases of a unilateral adrenocortical tumor producing cortisol that results in Cushing syndrome, the steroid secretion is autonomous and does not require ACTH activation. Following removal of the tumor, the patient is in a condition similar to the cessation of iatrogenic glucocorticoid therapy and should be provided with exogenous cortisol during the stress of surgery and during postsurgical period. The patient requires additional steroid coverage at times of intercurrent stress for the next period of 6–12 months.

RELATIVE ADRENAL INSUFFICIENCY DURING A CRITICAL ILLNESS

Critical illness can result in an increase in serum cortisol, changes in the circadian rhythm of serum cortisol, decrease in corticosteroid-binding proteins, and changes in the number and sensitivity of tissue glucocorticoid receptors. **Figure 82.1**, panel B, shows the initial response to stress. The early increase in CRH, ACTH, and cortisol levels are proportional to the degree of illness. However, due to multiple mechanisms with prolonged illness, there can be impairment of the glucocorticoid rise, which results in acute adrenal insufficiency (**Fig. 82.1**, panel C). This phenomenon has been called functional or "relative" adrenal insufficiency. Attempts to define relative adrenal insufficiency may require assessing the response to exogenous administration of ACTH.

Many factors can contribute to relative adrenal insufficiency seen in trauma, hemorrhagic shock, and following traumatic brain injury. Another factor that may contribute to relative adrenal insufficiency is being mechanically ventilated. Adrenal insufficiency was also described in patients who had end-stage liver disease.

Clinical Diagnosis of Relative Adrenal Insufficiency in the ICU

In the ICU, cortisol levels can be high or low. An ACTH stimulation test can be used as a diagnostic tool (**Fig. 82.2**). It can be performed using 250 μg of synthetic ACTH. It has been reported that <9 μg/dL increment from the baseline, 60 minutes after ACTH administration, is associated with mortality. High baseline with low increment probably means that the patient is maximally stressed, and not adrenally insufficient, although they may not respond appropriately to additional stress. Comparison of a low-dose (1 μg) corticotropin stimulation test with standard-dose (250 μg) for the diagnosis of relative adrenal insufficiency revealed that nonresponders to the low-dose test had a higher mortality rate than responders to both tests, which suggests that the low-dose test can identify patients in septic shock with inadequate adrenal function. These patients had poorer outcomes and would have been missed by the standard-dose test.

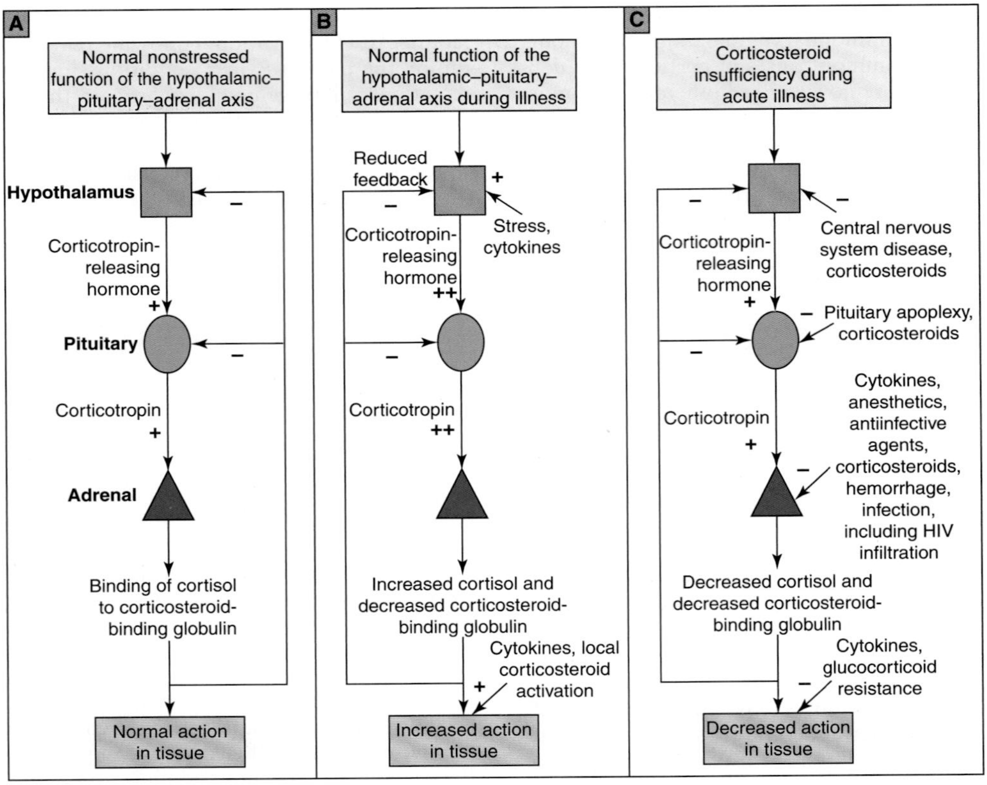

FIGURE 82.1. Activity of the HPA axis under normal conditions (panel A), during an appropriate response to stress (panel B), and during an inappropriate response to critical illness (panel C). A plus sign indicates a stimulatory effect, and a minus sign an inhibitory effect. (From Cooper M, Stewart P. Corticosteroid insufficiency in acutely ill patients. *N Engl J Med* 2003;348:727–34.)

ADRENAL HYPERFUNCTION

Cushing Syndrome

The most common cause of noniatrogenic Cushing syndrome in children is of adrenal origin. In adolescents who have Cushing disease, a central nervous system lesion, such as an ACTH-secreting adenoma, is more likely the cause of Cushing syndrome. In the ICU, Cushing syndrome in pediatrics is most often seen in patients who have received exogenous glucocorticoids. These patients may present with cushingoid appearance with moon-like facies, centripetal obesity, short stature, thin extremities, fragile capillaries, hirsutism, acne, delayed puberty, amenorrhea, hypertension, hyperglycemia, glucose intolerance, and osteopenia. In the ICU, the circadian rhythm of cortisol secretion is lost and cortisol levels at midnight and 8 a.m. are usually comparable. Diurnal blood samples from patients under conditions of stress in the ICU may demonstrate high levels of cortisol, making it difficult to differentiate these patients from those with Cushing syndrome. The treatment of pituitary-related Cushing disease in children is transsphenoidal pituitary microsurgery. Reoperation or pituitary irradiation is performed when relapses occurs. Patients with benign cortical adenoma can benefit from adrenalectomy.

Virilizing Tumors

Virilizing tumors are the most common pediatric adrenal tumor. Virilization is the presenting symptom and includes accelerated growth velocity, acne, muscular development, precocious development of axillary and pubic hair, and penile enlargement without testicular enlargement in males. In females, signs include hirsutism, masculinization with clitoral enlargement, and the precocious development of axillary and pubic hair with rapid growth. In addition to virilization, 20%–40% of the patients present with symptoms of cortisol excess. Patients have elevated levels of serum DHEA, DHEA-S, androstenedione, and testosterone. Cortisol and aldosterone levels are usually normal with normal serum electrolytes. Ultrasonography, CT scan, and MRI can be used to diagnose the tumor and metastasis. Surgery or laparoscopic removal of the tumor is the treatment of choice.

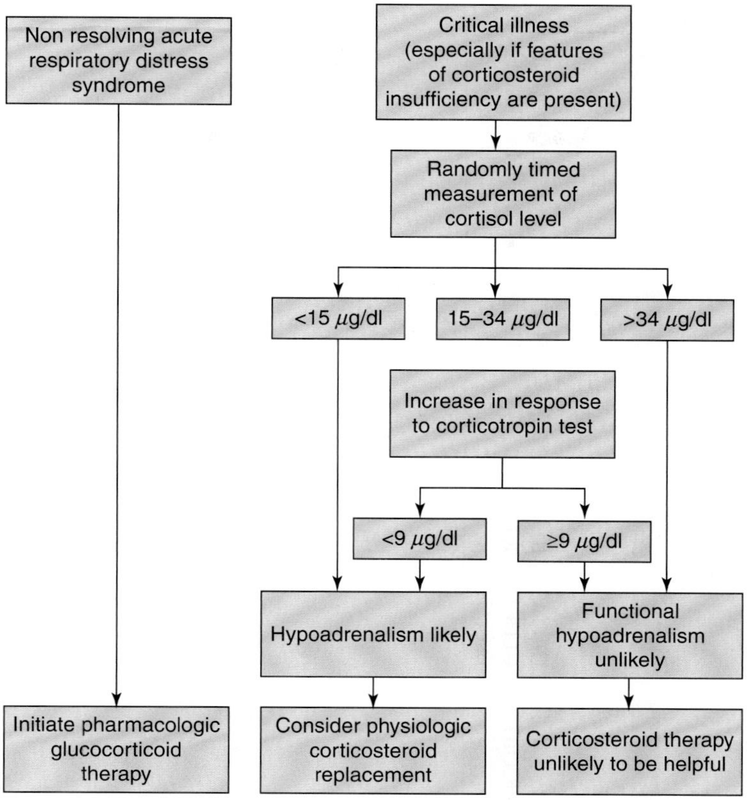

FIGURE 82.2. Investigation of adrenal corticosteroid function in critically ill patients on the basis of cortisol levels and response to the corticotropin stimulation test. The scheme has been evaluated for patients with septic shock. It must be borne in mind, however, that no cutoff value will be entirely reliable. (From Cooper M, Stewart P. Corticosteroid insufficiency in acutely ill patients. *N Engl J Med* 2003;348:727–34.)

STEROID SUPPLEMENTATION DURING STRESS OR IN THE PERIOPERATIVE PERIOD

In patients with acute glucocorticoid or adrenal insufficiency, treatment consists of supportive care, treatment of the underlying disease, and hydrocortisone replacement. Intubation should be prompt in unstable or obtunded patients. Etomidate can depress the adrenal cortical stress response and reduce cortisol and aldosterone production. Thiopental, propofol, and midazolam do not depress the adrenocortical response to stress, but inhibit steroidogenic enzymes. Children exposed to high doses of endogenous (Cushing syndrome) or exogenous steroids are susceptible to osteoporosis and pathologic fractures. These patients may have muscle weakness, so neuromuscular blocking drugs should be used with caution. Patients with adrenal insufficiency or receiving long-term steroid therapy need supplemental glucocorticoids in the perioperative period. A dose of 25 mg/m^2 of hydrocortisone sodium succinate is given IV just prior to anesthesia and is followed by a 50 mg/m^2 dose as a constant infusion during the surgical procedure, a third dose (~25–50 mg/m^2) is given as a constant IV infusion for the rest of the surgical day. This total of 100–125 mg/m^2 of hydrocortisone sodium succinate over a 24-hour period is ~10 times replacement therapy. This dosing can be followed the next day by three to four times replacement therapy (50 mg/m^2/day) of constant IV infusion. Eventually oral therapy is resumed.

THERAPEUTIC GUIDELINES/ STEROID PREPARATIONS

Various derivatives of steroids can be administered using multiple routes (**Table 82.3**). Hydrocortisone has the highest mineralocorticoid activity whereas dexamethasone has none. In adrenal crisis and hypovolemia, hydrocortisone is the best steroid to use whereas in patients with intracranial tumors or increased intracranial pressure, dexamethasone (which has no mineralocorticoid activity) is the most appropriate steroid to be used.

TABLE 82.3

Pharmacologic Characteristics of Various Steroids Relative to Cortisol

STEROID	ANTI-INFLAMMATORY GLUCOCORTICOID EFFECT	SALT-RETAINING MINERALOCORTICOID EFFECT	GROWTH-RETARDING GLUCOCORTICOID EFFECT	PLASMA HALF-LIFE (min)	BIOLOGIC HALF-LIFE (Hours)
Cortisone (Hydrocortisone, Cortef)	1.0	1.0	1.0	80–120	8
Cortisone acetate (oral)	0.8	0.8	0.8	80–120	8
Cortisone acetate (IM)	0.8	0.8	1.3		18
Prednisone	3.5–4	0.8	5	200	16–36
Prednisolone (Orapred, Pediapred)	4	0.8		120–300	16–36
Methylprednisolone (Medrol)	5	0.5	7.5		
Dexamethasone	30	0	80	150–300	36–54
9 α-Fluorocortisone (Fludrocortisone)		200			
Aldosterone	0.3	200–1000			

CHAPTER 83 ■ DISORDERS OF GLUCOSE HOMEOSTASIS

EDWARD VINCENT S. FAUSTINO, STUART A. WEINZIMER, MICHAEL F. CANARIE, AND CLIFFORD W. BOGUE

DIABETIC KETOACIDOSIS IN CHILDREN

Diabetic ketoacidosis (DKA) is defined as a blood glucose concentration >200 mg/dL, with ketonemia, and a venous pH <7.3 or bicarbonate <15 mEq/L. It is characterized by inadequate insulin action, hyperglycemia, dehydration, electrolyte loss, metabolic acidosis, and ketosis and is the most frequent cause of death in children with type 1 diabetes mellitus.

Pathophysiology

The primary abnormality in DKA is insulin deficiency that leads to increased gluconeogenesis, accelerated glycogenolysis, and impaired peripheral glucose utilization. When serum glucose levels exceed the renal threshold of 180 mg/dL, an osmotic diuresis occurs, resulting in dehydration and electrolyte loss. Physiologic stress caused by acidosis, dehydration, infection, or illness stimulates the release of counter-regulatory hormones (glucagon, catecholamines, and cortisol), which exacerbate hyperglycemia (increased hepatic glucose production and impaired peripheral glucose uptake) and promote lipolysis and free fatty acid release. Additionally, these hormones activate the β-oxidation of free fatty acids to ketone bodies, predominantly β-hydroxybutyrate and acetoacetate, which leads to ketoacidosis. Acetone is also formed (causes a fruity odor to the breath) but does not contribute to the acidosis. A vicious cycle of hyperglycemia, diuresis, dehydration, and acidosis ensues (**Fig. 83-1**). Poor peripheral perfusion can lead to lactic acidosis. Ketoacidosis leads to abdominal pain and vomiting, preventing hydration with oral fluids. The metabolic acidosis leads to potassium transport out of cells into the plasma and excretion in the urine. Patients are "total-body" potassium deficient (intra- and extracellular), often not reflected in serum level. Phosphate is affected similarly. A deficiency of 2,3-diphosphoglycerate may impair oxygen release from hemoglobin and further worsen lactic acidosis.

Clinical Presentation and Differential Diagnosis

DKA is not difficult to recognize in a child with known diabetes who is dehydrated, hyperventilating, and obtunded. In children not yet diagnosed with diabetes, it may be confused with gastroenteritis, pneumonia, sepsis, toxic ingestion, or a central nervous system (CNS) lesion. The diagnosis is suggested by a history of polyuria, polydipsia, polyphagia, nocturia, or enuresis in a previously toilet-trained child. Weakness and unexplained weight loss may also be present. Abdominal pain, tenderness, and guarding may mimic a surgical abdomen. Obtundation, vomiting, and abnormal breathing are related to the dehydration and acidosis. The physical findings include tachycardia, delayed capillary refill, dry mucous membranes, and poor skin turgor. Severe acidosis and dehydration may impair cardiac contractility, resulting in hypotension. Respiratory compensation for the metabolic acidosis induces hyperventilation, which may appear as deep sighing respirations (Kussmaul breathing). Acetone gives the breath a fruity odor, but it is not reliably detected. Most patients with severe metabolic derangements are lethargic but do not have severe CNS depression.

The laboratory evaluation includes blood glucose, plasma or urinary ketones, serum electrolyte concentration, blood urea nitrogen (BUN), creatinine, osmolarity, baseline calcium and phosphorus, and, if infection is suspected, complete blood count and blood culture. Although the definition of DKA presupposes hyperglycemia, ketoacidosis with normal or even low glucose levels may occur in patients with known diabetes who have taken insulin recently. Poor oral intake or vomiting may also present with near-normal glucose concentrations. Serum electrolyte concentrations may not reflect total body electrolyte disturbances. Because of the osmotic flux of water from the intracellular space to the extracellular space in the presence of hyperglycemia, serum sodium will be reduced. A normal or elevated sodium level in the setting of severe DKA suggests extreme free water losses. The degree of elevation of the BUN and creatinine, as well as the hematocrit, may also indicate

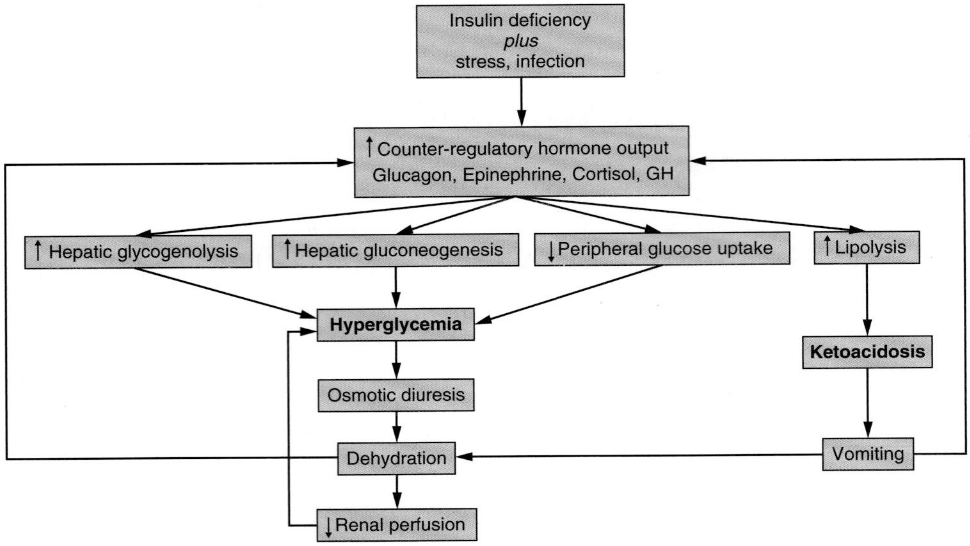

FIGURE 83.1. Pathophysiology of diabetic ketoacidosis. GH, growth hormone.

the extent of dehydration. The initial serum potassium may be low, normal, or high, depending on the degree of acidosis and urinary losses. However, total body potassium stores are almost always depleted, and severe hypokalemia may develop once treatment for DKA is initiated. Serum phosphate level may also decrease during therapy.

Clinical Management

Correction of Dehydration and Electrolyte Deficits

Overly rapid fluid administration should be avoided, and fluid deficits should be corrected over 48 hours. Hemodynamically unstable patients should receive isotonic fluid boluses in 10 mL/kg aliquots until improvement. Subsequent fluids should be isotonic or at least 0.45% saline to provide a gradual decline in serum osmolarity and prevent excessive free water administration. Hyperchloremic metabolic acidosis may develop. Early potassium replacement is needed to prevent a precipitous fall in serum potassium levels. Replacement with potassium phosphate also addresses the phosphate deficit. Serum calcium should be monitored when phosphate is given.

Correction of Acidosis and Reversal of Ketosis

Acidosis in DKA reverses with fluid replacement and insulin therapy but usually resolves more slowly than hyperglycemia. It is important to continue insulin therapy until acidosis resolves while supporting the patient with glucose to prevent hypoglycemia. Bicarbonate administration is not recommended in uncomplicated DKA.

Restoration of Blood Glucose to Near Normal

Insulin therapy, 0.05–0.1 U/kg/h without a bolus, should be initiated immediately after the patient has received initial volume expansion. The aim of therapy is gradual (50–100 mg/dL/h) correction of blood glucose. However, the serum glucose concentration often falls significantly with rehydration alone. Dextrose should be added to the IV fluid solution when the serum glucose level falls below 250 mg/dL and titrated to maintain blood glucose 100–150 mg/dL until DKA resolves. Insulin should be continued until the acidosis resolves. Many centers use two IV solutions that differ only in the dextrose concentration (10% and 0%). Independent manipulation of each infusion allows the dextrose infusion to be varied quickly and efficiently (the "two-bag" system).

Avoidance of Complications of Therapy

Cerebral edema carries a mortality rate of over 20% and occurs in ~0.5%–1% of pediatric DKA episodes. It is more common in patients during first diagnosis, in younger children, and in those with the most severe dehydration and metabolic derangement. It typically develops in the first 4–12 hours of treatment but may occur as late as 24–48 hours after the start of treatment. Symptoms include headache, confusion, slurred speech, bradycardia, hypertension, and signs of increased intracranial pressure. It is prudent to correct dehydration evenly over 48 hours (unless the patient is in shock), and monitor neurologic status and laboratory parameters closely. Treatment of cerebral edema is aimed at lowering intracranial pressure. IV mannitol may be beneficial if given early in the course. Hypertonic saline (3%) may be used as an alternative or in addition to mannitol.

Tracheal intubation may be needed for impending respiratory failure or airway protection. Although aggressive hyperventilation should be avoided as this decreases cerebral perfusion, care should be taken to match the level of hyperventilation the patient was spontaneously producing to avoid worsening acidosis. Intracranial imaging to exclude other pathologies, such as cerebral infarction or thrombosis, should be obtained but not at the expense of timely therapeutic interventions. Other less common complications of DKA include thrombosis (e.g., cerebral venous sinus thrombosis and catheter-associated deep venous thrombosis), cardiac dysrhythmias (related to electrolyte disturbances), pulmonary edema, renal failure, pancreatitis, rhabdomyolysis, and infection (e.g., aspiration pneumonia, sepsis, and mucormycosis).

Identification and Treatment of Precipitating Events

Infections are common precipitating events for DKA that should be worked up and treated. In children with known diabetes, additional education on insulin omission, or sick day or pump failure management, may be needed to prevent another episode of DKA.

HYPERGLYCEMIC HYPEROSMOLAR SYNDROME

Hyperglycemic hyperosmolar syndrome (HHS) is a potentially lethal disorder of decompensated glucose homeostasis, formerly known as hyperosmolar nonketotic coma or hyperglycemic hyperosmolar nonketotic syndrome. Patients with this syndrome suffer from the dangerous consequences of marked hyperglycemia and hyperosmolarity. The syndrome is increasingly described in younger patients.

Epidemiology

The syndrome affects known diabetics (particularly those with type 2 diabetes) but may also herald its onset. Precipitating factors include infections, coexisting medical problems (e.g., renal failure, pancreatitis), medications (notably, diuretics, steroids, anticonvulsants, and psychotropic drugs), and total parenteral nutrition, as well as conditions that lead to dehydration (e.g., burns and heat stroke). In contrast to the various etiologies described in the past, more recent reports noted a near-universal association with diabetic disorders (type 1 and 2 diabetes mellitus). Three-quarters of reported patients are obese. African Americans represent 70% of pediatric patients, consistent with the higher risk of type 2 diabetes in African Americans.

Pathophysiology

In HHS, insulin levels may be sufficient to suppress lipolysis and ketogenesis seen in DKA, but they are inadequate to promote normal anabolic function and inhibit gluconeogenesis and glycogenolysis. Thus, HHS presents as an unrecognized relative insulin deficiency triggered by intercurrent illness or medication. Regardless of the cause, the resulting surge of counter-regulatory hormones raises glucose levels by both enhanced hepatic glucose generation and worsening insulin resistance. This maladaptive milieu can precipitate massive osmotic diuresis and dehydration. Volume contraction reduces the glomerular filtration rate, further elevating glucose levels and hyperosmolarity. In HHS, ketoacidemia is generally neither the underlying nor the most extreme pathophysiologic disturbance. Because of the duration of symptoms and the extreme hyperosmolarity of patients with HHS, a much greater degree of volume depletion may be present. Typically DKA patients are 10% dehydrated, whereas HHS patients are15%–20% dehydrated. Greater electrolyte loss may be present and mortality is higher in HHS than DKA.

Clinical Presentation and Diagnosis

Patients with HHS commonly present with a history of weight loss, polydipsia, polyuria, and gastrointestinal distress. They are lethargic with neurologic impairments that range from a slightly altered sensorium, to focal neurologic deficits, to frank coma (the "nonketotic coma"). These patients are dehydrated, often with cardiovascular decompensation. The frequent absence of the symptoms and objective hallmarks of ketoacidemia may obscure the diagnosis. Laboratory findings show marked hyperglycemia (>600 mg/dL) and hyperosmolarity (>330 mOsm/kg). Glucose levels as high as 2580 mg/dL have been reported. The level of acidemia in these patients can be influenced by factors other than the degree of ketosis, such as severity of shock, effectiveness of respiratory compensation, and use of large quantities of normal saline. Laboratory evidence of end-organ injury is typically found, in particular acute kidney injury, as well as rhabdomyolysis and pancreatitis. Finally, patients with this disorder may have significant electrolyte imbalance.

Treatment

Volume resuscitation is the mainstay of therapy for HHS. Pediatric guidelines suggest an initial normal saline bolus of 20 mL/kg (repeating as necessary to restore peripheral perfusion), and an appropriate maintenance rate plus replacement of the remaining volume deficit over 24–48 hours, in addition to replacement of ongoing urinary losses, which can be exceedingly high. Central venous monitoring may assist volume status assessment and replacement. Isotonic fluid is generally recommended for the resuscitative phase of treatment, with half-normal saline employed later to complete rehydration.

Although insulin may have salutary, anti-inflammatory benefits, in the absence of significant ketoacidemia, it plays a secondary role in the initial management of HHS. Hyperglycemia can often be partially corrected by reestablishing renal perfusion and glomerular filtration, ensuring a more gradual correction of hyperosmolarity without rapid fluid and electrolyte shifts, and a lower insulin dose (0.025–0.05 U/kg/h) may be used in patients without severe acidemia. The blood glucose level should not decline by more than 100 mg/dL/h.

Electrolytes should be monitored carefully and replaced as indicated, with particular attention to potassium shifts with the initiation of insulin therapy. Volume contraction, the use of insulin, and copious amounts of normal saline commonly lead to hypernatremia. Finally, given the risk of rhabdomyolysis, serum creatinine phosphokinase should be monitored.

Outcomes

In pediatric patients, morbidity includes acute kidney injury, rhabdomyolysis, coma, malignant hyperthermia-type syndrome, and significant electrolyte disturbances. Neurologic findings are common. Adult mortality risk has been cited to be between 15% and 60%; newer estimates suggest a risk closer to 15%. In children, mortality risk ranges from 23% to 37%. Deaths have been attributed to cardiac arrest, refractory dysrhythmias, pulmonary thromboembolism, shock, and multisystem organ failure.

HYPERGLYCEMIA IN CRITICALLY ILL CHILDREN

Hyperglycemia has often been considered a marker of illness severity that required no significant intervention unless glucosuria occurred. A study that controlled blood glucose to normal levels with insulin and resulted in a survival benefit among critically ill surgical adults suggests a causal relationship between hyperglycemia and worse outcomes. Unfortunately, other studies have failed to replicate these results and management of hyperglycemia in the nondiabetic critically ill child remains unsettled. Despite the lack of a consensus definition for hyperglycemia, elevated glucose levels have been consistently associated with increased morbidity and mortality in critically ill children. Among all pediatric intensive care unit admissions, blood glucose >150 mg/dL is associated with a 2.5–10.9-fold increased risk of mortality. The intensity, timing, and duration of hyperglycemia are associated with outcome.

Normal Glucose Homeostasis

Noninsulin-mediated uptake of glucose by the CNS accounts for 80% of glucose utilization during basal conditions. Skeletal muscles remove the remaining 20%, half of which is insulin-mediated. After a meal, blood glucose is cleared in nearly equal amounts by the muscle, fat, hepatosplanchnic bed, and noninsulin-requiring tissues, including the CNS. The liver extracts as much as 40% of ingested glucose for conversion to glycogen. Although nearly all cells are involved in glucose uptake, glucose production occurs only in the liver and the kidneys. Two processes contribute to glucose formation: breakdown of glycogen in the liver and production of new glucose molecules from both the liver and the kidneys. Glycogenolysis provides most of the glucose after an overnight fast. However, with prolonged starvation, glycogen stores are depleted and other sources of energy are utilized. The balance of uptake and production of glucose is the result of an interaction between a number of hormonal, neural, and hepatic autoregulatory mechanisms. Insulin, glucagon, catecholamines, cortisol, and growth hormone are the major hormones involved. Insulin decreases blood glucose levels by enhancing glucose uptake and glycogenesis and inhibiting gluconeogenesis. In contrast, the counter-regulatory hormones inhibit glucose uptake and enhance glycogenolysis and gluconeogenesis.

Glucose Control during Critical Illness

Hyperglycemia results from the body's systemic response to stress. During stress, the hypothalamic–pituitary–adrenal axis and sympathetic system are activated, leading to increased cortisol and catecholamine secretion. Other counter-regulatory hormones and cytokines are secreted as well. This combination of factors leads to insulin resistance and elevated blood glucose. Studies indicate that stress hyperglycemia is a result of glucose overproduction rather than impairment of glucose uptake. Other gluconeogenic precursors, including lactate, alanine, glycerol, and glutamine, are produced during stress. The liver avidly extracts lactate from the circulation and converts it to glucose. The principal source of alanine is de novo synthesis from pyruvate in skeletal muscle rather than muscle breakdown, whereas glycerol is a by-product of adipocyte lipolysis. Fat mobilization significantly increases during stress. Finally, glutamine provides the primary source of carbon for glucose production in the kidneys. Counter-regulatory hormones and cytokines are responsible for the impaired glucose uptake in insulin-dependent tissues. Obesity, even in the absence of diabetes, is associated with insulin resistance. Hypothermia and hypoxemia can lead to insulin deficiency, whereas uremia and cirrhosis can increase insulin resistance. Glucocorticoid therapy and exogenous catecholamines produce hyperglycemia through a mechanism similar to their endogenous counterparts. Other underappreciated sources of hyperglycemia in the intensive care unit (ICU) are hypercaloric nutrition, infusion of dextrose-diluted medications, and the use of high glucose-containing dialysis solutions.

Pathologic Effects of Hyperglycemia

The data on the deleterious effect of hyperglycemia on the vasculature are derived mainly from adult studies. Hyperglycemic patients, both diabetic and nondiabetic, have worse outcomes after an acute cardiac or cerebral ischemic event, compared with normoglycemic patients. This finding has been attributed to impaired cardiac contractility, increased frequency of dysrhythmias, disruption of the blood–brain barrier, impaired endothelium-dependent vasorelaxation, and a prothrombotic state. Hyperglycemia, especially when prolonged, leads to nephropathy, neuropathy, and retinopathy. It is speculated that the effects of hyperglycemia are, at least in part, owing to endothelial dysfunction. High glucose concentrations also alter various components of the immune response. During hyperglycemia, vasodilation is decreased secondary to impaired endothelial nitric oxide generation, a dysfunctional kininogen–bradykinin system, and reduced mast cell secretion. Hyperglycemia-induced expression of adhesion molecules enhances the interaction between leukocytes and endothelium, preventing the white blood cells from migrating to the area of injury. Concentrations of complement cascade components increase with hyperglycemia, but complement-mediated functions such as phagocytosis and opsonization are depressed. Impairment in the immune response may explain the increased risk of cardiovascular dysfunction and infectious complications in hyperglycemic patients. Hyperglycemia also enhances coagulation by increasing the expression of tissue factor and activated factor VII. Multiorgan failure that is commonly associated with hyperglycemia is thought to result from increased coagulation activity leading to microthrombosis.

Management of Hyperglycemia Associated with Critical Illness

In the trial of mechanically ventilated adult surgical ICU patients randomized to tight glycemic control or conventional treatment the biggest decrease in mortality was seen in patients who stayed in the ICU longer than 5 days and in patients with multiorgan failure and a proven focus of infection. There was a significant reduction in bloodstream infections, acute kidney injury requiring dialysis or hemofiltration, and critical illness neuropathy in the treatment group. In a follow-up study that randomized critically ill adults who were anticipated to stay in the ICU for at least 3 days, there was no significant difference in the mortality between the two groups. However, there was a reduction in acute kidney injury, number of mechanical ventilator days, and duration of ICU and hospital stay in the treatment group. Subsequent multicenter trials failed to replicate these results. On the basis of the available studies, it is currently recommended to maintain blood glucose <180 mg/dL with a range that is more liberal than 80–110 mg/dL in critically ill adults.

A total of four randomized controlled trials on tight glycemic control in critically ill children have been completed. In one of the trials, only children who underwent repair of congenital heart disease were enrolled while in two other trials, the majority of those enrolled underwent cardiac surgery. In the fourth trial, only children with burns were enrolled. A meta-analysis of these trials did not show any survival benefit with tight glycemic control. However, the odds of infection were 0.76-fold lower with tight glycemic control, which was primarily driven by the trial of children with burns. The odds of hypoglycemia were sixfold higher with tight glycemic control. The risk of hypoglycemia, though, can be decreased with the use of continuous glucose monitoring. Tight glycemic control does not seem to provide any benefit in children who underwent repair of congenital heart disease. It is unknown if this is also true for children who did not undergo cardiac surgery, which is the subject of an ongoing trial. There are currently no formal recommendations to guide the treatment of hyperglycemia in critically ill children.

HYPOGLYCEMIA IN CHILDREN

Part of the difficulty in defining hypoglycemia results from the use of blood glucose measurement as a surrogate for symptomatic neuroglycopenia. Pediatric intensivists tend to use thresholds of 40–80 mg/dL to define hypoglycemia. Historically, the parameters for hypoglycemia were based on age and statistical rather than physiologic grounds. The infant brain may actually be more vulnerable to hypoglycemic injury and it is recommended that blood glucose <60 mg/dL deserves treatment. In the absence of insulin, hypoglycemia occurs in 7%–9.7% of children in the ICU.

Pathophysiology

With rare exceptions, hypoglycemia in infants and children is a failure of fasting adaptation. The elements of fasting include the four alternative fuel pathways: (a) hepatic glycogenolysis, (b) hepatic gluconeogenesis, (c) adipose tissue lipolysis, and (d) hepatic fatty acid oxidation and ketogenesis. These systems are under hormonal control by insulin (suppresses fasting systems) and the counter-regulatory hormones (stimulate fasting systems). Two to three hours after a meal, the circulating glucose derived from intestinal absorption of carbohydrates dissipates, and the first phase of fasting occurs. Insulin secretion is suppressed, and counter-regulatory hormones increase, allowing glucose to be released from hepatic glycogen stores. By 12–16 hours of fasting (earlier in sick or premature newborns), glycogen stores are depleted. Muscle and adipose stores are mobilized. Amino acids derived from muscle breakdown are the primary substrates for the production of new glucose by hepatic gluconeogenesis. Fatty acids released from lipolysis of adipose tissue are either utilized directly as a fuel (particularly in muscle) or further oxidized in the liver, generating the energy required for the process of hepatic gluconeogenesis and the formation of ketones, an alternate fuel for the brain. In insulin-induced hypoglycemia, lipolysis is inhibited and the reduced ketone production deprives the brain of an alternate energy source.

Causes of Hypoglycemia

Critically ill children may not have adequate glycogen stores as a result of malnutrition, prematurity, or prolonged illness. Renal and hepatic failure may impair gluconeogenesis. Renal failure may also impair insulin metabolism, leading to insulin accumulation and prolonged action of the drug. There may be a relative insufficiency of counter-regulatory hormones that is unable to counteract a drop in blood glucose. Sepsis and asphyxia induce a hyperinsulinemic state from cytokines. Other risk factors associated with hypoglycemia in critically ill children include age <1 year, high severity of illness, mechanical ventilation, or vasoactive drug support. Acute interruption of high-concentration IV dextrose infusion is one of the most common causes of hypoglycemia in hospitalized children. Supraphysiologic insulin secretion cannot be downregulated quickly enough when the infusion is abruptly stopped. Inappropriate elevated insulin levels at the time of hypoglycemia, along with suppression of free fatty acids and ketones, are consistent with this phenomenon of transient iatrogenic hyperinsulinism.

Medications may induce hypoglycemia and include insulin; sulfonylureas and other antidiabetic drugs (by stimulating insulin release); quinine, pentamidine, and disopyramide (through augmentation of insulin secretion); β-blockers (by blunting adrenergic response to hypoglycemia); and salicylates and octreotide (whose mechanism is unknown). Recreational drugs, such as ecstasy and alcohol intoxication, can also cause hypoglycemia. Finally, factitious hypoglycemia due to Munchausen syndrome, in which children or their caregivers surreptitiously administer insulin or an oral secretagogue, may mimic true hyperinsulinism. Other causes of hypoglycemia that are not specific to critically ill children include inborn errors of metabolism (e.g., glycogen storage disease, disorders of gluconeogenesis, and fatty acid oxidation disorders), liver failure, disorders of the hypothalamic–pituitary–adrenal axis, hyperinsulinism, and genetic syndromes (e.g., Beckwith–Wiedemann syndrome).

Clinical Presentation

Symptoms and signs of hypoglycemia either arise from autonomic responses to hypoglycemia (adrenergic) or from neurologic dysfunction (neuroglycopenic). Adrenergic symptoms include tremors, diaphoresis, tachycardia, hunger, weakness, and nervousness. Neuroglycopenic symptoms include lethargy, confusion, unusual behavior, and (with more severe decrements in blood glucose) seizures, and coma. Signs of hypoglycemia are less obvious, or absent, in infants and young children. Symptoms may include apnea, pallor, cyanosis, feeding difficulties, tachypnea, respiratory distress, hypothermia, or a sepsis-like state.

Diagnosis of Hypoglycemic Disorders

A normal child should not become hypoglycemic until all available fuel sources are depleted and counter-regulatory hormone stimulation is maximized. Analysis of the integrity of all of the control systems at the time of hypoglycemia is required to determine the etiology of the disorder, the so-called "critical sample." The critical sample, which should be obtained prior to treating the hypoglycemia, consists of the primary fuel (glucose), alternate fuels (lactate, ketones, and free fatty acids), and controlling hormones (insulin, cortisol, and growth hormone). Administration of glucagon, subcutaneously or intramuscularly, at the time of hypoglycemia provides valuable information, as a hyperglycemic response to glucagon signifies persistent hepatic glycogen stores, which is abnormal in the face of hypoglycemia. Additional studies to be obtained include electrolytes, ammonia, lactate, acylcarnitine and organic acid profiles, and urinalysis for ketones.

The duration of fasting tolerance (i.e., time to hypoglycemia from last carbohydrate consumed), amount of glucose required to restore and maintain euglycemia, serum bicarbonate, urinary ketones, and response to glucagon suggest the etiology of the hypoglycemia until the confirmatory critical sample results are known. The presence of acidosis with hypoglycemia indicates an accumulation of either ketones or lactate. Ketoacidosis is a normal response to prolonged fasting, while lactic acidosis generally indicates a block in the gluconeogenic pathway (failure to convert lactate to glucose). However, fasting tolerance of <4–6 hours, significant ketosis, and fatty acid breakdown in a child with hepatomegaly suggest one of the glycogen storage diseases, which are all characterized by the absence of glycemic response to glucagon and normal parenteral glucose requirements to restore and maintain euglycemia. Supraphysiologic glucose requirement, low or absent ketones, and glycemic response to glucagon (>30 mg/dL) are the hallmarks of hyperinsulinism, in which excessive insulin action inhibits glycogenolysis and promotes excessive peripheral glucose uptake. Disorders of fatty acid oxidation are also associated with low or absent ketones, but glucose requirements are normal and glycemic response to glucagon is absent. Hypopituitarism, either simple growth hormone deficiency or multiple pituitary hormone deficiency, is difficult to classify in this framework, as glucose requirements may be supraphysiologic and glycemic response to glucagon inconclusive.

Treatment of Hypoglycemia

In the acute setting, the immediate goal of treatment is to increase the plasma glucose to at least 70 mg/dL. Rapid improvement in blood sugar is normally seen after administration of 10% dextrose, 2 mL/kg by IV push, followed by continuous IV dextrose at a rate of at least 8 mg/kg/min, accompanied by frequent glucose levels and escalation if needed. Definitive treatment of hypoglycemia depends on the underlying condition.

Outcomes

The precise level and duration of hypoglycemia required to cause permanent neurologic dysfunction is unknown. Children with hyperinsulinism appear to be most vulnerable, with neurodevelopmental complications reported in 26%–44%. Younger age at presentation, longer duration of hypoglycemia, and unresponsiveness to medical therapy are associated with greater risk of neurologic sequelae.

CHAPTER 84 ■ DISORDERS OF WATER, SODIUM, AND POTASSIUM HOMEOSTASIS

JAMES SCHNEIDER AND ANDREA KELLY

Critically ill children are frequently admitted with, or develop, disorders of water, sodium (Na^+), or potassium (K^+).

NORMAL PHYSIOLOGY AND PATHOPHYSIOLOGY

Strict regulation of total body water, Na^+, and K^+ occurs through multiple, often redundant, pathways. Regulation of Na^+ is critical for maintaining extracellular fluid (ECF) volume, while regulation of K^+ is vital for maintaining cellular electrophysiology. Water regulation is primarily influenced by changes in serum osmolality and volume status. The kidney is the primary site for regulation of Na^+, K^+, and water (**Fig. 84.1**).

Renal Handling of Water and Solutes—an Overview

The glomerular filtration rate (GFR) dictates the maximum amount of fluid that can be delivered to the tubules. Vasoconstriction of afferent arterioles decreases glomerular blood flow, thereby decreasing glomerular pressure and filtration, while vasoconstriction of efferent arterioles increases glomerular pressure and filtration. A feedback mechanism, mediated by the macula densa, controls the vasoconstriction and vasodilation of the afferent and efferent arterioles to autoregulate the GFR. Afferent and efferent arterioles are regulated by the sympathetic nervous system and angiotensin II. Following filtration at the level of the glomerulus, the fluid is delivered to the

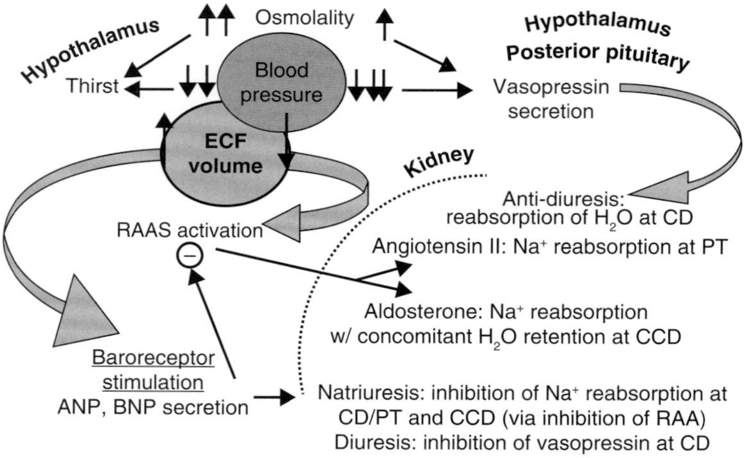

FIGURE 84.1. Regulation of extracellular fluid (ECF) osmolality and volume. Vasopressin secretion is primarily responsible for preserving plasma osmolality. Secretion of vasopressin by the hypothalamus occurs with as little as a 1% increase in plasma osmolality. Much larger increases in plasma osmolality are required to trigger thirst, the center for which is also located in the hypothalamus. This offsetting likely occurs to avoid simultaneously activating thirst and vasopressin secretion at the lower end of normal plasma osmolality, which would result in overcorrection. Significant decreases in blood pressure/effective ECF volume, communicated to the hypothalamus via cardiovascular baroreceptors, are required to trigger vasopressin secretion. Vasopressin recruits aquaporin-2 water channels in the renal collecting ducts (CD) to promote reabsorption of water and concentration of urine. ECF volume is primarily maintained through Na^+ homeostasis. Decreases in blood pressure/effective ECF volume also activate the renin–angiotensin–aldosterone system (RAAS). Aldosterone promotes reabsorption of Na^+ and water at the renal cortical-collecting duct (CCD), and angiotensin II stimulates Na^+ reabsorption at the proximal tubules (PT). Hypertension/fluid overload activates cardiovascular baroreceptors, leading to A-type natriuretic peptide (ANP) and brain natriuretic peptide (BNP) release. These peptides promote Na^+ and water excretion at the level of the kidney.

tubules. The proximal tubule accounts for 65% of filtrate reabsorption, including Na^+, K^+, and water. The descending thin limb of the loop of Henle is permeable to water, urea, and other solutes, while the ascending thin limb is relatively impermeable to water. The thick ascending limb (TAL) and the initial segment of the distal tubule avidly absorb Na^+ and other solutes but are impermeable to water regardless of the status of vasopressin and, hence, are referred to as the *diluting segment* of the kidney. The late distal tubule and cortical-collecting duct mediate the Na^+-retaining and K^+-wasting effects of aldosterone. In addition, like the collecting duct, they are permeable to water only in the presence of vasopressin. Na/K-ATPase pumps Na^+ into the renal interstitium and ultimately to the peritubular capillaries. Activity of this enzyme generates an Na^+ concentration gradient and an electrochemical gradient between the tubule lumen and the tubular cell.

Water Homeostasis

The human body is composed of 42%–75% water. Approximately two-thirds of the water is located intracellularly. The remaining estimated one-third is located extracellularly and is divided between the interstitium (three-fourths) and plasma (one-fourth). The solute content of these compartments differs significantly, with K^+ the primary constituent of intracellular fluid (ICF) and Na^+ the major electrolyte in ECF. Na/K-ATPase maintains the transcellular gradient, exchanging three molecules of intracellular Na^+ for two molecules of extracellular K. The normal range for blood osmolality is 280–290 mOsm/kg H_2O. Cell membranes are freely water permeable. As a result, when a concentration gradient develops between ECF and ICF, water passively moves from the compartment with the lower to the higher gradient, thus restoring equilibrium. ECF osmolality can be estimated based on the equation $2 \times Na + [\text{urea nitrogen (mg/dL)}/2.8] + [\text{glucose (mg/dL)}/18]$. Urea nitrogen and glucose (in the absence of hyperglycemia/insulin deficiency) freely permeate most cell membranes, with the exception of the blood–brain barrier (BBB), and are considered ineffective osmoles because they do not influence transcellular water flux. Plasma Na^+ effectively drives water homeostasis. Normally, insensible loss of water consists of ~300–500 mL/m^2/day.

Vasopressin

Arginine vasopressin (AVP), also referred to as antidiuretic hormone (ADH), is a peptide hormone produced in the hypothalamus. The distal axons of the neurons store AVP until its release into a plexus of capillaries and, together with the terminal axons of oxytocin-producing hypothalamic neurons, constitute the posterior pituitary. Plasma osmotic pressure is the major determinant of AVP release. In general, the threshold for AVP release is 280–285 mOsm/kg H_2O, and for every 1 mOsm/kg H_2O increase in plasma osmolality, plasma AVP increases by 0.4–1 pg/mL to a maximum of 4–5 pg/mL for maximal urinary concentration. Plasma osmolality is "monitored" via stretch-sensitive channels in osmo-sensitive cells. Changes in plasma osmotic pressure lead to changes in cell volume. Na^+ and mannitol are "effective" solutes because they do not freely permeate the cell membrane, leading to an osmotic gradient, shifts in osmosensor water content, and alterations in AVP release. Nonosmotic regulation of AVP includes blood pressure and ECF volume (**Fig. 84.2**), pain, nausea, and hypoglycemia. Normally, pressure receptors tonically inhibit AVP secretion. In contrast to the small increases in osmolality that stimulate AVP release, relatively large decreases in blood pressure (effective ECF volume) are required to mount an AVP response.

Activation of neural stretch-sensitive sensors in the cardiac atria, aorta, and carotid arteries leads to tonic inhibition of AVP secretion. Inflammatory mediators, such as IL-1β and IL-6, are stimulants of AVP release. Elevated levels of AVP are common in respiratory illness such as asthma and bronchiolitis. Further, high levels of AVP occur early in pediatric sepsis and septic shock (in contrast to deficiency of AVP in adults with septic shock). The primary antidiuretic activity of AVP occurs through recruitment of renal water channels (aquaporin-2) in the collecting duct. In the absence of vasopressin/aquaporin channels, urine is dilute (~50 mOsm/kg H_2O), reflecting

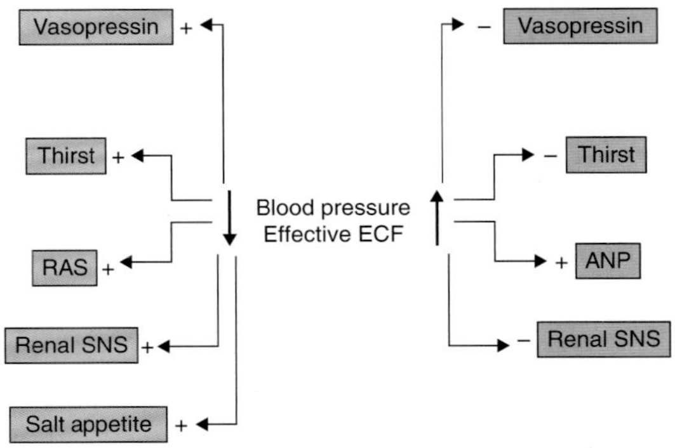

FIGURE 84.2. Responses to changes in blood pressure and effective extracellular fluid (ECF) volume. Detection of increased blood pressure or effective ECF volume by baroreceptors triggers suppression of vasopressin secretion, thirst, and the renal sympathetic nervous system (SNS), while stimulating secretion of A-type natriuretic peptide (ANP). Together, these mechanisms work to lower ECF volume and blood pressure. In contrast, detection of decreased blood pressure or effective ECF volume by baroreceptors triggers secretion of vasopressin, thirst, salt appetite, the renin-angiotensin system (RAS), and the renal SNS to affect water and salt retention and, ultimately, an increase in ECF volume. Discrepancies in blood pressure and effective ECF volume do occur; e.g., an increased ECF volume is ineffective, such as that occurs with congestive heart failure, and causes additional fluid retention.

the obligate solute losses by the kidney. With the provision of aquaporin channels, water is absorbed along the concentration gradient. Urine concentration increases linearly with increasing plasma AVP concentrations until a maximum above which urine can no longer be further concentrated.

Thirst

Thirst is one of the body's two main mechanisms to protect against the development of hyperosmolality. The thirst center is located in the preoptic medial nucleus in the anterior hypothalamus. As with AVP, thirst is regulated by plasma osmolality and blood pressure/volume status. Cardiovascular baroreceptors transmit their signals to the thirst center through the vagal and glossopharyngeal nerves via the medulla, while angiotensin II directly stimulates thirst. Hypoosmolality, increased arterial blood pressure, and increased gastric water all inhibit thirst. Following activation of thirst and consumption of fluids, AVP secretion is suppressed.

Sodium Homeostasis

Salt Appetite

Like the thirst center, the salt appetite center is located in the hypothalamus. It, too, is regulated by ECF Na^+ concentration and effective blood volume.

Renin–Angiotensin System

Two distinct renin–angiotensin systems (RASs) exist: one in the brain and the other in the periphery. The peripheral RAS only has access to the central nervous system (CNS) at sites where the BBB is absent, such as the posterior pituitary and the circumventricular structures. Decreases in circulating blood volume/blood pressure detected by baroreceptors in the renal arterioles, extrarenal baroreceptors, and the renal macula densa stimulate renin release from the renal juxtaglomerular cells. Renin release is inhibited by angiotensin II, vasopressin, and atrial natriuretic factor. Renin converts hepatically derived angiotensinogen to angiotensin I. Angiotensin-converting enzyme, located throughout the vasculature endothelium (particularly the lung), converts angiotensin I to the active hormone angiotensin II. Circulating angiotensin II has access to brain receptors, the activation of which stimulates thirst and AVP secretion. At the level of the kidney, angiotensin II stimulates Na^+ and water reabsorption. Angiotensin II is a potent vasoconstrictor, which is more potent for the efferent than for the afferent arterioles.

Aldosterone

Angiotensin II stimulates aldosterone secretion by the adrenal zona glomerulosa. Increased plasma K^+ and decreased plasma Na^+ also stimulate aldosterone release. Aldosterone binds to a specific mineralocorticoid cell-surface receptor in the late distal tubule, leading to enhanced Na^+ and water reabsorption and K^+ excretion. In addition, aldosterone increases Na^+/H^+ anti-porter activity in renal intercalated cells to enhance hydrogen (H^+) excretion in the urine.

Natriuretic Peptides

A number of natriuretic peptides have been identified, including *A-type natriuretic peptide* (ANP), *β-type natriuretic peptide* (BNP), *C-type natriuretic peptide* (CNP), and *urodilatin*. Both CNS and peripheral natriuretic systems exist (**Fig. 84.3**).

ANP is a hormone produced by both the hypothalamus and the cardiac atrial myocytes. Atrial myocytes release ANP in response to distention of the cardiac atria, as occurs in the setting of fluid

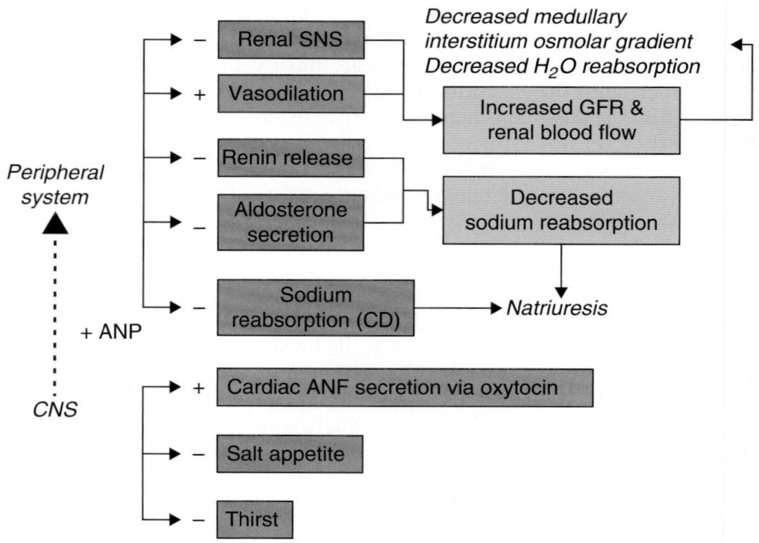

FIGURE 84.3. Activities of A-type natriuretic peptide (ANP). ANP acts both centrally and peripherally to mediate its effects. Centrally, ANP suppresses thirst and salt appetite while promoting additional atrial naturetic factor (ANF) release by the heart. Peripherally, ANP promotes vasodilation and inhibits the renal sympathetic nervous system (SNS) to increase glomerular filtration (GFR) and, ultimately, urine output. In addition, it directly inhibits renin and aldosterone secretion and Na^+ reabsorption at the collecting duct (CD) to promote natriuresis.

overload. β-Adrenergic stimulation also promotes ANP release. Through its effects on the renal vasculature, ANP increases the GFR, thereby promoting fluid excretion. It decreases renal Na^+ reabsorption by the distal convoluted tubules and collecting ducts, thereby promoting natriuresis. In addition, it inhibits renin and aldosterone secretion, relaxes vascular smooth muscle, and inhibits thirst. BNP is secreted by the ventricular myocardium in response to excessive stretching (i.e., fluid overload). Its mode of action is similar to that of ANP, although it binds to the natriuretic peptide receptor with much lower affinity. Its half-life is only 22 minutes, allowing it to dynamically reflect the state of the heart. Consequently, plasma BNP concentrations, or the biologically inactive *N*-terminal fragment (NT-proBNP), are used in the diagnosis and management of congenital or acquired heart disease and correlate with outcomes in those patients undergoing congenital heart surgery and in patients requiring extracorporeal membrane oxygenation. CNP is produced by vascular endothelial cells. CNP does not directly induce natriuresis and is thought to have an autocrine/paracrine effect at the level of the endothelium.

Cellular Responses to Disturbances in Plasma Osmolality

In response to an increase in plasma osmolality, water is shifted from the ICF to ECF in an attempt to maintain a balance in osmolality. A shift of inorganic osmoles, particularly Na^+, is accompanied by a shift of water to the ICF to help prevent cellular dehydration. Significant acute hyperosmolality can be accompanied by cellular shrinkage and likely accounts for the abrupt clinical symptomatology that accompanies such perturbations. In the brain, intracellular idiogenic organic osmoles (taurine, glycine, glutamine, sorbitol, and inositol) accumulate (by increased synthesis and decreased breakdown) over hours to days. These molecules offset increased plasma osmolality and reestablish normal intracellular volume without further increasing intracellular Na^+ and chloride, which can interrupt normal metabolism. Rapid correction of the hyperosmolar state in the presence of organic osmoles can lead to accumulation of ICF, leading to cellular swelling (i.e., cerebral edema). In response to a decrease in plasma osmolality, water is shifted to the intracellular compartment. The increase in cellular volume that accompanies these shifts activates Na/K-ATPase: Na^+ is exported extracellularly and is accompanied by water, minimizing the risk of cellular swelling. To compensate for chronic hypoosmolality, idiogenic osmoles are extruded and normal cell volume preserved.

Potassium Homeostasis

K^+ plays a key role in creating the resting membrane potential of the cell. The ICF contains nearly 98% of total body (40–50 mEq/kg) K^+ and has a K^+ concentration of 140–150 mEqL. The concentration of K^+ in the ECF, the site of the remaining 2% of total body K^+, ranges from 3.5 to 5.5 mEqL. Transport of K^+ with Na^+ occurs in the proximal tubule and TAL and accounts for over 90% of K^+ reabsorbed from glomerular filtrate. In addition, increases in ECF K^+ stimulate aldosterone secretion, thereby indirectly stimulating K^+ excretion in urine. Aldosterone interacts with the mineralocorticoid receptor in the late distal tubules and cortical-collecting ducts. Aldosterone also acts on the colon to stimulate Na^+ reabsorption and K^+ secretion. Other nonrenal regulators of K^+ include insulin, catecholamines, and acid–base balance. Insulin and stimulation of β_2-adrenergic receptors promote intracellular K^+ uptake through direct stimulation of Na/K-ATPase. Stimulation of α-adrenergic receptors triggers movement of K^+ to the ECF. Metabolic acidosis caused by mineral acids triggers a shift in K^+ to the extracellular space in exchange for hydrogen ions.

CLINICAL PRESENTATION AND DIFFERENTIAL DIAGNOSIS

Physical Examination

The physical examination must assess the degree of hydration as judged by vital signs, skin tone, and perfusion. An accurate weight as well as any recent change must be obtained. Examination should also include a search for the possibility of physical abuse.

Laboratory and Technical Studies

In addition to a basic metabolic panel, laboratory studies should include ionized calcium, serum magnesium, and studies of acid–base balance. A spot urinary Na^+ is extremely useful, with urinary Na^+ >20 mmol/L in conditions of hyponatremia indicative of high urinary Na^+ excretion. Direct measurements of plasma and urine osmolalities can be informative in diabetes insipidus (DI) and helpful in documenting salt-wasting polyuria. CT scan of the brain in those patients with potential cerebral edema or brain injury may be indicated. ECG is necessary for evaluation and for monitoring progress of all patients with water and electrolyte disturbances. Central venous pressure (CVP) is used to assess the degree of dehydration in selected patients.

Disorders of Sodium Balance

Differential Diagnosis of Hypernatremic Conditions

Hypernatremia is defined as the presence of serum Na^+ >145 mEq/L. Various factors contributing to the development of hypernatremia are commonly found in ICU patients (**Table 84.1**).

TABLE 84.1

Hypernatremic Conditions

Euvolemia (or Mild Hypervolemia)
Hypothalamic hypodipsia
Congenital central hypoventilation syndrome (CCHS)
Late-onset congenital hypoventilation syndrome (LOCHS)
Iatrogenic (excess Na^+ administration, e.g., hypertonic saline, medications, sodium bicarbonate, dialysis)
Hyperaldosteronism
Cushing syndrome
Hypovolemia (or Mild Hypovolemia to Euvolemia)
Water losses
Renal
Diabetes insipidus (central or nephrogenic)
Diuretics
Alcohol ingestion
Recovery after acute kidney injury
Hyperosmolality (e.g., hyperglycemia)
Gastrointestinal
Gastroenteritis
Osmotic diarrhea
Colostomy/ileostomy
Emesis
Insensible
Burns
Fever
High ambient temperature
Excessive sweating (overheating)
Decreased fluid intake
Neurologic impairment
Restricted access to fluids
Hypothalamic disorder
Fluid restriction

Hypernatremic Disorders Generally Associated with Euvolemia. Iatrogenic causes of hypernatremia are generally recognizable because such children are invariably being treated with IV solutions or tube feedings. Hypothalamic hypodipsia arises from loss of function of the hypothalamic thirst center incurred by brain injury or, less commonly, acquired congenitally. Affected children often have elevated Na^+ levels but remain asymptomatic. *Congenital central hypoventilation syndrome* (CCHS) is associated with hypothalamic hypodipsia and generally presents in the newborn period with periodic apnea and hypoventilation. This condition is often associated with Hirschsprung disease (20% of patients with congenital hypoventilation syndrome) and other autonomic nervous dysfunction, as well as tumors of the neural crest. The main issue with children with CCHS is hypoventilation during sleep, which results in hypercapnia and hypoxemia. In general, children with CCHS have normal growth and have intact hypothalamic function, including that of the thirst center (unlike late-onset central hypoventilation syndrome [LOCHS], which is frequently associated with hypothalamic dysfunction). Primary hyperaldosteronism is largely a disease of adulthood, whereas Cushing syndrome may occur in children (often due to primary adrenal tumors and less commonly due to pituitary adenoma). The more common cause of Cushing syndrome in pediatric intensive care unit (PICU) patients is iatrogenic, due to prolonged use of high-dose glucocorticoids.

Hypernatremic Conditions Associated with Hypovolemia (or Euvolemia). Many of the disorders that result in free water loss can be overcome with water intake, and relatively normal Na^+ levels and normal hydration can be preserved. However, if the fluid intake in response to free water loss contains significant electrolytes, hypernatremia is the outcome, despite normal hydration. Conversely, loss of free water without replacement will result in dehydration as well as hypernatremia. DI can arise from vasopressin deficiency (central DI) or vasopressin insensitivity (nephrogenic DI). The various causes of central DI are listed in **Table 84.2**. The most common reason for children with DI to be admitted to the PICU is for postoperative management of resection of a craniopharyngioma or other midline intracranial tumors such as astrocytoma. These resections are frequently accompanied by reversible injury or edema of the pituitary stalk, although complete and permanent transection can occur. A triphasic response follows severing of the pituitary stalk/injury, beginning with deficiency of vasopressin. This polyuric phase often lasts ~4–5 days. In the second phase, an unregulated release of stored vasopressin from necrotic vasopressin-secreting neurons occurs, which is often thought of as syndrome of inappropriate antidiuretic hormone (SIADH). Varying degrees of vasopressin deficiency then ensue, reflecting the extent of retrograde neuronal degeneration of vasopressin-secreting neurons.

Severe diarrhea or other forms of gastrointestinal loss of water, especially in very young children being treated with oral electrolyte fluid, can result in hypertonic dehydration. The child may be obtunded, with a doughy-like skin that will "tent" when pinched during assessment for degree of dehydration. The relatively high body surface areas of children predispose them to a higher risk of fluid loss than adults. For each degree elevation of core body temperature above 38°C, basal fluid requirements increase by ~12.5%. Diuretics, such as furosemide, that affect the loop of Henle in the kidney can result in mild hypernatremia. In addition, the accidental (or intentional) ingestion of alcohol will inhibit vasopressin release and cause excessive loss of free water.

Differential Diagnosis of Hyponatremic Conditions

The pediatric intensivist must be familiar with the diagnosis and management of hyponatremia, as it occurs in ~25% of hospitalized children, and is even

TABLE 84.2

Causes of Diabetes Insipidus

Central
Genetic
Autosomal-dominant inheritance
Autosomal-recessive inheritance
Wolfram syndrome (DIDMOAD syndrome) autosomal recessive
X-linked recessive inherited (associated with Xq2B)
Anatomic congenital malformation
Septo-optic dysplasia
Holoprosencephaly
Pituitary agenesis
Acquired
CNS tumors that involve hypothalamus or pituitary stalk (germinoma, craniopharyngioma)
Trauma—severing pituitary stalk
Surgery involving pituitary stalk (removal of craniopharyngioma or optic glioma)
Hypophysitis
Granulomatous disease—histiocytosis, sarcoid
Infection—meningitis, encephalitis
Vascular injury
Nephrogenic
Hereditary
X-linked (AVPR2 gene mutation)
Aquaporin-2 gene mutation (autosomal recessive, autosomal dominant)
Renal disorders
Sickle cell disease or trait
ADPCKD
Bartter syndrome
Bardet–Biedl syndrome
Cystinosis
Acquired
Hypercalcemia
Hypokalemia
Drugs
Lithium
Cidofovir
Foscarnet
Amphotericin B
Ifosfamide
Ofloxacin

DIDMOAD—DI, diabetes insipidus; DM, diabetes mellitus; OA, optic atrophy; D, deafness; CNS, central nervous system; AVPR2, arginine vasopressin receptor 2; ADPCKD, autosomal-dominant polycystic kidney disease.

TABLE 84.3

Hyponatremic Conditions

Associated with Euvolemia (or Mild Hypervolemia)
SIADH
Iatrogenic—water overload
Protein loss
Renal disease
Skin loss
Central adrenal insufficiency
Hypothyroidism
Associated with Hypovolemia
Salt wasting (cerebral, renal tubular)
Primary adrenal insufficiency
Nonketotic hyperosmolar coma
Drugs (diuretics)

more prevalent in PICU patients. After ensuring true hypoosmolality rather than dilutional hyponatremia (secondary to hyperlipidemia, hyperproteinemia, hyperglycemia, or elevation of some other effective osmole), hyponatremia can be separated into those with clinical euvolemia (or mild hypervolemia) and those with hypovolemia as outlined in **Table 84.3.**

Hyponatremia with Euvolemia. The SIADH, in which the concentration of AVP is pathologically elevated relative to the degree of hypoosmolality, is one of the most common causes of hyponatremia in the PICU. Due to the excess reabsorption of water, dilute urine cannot be produced, resulting in a urinary Na^+ level that is disproportionately elevated for the degree of hyponatremia. Nonphysiologic secretion of AVP is highly prevalent in PICU patients and is associated with a number of conditions, particularly brain injury (CNS surgery or radiation, traumatic brain injury), pulmonary injury, congenital malformations, and positive pressure mechanical ventilation. A number of chemotherapeutic agents used to treat childhood cancer, including vincristine and cyclophosphamide, have also been implicated as causing SIADH. In critically ill children, in whom the ability to self-regulate fluid intake is often compromised and for whom the renal handling of water is often impaired, free water overload can occur. The use of hypotonic maintenance fluids has been implicated in iatrogenic hyponatremia, prompting many to recommend isotonic solutions for maintenance therapy. In protein-losing disorders decreased intravascular oncotic pressure leads to interstitial fluid volume expansion, often resulting in symptoms of fluid overload, such as edema or ascites, but also may result in intravascular hypovolemia due to these fluid shifts. Decompensated heart failure, with compromised cardiac output, leads to hypervolemia (as evidence by edema) due to increased AVP levels as a result of carotid sinus baroreceptor stimulation.

Renal disease, both acute and chronic kidney injury, with reduced glomerular filtration and loss of tubular function, as well as after renal transplant, is a known cause of hyponatremia. The measure of the fractional excretion of sodium (FeNa) can identify the presence of abnormal renal Na^+ loss (if FeNa is greater than 2%) in patients with hyponatremia. FeNa can be calculated as

$$FeNa = 100 \times (UNa \times SCr)/(SNa \times UCr)$$

where U_{Na} is the urine concentration of Na^+, U_{Cr} the urine concentration of creatinine, S_{Na} the serum concentration of Na^+, and S_{Cr} the serum concentration of creatinine. Loss of Na^+ through skin can be substantial, especially in patients with cystic fibrosis or adrenal insufficiency during periods of excessive heat, in very febrile patients, or those with significant burns. Central adrenal insufficiency (i.e., secondary or tertiary corticotrophin-releasing hormone or adrenocorticotropic hormone [ACTH] deficiency) results in insufficient glucocorticoid production, especially during stress and can result in mild hyponatremia without hyperkalemia. Affected patients do not have the marked water and electrolyte problems of primary adrenal insufficiency because the adrenal zona glomerulosa is regulated by the RAS and not affected by ACTH deficiency.

Hyponatremia Associated with Hypovolemia. This clinical condition occurs as a result of the loss of both water and Na^+. Because salt wasting is associated with simultaneous water loss, it can result in severe hyponatremia and clinical dehydration. Prolonged use of diuretics, especially in the presence of concomitant salt restriction, can cause hypovolemic hyponatremia. Thiazides are associated with greater risk of hyponatremia than the loop diuretics. Primary adrenal crisis, or Addisonian crisis, causes the characteristic findings of hyponatremia and severe hyperkalemia and metabolic acidosis. Cerebral salt wasting (CSW) results in Na^+ and water losses from the kidney as a result of a CNS insult, despite normal renal function. The clue to differentiating CSW from SIADH is hydration status. The child with CSW will be dehydrated; the child with SIADH has normal-to-expanded blood volume (**Table 84.4**). The patient with type 2 diabetes who presents in the nonketotic hyperosmolar state can have significant urinary Na^+ loss from the osmotic diuresis and can have additional salt loss in vomitus. Nonrenal losses of sodium and water can occur in cases of diarrhea, emesis, gastrointestinal drains (i.e., ileostomies), or third-spacing (extravascular volume loss).

Disorders of Potassium Balance

Differential Diagnosis of Hyperkalemic Disorders

In general, mild hyperkalemia refers to plasma K^+ in the 5–6 mEq/L range, moderate hyperkalemia in the 6–7 mEq/L range, and severe hyperkalemia in the >7–8 mEq/L range. It is the intracellular content of K^+ that is of major concern. Initially, a mild elevation in the K^+ level is demonstrated by tall-peaked T waves, moderate elevations by a prolonged P-R interval, and severe elevations by flattened or absent P waves as well as widening QRS intervals (forming the classic sine wave), merging ST waves, and then bradycardia, all of which precede ventricular tachycardia.

Mild Elevations of Potassium Level. Routine electrolyte determinations often find mild elevations of K^+ secondary to hemolysis of red cells during blood sampling. Fasting or chronic starvation (e.g., anorexia nervosa) can result in suppression of insulin production and mild hyperkalemia. Drugs that result in mild hyperkalemia include β-blockers, angiotensin-converting enzyme inhibitors, and nonsteroidal anti-inflammatory drugs.

Moderate to Occasionally Severe Elevation of Potassium Levels. A number of drugs, including K^+-sparing diuretics, such as spironolactone, can raise K^+ levels. Other drugs that interfere with the RAS (including angiotensin-converting enzyme inhibitors, angiotensin receptor blockers, and heparin) may cause hyperkalemia. A single dose of succinylcholine will raise serum K^+ levels ~0.5 mEq/L. Those with neuromuscular disorders (i.e., muscular dystrophy), burns, and severe crush injuries will have a more profound release of intracellular K^+ and should not receive the drug. Massive cell death, such as that

TABLE 84.4

Differentiation of Disorders of Water and Sodium Balance Seen in Critical Care

	CLINICAL AND BIOCHEMICAL FINDINGS			
DISORDER	SERUM SODIUM	URINE SODIUM	URINE OUTPUT	VOLUME STATUS
DI (inadequate treatment)	High	Low	High	Hypovolemic
Excess DDAVP or water excess	Low	Low	Normal or low	Euvolemic/ hypervolemic
SIADH	Low	High	Low	Euvolemic/ hypervolemic
Salt wasting	Low	High	High	Hypovolemic

DI, diabetes insipidus; DDAVP, 1-deamino(8-D-arginine) vasopressin; SIADH, syndrome of inappropriate antidiuretic hormone.

occurs with tumor lysis or rhabdomyolysis, can cause hyperkalemia. Massive blood transfusion and red cell lysis during mechanical dialysis can similarly cause red cell breakdown and increase serum K^+ levels. Hyperkalemic periodic paralysis presents with attacks of disabling weakness and elevated serum K^+ levels. The average serum K^+ levels ranged between 4.9 and 6.1 mEq/L. A number of precipitants for these attacks are known, including cold, exercise, and hunger.

Potassium Disorders with Marked Elevation of Potassium. Renal disease, including chronic renal insufficiency, acute kidney injury, and end-stage renal failure, can be associated with significant hyperkalemia. Patients with primary adrenal crisis present in shock, dehydration, and often with cardiac dysrhythmias. Type IV renal tubular acidosis occurs in states of aldosterone deficiency or insensitivity and manifests as persistent hyperkalemia, reduced bicarbonate reabsorption, and potentially mild-to-moderate glomerular insufficiency.

Differential Diagnosis of the Hypokalemic Disorders. Hypokalemia, defined as a serum K^+ less than 3.5 mEq/L, is one of the most common electrolyte abnormalities faced in the PICU, and is less threatening than hyperkalemia. Nevertheless, low K^+ levels can be associated with cardiac dysrhythmias, particularly in the setting of preexisting cardiac dysfunction, or in patients receiving digoxin. ECG changes include flattening or inversion of T waves, ST depression, and development of U waves. Loop diuretics (furosemide, bumetanide, ethacrynic acid), particularly if used in conjunction with thiazides, are the most common cause of PICU-associated hypokalemia. Other drugs responsible for hypokalemia include glucocorticoids, chemotherapeutic agents, and laxatives. β-Adrenergic agonists and insulin cause an intracellular shift of K^+. Primary adrenal cortical disease (adrenal tumors or Cushing disease) occurs frequently in children, and the signs and symptoms are generally quite evident. Hypokalemic periodic paralysis arises from mutations in either the calcium (more common) or the Na^+ channel. Attacks are characterized by intermittent muscular weakness (particularly of the shoulders and hips) or generalized paralysis that lasts <24 hours. Bartter syndrome is clinically recognized by failure to thrive, developmental delay, increased renin levels, hypokalemia, and alkalosis. Hypertension and edema are absent. All subtypes of Bartter syndrome are autosomal recessive in inheritance and are characterized by abnormal NaCl reabsorption in the ascending limb of the loop of Henle. Gitelman syndrome arises from mutations in the thiazide-sensitive Na^+ chloride cotransporter. Affected children do not have growth failure or developmental delay.

MANAGEMENT OF SODIUM AND POTASSIUM DISORDERS

Regardless of the underlying electrolyte abnormality, the dehydrated child requires fluid resuscitation.

Hypernatremia

Hypernatremia with Hypovolemia

Following initial resuscitation with boluses and continuous infusions administered to restore perfusion and correct volume depletion, replacement therapy is required and must address the free water deficit. One can calculate the expected change in serum Na^+ with 1 L of a given fluid by the following equation:

$$\text{Change in serum } [Na^+] \text{ for each liter of given fluid} = (\text{serum } [Na^+] - \text{infusate } [Na^+])/(\text{liters of total body water} + 1)$$

In the child with known or presumed chronic hypernatremia, the subsequent goal of therapy is to decrease plasma Na^+ by ~0.5 mEq/L every hour (12 mEq/L/24 h) to reduce the risk of rapid shifts of free water into the intracellular space, causing cerebral edema. For patients with pure water loss (DI), the free water deficit can generally be calculated with the following equation:

$$\text{Free water deficit} = \text{TBWD} \times (\text{actual } [Na^+] - \text{desired } [Na^+])/\text{actual } [Na^+]).$$

An extremely obese adolescent may have a water distribution of 0.5; 0.6 is frequently used for the adult male, 0.5 for the adult female, and 0.7 for infants. After the free water deficit is calculated, a desired correction period needs to be determined. For the child with central DI, institution of vasopressin by continuous infusion (starting IV infusion dose of 0.5 mU/kg/h) will curb excessive losses. For some patients, vasopressin is not an option. In such circumstances, urine output must be replaced with water. One-sixth normal saline (0.15% NaCl) may initially be used to replace hourly urine output. Measurement of urine Na^+ should follow, adjusting the Na^+ content of the administered fluid to match the approximate tonicity to maintain stable serum Na^+ levels. If all urine output is to be replaced, then the maintenance component of the calculations must reflect insensible water losses only (300–500 mL/m^2/day) and daily electrolyte requirements. For children with hypotonic Na^+ loss (i.e., severe diarrhea, vomitus, nasogastric or drain output), the Adrogue–Madias formula calculates the amount that plasma Na^+ will drop following infusion of 1 L of fluid of varying components:

$$\frac{\text{Infusate } [Na^+] + \text{plasma } [Na^+]}{\text{TBWD} + \text{Wt (kg)} + \text{infusate volume (L)}}$$

Hypernatremia with Euvolemia or Hypervolemia

Treatment requires the withdrawal of the Na^+ source and the addition of water. For more severely compromised patients with fluid overload, the addition of furosemide to increase Na^+ excretion and water may be indicated. Determination of the hydration status will direct the evaluation as per **Figure 84.4.**

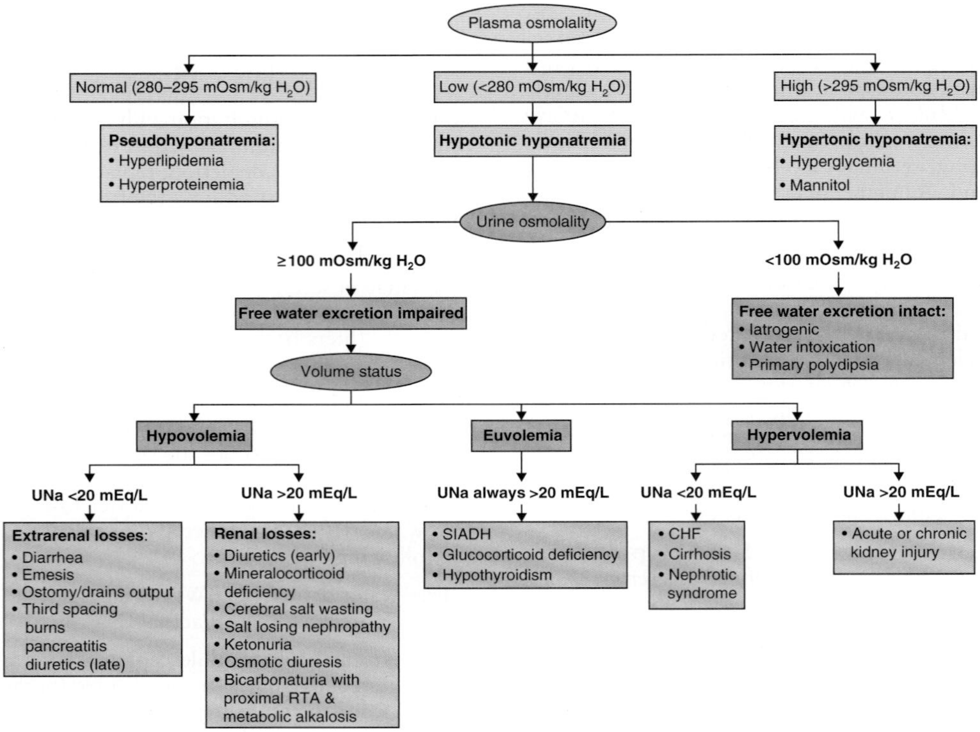

FIGURE 84.4. Diagnostic algorithm and differential diagnosis for hyponatremia (serum Na < 135 mEq/L). UNa, urine sodium concentration; RTA, renal tubular acidosis; SIADH, syndrome of inappropriate antidiuretic hormone secretion; CHF, congestive heart failure.

Hyponatremia

Hyponatremia with Hypovolemia

With hyponatremic dehydration, the Na^+ deficit exceeds the free water deficit. During an active seizure associated with acute hyponatremia, treatment considerations should include administration of 6 mL/kg of 3% NaCl to raise plasma Na^+ by ~5 mEq/L over 20–30 minutes. In general, if a patient has not had a seizure associated with the hyponatremia, it should be assumed that the development of hyponatremia has occurred over an extended period of time and thus should be corrected slowly. The total Na^+ deficit (in mEq/L) can be calculated as

$$(140 - \text{plasma } [Na^+]) \times (\text{TBWD} \times \text{Wt in kg}).$$

In an asymptomatic child, the target rate of rise should not exceed 0.5–1 mEq/L/h to avoid the risk of developing central pontine myelinolysis (CPM).

Hyponatremia with Salt-wasting and Known Central DI

After initial resuscitation, the Na^+ deficit should be determined and ongoing urinary Na^+ losses should be calculated by measuring urine Na^+ and volume. Vasopressin is withheld because it can potentiate hyponatremia. However, a vasopressin drip should be readily available at the bedside.

Hyponatremia with Euvolemia or Hypervolemia

This clinical scenario is almost always due to SIADH in critically ill children. It also arises in those with congestive heart failure, liver failure, or those on positive pressure ventilation. The child with symptomatic hyponatremia will require infusion of hypertonic saline. Following initial resuscitation in the symptomatic child, water restriction alone or in combination with hypertonic Na^+ chloride and a loop diuretic will increase Na^+ without exacerbating the fluid-overloaded state. Care must be taken not to attempt to correct a low plasma Na^+ level with sodium supplementation alone in the hypervolemic patient, such as with CHF or acute liver failure. AVP *receptor antagonists* (vaptans) enhance free water excretion while minimizing Na^+ loss. This new class of medications is FDA approved for the use in adults with euvolemic or hypervolemic hyponatremia. Although promising, subsequent clinical trials are necessary before routine use of vaptans will be recommended in children with hypervolemic or euvolemic hyponatremia.

Maintenance Fluids and Normal Serum Na^+

Children with illness requiring hospitalization have multiple nonosmotic factors leading to an excess in secretion of vasopressin. With the administration of hypotonic fluid according to the Holliday Segar formula, most hospitalized children are at significant risk for developing hyponatremia. The use of hypotonic fluids has been shown repeatedly to cause hyponatremia, and is the most important risk factor for the development of hospital-acquired hyponatremia. Therefore, it has been suggested that these solutions should only be reserved for patients with free water losses.

Hyperkalemia

Initial treatment of hyperkalemia in the setting of cardiac conduction abnormalities is two-pronged: stabilize the cell membrane electrical potential and acutely lower the plasma K^+ through redistribution. The former is achieved through administration of 10% (1 g calcium/10 mL) calcium gluconate, 1.0 mL/kg (100 mg/kg) IV over 2–3 minutes. Calcium infusion can be repeated in 5 minutes if ECG abnormalities persist. As to the second prong, rapid IV infusion of glucose (0.5–1 g/kg) and regular insulin (0.2 units/g glucose or 0.1–0.2 units/kg) will lower plasma K^+ within 10–20 minutes, with a peak effect between 30 and 60 minutes. IV dextrose should be continued and blood glucose tested. Treatment with inhaled β-adrenergic agonists is recommended in adults. A third prong to the treatment of hyperkalemia is the definitive removal of plasma K^+. This can be accomplished with sodium polystyrene sulfonate (Kayexalate), 1 g/kg orally or by rectum in sorbitol solution, if indicated and if not contraindicated by bowel pathology. Loop or thiazide diuretics are useful to increase renal excretion and thus should be considered early in therapy. Data on treatment of hyperkalemia with Na^+ bicarbonate are equivocal, and it is therefore not recommended as monotherapy.

Hypokalemia

The child with hypokalemia-induced paralysis or with hypokalemia-induced ECG changes requires urgent IV treatment (0.5 mEq/kg over 30–60 minutes by continuous IV infusion). The child who is on digoxin or has an underlying cardiac defect is at increased risk of dysrhythmias and may require IV treatment at higher doses (1 mEq/kg) and at higher plasma K^+ concentrations. Magnesium replacement may also be necessary to treat hypokalemia. The child with hypokalemia in the setting of DKA can be administered IV fluids as a combination of K^+ chloride and K^+ phosphate, as the child with DKA also has a phosphorus deficit.

CHAPTER 85 ■ DISORDERS OF CALCIUM, MAGNESIUM, AND PHOSPHATE

KENNETH J. BANASIAK

DISTRIBUTION OF CALCIUM, MAGNESIUM, AND PHOSPHATE

Approximately 99% of the total body calcium resides in the skeleton, with the remaining 1% in the soft tissues and extracellular spaces. Approximately 40% of plasma calcium is bound to protein, principally albumin, 10% is complexed with anions, and the remaining 50% exists in the unbound (ionized) form. Ionized calcium is the physiologically important circulating form of calcium. For magnesium, approximately 40%–50% lies within bone, 40% in the intracellular space, and only 1% in the extracellular space. Approximately 20%–30% of plasma magnesium is bound to protein, chiefly albumin, and 70%–80% is in the ionized form or is complexed to citrate, bicarbonate, and phosphate. The ionized form is the physiologically significant circulating form of magnesium. Approximately 85% of total body phosphorus is found in bones and teeth. The remaining total body phosphorus is distributed in the soft tissues (14%) and the extracellular space (1%). Approximately 60% of plasma phosphorous is in ionized forms of phosphate, hydrogen phosphate and dihydrogen phosphate. The remaining plasma phosphate is complexed to Ca^{2+}, Mg^{2+}, and Na^{+}, or is bound to plasma proteins.

REGULATION OF CALCIUM, MAGNESIUM, AND PHOSPHATE

Intestinal Absorption

Dietary calcium is passively absorbed in the small intestine and is actively transported in the duodenum and upper jejunum by mechanisms regulated by 1,25-dihydroxyvitamin D. Dietary magnesium is principally absorbed in the jejunum and the ileum by both active and passive mechanisms. Phosphate is absorbed in the duodenum and jejunum by passive processes and active mechanisms regulated by 1,25-dihydroxyvitamin D.

Renal Handling

Approximately 60%–70% of total plasma calcium is filtered by the kidneys, with <5% of filtered calcium being excreted in the urine. Most (~70%) of the filtered calcium is reabsorbed along with sodium and water in the proximal convoluted tubule (PCT). An additional 15%–20% of calcium is reabsorbed in the thick ascending limb of the loop of Henle (TALH). The remaining 10%–15% of filtered calcium is reabsorbed in the distal convoluted tubule (DCT), regulated by parathyroid hormone (PTH) and cyclic AMP. Approximately 70%–80% of plasma magnesium, in its ionized or complex forms, is filtered in the glomerulus. Approximately 3% of filtered magnesium is excreted in the urine, and 5%–15% is reabsorbed in the PCT. The majority of filtered magnesium (60%–70%) is reabsorbed in the TALH as the consequence of a voltage-dependent gradient generated by action of the Na^{+}-K^{+}-$2Cl^{-}$ cotransporter. The remaining 5%–10% of magnesium is reabsorbed in the DCT stimulated by PTH. The ionized and complexed forms of phosphate are filtered in the glomerulus and account for ultrafiltration of 85%–90% of the total plasma phosphate. The amount of phosphate excreted in the urine ranges from 3% to 20% of the filtered load. Nearly 80% of the filtered phosphate is reabsorbed in the PCT through the action of sodium–phosphate cotransporters, which are regulated by PTH. An additional 5% of phosphate is reabsorbed in the DCT. Thus, the kidney is the major site of regulation of total body phosphorous. Multiple factors can alter renal reabsorption or excretion of calcium, magnesium, and phosphate (**Table 85.1**).

Hormonal Regulation

The plasma concentrations of calcium, phosphate, and magnesium are regulated by hormones (**Table 85.2**).

Parathyroid Hormone

PTH tightly regulates ionized calcium and, to a lesser degree, phosphate levels in blood and extracellular fluids. PTH is synthesized in the parathyroid gland. PTH enhances reabsorption of calcium in the DCT and the cortical thick ascending loop of Henle. In contrast, PTH inhibits phosphate reabsorption in the proximal and distal tubules. Furthermore, PTH stimulates the conversion of 25-hydroxyvitamin D to $1,25(OH)_2D_3$ in the proximal tubule. PTH enhances release of calcium from bone. High blood concentrations of ionized calcium decrease PTH secretion,

TABLE 85.1

Factors Affecting Renal Excretion of Calcium, Magnesium, and Phosphate

FACTORS AFFECTING EXCRETION	CALCIUM		MAGNESIUM		PHOSPHATE	
	EFFECT ON RENAL EXCRETION	MECHANISM(S)	EFFECT ON RENAL EXCRETION	MECHANISM(S)	EFFECT ON RENAL EXCRETION	MECHANISM(S)
Volume expansion	↑	↓ reabsorption in PCT	↑	↓ reabsorption in PCT	↑	↓ reabsorption in PCT
Electrolyte Disturbances						
Hypercalcemia	↑	↓ reabsorption in PCT, TALH, DCT (↓ PTH)	↑	↓ tubular reabsorption	↓ (acute) ↑ (chronic)	↓ ultrafiltration, ↓ GFR and ↓ PTH (acute) ↓ tubular reabsorption via unknown mechanism (chronic)
Hypocalcemia	↓	↑ reabsorption in DCT due to ↑ PTH	↓	↑ reabsorption TALH	↑ or ↓ (chronic hypocalcemia)	↓ tubular reabsorption secondary to ↑ PTH
Hypermagnesemia	—	—	↑	↓ reabsorption in TALH	—	—
Hypomagnesemia	—	—	↓	↑ reabsorption in TALH	—	—
Hyperphosphatemia	↓	↑ reabsorption in DCT due to ↑ PTH	—	—	↑	↓ tubular reabsorption due to ↓ Na–P activity
Hypophosphatemia	↑	↓ reabsorption in DCT	↑	↓ reabsorption in TALH	↓	↑ tubular reabsorption due to ↑ Na–P activity
Acid–Base Disturbances						
Metabolic acidosis	↑	↓ reabsorption in DCT due to ↓ ECaC1 conductance	↑	↓ reabsorption in TALH	↑ (chronic metabolic acidosis)	↓ tubular reabsorption due to ↓ Na–P activity
Metabolic alkalosis	↓	↑ reabsorption in DCT due to ↑ ECaC1 conductance	↓	↑ reabsorption in TALH	↓	↑ tubular reabsorption due to ↑ Na–P activity
Respiratory acidosis	↑	—			↑	—
Respiratory alkalosis	—	—			↓	—
Metabolic acidosis	↑	↓ reabsorption in DCT due to ↓ ECaC1 conductance	↑	↓ reabsorption in TALH	↑ (chronic metabolic acidosis)	↓ tubular reabsorption due to ↓ Na–P activity
Medications						
Thiazide diuretics	↓		Minimal ↑	↓ reabsorption in DCT due to inhibition of Na–Cl cotransporter	↑	—
Loop diuretics	↑	↓ reabsorption in DCT due to altered inhibition of Na–K–2Cl cotransporter	↑	↓ reabsorption in DCT due to altered inhibition of Na–K–2Cl cotransporter	↑	Enhancement of phosphate excretion through inhibition of carbonic anhydrase
Aminoglycosides	—	—	↑	↓ reabsorption in TALH	—	—
Cisplatin	—	—	↑	↓ reabsorption in TALH	—	—
Cyclosporine	—	—	↑	↓ reabsorption in TALH	—	—

PCT, proximal convoluted tubule; TALH, thick ascending limb of the loop of Henle; DCT, distal convoluted tubule; PTH, parathyroid hormone; GFR, glomerular filtration rate; ECaC1, epithelial calcium channel type 1.
Modified from Suki WN, Lederer ED, Rouse D. Renal transport of calcium, magnesium, and phosphate. In: Brenner BM, ed. *Brenner and Rector's The Kidney*, 6th ed. Philadelphia, PA: WB Saunders, 2000:520–74.

TABLE 85.2

Hormonal Regulation of Calcium and Phosphate

	EFFECT ON SERUM LEVEL			
HORMONE	CALCIUM	MECHANISM OF ACTION	PHOSPHATE	MECHANISM OF ACTION
PTH	↑	↑ Reabsorption in DCT and TALH	↓	↓ Reabsorption in PCT and DCT
Vitamin D	↑	↑ Absorption in intestine and reabsorption in DCT	↑	↑ Absorption in intestine and reabsorption in DCT
Calcitonin	↓	↓ Bone resorption ↓ Reabsorption in renal tubules	—	—

PTH, parathyroid hormone; DCT, distal convoluted tubule; TALH, thick ascending limb of the loop of Henle; PCT, proximal convoluted tubule.

whereas low concentrations of ionized calcium increase PTH secretion. Elevated blood phosphate indirectly stimulates PTH secretion by reducing blood calcium and 1,25-dihydroxyvitamin D levels.

Vitamin D

Vitamin D is obtained from two primary sources: the skin and dietary supplementation. Vitamin D consumed in the diet is absorbed by the lymphatics and enters the circulation, where it is bound to vitamin D-binding protein and, to a lesser extent, albumin. In the liver, vitamin D undergoes 25-hydroxylation. Subsequently, the 25-hydroxyvitamin D undergoes 1-hydroxylation in the kidney to form the biologically active 1,25-dihydroxyvitamin D. 1,25-Dihydroxyvitamin D enhances calcium and phosphate absorption primarily in the intestine and, to some extent, in distal renal tubules. 1,25-Dihydroxyvitamin D also functions to promote osteoclast differentiation and bone resorption and to stimulate the synthesis of matrix proteins integral to normal bone mineralization.

Calcitonin

Calcitonin is secreted and stored in the C cells of the thyroid gland. Calcitonin inhibits renal tubular reabsorption of calcium and osteoclast-mediated bone resorption. The secretion of calcitonin is stimulated by increased blood calcium levels, glucocorticoids, calcitonin gene-related peptide, glucagon, enteroglucagon, gastrin, pentagastrin, pancreozymin, and β-adrenergic agents.

DISORDERS OF CALCIUM, MAGNESIUM, AND PHOSPHATE HOMEOSTASIS

Normal Values

Published normal values for total serum calcium range from 8.8 to 10.8 mg/dL. Because critically ill patients are frequently hypoalbuminemic and because ~40% of calcium is predominantly bound to albumin, one approach has been to calculate the corrected calcium level based on the serum albumin level using the following equation:

$$Ca_{corrected} = Ca_{measured} + [0.8\ (4.0 - albumin_{measured}\ mg/dL)]$$

However, it may be preferable for the clinician to obtain measurements of ionized calcium. Normal values for ionized calcium range between 4.2 and 5.5 mg/dL (1.0–1.4 mmol/dL). Reported normal values of magnesium are 1.5–2.3 mg/dL. Normal phosphate levels vary with age, with values ranging from 4.8 to 8.2 mg/dL in newborns and from 2.7 to 4.7 mg/dL in older adolescents.

Hypocalcemia

Hypocalcemia can occur due to inadequate calcium intake, malabsorption, hormonal imbalance or dysfunction, or chelation by anions (**Table 85.3**). Hypocalcemia in critically ill patients is commonly due to alterations in PTH secretion and action, vitamin D deficiency, administration of citrated blood products, and medication administration. PTH-deficient hypocalcemia may be due to impaired synthesis of PTH, inappropriate suppression of PTH secretion, or target organ resistance to PTH. Physiologic deficiency of PTH secretion occurs in neonates ("early neonatal hypocalcemia") during the first 4 days of life. Patients recover after several days of nutritional supplementation. Congenital agenesis or dysgenesis of the parathyroid glands occurs in a number of genetic defects, especially deletions in the chromosome 22q11 region, the locus for DiGeorge syndrome, velocardiofacial syndrome, and conotruncal face syndromes. A maldevelopment of the third and fourth branchial pouches causes thymic aplasia, facial anomalies (hypertelorism, antimongoloid slant of the eyes, short philtrum, low set ears, micrognathia),

TABLE 85.3

Causes of Hypocalcemia

Inadequate Intake or Malabsorption
PTH-related
Impaired parathyroid gland formation
Congenital agenesis or dysgenesis of the parathyroid glands
Digeorge syndrome
X-linked hypoparathyroidism
PTH gene mutations
Parathyroid gland destruction
Autoimmune polyglandular syndrome type 1
Inadvertent surgical destruction
Hemochromatosis
Thalassemia major
Wilson disease
Impaired secretion of PTH
Hypomagnesemia
Maternal hypercalcemia
Calcium-sensing receptor mutations
Cytokine release
Respiratory alkalosis
End-organ resistance to PTH (pseudohypoparathyroidism)
Vitamin D-related
Inadequate intake or absorption
Breast-feeding (without vitamin D supplementation)
Gastrectomy
Small-bowel surgery
Celiac disease
Inflammatory bowel disease
Cystic fibrosis
Increased catabolism
Phenobarbital
Phenytoin
Carbamazepine
Isoniazid
Rifampin
Theophylline
Decreased 25-hydroxylation (hepatic disease)
Decreased 1-hydroxylation (renal disease)
Vitamin D resistance
Chelation by Anions
Hyperphosphatemia
Red blood cell transfusions (citrate)
Lipid administration
Pancreatitis (fatty acids)
Other
Fluoride intoxication
"Hungry-Bone" syndrome
Critical illness

and aortocardiac anomalies (right-sided aortic arch, tetralogy of Fallot, truncus arteriosus).

Antibody-mediated destruction of the parathyroid glands has been detected in autoimmune polyglandular syndrome type 1 (APS1), resulting in hypoparathyroidism, primary adrenal insufficiency, and mucocutaneous candidiasis. Postsurgical destruction of the parathyroid glands is the most common cause of hypoparathyroidism. Destruction of the parathyroid glands is a rare complication of radioablative iodine therapy for Graves disease. Parathyroid destruction can rarely occur from deposition of iron in patients with hemochromatosis and thalassemia major and copper deposition in patients with Wilson disease.

In the initial stages of hypomagnesemia, PTH secretion is increased. However, as hypomagnesemia persists, intracellular depletion of magnesium develops and impairs PTH secretion. Pronounced suppression of PTH occurs in neonates of mothers with hyperparathyroidism. Disorders that contribute to macrophage-mediated cytokine release, such as gram-negative sepsis and toxic shock syndrome, have also been found to impair PTH secretion.

End-organ resistance to the action of PTH, or pseudohypoparathyroidism, results from defects in the PTH receptor–adenylate cyclase system. In these disorders, PTH levels are high in the face of hypocalcemia. In type 1 pseudohypoparathyroidism, decreased urinary excretion of cAMP and phosphate occurs in response to PTH. In type 1a, patients with this defect present with Albright hereditary osteodystrophy, characterized by round facies, short stature, short fourth metacarpal bones, obesity, subcutaneous ossifications, and developmental delay. Patients with type 1b pseudohypoparathyroidism do not exhibit the Albright phenotype, and it is believed that PTH resistance is confined to the kidneys in this disorder.

Hypocalcemia as the result of low 1,25-dihydroxyvitamin D can occur due to inadequate vitamin D intake or production, increased vitamin D catabolism, decreased 25-hydroxylation in the liver, decreased 1-hydroxylation in the kidney, and vitamin D resistance. Inadequate intestinal absorption of vitamin D is seen in patients with gastrectomy, celiac disease, extensive bowel surgery, inflammatory bowel disease, or pancreatic insufficiency due to cystic fibrosis. Enhanced catabolism of 1,25-dihydroxyvitamin D by activation of the cytochrome P450 system has been reported in patients receiving phenobarbital, phenytoin, carbamazepine, isoniazid, theophylline, rifampin, primidone, and glutethimide. Decreased 1-hydroxylation of 25-hydroxyvitamin D occurs in patients with renal disease due to decreased 1-hydroxylase synthesis. Vitamin D resistance occurs as the consequence of mutations that involve the vitamin D receptor gene.

Hyperphosphatemia as a consequence of massive tissue lysis (e.g., tumor lysis syndrome and rhabdomyolysis) or phosphate administration can induce hypocalcemia due to the formation of calcium phosphate precipitates in soft tissues. Hypocalcemia due to complex formation with citrate present in packed red blood cells is typically transient and not clinically significant unless large volumes are transfused rapidly (2 cc/kg/min) or with smaller volumes if liver dysfunction interferes with citrate metabolism. Administration of lipids or excess release of free fatty acids, as seen in pancreatitis, may also cause hypocalcemia.

Signs and Symptoms

The signs and symptoms of hypocalcemia are manifestations of altered function of calcium-dependent excitable tissues such as nerves and skeletal and cardiac muscle. Patients may present with myoclonic jerks and paresthesias of the perioral region, fingers, and toes or, in severe cases, with seizures, apnea, cyanosis, laryngospasm, tachypnea, tachycardia, and vomiting. On physical examination, percussion of the facial nerve below the zygomatic arch may result in facial muscle contraction (Chvostek sign). Compression of the arm or leg with a blood pressure cuff may result in carpopedal spasm (Trousseau sign). On electrocardiogram, prolongation of the QT interval and nonspecific ST–T-wave changes may be observed. Hypocalcemia rarely causes ventricular arrhythmias. Deficiency of vitamin D due to inadequate intake, 1-α-hydroxylase deficiency (vitamin D dependency type 1), or resistance to vitamin D (vitamin D dependency type 2) results in rickets. Rickets is characterized by abnormal mineralization of bone and growth-plate cartilage, resulting in widening, cupping, and fraying of the bone metaphysis. On clinical examination, skeletal changes include widened wrists, swelling of the costochondral junctions of the ribs (the "rachitic rosary"), and bowing of the legs.

Diagnosis and Treatment

Diagnosis begins with a thorough history of dietary intake (concentrating on sources of calcium and vitamin D). Physical examination includes a close evaluation of the bones and joints. Recommended laboratory studies include blood levels of total calcium, ionized calcium, albumin, phosphorus, magnesium, blood urea nitrogen, creatinine, alkaline phosphatase activity, PTH, 1,25-dihydroxyvitamin D, and 25-hydroxyvitamin D. On a random "spot" urine collection, urinary calcium excretion is best interpreted as a calcium/creatinine (mg/mg) ratio. Urinary phosphorous excretion is very dependent on diet and body phosphorous status. The ideal assessment is obtained with a fasting 2-hour urine collection, with a concomitant serum sample obtained midway through the urine collection. Serum phosphorus is usually low in patients with vitamin D deficiency and is elevated in renal failure, hypoparathyroidism, and pseudohypoparathyroidism. Serum alkaline phosphatase activity may be elevated in patients with long-standing vitamin D deficiency but usually not in early disease. A low or normal circulating PTH in the presence of hypocalcemia indicates an inappropriate parathyroid response to hypocalcemia (i.e., functional hypoparathyroidism). Increased PTH secretion is a normal physiologic response to hypocalcemia, such as in vitamin D deficiency or impaired vitamin D action.

For patients with acute symptomatic hypocalcemia (i.e., tetany, muscle twitching, carpopedal spasm, laryngospasm, or seizures), a bolus dose of calcium gluconate (100–200 mg/kg or 9–18 mg/kg elemental calcium to a maximum of 1–3 g in adults) should be administered over 10–20 minutes. A continuous infusion of calcium gluconate may be administered at starting dose of 10–30 mg/kg/h to maintain adequate calcium levels to prevent symptoms. We recommend administering IV calcium through a central venous catheter because of risk of tissue necrosis with peripheral administration. In hypocalcemic patients with hypomagnesemia, magnesium should be replenished with IV magnesium sulfate or oral magnesium oxide. In patients with concurrent hyperphosphatemia, the elevated phosphate should be corrected with phosphate binders, due to the risk of tissue deposition of calcium phosphate if the calcium–phosphate product exceeds 80 mg^2/dL^2. Once tetany resolves, oral preparations are available, including calcium carbonate (400 mg of elemental calcium/g), calcium glubionate (64 mg of elemental calcium/g), and calcium gluconate (90 mg of elemental calcium/g). A recommended starting dose is 50 mg/kg body weight/24 h of elemental calcium divided into three to four doses. In patients with hypocalcemia secondary to vitamin D deficiency or resistance, vitamin D replacement and adequate dietary calcium intake are the mainstays of therapy. Patients with malabsorption require doses of vitamin D as high as 25,000–50,000 IU/d to correct the deficiency. Similarly, patients on phenytoin therapy may require vitamin D supplementation. In patients with renal failure, vitamin D-dependent rickets type 1, hypoparathyroidism, or pseudohypoparathyroidism, reduced 1,25 $(OH)_2$ D synthesis may occur, requiring replacement with 1,25-dihydroxyvitamin D itself (calcitriol; 0.01–0.08 mcg/kg/d in children up to 10 kg; 0.25–1.0 mcg/d in adults).

Hypercalcemia

Hypercalcemia generally occurs as the consequence of excessive dietary calcium intake or increased intestinal absorption (**Table 85.4**). Hypercalcemia is uncommon in critically ill pediatric patients. Malignancy-associated and primary hyperparathyroidism have been found to be the most common causes. Less common causes include sarcoidosis, prolonged immobilization, and excessive thiazide diuretic use. The most common hormonal imbalance contributing to hypercalcemia is hyperparathyroidism. Primary hyperparathyroidism may occur as the result of mutations in *CASR* or tumors related to defects in the tumor suppressor genes in parathyroid cells. Familial hypocalciuric hypercalcemia is the consequence of heterozygous mutations in the *CASR* gene. Parathyroid adenomas can be seen as part of multiple endocrine neoplasia type 1 (hyperparathyroidism,

TABLE 85.4

Causes of Hypercalcemia

- Excessive intake
  - "Milk–alkali syndrome"
  - Oral calcium supplements
  - Parenteral nutrition
- PTH-related
  - Calcium-sensing receptor mutations
  - Multiple endocrine neoplasia type 1
  - Multiple endocrine neoplasia type 2a
  - Parathyroid adenoma
  - Transient neonatal hyperparathyroidism (parathyroid gland hyperplasia)
  - Chronic lithium toxicity
  - Chronic renal failure
  - Hyperparathyroidism–jaw tumor syndrome
- Humoral hypercalcemia of malignancy (PTHrP-, TNF-, or cytokine-mediated)
- Vitamin D intoxication
- Increased renal reabsorption
  - Thiazide diuretics
  - Calcium-sensing receptor mutations
- Increased bone resorption
  - Thyrotoxicosis
  - Vitamin A intoxication
  - Primary and metastatic tumors
  - Cytokine release
  - Immobilization
- Other
  - Williams syndrome
  - Subcutaneous fat necrosis

PTHrP, PTH-related peptide; TNF, tumor necrosis factor.

tumors of the anterior pituitary and pancreatic islets) and multiple endocrine neoplasia type 2a (hyperparathyroidism, medullary carcinoma of the thyroid, pheochromocytoma). Transient neonatal secondary hyperparathyroidism occurs in infants of mothers with hypoparathyroidism, due to prolonged fetal hypocalcemia that stimulates hyperplasia of the parathyroid glands. "Tertiary" hyperparathyroidism is seen in children with chronic renal failure, referring to the development of autonomous PTH secretion following chronic "secondary" or physiologic parathyroid gland hyperfunction. A number of malignancies, including rhabdoid tumors of the kidney, congenital mesoblastic nephroma, neuroblastoma, medulloblastoma, leukemia, Burkitt lymphoma, dysgerminoma, and rhabdomyosarcoma, are associated with hypercalcemia of malignancy. Thiazide diuretics stimulate calcium reabsorption in the DCT. Hypercalcemia secondary to increased bone resorption may accompany thyrotoxicosis and excess vitamin A ingestion. Other causes of hypercalcemia include Williams syndrome and immobilization.

Signs and Symptoms

Severe symptoms of hypercalcemia are observed in patients with serum calcium levels >15 mg/dL. Infants tend to present with gastrointestinal symptoms such as poor feeding, emesis, and failure to thrive. In older children, neurologic symptoms such as altered mental status, psychosis, and hallucinations may be present. Severe hypercalcemia contributes to a hyperpolarization across myocardial membranes, resulting in a shortened QT interval and ventricular dysrhythmias. Hypercalcemia impairs the renal response to antidiuretic hormone (ADH), causing nephrogenic diabetes insipidus and resulting in an inability to concentrate urine and polyuria.

Diagnosis and Treatment

The diagnosis of hypercalcemia should include a history of dietary intake, medications, vitamin intake, renal function, and familial disorders, including sarcoidosis and other granulomatous diseases, endocrine disorders, and hypercalcemia. Laboratory investigation should include blood levels of total calcium, phosphorus, blood urea nitrogen, creatinine, PTH, 1,25-dihydroxyvitamin D, and 25-hydroxyvitamin D, and alkaline phosphatase and urine levels of calcium, phosphorus, and creatinine (for calculation of the calcium/creatinine ratio and the tubular reabsorption of phosphorus). An elevated PTH is diagnostic for primary hyperparathyroidism, unless the history and physical examination suggest familial hypocalciuric hypercalcemia, malignancy, or lithium therapy.

The initial therapy should restore intravascular volume (as hypercalcemic patients are typically dehydrated) and to enhance renal excretion (administration of normal saline at two to three times maintenance fluid rate). Calcitonin and bisphosphonates, which inhibit bone resorption, are useful adjuncts in severe hypercalcemia. Glucocorticoids have been useful in treating hypercalcemia secondary to sarcoidosis and vitamin D deficiency. Indications for surgery for primary hyperparathyroidism include total calcium level >12 mg/dL, hyperparathyroid crisis, marked hypercalciuria, nephrolithiasis, impaired renal function, osteitis fibrosa cystica, reduced cortical bone density, bone mass greater than two standard deviations below age-matched controls, classic neuromuscular symptoms, proximal muscle weakness and atrophy, hyperreflexia, gait disturbance, and age <50 years.

Hypomagnesemia

Hypomagnesemia can occur from decreased dietary magnesium intake, malabsorption, decreased renal reabsorption, or redistribution from the extracellular to the intracellular space. The most common scenarios for nutritional magnesium deficiency are protein–calorie malnutrition, parenteral nutrition, and alcoholism. In patients with fat malabsorption, free fatty acids in the intestinal lumen chelate magnesium and prevent its absorption. Intestinal malabsorption or syndromes that are characterized by significant diarrhea (e.g., celiac disease, inflammatory bowel disease, and Whipple disease) are associated with increased magnesium loss in the stool. Decreased renal reabsorption of magnesium may occur as the consequence of congenital or acquired renal disorders, medications (loop diuretics, cisplatin, cyclosporine, amphotericin B, and aminoglycosides), or metabolic abnormalities. Inherited disorders associated with renal magnesium wasting include isolated familial hypomagnesemia, familial hypomagnesemia with hypercalciuria, primary hypomagnesemia with hypocalcemia, Bartter syndrome, and Gitelman syndrome. The movement of magnesium from extracellular to intracellular compartment occurs in insulin therapy for diabetic ketoacidosis and hyperinsulinism associated with the "refeeding syndrome" in chronic malnourishment. Enhanced intracellular uptake of magnesium has been observed in pancreatitis, hyperaldosteronism, respiratory alkalosis, and elevated plasma catecholamines. Hypomagnesemia can occur after cardiopulmonary bypass, massive transfusion, extensive burn injury, or excessive sweating.

Signs and symptoms of hypomagnesemia manifest when serum levels fall below 1 mg/dL. Symptoms are often due to the hypocalcemia from impaired PTH release or hypokalemia, which are associated with hypomagnesemia. Presenting neurologic signs include muscle weakness and tremors, tetany, Chvostek sign, Trousseau sign, and seizures. Hypokalemia consequent to hypomagnesemia lowers the myocardial action potential threshold, manifesting in nonspecific T-wave changes, U waves, a prolonged QT interval, and ventricular arrhythmias. Hypomagnesemia *per se* can predispose to cardiac dysrhythmias, particularly those of ventricular origin.

In addition to serum magnesium, calcium and potassium levels should be measured. If the cause of hypomagnesemia is unknown, calculation of the fractional excretion of magnesium (FE_{Mg}) using the equation below can assist in the differentiation between renal and nonrenal causes of hypomagnesemia:

$$FE_{Mg} = [(U_{Mg} \times P_{creatinine})/(0.7 \times P_{Mg} \times U_{creatinine})] \times 100$$

Normal values for FE_{Mg} range from 1% to 8%. In patients with hypomagnesemia due to nonrenal causes, the FE_{Mg} is <2%. In patients with renal magnesium wasting, the FE_{Mg} is >4%. If a renal cause of hypomagnesemia is suspected, an arterial blood gas should be obtained to assess for metabolic alkalosis. Symptomatic patients or asymptomatic patients with magnesium levels <1 mg/dL require IV replacement with a magnesium salt. Magnesium sulfate at a dose of 25–50 mg/kg (2.5–5.0 mg/kg of elemental magnesium) given as a slow IV infusion is recommended. For patients who require long-term therapy or for mild-to-moderate hypomagnesemia, oral supplementation with agents such as magnesium gluconate (5.4 mg elemental magnesium/100 mg), magnesium oxide (60 mg elemental magnesium/100 mg), and magnesium sulfate (10 mg elemental magnesium/100 mg) at doses of 20–40 mg/kg of elemental magnesium per day can be instituted. Patients with hypocalcemia and hypokalemia require replenishment of these minerals.

Critically ill patients with hypomagnesemia commonly have other coexisting electrolyte abnormalities, including hypocalcemia (most common), hypokalemia, hyponatremia, and hypophosphatemia. Common risk factors and causes include sepsis, cardiopulmonary bypass, and drug side effect (most commonly diuretic use). Hypomagnesemia has been associated with increased incidence of cardiac arrhythmias following cardiopulmonary bypass and increased ICU mortality.

Hypermagnesemia

Hypermagnesemia can be the result of increased intake or administration, decreased renal excretion, massive cellular release, or other causes. Hypermagnesemia most commonly occurs in the setting of excess administration of medications that contain magnesium (e.g., cathartics and antacids) or parenteral administration of magnesium to patients with preeclampsia. Patients with renal failure have impaired renal excretion of magnesium, but hypermagnesemia is uncommon unless the patient is receiving magnesium supplementation. Significant cellular lysis with release of intracellular magnesium and consequent hypermagnesemia has been reported in the setting of shock, trauma, and burns. Hypothyroidism and hypoaldosteronism are rare causes.

The signs and symptoms of hypermagnesemia usually do not manifest until the serum level is >4.0 mg/dL. The manifestations of hypermagnesemia are attributable, in part, to impaired release and binding of acetylcholine at the neuromuscular junction. Patients may develop muscle weakness, loss of deep tendon reflexes, lethargy, progression to coma, and respiratory failure. Magnesium-induced vasodilatation may cause hypotension. Ileus or decreased gastrointestinal motility may be a presenting sign. Hypermagnesemia also induces significant cardiac effects, including bradycardia, prolongation of the PR and QT intervals, heart block, and cardiac arrest.

Therapy for hypermagnesemia includes stopping magnesium intake and promoting magnesium excretion. Because hypermagnesemia may contribute to hypocalcemia, serum calcium levels should be measured and followed closely during therapy. Patients with significant neuromuscular or cardiac toxicity require measures to enhance magnesium excretion, which can be achieved by hydration with normal saline and administration of a loop diuretic or a non-magnesium-containing enema. Patients with refractory hypermagnesemia or with renal failure and severe hypermagnesemia may require hemodialysis or peritoneal dialysis to effectively reduce serum magnesium levels. Hypocalcemia should be corrected by calcium replacement.

Hypophosphatemia

Hypophosphatemia occurs as the consequence of decreased phosphate intake or malabsorption, decreased renal reabsorption, increased bone formation, or redistribution of phosphate from the extracellular to the intracellular space. Children with severe protein–calorie malnutrition and premature infants who ingest unsupplemented breast milk (which is low in phosphate content) may develop hypophosphatemia. Administration of carbohydrate in these patients enhances insulin release, which stimulates intracellular uptake of phosphate. Malabsorption due to intestinal disorders that affect the duodenum and jejunum (the primary sites for phosphate absorption) and ingestion of phosphate-binding acids are frequently encountered causes. Increased renal excretion of phosphate may occur by PTH-dependent and PTH-independent mechanisms. Hyperparathyroidism and tumor secretion of PTHrP decrease the renal TRP. PTH-independent mechanisms of hypophosphatemia include intravascular volume expansion, renal tubular disorders (e.g., X-linked hypophosphatemia and Fanconi syndrome), medications, and toxins. Acetazolamide, glucocorticoids, bicarbonate, ifosfamide, cisplatin, pamidronate, ethanol, and heavy metals also enhance renal excretion of phosphate. Redistribution of phosphate from the extracellular to the intracellular space is caused by increased endogenous insulin production following glucose infusion, insulin therapy for treatment of diabetic ketoacidosis, catecholamine administration, theophylline, and respiratory alkalosis.

Signs and symptoms of severe hypophosphatemia occur when serum phosphate levels are <1–1.5 mg/dL. Patients present with hemolysis, leukocyte dysfunction, platelet dysfunction, muscle weakness, paralysis, muscle atrophy, respiratory failure, rhabdomyolysis, and lethargy. Measurement of serum phosphate, total calcium, circulating PTH, and vitamin D levels is helpful. Patients with serum phosphate levels >2.2 mg/dL do not require aggressive therapy and can be treated with increased intake of milk. Patients with serum phosphate levels <1.5 mg/dL and/or symptomatic hypophosphatemia may require treatment with IV phosphate. It has been recommended that patients with asymptomatic severe hypophosphatemia (<1 mg/dL) receive 2.5 mg/kg of elemental phosphorus over 6 hours and that symptomatic patients receive 5 mg/kg of elemental phosphorus also over 6 hours.

In critically ill patients, hypophosphatemia is commonly due to phosphate depletion (malnutrition, antacid therapy, diuretic use) or cellular uptake of phosphate (insulin administration, cortisol administration, respiratory alkalosis). It occurs commonly following major surgical procedures including cardiac and hepatic surgery.

Hyperphosphatemia

Hyperphosphatemia is the result of increased intake, decreased renal excretion, or redistribution from the extracellular to the intracellular space. Increased intake is uncommon. Acute and chronic renal failure is the most common cause of hyperphosphatemia due to limitations of phosphate excretion. Other conditions with impaired renal excretion include acromegaly and tumoral calcinosis. Respiratory acidosis, metabolic acidosis, tumor lysis syndrome, rhabdomyolysis, hemolysis, crush injuries, and hyperthermia are associated with hyperphosphatemia.

Hyperphosphatemia alone generally does not result in physiologic manifestations. It may increase the calcium–phosphate product, which, when >80 mg/dL in infants (>60 in small children and >40 in older children and adults), promotes soft tissue calcification. Acute increases in serum phosphate levels result in a hypocalcemic response. Treatment goals are to improve renal filtration and excretion through volume expansion with normal saline and to stop intake of excess phosphate. Dialysis is effective in renal failure with severe hyperphosphatemia.

CHAPTER 86 ■ THYROID DISEASE

ORI EYAL AND SUSAN R. ROSE

NORMAL PHYSIOLOGY

Thyroid hormones play a key role in the regulation of energy expenditure, substrate metabolism, and growth and development. A classic feedback control loop exists between the thyroid gland, hypothalamus, and pituitary. Thyrotrophic-releasing hormone (TRH) is expressed in the hypothalamus and regulates thyroid-stimulating hormone (TSH) synthesis and secretion by the thyrotrophic cells in the pituitary. Serum TSH concentration exhibits a circadian pattern. After it reaches its nadir in the late afternoon, the serum TSH concentration rises to a peak around midnight, remains on a plateau for several hours, and then declines. TSH is the major regulator of the morphologic and functional states of the thyroid gland.

The substrate for the synthesis of thyroid hormone is circulating iodide. The thyroid gland traps iodide from the circulation by an energy-requiring mechanism. The formed triiodothyronine (T_3) and tetraiodothyronine (T_4) are stored in the thyroid gland in combination with thyroglobulin. Release of T_3 and T_4 from thyroglobulin occurs by proteolysis and is regulated by TSH. Under normal conditions, 10%–20% of T_3 and 100% of T_4 in the serum are directly secreted by the thyroid gland. The remaining 80%–90% of T_3 is derived from peripheral monodeiodination of T_4 by the enzyme 5′-monodeiodinase. Thyroxine (T_4) may also be metabolized peripherally to reverse T_3 (rT_3), which is largely metabolically inactive. Circulating T_3 is not active in the brain, and T_4 is not active in the brain without this enzyme. In the blood, thyroid hormones are mainly associated with carrier proteins: thyroxine-binding globulin (TBG), prealbumin or transthyretin, and albumin. The prolonged half-life of thyroid hormone is related to its protein binding. The most important carrier protein for T_4 is TBG. TBG and albumin are equally important as carrier proteins for T_3. The concentrations of free T_4 and free T_3 approximate 0.03% and 0.30%, respectively, of the total serum thyroid hormone concentration. The bound hormone acts merely as a serum reservoir. It is the free hormone that is available to the tissues for intracellular transport and feedback regulation.

CRITICAL NONTHYROIDAL ILLNESS

A decrease in serum T_3 and an increase in rT_3 levels are characteristic of the fasting state. These are also the most common changes in nonthyroidal illness (NTI) in response to a variety of acute and chronic illnesses, a condition that is referred to as the euthyroid sick syndrome, NTI, or the low-T_3 syndrome. The most rapid and consistent findings in NTI are decline in circulating total T_3 and free T_3 and an increase in the inactivated rT_3 concentrations. The greater the severity of the disease, the greater the decline in serum T_3 levels, greater the rise in rT_3, and the greater the reduction in the T_3/rT_3 ratio. The majority of patients with NTI have a normal or slightly decreased serum FT_4 level. Most commonly, serum total and free T_3 concentrations are low, whereas serum T_4 concentration remains within the normal range. However, with increasing severity of illness, both levels decrease. In severely ill patients, an additional suppression of the hypothalamic–pituitary hormone release is observed. The concentration of TSH typically remains within the low-to-normal range, but the circadian variation of TSH may be lost, and response of TSH to TRH is blunted. Low TSH level during critical illness is associated with poorer prognosis. Various agents, such as dopamine and corticosteroids, also decrease TSH levels (**Table 86.1**). In severe prolonged illness, the changes in thyroid function may be accompanied by a decline in secretion of growth hormone, gonadotropins, and adrenocorticotropic hormone (ACTH).

The treatment of NTI is controversial. In view of study results to date, critically ill patients with a low T_3 and T_4 should *not* be treated with thyroid hormone replacement unless there is also *clinical* evidence of hypothyroidism. A full thyroid function panel is needed to distinguish NTI from hypothyroidism. If the downregulation in NTI is an energy-saving neuroendocrine adaptation to disease, attempts to increase and thereby restore thyroid hormone concentrations may be disadvantageous. However, it is important to distinguish between patients with primary hypothyroidism and patients with NTI (**Table 86.2**). Patients with primary hypothyroidism almost always have a TSH level above 10 mU/L in parallel with a decreased T_4 level. In more severe stages, they also have a decreased T_3 level. Although elevated TSH may also occur in NTI upon recovery, it rarely exceeds 10 mU/L. In a situation in which TSH is mildly elevated (TSH 5–20 mU/L) with a low serum concentration of rT_3, a low thyroid hormone binding ratio, and especially a high ratio of serum T_3 to FT_4 ($T_3/FT_4 > 100$), the patient is more likely to have hypothyroidism with or without NTI. It is particularly difficult to distinguish between central hypothyroidism and NTI because, in both conditions, the TSH tends to be low-normal, and the FT_4 low. However, if the FT_4 is <0.4 ng/dL with a normal TSH, central hypothyroidism is more likely and T_4 therapy could be considered.

HYPOTHYROIDISM

Congenital hypothyroidism might be due to (in descending order of frequency) thyroid dysgenesis, thyroid dyshormonogenesis, and hypothalamic–pituitary hypothyroidism. In parts of the world where salt is not iodized, iodine deficiency is the most common cause of congenital hypothyroidism. *Hashimoto (autoimmune) thyroiditis* is the most common cause of acquired hypothyroidism in children older than 6 years of age in North America. Hypothalamic or pituitary disorders are frequently associated with TSH deficiency, producing *central hypothyroidism.* All patients with hypothalamic or pituitary disease should have thyroid function tests performed. In central hypothyroidism, the TSH is inappropriately low in relationship to low thyroid hormone concentrations. An increased frequency of primary hypothyroidism is associated with several chromosomal disorders, including Turner syndrome, Down syndrome, Klinefelter syndrome, and 18p or 18q deletions. The most common cause of hypothyroidism in these disorders is autoimmune thyroiditis.

TABLE 86.1

Medications Associated with Hypothyroidism

Decreased TSH secretion
Dopamine
Glucocorticoids
Octreotide
Decreased Thyroid Hormone Secretion
Lithium
Iodide
Amiodarone
Decreased T_4 Absorption
Colestipol
Cholestyramine
Aluminum hydroxide
Ferrous sulfate
Sucralfate
Increased Thyroid Hormone Metabolism
Phenobarbital
Rifampin
Phenytoin
Carbamazepine

TSH, thyroid-stimulating hormone.

Clinical Manifestations

Hypothyroidism should be considered in any child with subnormal growth and delayed bone age. Pubertal development is usually delayed. Affected girls may present with primary or secondary amenorrhea. Signs and symptoms include lethargy, cold intolerance, bradycardia, weight gain, slow and husky speech, dry coarse skin, spare dry and coarse hair, constipation, muscle pain, anorexia, and delayed deep tendon reflexes. In severe cases, the patient may exhibit myxedematous features (edema of periorbital tissues, hands and feet, macroglossia, and cool and dry skin). Pleural effusion, pericardial effusion, or bowel obstruction may be the first presenting symptom in previously unrecognized longstanding severe hypothyroidism.

Diagnosis

In primary hypothyroidism, serum TSH is usually elevated (>3 mU/mL), and is often the earliest laboratory finding. In secondary or tertiary (central) hypothyroidism, the TSH levels are low, normal, or slightly elevated (<10 mU/L). T_4 and FT_4 concentrations are low or low-normal. When the FT_4 is in the lowest third of the normal range and the TSH is low or normal, a TSH surge test is needed to confirm

TABLE 86.2

Changes in Thyroid Function Tests in Hypothyroidism and During Critical Illness

	TSH	T4	FT4	T3	RT3
Primary hypothyroidism	↑↑	↓	↓	↓ or =	↓
Central hypothyroidism	= or ↓	↓ or =	↓ or =	=	↓
NTI, acute phase	=	= or ↑	= or ↑	↓	↑
NTI, prolonged phase	↓	↓	↓	↓↓	↑ or =
Recovery phase	= or ↑	↓ or =	↓ or =	↓ or =	V

TSH, thyroid-stimulating hormone; T_4, tetraiodothyronine; FT_4, free T_4; T_3, triiodothyronine; rT_3, reverse T_3; NTI, nonthyroidal illness; V, variable; ↑, increased; ↓, decreased; =, normal range.

the diagnosis of central hypothyroidism. In central hypothyroidism, the TSH surge test shows blunting of the normal nocturnal surge.

Treatment

Most children require therapy with approximately 100 µg/m² body surface levothyroxine. Thyroid function tests should be checked 4–6 weeks after initiation of treatment and after a dose change has been made (sooner in newborn and infants), and the dose should be adjusted accordingly. In addition, thyroid function tests should be taken semiannually in children and annually in adolescents (more often in infants). A child with hypothyroidism who is admitted to the intensive care unit (ICU) should continue thyroid hormone therapy. If the patient cannot take oral medication, T_4 should be given intravenously in a dose that is approximately two-thirds of the oral dose.

HYPERTHYROIDISM (THYROTOXICOSIS)

The term *thyrotoxicosis* is often used to describe the hypermetabolic state that results from elevated circulating levels of thyroid hormones. Hyperthyroidism in childhood and adolescence is most commonly the result of *Graves disease*, an autoimmune disorder. Autoantibodies against the thyroid gland are often present, and autoantibodies against the TSH receptor play a key role. Other causes of hyperthyroidism include toxic multinodular goiter, toxic nodular goiter, exogenous thyroid hormone, iodine-induced thyrotoxicosis, excess release of thyroid hormone, struma ovarii, molar pregnancy, thyroid adenoma, destruction of thyroid tissue with excess hormone release as a result of trauma, subacute thyroiditis, chronic thyroiditis, or post-radiation thyroiditis. In rare cases, hyperthyroidism can be caused by increased TSH secretion as a result of pituitary adenoma. There is an association between idiopathic or heritable pulmonary arterial hypertension (PAH) and hyperthyroidism such that PAH patients should be routinely screened for hyperthyroidism. Generalized *resistance to thyroid hormone* (RTH) involves tissues throughout the body being resistant to the effects of thyroid hormone. In RTH, T_4 is high, TSH is normal, and the patients are euthyroid with a small goiter. Pituitary resistance to thyroid hormone (PRTH) is a rare non-neoplastic disorder caused by inherited mutations in the gene for the TRβ1. In this syndrome, T_4 is elevated, TSH is unsuppressed, and patients are clinically hyperthyroid.

Clinical Manifestations

The onset of thyrotoxicosis is usually insidious, with increasing nervousness, palpitations, increased appetite, and muscle weakness. A cardinal sign is loss of weight despite increased appetite. Other symptoms include fatigue with sleep disturbance, emotional instability, heat intolerance, excessive sweating, tremor, diarrhea, dyspnea, tachycardia, and atrial arrhythmia. On physical examination, findings may include thyroid enlargement; thyroid bruit (continuous murmur directly over the goiter); ophthalmopathy (retraction of the eyelids and lid lag); tremor; hyperactive reflexes; increased precordial activity; tachycardia; atrial fibrillation; warm, smooth, and moist skin; and separation of the end of the fingernail from the nail bed (onycholysis). Proximal muscle weakness is common and may be the dominant manifestation in some individuals. The hemodynamic changes of thyrotoxicosis mimic a hyperadrenergic state, caused by an increase in myocardial β-receptors, which is induced by excessive thyroid hormone. Supraventricular tachyarrhythmias are common. Severe hyperthyroidism may lead to cardiac failure secondary to atrial fibrillation. Uncontrolled hyperthyroidism with large goiter secondary to Graves disease may cause edema of the upper airway.

Diagnosis

Laboratory findings in patients with hyperthyroidism include increased serum concentrations of T_3 and T_4 because of increased production of these hormones. It is more valuable to measure the active thyroid hormone concentrations, free T_3 (FT_3) and FT_4, and to verify that either or both are elevated. The TSH is low and usually undetectable (except in the extremely rare cases of TSH-secreting tumors, TRH-secreting tumors, and selective PRTH). Quantitative human chorionic gonadotropin (hCG), which can cross-react at the TSH receptor level, is elevated in molar pregnancy.

Treatment

Management of hyperthyroidism includes medical treatment, radioactive iodine, or surgery. Previously, children with hyperthyroidism were treated with an antithyroid agent, such as propylthiouracil (PTU), methimazole, or carbimazole (used in Europe). These agents block synthesis of the thyroid hormone by inhibiting oxidation of iodide. However, due to association between PTU and severe liver failure in children and the subsequent black-box warning from the Food and Drug Administration, the use of PTU should be avoided in children. Methimazole should be the first-choice antithyroid medication, and in countries where it is not available, carbimazole, a drug that is biologically converted to methimazole, may be substituted. An initial dose of methimazole or carbimazole varies from 20 to 40 mg (0.4–0.6 mg/kg) daily PO, divided into two to three doses. In the initial state (before a euthyroid state is achieved), a β-adrenergic blocking agent, such as propranolol, may be added as 10–40 mg/dose (2 mg/kg/day) orally every 6 hours. After a euthyroid state is achieved, the methimazole dose should be decreased to maintenance dose (usually 1/3–2/3 of the initial dose given once or twice daily). The doses should be adjusted according to the FT_4 concentration, as TSH may remain suppressed for months.

A small percentage of patients develop hypersensitivity reactions to antithyroid drugs; they are usually mild and resolve when the drug is withdrawn, but a severe reaction may occur. The most common hypersensitivity reaction (10% of patients) is a rash that can take many forms, including hives. Among the serious reactions, agranulocytosis is the most common (<1% of patients) and accompanied by fever and sore throat. Hypersensitivity reaction usually occurs within the first few weeks of treatment. As these medications can affect blood count and liver function tests, it is advisable to perform complete blood count and liver function tests before initiation of an antithyroid drug treatment and to repeat them after the first few weeks of treatment, to help recognize these potential side effects.

Patients with hyperthyroidism admitted to the ICU should be monitored carefully for possible development of thyroid storm (see section Critical Hyperthyroidism: "Thyroid Storm"). Medical treatment should be continued and adjusted according to the thyroid function tests. As no parenteral preparations of antithyroid drugs are available, they must be administered orally or via a nasogastric tube. Rectal administration has also been used.

Radioactive iodine is used for treatment of older children and adolescents who fail medical treatment or in whom medical treatment is contraindicated owing to severe side effects. The main complication is primary hypothyroidism. Radioactive iodine may cause thyroid storm. Surgical treatment is used less often than in the past, but it is still an effective treatment option for hyperthyroidism. Surgery should be considered in patients with a large thyroid gland, severe ophthalmopathy, and a lack of remission with medical treatment. With proper surgical management most patients achieve a rapid remission; some may have recurrence of thyrotoxicosis or may develop hypothyroidism.

CRITICAL HYPOTHYROIDISM: "MYXEDEMA COMA"

The term myxedema coma is often used to describe clinically severe hypothyroidism. Critical hypothyroidism is characterized by progressive dysfunction of the cardiovascular, respiratory, and central nervous systems. Myxedema is related to organ hypofunction (e.g., cardiac, gastrointestinal [GI], skin, renal) and occurs with prolonged or severe hypothyroidism. If not recognized and treated, the mortality rate is exceedingly high. Typically, patients are older and have known hypothyroidism; however, it can be the initial presentation of hypothyroidism. Myxedema coma occurs most commonly in winter. Common precipitants include infection, trauma, hypothermia, and medications.

Clinical Manifestations

Cardinal findings include hypothermia and altered mental status. Additional features include bradycardia, hypotension, and hypoventilation. A reduction in hypoxic ventilatory drive results in a lowered respiratory rate, carbon dioxide narcosis, and progressive somnolence. Respiratory muscle weakness may also occur, further compromising the ability to ventilate. Presence of ascites, pleural effusion, or pericardial effusion may further impede effective ventilation. Cardiac contractility is reduced, resulting in a reduction of stroke volume and cardiac output. If present, myxedema is characterized by decreased metabolic clearance of all substances, reduced intravascular volume with fluid retention in tissues, generalized skin and soft tissue swelling, often with associated periorbital edema, ptosis, macroglossia, and cool, dry skin.

Diagnosis

The diagnosis of myxedema coma requires low levels of T_3 and of T_4 (total and free). TSH levels are usually elevated, but may be normal or low in the setting of hypothalamic–pituitary disease or critical illness. Additional laboratory findings include anemia, hyponatremia, hypoglycemia, azotemia, elevated liver enzymes, hypercholesterolemia, and elevated creatinine phosphokinase levels. Hypoxia, hypercapnia, and respiratory acidosis are common. The occurrence of pericardial effusion in hypothyroidism appears to be dependent on the severity of the disease. A chest radiograph may reveal cardiomegaly and pleural effusions. Echocardiography can reveal septal hypertrophy and hypertrophic subaortic stenosis in addition to the pericardial effusion. Electrocardiographic (ECG) findings include sinus bradycardia, decreased voltage with electrical alternans if a pericardial effusion is present, and nonspecific ST and T wave abnormalities. Other ECG abnormalities include prolongation of the QT interval and conduction abnormalities of varying degrees. A lumbar puncture may be indicated to exclude meningitis. An increased opening pressure and elevated protein levels in the cerebral spinal fluid are nonspecific findings associated with myxedema coma.

Treatment

The treatment of myxedema coma involves general supportive measures, correction of physiologic derangements, and immediate intravenous replacement of thyroid hormone. Patients should be treated in the ICU setting with careful monitoring. In patients who have severe hypotension, vasopressor therapy should be considered. Warm room temperature, blankets, and/or heating pad should be used to correct hypothermia. Rapid correction of hypothermia may cause hypotension and cardiovascular collapse owing to peripheral dilatation. Severe hyponatremia may be treated with hypertonic saline. Hypoglycemia should be treated with continuous dextrose infusion. Precipitating factors should be pursued and treated. Broad-spectrum antibiotics should be considered until infection has been excluded. The recommended initial therapy is with intravenous T_4 alone, with a loading dose of 200–500 µg (4 µg/kg if <50 kg), followed by 50–100 µg/day (1–2 µg/kg if <50 kg). Using T_4 alone allows a slow conversion of T_4 to T_3 in the periphery, thereby reducing the possible adverse cardiac effects that may occur with a large dose of T_3, especially in those with preexisting heart disease. If combination therapy is begun, a loading dose of 4 µg/kg of T_4 and 10 µg of T_3 (0.2 µg/kg) may be used, followed by maintenance doses of T_4 (50–100 µg daily; 1–2 µg/kg) and T_3 (10 µg; 0.2 µg/kg) every 8 hours until oral therapy is initiated. If intravenous T_3 alone is used, initial dose should be 10–20 µg (0.2–0.4 µg/kg), followed by 10 µg (0.2 µg/kg) every 4 hours for the first 24 hours, then 10 µg (0.2 µg/kg) every 6 hours for another 1–2 days. Rapid onset of action of T_3 can lead to adverse cardiovascular effects. Whatever the regimen, subsequent thyroid hormone dosing should be guided by frequent measurement of FT_4 concentrations. With the IV route, the peak level is reached within 3 hours, with subsequent gradual decline over a few days. Thus, it is recommended to check FT_4 twice daily when using the IV route to ensure that most levels are within the normal range. When the patient is converted to oral T_4, FT_4 can be measured once or twice per week.

Cortisol response to stress is blunted during severe hypothyroidism. Most investigators recommend the concurrent administration of "stress dose" corticosteroid therapy, in case of concurrent adrenal insufficiency. Hydrocortisone, 100 mg/m² IV, should be administered initially, followed by 25 mg/m² IV every 6 hours. Cortisol levels should be drawn before initiation of corticosteroid therapy. If the cortisol levels are low (<25 µg/dL), steroid therapy should be continued until the critical illness phase is resolved. At a later time, an ACTH stimulation test can be performed to exclude persistence of hypoadrenalism.

CRITICAL HYPERTHYROIDISM: "THYROID STORM"

Thyroid storm (or thyrotoxic crisis) is a life-threatening condition caused by the exaggeration of clinical manifestations of thyrotoxicosis. Thyroid storm most commonly occurs in Graves disease. The progression from thyrotoxicosis to life-threatening thyroid storm involves high fever, mental status changes, multiorgan dysfunction, adrenergic crisis (tachycardia, hypertension), and GI hypermotility. Early diagnosis and intervention are crucial to prevent morbidity and mortality. Precipitating factors include thyroid surgery, withdrawal of antithyroid drugs, radioiodine therapy, or the administration of iodinated radiocontrast dyes. In patients with preexisting thyrotoxicosis, thyroid storm can be precipitated by systemic insults (surgery, trauma, severe infection, and diabetic ketoacidosis). If left untreated, the mortality rate ranges between 20% and 30%. The sympathetic nervous system has been implicated in the pathogenesis of thyroid storm. The manifestations are similar to those seen in catecholamine excess and administration of β-blockers relieves the signs and symptoms. Thyroid hormones upregulate adrenergic receptor expression and thus affect tissue responsiveness to catecholamines. Another mechanism might be an enhanced cellular response to thyroid hormones as seen in conditions that precipitate thyroid storm (infection, hypoxemia, hypovolemia, and diabetic ketoacidosis).

Clinical Manifestations

Thyroid storm is characterized by four major features: fever, tachycardia, central nervous system dysfunction, and GI symptoms. The fever can progress to frank hyperpyrexia. Sinus tachycardia or a variety of supraventricular arrhythmias may be present (e.g., atrial fibrillation). Central nervous system manifestations range from agitation, restlessness, and emotional lability, to confusion, frank psychosis, and coma. GI symptoms include nausea, vomiting, and diarrhea. A useful scoring system for recognition of thyroid storm is presented in **Table 86.3.**

Diagnosis

Laboratory findings include elevated serum total and free thyroid hormonal levels (free T_3 and/or free T_4), with undetectable TSH. Liver function abnormalities, leukocytosis, or leucopenia may also be present.

Treatment

The aims of the treatment are to reduce the production and secretion of thyroid hormones, to antagonize the peripheral action of the thyroid hormones, to alleviate signs and symptoms, and to treat the precipitating factor. Supportive therapy includes respiratory support and management of hyperthermia. Phenobarbital may be used for sedation because it stimulates metabolic clearance of thyroid hormone by the liver. Hyperthermia may be treated with cool IV fluids, antipyretics, or cooling blankets. An early step in treatment must be the complete blockade of new thyroid hormone synthesis using either PTU or methimazole. Methimazole has a better safety profile and is given as a loading dose of 60–100 mg (1.2–2 mg/kg), followed by 20–30 mg (0.4–0.7 mg/kg) every 6–8 hours orally, but it does not provide inhibition of conversion of T_4 to T_3. PTU had been

TABLE 86.3

The Predictive Clinical Scale for Thyroid Storm (Burch and Wartofsky)

PARAMETER TAKEN INTO CONSIDERATION	SCORING POINTS
Thermoregulatory Dysfunction, Temperature (Oral; in F)	
99–99.9	5
100–100.9	10
101–101.9	15
102–102.9	20
103–103.9	25
≥104	30
CNS Effects	
Absent	0
Mild (agitation)	10
Moderate (delirium, psychosis, extreme lethargy)	20
Severe (seizures, coma)	30
GI–Hepatic Dysfunction	
Absent	0
Moderate (diarrhea, nausea/vomiting, abdominal pain)	10
Severe (unexplained jaundice)	20
Tachycardia (beats/min)	
99–109	5
110–119	10
120–129	15
130–139	20
≥140	25
Congestive Cardiac Failure	
Absent	0
Mild (pedal edema)	5
Moderate (bibasal rales)	10
Severe (pulmonary edema)	15
Atrial Fibrillation	
Absent	0
Present	10
Precipitating Event	
Absent	0
Present	10

A cumulative score of ≥45 is highly suggestive of thyroid storm, 25–44 is suggestive of "impeding" storm, and <25 is unlikely to represent thyroid storm.
From Rose SR. TSH above 3 is not usually normal. *The Endocrinologist* 2006;16.

considered the drug of choice because of its inhibition of peripheral conversion of T_4 to T_3 in addition to its inhibition of synthesis of thyroid hormone. However, PTU is now known to have more adverse effects, especially hepatotoxicity. PTU can be administered as a 600–1000-mg (12–20 mg/kg) loading dose, followed by 200–300 mg (4–6 mg/kg) every 4–6 hours orally. Both PTU and methimazole can be administered rectally, but no parenteral preparation for these drugs is available. To block the release of preformed thyroid hormone from the thyroid gland, inorganic iodine should be used. Ideally, iodine therapy should be administered 2 hours after initial thiourea dosing, to allow for initial blockade of iodine organification. Formulations for oral inorganic iodine that can be used include saturated solution of potassium iodide (children, five drops, 250 mg, two to four times per day; infants, two drops, four times per day) and

Lugol solution (four to eight drops, three times per day). Iodinated contrast dyes given intravenously are also effective. In addition to blocking thyroid hormone release, these radiocontrast agents interfere with peripheral conversion of T_4 to T_3 and may antagonize the binding of thyroid hormone to its receptors. Lithium therapy (300 mg or 6 mg/kg every 6 hours) may be used in addition to iodine to block thyroid hormone release. High-dose corticosteroids (hydrocortisone 50–100 mg, IV, every 6–8 hours or 25–50 mg/m^2 body surface) are also effective in blocking peripheral conversion of T_4 to T_3. Blocking the action of thyroid hormone is another mainstay of the treatment. In the absence of cardiac failure, a β-adrenergic blocking agent should be added. β-Blockers (e.g., propranolol, 40–80 mg, 0.5 mg/kg, orally, or 1–3 mg/dose IV, every 4–8 hours) are effective in reducing tachycardia, hypertension, and adrenergic symptoms associated with thyrotoxicosis. However, a short-acting β-blocker such as esmolol given IV may be safer in the critically ill patient by minimizing the risk of cardiovascular collapse and allowing better titration of the medication's effects because of the short half-life. In life-threatening cases in which medical therapy has been proven ineffective, plasmapheresis, plasma exchange, charcoal plasma perfusion, and peritoneal dialysis have all been used successfully to remove circulating thyroid hormone. Following initiation of therapy for thyroid storm, clinical and biochemical improvement should occur within 24 hours, although full recovery may take several days to weeks. In most cases, medical therapy should be used for weeks to months before definitive treatment with radioactive iodine or thyroidectomy.

CHAPTER 87 ■ ACUTE KIDNEY INJURY

CHRISTINE B. SETHNA, NATALIYA CHORNY, SMARIKA SAPKOTA, AND JAMES SCHNEIDER

DEFINITION OF ACUTE KIDNEY INJURY

Acute kidney injury (AKI), formerly known as acute renal failure (ARF), is defined as the abrupt onset of renal dysfunction resulting from injurious endogenous or exogenous processes characterized by a decrease in glomerular filtration rate (GFR) and an increase in serum creatinine. The RIFLE criteria, developed by the Acute Dialysis Quality Initiative group, consist of the acronym for the three graded levels of injury (risk, injury, and failure) based on either the degree of elevation in serum creatinine or urine output, and two outcome measures (loss and end-stage renal disease). The use of RIFLE criteria in the adult population has been validated, and there is a predictive correlation between the different degrees of AKI and mortality. For pediatric patients, a modified version of RIFLE criteria known as pRIFLE (**Table 87.1**) classifies the severity of AKI based on changes in estimated creatinine clearance and urine output. pRIFLE staging has been shown in several studies to be independently associated with morbidity and mortality. Another modified classification of RIFLE, introduced by The Acute Kidney Injury Network (AKIN), takes into account small variations in creatinine and has been validated in adults. More recently, the organization Kidney Disease: Improving Global Outcomes (KDIGO) released a definition and staging system for AKI that combines the RIFLE and AKIN criteria and includes pediatric measures (**Table 87.2**). However, the criteria have not yet been validated for use in children.

EPIDEMIOLOGY

AKI is common and increasing secondary to advances that have led to a growing population of more susceptible children. Specifically regarding critically ill children, the incidence of AKI has been reported to range from 10% to 46%. The incidence of AKI is even higher in specialized critically ill populations: those requiring mechanical ventilation or victims of trauma (58%–90%), those requiring extracorporeal membrane oxygenation support (64%), burn victims (45%), children undergoing congenital heart disease surgery (with incidence increasing as patients' age decreases) (30%–56%), and those requiring hematopoietic stem cell transplants (HSCTs) (17%–45%). Risk factors associated with development of HSCT-associated AKI are veno-occlusive disease, sepsis, and nephrotoxic medications. Unlike in adults, total body irradiation does not appear to significantly influence the development of AKI. Risk factors for AKI in developing countries include acute gastroenteritis, hypoxic/ischemia injury, and sepsis (hypoxic/ischemic injury is responsible for a much larger percentage in the neonatal population). AKI was identified more commonly in older children in US-based studies, with one-third of AKI patients being between 15 and

TABLE 87.1

pRIFLE Criteria

	■ PEDIATRIC-MODIFIED RIFLE (PRIFLE) CRITERIA	
	■ ESTIMATED CCI	■ URINE OUTPUT
Risk	eCCI decrease by 25%	<0.5 mL/kg/h for 8 h
Injury	eCCI decrease by 50%	<0.5 mL/kg/h for 16 h
Failure	eCCI decrease by 75% or eCCI < 35 mL/min/1073 m^2	<0.3 mL/kg/h for 24 h or anuric for 12 h
Loss	Persistent failure > 4 wk	
End	End-stage renal disease	
Stage	Persistent failure > 3 mo	

eCCI, estimated creatinine clearance; pRIFLE, pediatric risk, injury, failure, loss, and end-stage renal disease.
From Akcan-Arikan A, Zappitelli M, Loftis LL, Washburn KK, Jefferson LS, Goldstein SL. Modified RIFLE criteria in critically ill children with acute kidney injury. *Kidney Int* 2007;71(10):1028–35.

TABLE 87.2

KDIGO criteria

STAGE	SERUM CREATININE	URINE OUTPUT
1	1.5–1.9 times baseline or ≥0.3 mg/dL (≥26.5 μmol/L) increase	<0.5 mL/kg/h for 6–12 h
2	2.0–2.9 times baseline	<0.5 mL/kg/h for ≥12 h
3	3.0 times baseline or increase in serum creatinine to ≥4.0 mg/dL (≥26.5 μmol/L) or initiation of renal replacement therapy or, in patients <18 y, decrease in eGFR to <35 mL/min per 1.73 m^2	<0.3 mL/kg/h for ≥24 h or anuria for ≥12 h

From Kidney Disease. Improving Global Outcomes (KDIGO) Acute Kidney Injury Work Group. KDIGO clinical practice guideline for acute kidney injury. *Kidney Int Suppl* 2012;2:1–138.

18 years old. African Americans had the highest rate, accounting for 20% of all AKI hospitalizations. Currently, complications from systemic diseases, such as sepsis, multiple organ dysfunction, hematologic and oncologic (stem cell transplantation) complications, solid organ transplantation, pulmonary failure, congenital heart surgery, complications from neonatal care, and exposure to nephrotoxins, are responsible for the majority of AKI cases. Longer bypass and cross-clamp times, higher surgical complexity score, higher inotrope score, use of circulatory arrest, and younger age are all associated with the development of AKI after congenital heart surgery.

ESTIMATION OF GLOMERULAR FILTRATION RATE

GFR Estimation Equations

The gold standard for the measurement of GFR is the urinary clearance of inulin, but this method is expensive and cumbersome. Assessment of GFR using creatinine clearance estimation equations is more commonly utilized. The Schwartz equation is the traditional formula used to estimate GFR in children. The original Schwartz equation has been adapted to utilize enzymatically determined serum creatinine. This equation was derived from The Chronic Kidney Disease in Children (CKiD) Study. The formula is useful in the GFR range of 15–75 mL/min/1.73 m^2. The CKiD Schwartz formula:

$$\text{GFR (mL/min/1.73 m}^2\text{)} = 0.431 \times \text{height (cm)/serum creatinine (mg/dL)}$$

Children reach adult levels of GFR by the age of 2. Reference values for GFR are 110–120 mL/min/1.73 m^2 for children >2 years of age, <10 mL/min/1.73 m^2 for premature infants, and 10–40 mL/min/1.73 m^2 for term infants.

Creatinine

Serum creatinine is the most common laboratory test used to identify reduced GFR, but the measurement is inaccurate in those with fluctuating renal function and the rise in creatinine is often delayed. Creatinine is derived from the metabolism of creatine in skeletal muscle and from dietary meat intake. It is freely filtered across the glomerulus and is neither reabsorbed nor metabolized by the kidney. However, ~10%–40% of urinary creatinine is derived from tubular secretion in the proximal tubule, making it a suboptimal marker of estimated GFR. Additionally, serum creatinine is influenced by factors such as diet, hydration status, medications (cimetidine, trimethoprim), and hyperbilirubinemia. Normal creatinine values in pediatric patients vary with age and body mass. Reference values for serum creatinine by age are 0.3–1.0 mg/dL (27–88 μmol/L) for newborn, 0.2–0.4 mg/dL (18–35 μmol/L) for infant, 0.3–0.7 mg/dL (27–62 μmol/L) for child, and 0.5–1.0 mg/dL (44–88 μmol/L) for adolescent.

Cystatin C

Cystatin C is a protein produced at a constant rate by all nucleated cells. It is freely filtered by the glomerulus and reabsorbed, not secreted, but is catabolized in the tubules. Cystatin C blood levels are not significantly affected by age, gender, race, or muscle mass, and so it is effective as a marker of glomerular function in cachectic or pediatric patients, or in the case of early AKI where serum creatinine could underestimate the true renal function. Cystatin C may be superior to creatinine as a marker of GFR, but it should be noted that there are ongoing concerns related to the lack of standardization in cystatin C measurement.

Biomarkers

Significant renal damage has already occurred by the time the diagnosis of AKI has been made. Therefore, there has been a shift in focus to the early detection of AKI by novel biomarkers.

Neutrophil Gelatinase-Associated Lipocalin: Neutrophil gelatinase-associated lipocalin (NGAL) is a lipocalin secreted by activated neutrophils and expressed in many cells (e.g., kidney, lungs, stomach, and colon). Plasma NGAL is freely filtered by the glomerulus and is largely reabsorbed in the proximal tubules. After ischemia, it is secreted in the thick ascending limb and detected in the urine. In critically ill children, urine and plasma NGAL measurements predict AKI ~2 days prior to the rise in serum creatinine.

Kidney Injury Molecule-1: Human kidney injury molecule (KIM) is a glycoprotein receptor that is not detectable in normal kidney tissue or urine, but is expressed at very high levels in proximal tubule epithelial cells after ischemic or toxic injury. In 20 children after CBP surgery, urinary KIM-1 was elevated 6–12 hours following CBP, but not in children with normal renal function.

Interleukin 18: Interleukin 18 (IL-18) is a proinflammatory cytokine expressed in the intercalated cell of the late distal convoluted tubule and the collecting duct of the kidney. These cells have intracellular cysteine protease, which converts the proform of IL-18 to its active form, which then exits the cell and may enter the urine in AKI. When combined with NGAL, it predicted the duration of AKI in children after cardiac surgery.

Liver-type Fatty-Acid-Binding Protein: Liver-type fatty-acid-binding protein (L-FABP) is expressed in the proximal tubule of the kidney. It is an early biomarker in urine within 4 hours after surgery in children undergoing CPB who subsequently developed AKI.

***N*-Acetyl-β-Glucosaminidase:** NAG is a lysosomal enzyme, found predominantly in the proximal convoluted tubules. Increased activity of this enzyme in the urine suggests injury to tubular cells.

Combination of AKI Biomarkers: A combination of biomarkers may achieve the highest diagnostic and prognostic data in early prevention of AKI. Evaluation of serial measurements of multiple urinary biomarkers after pediatric cardiac surgery revealed a sequential appearance of AKI biomarkers, with NGAL and L-FABP being the earliest responders (2–4 hours) and KIM-1 and IL-18 being the intermediate responders (6–12 hours).

EVALUATION OF ACUTE KIDNEY INJURY

Once the diagnosis of AKI is established, a careful history, review of medications, and physical examination are needed to differentiate between prerenal, intrinsic renal, and postrenal etiologies of AKI. Initial testing generally includes serum creatinine, blood urea nitrogen (BUN), electrolytes, phosphorus, and albumin. Urine should be sent for general analysis, sodium, and creatinine. A complete blood count and renal ultrasound should also be performed (see **Table 87.3**).

Urinalysis: A key component of the urinalysis is assessment for proteinuria. The amount of protein can be further quantified by a protein-to-creatinine ratio sent on a random sample (normal is <0.2 mg/mg

TABLE 87.3

Laboratory Findings in Acute Kidney Injury

INDICES	PRERENAL AKI	INTRINSIC AKI: GLOMERULAR	INTRINSIC AKI: TUBULO-INTERSTITIAL	POSTRENAL AKI
BUN:creatinine	>20	<10	<10	<10
Urine sodium (mEq/L)				
Children	<10	>20	>20	>20
Neonates	<20–30	>30	>30	>30
FENa (%)				
Children	<1	>2	>2	>2
Neonates	<3	>3	>3	>3
Urine osmolality (mOSm/kg)	>500	<350	<350	<350
Urine specific gravity	>1.020	<1.010	<1.010	<1.010
Urine protein	Usually absent	May be absent or mild to moderate. Not nephrotic range	May be nephrotic range	Variable
Urine sediment	Hyaline casts	Dysmorphic red blood cells, red blood cell casts, lipid casts	Granular casts, muddy brown casts, white blood cell casts, epithelial casts, eosinophils	Variable

AKI, Acute Kidney Injury; BUN, Blood Urea Nitrogen; FENa, Fractional Excretion Of Sodium.

and nephrotic range is >2 mg/mg). The protein-to-creatinine ratio can be approximated to 24-hour protein by multiplying the ratio by a factor of 0.63 (normal is <4 mg/m²/h). Proteinuria is not typically found in prerenal or postrenal AKI, but can be significant in intrinsic renal disease. Urine sediment should be analyzed for the presence of casts, crystals, cellular debris, and red blood cell morphology. The urine dipstick can detect whole blood, hemoglobin, and myoglobin. The finding of dysmorphic RBCs or RBC casts indicates a glomerular origin of hematuria.

Urine Indices: In a state of volume depletion, urine sodium is usually <20 mEq/L. In acute tubular necrosis (ATN), the urine sodium is generally >20 mEq/L due to impaired tubular function. *Fractional excretion of sodium* (FENa) is a reliable test since it is a measure of sodium handling and is not altered by urine volume; it is calculated from a random urine specimen as follows:

$$\text{FENa } (\%) = (\text{Urine Sodium} \times \text{Serum Creatinine} / \text{Serum Sodium} \times \text{Urine Creatinine}) \times 100$$

The FENa is expected to be <1% in prerenal AKI and >2% in intrinsic and postrenal AKI. The ratio is normally higher in neonates due to decreased sodium reabsorption. A limitation of FENa is that it is inaccurate in patients receiving diuretics. The *fractional excretion of urea* (FE_{UN}) is not affected by diuretics. In states of hypovolemia, the FE_{UN} is <35%, while, in ATN, it is often >50%. *Urine osmolality* in prerenal AKI is >500 mOsm/kg, and specific gravity is >1.020. In contrast, intrinsic renal disease results in impairment of urine-concentrating ability, with urine osmolality <350 mOsm/kg and specific gravity <1.010.

BUN-to-Creatinine Ratio: BUN is preferentially reabsorbed along with sodium in the proximal tubule during hypovolemic states. The proximal tubule is impermeable to creatinine. A ratio of BUN to creatinine (mg/mg) >20 is suggestive of a prerenal etiology. This should be interpreted with caution as the ratio may be elevated with gastrointestinal bleeding, steroid use, and decreased muscle mass. A ratio <10–15 is common in ATN.

Ultrasound: Ultrasound is the imaging modality of choice in AKI. There is no need for radiation, contrast, or sedation. Doppler studies allow for the evaluation of the renal vasculature. The finding of obstruction on ultrasound is diagnostic for postrenal AKI. Increased echogenicity of the kidneys is seen in intrinsic AKI.

Prerenal Acute Kidney Injury

Etiology: Prerenal AKI is the result of decreased blood flow to the renal parenchyma from either volume depletion or ineffective circulating volume. Hypovolemic states that lead to prerenal AKI include hemorrhage; gastrointestinal, urinary, or cutaneous losses; and septic or myocardial shock. Ineffective circulating volume may also occur in hypervolemia (nephrotic syndrome, cardiac dysfunction, and liver disease).

Pathophysiology: A reduction in mean arterial pressure from decrease in cardiac output or systemic vascular resistance activates the cardiac and arterial stretch receptors and results in increased sympathetic tone and release of renin, angiotensin II, aldosterone, and antidiuretic hormone. Nephrons attempt to compensate for the decrease in GFR by releasing prostaglandins and angiotensin II, which dilate the afferent arterioles and constrict the efferent arterioles. Although there is a decrease in GFR, aldosterone reabsorbs sodium and antidiuretic hormone conserves water, leading to decreased urine output. When renal perfusion is restored, the GFR and urine flow return to normal. If diminished renal perfusion persists, prerenal AKI may convert to intrinsic AKI.

History and Physical Exam: Clinical findings include tachycardia, low blood pressure, poor skin turgor, dry mucous membranes, mental status changes, sunken eyes and fontanelle, reduced tears, and capillary refill greater than 2 seconds. Cardiac dysfunction, nephrotic syndrome, and liver disease may result in edema.

Diagnostic Evaluation: The BUN-to-creatinine ratio is >20. The urinalysis usually demonstrates no proteinuria, hematuria, or abnormal urine sediment, although hyaline casts may be present. The specific gravity is elevated with urine osmolality typically >500 mOsm/kg. The urine sodium concentration is expected to be <10 mEq/L and the FENa <1%. In neonates, these values are higher (urine sodium <20–30 mEq/L and FENa <3%).

Management: Management of prerenal AKI requires treatment of the underlying condition, volume resuscitation, and maintenance of renal perfusion.

INTRINSIC RENAL AKI

Intrinsic renal disease may arise from glomerular, tubulo-interstitial, or vascular components of the kidney. The most common cause is ATN due to ischemia, although in the ICU, intrinsic AKI is frequently multifactorial.

Glomerular Disease

Etiology: Glomerulonephritis (GN) is a renal disease characterized by inflammation and proliferation of glomeruli, with resulting renal dysfunction. The typical presentation of GN is nephritic syndrome, defined as glomerular hematuria, edema, azotemia, and hypertension. IgA nephropathy is the leading cause of GN worldwide, and poststreptococcal glomerulonephritis (PSAGN) is the most common cause in children. Rapidly progressive GN is a form of GN that presents with a rapid loss of renal function and is associated with the histologic presence of crescents in glomeruli.

Pathophysiology: Glomerular lesions are a result of immune deposits or in situ formation of immune complexes. Inflammation and proliferation lead to damage of the basement membrane, mesangium, or capillary wall endothelium, which creates a barrier to glomerular filtration.

History and Physical Examination: Patients with glomerular disease present with edema or tea-colored urine. A history of sore throat or skin infection preceding the onset of gross hematuria by 1–3 weeks is suggestive of PSAGN, while an upper respiratory illness at the time of hematuria is indicative of IgA nephropathy. Systemic symptoms such as joint aches, rash, and fever suggest an autoimmune disease or vasculitis. Pulmonary hemorrhage is associated with Goodpasture syndrome and anti-neutrophil cytoplasmic antibody (ANCA) vasculitis. Petechiae or purpura may be seen with Henoch–Schonlein Purpura and other vasculitides.

Diagnostic Evaluation: A hallmark of glomerular disease is hematuria and proteinuria on urinalysis. Urine osmolality is usually <350 mOsm/kg. The urine sodium concentration is expected to be >20 mEq/L and the FENa >2%. The BUN-to-creatinine ratio is <10. To obtain a specific diagnosis, serum complement levels (C3, C4), anti-streptolysin O antibody, streptozyme, antinuclear antibody, double-stranded DNA, anti-glomerular basement membrane antibody, and ANCA may be sent. Hypocomplementemia is suggestive of PSAGN, systemic lupus erythematosus, membranoproliferative GN, shunt nephritis, or bacterial endocarditis. On renal ultrasound, the kidneys may be enlarged and show increased echogenicity compared to the liver. Renal biopsy may aid in the diagnosis of glomerular disease.

Management: Treatment is geared toward the specific disease. PSAGN is a self-limited condition that requires supportive therapy. Immunosuppressive treatments and plasmapheresis may be needed for other forms of GN.

Tubular Disease: Acute Tubular Necrosis

ATN is the most common cause of AKI in the ICU. The majority of cases of ATN are due to renal ischemia, sepsis, and nephrotoxins.

Ischemic Renal Disease

Etiology: ATN is on a continuum with prerenal disease with progression when the ischemic insult persists. It frequently occurs with hypotension from sepsis and major surgery. Cardiac surgery with CPB, in particular, is a significant risk factor for AKI.

Pathophysiology: ATN occurs when ischemia persists long enough to induce cell injury and death. ATN generally follows three stages. In the initiation phase, ischemia and reperfusion lead to the release of calcium, reactive oxygen species, and phospholipases in the proximal tubule. In the maintenance phase, there is a sustained reduction in GFR of a variable time period, usually 1–2 weeks. In the recovery phase, the tubule cells regenerate, the obstruction of the tubule lumen resolves, and GFR returns to baseline.

History and Physical Examination: Patients with ischemic ATN present with a history of volume depletion similar to prerenal AKI (e.g., vomiting, diarrhea, hemorrhage, or sepsis). ATN may be oliguric or nonoliguric.

Diagnostic Evaluation: The classic finding on urinalysis is muddy brown granular casts of sloughed tubular cells. Mild-to-moderate proteinuria may be present, but hematuria is not significant. Urine osmolality is <350 mOsm/kg, urine sodium is >20 mEq/L, and FENa is >2% in ATN. The BUN-to-creatinine ratio is <10. On renal ultrasound, the kidneys may show increased echogenicity compared to the liver.

Management: Most cases of ischemic ATN are reversible if the underlying cause is treated; however, permanent damage with cortical necrosis may occur if the ischemia is severe.

Sepsis

Sepsis is an independent risk factor for the development of AKI and sepsis-induced AKI is associated with poor outcomes and increased risk of death. Immune-mediated injury, apoptosis, and alterations in intrarenal hemodynamics are thought to play a role in sepsis-induced AKI. The diagnostic evaluation and management of sepsis-induced AKI are similar to those of ischemic ATN.

Nephrotoxins

Drug-induced AKI is a significant preventable cause of AKI. Nephrotoxicity accounts for 16%–25% of AKI in the ICU. The primary mechanisms of nephrotoxicity include direct injury to the tubules, alteration of renal blood flow, and tubular obstruction. Aminoglycosides bind to tubular epithelial cells, are taken up by lysosomes, and cause rupture of the lysosomes with resultant necrosis of the tubule cell. The degree of injury is dose and duration dependent; therefore, monitoring of drug levels is essential. Nonsteroidal anti-inflammatory drugs (NSAIDs) inhibit prostaglandin synthesis, causing vasoconstriction of the afferent arteriole and reduced blood flow to the glomerulus. NSAIDs may also cause interstitial nephritis and nephrotic syndrome. Similarly, calcineurin inhibitors such as tacrolimus and cyclosporine cause vasoconstriction of the afferent arteriole by activating endothelin and thromboxane and inhibiting nitric oxide and prostaglandin activity. Angiotensin-converting enzyme inhibitors (ACEi) and angiotensin receptor blockers (ARBs) block the actions of angiotensin II and cause vasodilation of the efferent arteriole, which reduces glomerular pressure. The nephrotoxic effects of NSAIDs, calcineurin inhibitors, ACEi, and ARBs are potentiated in states of hypovolemia. Acyclovir precipitates in the distal tubules and results in tubular obstruction with trans-tubular back leak of glomerular filtrate. Alkalinization of the urine and adequate hydration may prevent nephrotoxicity from acyclovir. Contrast-induced nephropathy is caused by the administration of high osmolal ionic radiocontrast agents. The contrast is thought to induce renal vasoconstriction mediated by alterations in nitric oxide, endothelin, and/or adenosine. Preventive measures include use of lower doses of contrast, avoidance of volume depletion, and volume expansion prior to, and for several hours after, contrast administration. Studies of alkalinization of the urine with sodium bicarbonate and *N*-acetylcysteine (NAC) for the prevention of contrast-induced nephropathy are contradictory. However, NAC is thought to minimize vasoconstriction and oxygen-free radical generation.

Postrenal Acute Kidney Injury

Etiology: Postrenal AKI ensues when there is obstruction of the lower urinary tract or kidney. Obstruction may occur anywhere from the tubules to the ureters and beyond. The obstruction may be congenital or acquired.

Pathophysiology: Obstruction to the flow of tubular ultrafiltrate causes an increase in intratubular pressure and hydrostatic pressure in Bowman's space. As the pressure in Bowman's space rises, the overall difference in pressure that drives ultrafiltration is reduced and GFR is diminished. With bilateral obstruction or obstruction in a solitary kidney, the changes in renal function are significant and may lead to AKI.

History and Physical Examination: Significant obstruction may lead to oligohydramnios and immature development of the lungs in utero. Other congenital causes of obstruction may first be discovered during an evaluation for urinary tract infection. Children with postrenal AKI often present with a history of difficult urination, weak urine stream, or anuria. Nephrolithiasis, clots, or masses may present with abdominal or flank pain and/or gross hematuria. Abdominal examination may identify a palpable bladder or abdominal mass.

Diagnostic Evaluation: Renal ultrasound is highly useful for diagnosis of obstruction. A voiding cystourogram may aid in the diagnosis of posterior urethral valves, ureteropelvic junction obstruction, ureterovesical junction obstruction, and neurogenic bladder. The BUN-to-creatinine ratio is typically <10. The urinalysis may be variable, urine osmolality is usually <350 mOsm/kg, urine sodium >20 mEq/L, and FENa >1%.

Management: Relief of the obstruction by catheter drainage or intervention by urology is the treatment in postrenal AKI. Patients need to be monitored for postobstructive diuresis, manifested by polyuria and electrolyte abnormalities after the relief of obstruction. The inability to maximally concentrate urine due to a decreased medullary concentrating gradient and decreased response to ADH is thought to be a contributing factor for the development of postobstructive diuresis. Postobstructive diuresis is usually self-limited, lasting 24–36 hours, during which time creatinine clearance will improve rapidly and urinary replacement needs will taper off. Management focuses on avoiding severe volume depletion and electrolyte imbalances such as hypokalemia, hyponatremia, hypernatremia, and hypomagnesemia. As initial urine is isosthenuric, the starting fluid for replacement is 0.45% saline.

PREVENTION AND TREATMENT OF AKI

Current management is primarily supportive as there are no pharmacologic agents that can prevent or treat AKI. Early recognition of renal dysfunction and avoidance of nephrotoxins are the best preventive measures. The mainstays of treatment are restoration and maintenance of adequate fluid balance, correction of metabolic and electrolyte derangements, nutritional support, and limitation of further renal injury. When conservative therapy is unsuccessful, renal replacement therapy (RRT) becomes necessary.

Fluid Management

An accurate assessment of the patient's intravascular volume status is required to guide initial fluid management. Children with prerenal AKI presenting with dehydration, sepsis, or shock require immediate expansion of intravascular volume with boluses of 10–20 mL/kg of crystalloid fluid. After the initial phase of volume expansion, the remaining fluid deficit may be replaced over 24–48 hours while maintaining insensible and ongoing fluid losses. AKI due to prerenal etiologies is usually reversible and responsive to volume resuscitation. Volume expansion has also been successful in patients at risk for AKI in situations such as tumor lysis syndrome, contrast-induced AKI, and pigment nephropathy. However, once intrinsic AKI is confirmed by continued azotemia, oliguria (<1.0 mL/kg/h in infants, <0.5 mL/kg/h in children), or anuria (<0.2 mL/kg/h) after volume administration, fluid restriction is important in order to prevent volume overload. Some strongly suggest consideration of RRT when fluid overload exceeds 10% of body weight and definite initiation of RRT when fluid overload is greater than 15%. To maintain an even fluid balance, insensible water losses and ongoing losses need to be replaced. Insensible water losses can be estimated as a daily volume of 400 mL/m^2 (~1/3 "maintenance fluid" using Holliday Segar method) given as D5W or D10W at a constant rate. Of note, insensible losses are greater in febrile patients and lower in mechanically ventilated patients administered humidified air. Urine losses need to be replaced milliliter for milliliter with 0.45% normal saline. Other ongoing fluid losses (e.g., diarrhea, nasogastric output, and so on) should also be replaced with equivalent volumes.

Diuretics

Oliguric AKI is generally associated with worse outcomes when compared to nonoliguric AKI. Diuretic use to prevent AKI has not been proven and diuretics are not recommended as a prevention or treatment strategy. Diuretics can be used to manage volume overload. Patients with AKI do not respond normally to diuretics and usually require higher doses (furosemide 2–5 mg/kg/dose) to achieve a response. Diuretics should be quickly discontinued if there is no improvement, as they can cause ototoxicity. If there is a response, a continuous infusion of furosemide (0.1–0.3 mg/kg/h) may be superior to bolus dosing because overall less drug is needed.

Vasoactive Agents

The use of vasopressors is recommended in patients with vasomotor shock (not responsive to fluids) to maintain or restore renal perfusion in critically ill patients. Dopamine is thought to increase renal blood flow by promoting vasodilatation and improving urine output by promoting natriuresis. However, dopamine has not proven to alter the course of AKI, convert oliguric to nonoliguric AKI, decrease the need for dialysis, or improve survival in patients with AKI. Complications of dopamine include tachycardia, arrhythmias, myocardial ischemia, and intestinal ischemia. Norepinephrine is recommended as the first-line agent over dopamine for adults in vasomotor shock. In children with low cardiac output shock, vasoactive agents with greater inotropic support such as dopamine, epinephrine, and dobutamine are frequently utilized. Fenoldopam is a selective dopamine-1 receptor agonist that increases renal blood flow through systemic vasodilation. Results of adult studies are promising and studies to define the role of fenoldopam in children are warranted. Theophylline blocks the actions of adenosine, a potent renal vasoconstrictor released during ischemia. Given within the first hour of birth, theophylline was associated with improved fluid balance, higher GFR, and lower creatinine in severely asphyxiated newborns. It is recommended that a single dose of theophylline be given to these neonates who are at high risk for AKI. Other pharmacologic agents such as nesiritide (synthetic human brain natriuretic peptide), atrial natriuretic peptide, IGF-1, and NAC have not been beneficial and are not recommended for the prevention or treatment of AKI. An exception may be NAC for the prevention of contrast-induced AKI.

Electrolyte and Acid–Base Balance

Hyperkalemia in AKI results from reduced GFR, decreased secretion of potassium, and extracellular shifts of potassium during acidosis. Hyperkalemia is the most serious electrolyte abnormality associated with AKI with potential for arrhythmia and cardiac death. ECG changes usually do not occur until the plasma potassium concentration is above 6.5 mEq/L. Mild-to-moderate hyperkalemia (5–6.5 mEq/L) is treated with potassium restriction and medications that remove potassium from the body. Sodium polystyrene sulfonate eliminates potassium via the gastrointestinal tract. Caution should be used in neonates and premature infants. Loop diuretics may be given to patients who are not anuric to aid in excretion of potassium in the urine. Treatment of severe hyperkalemia includes calcium gluconate 10% solution (0.5–1.0 mL/kg intravenously over 5–15 minutes) to stabilize the cardiac membrane and the administration of medications that redistribute as well as remove potassium from the body. Albuterol, a β_2 agonist, is readily available in the ICU and works quickly (10–30 minutes) by transporting potassium into cells. Insulin stimulates beta-receptors on the cell membrane and works within 30 minutes. Insulin is given with glucose to prevent hypoglycemia, which requires large quantities of fluid (0.5–1.0 g of glucose/kg over 30 minutes and 0.1 unit/kg of insulin intravenously). Sodium bicarbonate (1–2 mEq/kg intravenously over 30–60 minutes) also shifts potassium into the cell and works within 30 minutes (lasts 1–2 hours). Hyperkalemia refractory to conservative measures may be treated with dialysis.

Acidosis is caused by the impaired secretion of titratable and nontitratable acids resulting in a consumption of bicarbonate as a buffer and the irregular tubular handling of bicarbonate. Supplementation with oral sodium citrate or sodium bicarbonate (oral or intravenous) may be given to treat the acidosis, although the use of intravenous sodium bicarbonate is controversial due to its adverse side-effect profile. Hyperphosphatemia is attributable to decreased phosphate excretion in the kidney during AKI. As a result, phosphorus binds to calcium resulting in hypocalcemia. Hypocalcemia is exacerbated by the inability of the kidney to generate active vitamin D and parathyroid hormone resistance. Restriction of phosphorus in the diet is recommended as well as the use of oral phosphate binders given with meals to bind phosphate in the gastrointestinal tract. Calcium carbonate is the first-line phosphate binder in children. Selvelamer is a non-calcium-containing phosphate binder. Aluminum-containing binders should be avoided in children due to the risk of neurotoxicity due to aluminum accumulation. Severe hypocalcemia can be treated with intravenous calcium preparations. Neuroendocrine axis changes in AKI cause altered carbohydrate metabolism, which may lead to hyperglycemia. Insulin therapy targets plasma glucose 110–149 in critically ill adults. Studies on insulin therapy in children require further exploration.

Dosing of Medications

Nephrotoxic medications should be avoided in patients at risk for AKI or with established AKI. For fungal infections, the lipid formulations of amphotericin B are suggested rather than conventional formulations. When appropriate, monitoring of drug levels is important as it allows for adjustment of drug dosing. Once AKI is established, medications that are excreted by the kidney require dosage adjustment based on the estimated GFR.

Hypertension

Hypertension in AKI usually results from volume overload although it may also be renin-mediated. To prevent sodium and fluid retention, sodium intake should be restricted to 2–3 mEq/kg/day. Hypertension that does not respond to fluid and sodium restriction requires treatment with antihypertensive medications (see **Table 87.4**). Nifedipine, labetalol, hydralazine, and clonidine are medications that work quickly. ACEi and ARBs are contraindicated in AKI because they reduce glomerular pressure and can lead to hyperkalemia. For hypertensive emergency and urgency, continuous infusion with short-acting medications such as nicardipine, labetalol, and sodium nitroprusside is recommended. The aim is to reduce blood pressure slowly, not more than 25% in the first hours of treatment and then gradually to normal over days.

Nutritional Support

The provision of adequate nutritional and metabolic support is essential in the care of the critically ill children with AKI as they are at increased risk for undernutrition. Alterations in physiologic metabolism in AKI lead to a state of hypercatabolism, hypoalbuminemia, loss of lean body mass, and increased utilization of fat stores. Patient energy requirements based on measured energy expenditure are estimated to be 0.20–0.26 mJ/kg/day, equal to a caloric intake of 50–60 cal/kg/day. In contrast to adults, protein intake is not restricted in children with AKI. Protein requirements are 2–3 g/kg/day for children 0–2 years and 1.5 g/kg/day for children and adolescents >2 years. Children on RRT require additional protein supplementation. Enteral feedings with renal formulas lower in solute load, phosphorus, and potassium are preferred over parenteral nutrition when feasible.

Renal Replacement Therapy

RRT will be covered briefly as it is discussed in further detail in Chapter 18. RRT is a life-supporting therapy that aids in the removal of fluid and solute

TABLE 87.4

Antihypertensive Medications

DRUG	CLASS	DOSE	COMMENTS
Furosemide	Loop diuretic	0.5–2 mg/kg oral or IV every 6–12 h, continuous infusion: start 0.05 mg/kg/h	Use only in nonoliguric AKI
Amlodipine	Calcium-channel blocker	Oral: 0.05–0.1 mg/kg/d Adult dose: 2.5–5 mg once daily	Avoid use with AV block, neonates, sick sinus
Clonidine	Central α_2 agonist	Oral: 5–25 µg/kg/d PO divided q 6–8 h	Rebound hypertension with abrupt withdrawal
		Transdermal: 0.1–0.3 mg patch	Start dose at 5–10 µg/kg/d and increase every 5–7 d
Nifedipine	Calcium-channel blocker (short acting)	Oral: 0.1–0.25 mg/kg/dose every 4–6 h	Side effects: flushing and tachycardia
Hydralazine	Direct arterial vasodilator (short acting)	Oral: 0.2–2 mg/kg every 6–12 h IV bolus: 0.1–0.5 mg/kg/dose every 3–4 h	Side effects: tachycardia, nausea, lupus-like reactions
Labetalol	α- and β-blocker	Oral: 0.5–1.5 mg/kg every 12 h IV bolus: 0.2–1.0 mg/kg every 10 min PRN, continuous infusion 0.25–3 mg/kg/h IV	Avoid use with bradycardia, AV block, bronchospasm, CHF
Nicardipine	Calcium-channel blocker	Continuous infusion 0.5–4 µg/kg/min	May require a large volume infused
Sodium nitroprusside	Arterial and venous vasodilator	Continuous infusion 0.3–10 µg/kg/min IV	Follow for cyanide toxicity. Risk is higher in AKI
Esmolol	β-blocker	Continuous infusion 100–500 µg/kg/min	Avoid use with asthma, IDDM, AV block

AKI, acute kidney injury; CHF, congestive heart failure
From Lexicomp Online, 2013.

waste when there is impaired kidney function. General indications for RRT are listed in **Table 87.5**. RRT modalities include peritoneal dialysis (PD), intermittent hemodialysis (iHD), and continuous renal replacement therapy (CRRT). PD is preferred in neonates because iHD and CRRT can be technically challenging due to difficult vascular access. For hemodynamically unstable patients, CRRT is the preferred modality. HD and CRRT are used to treat hyperammonemia and inborn errors of metabolism.

Peritoneal Dialysis

PD utilizes the capillaries of the peritoneal membrane as the conduit for dialysis. The surface area of the peritoneal membrane is larger in children relative to adults, which allows for rapid and efficient equilibration of solutes. A higher dextrose concentration achieves more fluid removal (1.5%, 2.5%, and 4.25% solutions). The dialysis prescription includes exchange volumes of 20–50 mL/kg (10 mg/kg at initiation to reduce risk of leak), dwell times of 25–50 minutes, and drain times of 5–15 minutes. Shorter dwell times result in increased clearance and fluid removal. The advantages of PD are that vascular access is not required and it is a simpler technique. Disadvantages are that PD may be less efficient than HD and CRRT for solute removal and the risk of peritonitis.

TABLE 87.5

Indications for Renal Replacement Therapy

Severe metabolic acidosis unresponsive to bicarbonate therapy
Electrolyte disturbance despite medical therapy
Fluid overload unresponsive to diuretics
Uremic complications(e.g., pericarditis, encephalopathy, coagulopathy)
Inborn errors of metabolism: urea cycle defects

Intermittent Hemodialysis

Intermittent HD is an extracorporeal blood purification treatment that utilizes a counter-current flow of blood and dialysate to allow diffusion of solutes across a semipermeable membrane of the dialyzer. Fluid removal is achieved by altering hydrostatic pressure within the dialyzer. Vascular access may be either temporary or permanent via the femoral or internal jugular vessels. The subclavian route is discouraged to prevent stenosis in a patient that may require long-term access for RRT. The advantages of intermittent HD are the short treatment times and accurate fluid removal. A disadvantage is that intermittent HD is not tolerated in a hemodynamically unstable patient.

Continuous Renal Replacement Therapy

CRRT is a slow, gentle treatment that is given continuously for 24 hours per day. The principles of CRRT are similar to that of HD with the exception that hemofiltration, through convection, may be used to aid in solute removal. Hemofiltration refers to the use of replacement fluid that is given either pre- or postfilter. The advantages of CRRT are that it can be used in unstable patients, it allows for administration of large daily volumes (nutrition and blood products), and it has accurate fluid removal.

PROGNOSIS

Children, as well as adults, demonstrate a clear increase in mortality, duration of mechanical ventilation, ICU length of stay, and hospital length of stay in the presence of AKI. There is limited data on long-term outcomes of children with AKI. There is a suggestion that AKI may increase the risk of developing chronic kidney disease. Children with known risk for AKI such as childhood cancer survivors, bone marrow transplant recipients, and premature infants have demonstrated increased risk of CKD after long-term follow-up.

CHAPTER 88 ■ CHRONIC KIDNEY DISEASE, DIALYSIS, AND RENAL TRANSPLANTATION

VINAI MODEM, ROBERT P. WORONIECKI, AND FANGMING LIN

DEFINITION AND RISK FACTORS FOR DEVELOPING CHRONIC KIDNEY DISEASE

Chronic kidney disease (CKD) can be diagnosed when there are pathologic abnormalities or markers of kidney damage such as persistent albuminuria (an indicator of ongoing renal injury), or reduced glomerular filtration rate (GFR) <60 mL/min/1.73 m^2 for ≥3 months. Chronic kidney condition is classified into five stages on the basis of the estimated GFR (**Table 88.1**). End-stage renal disease (ESRD) typically refers to stages IV and V, which require renal replacement therapy (RRT) in the form of either chronic dialysis or renal transplantation. Acute kidney injury (AKI) can become CKD when renal injury and dysfunction persist for >3 months. CKD staging can be used for adults and children ≥2 years of age. The prevalence of all stages of CKD has been increasing worldwide. Children with oncologic disease, hematopoietic stem cell transplantation, solid organ transplantation, congenital heart disease, and rheumatologic diseases are at a greater risk for developing CKD. Patients can also have primary renal disease that progresses to CKD. Common causes of primary renal disease in children include congenital anomalies of the kidney and urinary tract such as aplastic or hypodysplastic kidneys, obstructive uropathy (e.g., posterior urethral valves), and reflux nephropathy. Tubular disease (e.g., nephronophthisis and polycystic kidney disease), glomerular disease due to focal segmental glomerulosclerosis (FSGS), and vasculitis (e.g., lupus nephritis) also contribute to the development of CKD.

CHRONIC KIDNEY DISEASE IN PATIENTS WITH CRITICAL ILLNESS

Renal dysfunction affects multiple organ systems (**Fig. 88.1**). CKD stages I and II usually show evidence of renal injury and may have clinical manifestations of proteinuria and hypertension. The primary goal of CKD management for these stages is to prevent the progression by reducing proteinuria and controlling hypertension typically with angiotensin-converting enzyme inhibitors (ACEIs) and angiotensin receptor blockers (ARBs), which offer renal protection. As renal function deteriorates to stages III, IV, and V, patients will have multiple manifestations involving

TABLE 88.1

Chronic Kidney Disease Staging

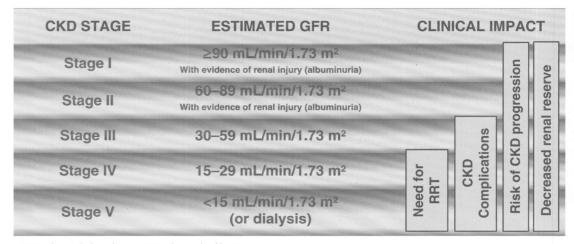

CKD STAGE	ESTIMATED GFR	CLINICAL IMPACT: Need for RRT	CLINICAL IMPACT: CKD Complications	CLINICAL IMPACT: Risk of CKD progression	CLINICAL IMPACT: Decreased renal reserve
Stage I	≥90 mL/min/1.73 m^2 With evidence of renal injury (albuminuria)			✓	✓
Stage II	60–89 mL/min/1.73 m^2 With evidence of renal injury (albuminuria)			✓	✓
Stage III	30–59 mL/min/1.73 m^2		✓	✓	✓
Stage IV	15–29 mL/min/1.73 m^2	✓	✓	✓	✓
Stage V	<15 mL/min/1.73 m^2 (or dialysis)	✓	✓	✓	✓

CKD, Chronic kidney disease; GFR, glomerular filtration rate.

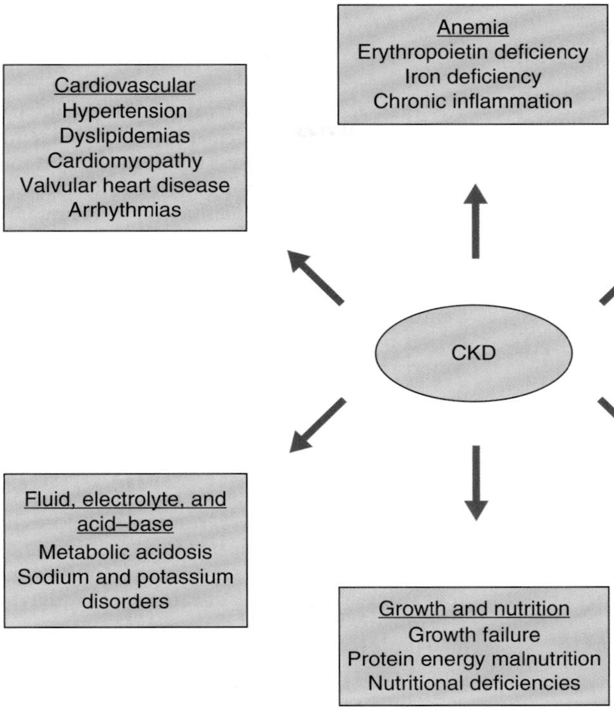

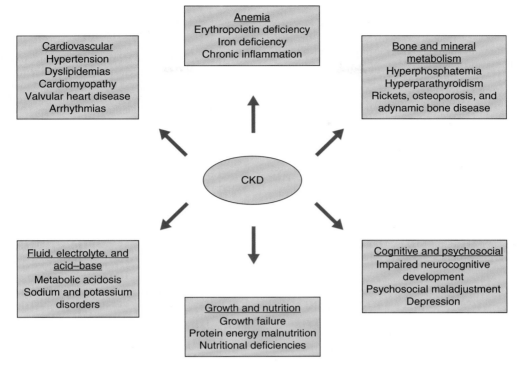

FIGURE 88.1. Multiorgan involvement in CKD.

various organ systems. Management focuses on the treatment of electrolyte and acid–base disturbances, anemia, hyperparathyroidism, malnutrition, and behavioral and psychological disorders.

Acute Kidney Injury on CKD

Normal kidneys have a significant functional reserve, primarily due to hyperfiltration at the level of individual nephrons. If the number of functional nephrons is reduced, this reserve is decreased. Chronic hyperfiltration is associated with hypertension and diabetes and can result in glomerular sclerosis and further loss of nephrons.

Impact of CKD on the Cardiovascular System

CKD can lead to cardiovascular pathology, including hypertension, vascular wall stiffness, cardiomyopathy, and valvular heart disease. These conditions increase the risk of developing congestive heart failure and dysrhythmias. Vascular complications of hypertension such as posterior reversible encephalopathy syndrome (PRES) (also called reversible posterior leukoencephalopathy syndrome [RPLS]) can occur. In addition to hypertension, uremia, vasculitis, immunosuppressant use, and organ transplant are risk factors for PRES/RPLS that may be seen with CKD or AKI. Vascular access is an important issue that deserves thoughtful management in CKD. Peripherally inserted central catheters (PICCs) have a high rate of venous thrombosis and stenosis limiting the vascular access options. There is an increased risk of dialysis catheter–related infection as well, with prior history of a PICC. Subclavian lines can lead to similar complications such as thrombosis and stenosis, rendering the vasculature on that arm unsuitable for dialysis access.

Hematologic and Immune Responses in CKD

Many patients with CKD have anemia and require erythropoiesis-stimulating agents (ESAs). During critical illness, there is increased red cell destruction and blood loss. In addition, systemic inflammation increases the resistance to ESAs. Therefore, severe anemia may develop in critically ill patients with preexisting CKD. Repeated blood transfusions increase the risk of developing anti-human leukocyte antigen antibodies, leading to difficulty in matching with future kidney donors. Every effort should be made to minimize iatrogenic blood loss and blood transfusions. The recommendation is to start recombinant human erythropoietin (or darbepoetin alfa) plus iron supplementation if the child's hemoglobin is $\leq$10 g/dL or if the child is symptomatic (e.g., fatigue, cognitive problems, left ventricular hypertrophy) with hemoglobin ≤ 5th percentile for age. The target hemoglobin range is 11–12 g/dL. Uremia can cause platelet dysfunction, which increases the risk of bleeding. In such patients, desmopressin (dDAVP, 0.3 μg/kg, intravenously) can be given 30 minutes prior to invasive procedures to promote clotting by stimulating endothelial release of von Willebrand factor multimers. Unfortunately, tachyphylaxis can develop after two doses, and alternative therapies to manage platelet dysfunction may be needed, including dialysis, estrogens, or cryoprecipitate.

The innate immune system is chronically activated with hypercytokinemia and increased levels of acute phase reactants such as C-reactive protein. Markers of chronic inflammation have been linked to complications of CKD and associated with mortality in patients with CKD. On the other hand, adaptive immunity is impaired with poor response to infections. Various factors such as uremic toxins, recurrent endotoxemia, and vitamin D deficiency have all been implicated in the pathogenesis of immune dysregulation in CKD.

UNIQUE CHALLENGES IN CHILDREN WITH ESRD

Children with ESRD require chronic dialysis or kidney transplantation. Common reasons for these patients to require intensive care unit (ICU) care include fluid overload, hypertensive crises, severe electrolyte imbalances (hyperkalemia), uremic complications, and catheter-related sepsis.

Differentiating ESRD from AKI

Previously unrecognized ESRD can present with uremia and its complications. When there is no history of kidney disease, the first step is to distinguish ESRD from AKI. The presence of features of CKD (anemia, growth failure, and hyperparathyroidism) is helpful with this. Renal sonogram can identify small, echogenic end-stage kidneys and structural abnormalities. The utility of renal biopsy to identify the underlying causes may be limited because end-stage kidneys usually show nonspecific changes such as sclerotic glomeruli, atrophic tubules, and fibrotic interstitium. In contrast, an urgent renal biopsy may be essential in some children with AKI, both from diagnostic as well as management perspective.

Fluid Overload

Fluid overload can present as systemic and pulmonary vascular congestion leading to congestive heart failure and hypertension. Most patients with chronic dialysis have an estimated "dry weight," and it serves as the goal for fluid removal. However, if hypertension continues despite reaching the goal, their dry weight needs to be challenged by removing more fluid until symptoms have improved and a new dry weight is established.

Infection of Vascular Access and Peritonitis

Vascular access is the primary site of infection in hemodialysis (HD) patients. Nontunneled temporary catheters have the highest risk for infection followed by tunneled catheters and arteriovenous grafts. Gram-positive bacteria (e.g., methicillin-resistant *Staphylococcus aureus* [MRSA]) account for the majority of infections. Vancomycin for gram-positive bacteria and aminoglycosides for gram-negative bacteria are usual treatment choices. The advantage of these antibiotics is that a single dose will maintain adequate blood concentration through the entire interdialytic period because renal failure limits their excretion. Catheter-related infections can lead to long-term issues such as vascular stenosis and thrombosis. Some of the preventive approaches to minimize infections include avoiding catheters with a "Fistula First" initiative, treating MRSA carriers, minimizing access of the catheter for nondialysis purpose (e.g., blood draws), and using thrombolytics (e.g., tissue plasminogen activator), antibiotic, or citrate locks for the catheter.

Similarly, peritoneal dialysis (PD) catheter–related infections occur at the exit site, at the subcutaneous tunnel, or in the catheter and can lead to life-threatening peritonitis and sepsis. Infection with gram-positive bacteria is the most common. Peritonitis can be treated with intraperitoneal antibiotics. Initial empiric regimen includes both cefazolin for gram-positive bacteria and ceftazidime for gram-negative bacteria, including pseudomonas. Other antibiotics that can be used intraperitoneally include vancomycin, aminoglycosides, carbapenems, and fluoroquinolones. There can be significant systemic absorption of antibiotics instilled into the peritoneum. The risk of fungal peritonitis is increased in patients who are malnourished and hypoalbuminemic. Fungal peritonitis, recurrent peritonitis by the same organism, and peritonitis with multidrug-resistant organisms are indications for catheter removal. These patients may need HD for a period of time until the peritoneum is cleared of infection. Repeated episodes of peritonitis can damage the peritoneum and lead to inadequate PD.

DIALYSIS AS A RENAL REPLACEMENT THERAPY

The primary goal of dialysis is to remove metabolic wastes (solute clearance) and fluid (ultrafiltration). Solute removal is measured in terms of clearance, which is defined as the volume of blood cleared in a unit time. The choice of using HD versus PD is influenced by patient condition, family preferences, institutional and family resources, dialysis goals, and the advantages or disadvantages of each modality.

Hemodialysis

HD uses an artificial semipermeable membrane (holofiber dialysis filter) for solute and water transport and requires an extracorporeal circuit. Blood flows inside the holofibers and dialysate flows outside the holofibers in a countercurrent fashion. Solute clearance occurs by diffusion driven by a concentration gradient between the blood and dialysate. The rate of diffusion depends on the size of solute molecules, concentration gradient, and surface area of the filter membrane. Blood flow rate, dialysate flow rate, surface area of the filter, and duration of HD session can be adjusted to achieve the goal clearance. The amount of fluid removed or ultrafiltration is controlled by adjusting the transmembrane pressure gradient across the dialysis membrane. The main advantage of HD is the rapid clearance of solutes and removal of fluid. But the extracorporeal volume and high blood flow rates can cause hemodynamic instability. *Dialysis disequilibrium syndrome*, which manifests with neurologic symptoms resulting from cerebral edema, could occur if clearance is rapid, especially on the first dialysis treatment. Therefore, it is advised that first dialysis provide no more than 25% urea reduction rate in a uremic patient. In CKD, the large urea (or other organic compound) gradient in the brain may pull fluid in and cause cerebral edema. The needs for vascular access, systemic anticoagulation, specialized equipment, and trained personnel are other considerations in determining whether to proceed with HD.

Peritoneal Dialysis

The peritoneal membrane is a semipermeable membrane made of mesothelial cells and capillaries of peritoneal cavity, across which water and solute transport occurs in PD. Water clearance occurs with ultrafiltration and is driven by an osmotic gradient. Solute clearance occurs primarily by diffusion and to a much less extent by ultrafiltration (convective clearance) when small molecules move along with the water, called solvent drag. Dwell volume is the amount of dialysate instilled with each cycle and dwell time is the duration for which the dialysate is left in the peritoneal cavity before draining. The rate of solute clearance depends on dwell volume, dwell time, number of cycles, and the characteristics of peritoneal membrane. The PD dialysate fluid typically consists of electrolytes (Na, Mg, Ca, and Cl), buffer (lactate), and an osmotic agent (e.g., dextrose, icodextrin). The concentration of osmotic agent (e.g., 1.5%–4.25% dextrose) can be adjusted to increase or decrease the rate of ultrafiltration. Additives such as heparin (used to prevent fibrin clots, especially in a new PD catheter or during peritonitis), bicarbonate (small amount to adjust the pH of dialysate and provide comfort to the patient), antibiotics, and electrolytes (e.g., potassium) can be added to the dialysate when needed.

PD has a role in acute setting in selected patients. One of its major advantages is that it can be performed continuously (it is considered a type of continuous RRT). It is better tolerated than intermittent HD in smaller infants and patients with hemodynamic instability. Technical simplicity, no requirement for systemic anticoagulation, and lower cost are other benefits. But, it does require a PD catheter placement and an accessible and functional peritoneum. Inadequate clearance and fluid retention are common problems associated with PD. These can occur in patients with constipation or when the tip of the PD catheter is malpositioned or occluded. In patients with respiratory distress or failure, the abdominal distension from instilling the dialysate can worsen the respiratory symptoms. Also, if the intra-abdominal pressure is greater than 18 cm H_2O, ultrafiltration can occur in the reverse direction with water moving from peritoneal space to intravascular space, resulting in fluid retention. Dextrose (the osmotic agent) absorption can lead to hyperglycemia over time.

RENAL TRANSPLANTATION

Renal transplantation is a form of RRT. Some patients may require special preparations such as removal of native kidneys (e.g., recurrent urinary tract infections, severe nephrotic syndrome), urologic surgery (e.g., bladder augmentation), and desensitization procedures (e.g., plasmapheresis, immunosuppression). Management around the time of transplant is crucial for kidney graft survival and requires collaboration between transplant surgeons, nephrologists, and critical care physicians.

Surgical and Anesthetic Management

Adequate hydration and stable hemodynamic status of the patient are essential before transplant surgery. In children, a disproportionately large adult donor kidney can take up >20% of the cardiac output, necessitating appropriate increase in cardiac output immediately after the donor kidney is connected. Adequate fluid resuscitation and continued vigilance to maintain effective circulating volume is the key. Some children may require vasopressor support such as dopamine to maintain adequate mean arterial pressure for perfusion of the kidney graft. Methods for kidney placement largely depend on the size of the patient. Younger children (usually <15 kg) require a transperitoneal approach with a large midline incision and intra-abdominal placement of the kidney graft. Older children (usually >15 kg) could take an extraperitoneal approach in the lower abdomen. Renal vessels are anastomosed with the abdominal aorta and inferior vena cava when the kidney is placed intra-abdominally and with the iliac vessels when the kidney is placed in the lower abdomen. The donor ureter is implanted into recipient's bladder. With adequate perfusion, the kidney graft will produce urine immediately after vascular anastomosis. The donor kidney undergoes warm and cold ischemia prior to anastomosis with the recipient vessels. Prolonged warm and cold ischemia times, especially >24 hours, increase the risk of delayed graft function largely due to acute tubular necrosis (ATN).

Respiratory Management

The majority of patients are extubated in the recovery room or soon after arriving in the ICU. Fluid overload is one of the main reasons causing delays in extubation. Most of these children have been given a large amount of fluid during the perioperative period while urine output has not increased enough to excrete excess amount of fluid. The patient may develop pulmonary edema with fluid overload.

Hemodynamic and Fluid Management

The primary goal for posttransplant management in the ICU is to ensure adequate perfusion of the new graft. Kidney injury from warm and cold ischemia as well as lack of intact renal innervation affects autoregulation. As a result, renal blood flow in the graft is blood pressure dependent. Also, most transplanted kidneys come from adult donors and require higher mean arterial pressure for perfusion. Adequate effective circulating volume is essential such that the central venous pressure should be maintained around 8–10 mm Hg. Vasopressors such as dopamine may be needed as well. Fluid requirement for the initial 24 hours after transplantation depends on the patient's urine output and hemodynamic status. Typically, patients are placed on a constant rate of dextrose-containing fluids to prevent hypoglycemia and to replenish insensible losses. In addition, they receive hourly urine replacement at a 1:1 ratio with 0.45% NaCl. Some patients may have exceedingly high urine output (>500 mL/h), and their urine replacement can be capped off at a maximal rate to prevent fluid overload and stop driving high urine output. After 24–48 hours, if patients continue to have good urine output and show improvement in renal function, urine replacement can be discontinued. The patients can be placed on a constant fluid rate to match the insensible, urinary, and other fluid losses. Patients may develop hypomagnesaemia and hypophosphatemia requiring supplementation. Calcitriol will be helpful to suppress parathyroid function and increase gastrointestinal absorption of phosphate.

Monitoring Renal Function

Urine output is a combination of urine produced by the transplanted kidney and patient's native kidneys if present. The transplanted kidney frequently lacks concentrating ability due to ATN, leading to polyuria. Decreased urine output, especially of sudden onset, should be investigated promptly. First, adequate blood pressure and intravascular volume should be ensured. Some patients have stents placed at the ureterovesical anastomosis, which can dislodge and cause obstruction. Other causes of urinary obstruction include lymphocele and kinking of the ureter. Urinary leak from the anastomotic site or bladder rupture (occurs rarely) can also lead to low urine output. This can result in urinary ascites or urinoma, both of which can be detected by sonogram and require surgical repair. If the patient continues to have poor urine output despite adequate hemodynamic status and no obstruction to urine flow, an urgent renal sonogram with Doppler flow study is required to assess renal blood flow and vascular anastomoses. Thrombosis of the vascular anastomotic site is a serious complication and can result in graft loss. Other important causes of poor urine output and graft dysfunction are acute rejection and recurrence of primary disease (e.g., FSGS, atypical hemolytic uremic syndrome), which might need a renal biopsy to confirm the diagnosis.

Pain Management

Good pain control is an important goal. It is usually achieved with an opioid and acetaminophen. However, one needs to be aware of impaired clearance of opioids and accumulation of their active metabolites with renal failure. Before allograft function is established, it is advised to use lower doses at reduced frequency. Patients who receive epidural anesthetic and analgesic infusions for pain control are at risk for vasodilation, especially in the lower extremities, which may lead to hypotension necessitating vasopressor support.

Immunosuppression

Induction of immunosuppression is initiated in the operating room. Common immunosuppressive agents include lymphocyte-depleting agents (polyclonal and monoclonal antibodies, IL-2 receptor antagonists), calcineurin inhibitors (tacrolimus, cyclosporine A), antiproliferative agents (mycophenolate), and corticosteroids. Acute rejection can occur in the immediate postoperative period. It requires a biopsy for diagnosis and needs to be treated immediately to prevent loss of the graft. Patients with immunosuppression are at risk for infections and need prophylaxis. In the immediate postoperative period, most patients receive antibacterial prophylaxis with cephalosporin. They require cytomegalovirus prophylaxis with ganciclovir, PCP prophylaxis with bactrim, and candida prophylaxis with nystatin or fluconazole for an extended period of time.

Other Postoperative Issues

The goal with anemia management is to minimize blood transfusions. Repeated transfusions can lead to sensitization to future donors. Depending on the etiology, hypertension can be managed with diuretics (in case of fluid overload), calcium-channel blockers, and clonidine. ACEIs and ARBs, which reduce glomerular filtration in the graft, are avoided. After transplant, most patients require phosphorus and magnesium supplements. Patients are also at risk for developing glucose intolerance and hyperglycemia from immunosuppressive medications (e.g., tacrolimus, prednisone).

CHAPTER 89 ■ HYPERTENSIVE CRISIS

GEORGE OFORI-AMANFO, ARTHUR J. SMERLING, AND CHARLES L. SCHLEIEN

INTRODUCTION AND DEFINITIONS

Hypertension occurs when there is an increase in blood flow or vascular resistance (or both) across a vascular bed. *Hypertensive crisis* is an acute, life-threatening elevation of blood pressure (BP). *Hypertensive emergency* is defined as sudden, severe hypertension complicated by acute end-organ damage; *hypertensive urgency* is characterized by severely elevated BP without end-organ damage. The organ systems most frequently involved are the central nervous system (CNS), cardiovascular system, and kidneys (**Table 89.1**).

Hypertensive encephalopathy manifests as insidious onset of headache, visual changes, nausea, and vomiting followed by altered mental status, focal neurologic deficits, and coma. Ocular involvement presents as retinal hemorrhages, exudates, and papilledema. Cardiac involvement leads to left ventricular (LV) failure, pulmonary edema, and acute myocardial ischemia. Renal effects result in hematuria, proteinuria, or azotemia. Patients experiencing hypertensive urgency may or may not develop severe headache, shortness of breath, epistaxis, or severe anxiety.

PATHOPHYSIOLOGY

Any disorder that causes hypertension can give rise to hypertensive crisis (**Table 89.2**). The endothelium in resistance vessels attempts to compensate for changes in vascular resistance through autocrine and paracrine release of vasodilator molecules, such as nitric oxide and prostacyclin. With sustained severe hypertension, vasodilator responses are overwhelmed. An abrupt increase in vascular resistance is likely related to a sudden surge in humoral vasoconstrictors. Activation of the renin–angiotensin system, nitric oxide (NO), endothelin, vasopressin, and catecholamines is also likely important.

The ensuing increase in BP generates mechanical stress and injury of the microvasculature, endothelial damage, activation of the renin–angiotensin system, and oxidative stress. The endothelial injury results in increased vascular permeability, activation of coagulation cascade, and platelet deposition of fibrin. Further progression leads to fibrinoid necrosis of the arterioles, resulting in ischemia and the release of additional vasoactive mediators, generating a vicious cycle of repeated injury. There is an increased

TABLE 89.1

Manifestations of Hypertensive Crises

■ HYPERTENSIVE CRISES
Hypertensive encephalopathy
Acute stroke
Retinopathy
Acute myocardial ischemia
Acute LV failure with pulmonary edema
Dissecting aortic aneurysm
Acute renal failure
Microangiopathic hemolytic anemia

TABLE 89.2

Causes of Hypertensive Crisis

■ DISORDER	■ CAUSE
Essential hypertension	
Primary CNS disease	Spinal cord injury
Renal parenchymal disorders	Reflux nephropathy
	Obstructive uropathy
	Glomerulonephritis
	Interstitial nephritis
	Hemolytic uremic syndrome
	Systemic lupus erythematosis
	Vasculitides
Renovascular disorders	Fibromuscular dysplasia
	Acute renal artery occlusion
	Polyarteritis nodosa
Endocrine disorders	Renin-secreting tumors
	Pheochromocytoma
	Thyroid crisis
	Cushing syndrome
	Conn disease
Ingestions/drugs	Cocaine
	Amphetamines
	Phencyclidine
	Cyclosporine
	Tacrolimus
	Sympathomimetic diet pills
Cardiovascular disorder	Coarctation of the aorta
	Midaortic syndrome
Preeclampsia/eclampsia	Pregnancy

production of proinflammatory cytokines (e.g., interleukin-6) and an increase in NADPH oxidase activity that generates the release of reactive oxygen species (ROS). The main characteristic of endothelial dysfunction present in arterial hypertension is the attenuated NO bioavailability. The increased ROS generated in the hypertensive patient act as potent NO scavengers and reduce NO bioavailability.

Other agents responsible for vasodilation include endothelial-derived hyperpolarizing factor (EDHF) and prostaglandin I_2 (PGI_2). EDHF is a potent non-NO, non–prostaglandin-mediated, endothelium-dependent vasodilator with a predominant effect on resistance vessels. PGI_2 is an eicosanoid of the cyclooxygenase pathway that causes vascular smooth muscle relaxation and inhibits platelet aggregation. Endothelin is another endothelium-derived agent that has a potent vasoconstrictor effect and may act alone or with other agents (e.g., thromboxane A_2, prostaglandin $F_{2\alpha}$, or endothelial-derived constrictor factor) to cause vasoconstriction.

Patients with chronic hypertension may have arterial wall hypertrophy and be relatively protected from acute BP elevation. Conversely, in patients without preexisting chronic hypertension, a hypertensive emergency can develop at a substantially lower BP.

Cerebral Autoregulation

Under conditions of normal intracranial and central venous pressures, cerebral blood flow (CBF) is related to mean arterial pressure (MAP) and inversely related to cerebrovascular resistance (CVR). In normotensive adults, CBF is constant over a wide BP range. The range of autoregulation shifts to the right in chronically hypertensive patients (**Fig. 89.1**; reversible with long-term BP control). This autoregulation is maintained by adjustments in CVR. Hypertensive encephalopathy occurs when MAP exceeds the upper limit of autoregulation.

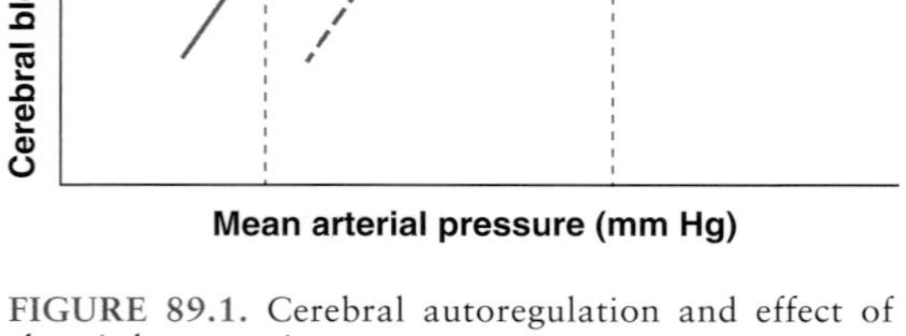

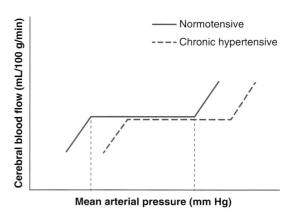

FIGURE 89.1. Cerebral autoregulation and effect of chronic hypertension.

CLINICAL PRESENTATION

The risk of development of hypertensive crisis is greater with secondary hypertension than with essential hypertension. The absolute BP is often not as important as the rate of elevation of the systemic BP. Acute elevations in BP are less well tolerated and more likely to produce symptoms than are chronic elevations.

In the neonate, symptoms and signs related to hypertension are lethargy and irritability; in the older child, they include severe headache, dizziness, blurred vision, and epistaxis. Physical examination findings such as altered mental status, papilledema, and pulmonary edema are related to the organs involved. It is difficult to apply an absolute BP level to define hypertensive emergencies and urgencies.

Neurologic Manifestations

Hypertensive Encephalopathy

Hypertensive encephalopathy is characterized by headache, nausea, vomiting, blurred vision, and altered mental status and may progress to focal or generalized seizures, focal neurologic deficits, and cortical blindness. If not treated, it may progress rapidly to cerebral hemorrhage, coma, and death. Fundoscopy may reveal evidence of papilledema, retinal hemorrhages, and exudates.

Differential Diagnosis of Hypertensive Encephalopathy. Hypertensive encephalopathy must be differentiated from other acute neurologic events that may be associated with hypertension, such as cerebral infarct or hemorrhage. Hypertension in response to cerebral ischemia can be caused by brainstem ischemia or increased intracranial pressure (ICP) (Cushing triad). Treatment of Cushing triad must be directed at managing increased ICP and not at lowering systemic BP (which will compromise cerebral perfusion pressure).

Pseudotumor cerebri, when associated with severe hypertension, may mimic hypertensive encephalopathy. Other causes of hypertension and altered mental status include primary renal disease (uremic encephalopathy), hepatorenal syndrome (hepatic encephalopathy), and steroid overdose (altered sensorium). Primary CNS disorders such as stroke and vasculitis may present with similar clinical findings.

Acute Stroke

Acute stroke with concomitant severe hypertension poses a diagnostic and management dilemma. The hypertension may be a reflex response to maintain cerebral perfusion or the cause of the stroke. In many patients in whom hypertension is secondary to stroke, the BP tends to resolve spontaneously within 48 hours.

Cardiovascular Manifestations

Myocardial Ischemia

The effects on the left ventricle of the sudden increase in afterload associated with a hypertensive crisis include increased oxygen demand and decreased oxygen supply. Myocardial ischemia results if there is no concurrent increase in coronary blood flow. A sustained increase in myocardial workload leads to LV failure, elevated LV end-diastolic pressure, and pulmonary edema. These pathophysiologic events manifest as acute chest pain, tachypnea, dyspnea, orthopnea, cough, and hemoptysis. Physical examination may reveal rales or gallop; chest x-ray may reveal pulmonary edema.

Aortic Dissection

Severe acute hypertension can cause aortic dissection, especially in patients with predisposing syndromes (Marfan, Loeys–Dietz, Ehler–Danlos type 4, Turner, and polycystic kidney disease). Severe chest or abdominal pain is the most common symptom. Syncope, paralysis, and blindness may result from carotid or innominate artery involvement. Dissection of the thoracic aorta may be associated with hemoptysis, orthopnea, and dyspnea. Involvement of the abdominal aorta may cause a variety of gastrointestinal and genitourinary disturbances. The diagnosis should be suspected in a hypertensive patient with abrupt onset of pain, pulse deficits, and signs of end-organ circulatory compromise.

Renal Manifestations

Acute renal dysfunction may be a cause or effect of hypertensive crisis. Among children, renal or renovascular disorders are the most common etiologies of severe hypertension. Mild proteinuria and elevated serum creatinine can be caused by primary renal disease or may be secondary manifestations of severe hypertension.

CLINICAL EVALUATION

BP must be obtained in all four extremities to exclude coarctation of the aorta. Fundoscopic examination can distinguish a true hypertensive emergency from hypertensive urgency. The cardiovascular assessment should include auscultation for new murmurs of aortic insufficiency (aortic dissection) or mitral insufficiency (myocardial infarction). The presence of parasternal heave or S3 gallop may reflect the presence of heart failure, and crackles in the lung fields may suggest pulmonary edema. Neurologic examination should evaluate level of consciousness, signs of meningeal irritation, visual fields, and focal neurologic deficits.

Initial laboratory investigations include serum electrolytes, urea, creatinine, full blood count with peripheral smear (for evidence of hemolysis), urinalysis, and chest radiograph. An electrocardiograph (ECG) may reveal LV hypertrophy and myocardial ischemia/infarction. Chest radiograph may demonstrate cardiac enlargement, widened mediastinum, or pulmonary edema. Measurement of plasma renin and aldosterone activity may be helpful. Once the patient is stabilized, investigations for secondary causes of severe hypertension should be performed, as guided by clinical presentation and laboratory findings (**Table 89.2**). Brain MRI, though not part of the initial work-up, may reveal posterior leukoencephalopathy affecting the white matter of the parieto-occipital, posterior frontal, and temporal regions of the brain (best appreciated on T2-weighted images). Pregnancy must be ruled out in female adolescents as this may impact on the approach to treatment and the choice of antihypertensive agents.

TREATMENT

General Principles

Management requires the immediate assessment of the airway, breathing, and circulation and initiation of appropriate interventions. The primary goal of therapy is to prevent end-organ injury, not solely to restore BP to normal. Reversible causes must be identified and treated appropriately. The recommended initial therapy is to reduce MAP by 20%–25% over a period of 15 minutes to 2 hours. Subsequent rate of reduction of the BP is dictated by clinical status and the rapidity with which the hypertension may have evolved. Too rapid a reduction in BP can worsen end-organ dysfunction and must be avoided. Volume depletion is common in patients with hypertensive crises and may lead to excessive fall in BP during treatment.

Aortic dissection is the most dramatic and most rapidly fatal complication of severe hypertension. Emergency surgery may be indicated. Medical management requires rapid reduction of systolic BP to 100–120 mm Hg or the normal range for age to avoid aortic rupture. Esmolol is often used as lowering heart rate is also helpful. Morphine is indicated for chest pain. If the systolic BP remains above the desired range despite an adequate esmolol infusion, then nitroprusside, nicardipine, or dilitiazem may be added.

Acute postoperative hypertension caused by pain, anxiety, bladder distension, hypothermia, or hypoxemia may present as a hypertensive urgency. If the BP remains significantly elevated after appropriate analgesia, bladder drainage, and normalization of O_2 saturation and body temperature, then a β-blocker or labetalol (combined α- and β-blocker) may be administered on the assumption the child has experienced an acute catecholamine surge from activation of the sympathetic nervous system.

Postcoarctectomy (paradoxical) hypertension in the first week after relief of coarctation of the aorta can occur with an incidence of 30%–56%. Provided a satisfactory repair the hypertension resolves after several days but initial treatment may be needed to avoid end-organ damage and risk of rupture of surgical suture lines.

Reflex, or rebound, hypertensive crisis is a condition that develops in patients who abruptly discontinue their antihypertensive medications, especially clonidine or β-blockers.

Pharmacologic Therapy

Hypertensive urgency can be treated in a non-ICU setting with oral medications over a 24–48-hour period. β-blockers, diuretics, ACE inhibitors, and calcium-channel blockers can be used in the inpatient setting. In the presence of acute end-organ damage, the patient should be admitted to the ICU and treated with IV medication.

The aim of drug therapy is to reduce BP in a controlled, predictable, and safe manner. This is best achieved with a continuous infusion of pharmacologic agents that have rapid onset, short half-life, and ease of titration. Drugs that significantly affect the CNS (clonidine and methyldopa) should be avoided in patients with hypertensive encephalopathy. Also, drugs that act by predominant β-receptor blockade must be avoided in pheochromocytoma crisis, as unopposed α-receptor stimulation may cause a paradoxical worsening of the hypertension. The most commonly used IV medications in children are sodium nitroprusside (SNP), fenoldopam, labetalol, and nicardipine (esmolol has been favored in postcoarctectomy hypertension). The most commonly used oral agents are calcium-channel blockers (nifedipine), ACE inhibitors (enalapril, captopril), and α_2-agonists (clonidine).

PARENTERAL ANTIHYPERTENSIVE AGENTS

Sodium Nitroprusside

SNP is a nonselective vasodilator with effect on both arterioles and venules. It decreases both systemic and pulmonary vascular resistance. Once infused, SNP interacts with oxyhemoglobin, dissociating immediately to form methemoglobin while releasing free cyanide and nitric oxide. Nitric oxide activates guanylate cyclase in the vascular smooth muscle, triggering an increase in intracellular cyclic guanosine monophosphate, followed by vasodilation. Each molecule of SNP metabolized results in the release of five cyanide radicals, some of which bind to methemoglobin, with the rest available to be converted to thiocyanate by the rhodanase enzyme in the liver and the kidneys. Free cyanide not converted to thiocyanate can inactivate tissue cytochrome oxidase and cause tissue hypoxia. Renal failure or prolonged SNP therapy can cause accumulation of thiocyanate.

SNP is particularly useful because of its rapid onset of action, ease of titration, rapid dissipation of its effects after discontinuation, and almost universal efficacy. It acts within 30 seconds, peak antihypertensive effect occurs within 2 minutes, and its effects persist for 2–4 minutes after cessation. Most patients respond to a starting dose of 0.3–0.5 μg/kg/min, which may be escalated as needed to 5 μg/kg/min. Doses as high as 10 μg/kg/min may be needed, but should be administered for no longer than 10 minutes to minimize toxicity. Reflex tachycardia usually occurs, and the addition of a small dose of β-blocker may improve BP control. When used in the treatment of aortic dissection, prior institution of β-blockade is imperative as the reflex tachycardia could be extremely deleterious.

The most common adverse effect of SNP is precipitous hypotension due to its potent vasodilator effect on both the venous and the arterial beds, particularly in the hypovolemic patient. It may also increase ICP, raising concern about its use when cerebral compliance is compromised. *Cyanide toxicity* is a rare, but potentially fatal complication. It presents as lactic acidosis, tachycardia, seizures, coma, and an almond smell on breath. Metabolic acidosis or an unexplained increase in venous oxygen saturation may be the first sign. Treatment is with immediate discontinuation of the infusion, administration of 100% oxygen, slow administration of sodium nitrite, sodium thiosulfate, and sodium bicarbonate (if acidotic). Hydroxocobalamin has also been used but is more controversial. Coadministration of SNP with sodium thiosulfate at a ratio of 10:1 (SNP:sodium thiosulfate) has been shown to increase the rate of CN^- processing and reduces the risk. *Thiocyanate toxicity* is the most common toxicity of SNP and results in nausea, confusion, muscle weakness, psychosis, and seizures. This occurs predominantly with renal dysfunction. Thiocyanate levels should be measured when SNP is used for >48 hours or at doses continuously >4 μg/kg/min. Methemoglobinemia can also be a complication of SNP use.

Fenoldopam

Fenoldopam is a selective dopamine agonist that results in vasodilation. It increases creatinine clearance, urinary flow, and sodium and potassium excretion. Peripheral DA_1 receptors are located postsynaptically in the systemic and renal vasculature and at various sites in the nephrons, parathyroid gland, the gastrointestinal tract, and the brain (fenoldopam does not cross the blood–brain barrier). Fenoldopam has a short half-life (5 minutes), a predictable dose response, and few drug interactions, is easily titrated, does not accumulate in organ failure, and is not associated with precipitous decline in BP. The onset is within 15 minutes of initiation. The recommended starting dose is 0.1 μg/kg/min, titrated to effect to a maximum of 1.6 μg/kg/min. Rebound hypertension after discontinuation is rare. Adverse effects are related to vasodilation and include headache, flushing, dizziness, and reflex tachycardia. ECG changes can occur but are not usually clinically important. Elevation of intraocular pressure has been reported; the effect on ICP is not well studied.

Nicardipine

Nicardipine is a nondihydropyridine derivative calcium-channel blocker that blocks calcium influx through voltage-sensitive channels in vascular smooth muscle cells and results in smooth muscle relaxation and vasodilation. It can be given as a continuous IV infusion and is easily titratable. Onset of action is 5–15 minutes. It is administered as a loading dose of 5–10 μg/kg, given over a minute, followed by a continuous infusion of 1–3 μg/kg/min. Adverse effects include orthostatic hypotension, tachycardia (reflex), and peripheral edema. Nicardipine undergoes considerable first-pass metabolism in the liver and excretion in the urine, so it requires careful use in patients with hepatic or renal dysfunction.

Labetalol

Labetalol is a competitive α_1-adrenergic and β-adrenergic receptor antagonist. The α_1-receptor blockade causes arterial smooth muscle relaxation, and the β-receptor antagonism contributes to the fall in BP by blocking reflex sympathetic stimulation of the heart. It also has sympathomimetic activity at β_2 receptors, which may contribute further to the peripheral vasodilation. It is available in oral and IV forms, but oral bioavailability varies. When given IV, the β-blocker effect is seven times greater than the α-blocker effect. The hypotensive effect of labetalol begins 2–5 minutes after an IV dose, peaks at 5–15 minutes, and persists for about 2–4 hours. The most common adverse effects associated with labetalol are precipitous hypotension and orthostatic hypotension. Bradycardia, heart block, and bronchospasm (all β-antagonist effects) may also complicate its use.

Esmolol

Esmolol is an intravenous, ultra-short-acting selective β_1-adrenergic antagonist. Significant bradycardia can be associated with its administration. Peak hemodynamic effect occurs in 6–10 minutes following an appropriate loading dose. Esmolol is administered as a bolus of 300–500 μg/kg IV over 1–3 minutes, then 25–200 μg/kg/min. Infusion dose may be titrated by 25–50 μg/kg/min q 5–10 minutes for optimal antihypertensive effect to a maximum infusion dose of 1000 μg/kg/min. Adverse effects include bradycardia, hypotension, congestive heart failure, and bronchoconstriction. It is contraindicated in second- or third-degree heart block or cardiogenic shock.

Enalaprilat

Enalaprilat is an ACE inhibitor that decreases circulating levels of angiotensin II, reduces serum aldosterone levels, and inhibits the indirect adrenergic effects of angiotensin II. The antihypertensive effect is the combined result of decreased vascular smooth muscle tone and its antiadrenergic properties. Effects are seen within 15 minutes of administration. Because of its potency and rapid onset of action, it must be administered over 5 minutes. Adverse effects are similar to captopril and rapid drop in BP may occur. It is contraindicated in pregnant patients because of the risk of fetal damage or death.

ORAL ANTIHYPERTENSIVE AGENTS

Nifedipine

Nifedipine is a dihydropyridine calcium-channel–blocking agent that induces peripheral vasodilation. It is administered either orally or sublingually. It reduces BP abruptly and therefore has an important role in the management of hypertensive urgencies. The usual dose is 0.25–0.5 mg/kg/dose; however, the lower end of this range is the preferred starting dose due to the risk of precipitous hypotension. The smallest commercially available dose is a 10-mg liquid-filled capsule, which can be punctured with a tuberculin syringe to administer either a 2.5-mg dose or a 5-mg dose. The dose may be repeated as needed to a daily maximum of 3 mg/kg. Onset of action is observed within 15–30 minutes and an elimination half-life may be as short as 1.5 hours. It must be used with caution since the peripheral vasodilation that follows its administration can trigger an intense reflex adrenergic stimulation with tachycardia as well as activation of the renin–angiotensin system.

Captopril

Captopril, an ACE inhibitor, reduces the levels of circulating angiotensin II. It lowers BP promptly without causing tachycardia. Captopril is very well absorbed; its antihypertensive effect begins within 15 minutes of administration and can last for up to 2 hours. Patients must be closely monitored after the first dose as an exaggerated hypotensive effect may be observed in patients presenting with acute severe hypertension associated with a high renin state. Adverse effects include cough, hyperkalemia, neutropenia, and, rarely, angioedema. In patients with bilateral renal artery stenosis or stenosis in a solitary kidney, captopril and other ACE inhibitors are contraindicated. Autoimmune renal disease with hypertension (e.g., scleroderma) is often associated with high renin states, and ACE inhibitors are to be used with utmost caution. Captopril is also contraindicated in severe renal failure.

Enalapril

Enalapril is an ACE inhibitor. It is a prodrug that is de-esterified in the liver and the kidneys to the active drug, enalaprilat. When administered orally, it is rapidly absorbed with a bioavailability of 60%, but peak plasma concentration of the active drug does not occur until after 4–5 hours. It is generally not a preferred drug if an acute drop in BP is necessary.

CHAPTER 90 ■ INBORN ERRORS OF METABOLISM

MICHAEL WILHELM AND WENDY K. CHUNG

PATHOPHYSIOLOGY

Inborn errors of metabolism (IEMs) result from the deficiency of enzymes involved in intermediary metabolism. They mainly have autosomal-recessive inheritance as partial activity is often sufficient for health. Since the mitochondrial genome is maternally inherited, mitochondrial disorders are often matrilineally transmitted. The X-linked disorders predominantly affect males. Manifestations may vary among family members for a given mutation. IEMs often present with nonspecific manifestations that culminate in critical illness. The pathophysiology of IEMs presenting in the pediatric intensive care unit can be categorized into the following processes: (a) intoxication from metabolites (e.g., ammonia, amino acid derivatives, or ketoacids), (b) reduced fasting tolerance, (c) derangements of energy metabolism, (d) derangement of neurotransmission, or (e) storage of nonmetabolizable substrates in vital organs or tissues.

CLINICAL PRESENTATION AND DIFFERENTIAL DIAGNOSIS

Historical Clues

IEMs presenting with mental status (lethargy, irritability, seizures, and coma) or cardiorespiratory changes can be confused with sepsis. Hypothermia is associated with metabolic decompensation (especially in the urea cycle defects). Some IEMs increase susceptibility to infection (*Escherichia coli* sepsis in galactosemia or neutropenia associated with organic acidurias). Infection often exacerbates metabolic derangements.

Infants can present with decreased appetite, recurrent episodes of lethargy, or difficulty recovering from minor illnesses. Children often demonstrate failure to thrive. Dietary intake may suggest the diagnosis (e.g., a high-protein meal inducing symptoms in urea cycle defects or fruits or sweet foods triggering decompensation in hereditary fructose intolerance). Children may (unknowingly) alter their diet to avoid foods that make them ill. Developmental delay, hypotonia, or seizures are associated with many IEMs.

Family history should include parental consanguinity, ethnicity (hepatorenal tyrosinemia in French Canadians and maple syrup urine disease (MSUD) in Pennsylvania Amish), fetal demise, unexplained deaths, sudden infant death syndrome, developmental delay, seizures, failure to thrive, or other unexplained chronic illness. Maternal liver disease or HELLP syndrome may suggest a long-chain fatty acid oxidation disorder.

Physical Examination Findings

The presence of an unusual body or urine odor might suggest a specific organic acidemia. The associate odors with IEMs include "sweaty feet" with glutaric acidemia (type II) and isovaleric acidemia, "maple syrup" with MSUD, "mousy" with phenylketonuria, "boiled cabbage" with hypermethioninemia and tyrosinemia type I, "swimming pool" with hawkinsinuria, "rotten fish" with trimethylaminuria and dimethylglycinuria, and "tomcat urine" with holocarboxylase synthetase deficiency.

Progressive hepatosplenomegaly occurs in IEMs when nonmetabolizable substrate accumulates (glycogen storage disorders and lysosomal storage disorders). Dysmorphic features are present at birth in peroxisomal biogenesis disorders, fatty acid oxidation disorders, congenital disorders of glycosylation, and pyruvate dehydrogenase deficiency or develop over time in the mucopolysaccharidoses (MPSs). Ophthalmologic examination may also provide clues (cataracts in galactosemia and retinal pigmentary changes in Tay–Sachs disease and some mitochondrial disorders).

Myopathy (hypotonia or cardiomyopathy) may herald a disorder of fatty acid oxidation, mitochondrial derangement, glycogen storage disorder, or rarely a congenital disorder of glycosylation. IEMs are important causes of cardiomyopathy to exclude since some etiologies can be treated.

Laboratory Findings

Laboratory results may suggest an IEM (**Table 90.1**). A primary respiratory alkalosis may be found with hyperammonemia caused by a urea cycle defect. A metabolic acidosis, particularly with an elevation in anion gap (AG) or in lactate, occurs in certain IEMs. Patients with an IEM may have lactate elevation out of proportion to their degree of illness.

TABLE 90.1

Results of Initial Laboratory Tests in Inborn Errors of Metabolisms

	■ UREA CYCLE DEFECT	■ AMINO ACIDOPATHY	■ ORGANIC ACIDURIA	■ FATTY ACID OXIDATION DISORDER	■ CARBOHYDRATE METABOLISM	■ ELECTRON TRANSPORT CHAIN
Blood pH	↑	↓/–	↓	↓/–	↓	↓
AG	WNL	↑/–	↑	↑/–	↑	↑
Glucose	WNL	+/–	WNL	↓↓	↓↓	+/–
Ammonia	↑↑	WNL	↑	↑	WNL	WNL
Lactate	WNL	WNL	↑/–	WNL	↑	↑↑
Ketones	Neg	↑	↑	↓↓	↑	Neg
LFTs	WNL	WNL	WNL	↑	↑	WNL
Serum amino acids	Abnormal	Abnormal	Abnormal	WNL	WNL	Alanine high
Urine organic acids	Some abnormal	Abnormal	Abnormal	Abnormal	WNL	Lactate in urine
Urine reducing substances	–	–	–	–	+/–	–

AG, anion gap; LFTs, liver function tests; WNL, within normal limits; Neg, negative.

The *lactate-to-pyruvate ratio* is helpful, with normal levels being about 20 when both concentrations are expressed in mmol/L. A consistent ratio <10 suggests a pyruvate dehydrogenase deficiency, whereas >25 occurs in tissue hypoxia, pyruvate carboxylase deficiency, and mitochondrial disorders.

The relationship of hypoglycemia to feeding can help identify specific diseases. Hypoglycemia immediately after the ingestion of fructose (fruit or foods containing sucrose) suggests hereditary fructose intolerance (usually detected when an infant transitions to solid foods). Further evidence for this disorder is the presence of reducing substance in the urine. In most other IEMs (glycogen storage diseases, fatty acid oxidation defects, disorders of gluconeogenesis, and some organic acidemias), hypoglycemia occurs with fasting. Nonketotic hypoglycemia suggests a defect in fatty acid oxidation or ketogenesis. Elevated ketone levels in the nonfasting/nonhypoglycemic patient suggest an organic acidemia or MSUD.

Hyperammonemia may occur in liver injury due to sepsis and toxins, but levels >400 μmol/L suggest a urea cycle defect. Disorders of mitochondrial metabolism, fatty acid oxidation disorders, and the organic acidemias can cause a lesser degree of secondary hyperammonemia because of interactions between these pathways and the urea cycle. During severe decompensation, several IEMs can present with elevated transaminases and coagulopathy. Mitochondrial disorders, neonatal hemochromatosis, Wilson disease, hepatorenal tyrosinemia, galactosemia, Crigler–Najjar syndrome, and Niemann–Pick disease can present with liver injury.

Initial labs help point to specific etiologies (**Fig. 90-1**). Once an IEM is suspected, metabolic testing should include urine organic acids, plasma amino acids, plasma carnitine levels, and acylcarnitine profile as well as specific tests depending on the suggested diagnoses. Pathognomonic metabolites may clear rapidly with resuscitative therapy. Molecular genetic testing is available to facilitate making some diagnoses.

CLINICAL MANAGEMENT PRINCIPLES

Many of the IEMs present with emesis, anorexia, and dehydration, but excess fluid can worsen cardiomyopathy or cerebral edema. Hypoglycemia should be corrected. If an IEM is suspected, patients should be made NPO and given sufficient IV glucose (~10 mg/kg/min or 6 cc/kg/h of a 10% dextrose solution) to prevent catabolism of amino acids and fatty acids. If glucose exacerbates lactic acidosis, there may be an error in the pyruvate dehydrogenase complex and may necessitate changing to a ketogenic diet.

Disease-specific therapies are often initiated empirically. Elimination of toxins (e.g., ammonia) with exchange transfusion or dialysis is rapidly done to prevent brain damage. A trial of IV pyridoxine and

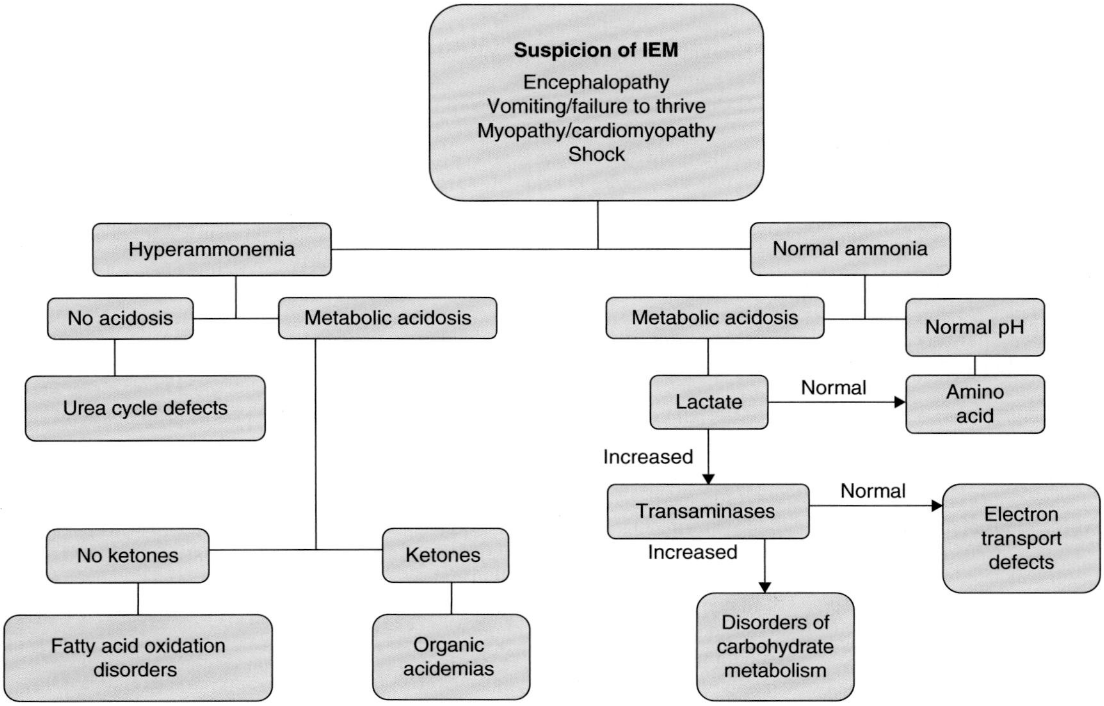

FIGURE 90.1. Categorization of IEMs based on laboratory results.

folinic acid may produce rapid and dramatic improvement in neonatal epileptic encephalopathy. A number of metabolic diseases require supplementation of specific vitamins or cofactors. Given the low toxicity of these agents, they should be initiated before a definitive diagnosis based on the differential diagnosis (**Table 90.2**). Early involvement of a metabolic disease specialist ensures optimal management.

Postmortem Evaluation

If a patient dies, a postmortem diagnosis can have significant implications for siblings and for genetic counseling of the parents. With advances in molecular genetic testing, samples as a source of DNA have become critical to making a definitive diagnosis. The earliest sample of urine obtained during the illness should be frozen, as should several milliliters of cerebrospinal fluid (CSF). Selected tissues can be helpful if the family refuses autopsy. A punch skin biopsy should be obtained pre- or postmortem for a fibroblast culture. Postmortem kidney, liver, muscle, and cardiac biopsies should also be performed. Tissues should ideally be obtained as soon as possible after death to preserve enzymatic activity. Careful discussion with the pathologist is important.

Newborn screening programs are administered on a state level, and online resources can identify the tests currently performed (http://genes-r-us.uthscsa.edu/7). Not all IEMs can be screened, and a normal neonatal screening test does not exclude an IEM in a critically ill child.

DISORDERS ASSOCIATED WITH LACTIC ACIDOSIS

Symptoms of lactic acidosis include poor feeding, failure to thrive, lethargy, change in mental status, seizures, hypotonia, ataxia, developmental delay, optic nerve atrophy, deafness, and dysfunction of the most energy-dependent organs (brain, heart, muscle, kidney, and liver). Lactic acidosis results from accumulation

TABLE 90.2

Supplemental Therapy for Metabolic Emergencies

SUSPECTED CATEGORY OF IEM	EMPIRIC THERAPY	RATIONALE
Urea cycle	L-Arginine 600 mg/kg IV over 90 min and 200–600 mg/kg/d	Essential amino acid in all but arginase deficiency
	Sodium benzoate 250 mg/kg IV over 90 min and 250 mg/kg/d	Condenses with glycine to enhance nitrogen excretion
	Sodium phenylacetate 250 mg/kg IV over 90 min and 250 mg/kg/d	Condenses with glutamine to enhance nitrogen excretion
	Sodium phenylbutyrate 100–200 mg/kg PO tid	Source of phenylacetate to enhance nitrogen excretion once patient is stabilized
Biotinidase deficiency and multiple carboxylase deficiency	Biotin 5–10 mg/d PO	Replaces biotin that is not adequately recycled
MMA and methionine synthase deficiency	Hydroxocobalamin 1–5 mg/d IM/IV	Enzymatic cofactor
Organic acidurias, carnitine transport defects, and fatty acid oxidation disorders	L-Carnitine 50–100 mg/kg/d divided bid IV/PO	Replace carnitine losses
Propionic academia	Metronidazole 15 mg/kg/d divided q8–12 h PO/IV	Inhibit production of propionate by intestinal bacteria
MSUD	Thiamine 150 mg/d IV/PO; >3 y, 300 mg/d	Enzymatic cofactor
Mitochondrial disorders	Coenzyme Q_{10} 25 mg tid PO	Cofactors and antioxidants
	Carnitine 50 mg/kg bid IV/PO	
	α-lipoic acid 100 mg q.d. PO/IV	
	B complex vitamins 100 mg each q.d. PO	
	Vitamin E 50 units q.d. PO	
Ketotic hyperglycinemia	Sodium benzoate 250 mg/kg IV over 90 min and 250 mg/kg/d	Condenses with glycine to enhance nitrogen excretion

MMA, methylmalonic acidemia; MSUD, maple syrup urine disease.

of pyruvate, which is converted into lactic acid and alanine. *Primary lactic acidemia* results from defects in gluconeogenesis or oxidative phosphorylation.

Secondary lactic acidemia results from either anaerobic metabolism or IEMs that produce less significant degrees of lactic acidosis (often detectable only during an acute metabolic crisis). In addition, liver injury or ischemia prevents the conversion of lactate into pyruvate. The differential diagnosis of IEMs causing secondary lactic acidosis includes many of the organic acidemias (propionic acidemia and methylmalonic acidemia [MMA]) readily identified by urine testing. Definitive diagnoses of the IEMs causing primary lactic acidosis are often challenging and frequently require tissue biopsies. Consideration should be given to measuring lactic acid from the CSF if any neurological symptoms are present even without elevated plasma lactate.

If a defect in mitochondrial oxidative phosphorylation is suspected, a muscle biopsy should be performed to look for ragged red fibers and to biochemically assess the respiratory chain complexes. In addition, specific genetic testing for conditions such as *MELAS (Mitochondrial Encephalopathy, Lactic Acidosis and Stroke)* and *MERRF* (*Mitochondrial Encephalopathy with Ragged Red Fibers*) is available. Complete mitochondrial sequencing and deletion analysis can be performed on a blood sample and avoid the need for a biopsy. Defects of the *pyruvate dehydrogenase complex* should be treated with a high-fat, low-carbohydrate diet and supplementation with thiamine and lipoic acid. Most of the other mitochondrial defects of oxidative phosphorylation are difficult to treat but can be empirically treated with thiamine, riboflavin, nicotinamide, vitamin E, and coenzyme Q10 while a definitive diagnosis is being established (**Table 90.2**). Sodium bicarbonate can be used to correct metabolic acidosis, but will not decrease lactic acid production.

METABOLIC ACIDOSIS WITHOUT INCREASED LACTATE

The organic acidemias and aminoacidopathies present with an AG acidosis that is *not* predominantly due to lactate. Classically, the organic acidurias present as massive ketosis and metabolic acidosis in a vomiting or lethargic neonate. Chronic treatment requires carefully balanced protein intake to provide adequate essential amino acids while minimizing the load of precursors that cannot be metabolized. The most common disorders within this category are MSUD, MMA, and propionic acidemia. Most present with episodes of encephalopathy and vomiting during catabolic stress, typically during the early neonatal period in an infant who initially appears well or has an intercurrent illness.

MSUD is a disorder of metabolism of the essential, branched-chain amino acids (BCAAs), valine, leucine, and isoleucine. Infants with the *classic* form present in the first few days of life with vomiting, encephalopathy, and severe metabolic acidosis. MSUD has an increased incidence in the Old Order Amish and Mennonites and Ashkenazi Jewish populations. Milder forms may present later in life during stress in a child with mild developmental delay or failure to thrive. Some patients respond dramatically to thiamine supplementation.

Isovaleric acidemia results from a deficiency of *isovaleryl CoA dehydrogenase*, which is further down the leucine degradative pathway. The acute form resembles MSUD but these patients have a characteristic odor of sweaty socks and may have associated neutropenia.

Propionic acid and *methylmalonic acid* are sequential catabolic products of isoleucine and valine as well as threonine, methionine, cholesterol, and odd-chain fatty acids. Deficiency of the enzymes responsible for their catabolism (*propionyl-CoA carboxylase* and *methylmalonyl CoA mutase*, respectively) results in *ketotic hyperglycinemia*. Disorders of cobalamin metabolism may also result in secondary MMA. These conditions present with vomiting, severe ketoacidosis, encephalopathy progressing to coma, and neutropenia. Because of secondary inhibition of the urea cycle, hyperammonemia may also occur. Sterilization of the intestinal tract with metronidazole minimizes production of propionic acid by intestinal bacteria. Carnitine supplementation may hasten resolution of metabolic acidosis. Biotin should be provided until a definitive diagnosis is established. Similarly, large doses of cobalamin should be provided to patients with suspected MMA.

Several other IEMs may present with metabolic acidosis, ketosis, and an intoxication syndrome. These include disorders affecting the four *biotin-dependent carboxylases*. Deficiency of *holocarboxylase synthetase* results in the most severe disorder and presents in the first few weeks of life. Patients have rashes that mimic eczema and a tomcat urine odor. *Biotinidase deficiency* presents similarly, may be associated with an eczematoid rash, and responds well to biotin supplementation.

Liver transplantation has been performed in MSUD and improves dietary protein tolerance and eliminates episodic decompensations. It has also been performed in patients with other organic acidemias unless irreversible neurocognitive deficits develop prior to transplantation.

HYPOGLYCEMIA

Although difficult, it is ideal to diagnostically evaluate the etiology at the time of hypoglycemia by assessing glucose, insulin, growth hormone, cortisol, serum chemistries, liver function tests (LFTs), ammonia, β-hydroxybutyrate, acetoacetate, free fatty acids, and lactate. During hypoglycemia insulin levels should be extremely low or undetectable and ketone bodies and free fatty acids should be elevated. Failure to produce ketone bodies during hypoglycemia suggests either hyperinsulinemia or a defect in the oxidation of fatty acids or ketone body production. Fatty acid oxidation disorders can then further be evaluated with an acylcarnitine profile, free and total carnitine, urine organic acids, and urine acylglycines.

Hypoglycemia immediately after a meal suggests provocation by the ingested substance. Infants with *hereditary fructose intolerance* present at 6 months of age during transition from breast milk or formula to solid foods, including introduction of fruits and vegetables. Within 30 minutes of ingesting foods containing fructose or sucrose they become hypoglycemic and have transient elevations of transaminases and lactic acid. Eliminating fructose and sucrose from the diet leads to normal health, growth, and development. Hypoglycemia associated with a high-protein diet can be provoked by high levels of leucine in deficiency of *glutamate dehydrogenase*, resulting in *hyperinsulinemic hyperammonemia*. Hypoglycemia and liver dysfunction in infancy can also be caused by ingestion of breast milk or cow's milk–based formulas in *galactosemia*, but most cases are now diagnosed by newborn screening and readily treated with a soy-based formula.

Hypoglycemia associated with fasting for ~8 hours is most characteristic of glycogen storage disorders such as glycogen storage disorder type I (glucose-6-phosphatase deficiency) or glycogen storage disorder type 0 (glycogen synthase deficiency). These disorders present when infants begin to sleep through the night (increased fasting interval) or during periods of intercurrent illness associated with anorexia or vomiting. Hypoglycemia associated with fasting for ~16 hours (after depletion of glycogen stores) is more characteristic of defects in gluconeogenesis (fructose-1,6-bisphosphatase deficiency, glycerol kinase deficiency, pyruvate carboxylase deficiency, or pyruvate kinase deficiency) or fatty acid oxidation disorders. Treatment for these disorders consists of avoiding fasting and dietary modifications.

HYPERAMMONEMIA

Newborns with hyperammonemia often present with progressive decreased feeding, hypothermia, lethargy, apnea, coma, and death within a period of hours in the most severe cases. Elevated concentrations of ammonia are extremely toxic to the brain and can cause respiratory failure. Blood samples should be placed on ice and analyzed immediately to avoid artifactual elevations. Mild hyperammonemia (<300 μmol/L) can be associated with *transient hyperammonemia of the newborn* as well as with IEMs (*organic acidurias, fatty acid oxidation defects, lysinuric protein intolerance,* and *hyperammonemia, hyperornithinemia*, and *homocitrullinuria syndrome)*. More severe degrees of hyperammonemia are typically observed with *urea cycle defects*. There is often an associated depression of the blood urea nitrogen (BUN) due to the inability to produce urea. These patients often initially demonstrate a respiratory alkalosis on their arterial blood gas (ABG). Secondary hyperammonemia can be associated with liver failure or overwhelming viral hepatitis. Initial treatment should consist of making the child NPO and keeping them anabolic with an infusion of dextrose and electrolytes.

Laboratory tests should include ABG, serum chemistries, liver function studies, urine organic acids (specifically tested for orotic acid), urinalysis, serum amino acids, acylcarnitine profile, and repeated and frequent measures of ammonia until the rate of rise can be determined. Metabolic acidosis or an increased AG suggests that the diagnosis is not a urea cycle defect. Urinary ketosis with mild hyperammonemia suggests an organic aciduria. *Fatty acid oxidation disorders* are not associated with urinary ketones, but are associated with hypoglycemia, elevated creatine phosphokinase (CPK), and *mild* hyperammonemia. *Ornithine transcarbamylase deficiency* is an X-linked disorder usually presenting in males in the neonatal period. A family history of neonatal deaths of unknown etiology is always suspicious.

Elevations of ammonia rapidly rising beyond 500 μmol/L should be treated with some form of hemodialysis (including CVVHD). Peritoneal dialysis and exchange transfusion are inadequate with such severe hyperammonemia. They should be given IV L-arginine to maintain the urea cycle and also loading doses and continuous infusions of sodium benzoate and phenylacetate to remove ammonia via alternative metabolic pathways to eliminate nitrogen (**Table 90.2**). To date, the best long-term treatment for children with urea cycle defects has been liver transplantation. However, significant hyperammonemia prior to transplant may result in irreversible brain damage and should be carefully considered by parents before pursuing transplantation. Females heterozygous for the X-linked *ornithine transcarbamylase deficiency* or patients with partial urea cycle defects may demonstrate only periodic metabolic crises associated with ingestion of large amounts of protein or a catabolic state induced by intercurrent illness.

LIVER FAILURE

Some inherited disorders cause direct hepatocyte damage, including *hepatorenal tyrosinemia, galactosemia, Wilson disease, α_1-antitrypsin deficiency*, peroxisomal disorders (*Zellweger syndrome* and *Refsum disease*), and defects in cholesterol and bile acid synthesis. Initially, it may be difficult to distinguish these IEMs from infectious causes of liver failure (hepatomegaly is more common with IEMs). A liver biopsy may be necessary to identify storage materials and enzymatic testing using fibroblasts or liver tissue for definitive diagnosis.

Neonatal liver failure can be caused by neonatal hemochromatosis, galactosemia, hepatorenal tyrosinemia, urea cycle defects, defects in oxidative phosphorylation, long-chain fatty acid oxidation disorders, and *Niemann–Pick types A and B*. *Galactosemia* is suggested by reducing substance in the urine (requires lactose ingestion within the previous 24 hours) and is associated with cataracts and *E. coli* sepsis. *Neonatal hemochromatosis* is a rare cause and abdominal MRI is useful to demonstrate increased liver iron stores. *Hepatorenal tyrosinemia* is suggested by rapid hepatic decompensation, greatly elevated α-fetoprotein, and is confirmed by demonstration of succinylacetone in the urine. *Defects of long-chain fatty acid oxidation* are suggested by the combination of hepatic necrosis, myopathy, and cardiomyopathy (these may occur in the neonatal period or throughout infancy). *Defects in oxidative phosphorylation* have multisystem involvement, are associated with increased lactic acid levels, and diagnosis requires a liver biopsy to demonstrate mitochondrial DNA depletion.

In many of the *lysosomal storage disorders*, liver function is intact although the liver can become extremely enlarged. Lysosomal storage disorders are suggested by short stature, failure to thrive, coarse facial features, developmental delay, hypotonia, or seizures. Many of the *glycogen storage diseases* produce hepatomegaly, with or without hypoglycemia, and are diagnosed by abnormal quantity or structure of glycogen on liver biopsy.

NONMETABOLIC CRITICAL ILLNESS IN INBORN ERRORS OF METABOLISM

Metabolic illness can impact ICU management. Lactate-containing fluids should be avoided for patients who may not metabolize exogenous lactate (mitochondrial disorders and pyruvate dehydrogenase complex deficiency). Propofol has been used in mitochondrial disorders but it should probably be avoided in fatty acid oxidation defects because of possible predisposition to propofol infusion syndrome. IEMs that have significant risk for *hyperkalemia* and *rhabdomyolysis* include glycogen storage diseases V (*McArdle disease*) and VII (*Tauri disease*). Mitochondrial disorders may predispose to malignant hyperthermia.

An increasing number of known contractile protein abnormalities cause *cardiomyopathy*. Any IEM that impairs energy metabolism, particularly disorders of the mitochondrial respiratory chain and fatty acid oxidation defects, may present with cardiomyopathy (usually dilated, not hypertrophic). The fatty acid oxidation disorders (including *fatty acyl-CoA dehydrogenase deficiencies* and *glutaric acidemia type II*) may present with arrhythmias and neonatal cardiomyopathy. Treatment is with a low-fat diet (minimal amounts of essential fatty acids), supplementation with medium-chain triglycerides, and carnitine replacement. *Primary carnitine deficiency* (due to a defect in the carnitine transporter in the heart, liver, and kidneys) presents with cardiomyopathy with or without skeletal myopathy beginning in late infancy or early childhood. *Carnitine-acylcarnitine translocase deficiency* and the severe form of *carnitine palmitoyltransferase-2 deficiency* also present with dilated cardiomyopathy. High-dose oral carnitine can be curative for primary carnitine deficiency.

Homocystinuria predisposes patients to thromboembolic disease. In the classic form (*cystathionine synthase deficiency*), patients present after 3 years of age with ectopia lentis, a Marfanoid habitus and developmental delay. A bleeding diathesis can be due to hypersplenism in storage diseases or to decreased liver function.

Type II glycogen storage disease (*Pompe disease*) results from deficiency of the enzyme *α-1,4-glucosidase* (acid maltase) and causes a hypertrophic cardiomyopathy syndrome with a short P–R interval, hypotonia, and macroglossia. The X-linked disorder, *Fabry disease* (*lysosomal α-galactosidase A deficiency*), causes disseminated glycosphingolipid deposition. Angiokeratomas are characteristic and result from deposition in the skin, typically in a "bathing suit distribution." The cardiovascular manifestations result from deposition causing obstructive vasculopathy, mitral valve thickening, and hypertrophic and eventually dilated cardiomyopathy. Mutations of the γ-subunit of AMP-activated protein kinase (*PRKAG2*) and X-linked lysosome-associated membrane protein (*LAMP2, Danon disease*) result in hypertrophic cardiomyopathy due to glycogen accumulation in the heart and are also associated with ventricular preexcitation.

Type I (*Hunter/Scheie*) and Type II (*Hurler*) MPSs result in varying degrees of myocardial and valvular diseases. Although the mucolipidoses, *I-cell disease* and *pseudo-Hurler polydystrophy*, share many features with the MPSs such as valvular disease, reports of cardiomyopathy are rare. Associated dysmorphisms and tracheal narrowing can make endotracheal intubation extremely challenging. Atlanto-axial instability, particularly in MPS IV (*Morquio syndrome*), must be considered during laryngoscopy as well.

There is increasing long-term experience with *enzyme replacement therapy* for a growing number of lysosomal storage disorders, including Gaucher disease, Pompe disease, Fabry disease, MPS I, and MPS VI. Therapy is effective only at treating the systemic disease, not the neurological component, and may not reverse damage already sustained. Direct intracerebroventricular infusion of enzyme is being considered for clinical trials. Bone marrow transplant and substrate inhibitors are also being used in some diseases.

CHAPTER 91 ■ CANCER THERAPY: MECHANISMS AND TOXICITY

DAVID M. LOEB AND MASANORI HAYASHI

Most pediatric malignancies are treated with multimodal therapy consisting of chemotherapy, radiation therapy, and surgery. Biologically based therapies include monoclonal antibodies, small-molecule kinase inhibitors, cytokines, differentiation therapies, and antiangiogenic therapies. Commonly used agents have implications for critical care. It is important to understand the mechanisms and toxicities of these treatments (**Table 91.1**).

ALKYLATING AGENTS

Most alkylating agents used in pediatric oncology are derivatives of nitrogen mustard, including cyclophosphamide and ifosfamide, or derivatives of methylnitrosourea, such as lomustine (CCNU) and carmustine (BCNU). These drugs form covalent bonds with DNA and other intracellular macromolecules. Following this initial alkylation reaction, the remaining reactive group interacts with a second macromolecule, to form either intrastrand or interstrand DNA cross-links. These cross-links may lead to cytotoxicity, by impeding DNA replication or by direct mutagenesis. Platinum-based antitumor compounds also create DNA cross-links. The two commonly used platinum-based compounds are cisplatin and carboplatin. As with classical alkylating agents, the relationship between DNA cross-links and cytotoxicity remains correlative, with proof of causality lacking.

Antimetabolites

The antimetabolites are classified based on the metabolic pathways with which they interfere. In pediatric oncology, antifolates and purine antimetabolites are most commonly used.

Antifolates

Methotrexate competitively inhibits dihydrofolate reductase. Inhibition of this key enzyme for synthesis of thymidine depletes intracellular thymidine triphosphate and arrests DNA synthesis. High doses of methotrexate decrease purine synthesis and lead to cell death. Methotrexate is also toxic to endothelial cells, and part of its effect (in both cancer and autoimmune diseases) may be through the inhibition of angiogenesis.

Purine Antimetabolites

Purine biosynthesis is critical for DNA synthesis and cell replication. Drugs that interfere with purine biosynthesis include 6-mercaptopurine and 6-thioguanine. Clofarabine is in a newer generation of purine antimetabolite, and is used to treat relapsed acute leukemias. These drugs are incorporated into growing DNA strands and inhibit DNA synthesis. Other mechanisms of their cytotoxicity include inhibition of enzymes needed for the synthesis of natural purines (adenine and guanine).

TABLE 91.1

Chemotherapeutics Organized by Class

■ CLASS	■ DRUGS
Alkylating agents	Cyclophosphamide, ifosfamide, lomustine (BCNU), carmustine (CCNU), cisplatin, carboplatin
Antimetabolites	Methotrexate, 6-mercaptopurine, 6-thioguanine, clofarabine
Topoisomerase inhibitors	Etoposide (VP16) and teniposide (VM26) inhibit Topo II Irinotecan and topotecan inhibit Topo I
Anthracyclines	Doxorubicin, daunorubicin, idarubicin, mitoxantrone
Antimicrotubule agents	Vincristine, vinblastine, vinorelbine, paclitaxel, docetaxel

Topoisomerase Inhibitors

Topoisomerases are enzymes involved in maintaining supercoiling of the DNA double helix. They are essential for DNA replication, transcription, and chromosomal segregation. Two classes of topoisomerase inhibitors are type I enzymes (make single-stranded cuts in DNA) and type II enzymes (make double-stranded cuts).

Inhibitors of Topoisomerase II

The two types of topoisomerase II inhibitors are podophyllotoxins and anthracyclines. Etoposide (VP16) is a commonly used podophyllotoxin; teniposide (VM26) is rarely used. Anthracycline antibiotics (doxorubicin, daunorubicin, and idarubicin) also inhibit topoisomerase II. Isolated from *Streptomyces peucetius*, anthracycline antibiotics act by intercalating between DNA base pairs in the intact double helix, through effects on nuclear helicases, and by generating iron free radicals.

Inhibitors of Topoisomerase I

Inhibitors of topoisomerase I are newer chemotherapeutic agents. The common agents, irinotecan and topotecan, are derivatives of camptothecin, a plant alkaloid.

Antimicrotubule Agents

Vinca Alkaloids

All vinca alkaloids (vincristine, vinblastine, and vinorelbine) are derived from the pink periwinkle plant. They produce cytotoxicity through interaction with tubulin, the major protein component of microtubules. The importance of microtubules in other cellular functions explains the noncytotoxic effects of these compounds. In particular, neurons require intact microtubules for axonal transport, and disruption of this function causes the well-known peripheral neuropathy associated with vincristine treatment.

Taxanes

The original taxane, paclitaxel, was found through screening plant extracts for anticancer activity, and isolated from the bark of the Pacific yew tree. The major source today is a semisynthetic derivative of the European yew. Docetaxel and paclitaxel are the two most commonly used taxanes; they bind to tubulin at sites distinct from those bound by the vinca alkaloids. Taxanes also inhibit angiogenesis.

Other Cytotoxic Drugs

Asparaginase

L-Asparaginase hydrolyzes asparagines to aspartic acid and ammonia. In sensitive tumor cells that lack adequate levels of asparagine synthetase, this enzyme depletes the cells of a critical amino acid, rapidly inhibiting protein synthesis. DNA and RNA syntheses are also inhibited, and cell death ensues.

Cytarabine

Cytarabine (araC) differs from cytidine by the substitution of arabinose for ribose. Uptake into the cell is via the same mechanisms responsible for other nucleosides. Once internalized, cytarabine is phosphorylated to generate araCTP by deoxycytidine kinase. Cytarabine decreases intracellular concentrations of deoxycytidine by competition for enzymes that activate cytidine, thereby inhibiting DNA synthesis. Gemcitabine is a cytidine analog and, like araC, is phosphorylated by nucleoside kinases. Gemcitabine triphosphate competes with dCTP for incorporation into DNA, inhibiting DNA polymerase and DNA synthesis.

THE BASICS OF RADIATION THERAPY

Radiation therapy is primarily used in the treatment of solid tumors as a means of local control. For some tumor types, such as Wilms tumor and most central nervous system (CNS) malignancies, radiation is a standard part of therapy. For others, such as Ewing sarcoma, radiation is used to treat patients for whom surgery is not an option or who have an inadequate resection. In the past, radiation was used for CNS prophylaxis for all leukemia patients, but due to long-term side effects, radiation is reserved for patients at high risk for CNS involvement. In addition, radiation therapy is sometimes incorporated into bone marrow transplant preparative regimens.

General Principles of Radiation Therapy

Radiation therapy delivers packets of energy to a target tissue with the intention of causing lethal damage to malignant cells while minimizing damage to normal cells. Radiation energy comes in different packets, the most commonly used being photons (e.g., X-rays), as well as other particles (e.g., protons or electrons). As the packets deposit their energy, ionization events occur in biologically important molecules and lead to tissue damage and cell death. The dose of energy delivered is measured in Gray (Gy), and 1 Gy = 1 J/kg. An older term, *rad,* is still used, and 1 rad = 1 cGy = 0.01 Gy. While multiple biologic macromolecules can be affected by ionizing radiation, induction of double-stranded DNA breaks is the proximate cause of cell death. It is estimated that a 1-Gy dose of X-rays will result in 40 double-stranded DNA breaks per cell. Ionizing radiation initiates a complex cascade of cellular responses that can result in cell-cycle arrest, induction of stress-response genes, induction of apoptosis, or repair of DNA damage.

These responses are not mutually exclusive. Several biologic characteristics of a tumor modify sensitivity to radiation. Oxygenation status of target tissue is a critical factor, and hypoxic tumors are more resistant to ionizing radiation than are normally oxygenated tumors. Another important determinant is position in the cell cycle. Cells in the G2 and M phases of cell cycle are most sensitive to radiation and, in late S phase, are relatively resistant. This differential sensitivity leads to a relative synchronization of tumor cells.

Types of External-Beam Radiation

Typical external-beam radiotherapy is delivered from a Cobalt-60 source and is composed of photons. To minimize delivery to normal tissue, perpendicular beams are used, with the area of overlap corresponding to the target. Because beams are rectangular but tumors are irregularly shaped, collimators, in the head of the radiation source, shape the beam to conform to the tumor shape (determined by CT scan). The beam can be further shaped with individually constructed blocks to shield body regions not in the target area. Photons typically deposit energy relatively deep into tissue, with higher-energy photons penetrating deeper than lower-energy photons. Electrons, in contrast, deposit their energy in a relatively shallow range, with a rapid drop-off of energy with increasing depth. Thus, a superficial tumor (such as leukemia cutis) will be more appropriately treated with electron-beam therapy. A proton beam can treat a target deeper than an electron beam, but with similar precision in the deposition of energy. Thus, proton-beam radiation is valuable when the target is located deep but adjacent to particularly sensitive normal tissue. Although photons and electrons are commonly available, a limited number of centers are capable of delivering proton-beam radiotherapy.

Targeted Radiation Therapy

Other means of delivering radiation therapy are brachytherapy and targeted radiation therapy. Brachytherapy is unlikely to result in complications requiring critical care. Physiologic targeting includes the use of iodine 131 metaiodobenzylguanidine (^{131}I-MIBG) to treat neuroblastoma, and samarium-153 ethylene diamine tetramethylene phosphonate (^{153}Sm-EDTMP) to treat osteosarcoma. Both agents are currently being studied in autologous peripheral blood stem cell support, making it likely that such patients will require critical care.

BIOLOGIC THERAPY

Biologic therapies include differentiation therapy, immunotherapy, small-molecule kinase inhibitors, and monoclonal antibody therapies. We emphasize agents that have significant toxicity.

Differentiation Therapy

The best-known example of differentiation therapy is the use of all-trans retinoic acid (ATRA) in the treatment of acute promyelocytic leukemia (APML). APML is known to the intensivist because of the characteristic profound bleeding diathesis seen at presentation. Prior to the routine use of ATRA, APML was associated with a high risk of death from hemorrhage during induction therapy. The malignant cells have a translocation between chromosomes 15 and 17 that produces a fusion protein that combines the retinoic acid receptor RARα with a nuclear protein called PML. Pharmacologic doses of ATRA overcome the block to differentiation caused by PML-RARα, and the malignant promyelocytes differentiate into granulocytes. ATRA therapy has improved the remission induction rate from 62% to greater than 90% and has significantly decreased the rate of hemorrhagic death. A second differentiation therapy is the use of 13-*cis*-retinoic acid to treat neuroblastoma.

Immunotherapy

The broad category of immunotherapy includes such diverse treatments as allogeneic hematopoietic stem cell transplantation, with or without infusion of donor lymphocytes, and treatment with various recombinant cytokines. Cytokine administration is rare in pediatric oncology; examples of this approach are efforts at inducing an immune response to metastatic melanoma and to renal cell carcinoma by infusions of interleukin (IL)-2. In neuroblastoma, a chimeric human–murine anti-GD2 monoclonal antibody has been used.

Small-Molecule Kinase Inhibitors

Gleevec treatment of chronic myelogenous leukemia (CML) is an example of targeted therapy based on a molecular understanding of tumorigenesis. CML is defined by the presence of a distinctive chromosomal translocation, t(9;22), or the Philadelphia chromosome. This translocation leads to the production of a fusion protein tyrosine kinase called BCR-ABL that drives the neoplastic process. Gleevec is a competitive inhibitor of the BCR-ABL tyrosine kinase and causes a complete hematologic response in 95% of CML patients. Many patients with CML achieve long-term remission with Gleevec, and second-generation tyrosine kinase inhibitors (TKIs) such as Dasatinib and Nilotinib are available for resistant disease.

Monoclonal Antibodies

Two frequently used monoclonal antibodies target antigens on the surface of lymphocytes. Rituximab is an antibody against CD20, a marker of B lymphocytes, and is used in non-Hodgkin lymphoma and autoimmune disorders, such as ITP and hemolytic anemia. Alemtuzumab, which is anti-CD52 (a pan-lymphocyte marker) results in a rapid, profound, and long-lasting depletion of circulating T cells, B cells, NK cells, and monocytes. Patients become lymphopenic within 2 weeks and remain lymphopenic for a year after treatment. Its primary use is in the context of bone marrow transplantation (BMT) as part of an immunoablative preparative regimen or in the prevention or treatment of graft-versus-host disease (GVHD). An appreciation of the profoundly immunosuppressive nature of this drug is critical to appropriately evaluate patients who have received it.

Antiangiogenic Therapy

The growth of solid tumors, such as sarcomas, is limited by the availability of oxygen and nutrients, which must be delivered by blood vessels. Aggregates of cancer cells are unable to grow into tumors of greater than 1–2 mm in diameter without an adequate blood supply. The major molecular driver of angiogenesis, vascular endothelial growth factor (VEGF), is overexpressed in multiple malignancies, and targeting of VEGF has been attempted through multiple approaches. One common VEGF-targeted therapy, bevacizumab, has been studied in CNS tumors and sarcomas. Common side effects include poor wound healing, thrombocytopenia, hypertension, proteinuria, and venous thrombosis.

Another antiangiogenic approach is the use of TKIs that target VEGF receptors, including Sunitinib and Cediranib. Sunitinib is an oral multitarget tyrosine kinase receptor inhibitor of the VEGF receptor as well as other targets such as the platelet-derived growth factor receptors. It is effective in renal cell carcinoma and gastrointestinal stromal tumors in adults, and is being studied for refractory solid tumors in children. Although generally well tolerated, cardiac toxicity has been reported in children. Cediranib, which is also a multi-targeted TKI, is known to be a VEGF receptor inhibitor and has been studied in children with refractory solid tumors. Common side effects such as hypertension and prolonged QTc have been reported as dose-limiting toxicities.

TOXICITIES

Table 91.2 lists typical toxicities caused by the commonly used chemotherapy drugs. The discussion below is organized by organ system, rather than by individual drug.

Fever in the Neutropenic Patient

The most common side effect of cytotoxic chemotherapy is myelosuppression, which leads to periods of neutropenia. Fever in a neutropenic cancer patient represents a true emergency due to the significant rate of gram-negative bacteremia in such patients.

Toxicities Related to Bone Marrow Transplantation

Children who have undergone BMT are subject to a number of unique toxicities, including veno-occlusive disease, cytokine storm/engraftment syndrome, and GVHD. Many of the immunosuppressive drugs used as prophylaxis or in treatment of GVHD can cause significant, difficult-to-control hypertension. Pneumonitis is a common problem encountered in the post-BMT setting.

TABLE 91.2

Typical Toxicities of Commonly Used Chemotherapy Drugs

■ DRUG	■ TOXICITIES
Ifosfamide	Renal tubular dysfunction, encephalopathy, hemorrhagic cystitis
Cyclophosphamide	Renal tubular dysfunction, hemorrhagic cystitis, myocardial necrosis
Cytarabine	Cerebellar syndrome, myelopathy, leukoencephalopathy, pulmonary edema, pneumonitis, *Streptococcus viridans* sepsis
Methotrexate	Skin sloughing, nephrotoxicity, encephalopathy, hepatic dysfunction
Anthracyclines	Severe mucositis, congestive heart failure
Bleomycin	Pneumonitis
ATRA	Capillary leak syndrome
L-asparaginase	Pancreatitis
Cisplatin	Renal tubular dysfunction, cardiotoxicity
Vincristine	Peripheral neuropathy, ileus, neuropathic pain
Sorafenib	Hand–foot rash syndrome, thrombocytopenia

ATRA, all-trans retinoic acid.
Most chemotherapeutic agents cause nausea, vomiting, mucositis, and pancytopenia; therefore, these are not included in this table. This table is *not* intended to be a comprehensive listing of chemotherapy side effects, but rather a list of the most common toxicities that may be encountered by the pediatric intensivist.

Toxicities of the Central Nervous System

A number of chemotherapeutic drugs cause CNS toxicity. *Ifosfamide* causes encephalopathy in 10%–30% of patients, ranging from mild (somnolence) to severe (coma or seizure); it occurs between 2 and 48 hours after administration. The mechanism for this toxicity is unclear. The management of ifosfamide-induced encephalopathy includes discontinuation of the drug and supportive measures. The use of methylene blue has been reported for the treatment of ifosfamide-induced encephalopathy, but the lack of controlled trials (and reports of spontaneous resolution) makes it difficult to determine if this agent is helpful. *AraC* also causes acute CNS toxicity. Intrathecal araC has been associated with a rapid-onset myelopathy (although this might be related to the use of benzyl alcohol as a diluent) or a slower-onset myelopathy, with symptoms beginning 2 days to 6 months after treatment. Seizures and leukoencephalopathy are rarely reported. Seizures have also been described in patients being treated with intravenous high-dose araC. In general, these have been self-limited and do not recur once therapy is stopped. *Cytarabine* causes an acute cerebellar syndrome. Onset of symptoms is 3–8 days after high-dose systemic treatment, and manifestations include dysarthria, dysdiadochokinesia, dysmetria, and ataxia. The outcome is variable, and ~30% of adults never regain normal function. The only effective therapy for this disorder is discontinuation of the drug and institution of supportive care as indicated. Finally, *methotrexate* is associated with CNS toxicities when administered intrathecally or at high doses intravenously. Common clinical presentation includes headache, confusion, disorientation, seizures, dysphagia, and weakness, including hemiparesis. The encephalopathy is usually self-limited. The pathophysiology of this neurotoxicity is unclear. Aminophylline (an adenosine receptor blocker) has been used in treatment since high adenosine levels have been observed in the CSF after methotrexate therapy, but there are no controlled trials.

Cardiac Toxicities

The *anthracyclines* are the best-known cardiotoxic chemotherapy drugs (doxorubicin, daunorubicin, and idarubicin). The mechanism of cardiotoxicity involves the generation of oxygen free radicals, which ultimately lead to irreversible loss of myocardiocytes and the development of cardiomyopathy. Anthracycline cardiotoxicity can be acute or delayed. Acute effects include transient arrhythmias and acute left ventricular failure. The acute effects are usually transient and attenuate after discontinuation of therapy. Cardiac injury can also present in a delayed fashion, years or decades after treatment. The most significant risk factor for cardiotoxicity is cumulative dose. Other than limiting total exposure, measures that have been investigated include the administration of liposome-encapsulated anthracyclines and the use of cardioprotectants, such as *dexrazoxane* (Zinecard). Dexrazoxane acts as an iron chelator, prevents the formation of an anthracycline–iron complex that is thought to be a critical mediator of myocardiocyte injury, and thus prevent cardiac damage. *Cyclophosphamide* has been associated with severe cardiotoxicity at high doses, as employed in BMT. The estimated incidence in children is 5% in patients treated with marrow ablative doses. Risk factors include prior anthracycline chemotherapy and chest irradiation. Severe hemorrhagic cardiac necrosis has been reported as well. Symptoms may be delayed by up to 2 weeks after administration, but can be rapidly fatal, with a 10% mortality rate. *Paclitaxel* has been associated with asymptomatic, reversible bradycardia in up to 29% of treated patients. Second- and third-degree heart blocks are also seen. Several cases of acute myocardial infarction after *cisplatin* therapy have also been reported. *Amsacrine*, an acridine derivative (not commercially available in the United States), can affect cardiac electrophysiology and cause a wide range of EKG changes, including ventricular tachycardia. *5-Fluorouracil* has also been reported to induce cardiotoxicity (including arrhythmias, silent ischemia, and even sudden death) in up to 18% of treated patients, occurring mostly in the setting of continuous infusion. Risk factors include preexisting coronary artery disease and concurrent radiotherapy.

Pulmonary Toxicities

Bleomycin is most frequently thought of for pulmonary toxicity, but other cytotoxic treatments can cause pulmonary fibrosis or edema, including *gemcitabine*, *cytarabine*, and *radiation therapy*. Additionally, a number of drugs (including carmustine, methotrexate, procarbazine, and bleomycin) have been linked with a hypersensitivity pneumonitis syndrome. Also referred to as inflammatory interstitial pneumonitis, this syndrome is characterized by an insidious progression of nonproductive cough, dyspnea, and low-grade fevers. Eosinophilia is noted in the peripheral blood and on lung biopsy, which often also reveals bronchiolitis obliterans with organizing pneumonia. This syndrome resolves with removal of the offending agent, although sometimes oral corticosteroids speed recovery. Bleomycin toxicity is primarily limited to lungs and skin because these organs lack bleomycin hydrolase. Most commonly, bleomycin causes an interstitial pneumonitis (bleomycin-induced pneumonitis, BIP) and has been reported in up to 46% of patients treated with bleomycin, with mortality seen in 3%. BIP is initially indolent, with a cough and dyspnea on exertion. Interstitial or alveolar infiltrates can be seen on plain film, and CT scan often shows small linear and subpleural nodular lesions in the lung bases. Lung biopsy may show characteristic lesions, such as squamous metaplasia of bronchiolar epithelium, inflammatory cells infiltrating into alveoli and alveolar septa, edema plus focal collagen depositions in these septa, and fibrotic areas. The pathogenesis appears to be related to initial endothelial damage, probably mediated through free radical production and release of cytokines. High-dose corticosteroids are frequently used to treat clinically significant BIP, but as yet, no randomized studies demonstrate the efficacy. Also of importance to the intensivist is the acute onset of pulmonary edema, often mimicking adult respiratory distress syndrome, in patients previously treated with bleomycin who are exposed to high concentrations of inspired oxygen, as may occur in conjunction with a surgical procedure, even years after chemotherapy is completed. This complication can be minimized by administering the lowest possible concentration of oxygen to patients with a history of treatment with bleomycin.

A *vascular leak syndrome*, leading to sometimes life-threatening pulmonary edema, has been described with infusions of *araC* or *IL-2*. The vascular leak is usually reversible with discontinuation of therapy and is treated with diuresis and oxygen. Prostaglandins or cyclooxygenase-2 may attenuate IL-2-induced vascular leak. Vascular leak has also been reported in patients treated with *ATRA* for APML. *Clofarabine* has been associated with a life-threatening capillary leak syndrome. Other chemotherapeutic agents associated with pulmonary toxicity include *Mitomycin-C*, which causes a delayed-onset interstitial pneumonitis, *actinomycin D*, which acts as a radiation sensitizer, and, rarely, *cyclophosphamide* or *ifosfamide*, which can cause pulmonary fibrosis.

Radiation therapy can damage capillary endothelial cells and type I pneumocytes, eventually leading to pneumonitis. Radiation pneumonitis is rare in patients treated with less than 20 Gy, but is highly likely in patients who receive greater than 60 Gy. Symptoms become evident 2–3 months following completion of therapy, and include dyspnea and a nonproductive cough. Permanent fibrosis evolves over 6–24 months, but usually stabilizes after this time period. No controlled trials have been conducted, but response to corticosteroids is seen. Symptomatic relief has been reported with pentoxifylline and vitamin E.

Retinoic Acid Syndrome

The retinoic acid syndrome is the major complication of ATRA treatment. It occurs in 25% of APML patients treated with ATRA. Improved recognition and treatment have decreased the mortality from 30% to 5%. The diagnosis requires at least three of the following signs and symptoms in the absence of alternative explanations: fever, weight gain, respiratory distress, pulmonary infiltrates, pleural or pericardial effusions, hypotension, and renal failure. The syndrome commonly manifests 10 days after the start of chemotherapy, but can occur as rapidly as 2 days into treatment. The pathogenesis is related to tissue infiltration, with newly differentiated granulocytes that produce cytokines. The endothelial damage leads to edema, hemorrhage, fibrinous exudates, and respiratory failure. The only specific therapy available is dexamethasone.

Pancreatitis

Treatment with L-*asparaginase* may cause acute pancreatitis. Management of asparaginase-induced pancreatitis is identical to idiopathic pancreatitis, including gut rest. Asparaginase-induced acute pancreatitis can progress to hemorrhagic pancreatitis and chronic pancreatitis.

Urinary Tract Toxicities

Both *ifosfamide* and *cyclophosphamide* can cause hemorrhagic cystitis. The degradation product acrolein is the major cause but other metabolites are also involved. Prophylaxis includes aggressive hydration (alkaline intravenous fluids at twice maintenance) and the use of mesna (sodium-2-mercaptoethanesulfonate). Mesna is rapidly oxidized to dimesna, which is filtered and excreted by the kidneys. It collects in the bladder, where it detoxifies acrolein and other oxazaphosphorine metabolites. Mesna is superior to placebo or hydration alone in the prevention of hemorrhagic cystitis. If prophylaxis fails, management includes cystoscopy and clot evacuation, aggressive bladder irrigation, and intravesicle instillation of formalin.

In addition to cystitis, *cyclophosphamide* and *ifosfamide* can also cause renal dysfunction, both tubular and glomerular. Proximal tubular dysfunction is the most common form of nephrotoxicity and manifests as Fanconi syndrome, with hypophosphatemia, renal tubular acidosis, hypokalemia, hypocalcemia, or hypomagnesemia. Any of these can be severe and require aggressive replacement therapy. Distal tubular dysfunction is less common, but nephrogenic diabetes insipidus has been reported. Glomerular toxicity is rare but can be severe enough to require dialysis and become chronic. Hypertension is also seen. Risk factors for ifosfamide nephrotoxicity include young age, total dose of ifosfamide (increased risk with total dose >60 g/m^2), prior or concurrent treatment with cisplatin, and preexisting renal impairment. *Cisplatin* is also nephrotoxic, through tubular necrosis caused by inhibition of protein synthesis and depletion of glutathione. Administration results in a dose-dependent reduction of glomerular filtration rate, hypomagnesemia, hypokalemia, and polyuria. Evidence suggests that aggressive hydration, including the use of mannitol, can attenuate the toxicity of cisplatin. The renal toxicity of cisplatin is usually reversible, but can become chronic and progressive.

Radiation Recall

Radiation recall is an inflammatory reaction in a previously irradiated body area, often in conjunction with a drug exposure. Most commonly, it manifests as an acute dermatitis. Reactions range from a mild maculopapular erythematous rash to severe necrosis and occur in a sharply demarcated area corresponding to the radiation field. The reaction can occur weeks to years after radiation exposure. Although skin is the most common organ involved, radiation recall has been reported in lung, esophagus, gut, and the CNS. In visceral organs, it manifests as inflammation of the target organ within a previous radiation field. Numerous hypotheses have been proposed but none have been proven to explain the process. About 50% of reported cases have been associated with the use of taxanes or anthracyclines. Treatment is with corticosteroids and withdrawal of the offending agent. Topical steroids are appropriate for skin reactions, but systemic steroids are necessary for visceral involvement.

Management of Chemotherapy Overdose

Overdose of chemotherapeutic agents is usually managed with aggressive supporting care, but there are a few specific therapies. With overdoses of *cisplatin*, plasmapheresis and sodium thiosulfate have been used. Hemodialysis has not been effective. The administration of *N*-acetylcysteine replenishes glutathione and allows the usual detoxification reactions to function. *Ifosfamide* overdose has been treated with methylene blue. Severe neurotoxicity experienced by one patient rapidly reversed. *Carboxypeptidase G2* (or Glucarpidase) is another recently developed "antidote" to chemotherapy overdose. It is a bacterial enzyme that hydrolyzes *methotrexate* to its inactive metabolites, 4-deoxy-4-amino-N10-methylpteroic acid and glutamate. It has been used to enhance methotrexate clearance and was used intrathecally in one patient with an accidental overdose. Hemodialysis is a nonspecific intervention often employed in the treatment of drug overdose. Paclitaxel pharmacokinetics is unaltered in anephric patients who are undergoing hemodialysis. Dialysis is effective in clearing *cisplatin* and *carboplatin* within a relatively short window after drug administration due to rapid and stable binding to proteins in serum (carboplatin) or peripheral tissues (cisplatin). *Methotrexate* and *cyclophosphamide* are readily dialyzable, with an increased rate of elimination, compared to renal clearance. *Ifosfamide* is also readily removed by hemodialysis, while etoposide, dactinomycin, vinca alkaloids, and anthracyclines are extensively protein bound and not cleared by hemodialysis.

CHAPTER 92 ■ ONCOLOGIC EMERGENCIES AND COMPLICATIONS

RODRIGO MEJIA, NIDRA I. RODRIGUEZ, JOSE A. CORTES, SANJU S. SAMUEL, FERNANDO F. CORRALES-MEDINA, REGINA OKHUYSEN, RIZA C. MAURICIO, AND WINSTON W. HUH

Cancer and toxicity from cancer treatment are associated with severe, life-threatening complications. Outcome may be improved with anticipation, recognition, and rapid intervention.

SEPTIC SHOCK

Children with cancer can have profound neutropenia, impaired mucosal barriers, and preexisting end-organ dysfunction that increases their vulnerability to sepsis and multiple organ system failure (MOSF). Critical interventions include the timely normalization of heart rate, cardiac output, perfusion pressures, and pursuit of a central venous oxygen saturation ($Scvo_2$) ≥70%. Aggressive fluid resuscitation (at least 60 mL/kg in the first hour with isotonic crystalloid, colloid, or blood products) in the absence of preexisting volume overload or congestive heart failure is the cornerstone of therapy. Patients with subclinical chemotherapy-induced myocardial dysfunction require close monitoring during fluid resuscitation because congestive heart failure may develop suddenly. Vasoactive agents are usually required to help achieve hemodynamic goals.

Appropriate antibiotic therapy must be implemented within the first hour of contact. Source control must be implemented if a focus of infection is identified. Corticosteroids are used frequently in pediatric oncology as part of chemotherapy and to control complications of cancer therapy (e.g., vomiting and graft-versus-host disease [GVHD]). Corticosteroid administration should occur early (particularly for catecholamine refractory shock) and be withdrawn as soon as practical. Extracorporeal support is appropriate for selected patients with underlying malignancies suffering from refractory shock.

CARDIAC DYSFUNCTION

Chemotherapy, particularly anthracyclines, may produce subclinical myocardial dysfunction that can rapidly deteriorate into florid cardiac failure with stress such as sepsis. Other agents (e.g., cytarabine, cyclophosphamide, 5-fluorouracil, and ifosfamide) can cause dysrhythmias or cardiac failure, particularly in the presence of electrolyte abnormalities. Persistent tachycardia, a narrow pulse pressure, a change in capillary refill, and other indicators of perfusion are important clues. The patient may develop a gallop, anasarca, pulmonary edema, and organ dysfunction. Biomarkers such as troponin and natriuretic peptide may help monitor children at risk.

Cardiac tumors are rare but may cause severe dysfunction in children of all ages. Most of the primary tumors (e.g., rhabdomyomas seen in tuberous sclerosis) are benign in histology but can cause significant hemodynamic compromise or dysrhythmias. Catecholamine-secreting tumors (pheochromocytoma) may cause cardiomyopathy or tachydysrhythmia.

PERICARDIAL EFFUSIONS AND CARDIAC TAMPONADE

Neoplasms and radiation-induced inflammation commonly cause pericardial effusions. These effusions can be exacerbated by thrombocytopenia and coagulopathy. If intrapericardial pressure exceeds transmural myocardial pressure, then diastolic filling and left ventricular output can be compromised. Classic signs of cardiac tamponade include tachycardia, jugular venous distension, pulsus paradoxus, Kussmaul sign (respiratory variation of jugular venous distension), muffled heart sounds, electrical alternans, generalized low voltages on electrocardiogram, and cardiomegaly with a bottle-shaped heart on a chest radiograph. Echocardiography can diagnose effusions and identify the extent of hemodynamic compromise.

Relative or functional hypovolemia requires appropriate fluid therapy. Sedation for procedures must be carefully administered. Fentanyl or ketamine may be less likely to precipitate cardiovascular collapse. Definitive treatment requires decompression of the pericardium.

FEBRILE NEUTROPENIA

Fever is defined as a single oral temperature ≥38.3°C (101 F) or a temperature ≥38°C (100.4 F) sustained over 1 hour. Axillary temperatures are discouraged, and rectal temperatures are contraindicated in neutropenic patients. The risk of sepsis or invasive bacterial infections increases with the extent and duration of neutropenia. The patients at increased risk for prolonged periods of neutropenia include those with hematologic malignancies (e.g., relapsed leukemia) and those who have undergone an allogeneic hematopoietic cell transplant (HCT).

Human granulocyte colony-stimulating factor (GCSF) and granulocyte-macrophage colony-stimulating factor (GM-CSF) are primarily used in patients at high risk for chemotherapy-associated neutropenia. GCSF stimulates the release of neutrophils, and GM-CSF enhances the release of both neutrophils and macrophages. These medications should be continued until neutrophil counts have recovered to more than 1000/mm^3 for 3 straight days. Bone pain, myalgia, and a flu-like syndrome are common side effects. The effect on long-term survival remains unclear. GCSF use for neutropenia and life-threatening infection has been better studied than the use of GM-CSF. Granulocyte transfusions are considered for neutropenic children with life-threatening bacterial or fungal infection. Systemic inflammatory response, acute lung injury, and fluid overload are common complications.

Specific Infectious Complications

Bacteremia

An infectious etiology is identified in 10%–45% of febrile neutropenia episodes. Clinical and laboratory features indicative of a high risk of infection in febrile neutropenia are listed in **Table 92.1.** Frequent sites of infection are central lines, the respiratory tract, the gastrointestinal tract, the skin, and the soft tissues. While the rate of gram-positive infections has increased, the rate of gram-negative infections remains unchanged. Current evidence supports empiric monotherapy with piperacillin-tazobactam or cefepime in intensive care units where antimicrobial susceptibility does not warrant a carbapenem (meropenem or imipenem/cilastin). Ceftazidime has decreasing activity against many gram-negative pathogens. Routine use of an aminoglycoside offers no survival advantage and is associated with increased toxicity. The addition of vancomycin is common for high-risk patients.

Neutropenic Enterocolitis and Typhlitis

Neutropenic enterocolitis is a complication that can involve the distal ileum, cecum, or ascending colon and is seen in patients with prolonged neutropenia. The pathogenesis may be related to direct cytotoxicity to the intestinal mucosal cells, overgrowth of specific bacterial flora, generalized immunodeficiency, production of bacterial endotoxins, or other causes. Cases that involve the cecum are referred to as *typhlitis*. The classic triad of fever, abdominal pain, and diarrhea is not always present and is not specific. Computed tomography imaging allows for differentiation from other diagnoses. Ultrasonography may be useful to assess bowel wall thickness. Sepsis and perforation are the most common complications. Current medical approach in patients without perforation consists of bowel rest, bowel decompression, broad-spectrum intravenous antibiotics (including antifungal agents), and sometimes G-CSF. Patients with perforation, obstruction, peritonitis, active gastrointestinal bleeding, or clinical deterioration may require surgery. Mortality directly from the colitis is uncommon.

Invasive Fungal Infections

Candida and *Aspergillus* are the most frequently isolated fungal organisms in cancer patients. Using fluconazole prophylaxis, the incidence of invasive candidiasis has dropped to <5% and shifted toward non-albicans species. The neutropenic patient with persistent fever for >3–5 days should have empiric coverage expanded to include fungal organisms. Amphotericin B has adverse effects including fever,

TABLE 92.1

Clinical and Laboratory High-Risk Factors in Febrile Neutropenia

CLINICAL RISK FACTORS	LABORATORY-BASED RISK FACTORS
Evidence of shock	Elevated C-reactive protein > 10 mg/L
Near-myeloablative chemotherapy (leukemia induction or delayed intensification)	Absolute neutrophil count < 200 cells/mm^3
Allogeneic hematopoietic stem cell transplant recipient	Absolute monocyte count < 100 cells/mm^3
Relapsed leukemia	Platelet count < 50,000/mm^3
Poorly controlled solid malignancies	Gram-negative bacteremia
Pneumonia	
Neutropenic enterocolitis	
Invasive fungal infection	
Severe oropharyngeal mucositis	
Prolonged neutropenia (>7 d)	
High presenting temperature (>39°C)	
High-dose cytosine arabinoside	
Age less than 1 y	

chills, hypokalemia, nausea, and vomiting. Newer preparations of amphotericin (AmBisome, Abelcet) as well as the azole antifungals (fluconazole, voriconazole, and posaconazole) have fewer side effects. The echinocandin class of antifungals, including caspofungin, micafungin, and anidulafungin, have activity against azole-resistant *Candida* species and *Aspergillus*.

Lower Respiratory Tract Infections

Pneumonia is an uncommon complication of febrile neutropenia. In stem cell transplant patients, pulmonary infections and noninfectious complications vary based on time following transplant (**Table 92.2**). *Pneumocystis jiroveci* pneumonia is rare due to trimethoprim-sulfamethoxazole use. Treatment is with IV trimethoprim-sulfamethoxazole (pentamidine is an alternative) and corticosteroids. Community-acquired infections in children (influenza, respiratory syncytial virus [RSV], and parainfluenza) can be devastating in immunocompromised hosts. Ribavirin, palivizumab, and RSV immune globulin may be of benefit in the management of HCT patients with RSV pneumonia. Mortality from cytomegalovirus (CMV) pneumonitis in HCT patients is high. Patients with antigenemia require preemptive therapy with ganciclovir or foscarnet.

HYPERLEUKOCYTOSIS

Hyperleukocytosis is a peripheral white blood cell (WBC) count greater than 100×10^9/L (100,000/mm^3). It occurs in 10%–30% of patients with acute lymphoblastic leukemia (ALL), 10%–20% patients with acute myeloid leukemia (AML), and the majority of patients with chronic myeloid leukemia (CML). Clinically significant hyperleukocytosis can be evident with WBC $\geq$200,000/mm^3 in AML and WBC $\geq$300,000/mm^3 in ALL and CML (i.e., myeloblasts are larger than lymphoblasts). The lungs and central nervous system (CNS) are the most common sites of leukostasis with vascular obstruction, although other organs can also be affected. CNS involvement is associated with intracranial hemorrhage. Disseminated intravascular coagulation (DIC) can also occur, as can acute tumor lysis syndrome (TLS).

The goal of hyperleukocytosis management is to rapidly lower the WBC count with chemotherapy, leukopheresis, exchange transfusion, or hydroxyurea. A goal WBC count $\leq$100,000/mm^3 seems to be acceptable. Leukopheresis should be avoided in patients with acute promyelocytic leukemia (APL) as it can worsen coagulopathy. Unnecessary red cell transfusions can increase blood viscosity and should be avoided until the blast count decreases.

ABNORMAL HEMOSTASIS IN CANCER

Thrombocytopenia is the most common hemostatic abnormality in pediatric cancer. Coagulation disturbances leading to hemorrhage may also be chemotherapy related. Cyclophosphamide, ifosfamide, methotrexate, and doxorubicin are known to cause hemorrhagic cystitis and mucositis. Radiation therapy may also cause bleeding secondary to blood vessel damage. Hemorrhage in cancer patients can result from defective hepatic clotting factor synthesis or hyperfibrinolysis. Patients can have decreased vitamin K availability or absorption with prolonged antibiotic use, poor oral intake, or diarrhea.

Bleeding in Acute Promyelocytic Leukemia

APL is a distinct subtype of AML characterized by severe coagulopathy. The release of tissue factor-like procoagulants from the leukemic blasts predisposes to DIC. Up to 40% of patients with DIC develop intracerebral or pulmonary hemorrhage during induction chemotherapy or before the diagnosis is established.

TABLE 92.2

Pulmonary Complications after Hematopoietic Stem Cell Transplant

■ PHASE	■ INFECTIOUS	■ NONINFECTIOUS
Neutropenic phase (0–30 d)	Bacteria (20%–50%) Fungal (12%–45%)	Pulmonary edema Drug toxicity DAH
Early phase (30–100 d)	CMV pneumonitis (40%) PCP	Idiopathic pneumonia syndrome
Late phase (>100 d)	Uncommon except in GVHD	Bronchiolitis obliterans Cryptogenic organizing pneumonia Chronic GVHD

DAH, diffuse alveolar hemorrhage; CMV, cytomegalovirus; PCP, *Pneumocystis jiroveci (carinii)* pneumonia; GVHD, graft-versus-host disease.

Children with APL treated with all-trans-retinoic acid (ATRA) show earlier normalization of coagulation.

THROMBOSIS IN CHILDHOOD CANCER

A major risk factor for thrombosis in childhood cancer is the presence of a central venous catheter. Other risk factors include chemotherapy, radiation, surgery, primary tumor type/size, the presence of metastatic disease, obesity, immobility, total parenteral nutrition, and inherited thrombophilia. Some chemotherapeutic agents (e.g., L-asparaginase) increase the risk of thrombosis by reducing antithrombin III levels. Other agents associated with thrombotic events include vincristine, the anthracyclines, and prednisone.

The management of thrombosis includes anticoagulation or thrombolysis. Anticoagulants used include unfractionated heparin (UFH), low-molecular-weight heparin (LMWH), and vitamin K antagonists. LMWH is most frequently used but UFH may be preferred perioperatively due to shorter half-life and reversibility. Thrombolysis is considered in selected cases and is associated with a significant risk of bleeding. Data on the use of inferior vena cava (IVC) filters to prevent pulmonary embolism in children are limited.

TUMOR LYSIS SYNDROME

TLS is a life-threatening emergency due to rapid tumor cell destruction that overwhelms metabolic and excretory pathways. TLS most often develops 12–72 hours after the initiation of cytolytic therapy and is characterized by hyperuricemia, hyperkalemia, and hyperphosphatemia. Precipitation of calcium phosphate causes symptomatic hypocalcemia. Precipitation of the urate or calcium phosphate crystals in the renal tubules may lead to renal failure. TLS occurs most frequently in patients with a large tumor burden or with tumors highly sensitive to chemotherapy (e.g., Burkitt lymphoma, lymphoblastic lymphoma, and leukemia).

Early, aggressive hydration to enhance urine flow is fundamental to the prevention and management of TLS. Uric acid control can be achieved with recombinant urate oxidase (rasburicase) or with a xanthine oxidase inhibitor (allopurinol). Urine alkalinization is not recommended if recombinant urate oxidase (rasburicase) is used. Rasburicase provides a more rapid reduction of uric acid and lower plasma levels compared with allopurinol (G6PD deficiency is a contraindication to rasburicase). Severe hyperkalemia should be treated with insulin, glucose, bicarbonate, calcium, β-adrenergic agents (hyperventilation to induce alkalosis can be used acutely), potassium exchange resins, and renal replacement therapy. The lowest calcium dose required to relieve hypocalcemic symptoms should be used because of the risk of calcium phosphate precipitation. Hyperphosphatemia is managed with oral phosphate binders, such as sevelamer hydrochloride, or aluminum hydroxide.

SPINAL CORD COMPRESSION

Malignant spinal cord compression (MSCC) is a true oncologic emergency. The epidural space is the most common area for spinal cord metastasis with the thoracic spine being the most common site. Back pain is a red flag in a patient with a history of malignancy and should be considered secondary to MSCC until proven otherwise. Common symptoms include sensory abnormalities (40%–90%), focal weakness (75%), and bowel and bladder dysfunction (40%–50%).

Craniospinal T1- and T2-weighted magnetic resonance imaging is the study of choice to demonstrate epidural involvement, intraparenchymal spread, or compression of nerve roots. Therapy (usually corticosteroids) should be initiated as soon as the diagnosis is considered. Later therapy may include radiation if the tumor is radiosensitive, surgery if there is severe spinal instability, rapidly progressive symptoms, or progressive symptoms in spite of radiation, and chemotherapy if the diagnosis is leukemia/lymphoma or neuroblastoma.

MEDIASTINAL MASSES

Patients with anterosuperior and middle mediastinal masses are at risk for life-threatening airway obstruction and vascular compression. Patients with posterior mediastinal masses are at risk for spinal cord compression. Lesions affecting the tracheobronchial tree may cause dyspnea, orthopnea, stridor, cough, and respiratory distress. Tumor masses compressing the great vessels may cause head and neck edema with or without neurological deficit. Tumors compressing the heart may cause syncope, cyanosis, and arrhythmias.

Supine position or sedation may worsen symptoms or lead to cardiopulmonary arrest, so careful planning of evaluation and management is necessary. Airway instrumentation should be performed in a controlled environment by experienced anesthesiologists with surgical and cardiopulmonary support available when possible. In most situations, endotracheal intubation takes place in conscious and spontaneously breathing patients employing topical anesthetic techniques with light sedation and avoiding neuromuscular blocking agents. Reinforced endotracheal tubes of decreased diameter but sufficient length to extend beyond the compression may be necessary. Extracorporeal membrane oxygenation or cardiopulmonary bypass back-up should be considered. Bone marrow biopsy, lymph node biopsy, or radiologic (ultrasound or CT-guided) percutaneous mediastinal biopsies may be safely performed with local anesthesia in many cases, avoiding the need for general anesthesia. Prebiopsy cytoreductive therapy using corticosteroids or radiation may be required in patients presenting with severe airway compromise (may reduce the ability to make a definitive diagnosis).

SUPERIOR MEDIASTINAL SYNDROME

Superior mediastinal syndrome (SMS) results from the compression of the tracheobronchial tree, the great vessels, and the heart by a growing mass or a thrombus. Progressive venous congestion and airway compression usually cause facial engorgement, headache, plethora, cyanotic facies, cough, dyspnea, orthopnea, hoarseness, stridor, and dysphasia with or without pleural and/or pericardial effusions. Most patients will not tolerate the supine position. Once the definitive diagnosis is reached, the appropriate chemotherapeutic plan will reduce tumor load rapidly with improvement of symptoms. Thrombolytic therapy should be considered in patients with extensive thromboembolism if no contraindications.

MASSIVE HEMOPTYSIS

The most common cause of massive hemoptysis in the pediatric cancer patient is invasive pulmonary aspergillosis (IPA). IPA usually presents after myeloablative chemotherapy for HCT or during the recovery phase of prolonged neutropenia after chemotherapy. Other infections to be considered include invasive fungi (mucormycosis), bacterial necrotizing pneumonias due to *Staphylococcus aureus*, *Pseudomonas aeruginosa*, *Klebsiella,* and tuberculosis. Noninfectious etiologies include primary endobronchial tumors, diffuse alveolar hemorrhage, bronchiectasis, and foreign bodies. CT imaging is the most sensitive radiologic test available for the early diagnosis of IPA. The *halo sign*, a dense nodular lesion surrounded by ground glass attenuation (>180°), may be seen. Tissue may be obtained by CT-guided percutaneous lung biopsy, transbronchial biopsy, or open lung biopsy.

Early intubation and ventilation should be considered. Aggressive treatment of associated coagulopathy, thrombocytopenia, and anemia and appropriate antibiotics or antifungals are warranted. Bronchoscopy should be considered if endoluminal control of the bleeding is feasible. Other options include bronchial arteriography with transcatheter embolization in nonsurgical candidates, wedge resection of the affected lung segment, or lobectomy.

BOWEL OBSTRUCTION

Bowel obstruction from primary malignancy is not as common in children as in adults because of a lower frequency of colon and ovarian cancer. Conditions that increase the risk of bowel obstruction include surgery, radiation therapy, opioid use, prolonged bed rest, malnutrition, and electrolyte abnormalities. CT imaging is sensitive and specific in identifying small bowel obstruction. Patients with partial obstruction can often be managed medically. Dexamethasone and octreotide are effective in relieving symptoms in most patients with malignant bowel obstruction. Surgery is indicated for patients with complete mechanical obstruction, partial mechanical obstruction not responding to medical treatment, peritonitis, and frank perforation. Palliative measures (e.g., a venting gastrostomy or jejunostomy tube) are appropriate in end-stage, inoperable disease. Primary intestinal neoplasms or intestinal metastatic tumors (e.g., carcinomas or lymphomas) may serve as lead points for intussusception. The "classic triad" of intussusception includes colicky pain, abdominal mass, and bloody stools. Most children present with abdominal pain and vomiting. Ultrasonography is more accurate than abdominal radiographs and can detect the lead point and other intra-abdominal pathology. The treatment of choice is surgical reduction of the intussusception and resection of the inciting pathology rather than radiologic reduction using contrast enema.

CHAPTER 93 ■ HEMATOLOGIC EMERGENCIES

MICHAEL C. MCCRORY, KENNETH M. BRADY, CLIFFORD M. TAKEMOTO, AND R. BLAINE EASLEY

RED BLOOD CELL ABNORMALITIES

Anemia

Anemia (erythropenia) is the most common hematologic abnormality in the pediatric intensive care unit (PICU). The most common etiologies that require emergent evaluation include hemorrhage, hemolysis, and splenic sequestration. Anemia, regardless of etiology, results in a decreased O_2-carrying capacity and, when severe, decreased O_2 delivery. The differential diagnosis of anemia based on mean corpuscular volume (MCV) is summarized in **Figure 93-1**.

Iron-deficiency anemia is the leading cause of anemia in early childhood. Iron-deficiency anemia has low hemoglobin (Hb), low red blood cell (RBC) count, low MCV, low reticulocyte count, elevated free erythrocyte protoporphyrin, and increased red-cell distribution width. Ferritin and serum iron are low, and total iron-binding capacity and transferrin are increased. Iron deficiency is most common in children <3 years and results from inadequate iron intake during a period of rapid growth. It is often complicated by other clinical findings of poor nutrition, neglect, or excessive intake of cow's milk. In older children and adults with iron deficiency, occult blood loss should be suspected and should prompt a gastrointestinal evaluation. Optimal *treatment* is obtained with 3–6 mg/kg/day of elemental iron. Enteral ferrous sulfate is preferred; parenteral administration (with iron dextran) is an option if compliance or tolerance is an issue. *Prevention* of iron-deficiency anemia includes iron supplementation (1–2 mg/kg/day) for breastfed infants after 4 months of age, use of iron-fortified formulas (containing 12 mg iron as ferrous sulfate per liter), iron supplement (2–3 mg/kg/day) to preterm infants after the first month of life, and delayed introduction of cow's milk until >1 year. Transfusion is usually recommended for children with or without cardiorespiratory symptoms when Hb is ≤4 g/dL. In children who have Hb values between 4 and 6 g/dL, treatment practices vary and the decision to transfuse can be based on symptoms, available resources, comorbid conditions (malaria, fever), and end-organ manifestations. Typically, packed RBCs (5 mL/kg) are administered over 4 hours, followed by another 5 mL/kg transfusion over 4 hours. Diuretics

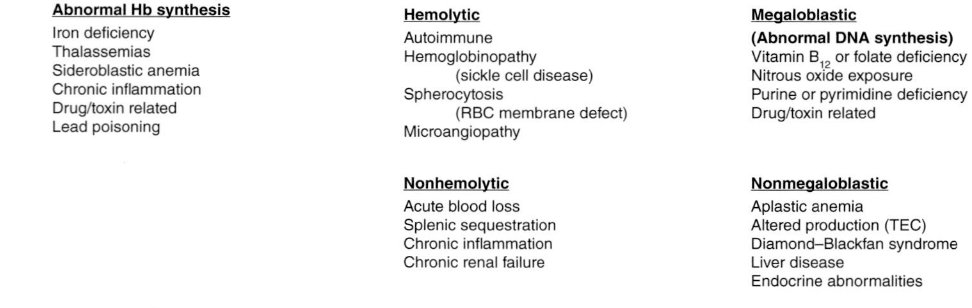

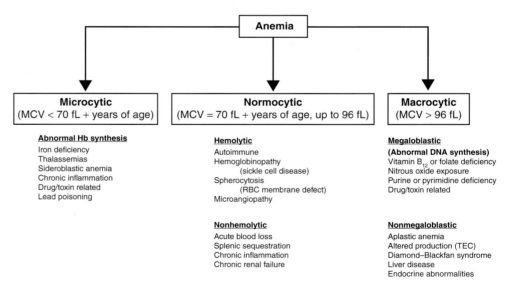

FIGURE 93.1. The differential diagnosis of anemia. MCV, mean corpuscular volume; fL, femtoliter; TEC, transient erythropenia of childhood. (Adapted from Sadowitz PD, Amanullah S, Souid AK. Hematologic emergencies in the pediatric emergency room. *Emerg Med Clin North Am* 2002;20(1):177–98, vii.)

may also be required to avoid volume overload in an anemic patient's volume-expanded state.

Hemolytic anemia and autoimmune hemolytic anemia can be caused by either intracellular or extracellular disorders. Intracellular disorders consist of RBC membrane defects, abnormal erythrocyte metabolism, or hemoglobinopathies. Extracorpuscular disorders include immune-mediated destruction, mechanical fragmentation, infections, drugs, chemicals, and venoms. Tests used to diagnose a hemolytic process include evaluation of peripheral blood smear for irregular RBCs (spherocytes or schistocytes) and Heinz bodies (denatured Hb), elevated reticulocyte count, positive Coombs test (direct and indirect), elevated serum aspartate aminotransferase, lactate dehydrogenase, and serum bilirubin, with lowered serum haptoglobin.

G6PD deficiency is the most common RBC-associated enzyme disorder and has X-linked inheritance. The Mediterranean variety is the most severe and has the lowest G6PD activity. The African variety is unique because only mature RBCs are enzyme-deficient. Lack of this enzyme allows rapid depletion of antioxidants and subsequent denaturation of the Hb unit. Unripe peaches, fava beans, methylene blue, naphthalene, phenazopyridine, nitroglycerin, prilocaine, benzocaine, and sulfamethoxazole are agents that result in hemolysis in G6PD-deficient patients. Salicylates pose a risk for hemolysis in high doses. Avoidance of oxidants (e.g., sulfa drugs) and careful observation during stress (e.g., infection and surgery) are necessary.

Antibody-mediated (autoimmune) hemolytic anemia is an extracellular process of RBC destruction. Evaluation reveals a rapidly falling Hb, low haptoglobin, increased bilirubin metabolites in the urine, positive Coombs tests, and abundant spherocytes on smear. The direct Coombs test confirms antibody bound to the RBCs. The indirect Coombs test detects free antibody in the serum. Clinically significant hemolysis can occur with either IgG or IgM antibodies, but usually with IgG. IgG antibody-coated RBCs are destroyed in the spleen. Treatment involves careful observation, high-dose steroids, and, if necessary, RBC transfusion with the most compatible blood. Plasmapheresis and splenectomy are options for refractory patients.

Transient erythrocytopenia of childhood (TEC) has a gradual onset of normocytic anemia and reticulocytopenia caused by temporary suppression of RBC production. It usually occurs in children 6 months to 3 years and is commonly preceded by a viral illness. Full recovery usually occurs in 4–6 weeks. TEC must be distinguished from a rare disease, *pure red-cell aplasia,* or *Diamond–Blackfan syndrome*. Patients with Diamond–Blackfan syndrome typically have macrocytic erythrocytes (elevated MCV), dysmorphic features, and persistent anemia. Bone marrow recovery occurs in TEC and rules out Diamond–Blackfan syndrome.

Bone marrow infiltration can result from malignant cells, inherited metabolic disorders, or infections (fungus, tuberculosis). Regardless of the process, the result is a normocytic anemia with a low reticulocyte count. These patients can have lymphadenopathy, hepatomegaly, splenomegaly, reticulocytopenia, neutropenia, thrombocytopenia, and circulating immature cells (e.g., nucleated RBCs, promyelocytes, metamyelocytes, and myelocytes). Bone marrow examination is essential in this setting to establish the correct diagnosis.

Acquired aplastic anemia is defined as peripheral blood pancytopenia with bone marrow hypocellularity in the absence of underlying malignant or myeloproliferative disease. The principal pathophysiologic mechanism is thought to be immune-mediated destruction of hematopoietic stem cells by cytotoxic T lymphocytes. Drug-induced causes account for 50% of all cases and result from either toxic effects or immune-mediated phenomena. Progenitor stem cells are most commonly affected. Common toxic agents include ionizing radiation, chemotherapeutic drugs, antibiotics (chloramphenicol), hydrocarbons (benzene), anti-inflammatory medications (phenylbutazone, indomethacin), and metals (gold). Other drugs with a risk for aplastic anemia are anticonvulsants (fosphenytoin, phenytoin, carbamazepine) and quinacrine. Supportive care is typically required, with recovery of the RBC counts occurring over time once the causative agent is discontinued.

Megaloblastic anemia may be caused by decreased vitamin absorption or impaired metabolism. Vitamin B_{12} and folate deficiencies impair cellular DNA synthesis. Decreased vitamin B_{12} absorption in children results from limited nutritional intake or intestinal malabsorption. Agents that impair B_{12} absorption include metformin, colchicine, neomycin, para-aminosalicylic acid, and slow-release potassium chloride. Causes of folate deficiency include sepsis, pregnancy, malignancy, chronic hemodialysis, and medications. Anticonvulsants can limit folate absorption. Approximately 50% of patients on long-term phenytoin have low folate levels, and 30% have red-cell macrocytosis, and megaloblastic changes in the bone marrow. Folate replacement improves the anemia. Methotrexate, trimethoprim, triamterene, and pyrimethamine inhibit dihydrofolate reductase and cause megaloblastic anemia that is not folate responsive during long-term and high-dose therapy. Acute megaloblastic anemia may also be caused by prolonged or repeated nitrous oxide anesthesia.

Hemoglobinopathies

Primary hemoglobinopathy describes structural abnormalities of Hb that are often inherited. In normal human maturation, HbA ($\alpha 2\beta 2$) becomes the dominant form, taking over from the HbF ($\alpha 2\gamma 2$) during the first year of life. The thalassemias are the most common worldwide genetic disorder. Examples of common beta-chain mutations that result in hemoglobinopathies include S (sickle) and C, which can result in symptomatic anemia syndromes. Other structurally abnormal Hbs result in increased O_2 affinity and relative tissue hypoxia that leads to polycythemia. Erythropoietin levels are often elevated. *Familial methemoglobinemia* (HbM) is a rare autosomal-dominant disorder, and affected individuals present with cyanosis at birth. HbM and other clinically significant hemoglobinopathies are detectable by newborn screening using liquid chromatography or electrophoresis (as in HbS). The "secondary" causes of methemoglobinemia (MetHb) are more common.

Secondary hemoglobinopathies result from conditions that induce abnormal Hb production or adversely affect Hb function. Dyshemoglobinemias are conditions that produce abnormal O_2 binding of structurally normal Hb. All dyshemoglobinemias shift the oxygen disassociation curve, impair binding of O_2 by Hb, and impair O_2 delivery to the tissues (**Fig. 93-2**). Diagnosis is made with routine co-oximetry, which measures the fraction of abnormal Hb. Iatrogenic causes in the PICU may result from inhaled nitric oxide therapy (MetHb) and nitroprusside infusions (cyanohemoglobinemia). If the dyshemoglobinemia is potentially life-threatening from a toxic exposure, treatment involves removal of the cause and antidote treatment when appropriate. Exchange transfusion and hyperbaric oxygen therapy are considerations for acute and life-threatening causes of dyshemoglobinemia with clinically impaired O_2 delivery. A normal individual has up to 1.5% MetHb, and <1% of sulfhemoglobin (SulfHb), cyanohemoglobin (CyanoHb), and carboxyhemoglobin (COHb). MetHb and COHb, the most common acquired dyshemoglobinemias, are detectable on routine co-oximetry. Common dyshemoglobinemias and treatment options are listed in **Table 93.1**. MetHb causes chocolate-brown discoloration of blood, cyanosis, and functional "anemia" in high enough concentrations. Cyanosis becomes apparent at a MetHb of 1.5 g/dL (~10% of total Hb). Infants may be at a greater risk to the toxic effects of MetHb because they have lower MetHb-reductase levels and altered oxygen–Hb dissociation properties. Additionally, fetal Hb is more susceptible to oxidant stresses with a more rapid conversion of MetHb.

MetHb concentrations <25% may be asymptomatic, levels of 35%–50% result in mild symptoms (exertional dyspnea and headaches), and levels >70% are lethal. Therapy with ascorbic acid or methylthioninium chloride (methylene blue) reduces the level of oxidized Hb, the latter by the NADPH-MetHb-reductase system.

SulfHb is a mixture of oxidized and partially denatured Hb that forms during oxidative hemolysis. The normal SulfHb is ≤1% and, even in disease states, seldom exceeds 10%. Unlike MetHb, SulfHb cannot be reduced back to Hb and results in a mild, asymptomatic cyanosis. Blood samples have a mauve-lavender color. SulfHb has been reported from treatment with sulfonamides or aromatic amine medications (phenacetin, acetanilide), and from severe constipation complicated by bacteremia due to *Clostridium perfringens* (*enterogenous cyanosis*). SulfHb is not detected on routine co-oximetry; it is incorrectly measured as MetHb. SulfHb is best detected using differential Hb spectrophotometry or gas chromatography. Sulfhemoglobinemia should be suspected for environmentally acquired cyanosis that fails to respond to MetHb therapy.

CyanoHb forms when Hb combines with cyanide. Cyanide can be inhaled, absorbed transcutaneously,

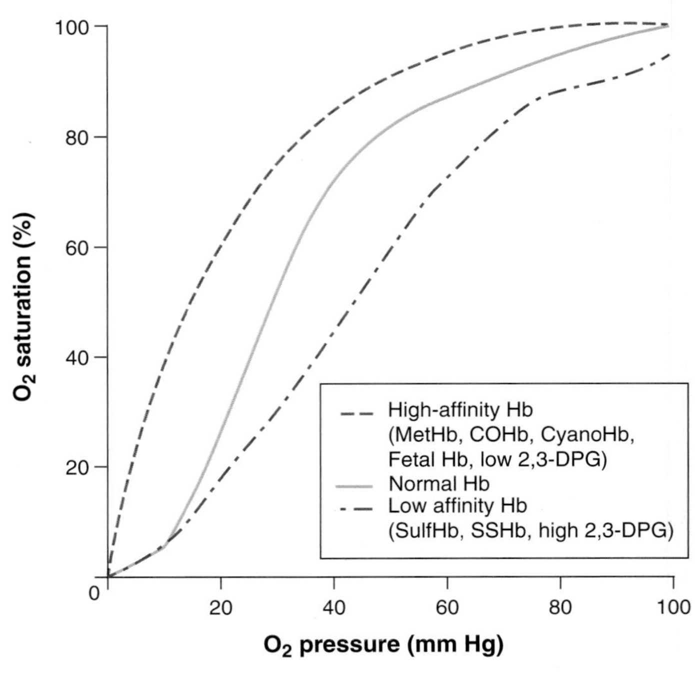

FIGURE 93.2. Dyshemoglobinemia and effect on the oxygen–hemoglobin disassociation curve. Environmental exposures impact not only the ability of O_2 to bind to hemoglobin but the ability to effectively deliver O_2 to the tissues. Shift of the O_2 dissociation curve to the left results in impaired delivery of O_2. Cyanohemoglobin (CyanoHb), methemoglobin (MetHb), and carboxyhemoglobin (COHb) result in a leftward shift. While sulfhemoglobin (SulfHb) results in cyanosis, higher concentrations are tolerated because of the rightward shift of the O_2 dissociation curve. Other forms of hemoglobin and their relative effect on O_2 dissociation curve are also shown. 2,3-DPG, 2,3-diphosphoglycerate; HbF, fetal Hb; HbSS, sickle cell disease hemoglobin.

TABLE 93.1

Treatment of Acquired Dyshemoglobinemias

HB VARIANT	MEASUREMENT	TREATMENT
MetHb	Routine co-oximetry	1. Determine source 2. IV methylene blue 3. Consider SulfHb if fails to resolve with treatment
SulfHb	Hb spectrophotometry Gas chromatography	1. Determine source 2. Irreversible 3. Consider exchange transfusion if severe
CyanoHb	Hb spectrophotometry RBC cyanide level	1. Determine source 2. IV sodium nitrate or inhaled amyl nitrate with IV thiosulfate 3. IV hydroxycoalbumin 4. IV dicobalt edetate 5. Consider exchange transfusion if severe
COHb	Routine co-oximetry	1. Determine source 2. Provide F_{IO_2} 1.0 via non-rebreather/high-flow breathing mask 3. Consider HBO_2 therapy, if severe 4. Consider exchange transfusion if HBO_2 unavailable

HBO_2 and/or exchange transfusion may be useful treatments if severe impairment to O_2 delivery is present. Contacting local poison control authorities will help to identify local resources and latest treatment information.
MetHb, methemoglobin; SulfHb, sulfhemoglobin; Hb, hemoglobin; CyanoHb, cyanohemoglobin; RBC, red blood cell; COHb, carboxyhemoglobin; HBO_2, hyperbaric oxygen.

or ingested. Toxic effects arise because of the greater affinity of Hb for cyanide than for O_2, decreased O_2 delivery, inhibition of mitochondrial cytochrome oxidase, and decreased cellular oxidative metabolism. In children, CyanoHb formation and toxicity have resulted from holistic drugs (laetrile), cyanogenic foods (fava beans, apricot pits), and medications (nitroprusside infusions). CyanoHb and O_2Hb are responsible for the "cherry red" appearance of mucous membranes in cyanide poisoning. Other laboratory test results (high anion gap metabolic acidosis, elevated lactate, elevated venous O_2) support the diagnosis of cyanide toxicity. Critically ill children and those receiving rapid infusions of sodium nitroprusside may not eliminate the cyanide formed quickly enough to avert toxic effects. Excessive light exposure of nitroprusside causes a premature and excessive release of cyanide. Treatment for cyanide toxicity involves inducing MetHb (with nitrites) to attract the cyanide ion from cytochrome oxidase (MetHb has a high affinity for cyanide and readily combines to form CyanoMetHb), a safe but non–oxygen-carrying form of Hb. Because of reduced MetHb-reductase activity in children and concern about their susceptibility to thiocyanate toxicity, alternative strategies for the treatment of cyanide toxicity are being investigated.

Endogenous CO produced in the degradation of heme to bilirubin normally accounts for about 0.5% COHb in the blood and is increased in hemolytic anemia. COHb cannot bind to O_2, and increasing concentrations of COHb shift the Hb–oxygen dissociation curve further to the left, adding to the anoxia. If a patient poisoned with CO receives pure O_2, the conversion of COHb to O_2Hb is greatly enhanced. COHb may be quantitated with most routine co-oximetry monitors.

Erythrocytosis

Polycythemia: Polycythemia is synonymous with *erythrocytosis*. Increased red-cell mass and Hb content (>2 SD of normal) occur in PICU patients from dehydration, chronic hypoxia, and overtransfusion. The complications of elevated RBC mass include hyperviscosity, hypercoagulability, and thrombosis. Polycythemia can be primary or secondary based on the respective low or high levels of erythropoietin. Primary causes (*primary absolute erythrocytosis* and *polycythemia vera*) are rare in children. Acute intervention is phlebotomy. Maintenance treatment and evaluation should include a pediatric hematologist.

Secondary absolute erythrocytosis: Secondary absolute erythrocytosis is more common, but rare in critically ill patients. An increase in erythropoietin production results in an elevation of the RBC mass. This condition is an appropriate response to hypoxemia (cyanotic congenital heart disease, chronic pulmonary disease, severe obstructive sleep apnea [Pickwickian syndrome], and hemoglobinopathies with increased O_2 affinity). Inappropriate overproduction of erythropoietin should also be considered. The evaluation includes a hemogram with red-cell parameters, measurement of erythropoietin levels, and arterial oxygen saturation. In uncorrectable causes of erythrocytosis, chronic phlebotomy to keep the Hct <60% is used to prevent hyperviscosity and microcirculatory congestion.

Neonatal polycythemia and hyperviscosity: Approximately 1%–5% of newborns are polycythemic. Polycythemia can be associated with increased blood viscosity. Hct levels >65%–70% are associated with diminished blood flow, especially in the cerebral, hepatic, renal, and mesenteric microcirculations. Clinical symptoms include lethargy, cyanosis, respiratory distress, jitteriness, hypotonia, feeding intolerance, hypoglycemia, and hyperbilirubinemia. Treatment of neonatal polycythemia and hyperviscosity remains controversial as data do not show long-term benefits. In the symptomatic polycythemic newborn, the total exchange volume for partial exchange transfusion (PET) is generally calculated using the following formula:

$$\text{PET volume} = \text{Circulating blood volume} \times [(\text{Hct}_{\text{current}} - \text{Hct}_{\text{desired}})/\text{Hct}_{\text{current}}]$$

Circulating blood volume refers to the infant's weight in kilograms multiplied by the expected intravascular volume in milliliter per kilogram of body weight (80–90 mL/kg in term infants; 100 mL/kg in preterm infants). During and up to 4 hours after PET, enteral feedings should be held. Typical Hct goals from PET are <55%.

WHITE BLOOD CELL ABNORMALITIES (NONMALIGNANT)

Leukopenia

Leukopenia is a total white blood cell (WBC) count $<4000/\text{mm}^3$. In children, a WBC count 2 SDs below an age-appropriate mean is often used. Evaluation requires a careful history, physical examination, and review of the complete blood count (CBC) with differential. *Lymphopenia* is a decline in total lymphocytes below the lower range of normal ($1000/\text{mm}^3$ in adults and $4500/\text{mm}^3$ in infants). Most often, it results transiently from viral, fungal, or parasitic infections. Human immunodeficiency virus, with or without AIDS, is a common, worldwide infectious disease associated with lymphopenia. If lymphopenia persists, multiple cell lines are deficient, or common transiently acquired etiologies are not found, immunoglobulin measurements, flow cytometry, and CD4 and CD8 T-lymphocyte subset quantification are warranted. *Neutropenia* is "mild" if circulating WBC counts are $1000–1500/\text{mm}^3$, "moderate" if $500–1000/\text{mm}^3$, and "severe" (with increased risk for a life-threatening infection) when the absolute neutrophil count (ANC) is $<500/\text{mm}^3$. Evaluation of neutropenia in children involves a tiered approach including serial neutrophil counts, peripheral blood smear, withdrawal of a potential inciting medication, further laboratory testing (kidney and liver function tests, electrolytes, c-reactive protein, blood pH, immunoglobulin, screening for autoimmune or infectious etiologies), or bone marrow investigation.

General Management of Neutropenia Not Associated with Malignancy

Children with neutropenia are at increased risk for infectious complications because of their weakened defense system. Most infections result from organisms that are normal flora (gram-negative bacteria, *Candida albicans*, varicella, and *Pneumocystis*). Other exogenously acquired infective agents are *Pseudomonas* or *Aspergillus* species. *Escherichia coli*, *Pseudomonas*, and *Klebsiella* species represent the most common gram-negative organisms that infect immunocompromised children and coagulase-negative staphylococci are the predominant gram-positive organisms that cause infection, especially in patients with central venous catheters (CVCs). Anaerobic infections are uncommon. *Candida* and *Aspergillus* species are the most common fungal infections. The most common viral pathogens include herpes simplex, varicella zoster, cytomegalovirus (CMV), Epstein–Barr virus (EBV), and adenovirus. *Pneumocystis* and *Toxoplasma* represent the major protozoan infections in this group. The standard approach for neutropenic patients with fever and no focus of infection is combination therapy to cover gram-positive and gram-negative bacteria. Ceftazidime (or Piperacillin/Tazobactam) and vancomycin are used as initial therapy (especially in patients with a CVC). Children with pneumonia or perirectal infections may require antibiotics that cover pathogens such as *Pneumocystis* and *Clostridium*. Culturing strategies are also controversial. We advocate culturing from all central-line ports, as well as percutaneously ("peripheral blood culture"). Additional tests include a CBC with differential, urine analysis with Gram stain and culture, and chest x-ray. A tracheal aspirate with a culture should be considered in patients who are tracheally intubated. Most simple catheter infections can be cleared with antibiotics without catheter removal. Tunnel-site infections (infections where the catheter enters the skin) represent a more difficult problem. Despite appropriate antibiotics, many catheters must be removed to clear the infection. Treatment to stimulate neutrophil recovery should be considered. Recombinant human granulocyte colony-stimulating factor (rhGCSF or GCSF) stimulates the production of neutrophils from committed progenitor cells in the marrow, and is often used for chemotherapy-related neutropenia. The dose is 5–10 μg/kg administered subcutaneously. An improvement is generally noted in 10–14 days to an ANC above $1500/\text{mm}^3$.

Autoimmune neutropenia is caused by the production of antibodies against neutrophil antigens. This entity is usually self-limited, with recovery over several months. Appropriate antibiotics should be given to febrile, neutropenic patients, as noted previously. Treatment with rhGCSF is usually reserved for active bacterial infections or for prophylaxis against recurrent infections. Alternative treatments with corticosteroids (prednisone, 1–2 mg/kg/day for 1 week) and IV immunoglobulin (IVIG) (a single dose of 1 g/kg) hasten recovery of the ANC. The use of these modalities should be done in consultation with a pediatric hematologist.

Severe congenital neutropenia (SCN) is severe neutropenia (ANC <200 per mm^3) from birth. Omphalitis, recurrent cellulitis, and abscesses are common. SCN is most commonly secondary to heterozygous mutations in the elastase-neutrophil expressed (ELANE) gene. *Congenital cyclical neutropenia* is caused by a defect in stem cell development, with ELANE gene mutations in 80%–100%. The duration of each cycle is usually 21 days. The most common manifestations are oral ulcers, stomatitis, pharyngitis, tonsillitis, lymphadenitis, cellulitis, otitis media, and sinusitis. Presentation usually occurs in early childhood. Infectious episodes should be treated promptly with appropriate antibiotics and rhGCSF (5 μg/kg daily subq until the WBC count is ≥10,000/mm^3).

Leukocytosis

Abnormally high (>2 SDs for age) circulating WBC counts are regarded as "leukocytosis." Primary leukocytosis is an extremely rare event and is often hereditary. Secondary leukocytosis may occur from stress, infection, inflammation, endocrinopathies, drugs, and toxins. WBC counts >50,000/mm^3 are classified as *leukemoid reactions*. Stress-induced demargination in the setting of trauma, burns, surgery, hemolysis, and hemorrhage will result in elevation of multiple WBC subtypes (neutrophils, monocytes, lymphocytes). Acute leukocytosis with a neutrophil predominance is suggestive of a serious bacterial infection, while elevation in WBC with a majority of eosinophils is suggestive of an allergic reaction or parasitic infection.

Neutrophilia in adults and older children is a neutrophil count >8000/mm^3. An acute transient increase in circulating neutrophils can result from inflammation, stress, infection, or injury. Common intensive care medications that induce neutrophilia are epinephrine, corticosteroids, and rhGCSF. Chronic inflammatory diseases (autoimmune, tuberculosis, sarcoidosis, and so on) and chronic drug exposure (corticosteroids) can result in chronic neutrophilia. Potential nonmalignant causes of persistent neutrophilia include congenital asplenia, familial myeloproliferative disease, and genetic disorders of leukocyte adhesion.

Eosinophilia is related to acute or chronic disease in adults and children and is classified as mild (351–1500/mm^3), moderate (>1500–5000/mm^3), or severe (>5000/mm^3). The most common cause of eosinophilia worldwide is helminthic infections, and in industrialized nations it is atopic disease. Eosinophilic disorders are categorized as reactive, disease-associated, clonal, or idiopathic. Reactive causes of eosinophilia include life-threatening allergic reactions (anaphylaxis, status asthmaticus), parasitic infections (helminths), and drug reactions. Secondary (disease-associated) eosinophilia occurs in gastroenteritis/esophagitis, autoimmune (connective tissue diseases), paraneoplastic (Hodgkin lymphoma), immunologic (hyper-IgE syndrome), vasculitic (Churg–Strauss syndrome, Wegener granulomatosis), pulmonary (Loeffler syndrome, cystic fibrosis), and endocrine (adrenal insufficiency) disorders. Clonal eosinophilia includes lymphoproliferative and myeloproliferative variants. Bone marrow biopsy and consultation with a pediatric hematologist or immunologist is necessary to evaluate nonreactive or persistent eosinophilia. In the cases of reactive or secondary eosinophilia (which represent the majority of pediatric eosinophilia cases), episodes resolve spontaneously or with treatment of the underlying condition. In scenarios with no diagnosis, clonal causes excluded, and eosinophilia persists, treatment remains controversial. Regardless of treatment, patients with persistent eosinophilia should have periodic evaluations, including pulmonary, cardiac (echocardiographic), and ophthalmologic examinations to detect eosinophil-mediated tissue damage.

Lymphocytosis in children is usually caused by leukemia or lymphoma. The most common nonmalignant cause is a viral infection. Hyperthyroidism and adrenal insufficiency are also associated with lymphocytosis in the critically ill. Pertussis infection in infants <6 months results in lymphocytosis in 25% of cases. WBC count >100,000 is a predictor of mortality. Hyperviscosity and microvascular obstruction can cause widespread tissue necrosis and pulmonary arteriolar thromboses. Pulmonary hypertension resistant to conventional therapy and multiorgan failure may occur. In infants with cardiorespiratory failure from pertussis, double volume exchange transfusion or leukapheresis can be used for leukoreduction, with a goal of lowering WBC count to <15,000.

Monocytosis is often described in children recovering from myelosuppressive chemotherapy preceding recovery from neutropenia. Primary causes of monocytosis include juvenile myelomonocytic leukemia (JMML), with thrombocytopenia, anemia, and splenomegaly. Prognosis is poor, but bone marrow transplant can be curative. Individuals with Noonan syndrome can also have features similar to JMML that improves without treatment.

PLATELET ABNORMALITIES

Thrombocytosis

In children, the classifications used include mild thrombocytosis, platelet count is 500,000–700,000/mm^3; moderate thrombocytosis, 700,000–900,000/mm^3; severe thrombocytosis, 900,000/mm^3–1,000,000/mm^3; and extreme thrombocytosis, if the platelet count is >1,000,000/mm^3.

Essential (or primary) thrombocytosis is rare in children and is a form of myeloproliferative disease resulting from either monoclonal/polyclonal expansion of megakaryocytes or abnormalities in thrombopoietin.

Reactive (or secondary) thrombocytosis (RT) is the most common cause of thrombocytosis. These are associated with inflammation or iron deficiency. Agents associated with RT in children include epinephrine, corticosteroids, vinca alkaloids, penicillamine, imipenem, and meropenem. Complications are rare, and risk factors for thromboembolic disease in children are young age (neonate/infant), CVC, cardiac malformations, and septicemia. Treatment should focus on diagnosis and management of the underlying disease process.

Thrombocytopenia

Thrombocytopenia (a platelet count <150,000/mm^3) affects 15%–58% of PICU patients. Spontaneous bleeding rarely occurs until the platelet count is <20,000/mm^3. Platelets are usually transfused to maintain platelet counts >50,000/mm^3 in the presence of an associated risk of bleeding. True thrombocytopenia can have an inherited or acquired cause. Primary (inherited) thrombocytopenias are less common than acquired disorders in children.

Secondary (or acquired) thrombocytopenia is acute onset and described by the mechanism: impaired production, increased destruction, dilution, or sequestration (differential diagnosis in **Fig. 93-3**).

Medication-induced (iatrogenic) thrombocytopenia may be due to impaired platelet production from myelosuppression or destruction by drug-dependent antibodies. Thrombocytopenia is the most common drug-induced hematologic abnormality. Common medications such as cardiovascular drugs, antibiotics, sedative/anesthetic agents, neuroleptics, antiepileptics (carbamazepine, valproate, and phenytoin), and antidepressants (lithium, fluoxetine, sertraline, paroxetine, and citalopram) can cause thrombocytopenia. Heparin can cause very severe antibody-dependent immune thrombocytopenia (ITP). More common in adults, *heparin-induced thrombocytopenia* (HIT) is important to recognize. Quinidine can also cause antibody-mediated thrombocytopenia.

ITP (previously called "idiopathic") is caused by the production of antibodies against platelet antigens. These antibody-coated platelets are destroyed in the reticuloendothelial system (primarily the spleen). The typical history is sudden onset of petechiae and bruising in a previously healthy child with a preceding viral illness. The CBC and blood smear are normal except for isolated thrombocytopenia. Children with excessive skin and mucosal bleeding or with platelet counts of <10,000/mm^3 may be at increased risk for life-threatening bleeding. Treatment remains controversial. Current treatment options include corticosteroids, IVIG, and anti-Rh (D) immunoglobulin. Corticosteroids (prednisone 2 mg/kg/d) increase vascular stability, enhance platelet production, decrease antibody production, and impair clearance of antibody-coated platelets. IVIG (1 g/kg/day for two consecutive days) binds to receptors in the reticuloendothelial system, preventing platelet destruction. IV anti-D (a single dose of 50 μg/kg

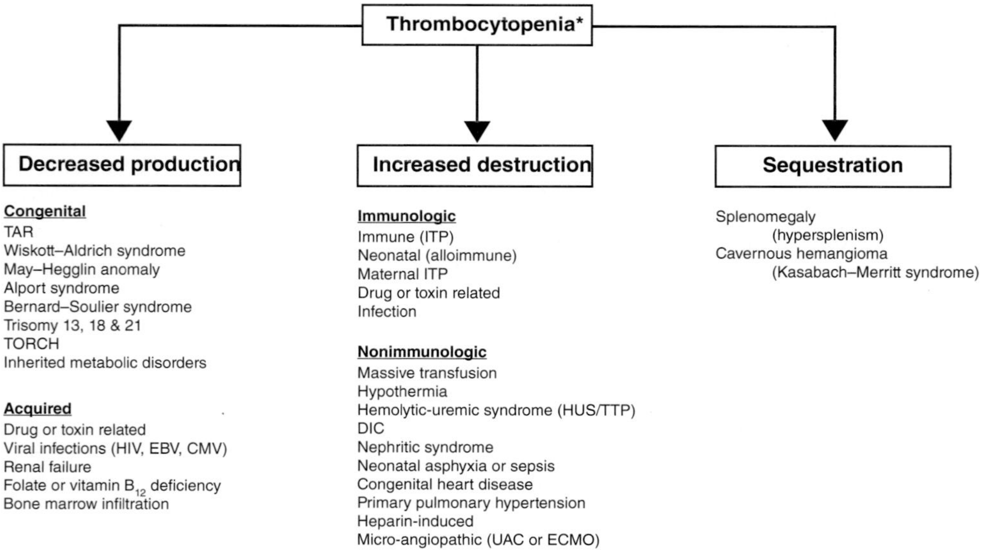

FIGURE 93.3. Differential diagnosis of thrombocytopenia.
**Note*: "Pseudo-thrombocytopenia" occurs with platelet clumping, either spontaneously or from collection-tube preservatives (EDTA or citrate). TAR, thrombocytopenia with absent radius; TORCH, toxoplasmosis, other infections, rubella, cytomegalovirus infection, and herpes simplex; HIV, human immunodeficiency virus; EBV, Epstein–Barr virus; CMV, cytomegalovirus; ITP, immune thrombocytopenic purpura; DIC, disseminated intravascular coagulopathy; UAC, umbilical artery catheter; ECMO, extracorporeal membrane oxygenation. (Adapted from Sadowitz PD, Amanullah S, Souid AK. Hematologic emergencies in the pediatric emergency room. *Emerg Med Clin North Am* 2002;20(1):177–98.)

[250 IU/kg]) is effective in Rh-positive patients. Aspirin and nonsteroidal anti-inflammatory drugs (NSAIDs) should be avoided in all thrombocytopenic patients.

Hypersplenism (enlarged spleen or accessory spleens) causes thrombocytopenia by sequestration or destruction of circulating cells. The differential diagnosis for a chronically enlarged spleen includes portal hypertension, storage cell disease, lymphoproliferative disease and hematologic malignancy, and hemolytic anemia.

Postoperative (dilutional) thrombocytopenia occurs with massive blood loss and volume replacement. Surgeries associated with higher bleeding complications (e.g., neurosurgery, cardiac surgery, or organ transplantation) may require a higher threshold for treatment.

Neonatal thrombocytopenia occurs in infants between birth and 2 months. Neonatal conditions that impact platelet production are viral infections (TORCH), medication (ranitidine, milrinone), hepatic disease, maternal factors (pregnancy-induced hypertension and gestational diabetes), leukemia, and intrauterine growth retardation. Causes due to consumptive processes are thrombosis (catheter-related), infections (disseminated intravascular coagulopathy), vascular malformations (hemangiomas with Kasabach–Merritt syndrome), and hypoxia/asphyxia. Thrombocytopenia in other conditions may be secondary to both decreased production and consumption and include infectious processes (viral, bacterial, fungal) or stress (necrotizing enterocolitis, surgery). Finally, thrombocytopenia that occurs less than 24 hours after birth often represents immune-mediated destruction or inherited platelet abnormality. Maternal transfer of antiplatelet antibodies can cause ITP and *neonatal alloimmune thrombocytopenia* (NAIT). Other conditions that cause thrombocytopenia at birth include congenital infections (TORCH—toxoplasmosis, other infections, rubella, CMV infection, and herpes simplex) and congenital thrombocytopenia due to inherited genetic mutations. A careful family history that evaluates for bleeding problems and/or platelet abnormalities should be obtained. Physical exam should include neurologic examination and search for evidence of bruising or abnormal bleeding. The size of the liver and spleen should be noted. When platelet counts are <30,000/mm^3, a head ultrasound to evaluate for intraventricular hemorrhage is common. For persistent cases of neonatal thrombocytopenia, imaging with magnetic resonance imaging (MRI), computed tomography (CT), or angiography of the head, chest, and abdomen may be necessary to evaluate for hemangiomas and/or vascular malformations. NAIT often begins in utero and may necessitate fetal therapy in future pregnancies. Over the 2–3 days following birth, intracranial bleeding and severe thrombocytopenia (<20,000/mm^3) may occur. These neonates are transfused with matched (antigen-negative) platelets. In the emergent setting, random donor platelets are often used. Prompt recognition and consultation with a pediatric hematologist is crucial. Newborns with NAIT should undergo urgent neuroimaging to assess for intracranial bleeding. If platelets cannot be maintained at >20,000/mm^3 with transfusion, consideration should be given to IVIG (0.4–1 g/kg/d for 1–5 days) and (1 mg/kg IV every 8 hours) until platelet counts improve (>30,000–50,000/mm^3).

Thrombocytopathy (Platelet Dysfunction)

Thrombocytopathy implies a normal number of platelets with impairment in their biochemical functionality. These disorders can result in increased bleeding or hypercoagulability. Inherited rare forms include gray platelet syndrome (reduction or absence of platelet α granules) and Glanzmann thrombasthenia (absent or defective platelet fibrinogen receptor). In the ICU, the most common problems with platelet function are the acquired forms. Causes of acquired functional platelet disorders include uremia, autoimmune disorders, infections, liver disease, nutritional deficiencies, and drugs. Salicylates, NSAIDs, and antibiotics are medications that affect platelet function. NSAIDs inhibit platelet COX, but, in contrast to salicylates, their effects last <4–8 hours depending on the half-life of the medication. High-dose penicillin and cephalosporin antibiotics prolong bleeding time by reducing platelet adhesion and activation. Heparin, organic nitrates (nitroprusside and nitroglycerin), fish oils, and herbal medications (garlic) also affect platelet function. Quantitative tests to assess platelet function are available, such as whole-blood platelet aggregation testing, and the PFA-100.

THROMBOTIC DISEASES

Pathophysiology

The coagulation system attempts to confine thrombin generation to the site of an injury and avoid thrombotic events (**Fig. 93-4**). Endothelial-dependent inhibition of coagulation includes protein C (and its cofactor, protein S) and tissue factor pathway inhibitor (TFPI). The proteolytic site of thrombin cleaves a peptide from protein C, converting it to activated protein C (APC). APC enzymatically cleaves factors Va and VIIIa. The function of APC in the inactivation of factors Va and VIIIa is facilitated by protein S. TFPI is the major inhibitor of the tissue factor pathway that regulates the conversion of factor VII to VIIa after tissue factor has been exposed at the site of tissue injury. Hepatic-dependent aspects of the anticoagulant system include antithrombin III (AT-III), heparin cofactor (HC) II, and plasminogen. AT-III irreversibly inhibits the function of several activated coagulation factors, including IIa, IXa, Xa, XIa, and XIIa. AT-III activity is enhanced by administration of therapeutic heparin concentrations and by endogenous glycosaminoglycans, such as heparin sulfate, found on the endothelial surface. HC II is

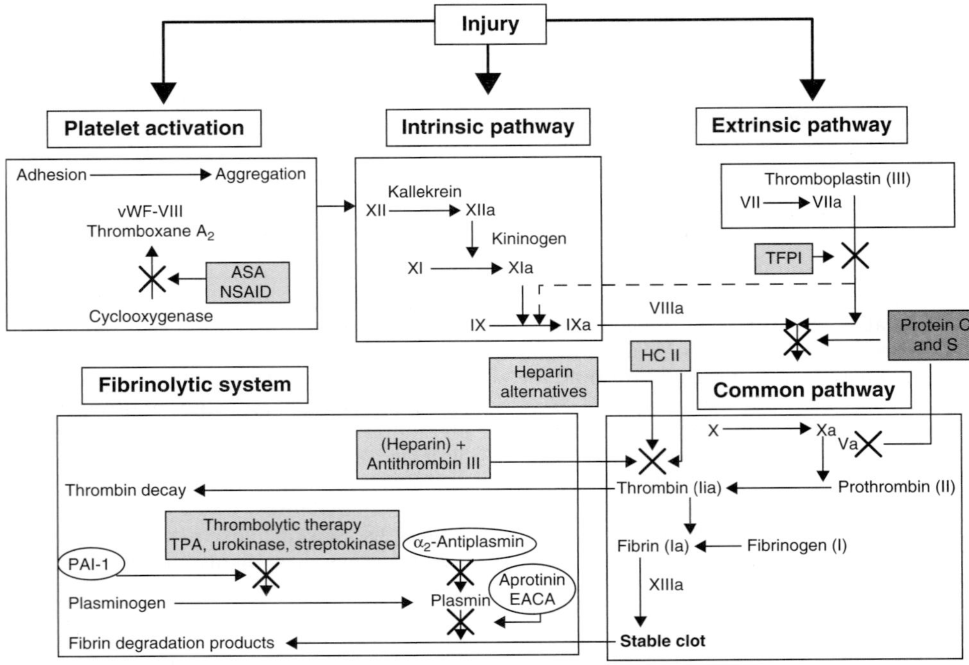

FIGURE 93.4. Coagulation cascade. "X" indicates sites of inhibition/inactivation. Anticoagulants are indicated in *gray*. Proteins C and S, antithrombin III, HC II, and TFPI are considered "natural anticoagulants" (inhibitors). Antifibrinolytics are indicated in *circles*. PAI-1 and α_2-antiplasmin are "natural antifibrinolytics." vWF, von Willebrand factor; ASA, aspirin; NSAID, nonsteroidal anti-inflammatory drug; TFPI, tissue factor pathway inhibitor; HC II, heparin cofactor II; PAI-1, plasminogen activator inhibitor; tPA, tissue plasminogen activator; EACA, ε-aminocaproic acid.

a hepatic-synthesized plasma protein that inhibits thrombin and is stimulated by dermatan sulfate and heparin sulfate. Plasminogen is converted to the proteolytic enzyme plasmin whose major function is to dissolve fibrin clots and restore patency to the vascular system. The two physiologic activators of plasminogen are tissue plasminogen activator (tPA) and urinary-type plasminogen activator (*urokinase*). Thrombin generation by the coagulation cascade stimulates release of tPA from endothelial cells. tPA forms a complex with fibrin and converts plasminogen to plasmin. Kallikrein, a protein component of the plasma contact activation system, stimulates the release of urokinase from the kidney. Exogenously produced forms of tPA, urokinase, and streptokinase (another plasminogen activator, produced by α-hemolytic streptococci) have been used as therapeutic agents in the treatment of thrombotic disease.

Reported incidence of venous thrombosis in hospitalized children has increased to 22–58 per 10,000 hospital admissions. The highest rates of thrombotic disease occur in infants with a second peak during adolescence. Various acquired or inherited disorders place the pediatric patient at risk for thrombotic diseases. The majority of children (70%–95%) possess one or more comorbid features that place them at risk. In adults ~50% of venous thromboses are idiopathic. Arterial thrombotic disease is less common in children, but is associated with significant morbidity and mortality. Age is an important risk factor for arterial thrombosis (45% occur in children <6 months). Risk factors for arterial thrombosis include arterial catheters, cardiac disease, infection, vascular abnormalities, autoimmune/inflammatory disease, malignancy, HIT, and thrombophilia (especially AT deficiency, protein C deficiency, elevated lipoprotein a, and antiphospholipid antibody syndrome [APS]).

Acquired Diseases

The majority of pediatric thrombosis have at least one risk factor, with many having multiple risk factors. Common risk factors for PICU patients include vascular catheters, oncologic disease, nephrotic syndrome, autoimmune disease, HIT, hemoglobinopathies, and congenital heart disease.

CVCs represent the most common acquired risk factor for thrombotic events. The femoral location is consistently associated with a higher risk of thrombosis compared to other locations in children, subclavian location is associated with increased risk in some studies, and jugular location has the lowest risk. Percutaneous insertion is associated with a higher risk of thrombosis than tunneled lines. Multilumen CVCs have been reported to have a higher risk.

Oncologic diseases may predispose to thrombotic events because of endothelial damage induced by the malignancy, by effects of chemotherapy on proteins involved in hemostasis, by hyperleukocytosis and hyperviscosity, or by inflammation related to infection or the oncologic process. One example is the prothrombotic state produced by the chemotherapeutic agent, L-asparaginase, which depresses AT-III levels.

Nephrotic syndrome has a prevalence of thrombosis of 3%–30%, with adolescents at highest risk. The most common thrombotic events included renal vein thrombosis, DVT, and pulmonary embolism (PE). Hematologic abnormalities in nephrotic syndrome include increased plasma concentrations of fibrinogen, V, and VIII; increased von Willebrand factor (vWF); low AT-III levels; increased platelet aggregation; and depressed fibrinolysis. The severity of the changes correlates with the severity of the nephrotic syndrome and serum albumin concentrations.

Systemic lupus erythematosus (SLE) and autoimmune disorders may predispose patients to thromboembolic diseases, and increased risk is associated with the APS. Antiphospholipid antibodies (aPLs) have prothrombotic effects related to their effects on phospholipids located on the vascular endothelium or the surface of platelets. Testing for lupus anticoagulant often starts with testing for prolongation of the activated partial thromboplastin time (aPTT) and/or dilute Russell's viper venom time. A mixing test can be conducted to identify whether any prolongation of the clotting time is a result of coagulation factor deficiency or inhibition from the lupus anticoagulant. Additional laboratory testing for aPLs typically includes assessment for IgM and IgG directed against the phospholipid cardiolipin, as well as the cofactor plasma protein β_2-glycoprotein 1. The constellation of recurrent arterial or venous thrombosis, recurrent fetal losses, thrombocytopenia, and aPLs is known as the APS. Treatment of APS remains controversial, with limited prospective data on which to base clinical decisions. Treatment strategies aimed at reducing the aPLs include corticosteroids, immunosuppressive agents, IVIG, and plasmapheresis. Perioperative measures may include the use of heparin prophylaxis, maintenance of adequate hydration, early ambulation, and sequential compression devices for the lower extremities.

HIT occurs when antibodies are formed against an antigenic complex composed of heparin and platelet factor 4. Platelet factor 4, a protein stored in the α-granule, binds heparin. The platelet factor 4/heparin complex binds heparin antibodies and activates platelets, leading to their clearance from the circulation. HIT can develop after exposure to either unfractionated (UFH) or low-molecular-weight heparin (LMWH), although the incidence is highest with UFH. Exposure to heparin can occur from a bolus or an infusion, through the IV or subcutaneous route. The platelet count decreases 5–14 days after exposure to heparin. If circulating anti-heparin IgG antibody is already present, the platelet count may fall immediately on re-exposure to heparin. Thrombotic complications occur in a minority of children with laboratory evidence of HIT; however, thromboses may be life- or limb-threatening. The commonly available ELISA test for anti-PF4/heparin antibodies is highly sensitive (>95%) but has limited specificity (75%–90%). A functional assay, the ^{14}C serotonin release assay, is highly sensitive and specific (>95% for each), but is not widely available. Clinical scoring systems are available to assist with diagnosis; however, none have been validated in children. Treatment of HIT includes the cessation of heparin administration, evaluation for thrombosis in the upper and lower extremities, and use of alternative anticoagulants (direct thrombin inhibitors, see below).

Hemoglobinopathies (SCD) are associated with venous and arterial thrombotic events. Patients with SCD have depressed levels of protein S, protein C, factor V, and factor VII, elevated levels of vWF and factor VIII, increased adherence of sickle cells to endothelium, and platelet activation due to abnormal endothelial function.

Congenital heart disease in critically ill children is associated with thrombosis. Risk of thrombosis in these children is associated with young age (<6 months), severity of illness, mechanical ventilation, use of CVCs, oxygen saturation <85%, heart transplantation, hypothermic circulatory arrest, and extracorporeal support. Coexisting disorders of enhanced coagulation function, depressed antithrombotic function, or predisposition for thrombotic events (including factor V Leiden, protein C deficiency, and elevated levels of lipoprotein A) may further increase the incidence of thrombotic complications in patients with CHD.

Other acquired diseases associated with thrombosis include meningitis, mastoiditis, and otitis media. In these diseases the thrombotic complications occur in the direct vicinity of the disease process due to a localized vasculitis associated with the infection. Thromboses may occur at sites distal to the infection in patients with systemic bacteremia. In addition to SLE, other disease processes (Takayasu arteritis, Kawasaki disease) that result in vasculitis may also lead to thrombotic complications. Prothrombotic changes occur in patients with inflammatory bowel disease (ulcerative colitis), including increased fibrinogen and factor VIII, accelerated thromboplastin generation, and decreased protein C. Severe dehydration or shock may predispose children to thrombotic sequelae. Pregnancy, smoking, or medications (oral contraceptives) are risk factors. Metabolic diseases, either acquired or inherited, including diabetes mellitus, homocystinuria, increased lipoprotein A, and galactosemia, may also be associated with an increased risk of thrombotic complications.

Inherited/Congenital Diseases

Protein S/C and Resistance to APC (Factor V Leiden). Defects may involve protein S, protein C, or a mutation in the factor V gene, which confers resistance to the effects of APC. Protein C deficiency may result from a low concentration of normally functioning protein C (type I) or normal concentration of a defective protein C molecule (type II). Treatment involves acute therapy, including heparin, LMWH, or thrombolytic agents, or prophylactic therapy, to prevent recurrent thrombotic complications. In the homozygous state, treatment necessitates providing a source of protein C by the administration of fresh frozen plasma. In the adult Caucasian population, protein S deficiency is present in 1%–5% of patients who have a thrombotic event. Acquired protein S deficiency may also occur associated with inflammation, estrogen administration, or pregnancy. Factor V Leiden is relatively common, especially in the northern European populations.

Antithrombin-III Deficiency May be an Acquired or Inherited Defect. Acquired AT-III deficiency can result from medications (L-asparaginase) or comorbid disease (hepatic failure, nephrotic syndrome, preeclampsia, shock, disseminated intravascular coagulation, and the use of extracorporeal circulation). AT-III levels <50% during septic shock are associated with morbidity and mortality (mortality approaches 100% when levels are <20%). Treatment includes elimination of risk factors and consideration for long-term anticoagulation in patients with recurrent thrombotic disease. The use of AT-III concentrate is considered prior to major surgery, during pregnancy, and to allow for therapeutic heparinization during extracorporeal support.

Homocystinuria. Homocystinuria is an inherited defect of amino acid metabolism that results in mental retardation, skeletal involvement, lens dislocation, and arterial or venous thrombosis. Depending on the enzymatic defect, the administration of folate, B_{12}, and B_6 may provide effective therapy and control plasma levels.

Prothrombin Gene Mutation (Prothrombin Mutation, Prothrombin Variant, Prothrombin G20210A, or Factor II Mutation). Prothrombin gene mutation results in the increased expression of prothrombin. The prevalence is 2% of Caucasians and 0.5% of African Americans are heterozygous for the prothrombin mutation.

Lipoprotein A. Lipoprotein A is a cholesterol-containing protein with a composition similar to low-density lipoproteins. There is an increased risk of coronary artery disease and stroke in adults with elevated lipoprotein A concentrations. Increased lipoprotein A concentrations (≥50 mg/dL) are seen in 22% of children with arterial disease and 13.8% of children with venous involvement.

Platelet disorders. Platelet disorders may manifest as a prothrombotic state. They may manifest as peripheral venous/arterial thrombosis, but more commonly result in early myocardial infarction in otherwise normal coronary arteries.

Diagnosis

Symptoms of arterial thromboses are straightforward with total occlusion, a painful, cold, and pulseless extremity. Symptoms of venous thromboses depend on the site (unilateral swelling with extremity involvement, superior vena cava syndrome or chylothorax with superior vena cava involvement, and hepatomegaly and ascites with inferior vena cava involvement). Loss of patency of a CVC may be the first indication.

Radiologic Imaging

Doppler ultrasonography is used for thrombus evaluation to identify the following features: an echogenic filling defect, noncompressibility of the vein, loss of respiratory variability in vessel pulsation, and lack of flow or abnormal waveforms distal to the occlusion. CT with contrast or magnetic resonance venography has greater sensitivity and specificity to detect thromboses of central veins (intrathoracic vessels or the CNS). Fluoroscopic-guided contrast studies offer the prospect of direct intervention to recanalize an occluded vessel.

Laboratory Evaluation

A high index of suspicion for a prothrombotic condition should be entertained in patients who lack associated risk factors or comorbid diseases when thrombotic disease involves unusual locations (CNS, mesentery), with arterial occlusion, recurrent thrombotic events, or a family history of thrombotic disease in first-degree relatives. A suggested laboratory evaluation for children with thrombosis is summarized in **Table 93.2**.

Treatment

Thrombus treatment includes regimens to prevent thrombus extension and therapies to dissolve thrombus.

Heparin, LMWH, and Warfarin

The most commonly used medications to treat or prevent thrombosis are heparin preparations that activate AT-III to inhibit thrombin and factor Xa. For UFH, Xa assays are preferred or used in addition to aPTT monitoring (especially for children <1 year or with critical illness) due to inconsistent correlation between the anti-Xa and the aPTT. For monitoring, anti-Xa or aPTT is measured 4–6 hours following the initiation of therapy and maintained at 0.35–0.70 for anti-Xa or 60–85 seconds for aPTT. Unlike UFH, which acts against both Xa and thrombin, LMWH preferentially targets Xa activity. The most commonly used agent is enoxaparin, with treatment dosing of 1.5 mg/kg/dose every 12 hours for infants <2 months, and 1.0 mg/kg/dose every 12 hours for children >2 months (doses are halved for prophylaxis). Goal range for monitoring is an anti-Xa level of 0.5–1.0 units per mL for treatment and 0.1–0.3 for prophylaxis. When long-term anticoagulation therapy is planned and an oral agent is preferred, vitamin K antagonist warfarin (Coumadin) may be started at 0.2 mg/kg (maximum dose of 7.5 mg) and adjusted according to the international normalized ratio (INR) of the PT. Once a therapeutic INR level is achieved, heparin or LMWH is discontinued, but should overlap for at least 5 days.

TABLE 93.2

Diagnostic Evaluation of Hypercoagulability in Children

Level I—Initial Evaluation
CBC with differential
PT, PTT, fibrinogen
Factor V Leiden (activated protein C resistance)[a]
Antithrombin activity[b]
Prothrombin 20210 mutation
Protein C activity[b]
Protein S—free and total antigen[b]
Antiphospholipid antibodies (DRRVT, anticardiolipin, lupus anticoagulant, anti-β_2 glycoprotein)[b]
MTHFR T677T and/or fasting homocysteine level[b]
Lipoprotein (a)[a]
Consider: [HIT type 2[b], sickle cell screen/hemoglobin electrophoresis, factor VIII]
Level II—Extended Evaluation
Dysfibrinogenemia evaluation[a] (FDP, fibrinogen activity, thrombin and reptilase time, consider immunoelectrophoresis)
Heparin cofactor II[c]
Plasminogen activity[c]
PAI: plasminogen activator inhibitor[c]
Factor IX, XI, XII[c]
Von Willebrand factor level[c] and multimers [ADAMTS13[b]]
Spontaneous platelet aggregation
Tissue plasminogen activity
Tissue factor pathway inhibitor

[a]Indicates lower risk factors.
[b]Indicates high-risk factors with therapeutic and/or prognostic relevance.
[c]Potential thrombotic risk factors.
Level I tests are often performed in children with thrombosis. Level II tests are recommended in those children with normal Level I values and/or in the settings of recurrent thrombosis or strong family history of thrombotic disease. [] indicates studies to be done when clinical scenarios implicate their involvement.
CBC, complete blood count; PT, prothrombin time; PTT, partial thromboplastin time; APC, activated protein C; HIT, heparin-induced thrombocytopenia; FDP, fibrin degradation products.
Adapted from Manco-Johnson MJ, Grabowski EF, Hellgreen M, et al. Laboratory testing for thrombophilia in pediatric patients. On behalf of the Subcommittee for Perinatal and Pediatric Thrombosis of the Scientific and Standardization Committee of the International Society of Thrombosis and Haemostasis (ISTH). *Thromb Haemost* 2002;88(1):155–6; Schneppenheim R, Greiner J. Thrombosis in infants and children. *Hematology Am Soc Hematol Educ Program* 2006;86–96; and Raffini L. Thrombophilia in children: who to test, how, when, and why? *Hematology Am Soc Hematol Educ Program* 2008;2008:228–35.

Heparin Alternatives

The most commonly used alternative anticoagulants are the direct thrombin inhibitors (argatroban, lepirudin, bivalirudin). Argatroban is metabolized in the liver, with an elimination half-life of 40–60 minutes. Significant increases in the elimination half-life are seen with hepatic dysfunction. Lepirudin undergoes renal clearance with an elimination half-life of 80 minutes (significant prolongations in renal insufficiency). Unlike lepirudin, the binding of bivalirudin to thrombin is reversible. Bivalirudin has a short plasma half-life of ~25 minutes and is cleared by enzymatic breakdown by plasma proteases as well as renal clearance (20% of dose recovered in the urine). No reversal agent exists for DTIs, although modified ultrafiltration can enhance elimination. Monitoring of DTIs involves a target aPTT at 1.5–2.5 × control values. The "new oral anticoagulants" or "NOACs" include the direct thrombin inhibitor dabigatran and the factor Xa inhibitors rivaroxaban and apixaban. Further studies are needed prior to clinical use in the PICU.

Fibrinolytic Therapy

The thrombolytic agents include tPA, streptokinase, and urokinase. These agents activate plasminogen to plasmin, which degrades fibrin. Dosing protocols for central-line occlusions are listed in **Table 93.3**. Medical thrombolysis results in complete resolution of clot in 39%–70% with no difference between agents. Bleeding is a significant risk, including intracranial hemorrhage. Major bleeding requiring transfusion occurs in ~20% of children treated systemically with thrombolytics, and minor bleeding in 25%–70%. Infusions of tPA should be used in conjunction with a hematologist. Systemic low-dose heparin infusion is often used during thrombolysis, with subsequent therapeutic heparinization. Supplementation with fresh frozen plasma, especially for neonates whose plasminogen levels are only 25%–50% of adult levels, may be considered prior to therapy. Hypofibrinogenemia is common during thrombolysis and should be corrected with cryoprecipitate when fibrinogen is <100–150 mg/dL. Maintaining a platelet count >100,000/mm^3 also may help attenuate the bleeding risk. Thrombolytic therapy may be indicated for life- or limb-threatening thrombosis when the risks of morbidity and mortality from the thrombotic process outweigh the risks of thrombolytic therapy.

Thromboprophylaxis

PICU clinicians may use mechanical methods for thromboprophylaxis, such as pneumatic compression devices, with or without pharmacologic prophylaxis such as subcutaneous LMWH or heparin. Available guidelines suggest consideration of longer-term prophylaxis in select high-risk groups including oral vitamin K antagonists for children with long-term home total parenteral nutrition, cardiomyopathy awaiting transplant, cavopulmonary anastomosis, mechanical heart valves, and primary pulmonary hypertension.

TABLE 93.3

Treatment of Central Catheter Occlusion

AGE/WEIGHT	TYPE OF CATHETER AND NO OF LUMENS	UROKINASE DOSE AND VOLUME	ALTEPLASE (tPA) DOSE AND VOLUME
Newborn (≤4 weeks)	Single-lumen Hickman	0.5 mL/2500 U	0.5 mg/0.5 mL
≤10 kg	Single-lumen Hickman	1 mL/5000 U	1 mg/1 mL
≤10 kg	Double-lumen Hickman	1 mL/5000 U each lumen	1 mg/1 mL each lumen
≥10 kg	Single-lumen Hickman	1.5 mL/7500 U	1.5 mg/1.5 mL
≥10 kg	Double-lumen Hickman	1 mL/5000 U small lumen, 1.5 mL/7500 U in large lumen	1 mg/1 mL small lumen, 1.5 mg/1.5 mL large lumen
Any weight	Small/low-volume Infusaport	1.5 mL/7500 U	1.5 mg/1.5 mL
Any weight	Large/high-volume Infusaport	3 mL/15,000 U	3 mg/3 mL
Any weight	3.0 and 4.0 Fr. PICC	1 mL/5000 U	1 mg/1 mL
Any weight	≤2.0 Fr. PICC	Manufacturer does not recommend declotting	

General Recommendations: Urokinase or alteplase (tPA) are the drugs of choice for bolus administration to indwell in the catheter. Length of time urokinase or tPA should indwell in catheter: First dose of urokinase or tPA should indwell for at least 2 h before blood withdrawal is attempted. After 2 h, attempts to withdraw blood may be made every 2 h for three attempts. The second dose of urokinase or tPA should indwell in the catheter for 3–4 h before blood withdrawal is attempted. After 3–4 h, blood withdrawal should be attempted every 2 h for three attempts. If the catheter remains difficult to flush after 2 bolus urokinase doses or 2 bolus tPA doses, a 24-h continuous urokinase infusion can be considered. Urokinase and streptokinase continuous infusion doses:
(a) The dose of streptokinase for a continuous infusion is 80 U/kg/h (per lumen).
(b) The dose of urokinase for a continuous infusion is 200 U/kg/h (per lumen).
Note: tPA is not routinely utilized as a continuous infusion for catheter clearance due to limited data in pediatrics. The urokinase and streptokinase should be mixed in solutions of normal saline or dextrose and water for IV infusion. In patients with a recent streptococcal infection or signs and symptoms of an allergic response to streptokinase, an alternative agent is selected. Unsuccessfully declotted catheters should be considered for removal.
PICC, peripherally inserted central catheter.
Adapted from Children's Center Care Protocol, Johns Hopkins Hospital, Baltimore, MD.

Select Thrombotic Emergencies

PE is a potentially devastating thrombotic disease that accounts for an estimated 8%–16% of total venous thromboses in pediatrics. The electrocardiogram may show signs of right ventricular strain such as Q-wave and T-wave inversion in lead 3, with a deep S in lead 1 (S1-Q3-T3 pattern). Diagnosis is often made by helical CT scan with contrast. Ventilation-perfusion scans or MRI also provides excellent predictive value. Available pediatric guidelines suggest initial therapy with either UFH or LMWH for at least 5 days, followed by ongoing anticoagulation with heparin, LMWH, or oral vitamin K antagonists for a minimum of 3 months after resolution of an inciting risk factor or longer if an identified major risk factor (such as malignancy or nephrotic syndrome) is ongoing. Idiopathic PE or other venous thromboses are typically treated with 6–12 months of systemic anticoagulation. In massive, life-threating PE, further therapies may include systemic thrombolysis, pulmonary embolectomy, and/or emergent extracorporeal life support.

Deep venous thrombosis may occur in the large veins of the upper or lower venous system, primarily in patients with CVCs or immobility, often concurrent with additional risk factors as detailed above. Thrombosis recurrence may occur in 7.5% of patients while postthrombotic syndrome (chronic venous insufficiency with pain, edema, dermatitis) occurs in approximately 26% of cases of DVT. The diagnosis of DVT in the PICU setting is most often confirmed by Doppler ultrasound. CT with contrast, MRI, echocardiography, or interventional contrast venography may also be used when deeper venous structures are involved or the need for intervention is anticipated. Similar to PE, acute anticoagulant therapy with UFH or LMWH is recommended for at least 5 days with ongoing therapy for at least 3 months (typically with LMWH or oral vitamin K antagonist) if a precipitating factor is removed, or 6–12 months after idiopathic DVT. For CVC-related DVT, 3–5 days of anticoagulation is recommended prior to removal followed by at least 3 months of therapy. Thrombolysis or thrombectomy is typically reserved for those with life or limb-threatening thrombosis. Inferior vena cava filters may be considered, especially for children weighing >10 kg with recurrent lower-extremity thrombosis and/or contraindications to anticoagulation.

Arterial thromboses outside of the CNS in children are commonly associated with an arterial catheter. Clinical presentation may include paresthesia (often the first symptom), pallor, diminished pulses, decreased skin temperature, and prolonged capillary refill time. Other categories of nonstroke arterial thrombosis typically include complications of congenital heart disease (e.g., related to mechanical valves, Blalock–Taussig shunt, or post-Fontan procedure), transplanted organ thrombosis (such as renal or hepatic artery), Takayasu's arteritis, and Kawasaki disease-related aneurysms. The diagnosis of arterial thrombosis outside of the CNS is most often made by Doppler ultrasound, with CT, MRI, echocardiography, or contrast arteriography also potentially useful depending upon the site of thrombosis. Management of femoral artery thrombosis consists of UFH or LMWH with subsequent conversion to LMWH or continuation of UFH to complete 5–7 days of therapy. The majority of femoral artery thromboses after cardiac catheterization will resolve with heparin alone within 24–48 hours. Asymptomatic peripheral arterial catheter-related thrombosis may resolve with removal of the catheter, while UFH is recommended for symptomatic peripheral arterial thrombosis, and thrombolysis and/or surgical thrombectomy with microvascular repair may be indicated when significant ischemia is present.

Thrombotic thrombocytopenic purpura (TTP) presents with thrombocytopenia, microangiopathic hemolytic anemia, fever, and disseminated microvascular thrombi causing organ dysfunction, most prominently in the brain and kidneys. Microthrombi in the heart, adrenal glands, gastrointestinal tract, liver, and spleen may also occur. Deficiency in the metalloprotease ADAMTS13, which normally cleaves vWF, is associated with both congenital and acquired forms of TTP. Congenital ADAMTS13 deficiency may manifest as symptomatic TTP in early childhood. Acquired TTP may occur with autoimmune diseases (SLE), bone marrow transplant, or with systemic infections. Treatment for congenital TTP typically involves administration of fresh frozen plasma or cryoprecipitate, while acquired TTP warrants plasma exchange, often repeated daily until clinical symptoms improve. The addition of steroids or rituximab may be beneficial.

CHAPTER 94 ■ HEMATOPOIETIC CELL TRANSPLANTATION

MONICA BHATIA AND KATHERINE V. BIAGAS

Hematopoietic cell transplantation (HCT) has been a successful treatment for a variety of childhood and adolescent diseases (malignant conditions, immune deficiencies, inborn errors of metabolism, genetic disorders, hematopoietic disorders, and autoimmune conditions).

SOURCES OF HEMATOPOIETIC PROGENITOR CELLS

Hematopoietic progenitor cells (HPCs) may be obtained from three donor locations: bone marrow (BM), peripheral blood, and cord blood (CB). *Autologous HPCs* are progenitor cells obtained from the recipient (self). *Syngeneic HPCs* are obtained from an identical twin and are genetically identical. *Allogeneic HPCs* are cells obtained from a human being other than an identical twin. Selection of allogeneic donors is determined by histocompatibility testing between the donor and the recipient.

Histocompatibility leukocyte antigens (HLAs) comprise a highly polymorphic, closely linked group of genes that regulate T-cell recognition and are critical to both immunocompetence and self-tolerance. The two major classes include HLA class I antigens (A, B, C) and class II antigens (DR, DQ, DP). The preferred allogeneic donor source is a matched sibling donor at the HLA-A, -B, and DR loci (6 out of 6 matches). Additional allogeneic donor sources include related mismatched family members. If a closely matched family donor is not available, unrelated adult donors and unrelated CB donors are sought, preferably matching at 7 or 8 out of 8 antigens at the HLA-A, -B, -C, and DRB1 loci.

Less than 25% of potential recipients have an HLA-identical related sibling or parental donor. The Bone Marrow Donor Worldwide program has over 22 million potential unrelated adult donors available. Additionally, a number of umbilical CB banks have been established throughout the world. To date, the use of unrelated CB donor transplantation has been associated with delayed hematopoietic reconstitution, decreased severe acute graft-versus-host disease (aGVHD), and decreased chronic GVHD (cGVHD).

PREPARATIVE THERAPY OR CONDITIONING

Most patients receive conditioning or preparative therapy that commonly includes total-body irradiation (TBI) with additional high-dose chemotherapy (chemoradiotherapy). Myeloablative conditioning is uniform for autologous transplantation because of the need to eradicate tumor cells. The HPC infusion rescues the patient from hematopoietic toxicity and reduces the time to hematopoietic reconstitution. Complications following conditioning include mucositis, infection, bleeding, pain, nausea, and vomiting. Some centers have used nonmyeloablative conditioning to reduce the acute and long-term effects that usually follow HCT. Reduced-intensity conditioning regimens work best in diseases that have an unusual sensitivity to a graft-versus-tumor effect, diseases with a genetic defect, and diseases that may benefit from a graft-versus-autoimmune effect.

PROCESSING AND INFUSION OF HEMATOPOIETIC PROGENITOR CELLS

Allogeneic HPCs may require red blood cell depletion because of ABO blood group incompatibility between the donor HPCs and the recipient. Depletion may prevent a hemolytic reaction and may be lifesaving. Transplants from haploidentical donors (siblings or parents matched at 3 out of 6 HLA loci) and HLA disparate, unrelated, adult donors are associated with a high incidence of serious aGVHD. Some require a depletion of total or subpopulations of T cells to prevent severe aGVHD. T-cell depletion may result in delay in hematopoietic and immunologic reconstitution and an increased incidence of Epstein–Barr virus (EBV)-related posttransplant lymphoproliferative syndrome (PTLD).

Most recipients are premedicated with hydrocortisone, diphenhydramine, and acetaminophen before HPC infusion. Infusion may result in acute reactions, including fever, chills, tachycardia, bradycardia, hypotension, respiratory distress, allergic reactions, hemolytic reactions, sepsis, and, on rare occasions, anaphylaxis.

GRAFT-VERSUS-HOST DISEASE PROPHYLAXIS

AlloHCT is associated with a risk of developing GVHD (donor-derived cells attack the patient's tissues). Risk factors for GVHD include an abnormal immune system in the recipient, donor cells that are immunocompetent, and HLA disparity. The highest risk of GVHD follows haploidentical family donor transplants, adult unrelated donor transplants, and unrelated CB transplants. The lowest risk occurs in transplants using matched, related family donors. GVHD prophylaxis regimens have used steroids, cyclosporine, and methotrexate. Recent regimens incorporate tacrolimus, mycophenolate mofetil, sirolimus, antithymocyte globulin, and alemtuzumab. Although immunosuppressive medications may result in a decreased incidence or severity of GVHD, such therapies increase the risk of serious opportunistic infections.

RECONSTITUTION OF HEMATOPOIETIC CELLS

Hematopoietic reconstitution is accelerated using hematopoietic growth factors, either granulocyte colony-stimulating factor (GCSF) or granulocyte macrophage colony-stimulating factor (GM-CSF). It is not clear that improved neutrophil recovery improves survival or decreased morbidity.

RESPIRATORY FAILURE ASSOCIATED WITH TRANSPLANTATION

Respiratory failure is the leading cause of mortality and morbidity in HCT. Improvements in ventilator management have reduced complications, severity of GVHD, and severity of MODS and improved outcomes.

Infections That Cause Respiratory Failure

In the early posttransplant period (up to 30 days), patients are neutropenic and susceptible to bacterial and fungal infections, especially *Aspergillus* and *Candida* species. *Aspergillus* infections may be particularly severe, with angioinvasive disease. Noninfectious early posttransplant complications include pulmonary edema, fluid overload, drug reactions, congestive heart failure, and aGVHD. Peri-engraftment respiratory distress syndrome (PERDS), previously referred to as engraftment syndrome, is characterized by fever, rash, and pulmonary edema. PERDS is generally mild and resolves with white blood cell recovery.

In the second posttransplant phase (30–100 days post-HCT), viral infections predominate, particularly CMV. The CMV pneumonitis fatality rate is higher in recipients of HCT than in solid-organ transplants. The use of leukocyte-depleted (CMV is an intracellular organism that is latent in lymphocytes) and seronegative blood products has reduced the incidence. Prophylaxis (with ganciclovir or valganciclovir) has decreased incidence and treatment with ganciclovir and CMV-specific immunoglobulin has reduced mortality. Patients in this stage are also at risk for infection with community-acquired viruses and opportunistic organisms, particularly *Pneumocystis jiroveci*. The use of low-dose trimethoprim-sulfamethoxazole (TMP-SMX) or pentamidine greatly reduces the incidence. IV pentamidine can be used in patients unable to tolerate TMP-SMX.

In the late posttransplant phase (more than 100 days post-HCT), noninfectious pulmonary complications predominate, such as bronchiolitis obliterans (BO), cryptogenic-organizing pneumonia, and cGVHD. CMV reactivation, as well as adenovirus infection, should be considered.

Respiratory Failure from Noninfectious Causes

The hallmarks of noninfectious pulmonary diseases are interstitial disease, restrictive changes, and chronic airflow obstruction. These result from radiation, cytotoxic therapy, and ongoing injury.

Pulmonary edema is a common early complication of HCT that is worsened by fluid administration, renal or cardiac dysfunction, and concurrent processes that cause systemic inflammatory response syndrome (SIRS).

Idiopathic Pulmonary Syndrome is an "idiopathic pneumopathy after HCT with evidence of widespread alveolar injury and in which an infectious etiology, cardiac dysfunction, acute renal failure, or iatrogenic fluid overload have been excluded." Onset is generally 50–100 days after HCT. Possible etiologies include HCT conditioning, inflammation, GVHD, and latent viral infection.

Diffuse alveolar hemorrhage presents with progressive hypoxemia, dyspnea, and diffuse infiltrates on chest X-ray. Hemoptysis is rare, although BAL fluid demonstrates hemosiderin-laden macrophages. High doses of corticosteroids may be effective in reducing mortality.

BO affects 10% of transplant survivors. It is due to chronic GVHD, infection, or chemotherapy toxicity. Patients present with progressive dyspnea on exertion, nonproductive cough, and an obstructive lung disease pattern. Biopsy shows occlusion of respiratory and terminal bronchioles with inflammatory and fibrous material. In extreme cases, scarring is present, with obliteration of distal airways. Open biopsy is required for pathologic confirmation. Therapy consists of immunosuppression and bronchodilators.

Management of Respiratory Failure

The need for mechanical ventilation is no longer indicative of certain death. Noninvasive ventilation may avoid complications of endotracheal intubation. Normal gas exchange is not necessary; and respiratory acidosis (pH $\geq$ 7.15) and moderate hypoxemia are tolerated. Treatment of cardiac failure, supportive care for renal and liver failure, and management of fluid overload are important adjunctive therapies. Unproven therapies for ARDS in HCT include surfactant, inhaled nitric oxide, and other pulmonary vasodilators. The use of extracorporeal membrane oxygenation (ECMO) is controversial because of the high patient mortality. Decisions about ECMO should consider the likelihood of disease being reversible and the burden of associated MODS.

RENAL FAILURE ASSOCIATED WITH TRANSPLANTATION

Renal dysfunction occurs in 25%–50% of children in the first 3 months after transplantation, and >10% require renal replacement therapy (RRT). Patients who require dialysis for severe acidosis or electrolyte disturbances have an 80% mortality. Preexisting renal dysfunction may be worsened by conditioning regimens. In a few cases, nephrotoxicity is seen with HPC infusion. Release of free hemoglobin and cytotoxins from cell lysis during storage of HPC may cause tubular obstruction and damage.

Sepsis, with or without hypotension, is a common cause of acute kidney injury (AKI). AKI develops in 25%–40% of patients with sepsis in the early posttransplant phase. Glomerular and tubular injury may be induced by cytokines and inflammatory cascades. Renal infection is rare, but renal abscesses with fungal or gram-negative bacteria occur. Adenoviruses and BK virus can cause primary nephritis while hepatitis B or C infection may cause membranous glomerulonephropathy. Vancomycin, aminoglycosides, amphotericin B, and β-lactam antibiotics may worsen function and empiric courses should be as short as possible.

Hepatorenal syndrome is hepatic dysfunction, poor GFR, sodium retention, peripheral edema, weight gain, and ascites. Patients have pulmonary edema, hypotension, and preserved urine output, especially early in the condition. Urine output falls later and hypotension worsens. Hemorrhagic cystitis may cause bladder obstruction and postrenal failure. Maintenance of brisk urine output is essential in such cases. "BMT nephropathy" occurs more than 3 months after HCT, most often after TBI. BMT nephropathy is similar to hemolytic uremic syndrome or thrombotic thrombocytopenic purpura syndrome. Renal dysfunction may be rapidly progressive. Plasma exchange and immunoadsorption have been attempted but are unproven.

Management of Renal Failure

Prevention of further injury is important and chemotherapy should be adjusted in children with reduced GFR. Intravascular volume must be maintained, despite vomiting, diarrhea, or "third spacing" of fluids. The use of angiotensin-converting enzyme inhibitors should be avoided. Diuretic therapy may diminish fluid overload. Continuous infusions may be better tolerated in patients with hemodynamic compromise. Extracorporeal continuous venovenous hemofiltration (CVVH) is the most common form of RRT. Therapy can be tailored to achieve fluid removal, hemofiltration, dialysis, or solute removal.

FLUID AND ELECTROLYTE PROBLEMS

Fluid overload in HCT patients occurs from excess IV fluid, SIRS, cardiac failure, or AKI. Electrolyte disorders can be seen without AKI. Sodium overload is common. Hyponatremia is seen in congestive heart failure and treated with fluid restriction rather than sodium supplementation. Hyponatremia and hyperkalemia are seen with tacrolimus from altered renal handling of univalent cations. Ifosfamide may induce phosphate wasting and Fanconi syndrome. Foscarnet can cause loss of cations and phosphate.

Parenteral nutrition is often used peritransplant as patients have gut dysfunction, loss of mucosal integrity, vomiting, or diarrhea. Patients should resume enteral intake as soon as possible. Even small-volume, nonnutritive feedings may ameliorate barrier dysfunction. Control of serum glucose levels is recommended, but there is no consensus on serum glucose goal.

GRAFT-VERSUS-HOST DISEASE

The incidence and severity of GVHD following alloHCT depend on donor source, HLA disparity between donor and recipient, sex of donor, multiparity status of donor, type of graft-versus-host prophylaxis, CMV status of donor and recipient, age of donor, and other factors. It occurs in 40% to 60% of patients. It is subdivided into hyperacute, acute, and chronic types. Hyperacute GVHD usually occurs within the first week after alloHCT and before full HPC engraftment but with early engraftment of donor T cells into targeted affected tissues. aGVHD commonly develops between day +7 and day +100 following alloHCT. cGVHD is defined as GVHD occurring after day +100, diagnosed as long as 2–3 years post-alloHCT.

aGVHD involves the skin (81%), GI tract (54%), and liver (50%). Skin aGVHD usually presents around engraftment as a macular–papular rash, commonly on the palms and soles. It can be asymptomatic, pruritic, or painful. It is graded into four stages. The differential diagnosis includes reactions secondary to conditioning regimens, antibiotics, or skin manifestations of disseminated infections. It may be difficult to distinguish from Stevens–Johnson syndrome or toxic epidermal necrolysis. A skin biopsy may be necessary.

GI GVHD presents as diarrhea, abdominal pain, nausea, vomiting, and anorexia. Severe intestinal GVHD may lead to significant mucosal damage, electrolyte abnormalities, protein-losing enteropathy, bloody diarrhea, and massive losses of fluid to the extravascular space. Staging is based on the volume of diarrhea per day and severity of abdominal pain. The differential diagnosis includes *Clostridium difficile* colitis, CMV enteritis, herpes simplex or *Candida* esophagitis, gastritis, ulcers, and post–chemo radiation effects. Histologic features include apoptotic bodies in the base of crypts, crypt abscesses, and loss and flattening of surface epithelium.

Hepatic GVHD is due to damage to bile canaliculi leading to cholestasis, hyperbilirubinemia, and elevated alkaline phosphatase. Staging is based on serum bilirubin level. Hepatic GVHD is the most difficult form to treat. Hepatic sinusoidal obstructive syndrome (SOS), also known as veno-occlusive disease, may be difficult to distinguish from hepatic GVHD. Drug toxicity, infection, and cholelithiasis can appear similarly.

Treatment of aGVHD usually requires systemic immunosuppression with glucocorticoids. Corticosteroid treatment results in complete or partial response in 50%–60% of patients. Only 25%–35% of patients develop complete resolution of aGVHD while another 15%–20% improve, usually with multiple exacerbations. aGVHD resistant to corticosteroids has poor long-term survival.

SINUSOIDAL OBSTRUCTIVE SYNDROME

SOS is characterized by rapid weight gain, ascites, painful hepatomegaly, and jaundice. It begins with right upper-quadrant tenderness and hepatomegaly within 7–20 days after HCT. Ultrasound and CT demonstrate hepatomegaly, ascites, and attenuated venous flow. The mechanism is chemotherapy or radiation injury leading to inflammation, microvascular thrombosis, and sinusoidal obstruction. Liver biopsy may be helpful and the transjugular approach may decrease the risk of bleeding.

For patients with prior liver disease, nonmyeloablative or reduced-intensity conditioning regimens may decrease the risk of SOS. Ursodeoxycholic acid is used as a prophylactic agent. Mild SOS does not require medical intervention while moderate and severe SOS require close fluid and electrolyte monitoring, aggressive diuretic use, reduction of weight gain, and nutrition support. Defibrotide, a polydeoxyribonucleotide, binds to adenine C receptors on the surface of vascular endothelium, alters endothelial cell response to injury, and increases prostacyclin, prostaglandin E_2, and thrombomodulin. Thrombolytic therapies carry a risk of severe or fatal bleeding. Surgically or radiologically placed peritoneal venous shunts or transhepatic and intrahepatic portal systemic shunting have some success. Occasionally, liver transplantation is required.

INFECTIONS

In early recovery, neutropenia and alteration of mucosal and integument barriers make the patient susceptible to bacterial infections. In the mid-recovery period, the patient is susceptible to infection because of decreased cellular immunity, skin barrier compromise by central venous catheters, and disruption of the GI mucosal barrier due to GVHD. In the late-recovery period, impaired mucosal defenses, chemotactic defects, functional asplenia, and qualitative and quantitative B- and T-cell abnormalities associated with cGVHD are seen. During the mid- and late-recovery phases, viral and fungal infections predominate (**Table 94.1**).

Bacteria account for >90% of infections during the neutropenic phase. Gram-positive infections occur with central venous catheters and severe mucositis. Gram-negative infections occur with severe GI mucosal damage. Despite appropriate therapy, infection-related mortality remains high. *Streptococcus mitis* is associated with ARDS and septic shock. Gram-negative bacilli can cause overwhelming sepsis and toxemia. A serious localized infection, ecthyma gangrenosum, is often caused by *P. aeruginosa*.

Viral infection is the leading cause of morbidity and mortality following HCT. Patients encounter viruses through exposure or reactivation. The herpes viruses, including herpes simplex virus (HSV), cytomegalovirus (CMV), varicella zoster virus (VZV), EBV, and human herpes virus 6 (HHV-6), account for the majority of posttransplant viral infections. HSV skin lesions may be atypical and present in unusual sites. Esophagitis is common, and pneumonia can develop. CMV infection can develop early or late after transplantation and occurs in ~60%–70% of CMV-positive patients or in CMV-seronegative patients who receive a transplant from a CMV-positive donor. Patients present with fever, fatigue, leukopenia, or multiorgan disease including pneumonia, hepatitis, gastroenteritis, chorioretinitis, and encephalitis. Pneumonia is often fatal. VZV can present as shingles or as disseminated disease. HHV-6 infection, although rare, manifests as encephalitis, pneumonitis, or graft suppression. Infection with EBV can cause B-cell PTLD. Patients present with fever, lymphadenopathy, diarrhea, or elevated liver enzymes depending on organ involvement. Adenovirus infection presents with diarrhea, hemorrhagic cystitis, and pneumonia. Infections with RSV, influenza A and B, or parainfluenza coincide with community outbreaks.

Risk factors for *invasive fungal disease* include prolonged neutropenia, HLA-mismatched transplant, GVHD or its treatment, steroid therapy, and graft

TABLE 94.1

Phases of Predictable Opportunistic Infections Among Recipients of Hematopoietic Stem Cells

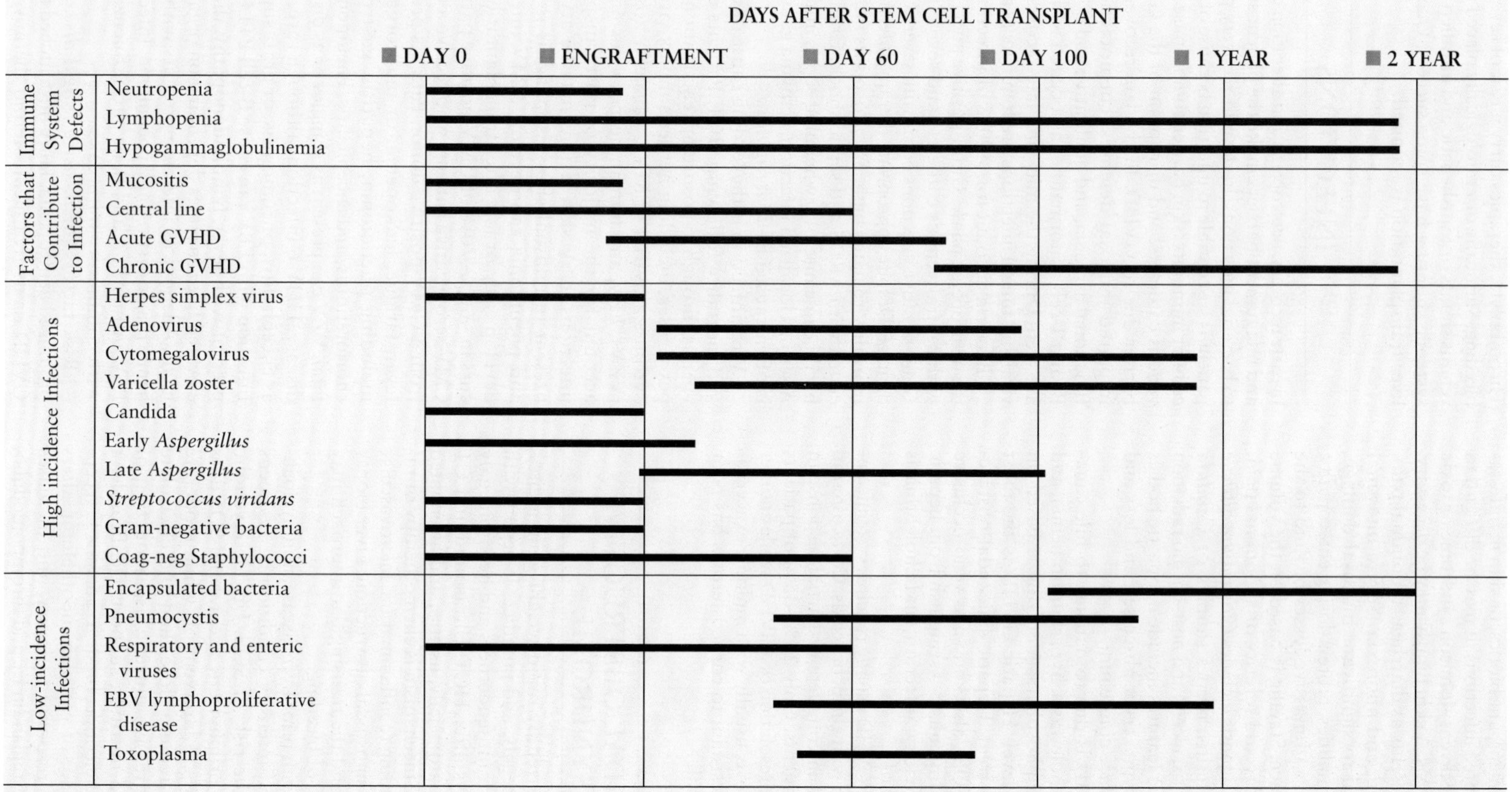
DAYS AFTER STEM CELL TRANSPLANT
DAY 0
ENGRAFTMENT
DAY 60
DAY 100
1 YEAR
2 YEAR
Immune System Defects
Neutropenia
Lymphopenia
Hypogammaglobulinemia
Factors that Contribute to Infection
Mucositis
Central line
Acute GVHD
Chronic GVHD
High incidence Infections
Herpes simplex virus
Adenovirus
Cytomegalovirus
Varicella zoster
Candida
Early *Aspergillus*
Late *Aspergillus*
Streptococcus viridans
Gram-negative bacteria
Coag-neg Staphylococci
Low-incidence Infections
Encapsulated bacteria
Pneumocystis
Respiratory and enteric viruses
EBV lymphoproliferative disease
Toxoplasma

Opportunistic infections occurring in HCT recipients and the time period they are at highest risk. Immune system defects and transplant-related factors that occur at these time periods to contribute to infection.

Adapted from Van Burik J, Weisdorf D. Infections in recipients of hematopoietic stem cell transplantation. In: Mandell GL, Bennett JE, Dolin R, eds. *Mandell, Douglas, and Bennett's Principles and Practice of Infectious Diseases,* 6th ed. Philadelphia, PA: Elsevier Churchill Livingstone, 2005:3486–97.

failure. Diagnosis relies on culture of the organism by histologic methods. Various antibody and antigen tests have been developed for invasive candidosis and aspergillosis (the most common organisms isolated). *Candida* infections may be superficial, mucocutaneous, or deep-seated. *Aspergillus* is the leading cause of death from infection after alloHCT. The usual site for *Aspergillus* infection is the lung. Dissemination to the brain, liver, and skin is common. Cryptococcosis is rare and results in meningitis or pulmonary infection. Zygomycosis or mucormycosis often presents as sinus disease, but pulmonary and disseminated disease may occur.

Pneumocystis jiroveci pneumonia, a protozoan infection, occurs post engraftment. Patients present with progressive dyspnea with a dry cough but can also present with a fulminant course. Hypoxia is present in >90% of patients. Chest X-ray often shows interstitial acinar infiltrates.

Tuberculous and nontuberculous Mycobacterium (NTM) infections can occur any time after HCT. Diagnosis is difficult because of the lag in development of symptoms and isolation of the organism. Patients present with fever, pneumonia, and, in some instances, diarrhea. Primary skin infection and central nervous system disease have been reported.

Prophylactic therapies and empiric therapy started at the onset of fever have improved outcome. Once disseminated disease develops, the risk of mortality increases significantly despite appropriate therapy. Additional strategies include decreasing risk by reduced-intensity preparative regimens, withdrawing immune suppression earlier, and administering immunoregulatory therapy in the form of donor lymphocytes or specific cytotoxic T cells.

MUCOSITIS

Approximately 75%–90% of HCT recipients experience oral or GI mucositis, 50% develop grade III–IV (grade III is extreme sensitivity to swallowing and grade IV is inability to swallow). Oral mucositis (OM) usually begins 5–10 days after myeloablative therapy with asymptomatic redness, ultimately becoming large, painful, contiguous pseudomembranous lesions and mucosal edema, dysphagia, and decreased oral intake. Severe mucositis can cause airway obstruction. Bacteremia may be related to mucosal breakdown. Intestinal involvement often begins in the small intestine and progresses to the large intestine. It is important to distinguish mucosal tissue injury that results from infection. Biopsy may be required to make this determination.

Management is largely with supportive care to control symptoms. Oral regimens incorporate a combination of agents that coat and anesthetize the mucosa and reduce the risk for mucosal infection. IV pain medication may be required. Palifermin (keratocyte growth factor) has been approved for use in patients with mucositis and hematologic malignancies who require myeloablative therapy.

CHAPTER 95 ■ COAGULATION ISSUES IN THE PICU

ROBERT I. PARKER AND DAVID G. NICHOLS

The coagulopathic conditions encountered in the PICU can be divided (by relative importance) into conditions associated with serious bleeding or a high probability of bleeding, thrombotic syndromes or conditions associated with a higher probability of thrombosis, and systemic diseases associated with selective coagulation factor deficiencies (**Table 95.1**).

TABLE 95.1

Overview of Coagulation Disorders

Conditions Associated with Serious Bleeding or a High Probability of Bleeding
Disseminated intravascular coagulation
Liver disease/hepatic insufficiency
Vitamin K deficiency/depletion
Massive transfusion syndrome
Anticoagulant overdose (heparin, warfarin)
Thrombocytopenia (drug induced, immunologic)
Acquired platelet defects (drug induced, uremia)
Thrombotic Conditions
Thrombotic thrombocytopenia purpura/hemolytic uremic syndrome
Deep venous thrombosis
Pulmonary embolism
Coronary thrombosis/acute myocardial infarction
Systemic Conditions Associated with Selective Coagulation Factor Deficiencies
Hemophilia (A and B)
Specific factor deficiencies associated with specific diseases
Amyloidosis–factor X, Gaucher disease–factor IX, nephritic syndrome–factor IX, antithrombin III
Cyanotic congenital heart disease (polycythemia, qualitative platelet defect)
Depressed clotting factor levels (newborns)
Laboratory Abnormalities Not Associated with Clinically Significant Bleeding
Lupus anticoagulant
Reactive hyperfibrinogenemia

OVERVIEW OF COAGULATION

Traditionally, blood clotting has been presented as the "intrinsic" (contact activation), "extrinsic" (*tissue factor* [TF]), and "common" pathways (**Fig. 95-1**). Once initiated, clot production and clot destruction (fibrinolysis) occur simultaneously with contributions from inflammation, platelets, and endothelium. After damage to vascular endothelium, blood comes in contact with TF expressed on fibroblasts and leukocytes. TF triggers a cellular component of hemostasis (by activating platelets to form a primary platelet plug) and a soluble (protein) component by binding with activated F.VII (F.VIIa). The TF-F.VIIa complex unleashes a cascade of protein reactions that ultimately result in the production of fibrin strands, which reinforce the platelet plug. The "intrinsic" pathway begins with the activation of F.XII to activated factor XII (F.XIIa) through contact with a biologic or foreign surface. However, the activation of F.X to activated F.X (F.Xa) through the action of the TF-F.VIIa complex plays a more central role in coagulation, referred to as the extrinsic tenase complex; the F.IXa/F.VIIIa complex is referred to as the intrinsic tenase complex. The term *prothrombinase* describes the F.Xa/F.Va complex, which cleaves prothrombin (F.II) to form thrombin (F.IIa). *Cross talk* occurs between the two arms of the clotting cascade, such that F.VIIa (from the extrinsic pathway) enhances the activation of F.IX (to F.IXa) and of F.XI (to F.XIa) (from the intrinsic pathway), further highlighting the central role of F.VIIa and TF in vivo (**Fig. 95-1**). Furthermore, thrombin initiates various *positive feedback loops* to enhance the "upstream" activation of the clotting process.

Platelets initiate clot formation through the formation of a platelet plug, but more importantly, they also bring proteins that regulate the clotting response (e.g., F.VIII, inhibitors of fibrinolysis, etc.) to the area of bleeding and provide a surface for efficient clot formation. Under unstimulated conditions, platelets do not adhere to the vascular endothelium, but when the endothelium is disrupted (e.g., cut) or activated by inflammation, platelets adhere to the endothelial cell or subendothelial matrix via a von Willebrand factor–dependent mechanism. Once adherent, platelets become activated and secrete various molecules that further enhance platelet adherence and aggregation, vascular contraction, clot formation, and wound

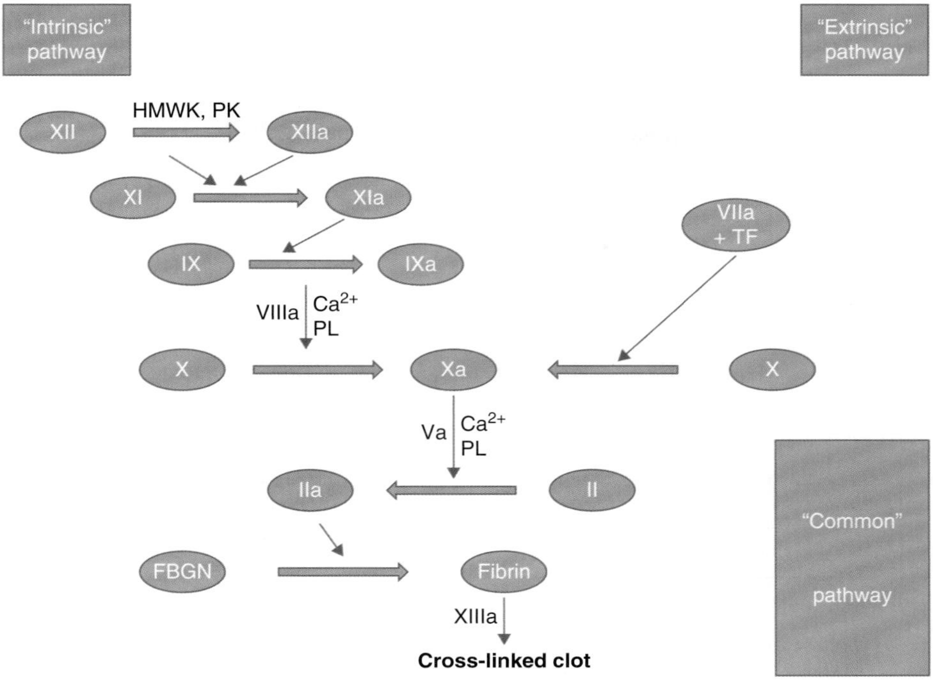

FIGURE 95.1. "Classical" coagulation cascade with cross talk. Thin lines with "+" indicate enhancement of generation of F.XIa and F.IXa by the F.VIIa/TF complex. HMWK, high-molecular-weight kininogen; PK, prekallekrein; TF, tissue factor; PL, phospholipid; Ca, calcium; Clotting factors: XII, factor XII; XIIa, activated factor XII; XI, factor XI; XI, activated factor XI; IX, factor IX; IXa, activated factor IX; VIIIa, activated factor VIII; VIIa, activated Factor VII; X, factor X; Xa, activated factor Xa; Va, activated factor V; II, prothrombin; IIa, thrombin; FBGN, fibrinogen; XIIIa, activated factor XIII.

healing. The normal endothelium produces inhibitors of coagulation and platelet activation and modulates vascular tone and permeability (**Fig. 95-2**). Endothelial cells also synthesize and secrete components of the subendothelial extracellular matrix, including adhesive glycoproteins, collagen, fibronectin, and von Willebrand factor (vWf). When this system is disrupted, bleeding occurs. However, when inflamed, the endothelium becomes prothrombotic.

Interaction of Coagulation and Inflammation

In disseminated intravascular coagulation (DIC), coagulation pathways are activated, inhibitory pathways of coagulation are dysfunctional, and the fibrinolytic system is dysregulated. All of these are consequences of the inflammatory response. During sepsis, TF expression is upregulated in activated monocytes and endothelial cells as a response to endotoxin and other pathogen-associated/pathogen-initiated events. The upregulated TF expression results in the secretion of proinflammatory cytokines and activation of the coagulation cascade including increased thrombin generation. Prior to neutralization by *antithrombin III* (AT-III), thrombin generation produces a procoagulant state that leads to the formation of fibrin; activation of factors V, VIII, IX, and XI; expression of TF and vWf; and aggregation of platelets. Thrombin has anti-inflammatory effects through the production of *activated protein C* (APC) (see **Fig. 95-2**). Concurrent with coagulation activation, there is depression of natural anticoagulant systems, involving antithrombin and protein C (PC), and there is inhibition of fibrinolysis through the production of *plasminogen activator inhibitor type-1* (PAI-1) and *thrombin-activatable fibrinolysis inhibitor* (TAFI) (**Figs. 95-2 and 95-3**). Other causes of reduced levels of AT-III and PC include decreased production (hepatic dysfunction), loss from the vascular space (capillary leakage), immaturity (both levels are decreased at birth and do not achieve "near-adult" levels until 3–6 months), and consumption (conversion of PC to APC).

The Role of the Protein C System

Components of the PC system regulate coagulation as natural anticoagulants. Decreased activity of this pathway results in pathologic thrombosis. PC activation in sepsis and inflammation is downregulated

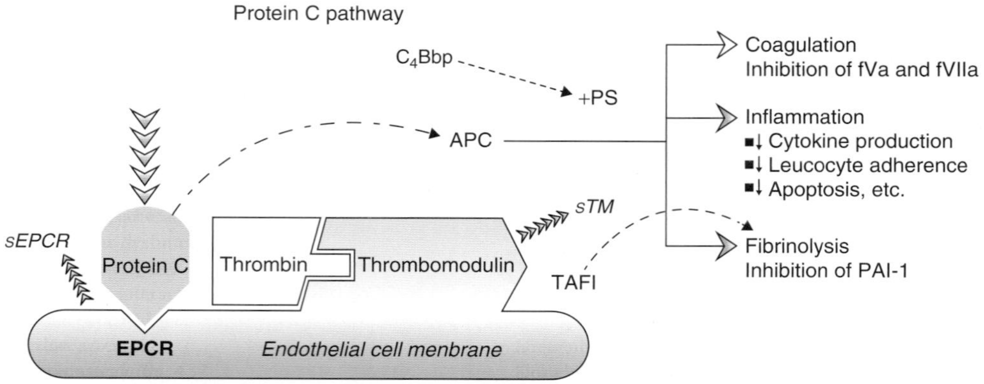

FIGURE 95.2. The interaction of the protein C system with the endothelium. Thrombin bound to thrombomodulin (TM) modifies protein C bound to the endothelial protein C receptor on the cell surface to generate activated protein C (APC). APC acts as a natural anticoagulant by inactivating activated factors V (fVa) and VIII (fVIIIa), modulating inflammation by downregulating the synthesis of proinflammatory cytokines, leukocyte adherence, and apoptosis and enhancing fibrinolysis by inhibiting thrombin-activatable fibrinolysis inhibitor (TAFI) and plasminogen activator inhibitor type-1 (PAI-1). C4Bbp, C4b binding protein; +PS, in the presence of protein S; sTM, soluble thrombomodulin; sEPCR, soluble endothelial cell protein C receptor.

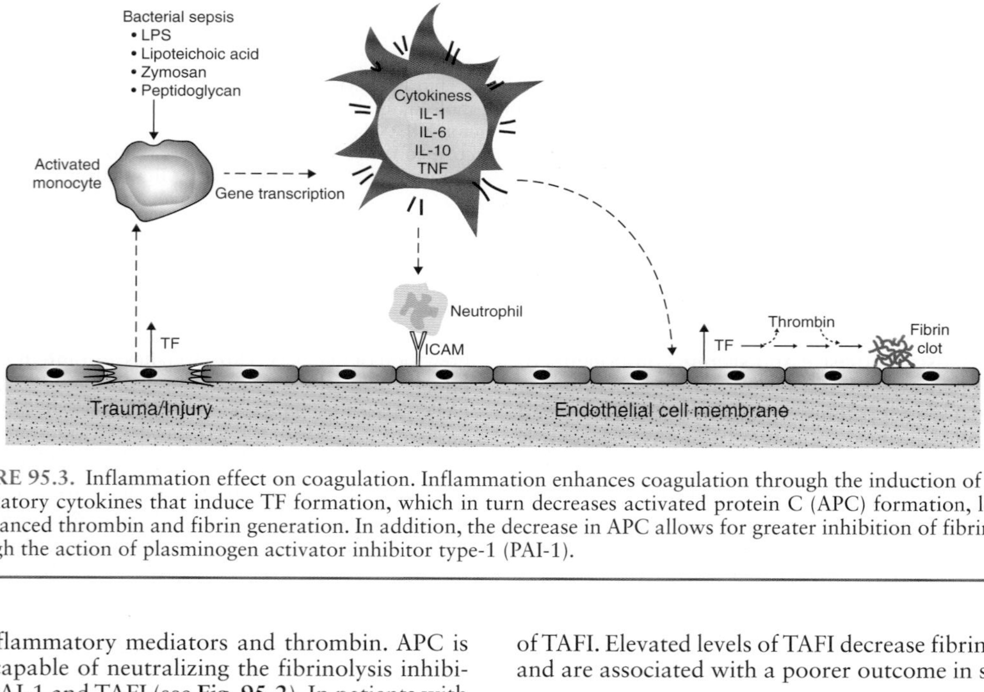

FIGURE 95.3. Inflammation effect on coagulation. Inflammation enhances coagulation through the induction of proinflammatory cytokines that induce TF formation, which in turn decreases activated protein C (APC) formation, leading to enhanced thrombin and fibrin generation. In addition, the decrease in APC allows for greater inhibition of fibrinolysis through the action of plasminogen activator inhibitor type-1 (PAI-1).

by inflammatory mediators and thrombin. APC is also capable of neutralizing the fibrinolysis inhibitors PAI-1 and TAFI (see **Fig. 95-2**). In patients with sepsis, increased levels of PAI-1 are associated with increased levels of cytokines and acute-phase proteins, abnormal coagulation parameters, increased severity of disease, and poorer outcomes. APC stimulates fibrinolysis by forming a tight 1:1 complex with PAI-1 that inactivates PAI-1. High levels of thrombin lead to increased levels of APC, which can complex to PAI-1. The increased formation and clearance of these complexes result in PC depletion that results in an increased risk for microvascular thrombus formation. Thrombin generation also increases the levels of TAFI. Elevated levels of TAFI decrease fibrinolysis and are associated with a poorer outcome in sepsis.

APPROACH TO THE PATIENT WITH AN ACTUAL OR SUSPECTED COAGULATION DISORDER

Clinical History

A history of excessive bleeding or recurrent thrombosis may direct laboratory investigation and guide emergency therapy. Numerous aspirin-containing medications interfere with platelet-mediated hemostasis. Herbal medications may contribute to impaired clot formation or abnormal bleeding (e.g., garlic, ginko, senna, cascara). A prior history of the patient or family member having significant thrombosis (e.g., deep venous thrombosis, pulmonary embolus, stroke) suggests the possibility of a hypercoagulable condition. Patients with *primary hemostasis* defects (platelet plug abnormality) manifest "capillary-type bleeding" including oozing from cuts, mucous membrane bleeding, or excessive bruising. This type of bleeding is seen in patients with quantitative or qualitative platelet defects or von Willebrand disease. In contrast, patients with dysfunction of *secondary hemostasis* (addition of fibrin to the platelet plug) display "large-vessel bleeding," characterized by hemarthrosis, intramuscular hematomas, and intracranial hemorrhage. This type of bleeding is often associated with coagulation factor deficiencies or inhibitors. Patients with severe platelet-type defects may also manifest this type of bleeding.

Physical Examination

Common causes of generalized bleeding in critically ill children include sepsis-related DIC, massive transfusion syndrome, severe liver dysfunction, undiagnosed hemophilia, battered child syndrome, and vitamin K deficiency. Splenomegaly accompanied by prolongation of the PT and/or aPTT may be due to liver disease, while splenomegaly with a normal PT and aPTT may indicate a marrow infiltrative process. Evidence of liver disease (e.g., varices, ascites) points to decreased factor synthesis as a possible etiology of a prolonged PT or aPTT. When lymphadenopathy, splenomegaly, or other findings suggest disseminated malignancy, acute or chronic DIC should be suspected. Palpable purpura suggests capillary leak from vasculitis, whereas nonpalpable purpura suggests thrombocytopenia or qualitative platelet defects. Venous or arterial telangiectasia are seen in von Willebrand disease and liver disease, respectively.

Laboratory Evaluation

Heparin in the infusing fluid of a vascular catheter can cause fibrin degradation products (FDPs) to be falsely elevated and fibrinogen falsely low. Likewise, heparin contamination spuriously prolongs PT, aPTT, and thrombin time (TT). Therefore, 20 mL of blood in adolescents and adults (10 mL of blood in younger children) should be withdrawn through the cannula before obtaining a specimen for laboratory hemostasis analysis. The presence of most bleeding disorders can be confirmed using the peripheral blood smear, PT, aPTT, TT, fibrinogen level, FDPs, and D-dimer fragment of polymerized fibrin (**Table 95.2**). Patients with a thrombotic event generally do not have abnormalities

TABLE 95.2

Coagulation Disorders and Associated Laboratory Findings

CLINICAL SYNDROME	SCREENING TESTS	SUPPORTIVE TESTS
Disseminated intravascular coagulation	Prolonged PT, aPTT, TT; decreased fibrinogen, platelets; microangiopathy	(+) FDPs, D-dimer; decreased factors V, VIII, and II (late)
Massive transfusion	Prolonged PT, aPTT; decreased fibrinogen, platelets; ± prolonged TT	All factors decreased; (−) FDPs, D-dimer (unless DIC develops); (+) transfusion history
Heparin overdose	Prolonged aPTT, TT; ± prolonged PT	Toluidine blue/protamine corrects TT; reptilase time normal
Warfarin overdose (same as vitamin K deficiency)	Prolonged PT; ± prolonged aPTT (severe); normal TT, fibrinogen, platelets	Vitamin K-dependent factors decreased; factors V, VIII normal
Liver disease, early	Prolonged PT	Decreased Factor VII
Liver disease, late	Prolonged PT, aPTT; decreased fibrinogen (terminal liver failure); normal platelet count (if splenomegaly absent)	Decreased factors II, V, VII, IX, and X; decreased plasminogen; ± FDPs unless DIC develops
Primary fibrinolysis	Prolonged PT, aPTT, TT; decreased fibrinogen: ± platelets decreased	(+) FDPs, (−) D-dimer; short euglobulin clot lysis time
Thrombotic thrombocytopenic purpura	Thrombocytopenia, microangiopathy with mild anemia; PT, aPTT, fibrinogen generally within normal limits/mildly abnormal	ADAMTS-13 deficiency/inhibitor, unusually large von Willebrand factor multimers between episodes; mild increase in FDPs or D-dimer
Hemolytic uremic syndrome	Microangiopathic hemolytic anemia, ± thrombocytopenia; PT, aPTT generally within normal limits	Renal insufficiency; FDPs and D-dimer generally (−)

PT, prothrombin time; aPTT, activated partial thromboplastin time; TT, thrombin time; FDPs, fibrin degradation products.

of usual "clotting" studies. While *hyperfibrinogenemia* (>400 mg/dL) and persistent elevations of F.VIII (>400%) have been associated with an increased risk of thrombosis in adults, both may be elevated by acute inflammation. When a thrombotic event is suspected, prior to the initiation of anticoagulation, plasma levels of protein C (antigen and activity), protein S (antigen and activity; total and free), and AT-III (antigen and activity) should be obtained. In addition, PCR analysis for mutations in the F.V (F.V Leiden; R506Q) and prothrombin (G20210A) genes should be performed. A homocysteine level may be obtained as the thrombosis risk of the MTHFR mutation may be related to elevations of homocysteine caused by alterations in the metabolism of folic acid. The intensive care physician must look for confounding clinical conditions, such as dehydration (in cerebral venous sinus thrombosis), indwelling catheters, vascular compression (e.g., cervical ribs), and type II heparin-induced thrombocytopenia (see below) in evaluating children with thrombosis.

CONDITIONS ASSOCIATED WITH SERIOUS BLEEDING OR SERIOUS HEMOSTATIC SEQUELAE

Disseminated Intravascular Coagulation

DIC is one of the most serious hemostatic abnormalities seen in the PICU (**Table 95.3**). It is caused by an abnormal activation of blood coagulation, leading to excessive thrombin generation, widespread formation of fibrin thrombi in the microcirculation, and the consumption of clotting factors and platelets. Ultimately, this consumption of clotting factors and platelets causes significant bleeding when consumption exceeds production. DIC represents an imbalance between coagulation and fibrinolysis. Thrombin generation or release of tissue plasminogen activator (tPA) initiate fibrinolysis by converting plasminogen to plasmin, which digests fibrinogen and fibrin clots as they form (**Fig. 95-4**). Plasmin also inactivates several activated coagulation factors and impairs platelet aggregation. In addition to bleeding complications, the fibrin thrombi in the microcirculation lead to ischemic tissue injury. In most DIC, bleeding is the predominant problem, with only 10% exclusively thrombotic. Regardless of presentation, microthrombosis likely contributes to the development and progression of multiorgan failure.

While infection and multiple trauma are the most common conditions associated with the development of DIC, multiple organ system dysfunction syndrome (MODS) and acute respiratory distress syndrome are associated with severe forms of DIC. The triad of a prolonged PT, hypofibrinogenemia, and thrombocytopenia in an appropriate clinical setting is sufficient to suspect DIC. Severe hepatic insufficiency (with splenomegaly and splenic sequestration of platelets) can yield a similar laboratory profile and must be ruled out. Other conditions in the differential diagnosis include massive transfusion syndrome, primary fibrinolysis, thrombotic thrombocytopenic purpura (TTP), hemolytic uremic syndrome (HUS), heparin therapy, and dysfibrinogenemia. To confirm a diagnosis of DIC, the D-dimer assay is both sensitive and specific for proteolytic degradation of polymerized fibrin. A modest elevation of D-dimer must be interpreted with caution in a postoperative or trauma patient because thrombin is produced whenever coagulation is activated in the presence of bleeding. Other causes for elevated D-dimer test include pregnancy, liver disease, and some cancers. Hyperbilirubinemia or a hemolyzed blood specimen may lead to a false-positive D-dimer test.

TABLE 95.3

Conditions Associated with Disseminated Intravascular Coagulation

Sepsis	Retained placenta
Liver disease	Hypertonic saline abortion
Shock	Amniotic fluid embolus
Penetrating brain injury	Retention of a dead fetus
Necrotizing pneumonitis	Eclampsia
Tissue necrosis/crush injury	Localized endothelial injury
Intravascular hemolysis	(aortic aneurysm, giant hemangiomata, angiography)
Acute promyelocytic leukemia	Disseminated malignancy (prostate, pancreatic)
Thermal injury	
Freshwater drowning	
Fat embolism syndrome	

Meningococcal Purpura Fulminans

Purpura fulminans is a systemic coagulopathy similar to DIC that accompanies meningococcal sepsis or other severe infections. The hallmark of this syndrome is tissue ischemia and necrosis due to marked microvascular thrombosis. Patients have severely depressed levels of PC (the degree of suppression correlates with mortality). The use of APC does not affect mortality, but is associated with increased bleeding and should not be used outside of clinical trials.

DIC Management

Therapy primarily addressing the hemostatic dysfunction in DIC should not be undertaken unless the patient has significant bleeding or organ dysfunction, significant thrombosis has occurred, or treatment of the underlying disorder (i.e., acute promyelocytic leukemia) is likely to increase the severity of DIC. Fresh whole blood (i.e., <48 hours old) may replete both volume and oxygen-carrying capacity, as well as provide coagulation

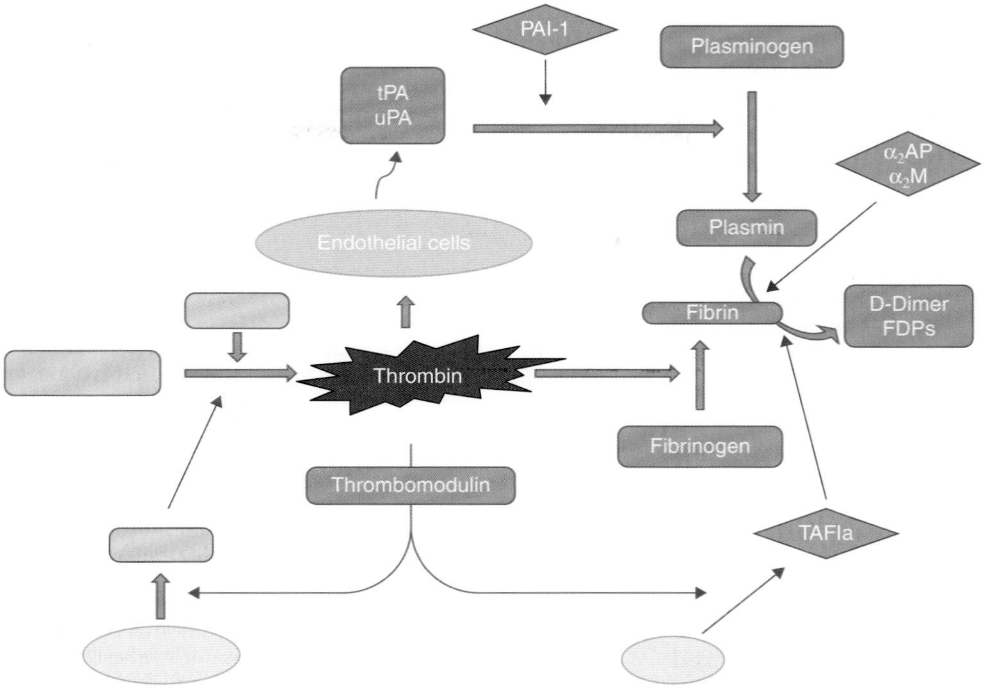

FIGURE 95.4. Fibrinolysis. Thrombin, generated from prothrombin by the action of the Xa/Va prothrombinase complex activates endothelial cells to produce plasminogen activators. These, in turn, cleave plasminogen to form plasmin, which degrades fibrin (formed by the action of thrombin on fibrinogen) to D-dimer fragments and other fibrinogen degradation products. Inhibitors of fibrinolysis (in diamonds) include PAI-1, which inhibit the actions of tPA and uPA, and α_2AP, α_2M, and TAFI, which inhibit plasmin. Thrombin, when bound to thrombomodulin on the surface of endothelial cells, activates TAFI to its active form and produces activated Protein C an important vitamin K-dependent protein with anticoagulant and anti-inflammatory properties. α_2AP, alpha-2-antiplasmin (alpha-2-plasmin inhibitor); α_2M, alpha-2-macroglobulin; tPA, tissue-type plasminogen activator; uPA, urine-type plasminogen activator; PAI-1, plasminogen activator inhibitor type-1; FDPs, fibrin degradation products; Xa, activated factor X; Va, activated factor V; APC, activated Protein C; TAFI, thrombin-activatable fibrinolysis inhibitor; TAFIa, activated TAFI.

proteins, fibrinogen, and platelets. Cryoprecipitate contains significantly more fibrinogen than whole blood or fresh frozen plasma (FFP) and is more likely to provide the quantity necessary to replete the fibrinogen that is consumed by DIC. FFP infusions (10 mL/kg BID or QD) may replete other procoagulant and anticoagulant factors (e.g., PC) consumed with DIC. If the serum fibrinogen level is <50–75 mg/dL in patient with DIC, infusion of cryoprecipitate to raise plasma levels to ≥100 mg/dL should be attempted as a first step. A reasonable starting dose is 1 bag of cryoprecipitate for every 10 kg of body weight every 8–12 hours. Platelet transfusions in patients with DIC should be considered to maintain platelet counts up to 40,000–80,000/mcL, depending on the severity of bleeding. Pharmacologic therapy for DIC has two aims, to "turn off" ongoing coagulation so that repletion of factors may begin and to impede thrombus formation that leads to ischemic injury. Recombinant activated Factor VII (rhF.VIIa) has been used to treat life-threatening bleeding in DIC refractory to other therapies.

Microangiopathies with Microvascular Thrombosis

Hemolytic uremic syndrome is a multisystem disease with renal injury and less commonly central nervous system (CNS) dysfunction (seizures, coma, stroke), GI dysfunction (colitis, intussusception, bowel perforation), as well as pancreatic and hepatic involvement. The diagnosis is made on the basis of prodromal diarrhea and the triad of microangiopathic hemolytic anemia, thrombocytopenia, and acute kidney injury. Endemic cases of HUS are generally caused by verotoxin expressing strains of enteropathic *Escherichia coli* (O157:H7) or shigatoxin-expressing strains of *Shigella*. Therapy is supportive and includes renal replacement measures when indicated. Neither plasma infusion nor plasma exchange has been beneficial. In atypical HUS (characterized by genetic abnormalities in the complement pathway) with severe CNS involvement the monoclonal antibody, eculizumab, may be beneficial. Platelet transfusion in HUS is not recommended due to an increased risk of thrombosis.

Thrombotic thrombocytopenic purpura is characterized by the pentad of microangiopathic hemolytic anemia, thrombocytopenia, neurologic symptoms, fever, and renal dysfunction. While only 40% of patients display the full pentad, 75% manifest a triad of microangiopathic hemolytic anemia, neurologic symptoms, and thrombocytopenia. In many instances, this disorder is due to the absence or deficiency of the von Willebrand factor–cleaving protease *ADAMTS-13*, resulting in the circulation of large vWf multimers that enhance adhesion of platelets to the endothelium. The therapy of choice for TTP is plasma exchange by apheresis, which both replaces plasma ADAMTS-13 and removes inhibitory antibodies from circulation. Platelet transfusions are generally not recommended, except in the case of major bleeding.

Thrombocytopenia-associated multiple organ failure (TAMOF) also involves decreases in ADAMTS-13 in septic patients. Intensive plasma exchange by apheresis has been shown to reverse the course of disease and multiorgan failure in many of these children.

Liver Disease and Hepatic Insufficiency

Abnormal Hemostasis in Liver Disease

The hemostatic defects associated with liver disease involve impaired synthesis of coagulation factors II, V, VII, IX, and X. Fibrinogen synthesis is generally maintained at levels that prevent bleeding until liver failure is terminal. Factor VIII and vWf levels are normal or increased in liver disease because they are acute-phase reactants and are synthesized by endothelial cells (FVIII, vWf) and megakaryocytes (vWf). Many patients with cirrhosis or portocaval shunts also have increased fibrinolytic activity. In liver disease, FDP levels can be elevated because of increased fibrinolysis and decreased hepatic clearance. Thrombocytopenia may be present due to splenic sequestration. Liver disease may cause decreased synthesis of the vitamin K-dependent anticoagulants protein C and protein S, as well as AT-III (synthesized in the liver but not vitamin K-dependent). Decreased levels of these natural anticoagulants increase the risk of thrombosis. The PT, aPTT, and TT will not be affected by the levels of any of these naturally occurring anticoagulants. The INR evaluates the intensity of *vitamin K antagonist* (VKA) anticoagulant therapy. There are no data to show that the presence of an elevated INR (or PT) in liver disease indicates an increased risk for bleeding. This is contrast to the patient receiving VKA therapy, where an elevated INR does indicate an increased risk of bleeding. Patients with liver disease may experience significant bleeding due to severe thrombocytopenia, uncompensated decreases in procoagulant clotting factors or increased fibrinolysis. Esophageal varices due to portal hypertension also represent a significant risk for upper gastrointestinal hemorrhage in these patients.

Presentation of Hemostatic Defects in Liver Disease

In patients with liver disease and impaired synthetic capabilities, F.VII activity levels are the first to decrease due to its short half-life of 4–6 hours. The resulting prolonged PT can occur before markers of hepatocellular injury/hepatic insufficiency increase. As the severity of liver disease increases, the aPTT may also be affected, reflecting more severely impaired synthetic function with decreased plasma concentrations of the vitamin K-dependent coagulation proteins and F.V. When fibrinogen levels are severely depressed as a consequence of decreased synthesis and not degradation or consumption, liver failure has reached the terminal phase. The differentiation of concomitant DIC from fibrinolysis attributable to liver disease may be difficult. D-dimer may be elevated in hepatic failure due to decreased hepatic clearance. The presence of multiorgan ischemic disease secondary to microvascular thrombosis combined with a low F.VIII level (which is not synthesized in the liver) would be more suggestive of DIC.

Management of Abnormal Hemostasis in Liver Disease

Minor invasive procedures such as central line placement can be performed safely without correction of a prolonged PT. When a correction of the coagulation abnormalities is desired prior to surgery in the nonbleeding patient with liver disease, a reasonable approach includes administration of vitamin K and FFP to decrease the PT value to within ≤3 seconds of the upper limit of normal for the testing lab and platelet transfusion to >50,000.

A comprehensive therapeutic approach is required for active bleeding as a result of liver disease. Vitamin K should be empirically administered on the presumption that part of the synthetic defect may result from a lack of this cofactor. The following management algorithm is suggested: Transfuse platelets to >50,000/mL. Infuse cryoprecipitate to fibrinogen levels >100 mg/dL. Administer FFP 10 mL/kg every 6–8 hours until bleeding slows significantly. Continuous infusions of FFP (starting dose 2–4 mL/kg/h) have also been used with success to control bleeding following a bolus infusion. Transfuse packed cells as appropriate to maintain hemodynamic stability and adequate O_2-carrying capacity. Consider rhF.VIIa in those patients with *life-threatening* hemorrhage who are unresponsive to the above steps. With the Food and Drug Administration (FDA) approval of a 4-factor prothrombin complex concentrate (4-PCC) in the United States, this agent is now preferred for the front-line treatment of bleeding in patients with either liver disease of VKA therapy–associated bleeding.

Vitamin K Deficiency

Vitamin K is necessary for the γ-carboxylation of factors II, VII, IX, and X, without which these factors cannot bind calcium and are not efficiently converted into activated forms. Vitamin K deficiency can occur due to the use of broad-spectrum antibiotics, poor nutrition, and the use of parenteral nutrition without vitamin K supplementation. Neonates who fail to receive vitamin K may develop a systemic coagulopathy, bruising, and gastrointestinal bleeding, between 1 and 2 weeks of age. Infants with malabsorption or breastfed infants who ingest medications that interfere with vitamin K in breast milk may develop similar manifestations beyond 2 weeks of age. Fat malabsorption states, including cystic fibrosis, are also associated with vitamin K deficiency. The differential diagnosis of an isolated prolonged PT includes vitamin K deficiency, liver disease, VKA administration (or intoxication), and either acquired or congenital deficiency of F.VII. VKA (e.g., warfarin) administration (either overt or covert) should be excluded. The laboratory findings of an isolated vitamin K deficiency include a prolonged PT with normal fibrinogen, platelet count, and F.V level.

The management of vitamin K deficiency consists of repletion by IV or subcutaneous routes in critically ill patients. The risk of anaphylactoid reactions with the IV use is minimized by slow administration over 30–45 minutes. The usual dose of vitamin K in children is 1–5 mg IV or subcutaneously (up to 10 mg in large children/adults). If the PT does not correct within 72 hours after three daily doses of vitamin K, intrinsic liver disease should be suspected. During active bleeding, 10–15 mL/kg of FFP is typically restores hemostasis to acceptable levels (30%–50% of normal enzyme activity). A similar approach is used to reverse warfarin. The use of 4-PCC is preferred over FFP, 3-factor PCC or rhF.VIIa infusion to treat warfarin-induced bleeding. If rhF.VIIa is to be used, it should be reserved for life-threatening cases refractory to all other therapeutic measures.

IATROGENIC COAGULOPATHY

Massive Transfusion Syndrome

Transfusion of large quantities of blood can result in a hemostatic defect due to "washout" of coagulation proteins and platelets, and exacerbated by DIC-induced factor consumption, hypothermia, acidosis, citrate toxicity, or hypocalcemia. A washout syndrome results from transfusion of large volumes of packed red blood cells without FFP and platelets. Massive transfusion presents with diffuse oozing and bleeding from surgical and puncture sites. Laboratory abnormalities include prolonged PT, aPTT, and TT. Fibrinogen levels and platelet counts are decreased; FDPs are not increased unless concurrent DIC is present (see **Table 95.2**).

When the magnitude of insult and the need for blood are large, both platelets and FFP should be given before a coagulopathy develops. In trauma centers, a fixed ratio of 1 unit of FFP for every unit of packed RBCs transfused effectively replaces plasma clotting factors. In large children (weight ≥30–40 kg or body surface area ≥1.0 m^2), half a unit of apheresis-collected platelets (equivalent to 4–5 units of platelets from whole blood donation) and 1 unit of FFP should be given for each 3–5 units of whole blood or packed cells transfused. In smaller children, 10 mL/kg of platelets and 10–15 mL/kg FFP should be given for each 40–50 mL/kg of blood transfused. Hypothermia is prevented by warming blood products. Electrolyte abnormalities (hypocalcemia, hyperkalemia, hypokalemia, or acidosis) are anticipated and corrected.

Anticoagulant Overdose

Heparin Overdose

Heparin is found in two forms: unfractionated heparin (UH) and low-molecular-weight heparin (LMWH). UH has an immediate effect on coagulation mediated through AT-III. The resulting heparin–AT-III complex inactivates thrombin and slows clot formation. Heparin also has a minor direct effect through inhibition of activated F.X (F.Xa). Because the effect on F.Xa is minor, achieving a therapeutic aPTT with UH is difficult if levels of AT-III are low. In contrast, LMWH effects anticoagulation almost exclusively through inhibition of F.Xa. While this process is also AT-III mediated, it is much less sensitive to low levels of AT-III. Due to its longer half-life (~3–5 hours) and biologic activity (~24 hours), LMWH allows for intermittent bolus therapy (12 or 24 hours) while maintaining a steady-state effect. As the rate of heparin administration is increased, the half-life of the drug is prolonged due to increase in the percentage of the drug excreted by the kidney. The risk of pathologic bleeding increases when the prolongation of the aPTT is beyond the therapeutic window (1.5–2.5 times the patient's baseline aPTT, plasma heparin concentration of 0.2–0.4 units/mL, or anti-Xa level of 0.3–0.7 units/mL).

Serious bleeding from heparin overdose can be rapidly reversed by protamine sulfate. As a general rule, 1 mg of protamine neutralizes ~100 U of heparin. The protamine dose is calculated from the number of units of active heparin remaining in the patient's system (which is estimated from the original heparin dose and the half-life for that infusion rate). Protamine has several adverse effects including hypotension, anaphylactoid reactions, and anticoagulation. The first rule is never give protamine unless there is significant bleeding caused by heparin overdose. Protamine should be given by **slow** IV administration over 8–10 minutes. A single dose should not exceed 1 mg/kg (50 mg maximum dose). *Because of the many risks of protamine, it is rarely used outside of the cardiac operating room.* LMWH is not consistently neutralized by protamine, so elective invasive procedures should not be performed within 24 hours of LMWH administration.

Warfarin Overdose

Warfarin acts through competitive inhibition of *vitamin K epoxide reductase*, which is necessary to regenerate the reduced form of vitamin K. The INR is an accurate indicator of the effects of warfarin once the INR is near target value for 2–3 days. In severe cases of warfarin overdose, the aPTT also becomes prolonged as a result of a marked reduction of the active forms of factors II, IX, and X. Many drugs prolong the effects of warfarin, especially antibiotics. Aspirin does not influence warfarin metabolism, but so profoundly inhibits platelet function that it increases the bleeding risk in patients receiving warfarin (same for clofibrate). Warfarin is metabolized by the liver. The initial dose should be lowered from 0.2 mg/kg (maximum dose 10 mg) in the child with a normal INR and liver function to 0.1 mg/kg in the child with liver dysfunction or other conditions that enhance the warfarin anticoagulant effect. A syndrome referred to as "warfarin (coumadin) necrosis" occurs during the initial anticoagulation with a VKA, characterized by the development of skin and subcutaneous necrosis in areas of subcutaneous fat. This syndrome is caused by the rapid depletion of the vitamin K-dependent, protein C prior to achieving depletion of procoagulant proteins and occurs in individuals who are heterozygous for PC deficiency. This syndrome can be avoided if heparin and warfarin therapy overlap until "coumadinization" is complete (usually 4–5 days), and if large loading doses of warfarin (>10–15 mg) are avoided.

When excessive anticoagulation with warfarin causes bleeding, immediate reversal is usually mandated. The use of 4-PCC is preferred over FFP, 3-factor PCC or rhF.VIIa infusion to treat warfarin-induced bleeding. Ten to 15 mL/kg of FFP is usually produces significant correction of the PT, repeat infusions may be necessary. Vitamin K also may be administered although this will make re-coumadinization more difficult. For severe bleeding or bleeding not controlled by 4-factor prothrombin complex concentrate (4PCC) or FFP, rhF.VIIa has been successful. Treatment of poisoning with long-acting VKA rodenticides ("superwarfarin") requires aggressive, prolonged use of vitamin K, FFP infusions, or 4PCC.

Tissue Plasminogen Activator and Urokinase Overdose

Vascular or device thrombosis or thromboembolism can be treated with thrombolytic agents (tissue plasminogen activator [tPA] or urokinase) that accelerate the conversion of plasminogen to plasmin and enhance fibrinolysis. Newborns and patients with low fibrinogen levels are likely to have reduced endogenous plasminogen, which can be restored through administration of FFP.

The management of bleeding due to thrombolytic therapy includes cessation of all anticoagulant therapy, application of pressure to the bleeding site, and correction of hemostatic defects (e.g., thrombocytopenia or vitamin K deficiency). Topical thrombin may effectively treat localized minor bleeding. Significant bleeding from multiple sites requires FFP transfusion. Aminocaproic acid (Amicar) or tranexamic acid (Lysteda; Cyklokapron) may be used in significant hemorrhage following thrombolytic therapy. These agents inhibit plasminogen-binding sites and decrease plasmin formation.

Platelet Disorders

Platelets are critical for "primary hemostasis" (interaction of platelets with the endothelium).

Quantitative Platelet Disorders

A decreased number of circulating platelets reflects increased peripheral destruction or sequestration, decreased marrow production, or a combination. Causes of increased peripheral destruction include immune-mediated processes (autoimmune or drug induced), abnormal consumption (DIC), and mechanical destruction (cardiopulmonary bypass, hyperthermia). Autoimmune processes such as idiopathic thrombocytopenic purpura (now referred to as Immune Thrombocytopenia; ITP), systemic lupus erythematosus, or AIDS result in increased peripheral destruction and splenic sequestration. Autoimmune destruction also may occur in lymphocytic leukemia or lymphoma.

Immune thrombocytopenia (ITP) involves immunoglobulin (generally IgG) directed against specific platelet antigens resulting in platelet destruction via the reticuloendothelial system. Acute ITP is a self-limited, viral-induced condition in children. In contrast, chronic ITP generally occurs in women and requires immunosuppressive therapy to maintain an acceptable platelet count. Neither condition is likely to have life-threatening bleeding; the frequency of CNS hemorrhage in ITP is approximately 0.2% of patients. Corticosteroids may be given (2–4 mg/kg day of prednisone for 4 days). High-dose IV γ-globulin (IVIG 400 mg/kg q day for 5 days or IVIG1000 mg/kg as a single infusion), infusions of anti-RhD antigen antibody in Rh-positive patients (WinRho; 25–50 mcg/kg as a single infusion) or high-dose pulse methylprednisolone (30mg/kg/day × 3 days; max dose 1500mg/day) are equally efficacious in transiently elevating the platelet count. Splenectomy may be required in patients with serious bleeding who do not respond to medical management, and this approach is chosen less often in children than in adults.

Drug-induced, immune-mediated platelet destruction is usually reversible, and withdrawal of the offending drug prevents further platelet destruction. Drugs used in the ICU associated with this include quinidine, quinine, heparin, penicillins, cephalosporins, vancomycin, and sulfonamides.

Drug-induced, nonimmune thrombocytopenia occurs with most cancer chemotherapeutic agents that produce marrow suppression. The thiazide diuretics, cimetidine, ethanol, and several cephalosporin and penicillin antibiotics may suppress platelet production. Generalized infection and many viral illnesses cause bone marrow suppression or immune platelet destruction. Gaucher disease causes thrombocytopenia by replacing marrow with nonhematopoietic cells.

Platelet consumption and destruction is the cause of thrombocytopenia in DIC. Mechanical destruction occurs during cardiopulmonary bypass (CPB) and cause a 50% drop in platelet count. Platelet counts generally recover toward preoperative levels by 48–72 hours after CPB. Platelets may also be destroyed by high body temperatures seen in severe hyperthermic syndromes.

Acute nonidiosyncratic *heparin-induced thrombocytopenia* occurs in 10%–15% of patients who receive heparin. The degree of thrombocytopenia is usually mild, is not associated with thrombotic complications, remits despite continued use of the drug, and heparin administration need not be stopped (type I HIT). In contrast, idiosyncratic HIT occurs in <5% of patients receiving heparin, and the most significant risk of this form of HIT (type II HIT) is arterial thrombosis, which may cause myocardial infarction, cerebrovascular accident, pulmonary embolism, or renal infarction. The incidence of type II HIT is rare in children (0.33% after cardiopulmonary bypass). Thrombocytopenia in this disorder involves a specific antibody, directed against a heparin–*platelet factor 4* (PF4) complex that mediates the formation of platelet aggregates in the presence of heparin. Clinical scoring systems are useful to exclude the diagnosis of HIT but have not been validated in children. The clinical profile of type II HIT includes thrombocytopenia (or >30% decrease in platelet count from baseline) 5–14 days after heparin exposure (sooner with a history of prior heparin exposures) with a coincident thrombotic event and exclusion of other causes of thrombocytopenia. Diagnostic markers (e.g., heparin-dependent platelet antibodies, aggregation, or serotonin release) are at best confirmatory and not exclusionary. An ELISA assay for heparin-dependent platelet antibodies has a relatively high "false-positive" rate. The more specific heparin-induced platelet injury assay (serotonin release assay) is recommended for confirmation.

When type II HIT is suspected, all exposure to heparin, including heparin in flushes, in total parenteral nutrition, and heparin-coated catheters, must be removed pending the confirmatory test. Anticoagulation with an alternate agent must be initiated because delayed thrombosis can occur up to 30 days after removal of heparin exposure. Continued anticoagulation for type II HIT is provided with direct thrombin inhibitors (argatroban, lepirudin, bivalirudin) or with the heparinoid danaparoid (currently not available in the United States). The direct thrombin inhibitors are preferred, as they carry no risk of cross-reacting with the heparin-dependent antibodies. Of the members of this class of anticoagulants, bivalirudin is gaining increasing preference for anticoagulation in children at high risk for or with documented HIT. Warfarin alone is contraindicated for suspected type II HIT because of the risk of thrombosis from depression of PC levels, which may lead to skin necrosis, gangrene, and amputation.

Qualitative Platelet Disorders

In most cases, discontinuing offending drugs restores platelet function. Aspirin is an exception, as it irreversibly inhibits cyclooxygenase, lasting the platelet's life span (8–9 days). Ideally, aspirin is avoided at least 7 days prior to an invasive procedure. New drugs that target the adenosine diphosphate P_2Y_{12} receptor on the surface of platelets (e.g., clopidogrel, prasugrel, ticagrelor) produce an inhibition of platelet reactivity that may last up to 2 weeks following discontinuance of the drug depending on the duration of therapy. Nonsteroidal anti-inflammatory (NSAID) effects are reversible, and normal platelet function is restored within 24 hours of the last dose. The β-lactam antibiotics hinder the binding of a platelet aggregation agonist (e.g., adenosine diphosphate) to its platelet receptor, resulting in impaired platelet aggregation. Rare inherited disorders include Glanzmann thrombasthenia (abnormal platelet GPIIb/IIIa), Bernard–Soulier syndrome (abnormal GP Ib/IX), Wiskott–Aldrich syndrome, platelet storage pool deficiency (abnormal platelet-dense bodies), and the Gray platelet disorder (abnormal platelet α-granules).

Because many of the adverse drug-related platelet effects are reversible, medications should be discontinued promptly (if not essential for treatment) or substituted for drugs not associated with platelet dysfunction. In thrombocytopenia seen with cancer chemotherapy and bone marrow aplasia, platelet transfusion may not be required until counts fall below 10,000–20,000/mm^3. Current practice sets the threshold for routine prophylactic platelet transfusions at <10,000/µL. Autoimmune disorders associated with increased peripheral platelet destruction, disorders of splenic sequestration, and drug-related thrombocytopenia are unlikely to benefit from platelet transfusion as transfused platelets may be rapidly removed from circulation or exhibit impaired function upon exposure to drugs in circulation. An exception is that children who are to have invasive procedures may benefit from platelet transfusion immediately before the procedure.

Uremia causes a reversible impairment of platelet function. Thrombotic events are also increased reflecting increased renal loss of antithrombin III and protein S from proteinuria. The primary therapy in this setting is dialysis and resolution of uremia. Cryoprecipitate, 1-deamino-8-D-arginine vasopressin (DDAVP; 0.3 mcg/kg IV over 15–30 minutes, maximum dose 21 mcg), and conjugated estrogens (10 mg/day in adult patients) have good results with severe uremia and defective hemostasis. Cryoprecipitate and DDAVP improve platelet adhesion by increasing the plasma concentration of the large multimers of vWf. Up to 50% of patients will exhibit tachyphylaxis to DDAVP and may require 48–72 hours before responding again. The effect of estrogen is protracted and does not diminish with repeat dosing, although a benefit is not noted until 3–5 days after therapy starts.

THROMBOTIC SYNDROMES

Thrombotic syndromes seen in the PICU include deep venous thrombosis (specifically in association with a central venous catheter), HIT, pulmonary embolism syndrome, TTP/HUS, thrombotic DIC, stroke, and cerebral venous sinus thrombosis (most commonly seen in infants with marked dehydration). Both inherited and acquired risk factors have been identified in children who subsequently develop thromboembolic phenomena (**Table 95.4**).

Thromboprophylaxis

There is no consensus for thromboprophylaxis in children and actual practice varies greatly. Pneumatic compression devices are suggested for adolescents who will be immobilized in the PICU for more than 1–2 days because their risk of thrombosis may closely conform to that of the adult population. Prophylactic administration of antithrombotic therapy (e.g., LMWH) is not recommended unless the patient is considered at very high risk for thrombosis.

Management

The initial management for documented (or highly suspected) thrombotic events is anticoagulation with either UH or LMWH. Infants require relatively more heparin (UH) than young children, who require more than older children and adults due to greater volume of distribution, shorter half-life, and age-dependent differences in the ability of UH to inhibit thrombin. Irrespective of the age, anticoagulation is adjusted to keep the aPTT roughly 1.5–2.5 times baseline values (corresponds to a heparin concentration of 0.2–0.4 units/mL in adults, or an anti-Xa level of 0.3–0.7 units/mL). Children <2 months of age with thromboembolism should receive larger doses of LMWH (1.5 mg/kg q 12 h) than children >2 months (1 mg/kg q 12 h) with subsequent adjustment targeted to anti-Xa levels of 0.5–1 units/mL. Warfarin (coumadin) therapy is weight related, with a loading dose of ~0.2 mg/kg/day PO for 1–3 days followed by a maintenance dose of ~0.1 mg/kg/day PO. Congenital heart disease patients who have undergone the Fontan operation are sensitive to warfarin and lower doses should be used. Thrombolytic therapy is not recommended as first-line therapy for thrombosis in newborn infants because of the high risk of hemorrhage. Data for children are lacking, and so adult dosing guidelines are generally followed. Consultation with the pediatric hematologist is recommended before initiating thrombolytic therapy. Newer anticoagulants include direct thrombin inhibitors (discussed above) and anti-Xa agents fondaparinux, rivaroxaban, and apixaban. Argatroban, lepirudin, bivalirudin, and fondaparinux are used as alternate anticoagulants for documented or suspected HIT.

TABLE 95.4

Inherited and Acquired Prothrombotic Conditions

INHERITED	ACQUIRED
Protein C deficiency	Central venous lines (majority of cases)
Protein S deficiency	Congenital heart disease
Antithrombin III deficiency	Atrial fibrillation
Plasminogen deficiency	Systemic lupus erythematosus (and other vasculitis syndromes)
Dysfibrinogenemia	Nephrotic syndrome
Factor V Leiden mutation	Leukemia (and chemotherapy)
Prothrombin G20210A mutation	Trauma
4G PAI-1 genotype (elevated PAI-1)	Prolonged immobilization (>5 d)
Homocysteinemia	Morbid obesity
Lipoprotein (a) (increased)	

CHAPTER 96 ■ SICKLE CELL DISEASE

KEVIN J. SULLIVAN, ERIN COLETTI, SALVATORE R. GOODWIN, CYNTHIA GAUGER, AND NIRANJAN "TEX" KISSOON

NORMAL HEMOGLOBIN STRUCTURE AND FUNCTION

Normal hemoglobin is composed of two α and two β chains, and each chain is composed of an iron-containing protoheme moiety (binds oxygen) and a globin chain of amino acids. The heme groups are identical, but the amino acid sequences of the globin chains differ imparting unique functional characteristics (including oxygen affinity). Hemoglobin consists of two α and two non-α chains. *Hemoglobin A* (95% of adult hemoglobin) contains two α and two β chains (HbA: α_2, β_2). *Hemoglobin A$_2$* (1%–4% of adult hemoglobin) is composed of two α and two δ chains (HbA_2, α_2, δ_2). *Fetal hemoglobin* is composed of two α and two λ chains (HbF: α_2, λ_2). At birth, erythrocytes contain 70%–90% HbF, which predominates until 2–4 months of age. The persistence of HbF offers a protective effect in patients with certain hemoglobinopathies. *Sickle cell disease* (SCD) refers to a variety of genotypes that produce sickled erythrocytes upon hemoglobin deoxygenation, leading to chronic hemolysis, recurrent vaso-occlusion, and ischemic end-organ injury. Patients with the SCD phenotype inherit a mutant allele in which valine is substituted for glutamine at the sixth amino acid position of the β-globin chain. Hemoglobin that incorporates this mutant β^S-globin chain is referred to as HbS, and homozygotes for the β^S allele are said to have *sickle cell anemia* (SCA, HbSS), while heterozygotes for the β^S allele are said to have *sickle cell trait* (SCT, HbAS). Patients with SCT do not express the SCD phenotype because of the protective effects of HbA. Heterozygous genotypes coding for HbS, together with other alterations in β-chain production (non-HbA), can also result in the SCD phenotype. The most common heterozygous SCD genotypes are HbSC and the sickle β thalassemias. Approximately 70% of the SCD patients in the United States are homozygous for β^S (SCA), while HbSC (~20%) and sickle β thalassemias (10%) comprise the remainder. Patients with HbSC or HbS–β^+ thalassemia have less severe symptoms than with HbSS because of the protective effects of HbF (in patients with HbSC) or hemoglobins A and F (patients with HbS–β^+ thalassemia produce a reduced amount of β chains of HbA). Patients with HbS–β^0 thalassemia produce no β chains of HbA and exhibit a clinical course similar in severity to that of patients with HbSS (**Table 96.1**).

TABLE 96.1

Severity and Diagnostic Testing for Relevant Sickle Cell Syndromes

■ SYNDROME	■ GENOTYPE	■ SEVERITY	■ NEONATAL SCREENING[a]	■ HEMOGLOBIN ELECTROPHORESIS IN OLDER CHILDREN (%)				
				HbA	HbS	HbF	HbA_2	HbC
Sickle cell anemia	S-S	++++	FS	0	80–95	2–20	<3.5	0
Sickle β^0 thalassemia[b]	S-b^0	+++	FS	0	80–92	2–15	3.5–7	0
Hemoglobin SC disease	S-C	++	FSC	0	45–50	1–5	NA[c]	45–50
Sickle β^+ thalassemia[b]	S-β^+	+	FSA or FS[d]	5–30	65–90	2–10	3.5–6	0
Sickle cell trait	A-S	0	FAS	50–60	35–45	<2	<3.5	0

[a]Hemoglobins reported in order of decreasing quantity (e.g., FS = F > S); F, fetal hemoglobin; S, sickle hemoglobin; C, hemoglobin C; A, hemoglobin A.
[b]β^0 indicates thalassemia mutation with absent production of β-globin; β^+ indicates thalassemia mutation with reduced production of β-globin.
[c]Quantity of HbA_2 cannot be measured in the presence of HbC.
[d]Quantity of HbA at birth sometimes insufficient for detection.
Adapted from Lane PA. Sickle cell disease. *Pediatr Clin N Am* 1996;43(3):639–64, table 1 on page 642, with permission.

SCA affects 1 in 600 African Americans and 1%–4% of infants in sub-Saharan Africa. SCD inheritance is autosomal recessive.

RELEVANCE TO PEDIATRIC CRITICAL CARE

The complications of SCD that require pediatric intensive care include splenic sequestration, aplastic crisis, sepsis, acute chest syndrome (ACS), stroke, and perioperative management. Chronic injury of the circulatory, respiratory, nervous, renal, and immune systems may already be present in children with SCD requiring intensive care. The fundamental defect in SCD is an abnormality of the β-globin gene that results in the tendency for hemoglobin to irreversibly polymerize, forming a gel that decreases erythrocyte flexibility, resulting in microvascular occlusion, hemolysis, and chronic anemia. The contributions to the pathogenesis of SCD by environmental factors are listed in **Table 96.2**.

BIOLOGIC PRECIPITANTS OF SICKLE CELL COMPLICATIONS

SCD complications are related to interactions between abnormal hemoglobin and the circulatory system. Major contributors to the pathophysiology include the erythrocytes and hemoglobin, endothelial cells, leukocytes, platelets, the coagulation cascade, NO, oxidant-mediated injury, and systemic inflammation.

Erythrocytes and Hemoglobin: The substitution of valine for glutamine in the β-globin chain destabilizes oxygenated hemoglobin (accelerated denaturation), and reduces the solubility of deoxygenated hemoglobin. HbS polymerization results in precipitation and formation of a gel. These changes damage the erythrocyte cell membrane, reduce membrane flexibility and the ability to traverse capillary beds, and result in ischemic injury. The destruction of globin chains results in oxidation of iron to the ferric state and increased generation of superoxide, hydrogen peroxide, and hydroxyl radicals. These potent oxidants combined with liberated iron, denature erythrocyte surface proteins, alter cation permeability, and disrupt phospholipid membrane structure. Disruption of ion transport mechanisms results in erythrocyte dehydration, increased corpuscular hemoglobin concentration, accelerated hemoglobin polymerization, and intracellular oxidant injury. A vicious cycle is initiated within the erythrocyte that disturbs flow characteristics and results in stagnant microvascular blood flow, blood vessel obstruction, and distal tissue ischemia.

Endothelium: The endothelium is active in the pathogenesis of SCD with increased expression of adhesion molecules such as vascular cell adhesion molecule-1 (VCAM-1), intercellular adhesion molecule-1 (ICAM-1), E-selectin, and P-selectin. These adhesion molecules and activated endothelial cells potentiate vascular inflammation. Activated endothelial cells promote thrombosis and vasculopathy through increased interactions with abnormal erythrocytes, activated leukocytes, the hemostatic pathway, and activated platelets. The abnormality of von Willebrand factor (VWF) protease (ADAMTS-13) activity in SCD suggests overlap with the thrombosis mechanism in thrombotic thrombocytopenic purpura (TTP). VCAM-1 expression causes sickle reticulocytes to adhere to endothelial cells. The degree of affinity between erythrocytes and endothelium correlates with clinical severity. Endothelin-1, produced in activated endothelial cells, is implicated in pulmonary hypertension in ACS.

TABLE 96.2

Factors That May Promote Sickling

Hemoglobin Desaturation

1. Failure to oxygenate in the lungs
   a. Atelectasis
   b. Infection
      i. Bacterial
      ii. Viral
   c. Chronic lung disease
   d. Pulmonary vascular disease
   e. High altitude
2. Diminished tissue oxygen delivery
   a. Diminished cardiac output
      i. Hypovolemia (dehydration, sequestration, sepsis)
      ii. Septic shock
      iii. Diminished cardiac contractility
      iv. Pericardial disease
      v. Increased systemic vascular resistance
      vi. Anesthetics/drugs
   b. Severe anemia
   c. Hypoxemic cardiac output (see 1.a)
3. Increased tissue extraction of oxygen
   a. Increased tissue demands
      i. Vigorous exercise
      ii. Thyrotoxicosis
      iii. Malignant hyperthermia
      iv. Seizures
      v. Sepsis
      vi. Shivering
   b. Factors accelerating tissue oxygen extraction
      i. Acidosis
      ii. Hyperthermia

Increased Microvascular Transit Time

1. Increased viscosity
   a. Excessive transfusion
   b. Dehydration
2. Vasoconstriction
   a. Hypothermia
   b. Vasoconstrictor drugs
   c. Tourniquet use (orthopedic surgery)

Leukocytes: Leukocyte adherence to endothelial cells and release of proteolytic enzymes propagate vascular injury in SCD. Monocytes from patients with SCD contain more IL-1β and tumor necrosis factor (TNF)-α. These changes are secondary to a chronic inflammatory state in patients with SCD. Monocytes from SCD patients cause translocation of nuclear factor-κB in endothelial cells. Neutrophils from patients with SCA demonstrate increased endothelial cell adhesion.

Platelets: Platelet activation is prominent in SCD. Hemolysis and cell-free hemoglobin activate platelets. Hemolysis-associated defects in NO activate platelets, and sildenafil decreases platelet activation. Platelets in SCD are in a chronic state of heightened activity, resulting in fatigue of platelet response. Circulating platelet-derived factors such as thrombospondin facilitate erythrocyte adherence to endothelial cells.

Coagulation Cascade: Extracellular hemoglobin inhibits the protease activity of ADAMTS-13 generating multimers of VWF that contribute to vascular complications in SCD. There is enhanced thrombin generation, reduced protein C and protein S activity, decreased factor V, elevated factor VIII, decreased plasminogen levels, shorter thrombin times, and higher serum fibrinogen degradation products. Autopsy studies demonstrate diffuse arteriolar thrombosis and interstitial fibrotic lesions unrelated to large-vessel thrombotic or embolic disease.

Nitric Oxide Scavenging: NO coordinates vascular regulation by inhibiting platelet activation, vascular smooth muscle constriction, release of procoagulant proteins, inflammatory mediators, cell membrane adhesion molecules, and proliferative factors. Free hemoglobin reaction with NO produces nitrate and reduces available NO. Release of arginase from the erythrocyte magnifies this effect. Plasma arginase activity is associated with pulmonary hypertension and mortality. Inhibitors of NO synthase are also increased, particularly asymmetric dimethylarginine (ADMA). Vaso-occlusion results from diminished inhibition of NO on VCAM expression, on leukocyte adhesion, on platelet activation, and diminished NO-mediated vasodilation. Diminished NO levels in the lungs may result in ventilation–perfusion mismatch, regional hypoxemia, and intrapulmonary erythrocyte sickling.

Oxidative Stress: Free hemoglobin can induce oxidative stress. Depletion of glutathione, the major antioxidant of the erythrocyte, is linked to hemolytic rate and the development of pulmonary hypertension. Plasma from patients with vaso-occlusive crisis (VOC) and ACS is oxidative in nature, depleting cellular glutathione and promoting the formation of injurious peroxynitrite.

Perioperative and Physiologic Precipitants of Sickle Cell Disease

Hemoglobin deoxygenation is a potent precipitant of vaso-occlusive phenomena in patients with SCD. Close monitoring and maintenance of oxygenation by administration of supplemental oxygen are recommended. Patients with SCD are accustomed to anemia and preserve oxygen delivery by increasing cardiac output and erythrocyte 2,3-diphosphoglycerate concentrations. Transit time through the circulation is affected by dehydration, systemic hypotension, tourniquet use, and vasoconstriction. Dehydration is also a precipitant of SCD-related complications. Intracellular erythrocyte dehydration especially promotes hemoglobin polymerization in the presence of the cellular, inflammatory, oxidant, and NO abnormalities. Fluid management should provide generous intravascular hydration to preserve euvolemia. Hypothermia restricts oxygen unloading, promotes cutaneous vasoconstriction, increases red cell tissue–lung transit time, and promotes erythrocyte sickling. The benefits of mild therapeutic hypothermia for neurologic protection after ischemic brain injury must be weighed against the potential for hypothermia to promote SCD-related complications. Hyperthermia shifts the hemoglobin–oxygen dissociation curve to the right, favoring the release of oxygen to the tissues and hemoglobin desaturation. No definitive work has related the presence of pyrexia to the development of SCD-related complications. Acidosis has been linked to the development of SCD-related complications. The administration of sodium bicarbonate does not prevent perioperative pain crises. It can be difficult to separate the effects of acidosis from the underlying cause but it is prudent to maintain acid–base status in a reasonable physiologic range.

SICKLE CELL DISEASE COMPLICATIONS

Patients with SCD suffer a lifetime of indolent, ischemic injury to all organ systems combined with periodic acute crises that cause considerable morbidity or premature mortality.

Vaso-occlusive Crisis

VOC is the most common crisis in children with SCD. It rarely requires PICU admission, but may precede serious SCD complications. The most common type of VOC is bony crisis that affects long bones, ribs, vertebrae and in children <3 years, the hands and feet (dactylitis). Symptoms of bone pain can be associated with fever, leukocytosis, and malaise. The differential diagnosis includes trauma and osteomyelitis (common in SCD due to susceptibility to bacteremia). Differentiation may require blood and bone cultures, radiographs, MRI, or bone scan. The white blood cell count and differential do not help distinguish between infection and infarction. If osteomyelitis is suspected, antimicrobials effective against *Staphylococcus aureus* and *Salmonella* species should be started while awaiting bone biopsy.

VOC involving the abdominal viscera blood vessels produces abdominal pain, fever, malaise, anorexia, nausea, diminished bowel sounds, and abdominal tenderness resembling a surgical cause of abdominal symptoms. Chronic hemolysis makes cholelithiasis and cholecystitis more frequent. Evaluation may require X-ray, CT of the abdomen, liver function tests (total and fractionated bilirubin), amylase, lipase, urinalysis, serial examinations of the abdomen, and surgical consultation.

Treatment of VOC is supportive with analgesia, oxygen, antibiotics, and hydration (1.5 times maintenance fluid). Simple transfusion is seldom used, but frequent recurrence of VOC may require chronic transfusions. Successful pain management modalities include acetaminophen, nonsteroidal anti-inflammatory medications, opioids (intermittent or patient-controlled administration), and regional anesthesia (epidural analgesia or nerve blocks). Ketorolac may be useful but is contraindicated if hemorrhagic stroke is suspected. Expert titration of opioid therapy is essential to achieve pain relief, allow deep breathing exercises, promote ambulation, minimize splinting and avoid respiratory depression. Psychology and psychiatry services should assist with identification and treatment of depression and pain-coping strategies.

Transfusion Therapy in Sickle Cell Disease Patients

Transfusion therapy for SCD minimizes vaso-occlusion by decreasing the percentage of HbS-containing erythrocytes in the circulation and improves hemoglobin concentration to restore reduced oxygen delivery. *Simple transfusion* refers to the administration of sickle-free red blood cells, while *exchange transfusion* involves the administration of sickle-free red blood cells with simultaneous removal of the patient's blood. The type of transfusion is based on the desired effect(s) and desired speed of improvement of hemoglobin concentration and hemoglobin S fraction. During transfusions, hemoglobin concentration should be closely monitored as elevations in hematocrit to >33% are associated with increased blood viscosity and central nervous system (CNS) thrombotic injury. Exchange transfusion therapy can be accomplished in infants using an arterial catheter for blood withdrawal and venous access for infusion of blood. Alternatively, a large-bore central venous catheter can be used for withdrawal and infusion. Exchange transfusion can be performed manually or, in larger children, by automated erythrocytapheresis. To quickly reduce HbS percentage to 30%, roughly twice the circulating blood volume is replaced with a solution of sickle-free erythrocytes and fresh frozen plasma (or saline) over 4–6 hours. If the hematocrit increases to >30%–33%, a nonerythrocyte volume expander (i.e., fresh frozen plasma) is substituted for blood cells until the hematocrit falls to an acceptable level. With rapid transfusions or hepatic dysfunction, ionized hypocalcemia may result from citrate toxicity and must be closely monitored. Given the volume and rate of the transfusion, an approved and monitored blood warmer should be used for exchange transfusions. For VOC, ACS, and acute splenic sequestration crisis (ASSC) simple transfusion is offered and exchange transfusion is reserved for aggressive disease and physiologic instability. For an acute cerebrovascular accident (CVA), exchange transfusion restores cerebral circulation as soon as possible. Transfusion therapy, while lifesaving, may have adverse events. Febrile nonhemolytic reactions can be prevented by filtering leukocytes from the blood before administration. Strategies to minimize the development of alloimmunization include extended crossmatching of red blood cell units to minor antigen loci, and use of a limited donor program. Leukoreduced blood specifically crossmatched against minor antigens C, E, and Kell helps reduce the risk of alloimmunization. Corticosteroids, with or without intravenous immunoglobulin, can help prevent posttransfusion hemolysis of both autologous and transfused blood cells seen uncommonly in SCD patients who develop autoantibodies to their, and transfused, red blood cells. Leukocyte reduction of transfused blood products is recommended to prevent alloimmunization to human leukocyte antigens (HLAs) and platelet-specific antibodies that limit the efficacy of platelet transfusion support in patients who subsequently undergo hematopoietic stem cell transplantation (HSCT). Nonimmune complications of transfusion include iron overload (treated with deferoxamine or deferasirox) and blood-borne infections.

Acute Chest Syndrome

ACS is characterized by fever, cough, pleuritic chest pain, tachypnea, hypoxemia, and new or rapidly progressive pulmonary infiltrate(s) on chest radiograph. Patients with ACS demonstrate an abrupt decrease in platelet count and hematocrit. Risk factors for ACS include younger age, higher hemoglobin level, lower HbF percentage, increased neutrophil count, history of asthma in children, active smoking, and environmental smoke exposure. ACS can progress rapidly to acute respiratory failure resembling acute respiratory distress syndrome (ARDS) and resulting in substantial morbidity and mortality. ACS is a leading cause of premature death; mortality is associated with acute lung injury (ALI) combined with pulmonary hypertension and right ventricular (RV) dysfunction. The etiology of ACS includes pulmonary or systemic infection, embolism, and direct pulmonary infarction. ACS occurs within 1–3 days in 10%–20% of patients admitted for severe VOC. An infectious agent (mostly atypical bacteria or viruses) is identified in 54% of ACS admissions (including respiratory syncytial virus, parvovirus, rhinovirus, parainfluenza virus, influenza A and B, and the H1N1 virus) (**Fig. 96.1**). Encapsulated bacteria are rarely isolated despite functional asplenia (*Staphylococcus*

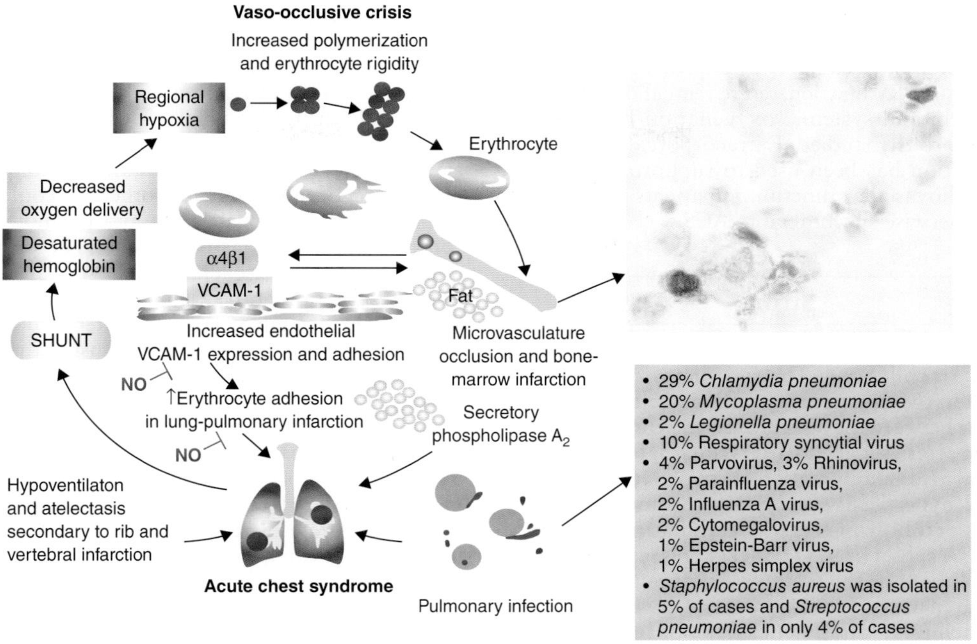

FIGURE 96.1. Vicious cycle of vaso-occlusive crisis and acute chest syndrome. (From Gladwin MT, Vichinsky E. Pulmonary complications of sickle cell disease. *NEJM* 2008;359(21):2254–2265.)

aureus, 5% and *Streptococcus pneumoniae*, 4%). Fat embolization leads to ACS as a result of pulmonary vascular occlusion by marrow contents, lung injury, hypoxemia, inflammation, and pulmonary artery hypertension. It presents with rapid deterioration, acute increase in pulmonary artery pressure (PAP), liver dysfunction, CNS dysfunction, thrombocytopenia, and coagulopathy. The diagnosis is further suggested by the presence of oil red O–positive lipid accumulation in the sputum. Direct adhesion of sickled cells in the pulmonary vasculature has been proposed for pulmonary infarction leading to the development of ACS. Patients with ACS usually have a decrease in hemoglobin and platelets along with an increase in lactate dehydrogenase suggesting intravascular hemolysis, and thrombosis. Echocardiography to assess tricuspid valve regurgitant jet velocity, RV function, left ventricular function, and estimated PAP is recommended to stratify severity of illness. Tricuspid regurgitant jet velocity (TRV) $\geq$ 2.5–3 m/s is an indicator of poor prognosis and associated with pulmonary hypertension, RV failure, elevated B-type natriuretic peptide, and troponin I levels.

Treatment of ACS begins with general supportive care. Hydration is liberal and modified based on cardiovascular status, renal function, atrial filling pressures, and estimated RV pressure. Supplemental oxygen is administered with a goal of keeping Pao_2 and Sao_2 in an acceptable range ($Pao_2 \geq$ 80–100 mm Hg and $Sao_2 \geq 95\%$). For milder disease, ambulation should be encouraged. Analgesia should be provided to minimize reduced respiratory efforts from pleuritic chest pain, and exercises that promote pulmonary toilet such as incentive spirometry are encouraged. Regional anesthetic techniques, including central neuraxial blockade and continuous nerve block techniques, have also been employed with good results. The role of corticosteroids in ACS is unclear, but may be used to treat wheezing if the patient has a comorbid asthma history. The most effective therapeutic modality is transfusion therapy to dilute the HbS-containing erythrocytes, attenuate microvascular occlusion of the pulmonary circulation, and increase systemic oxygen delivery. For mild-to-moderate ACS, many clinicians provide simple transfusion to increase hemoglobin concentration to 10 g/dL. For more severe or rapidly progressive disease, exchange transfusion rapidly decreases the percentage of HbS to <30%, with total hemoglobin and hematocrit of 10 g/dL and 30%, respectively. Empiric antibiotic therapy with a third-generation cephalosporin and a macrolide antibiotic, with or without vancomycin, is a reasonable initial antibiotic regimen to cover organisms that cause atypical pneumonia, community-acquired pneumonia, and resistant staphylococcal and streptococcal infections. Appropriate serologic, nuclear amplification, and culture material is collected. Antibiotic coverage may be narrowed when microbiology results become available. ACS can progress in severity to severe ALI or ARDS. Noninvasive mechanical ventilation is commonly offered and improves gas exchange but not transfusion requirements, pain scores, narcotic use, hypoxemia resolution by day 3, or speed of discharge. Mechanical ventilation should use lung protective strategies. The administration of inhaled NO to patients with severe ACS has resulted in favorable outcomes, presumably by improving pulmonary hypertension, RV function, severe ventilation–perfusion mismatch, and systemic oxygenation but has not been rigorously studied. Extracorporeal membrane oxygenation has been used to support pulmonary and cardiovascular function in patients who would have otherwise succumbed to ACS.

Stroke

SCD is one of the most common causes of stroke (CVAs) in childhood. The risk of stroke in SCD is highest in the first decade, with an incidence of 1% per year between the ages of 2 and 5 years. Occlusion of large arteries (carotid artery, internal carotid, and cerebral arterial bifurcation points) may result from intimal hyperplasia, secondary thrombosis, distal thromboembolization, or combinations of these factors. A subset of SCD patients present with small-vessel disease in the CNS vasculature. Most CVAs in children are ischemic infarcts. Hemorrhagic CVA (subarachnoid, intraparenchymal, or intraventricular hemorrhage) are less common in children (3%) than adults (33%). Recurrence of cerebral infarction occurs in two-thirds of patients who do not receive chronic transfusion therapy, most within 2–3 years. The risk of recurrent stroke is even greater in SCD patients with moyamoya vasculopathy. Other risk factors include an acute decrease in hemoglobin concentration (as seen in aplastic crises due to parvovirus B19), a history of transient ischemic attack, ACS within the two previous weeks, more than two ACS events per year, the degree of anemia, and systolic hypertension. Silent cerebral infarction (ischemic MRI changes in the absence of clinical evidence of stroke) is the most common form of CNS injury in SCD. It occurs in 15%–25% of children <14 years and predicts subsequent neurologic injury. The diagnosis of CVA is made on the usual signs and symptoms. The differential diagnosis includes CNS infections and toxic ingestion. Emergent CT scan or MRI is used to define CNS abnormalities and to exclude the presence of lesions amenable to neurosurgical intervention (parenchymal, epidural, or subdural hematoma). MRI more clearly defines the CNS vasculature and detects ischemic parenchymal changes. The increased diagnostic potential of MRI must be weighed against the need for sedation. In ambiguous clinical presentations, lumbar puncture, antibiotic therapy, and toxicologic studies should be performed. The new onset of seizure activity should be considered indicative of cerebral ischemic injury until proven otherwise. Seizure control should is implemented as described for status epilepticus (Chapter 40), with particular care to ensure arterial oxygenation. The most urgent therapeutic intervention is an exchange transfusion (decreasing HbS to <30% and maintaining the hemoglobin at 10 g/dL) to reverse, or prevent progression of, ischemic CNS injury. Therapy for children with SCD and CVA is otherwise supportive, with careful attention to protection of the airway, suppression of seizure activity, and preservation of respiratory and hemodynamic function. In the setting of a large cerebral infarction, the patient is monitored for intracranial hypertension, and neurosurgical consultation is obtained. The application of therapeutic hypothermia could result in peripheral vasoconstriction and promote erythrocyte sickling and vaso-occlusion. The protective effects of aggressive exchange transfusion therapy in the setting of therapeutic hypothermia (33°C for 24 hours) in an adult SCD patient after cardiac arrest have been reported. Chronic transfusion therapy, is effective in preventing progressive neurologic injury but represents a considerable physiologic (systemic iron overload and alloimmunization) and financial burden. HSCT represents an alternative but is associated with obvious morbidity and the need for a suitable marrow donor. Hydroxyurea has an increased (but noninferior) rate of recurrent stroke (10% vs. 0% in the transfusion group).

Acute Splenic Sequestration Crisis

ASSC refers to a sudden drop in hemoglobin concentration associated with development of splenomegaly, reticulocytosis, intravascular volume depletion, and shock. The spleen becomes massively enlarged and tender. ASSC is rare in older children related to autosplenectomy. Patients with HbSC and HbS– β thalassemia undergo autosplenectomy later and experience ASSC later. Children with ASSC are anemic, pale, and have inadequate oxygen delivery. In severe cases, shock is present and patients present in extremis. Therapy involves restoration of blood volume with crystalloid and sickle-free red blood cells. Hemoglobin level should be closely monitored during transfusion because sequestered blood may reenter the circulation (autotransfusion) and result in hyperviscosity leading to stroke. In severe heart failure or shock, rapid exchange transfusion can rapidly restore oxygen-carrying capacity and avoid fluid overload. Patients who do not respond to aggressive medical therapy require splenectomy. Patients with ASSC may experience recurrent episodes, and splenectomy may be recommended after an episode of ASSC.

Aplastic Crisis

Aplastic crisis is an acute suppression of bone marrow function, commonly caused by parvovirus B19. Platelet and leukocyte counts are also decreased. Treatment is supportive with erythrocyte transfusion. The hemoglobin target for ASSC and aplastic crisis depends on oxygen supply and demand, lactic acid levels, mixed venous oxygen saturation, and arteriovenous oxygen gradient. These patients tolerate chronic anemia, and a hemoglobin level of 7–9 g/dL is usually adequate.

Sepsis

Because of impaired splenic function and decreased opsonic activity, children with SCD are at increased risk for serious bacterial infections with encapsulated organisms such as *S. pneumoniae* and *N. meningitidis*. Use of penicillin prophylaxis, vaccinations against *S. pneumoniae*, *H. influenza*, *and N. meningitides*, and aggressive antibiotic therapy in febrile SCD patients has improved sepsis-related mortality. Ceftriaxone is often the initial antibiotic for SCD patients with suspected sepsis; however, repeated doses are associated with fatal immune-mediated hemolytic anemia in SCD and antibiotics should be switched if the patient requires a full course. In patients with SCD and sepsis, mechanical ventilation, vasopressor support, steroid therapy (when appropriate), and other sepsis-specific therapies are implemented as indicated.

Chronic Injury of the Cardiovascular System

Older children needing critical care for complications of SCD may have significant preexisting dysfunction of the respiratory, cardiovascular, or renal systems that can affect their morbidity and mortality. Chronic complications of cardiovascular disease include systolic and diastolic dysfunction of the left or right heart, sudden death, and pulmonary hypertension. The chronic anemia of SCD leads to an increase in cardiac output primarily by an increased left ventricular (LV) stroke volume that results in LV dilation. The dilated LV adapts to increased wall stress by developing eccentric hypertrophy which helps maintain normal filling pressures and diastolic compliance. LV diastolic dysfunction, common in SCD, increases mortality (even further in combination with pulmonary hypertension). Half of SCD patients with pulmonary hypertension have diastolic dysfunction. LV systolic dysfunction in SCD is rare, found in older patients and those with hypertension and renal disease. SCD patients without pulmonary hypertension tend to have dilated right heart chambers without significant RV dysfunction. RV dysfunction may rapidly develop with the acute increase in afterload seen in ACS. In hospitalized SCD patients, RV dysfunction was present in 13%: they all had a TRV >3 m/s and an increased risk for multiorgan failure and sudden death. Sudden death is associated with underlying cardiac disease, pulmonary disease, or pulmonary vascular disease and is increasingly recognized in the aging SCD population. Sudden unexpected death occurs in 40% of SCD patients, usually associated with an acute event. Sudden death/pulseless electrical activity (PEA), heart failure, myocardial infarction, pulmonary embolism, and pulmonary hypertension are common at the time of death.

Pulmonary hypertension should be considered in SCD patients with acute lung pathology and in older SCD patients. Risk factors include deranged arginine/NO metabolism, surgical splenectomy, functional asplenia, thromboembolism, lung fibrosis, hypoxemia, increase in vasoactive mediators (i.e., endothelin-1), renal insufficiency, biochemical indices of hemolysis, biochemical markers of cholestatic liver dysfunction, and genetic factors (**Fig. 96.2**). Pulmonary hypertension is the most potent predictor of premature mortality in SCD. Noninvasive assessment of PAP relies on echocardiographic assessment of TRV. A TRV of 2.5 m/s is present in 30%, and 3 m/s in 10%, of patients. A mild-to-moderate elevation in Doppler-estimated RV systolic pressure is associated with early death. The development of pulmonary hypertension may be due to left heart dysfunction (50%—pulmonary venous hypertension) with a pulmonary arterial occlusion pressure (PAOP) >15 mmHg or intrinsic elevation of pulmonary vascular resistance with normal left-sided function (50%—pulmonary arterial hypertension) with a PAOP <15 mmHg. The etiology of pulmonary hypertension in SCD is multifactorial. It arises as a result of chronic hemolytic anemia and is associated with concomitant end-organ dysfunction, but is not a direct consequence of repeated episodes of vaso-occlusion and ACS. Pulmonary hypertension should be considered in any critically ill patient with lung disease, shock, acidosis, and other stressors of cardiovascular reserve. Patients should be evaluated for thromboembolic disease, sleep apnea, human immunodeficiency virus, liver disease, collagen vascular disease, renal insufficiency, and other conditions that could contribute to pulmonary hypertension.

Critical care support for right heart decompensation includes maintenance of functional residual capacity, supplemental oxygen, adequate ventilation, treatment of metabolic acidosis, monitoring right and/or left atrial pressures, fluid management, inotropic support, and the administration of pulmonary artery vasodilators. Chronic treatment begins with hydroxyurea titrated to maximize fetal hemoglobin levels with minimal side effects. Patients not responding to (or tolerating) hydroxyurea or with significant pulmonary hypertension should begin chronic transfusions targeting a hemoglobin S <20%. Pulmonary hypertension–specific therapies are considered in patients with pulmonary hypertension without left heart failure (mPAP > 25 mm Hg, PAOP < 15 mm Hg, and a transpulmonary gradient of >10–12 mm Hg). In these patients the endothelin receptor antagonist (ERA) ambrisentan (once daily PO dosing and less hepatotoxicity than bosentan) may be considered with diuresis to control right heart failure, while phosphodiesterase-5 (PDE-5) inhibitors and prostanoids are reserved for more severe disease already optimized with chronic transfusion therapy. PDE-5 inhibition therapy seems to be effective in both pulmonary arterial and pulmonary venous hypertension related to diastolic dysfunction. Sildenafil (a PDE-5 inhibitor) in patients with taking maximal hydroxyurea therapy or transfusions improves TRV, NT-proBNP levels, and functional exercise status. A large multicenter study of SCD patients using sildenafil was stopped because of an increased frequency of hospital admission secondary

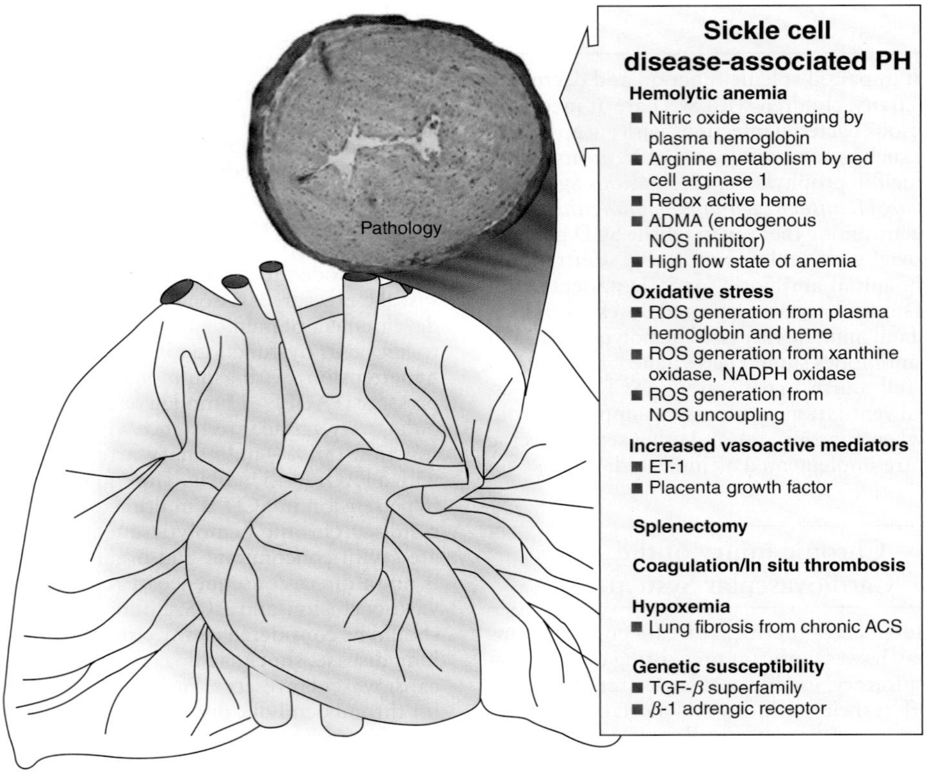
Pathology
Sickle cell disease-associated PH
Hemolytic anemia
■ Nitric oxide scavenging by plasma hemoglobin
■ Arginine metabolism by red cell arginase 1
■ Redox active heme
■ ADMA (endogenous NOS inhibitor)
■ High flow state of anemia
Oxidative stress
■ ROS generation from plasma hemoglobin and heme
■ ROS generation from xanthine oxidase, NADPH oxidase
■ ROS generation from NOS uncoupling
Increased vasoactive mediators
■ ET-1
■ Placenta growth factor
Splenectomy
Coagulation/In situ thrombosis
Hypoxemia
■ Lung fibrosis from chronic ACS
Genetic susceptibility
■ TGF-β superfamily
■ β-1 adrengic receptor

FIGURE 96.2. Mechanisms of pulmonary hypertension in SCD patients. (From Rudski LG, Lai WW, Afilalo J, Hua L, Handschumacher MD, Chandrasekaran K, et al. Guidelines for the echocardiographic assessment of the right heart in adults: A report from the American Society of Echocardiography endorsed by the European Association of Echocardiography, a registered branch of the European Society of Cardiology, and the Canadian Society of Echocardiography. *J Am Soc Echocardiogr* 2010;23(7):685–713; quiz 786–8; Gladwin MT, Sachdev V. Cardiovascular abnormalities in sickle cell disease. *J Am Coll Cardiol* 2012;59(13):1123–33.)

to myalgia and back pain. Other therapies that have been attempted with minimal efficacy include inhaled NO and arginine supplementation.

Chronic Injury of the Respiratory System

Chronic lung injury (sickle cell chronic lung disease, SCCLD) and airway hyperreactivity may develop in the SCD patients. Severe interstitial disease associated with SCCLD is rare, but mild spirometric abnormalities are common. In the pre–hydroxyurea treatment era, 90% of the SCD population demonstrated spirometric abnormalities including mild restrictive defects, isolated reduction in the DLCO, and low normal FEV_1 and FVC with a normal FEV_1/FVC ratio. Obstructive disease is uncommon. The prevalence of asthma among children with SCD is similar to normal children of African descent. Airway hyperresponsiveness to methacholine challenge is common in children with SCD and associated with younger age, elevated serum IgE levels, and markers of hemolysis. Asthma is associated with increased rates of ACS. Children admitted for VOC with a previous diagnosis of asthma are more likely to develop ACS, to be hospitalized longer, and to be readmitted within 3 days after discharge. Children with a history of asthma suffer twice as many ACS episodes, develop ACS at a younger age, have more painful episodes, and require more blood transfusions than patients without asthma. A history of asthma is also associated with increased (twofold) mortality in SCD. Management of asthma in SCD patients follows the same pathway as described in Chapter 23 with a few caveats. Given the increased potential for severe VOC and ACS the threshold for hospital admission should be low. The importance of provision of and compliance with controller medications must be stressed to avoid the morbidity and mortality associated with asthma in this high-risk patient population.

Chronic Injury to the Kidney

The kidney, like the spleen, suffers significant functional impairment from repeated ischemic insults. Older patients may require dialysis or renal transplantation.

Patients with SCD or SCT demonstrate *isosthenuria*, an impairment in the ability to concentrate urine and preserve free water, making SCD patients more susceptible to dehydration. The potential of renal dysfunction must be considered when managing fluids, acid–base balance, electrolytes, and medications.

PERIOPERATIVE MANAGEMENT OF SCD PATIENTS

Perioperative care must consider the risks of the proposed surgery, the patient, and the patient's clinical course of SCD. Preoperative preparation includes attention to preoperative hydration, optimization of vital organ function, and consideration of preoperative red blood cell transfusions. Patients with SCD should be well hydrated throughout the perioperative course. Many procedures are performed as outpatients, with SCD patients scheduled early in the day and with attention to *nil per os* guidelines to limit dehydration. Subsequent overhydration does not correct the intracellular dehydration present in sickled cells. Major organ systems should be evaluated for dysfunction that may adversely impact the intraoperative and postoperative course.

Perioperative transfusion therapy is a controversial topic. The usual reasons for transfusion are correction of anemia, improvement of oxygen-carrying capacity, and dilution of HbS- with HbA-containing erythrocytes. Prophylactic transfusion therapy is effective in reducing perioperative SCD complications. Postoperative complications develop in 26% of children with SCD who undergo surgical procedures without preoperative transfusion (most are minor and self-limited). The mortality rate within 30 days of surgery for SCD is 1:100 compared with 1: 300,000 in adults and 1: 80,000 in children. Perioperative blood transfusion confers protection against complications for low-risk procedures in HbSS patients, and low- and moderate-risk procedures in HbSC. Conservative transfusion strategies may be as effective as aggressive transfusion and result in fewer transfusion-related complications. The goal of aggressive transfusion is a HbS of 30% by either serial transfusion or exchange transfusion and for conservative transfusion it is a hemoglobin level of 10 g/dL by simple transfusion. There are no high-quality data to guide the performance of elective surgery without preoperative transfusion. For patients with high-risk SCD and those undergoing procedures with high potential for CNS injury and ACS (i.e., cardiac surgery with cardiopulmonary bypass, deep hypothermia with circulatory arrest, and neurosurgical procedures), consultation with the anesthesiologist, surgeon, and hematologist caring for the patient is recommended, and consideration given to more aggressive transfusion preparation.

Operative management requires attention to the precipitants of SCD complications (oxygenation, hydration, acid–base balance, and thermoregulation). Anesthetic technique (general anesthesia, regional anesthesia, or combined) is not related to risk of complications. The type of procedure impacts the probability of complications with thoracotomy, laparotomy, and obstetrical, intracranial, and airway procedures having the greatest risk. Cardiac surgery (requiring cardiopulmonary bypass, hypothermia, or aortic cross-clamping) and revascularization procedures for the CNS have significant risk. Consideration should be given to perioperative transfusion practices, temperature management that confers myocardial or CNS protection without provoking sickling phenomenon, and respiratory and metabolic operative management of acid–base status to optimize myocardial and CNS perfusion.

Postoperative management requires continuation of the previous principles. Whether SCD patients should be managed as outpatients is controversial with a lack of data. Analgesia should be optimized to facilitate respiratory function without depressing respiratory drive. Pulmonary toilet and early ambulation are important. Attention is still needed to fluid intake and output, including insensible losses, urine output, and losses from drains and catheters.

OUTCOMES

SCD patients are living longer due to penicillin prophylaxis, vaccinations against *H. influenzae* and *S. pneumoniae*, surveillance measures (echocardiography and TCD) for early identification of serious complications, and therapies such as hydroxyurea, stem-cell transplantation, and chronic transfusion therapy. Pulmonary complications (ACS often superimposed on pulmonary hypertension), remain the leading cause of morbidity and mortality. Stroke is an increasingly important cause of morbidity and mortality with a peak incidence between 2 and 8 years of age.

INDEX

Note: Page numbers followed by *f* indicate figures; page numbers followed by *t* indicate tabular material